Human Blood Groups

Human Blood Groups

Geoff Daniels
BSc, PhD, MRCPath
Senior Research Fellow
Bristol Institute for Transfusion Sciences
Molecular Diagnostics Manager
International Blood Group Reference Laboratory
UK

Foreword by
Ruth Sanger

SECOND EDITION

Blackwell
Science

First published 1995
Second edition 2002

2   2007

ISBN 978-0-6320-5646-0

Catalogue records for this title are available from the Library of Congress and the British Library

For further information on Blackwell Science, visit our website:
www.blackwell-science.com

Contents

Foreword

It is a particular pleasure for me to welcome this new book on human blood groups, the more so since it emanates from the Medical Research Council's Blood Group Unit. For 25 years this Unit devoted its energies to the search for new red cell antigens and the application of those already known to various problems, particularly to human genetics. During these years Rob Race and I produced six editions of Blood Groups in Man.

Dr Geoff Daniels joined the Unit in 1973 on Dr Race's retirement; soon after, concurrently with the Unit's move from the Lister Institute to University College, the scope of the Unit's interest was broadened.

Having been divorced from blood groups and otherwise occupied in 12 years of retirement, I am delighted and astonished at the rapid advances made in recent years. The number of blood group loci have increased to 23 and all except one have found their chromosomal home. The biochemical backgrounds of most of the corresponding antigens are defined and hence several high and low incidence antigens gathered into systems. The molecular basis of many red cell antigens has provided an explanation for some confusing serological relationships which were observed many years before.

Dr Daniels is to be congratulated on his stamina in producing a comprehensive text and reference book on human blood groups, for which many scientists will be grateful.

Ruth Sanger
December 1994

Preface

As with the first edition, the primary purpose of this book is to describe human blood group antigens and their inheritance, the antibodies that define them, the structure and functions of the red cell membrane macromolecules that carry them, and the genes that encode them or control their biosynthesis. In addition, this book provides information on the clinical relevance of blood groups and on the importance of blood group antibodies in transfusion medicine in particular.

The first edition of *Human Blood Groups* was published in 1995; this new edition will appear seven years later. There have been many new findings in the blood group world over those seven years, so much of the first edition has been rewritten. In order to prevent the book from becoming too cumbersome, my goal has been to produce a second edition roughly the same size as the first. I have tried to do this without eliminating anything too important, although this has not been easy, with so much new material to include.

During the last seven years, the major advances that have occurred in the science of human blood groups have mostly involved molecular genetics. With the exception of Scianna, RAPH, and possibly P, the genes for all the blood group systems have been cloned and the molecular bases for almost all the polymorphisms are known. Most chapters now have the biochemistry and molecular biology section at the beginning, so that when the serological polymorphisms and variants are subsequently explained, they can be described together with the genetic changes that cause them. Another topic that has progressed apace is the biological significance of red cell surface proteins. Consequently, I have placed a greater emphasis on functional aspects of blood groups than in the first edition.

I wish to thank again all the people who helped me produce the first edition, in particular Patricia Tippett, Carole Green, and Joan Daniels. Since the first edition was published, the Medical Research Council Blood Group Unit has closed and I have moved to the Bristol Institute for Transfusion Sciences. I would like to thank David Anstee for his support while I prepared this new edition. I am proud to keep the foreword to the first edition written by Ruth Sanger, author of six editions of *Blood Groups in Man*, who sadly died just a few weeks before the manuscript of this second edition was submitted for publication.

Some abbreviations used

ADP   Adenosine diphosphate
ATP   Adenosine triphosphate
AET   2-aminoethylisothiouronium bromide
AIDS   Acquired immune-deficiency syndrome
AIHA   Autoimmune haemolytic anaemia
BFU-E   Burst-forming unit — erythroid
bp   Basepair
CDA   Congenital dyserythropoietic anaemia
CGD   Chronic granulomatous disease
cDNA   Complementary deoxyribonucleic acid
CFU-E   Colony-forming unit — erythroid
CFU-GM   Colony-forming unit — granulocyte/macrophage
CFU-MK   Colony-forming unit — megakaryocyte
DAT   Direct antiglobulin test (or direct antiglobulin reaction)
DHTR   Delayed haemolytic transfusion reaction
DL   Donath-Landsteiner
DNA   Deoxyribonucleic acid
DTT   Dithiothreitol
EBV   Epstein—Barr virus
EST   Expressed sequence tag
GDP   Guanosine diphosphate
GPI   Glycosylphosphatidylinositol
HCF   Hydatid cyst fluid
HDN   Haemolytic disease of the newborn (also used for haemolytic disease of the fetus)

IHTR   Immediate haemolytic transfusion reaction
ISBT   International Society of Blood Transfusion
kb   Kilobase
LISS   Low ionic-strength solution
MAIEA   Monoclonal antibody-specific immobilization of erythrocyte antigens
M_r Relative molecular mass (molecular weight)
mRNA   Messenger ribonucleic acid
PAS   Periodic acid–Schiff
PCH   Paroxysmal cold haemoglobinuria
PCR   Polymerase chain reaction
PNH   Paroxysmal nocturnal haemoglobinuria
RFLP   Restriction fragment-length polymorphism
RNA   Ribonucleic acid
RT-PCR   Reverse transcriptase-polymerase chain reaction
SAO   South-East Asian ovalocytosis
SDS PAGE   Sodium dodecyl sulphate polyacrylamide gel electrophoresis
SNP   Single nucleotide polymorphism
SSEA   Stage-specific embryonic antigen
UDP   Uridine diphosphate

1 Human blood groups: introduction, terminology, and function

1.1 Introduction

What is the definition of a blood group? Taken literally, any variation or polymorphism detected in the blood could be considered a blood group. However, the term blood group is usually restricted to blood cell surface antigens, and generally to red cell surface antigens. This book focuses on the inherited variations in human red cell membrane proteins, glycoproteins, and glycolipids. These variations are detected by alloantibodies, which occur either 'naturally', as a result of immunization by ubiquitous antigens present in the environment, or as a result of alloimmunization by human red cells, usually introduced by blood transfusion or pregnancy. Although it is possible to detect polymorphism in red cell surface proteins by other methods, such as DNA sequence analysis, such variants cannot be called blood groups unless they are defined by an antibody.

Blood groups were discovered at the beginning of the twentieth century when Landsteiner [1,2] noticed that plasma from some individuals agglutinated the red cells from others. For the next 45 years, only those antibodies that directly agglutinate red cells could be studied. With the development of the antiglobulin test by Coombs, Mourant, and Race in 1945 [3,4], non-agglutinating antibodies could be detected and the science of blood group serology blossomed: there are now about 270 authenticated blood group antigens. Many of these blood group antigens fall into one of 26 blood group systems, genetically discrete groups of antigens controlled by a single gene or cluster of two or three closely linked homologous genes (Table 1.1). Some of these systems, notably Rh and MNS, are highly complex.

Most blood group antigens are synthesized by the red cell, but the antigens of the Lewis and Chido/Rodgers systems are adsorbed onto the red cell membrane from the plasma. Some blood group antigens are detected only on red cells, others are found throughout the body and should, more precisely, be called histo-blood group antigens.

Biochemical analysis of blood group antigens has shown that they fall into two main types: (i) protein determinants, which represent the primary products of blood group genes; and (ii) carbohydrate determinants on glycoproteins and glycolipids, in which the products of the genes controlling antigen expression are glycosyltransferase enzymes. Some antigens are defined by the amino acid sequence of a glycoprotein, but are dependent on the presence of carbohydrate for their recognition serologically.

In recent years, molecular genetical techniques have been introduced into the study of human blood groups and now most of the genes governing blood group systems have been cloned and sequenced (Table 1.1). Many serological complexities of blood groups are now explained at the gene level by a variety of mechanisms, including point mutation, unequal crossing-over, gene conversion, and alternative RNA splicing.

Discovery of the ABO blood groups first made blood transfusion feasible and disclosure of the Rh antigens led to the understanding and subsequent prevention of haemolytic disease of the newborn (HDN). Although ABO and Rh are the most important systems in transfusion medicine, many other blood group antibodies are capable of causing haemolytic transfusion reactions or HDN. Red cell groups have been important tools in forensic science, although this role was diminished with the introduction of HLA testing and has recently been displaced by DNA 'fingerprinting'. For many years blood groups were the best human genetic markers and have played a major part in the mapping of the human genome.

Blood groups still have much to teach us. Because red cells are readily available and haemagglutination tests relatively easy to perform, the structure and genetics of the red cell membrane proteins and lipids are understood in great detail. With the unravelling of the complexities of blood group systems by molecular

1

Table 1.1 Blood group systems.

No.	Name	Symbol	No. of antigens	Associated membrane structures	Gene name(s)	Chromosome
001	ABO	ABO	4	Carbohydrate	ABO	9
002	MNS	MNS	43	GPA (CD235A), GPB (CD235B)	GYPA, GYPB GYPE	4
003	P	P1	1	Carbohydrate	P1	22
004	Rh	RH	46	RhD (CD240D), RhCcEe (CD240CE)	RHD, RHCE	1
005	Lutheran	LU	18	CD239, IgSF	LU	19
006	Kell	KEL	24	CD238, endopeptidase	KEL	7
007	Lewis	LE	6	Carbohydrate	FUT3	19
008	Duffy	FY	6	CD234, chemokine receptor	FY	1
009	Kidd	JK	3	Urea transporter	SLC14A1	18
010	Diego	DI	21	Band 3, anion exchanger (CD233)	SLC4AE1 (AE1)	17
011	Yt	YT	2	Acetylcholinesterase	ACHE	7
012	Xg	XG	2	Glycoproteins, including CD99	XG, MIC2	X/Y
013	Scianna	SC	3	Glycoprotein	SC	1
014	Dombrock	DO	5	ADP-ribosyltransferase?	DO	12
015	Colton	CO	3	Aquaporin-1	AQP1	7
016	Landsteiner-Wiener	LW	3	ICAM-4, IgSF, CD242	LW	19
017	Chido/Rodgers	CH/RG	9	C4A, C4B (C′)	C4A, C4B	6
018	Hh	H	1	CD173 (Type 2 H), carbohydrate	FUT1	19
019	Kx	XK	1	Protein	XK	X
020	Gerbich	GE	7	GPC, GPD (CD236)	GYPC	2
021	Cromer	CROM	10	CD55, DAF, C′ regulator	DAF	1
022	Knops	KN	7	CD35, CR1, C′ regulator	CR1	1
023	Indian	IN	2	CD44	CD44	11
024	Ok	OK	1	CD147, EMMPRIN, IgSF	CD147	19
025	Raph	RAPH	1	Glycoprotein	MER2	11
026	John Milton Hagen	JMH	1	CDw108, semaphorin	SEMA7A	15

C′, complement; IgSF, immunoglobulin superfamily.

genetical techniques, much will be learnt about the mechanisms responsible for the diversification of protein structures and the nature of the human immune response to proteins of different shapes resulting from variations in amino acid sequence.

1.2 Blood group terminology

'Last come the Twins, who cannot be described because we should be sure to be describing the wrong one.' (J.M. Barrie)

The problem of providing a logical and universally agreed nomenclature has dogged blood group serologists almost since the discovery of the ABO system. Before going any further, it is important to understand how blood groups are named and how they are categorized into systems, collections, and series.

1.2.1 An internationally agreed nomenclature

The International Society of Blood Transfusion (ISBT) Working Party on Terminology for Red Cell Surface

Antigens was set up in 1980 to establish a uniform nomenclature that is 'both eye and machine readable'. Part of the brief of the Working Party was to produce a nomenclature 'in keeping with the genetic basis of blood groups' and so a terminology based primarily around the blood group systems was devised. First the systems and the antigens they contained were numbered, then the high and low frequency antigens received numbers, and then, in 1988, collections were introduced. Numbers are never recycled: antigens that become part of a system or collection are given a new number and their original number becomes obsolete.

Blood group antigens are categorized into 26 systems, five collections, and two series. The significance of these categories, and the general principles on which the ISBT terminology is based, will be described below. The Working Party produced a monograph in 1995 to describe the terminology [5], which has been updated [6], and has a website (http://www.iccbba.com/page25.htm).

1.2.2 Antigen, phenotype, gene, and genotype symbols

Every authenticated blood group antigen is given a six-digit identification number. The first three digits represent the system (001–026), collection (205–210), or series (700 for low frequency, 901 for high frequency); the second three digits identify the antigen. For example, the Lutheran system is system 005 and Lu^a, the first antigen in that system, has the number 005001. Each system also has an alphabetical symbol: that for Lutheran is LU. So Lu^a is also LU001 or, because redundant sinistral zeros may be discarded, LU1.

For phenotypes, the system symbol is followed by a colon and then by a list of antigens present, each separated by a comma. If an antigen is known to be absent, its number is preceded by a minus sign. For example, Lu(a–b+) becomes LU:–1,2. Genes have the system symbol followed by a space or asterisk followed in turn by the antigen number representing that gene. For example, Lu^a gene becomes *LU 1* or *LU*1*. Genotypes have the symbol followed by a space or asterisk followed by the two alleles or haplotypes separated by a stroke. For example, Lu^a/Lu^b becomes *LU 1/2* or *LU*1/2*, and Lu^aLu^6/Lu^bLu^9 would be *LU 1,6/2,9* or *LU*1,6/2,9*. Genes and genotypes are always italicized or underlined. Some examples of antigens, phe-

Table 1.2 Some examples of Kell system terminology.

	Original	Numerical
Antigen	K, k, Kp^a, Kp^b	KEL1, KEL2, KEL3, KEL4
Phenotype	K–k+ Kp(a–b+)	KEL:–1,2,–3,4
Gene	*K, k, Kp^a, Kp^b*	*KEL 1, KEL 2, KEL 3, KEL 4*
	K^0	*KEL 0*
Genotype	*kKp^b/kKp^b*	*KEL 2,4/2,4*
	Ul^a/Ul	*KEL 10/–10*
	kKp^a/K^0	*KEL 2,3/0*

An asterisk may occupy the space following the system symbol in genes and genotypes, e.g. *KEL*1*.

notypes, genes, and genotypes within the Kell system are given in Table 1.2.

1.2.3 Blood group systems

A blood group system consists of one or more antigens. These are governed by a single gene locus or by a complex of two or more very closely linked homologous genes with virtually no recombination occurring between them. Each system is genetically discrete from every other blood group system. Any two systems may be shown to be different either by demonstrating that the genes segregate at meiosis through the analysis of families, or by the gene loci being allocated to different chromosomes or to clearly distinct parts of the same chromosome. New antigens should only be assigned to a system when it is proven that the antigen is controlled by a gene at the blood group system locus.

In some systems the gene directly encodes the blood group determinant, whereas in others, where the antigen is carbohydrate in nature, the gene encodes a transferase enzyme that catalyses biosynthesis of the antigen. A, B, and H antigens, for example, may all be located on the same macromolecule, yet H-glycosyltransferase is produced by a gene on chromosome 19 while A- and B-transferases, which require H antigen as an acceptor substrate, are products of a gene on chromosome 9. Hence H belongs to a separate blood group system from A and B. Regulator genes may affect expression of antigens from more than one system: *In(Lu)* down-regulates expression of antigens from both Lutheran and P systems; mutations in *RHAG* are responsible for Rh$_{null}$ phenotype, but may also cause absence of U (MNS5) and Fy5 antigens. So absence of an antigen from cells of a null-phenotype is never sufficient evidence for allocation to a system. Four systems consist of more than one gene locus: MNS comprises three loci, Rh, Xg and Chido/Rodgers have two each.

1.2.4 Collections

Collections were introduced into the terminology in 1988 to bring together genetically, biochemically, or serologically related sets of antigens that could not, at that time, achieve system status. For example, before setting up the Cromer collection the allelic antigens Tc^a, Tc^b, and Tc^c had the numbers 900020, 700035, and 700036, respectively, and WES^a and WES^b had the numbers 700042 and 900033; yet all five reside on the same macromolecule. Together with five other biochemically and serologically related antigens, these antigens became the Cromer collection. Initially they could not become the Cromer system as they had not been shown to be genetically distinct from all existing systems; that required another couple of years.

Eleven collections have been created, six of which have subsequently been declared obsolete: the Gerbich (201), Cromer (202), and Indian (203) collections have now become systems; Auberger (204), Gregory (206), and Wright (211) have been incorporated into the Lutheran, Dombrock, and Diego systems, respectively (Table 1.3).

1.2.5 Low frequency antigens, the 700 series

Red cell antigens that do not fit into any system or collection and have an incidence of less than 1% in most populations tested are given a 700 number (see Table 27.1). The 700 series currently consists of 22 antigens.

Table 1.3 Blood group collections.

No.	Name	Symbol	No. of antigens
205	Cost	COST	2
207	Ii	I	2
208	Er	ER	2
209	Globoside	GLOB	3
210	(Le^c and Le^d)		2

Thirty-two 700 numbers are now obsolete as the corresponding antigens have found homes in systems, or can no longer be defined because of a lack of reagents.

1.2.6 High frequency antigens, the 901 series

Originally, antigens with a frequency greater than 99% were placed in a holding file called the 900 series, equivalent to the 700 series for low frequency antigens. With the establishment of the collections, so many of these 900 numbers became obsolete that the whole series was abandoned and the remaining high frequency antigens were relocated in a new series, the 901 series, which now comprises 11 antigens (see Table 28.1).

1.2.7 Blood group terminology used in this book

The ISBT terminology provides a uniform nomenclature for blood groups that can be continuously updated and is suitable for storage of information on computer databases. The Terminology Working Party does not expect, or even desire, that the numerical terminology be used in all circumstances, although it is important that it should be understood so that the genetically based classification is understood. In this book, the alternative, 'popular' nomenclature, recommended by the Working Party [5], will generally be used. This does not reflect a lack of confidence in the numerical terminology, but is simply because most readers will not be well acquainted with blood group numbers and will find the contents of the book easier to digest if familiar names are used. The numerical terminology will be provided throughout the book in tables and often, in parentheses, in the text.

The order of the chapters of this book is based on the order of the blood group systems, collections, and series. However, there are a few exceptions, the most notable of which are the ABO, H, and Lewis systems, which appear in one mega-chapter (Chapter 2), because they are so closely related, biochemically.

1.3 Structures and functions of blood group antigens

For the half-century following Landsteiner's discovery, human blood groups were understood predominantly as patterns of inherited serological reactions.

From the 1950s some structural information was obtained through biochemical analyses, first of the carbohydrate antigens and then of the proteins. In 1986, *GYPA*, the gene encoding the MN antigens, was cloned and this led into the molecular era of blood groups. A great deal is now known about the structures of many blood group antigens, yet remarkably little is known about their functions and most of what we do know has been deduced from their structures. Functional aspects of blood group antigens are included in the appropriate chapters of this book; provided here is a brief synopsis of the relationship between their structures and putative functions. The subject is also reviewed by Daniels [7].

1.3.1 Membrane transporters

Membrane transporters facilitate the transfer of biologically important molecules in and out of the cell. In the red cell they are polytopic, crossing the membrane several times, with cytoplasmic N- and C-termini, and are *N*-glycosylated on one of the external loops. Band 3, the Diego blood group antigen (Chapter 10) is an anion transporter, the Kidd glycoprotein (Chapter 9) is a urea transporter, and the Colton glycoprotein is a water channel (Chapter 15). The Rh proteins and the Rh-associated glycoprotein (RhAG) have structure characteristic of membrane transporters (except the Rh proteins are not glycosylated). There is some evidence to suggest that the Rh complex could be involved in ammonium transport (Chapter 5).

1.3.2 Receptors and adhesion molecules

The Duffy glycoprotein is polytopic, but has an extracellular N-terminus. It is a member of the G protein-coupled superfamily of receptors and might function as a receptor for chemokines (Chapter 8).

The Lutheran glycoproteins (Chapter 6), LW glycoprotein (Chapter 16), and CD147, the Ok glycoprotein (Chapter 22), are members of the immunoglobulin superfamily (IgSF). The IgSF is a large family of receptors and adhesion molecules with extracellular domains containing different numbers of repeating domains with sequence homology to immunoglobulin domains. CD47 (Chapter 5) and CD58 (Chapter 19) are also red cell IgSF glycoproteins, but do not express blood group activity. The functions of these structures on red cells are not known, but their primary functional activity may occur during erythropoiesis.

Some other red cell surface antigens with structures that suggest they could function as receptors and adhesion molecules are CD44, the Indian antigen (Chapter 21), the Xg and CD99 glycoproteins (Chapter 12), CDw108, the JMH blood group antigen (Chapter 24), and CDw75 (Chapter 6).

1.3.3 Complement regulatory glycoproteins

Red cells have at least three glycoproteins that exist, at least in part, to protect the cell from destruction by autologous complement. Two, decay-accelerating factor (DAF, CD55), the Cromer glycoprotein (Chapter 19), and complement receptor-1 (CR1, CD35), the Knops glycoprotein (Chapter 20), belong to the complement control protein superfamily. CD59, the most important of these for protecting against autologous complement, is not polymorphic and does not have blood group activity (Chapter 19). The major function of red cell CR1 is to bind and process C3b/C4b-coated immune complexes and to transport them to the liver and spleen for removal from the circulation.

1.3.4 Enzymes

Two blood group glycoproteins have enzymatic activity. The Yt glycoprotein is acetylcholinesterase, a vital enzyme in neurotransmission (Chapter 11). The Kell glycoprotein is an endopeptidase that can cleave a biologically inactive peptide to produce the active vasoconstrictor, endothelin (Chapter 7). The red cell function for both of these enzymes is unknown. The structure of the Dombrock glycoprotein suggests that it belongs to a family of ADP-ribosyltransferases (Chapter 14).

1.3.5 Structural components

The shape and integrity of the red cell is maintained by the membrane skeleton, a network of glycoproteins beneath the plasma membrane. At least two red cell membrane glycoproteins have an extended cytoplasmic domain, which functions to link the membrane with its skeleton. These proteins are band 3, the Diego antigen (Chapter 10), and glycophorin C and its isoform glycophorin D, the Gerbich blood group antigens (Chapter 18). Mutations in the genes encoding these proteins can result in abnormally shaped red cells.

1.3.6 Components of the glycocalyx

Band 3 and glycophorin A, the MN antigen (Chapter 3), are the two most abundant glycoproteins of the red cell surface. The N-glycans of band 3, together with those of the glucose transporter, provide the majority of red cell ABH antigens, which are also expressed on some other glycoproteins and on glycolipids (Chapter 2). The extracellular domains of glycophorin A and other glycophorin molecules are heavily O-glycosylated. Carbohydrate at the red cell surface constitutes the glycocalyx, or cell coat, an extracellular matrix of carbohydrate that protects the cell from mechanical damage and microbial attack.

1.3.7 What is the biological significance of blood group polymorphism?

Very little is known about the biological significance of the polymorphisms that make blood groups alloantigenic. In any polymorphism one of the alleles is likely to have, or at least had in the past, a selective advantage in order to achieve a frequency of >1% in a large population. Glycoproteins and glycolipids carrying blood group activity are often exploited by pathogenic microorganisms as receptors for attachment to the cells and subsequent invasion. This may have nothing to do with red cells; the target for the parasite could be other cells that carry the protein. It is likely that most blood group polymorphism is a relic of the selective balances that can result from mutations making cell surface structures less suitable as pathogen receptors and resultant adaptation of the parasite in response to these selective pressures. It is important to remember that while blood group polymorphism undoubtedly arose from the effects of selective pressures, these factors may have disappeared long ago, so that little hope remains of ever identifying them. To quote Charles Darwin in *The Origin of Species* (1859), 'The chief part of the organization of any living creature is due to inheritance; and consequently, though each being assuredly is well fitted for its place in nature, many structures have now no very close and direct relations to present habits of life.'

References

1 Landsteiner K. Zur Kenntnis der antifermentativen, lytischen und agglutinietenden Wirkungen des Blutserums und der Lymphe. *Zbl Bakt* 1900;**27**:357–66.

2 Landsteiner K. Über Agglutinationserscheinungen normalen menschlichen Blutes. *Wien Klin Wschr* 1901;**14**: 1132–4.

3 Coombs RRA, Mourant AE, Race RR. Detection of weak and 'incomplete' Rh agglutinins: a new test. *Lancet* 1945;**ii**:15.

4 Coombs RRA, Mourant AE, Race RR. A new test for detection of weak and 'incomplete' Rh agglutinins. *Br J Exp Pathol* 1945;**26**:255–66.

5 Daniels GL and members of the ISBT Working Party on Terminology for Red Cell Surface Antigens. Blood group terminology 1995. *Vox Sang* 1995;**69**:265–79.

6 Daniels GL and members of the ISBT Working Party on Terminology for Red Cell Surface Antigens. Reports and guidelines. *Vox Sang* 2001;**80**:193–6.

7 Daniels G. Functional aspects of red cell antigens. *Blood Rev* 1999;**13**:14–35.

2 ABO, Hh, and Lewis systems

Part 1: History and introduction

Described in this chapter are three blood group systems, ABO, Hh, and Lewis (Table 2.1), although Lewis is really an 'adopted' blood group system because the antigens are not intrinsic to the red cells, but introduced into the membrane from the plasma. These three systems are genetically discrete, but are discussed in the same chapter because they are phenotypically and biochemically closely related. A complex interaction of genes at several loci controls the expression of ABO, H, Lewis, and other related antigens on red cells and in secretions.

The science of immunohaematology came into existence in 1900 when Landsteiner [1] reported that, 'The serum of healthy humans not only has an agglutinating effect on animal blood corpuscles, but also on human blood corpuscles from different individuals.' The following year Landsteiner [2] showed that by mixing together sera and red cells from different peo-

ple three groups, A, B, and C (later called O), could be recognized. In group A, the serum agglutinated group B, but not other A cells; in group B, the serum agglutinated A, but not B cells; and in group C (O), the cells were not agglutinated by any serum, and the serum appeared to contain a mixture of two agglutinins capable of agglutinating A and B cells. Decastello and Sturli [3] added a fourth group (AB), in which the cells are agglutinated by sera of all other groups and the serum contains neither agglutinin. Healthy adults always have A or B agglutinins in their serum if they lack the corresponding agglutinogen from their red cells (Table 2.2).

Epstein and Ottenberg [4] suggested that blood groups may be inherited and, in 1910, von Dungern and Hirschfeld [5] confirmed that the inheritance of the A and B antigens obeyed Mendel's laws, with the presence of A or B being dominant over their absence. Bernstein [6,7], in 1924, showed that only three alleles at one locus were necessary to explain ABO inheritance (Table 2.2).

Table 2.1 Numerical notation for the ABO, Lewis, and Hh systems, and for Le^c and Le^d.

ABO (system 001)		Lewis (system 007)		Hh (system 018)		Collection 210	
ABO1	A	LE1	Le^a	H1	H	210001	Le^c
ABO2	B	LE2	Le^b			210002	Le^d
ABO3	A,B	LE3	Le^{ab}				
ABO4	A$_1$	LE4	Le^{bH}				
		LE5	ALe^b				
		LE6	BLe^b				

Obsolete: ABO5, previously H.

Table 2.2 The ABO system at its simplest level.

ABO group	Antigens on red cells	Antibodies in serum	Genotype
O	None	Anti-A,B	*O/O*
A	A	Anti-B	*A/A* or *A/O*
B	B	Anti-A	*B/B* or *B/O*
AB	A and B	None	*A/B*

Some group A people produce an antibody that agglutinates the red cells of most other A individuals. Thus A was subdivided into A$_1$ and A$_2$, and the three allele theory of Bernstein was extended by Thomsen *et al.* [8] to four alleles: *A^1*, *A^2*, *B* and *O* (Section 2.4). Many rare subgroups of A and B have now been identified (Sections 2.7 and 2.8).

The structure and biosynthesis of the ABO, H, and Lewis antigens is well understood, thanks mainly to the pioneering work in the 1950s of Morgan and Watkins [9,10] and of Kabat [11]. A and B red cell antigens are carbohydrate determinants of glycoproteins and glycolipids and are distinguished by the nature of an immunodominant terminal monosaccharide: *N*-acetylgalactosamine in group A and galactose in group B. The *A* and *B* genes encode glycosyltransferases, which catalyse the transfer of the appropriate immunodominant sugar from a nucleotide donor to an acceptor substrate, the H antigen. The *O* gene produces no active transferase (Sections 2.2 and 2.3). The sequences of the *A* and *B* genes demonstrate that A- and B-transferases differ by four amino acid residues; the most common O gene contains a nucleotide deletion and encodes a truncated protein.

H antigen is synthesized by a glycosyltransferase produced by a gene (*FUT1*) independent of *ABO*. Very rare individuals lacking the *H* gene have no H antigen on their red cells and, consequently, are unable to produce A or B antigens, even when the enzyme products of the *A* or *B* genes are present (Section 2.13).

H antigen is present in body secretions of about 80% of people. The presence of H in secretions is governed by a gene (*FUT2*) separate from, but closely linked to, the *H* (*FUT1*) gene. Individuals who secrete H also secrete A or B antigens if they have the appropriate *ABO* genes. Non-secretors of H do not secrete A or B, even when those antigens are expressed on their red cells (Section 2.6). Secretion of H is also important in determining Lewis phenotypes.

The first two examples of anti-Lewis, later to be called anti-Le^a, were described by Mourant [12] in 1946. These antibodies agglutinated the red cells of about 25% of English people. Andresen [13] found an antibody, later to become anti-Le^b, that defined a determinant only present on Le(a–) cells of adults. Six per cent of group O adults lacked both antigens. Although Le^a and Le^b are not synthesized by the red cells, but are acquired from the plasma, they are considered blood group antigens because they were first recognized on red cells. The terminology Le^a and Le^b is misleading as these antigens are not allelic.

The Lewis gene (*FUT3*) encodes a glycosyltransferase that catalyses the addition of a fucose residue to H antigen in secretions to produce Le^b antigen or, if no H is present (non-secretors), to the precursor of H to produce Le^a. Consequently, as these structures are acquired from the plasma by the red cell membrane, red cells of most H secretors are Le(a–b+) and those of most H non-secretors are Le(a+b–). The Lewis-transferase can also convert A to ALe^b and B to BLe^b. About 6% of white people and 25% of black people are homozygous for a silent gene at the Lewis locus and, as they do not produce the Lewis enzyme, have Le(a−b−) red cells and lack Lewis substances in their secretions (Sections 2.3 and 2.16). In Asia the red cell phenotype Le(a+b+) is common, as a result of a weak secretor allele (Section 2.6.3).

The antigens Le^c and Le^d represent precursors of the Lewis antigens and are present in increased quantity in the plasma of Le(a−b−) individuals. Le^c is detected on the red cells of Le(a−b−) non-secretors of H, and Le^d is detected on the red cells of Le(a−b−) secretors of H. Le^x and Le^y antigens, isomers of Le^a and Le^b, are not present in substantial quantities on red cells (Section 2.19).

ABH and Lewis antigens are often referred to as histo-blood group antigens [14] as they are ubiquitous structures, occurring on the surface of endothelial cells and most epithelial cells. Because of the intricacy of the gene interactions involved, the precise nature of the histo-blood group antigens expressed varies between tissues within the same individual (Section 2.20).

ABO is on chromosome 9; *FUT1*, *FUT2*, and *FUT3* are on chromosome 19 (Chapter 32).

Part 2: Biochemistry, inheritance, and biosynthesis of the ABH and Lewis antigens

2.2 Structure of ABH, Lewis, and related antigens

ABH and Lewis antigens are carbohydrate structures. These oligosaccharide chains are generally conjugated with polypeptides to form glycoproteins, or with ceramide to form glycosphingolipids. Oligosaccharides are synthesized in a stepwise fashion, the addition of each monosaccharide being catalysed by a specific glycosyltransferase enzyme. The oligosaccharide moieties responsible for expression of ABH, Lewis, and related antigens are shown in Table 2.3 and abbreviations for monosaccharides are given in Table 2.4. The biosynthesis of these structures is described in Section 2.3 and represented diagrammatically in Fig. 2.1. There is a vast literature on the biochemistry of these blood group antigens and only some of the relevant references can be given in this chapter. The following reviews are recommended [10,14–24].

2.2.1 Glycoconjugates expressing ABH and Lewis antigens

Two major classes of carbohydrate chains on glycoproteins express ABH antigens:

1 *N*-glycans, highly branched structures attached to the amide nitrogen of asparagine through *N*-acetylglucosamine; and

2 *O*-glycans, simple or complex structures attached to the hydroxyl oxygen of serine or threonine through *N*-acetylgalactosamine.

Glycosphingolipids consist of carbohydrate chains attached to ceramide. They are classified as lacto-, globo-, or ganglio-series according to the nature of the carbohydrate chain. Glycosphingolipid-borne ABH and Lewis antigens are present predominantly on glycolipids of the lacto-series, although ABH antigens have also been detected on globo- and ganglio-series glycolipids. The carbohydrate chains of most ABH-bearing glycoproteins and of lacto-series glycolipids are based on a poly *N*-acetyllactosamine structure; i.e. they are extended by repeating Galβ1→4GlcNAcβ1→3 disaccharides (see Table 2.5 for examples).

Before 1980 it was generally considered that most ABH determinants on red cells were carried on glycosphingolipids [10,15], but in 1980 several reports were published showing that glycolipids have a minor role compared with glycoproteins [25–29]. On red cells, most ABH antigens are on the single, highly branched, poly-*N*-acetyllactosaminyl *N*-glycans of the anion exchange protein, band 3, and the glucose transport protein, band 4.5 [30]. There are about 1 million monomers of band 3 protein and half a million monomers of band 4.5 protein per adult red cell [31]. The other major red cell glycoprotein, glycophorin A, does not appear to carry any ABH antigen [29,32], but ABH determinants have been detected on the Rh-associated glycoprotein [33]. Lewis antigens on red cells are not expressed on glycoproteins; they are not intrinsic to red cells, but are acquired from the plasma.

Red cell glycosphingolipids of the poly *N*-acetyllactosaminyl type that express ABH antigens may have relatively simple linear or branched carbohydrate chains [15] (Table 2.5) or may be highly complex, branched structures called polyglycosylceramides, with up to 60 carbohydrate residues per molecule [34].

Table 2.3 Structures of A, B, H, Lewis, and related antigens (for abbreviations see Table 2.4).

	Type 1		*Type 2*
Precursor (Le^c)	Galβ1→3GlcNAcβ1→R*	**Precursor**	Galβ1→4GlcNAcβ1→R
H (Le^d)	Galβ1→3GlcNAcβ1→R* 2 ↑ Fucα1	**H** (CD173)	Galβ1→4GlcNAcβ1→R† 2 ↑ Fucα1
A	GalNAcα1→3Galβ1→3GlcNAcβ1→R* 2 ↑ Fucα1	**A**	GalNAcα1→3Galβ1→4GlcNAcβ1→R† 2 ↑ Fucα1
B	Galα1→3Galβ1→3GlcNAcβ1→R* 2 ↑ Fucα1	**B**	Galα1→3Galβ1→4GlcNAcβ1→R† 2 ↑ Fucα1
Le^a	Galβ1→3GlcNAcβ1→R* 4 ↑ Fucα1	**Le^x**	Galβ1→4GlcNAcβ1→R 3 ↑ Fucα1
Le^b	Galβ1→3GlcNAcβ1→R* 2 4 ↑ ↑ Fucα1 Fucα1	**Le^y**	Galβ1→4GlcNAcβ1→R 2 3 ↑ ↑ Fucα1 Fucα1
ALe^b	GalNAcα1→3Galβ1→3GlcNAcβ1→R* 2 4 ↑ ↑ Fucα1 Fucα1	**ALe^y**	GalNAcα1→3Galβ1→4GlcNAcβ1→R 2 3 ↑ ↑ Fucα1 Fucα1
BLe^b	Galα1→3Galβ1→3GlcNAcβ1→R* 2 4 ↑ ↑ Fucα1 Fucα1	**BLe^y**	Galα1→3Galβ1→4GlcNAcβ1→R 2 3 ↑ ↑ Fucα1 Fucα1
sialyl-Le^a	Galβ1→3GlcNAcβ1→R 3 4 ↑ ↑ NeuAcα2 Fucα1	**sialyl-Le^x**	Galβ1→4GlcNAcβ1→R 3 3 ↑ ↑ NeuAcα2 Fucα1

Type 3: O-linked mucin type

Precursor (T antigen)	Galβ1→3GalNAcα1→O-Ser/Thr	**H**	Galβ1→3GalNAcα1→O-Ser/Thr 2 ↑ Fucα1
A	GalNAcα1→3Galβ1→3GalNAcα1→O-Ser/Thr 2 ↑ Fucα1	**B**	Galα1→3Galβ1→3GalNAcα1→O-Ser/Thr 2 ↑ Fucα1

Continued

Table 2.3 *Continued*

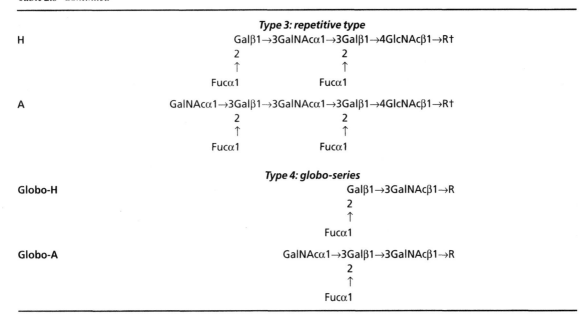

*Adsorbed onto red cells from plasma in individuals of appropriate genotype.
†Intrinsic to red cells and detected in significant quantity on red cells of individuals of appropriate genotype.

Table 2.4 Some abbreviations for monosaccharides and the structures they are linked to.

Asp	Asparagine
Cer	Ceramide
Fuc	L-Fucose
Gal	D-galactose
GalNAc	N-acetyl-D-galactosamine
Glc	Glucose
GlcNAc	N-acetyl-D-glucosamine
Man	Mannose
NeuAc	Sialic acid (N-acetylneuraminic acid)
R	Remainder of molecule
Ser	Serine
Thr	Threonine

All the early work establishing the structures of the ABH and Lewis determinants was carried out on body secretions, especially the pathological fluid from human ovarian cysts, which was found to be an abundant source of soluble A, B, and H substances [35]. ABH and Lewis antigens in secretions are glycoproteins; oligosaccharide chains attached to mucin molecules by O-glycosidic linkage to serine or threonine (for reviews see [9,10]). These macromolecules have molecular weights varying from 2×10^5 to several millions. In milk and urine, free oligosaccharides with ABH and Lewis activity are also found [36,37]. ABH and Lewis determinants are present in plasma on glycosphingolipids, some of which may become incorporated into the red cell membrane (Section 2.16.4).

2.2.2 Carbohydrate determinants

Expression of H, A, and B antigens is dependent on the presence of specific monosaccharides attached to various precursor disaccharides at the non-reducing end of a carbohydrate chain. There are at least six precursor disaccharides, also called peripheral core structures (for reviews see [14,18,21,24,38]):

Type 1 Galβ1→3GlcNAcβ1→R
Type 2 Galβ1→4GlcNAcβ1→R
Type 3 Galβ1→3GalNAcα1→R
Type 4 Galβ1→3GalNAcβ1→R
Type 5 Galβ1→3Galβ1→R
Type 6 Galβ1→4Glcβ1→R.

Types 1–4 and Type 6 occur in humans; Type 5 has only been chemically synthesized.

H-active structures have L-fucose α-linked to C-2 of the terminal galactose [39,40]; A- and B-active struc-

11

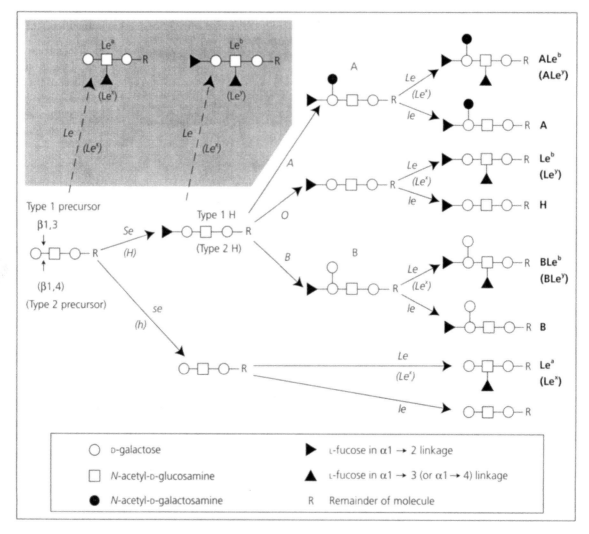

Fig. 2.1 Diagram representing the biosynthetic pathways of ABH, Lewis, Le[x], and Le[y] antigens derived from Type 1 and 2 core chains. Genes controlling steps in the pathway are shown in italics and the gene products are listed in Table 2.6. Type 1 and 2 precursors differ in the nature of the linkage between the non-reducing terminal galactose and N-acetylglucosamine: $\beta1 \rightarrow 3$ in Type 1 and $\beta1 \rightarrow 4$ in Type 2. Type 2 structures and the genes acting on them are shown in parentheses. Dashed lines show how Le[a] (Le[x]) and Le[b] (Le[y]), produced from the precursor and H structures, respectively, are not substrates for the H, Se, or ABO transferases and remain unconverted.

tures have N-acetyl-D-galactosamine and D-galactose, respectively, attached in α-linkage to C-3 of this $\alpha1 \rightarrow 2$ fucosylated galactose residue (Table 2.3). Although fucose does not represent the whole H determinant, it is the H immunodominant sugar because its loss results in loss of H activity. Likewise, N-acetylgalactosamine is the A immunodominant sugar and galactose is the B immunodominant sugar.

Le[a] and Le[b] antigens are expressed when fucose is attached to the N-acetylglucosamine of the Type 1 precursor and of Type 1 H, respectively [41–45]. Le[x] and Le[y] are the Type 2 isomers of Le[a] and Le[b] [40,44,46,47]. Fucose is linked $\alpha1 \rightarrow 4$ to the N-acetylglucosamine of a Type 1 chain in Le[a] and Le[b] and $\alpha1 \rightarrow 3$ to the N-acetylglucosamine of a Type 2 chain in Le[x] and Le[y]. Le[x] and Le[y] are not present in substantial

Table 2.5 Examples of H-active glycoconjugates with Type 2 precursor chains (for abbreviations see Table 2.4).

Glycosphingolipid (simple linear)
Fucα1→2Galβ1→4GlcNAcβ1→3Galβ1→4Glcβ1→Cer

Glycosphingolipid (branched)
Fucα1→2Galβ1→4GlcNAcβ1→3(Galβ1→4GlcNAcβ1→3)$_n$Galβ1→4Glcβ1→Cer
                                          6
                                          ↑
        Fucα1→2Galβ1→4GlcNAcβ1

N-linked glycoprotein
        Fucα1→2Galβ1→4GlcNAcβ1
                      ↓
                      6
Fucα1→2Galβ1→4GlcNAcβ1→3(Galβ1→4GlcNAcβ)$_n$1→2Man
                                                      Man-GlcNAc-GlcNAc-Asn
Fucα1→2Galβ1→4GlcNAcβ1→3(Galβ1→4GlcNAcβ)$_n$1→2Man
                                          6
                                          ↑
        Fucα1→2Galβ1→4GlcNAcβ1

O-linked glycoprotein (complex mucin type)
                Fucα1→2Galβ1→4GlcNAcβ1
                                ↓
                                6
Fucα1→2Galβ1→4GlcNAcβ1→3(Galβ1→4GlcNAcβ1→3)$_n$GalNAcα1→Ser/Thr
                          6
                          ↑
        Fucα1→2Galβ1→4GlcNAcβ1

$n = 0$–5 or more.

quantities on red cells [48]. The monofucosylated Le^a and Le^x structures may be sialylated at the C-3 of galactose [49–51] (Table 2.3).

Type 1 ABH and Lewis structures are present in secretions, plasma, and endodermally derived tissues [21]. They are not synthesized by red cells, but are incorporated into the red cell membrane from the plasma [52]. Lewis antigens (Le^a and Le^b) are only present on Type 1 structures. Elongated carbohydrate chains with Type 1 peripheral structures are generally extended by repeating poly N-acetyllactosamine disaccharides with the Type 2 (β1→4) linkage [53] (Table 2.5). Extended Type 1 structures with Le^a and Le^b activity have been detected in plasma, particularly in persons with Le(a+b+) red cells [54–56], and in carcinoma cell lines [57,58].

Type 2 chain antigens represent the major ABH-active oligosaccharides on red cells and are also detected in secretions and various ectodermally or mesodermally derived tissues [15,21]. Type 2 structures in secretions are probably more often difucosylated (Le^y, ALe^y, BLe^y) than monofucosylated (H, A, B) [59,60].

There are two forms of Type 3 ABH antigens: the O-linked mucin type and the repetitive A-associated type. In the O-linked mucin type the precursor exists as a disaccharide linked directly, by O-glycosidic bond, to a serine or threonine residue of mucin [61]. This precursor represents the T cryptantigen (see Section 3.18.2), but is not usually expressed because it is masked by substitution with sialic acid residues or other sugars. Type 3 ABH antigens of the O-linked mucin type are not found on red cells [62]. Repetitive Type 3 chains are present on red cell glycolipids and secreted mucins from group A individuals. They are restricted to group A because they are biosynthesized by the addition of galactose in β1→3 linkage to the terminal N-acetylgalactosamine of an A-active Type 2 chain

[48,62–65]. This A-associated form of Type 3 chain is discussed more fully in Section 2.4.

Type 4 ABH structures are only located on glycolipids. Type 4 precursor chain of the globo-series results from the addition of terminal galactose to globoside [66] (P antigen, see Chapter 4). Type 4 globo-H and globo-A have been detected in small quantities on red cells [66,67], but are more abundant in kidney [68]; Type 4 globo-B has only been found, in minute quantities, in kidney [69]. Kidney from a group A person with the p phenotype, which prevents extension of the globoseries structure, lacked Type 4 A [70] (see Chapter 4).

Type 6 chains have been found as free oligosaccharides in milk [36] and urine [37].

The internal carbohydrate chains express I and i antigens. In fetal cells linear chains predominate and i antigen is expressed, whereas in adult glycoproteins and glycolipids there is far more branching of the inner core chains and I antigen is expressed (see Chapter 25).

2.3 Biosynthesis, inheritance, and molecular genetics

Antigens of the ABO, Hh, and Lewis blood group systems are carbohydrates and are not the primary products of the genes governing their expression. Carbohydrate chains are built up by the sequential addition of various monosaccharides, each extension of the chain being catalysed by a specific glycosyltransferase enzyme. These enzymes catalyse the transfer of a monosaccharide from its nucleotide donor, and its attachment, in a specific glycosidic linkage, to its acceptor substrate. Glycosyltransferases represent the primary products of the ABO, H (*FUT1*), secretor (*FUT2*), and Lewis (*FUT3*) genes (Table 2.6).

It has been estimated that at least 100 glycosyltransferases are required for synthesis of the known human carbohydrates. The genes producing many of them have been cloned and sequenced, including those for the ABO, H, and Lewis blood groups, and for secretion of H. The gene products are *trans*-membrane proteins of the Golgi apparatus. They share a common domain structure comprising a short N-terminal cytoplasmic tail, a 16–20 amino acid membrane-spanning domain, and an extended stem region followed by a large C-terminal catalytic domain. Soluble glycosyltransferases present in secretions may result from the release of membrane-bound enzymes by endogenous proteases or they may lack the membrane-spanning domain as a result of mRNA translation-initiation at an alternative site (for reviews see [22,71,72]).

The regulation mechanisms required to assure that carbohydrate chains with the appropriate sequences are produced are complex. They involve the presence or absence of certain enzymes according to the genes expressed in various tissues and at different stages of development, and according to the genotype of the individual. Competition between different transferases for the same donor or acceptor substrate is also important in determining the carbohydrate chain produced (review in [16]).

2.3.1 H antigen

H antigen is produced when an α1,2-L-fucosyltransferase catalyses the transfer of L-fucose from a guanosine diphosphate (GDP)-L-fucose donor to the C-2 position of the terminal galactose of one of the precursor structures shown in Section 2.2.2 (Table 2.3, Fig. 2.1). Two α1,2-L-fucosyltransferases, produced by two genes, *FUT1* (*H*) and *FUT2* (*SE*), catalyse the biosynthesis of H-active structures in different tissues. H-transferase, the product of *FUT1*, is active

Table 2.6 Some glycosyltransferase genes and the enzymes they produce.

Locus	Allele	Transferase
FUT1 (*H*)	*H*	α1,2-L-fucosyltransferase
	h	None
FUT2 (*SE*)	*Se*	α1,2-L-fucosyltransferase
	se	None
ABO	*A*	α1,3-*N*-acetyl-D-galactosaminyltransferase
	B	α1,3-D-galactosyltransferase
	O	None
FUT3 (*LE*)	*Le*	α1,3/4-L-fucosyltransferase
	le	None
FUT4		
FUT5		α1,3-L-fucosyltransferase
FUT6		
FUT7		
FUT8		α1,6-L-fucosyltransferase

in tissues of endodermal and mesodermal origin, and synthesizes red cell H antigen; secretor-transferase, the product of *FUT2*, is active in tissues of ectodermal origin, and is responsible for soluble H antigen in secretions (for review see [72]). *FUT1* has a higher affinity for Type 2 acceptor substrate than Type 1, whereas *FUT2* shows a preference for Type 1 acceptor substrate [73–76]. *FUT1* and *FUT2* share about 70% sequence identity and are 35 kilobases (kb) apart on the long arm of chromosome 19 [77,78] (see Chapter 32), suggesting that they were generated by duplication of an ancestral gene. *FUT1* consists of four exons and *FUT2* of two exons, but in both genes only one exon (exon 4 in *FUT1*, exon 2 in *FUT2*) encodes the protein product [79,80].

2.3.1.1 Red cells

Ernst, Rajan, Larsen *et al.* [81–83] used a gene-transfer method to isolate *FUT1* (*H*), because of difficulties in purifying the very small quantities of H-transferase present in tissues. Human genomic DNA was transfected into cultured mouse cells, which have all of the apparatus necessary to produce H-active carbohydrate chains apart from the *H*-gene-specified α1,2-fucosyltransferase. Transfected cells expressing H antigen were isolated with H-specific monoclonal antibodies and the human DNA in those cells used to produce secondary transfectants in mouse cells. Again, cells producing H antigen were isolated immunologically. With an *Eco*RI restriction fragment common to all secondary transfectants expressing H as a probe, a mammalian cDNA library was screened; the *H* gene was isolated, cloned, sequenced, and expressed in cultured monkey (COS-1) cells [81,82]. The expressed enzyme was an α1,2-L-fucosyltransferase with an apparent K_m very similar to that of H-transferase and different from the putative *Se* gene product (see below). Southern analysis showed that cDNA corresponded to genomic sequences syntenic to the *FUT1* locus on chromosome 19 [83].

Stable transfection of Chinese hamster ovary (CHO) cells with human *FUT1* cDNA revealed that H-transferase acts preferentially to fucosylate polylactosamine sequences [84]. The enzyme therefore does not indiscriminately act on all glycoprotein glycans, but favours glycoproteins containing polylactosamine sequences. This explains why ABH expression is restricted to relatively few red cell surface glycoproteins.

Most people have H antigen on their red cells. Rare alleles at the *FUT1* locus produce little or no active transferase and individuals homozygous for these alleles have little or no H on their red cells (see Section 2.13).

2.3.1.2 Secretions

Almost everybody expresses H antigen on their red cells, but only about 80% of Europeans have H antigen in their body secretions. These people are called ABH secretors because, if they have an *A* and/or *B* gene, they also secrete A and/or B antigens. The remaining 20% are called ABH non-secretors as they do not secrete H, A, or B regardless of *ABO* genotype. In people of European origin, ABH secretor status appears to be controlled by a pair of alleles, *Se* and *se*, at the secretor locus (*FUT2*). *Se*, the gene responsible for H secretion, is dominant over *se* [85,86] (see Section 2.6).

Before 1980 it was generally thought that secretor behaved as a regulator gene, which controlled expression of the *H* gene in secretory tissues. The very different conformations of Type 1 (Galβ1→3GlcNAc) and Type 2 (Galβ1→4GlcNAc) disaccharides in two-dimensional models led Lemieux [87] to suggest the probable existence of two distinct fucosyltransferases, one specific for a Type 1 chain and the other for a Type 2 chain. It was well established that red cells produce only Type 2 H structures, whereas secretions of ABH secretors contain both Type 1 H and Type 2 H [11]. Oriol *et al.* [88–90] proposed that the *H* gene codes for an α1,2-fucosyltransferase specific for Type 2 substrate and present in haemopoietic tissues, and that the *Se* gene codes for an α1,2-fucosyltransferase that utilizes both Type 1 and 2 substrate and is present in secretory glands. Identification of two human α1,2-fucosyltransferases with slightly different properties and subsequent cloning of two α1,2-fucosyltransferase genes has confirmed the concept of two structural genes.

Le Pendu *et al.* [73] compared α1,2-fucosyltransferase from the serum of non-secretor individuals with that from the serum of rare ABH secretors who lack H from their red cells (para-Bombay phenotype, see Section 2.13.3). The former transferase mostly originates from haemopoietic tissues and is the product of the *H* gene; the latter is believed to be the *Se* gene product [73,91]. Fucosyltransferases from these two sources differed from each other in various physicochemical characteristics, such as K_m for GDP-fucose and sensitivity to heat inactivation. The transferase present in the serum of the non-secretors (*H* product) favoured Type 2 acceptors, whereas that in serum from the secretors with H-deficient red cells (*Se* product) showed a definite preference for Type 1 substrate. Other, similar studies produced comparable results [74,75] and two α1,2-fucosyltransferases with different K_m values and electrophoretic mobilities were purified from pooled human serum [92].

In 1995, Rouquier *et al.* [77] exploited the close homology between the two α1,2-fucosyltransferase genes to clone *FUT2* (*Se*) from a human chromosome 19 cosmid library by cross-hybridization with *FUT1* cDNA. *FUT2* encodes a 332 amino acid polypeptide, with substantial sequence homology to the product of *FUT1*, plus an isoform with 11 extra residues at the N-terminus [78]. The expressed product had α1,2-fucosyltransferase activity with a pH optimum and K_m similar to that ascribed to the secretor-transferase. A nonsense mutation (Trp143Stop) was associated with an allele commonly responsible for the non-secretor phenotype [78]. In addition to *FUT2*, a pseudogene, *Sec1*, was isolated [77,78]. *Sec1* and *FUT2* are separated by 12 kilobases and share over 80% sequence identity, but *Sec1* contains translation termination codons, which disrupt potential open reading frames. The two α1,2-fucosyltransferase genes, *FUT1* and *FUT2*, and the pseudogene, *Sec1*, are located within about 50 kb on chromosome 19, and probably arose by gene duplication [72].

Se gene specified α1,2-fucosyltransferase is capable of activity on red cells *in vitro*. Bombay phenotype red cells, which are deficient in H-transferase and have no H, A, or B antigens (Section 2.13), become H-active after treatment, in the presence of GDP-fucose, with fucosyltransferase prepared from human gastric mucosa of a group O secretor, but not with that from a non-secretor [93]. Conversion was only achieved with sialidase-treated red cells, suggesting that the H precursor molecules on Bombay cells are masked by sialyl residues. The resulting H-active 'Bombay' cells could then be further converted to A activity with A-transferase in the presence of the appropriate nucleotide sugar donor [93].

The common non-secretor allele of *FUT2* in people of European and African origin (*se428*) contains a G428A nonsense mutation converting the codon for

Trp143 to a translation stop codon, so no active enzyme is produced [78,94–96] (Table 2.7). The *se428* allele also encodes a Gly247Ser substitution, but that change alone does not affect α1,2-fucosyltransferase activity [76,78]. The *se428* allele has not been found in Japan and Taiwan [95,98,99,102], but six other non-secretor alleles, four containing nonsense mutations and two containing three-nucleotide deletions, have been identified in Oriental, Polynesian, and Filipino non-secretors [76,94,98,101–104] (Table 2.7). An allele with a single base deletion was found in two of 101 black South Africans (Xhosa) [96].

Another non-secretor allele found in Japanese is a fusion gene comprising the 5′ region of the pseudogene *Sec1* and the 3′ region of *FUT2* [98]. COS cells transfected with the fusion gene had about 20% of the α1,2-fucosyltransferase activity of those transfected with the normal gene, yet expressed no H antigen. Although the sequence of the fusion gene suggests that it encodes a structurally functional protein, the promoter region of the fusion gene is expected to be identical to that of the pseudogene. This might explain why the gene is expressed in transfected COS cells, but not in native tissues [98].

Indian people with the rare Bombay phenotype have no H antigen on their red cells or in their secretions (Section 2.13.1). This phenotype results from homozygosity for an inactivating missense mutation in *FUT1* together with a deletion of exon 2 of *FUT2*, the whole of the coding region of the gene [105,106]. In one family of Indian people living in Réunion Island, a haplotype was identified in which a deleted *FUT2* was in *cis* with an apparently active *FUT1* [106]. It is probable that the *FUT2* deletion is not uncommon among non-secretors in India.

An allele of *FUT2* (*Sew385*), common in the Far East and South Pacific, encodes an Ile129Phe substitution in the stem region of the α1,2-fucosyltransferase [76,97–100]. This enzyme has identical substrate specificities to the normal *FUT2* product, but has at least a fivefold reduction in enzyme activity [76,98,99]. *Sew385* has a gene frequency of 44% in Japanese [98], but has not been detected in Europeans or Africans [76,96]. Homozygosity for *Sew385* (or heterozygosity for *Sew385* and a non-secretor allele) results in reduced levels of secreted H and the Le(a+b+) red cell phenotype, common in Far East and Pacific regions (Section 2.6.3).

A single, multiplex polymerase chain reaction

Table 2.7 *FUT2* alleles responsible for ABH non-secretor phenotypes (*se*) or partial-secretor phenotype (*Se^w*).

Allele	Mutation	Amino acid substitution	Population	Reference
Se^{w385}	A385T	Ile129Phe	Taiwan Chinese, Japanese, Indonesian, Polynesian, Filipino	[76,97–101]
se^{428}	G428A	Trp143Stop	European, African	[78,96,99]
se^{571}	C571T	Arg191Stop	Polynesian, Taiwanese, Japanese, European, Filipino	[76,94,96,98,101,102]
se^{628}	C628T	Arg210Stop	Japanese	[98]
se^{658}	C658T	Arg220Stop	Chinese	[103]
se^{685}	del GTG 685–689	del Val229 or 230	Taiwanese	[104]
se^{688}	del GTC 688–690	del Val230	Filipino	[101]
se^{778}	del C778	RFS Pro260, Stop at 275	African	[96]
se^{849}	G849A	Trp283Stop	Taiwanese, Filipino	[101,102]
se^{del}	del exon 2		Indian	[105,106]
se^{fus}	Sec1-FUT2 fusion		Japanese	[98]

del, deletion; RFS, reading frameshift.

(PCR) technique followed by restriction fragment-length polymorphism (RFLP) analysis has been devised to detect most of the known *FUT2* mutations [107].

Four *FUT2* alleles encoding amino acid substitutions appear to be responsible for between 50% and 80% reduction in enzyme activity [96]. Three of the alleles were found in black South Africans: *Se^{40}* Ile14Val; *Se^{481}* Asp161Asn; *Se^{40,481}* Ile14Val, Asp161Asn. The other allele, *Se^{379}* Arg127Cys, was present in a white South African [96].

2.3.1.3 Other tissues

Control of expression of H antigen in various human tissues follows a general trend, summarized as follows: H antigens on tissues of ectodermal and mesodermal origin (e.g. primary sensory neurones, skin, vascular endothelium, and bone marrow) are Type 2 structures and produced by *FUT1* (*H*) gene-specified α1,2-fucosyltransferase; those on tissues of endodermal origin (digestive and respiratory mucosae, salivary glands) are Type 1 and 2 structures and produced by the *FUT2* (*Se*) gene-specified enzyme [21]. However, there are a number of exceptions to these rules (Section 2.20.3). Plasma α1,2-fucosyltransferase is predominantly haemopoietic in origin [108] and may originate from circulating red cells and platelets [109].

FUT2 transcript was detected strongly in colon and small intestine and weakly in lung; no *FUT2* transcript was detected in liver or kidney [77].

2.3.2 ABO antigens

2.3.2.1 A- and B-transferases

H antigen, whether produced by H-transferase or Se-transferase, is the acceptor substrate for the *A* and *B* gene-specified glycosyltransferases (Fig. 2.1). The *A* gene product is an α1,3-N-acetyl-D-galactosaminyltransferase, which transfers N-acetyl-D-galactosamine from a uridine diphosphate (UDP)-N-acetylgalactosamine donor to the fucosylated galactosyl residue of H antigen. The *B* gene product, an α1,3-D-galactosyltransferase, transfers D-galactose from UDP-galactose to the fucosylated galactose of H. *A* and *B* are alleles at the *ABO* locus on chromosome 9. A third allele, *O*, does not produce an active enzyme and in persons homozygous for *O* the H antigen remains unmodified. If, because of the absence of H-transferase or Se-transferase, no H structure is available, A and B antigens cannot be produced despite the presence of the appropriate A- or B-transferase. This situation occurs in the secretions of ABH non-secretors and on red cells of the rare H-deficient (Bombay) phenotypes. The different species of A-

17

transferase associated with A_1 and A_2 phenotypes are described in Section 2.4.1.

Anti-H reagents agglutinate group O cells far more readily than most A and B cells as H antigen activity is masked by N-acetylgalactosamine and galactose in A- and B-active structures.

A-, B-, and H-transferase activity has been demonstrated *in vitro*. A-transferase prepared from human gastric mucosa converts O or B cells to A or AB activity in the presence of UDP-N-acetylgalactosamine [110]. Gastric mucosa, serum, saliva, and milk from group B individuals have all been used as sources of B-transferase for converting O cells to B-active cells in the presence of UDP-galactose [110–113]. Bombay phenotype cells, which lack the H-active substrate, could not be converted to B cells with α-galactosyltransferases [111].

Glycosyltransferases are antigenic structures. Human antibodies to blood group transferases are often produced following organ transplantation [114–117]. B, H, Le^a, Le^x, and Le^y determinants have all been detected on the carbohydrate chains of galactosyltransferase from human milk [118]. Rabbit antibodies [119] and murine monoclonal antibodies [120] raised to A-transferase cross-react with B-transferase.

2.3.2.2 Molecular genetics

A-transferase was purified to homogeneity from human lung and gastric tissues, and partial amino acid sequences were obtained [121,122]. Degenerate synthetic oligodeoxynucleotides based on the A-transferase partial amino acid sequence were employed by Yamamoto *et al.* [123] in the isolation and cloning of cDNA representing the *A* gene. The cDNA library was constructed from RNA isolated from a human gastric carcinoma cell line that expressed high levels of A antigen. The 1062 basepair (bp) sequence predicted a 353 amino acid protein with the three-domain structure characteristic of a glycosyltransferase. After the initial publication [123], it became apparent that the original clone from a gastric carcinoma contained a unique 3 bp deletion [124]. The numbering of nucleotides and encoded amino acids used in this chapter and in most publications reflects the usual sequence of the gene.

Based on the cDNA clone encoding A-transferase, *B* and *O* cDNA was also cloned and sequenced

[125,126]. *A* and *B* cDNAs were found to differ by seven nucleotides, four of which were responsible for amino acid substitutions at positions 176, 235, 266 and 268 (Figs 2.2 and 2.3). The *O* (or *O¹*) sequence is identical to the *A* (or *A¹*) sequence apart from a deletion of nucleotide 261 causing a shift in the reading frame and generation of a premature translation stop signal at the codon for amino acid residue 116. This allele encodes a truncated protein with no catalytic domain (Fig. 2.3) and may produce a mRNA transcript of reduced stability [127]. Cloned A and B cDNA was transfected into recipient cells expressing H antigen and the resulting A and B phenotypes could be detected immunologically. The common *A* sequence (*A¹*) is often referred to as the 'consensus sequence' and is used as a reference for the sequences of all other *ABO* alleles. The *A²* allele has a single nucleotide deletion in the codon before the translation stop codon of an *A¹* allele, resulting in disruption of that stop codon and an A-transferase product with an extra 21 amino acids at the C-terminus [128] (see Section 2.4.1).

The *O* allele described by Yamamoto *et al.* [125,126], with an *A¹* sequence disrupted by a single base deletion at position 261, is now named *O¹*. There are two other O alleles of significant frequency. A very common allele, *O¹ᵛ* (for *O¹*-variant), has the single base deletion of *O¹* at position 261, preventing the production of any active transferase, but contains at least nine other nucleotide differences from *O¹* and *A¹* [129]. The proportions of O alleles with the G261 deletion that are *O¹ᵛ* are as follows: Swedes, 42% [129]; Australians, 42% [130]; black Brazilians, 31% [131]; native Brazilians, 91% [131]; Japanese, 49–55% [132,133]; and Chinese, 39% [134]. Another O allele, *O²*, lacks the G261 nucleotide deletion, but has two nucleotide differences from the *A¹* sequence that encode amino acid changes: Arg176Gly (identical to that of B-transferase) and Gly268Arg [135,136] (Fig. 2.2). The substitution at position 268 exchanges a charged arginine residue for a non-charged glycine, presumably disrupting the catalytic site (Fig. 2.3). *In vitro* expression of an *A¹* cDNA construct with the codon for glycine at position 268 changed to an arginine codon by site-directed mutagenesis resulted in no A-transferase activity or A antigen expression [137]. Between 2% and 6% of *O* alleles in white donors from Europe, Australia, and the USA are *O²* [130,136,138–141]; *O²* has not been found in Japanese or Chinese [132–134]. The symbols *O101*

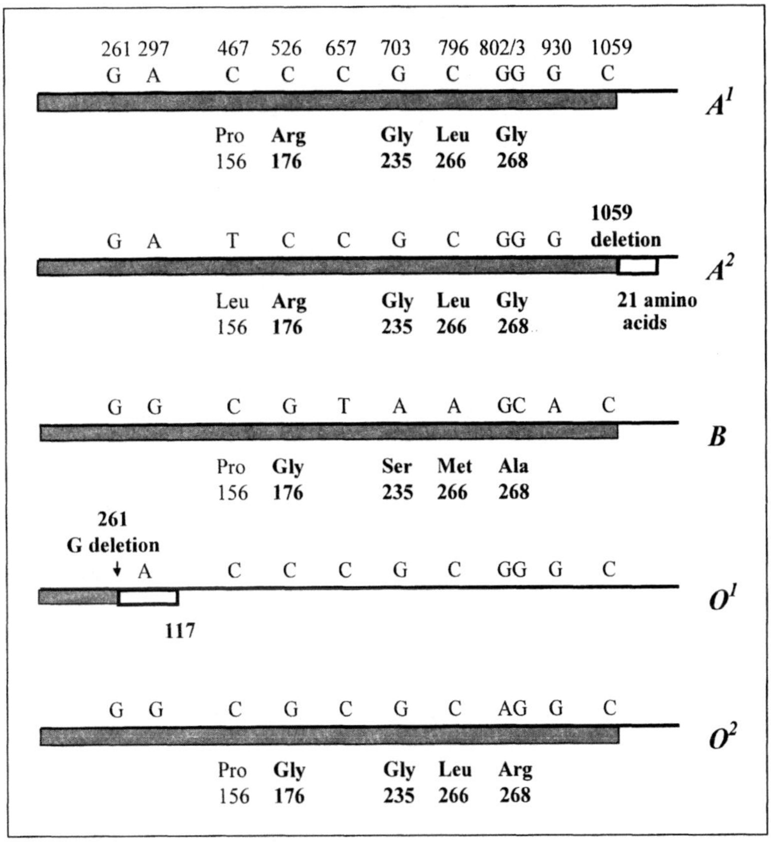

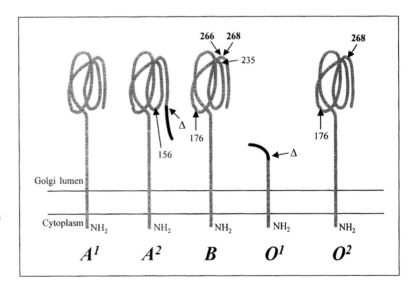

Fig. 2.2 Diagram representing cDNA and protein products of five common ABO alleles. Seven nucleotide changes distinguish A and B alleles and result in four amino acid differences between A- and B-transferases. Single base deletions in A^2 and O^1 result in reading frameshifts and introduction and abolition of stop codons in O^1 and A^2, respectively. Amino acid substitution at position 268 is responsible for inactivation of the O^2 product.

Fig. 2.3 Diagrammatic representation of the products of five *ABO* alleles located in the membrane of the Golgi apparatus (modified from Clausen *et al.* [20]), showing the positions of amino acids that differ from those of the A_1-transferase and the positions of the nucleotide deletions (Δ) in the A^2 and O^1 genes. Regions shown in black are the extra 21 amino acids in the A_2-transferase and the sequence encoded between the nucleotide deletion and the stop codon in the product of O^1.

and *O201 have also been used for O^1 and O^{1v}, respectively [133].

Yamamoto and Hakomori [126] constructed A-B cDNA chimeras representing all 16 possible combinations of the four amino acid substitutions distinguishing A and B cDNA. Transfection experiments, in a group O human cell line, demonstrated that the third (266) and fourth (268) amino acid substitutions (Fig. 2.2) are the most important in determining the specificity of the transferase. An enzyme with Met266 and Gly268 had dual A- and B-transferase activity. In vitro mutagenesis experiments, in which cDNA constructs encoding every possible amino acid residue at position 268 were expressed, led to the conclusion that the side chain of the amino acid residue at position 268 is responsible for determining both activity and donor-substrate specificity of the transferase product [137].

The coding region of the ABO gene is organized into seven exons, spanning 18 kb. Exons 6 and 7 constitute 77% of the coding sequence [124,142] (Fig. 2.4). The G261 deletion of O^1 and O^{1v} genes is in exon 6; the nucleotide changes that distinguish A, B, and O^2 are in exon 7.

Several GC boxes were found in a region just upstream of the transcription-initiation codon, but no sequence motifs for tissue-specific DNA-binding proteins [124]. However, DNA methylation of a CpG island within the gene promoter may have an important role in regulation of ABO expression in different tissues [143]. Transcription regulation of the ABO gene is dependent on a minisatellite almost 4 kb upstream of the start of the translated sequence, that contains a CBF/NF-Y transcription factor-binding motif [144]. This minisatellite consists of four copies of a 43-bp repeat sequence in A^2, B, O^1, and O^{1v} alleles, but only one copy in A^1 and O^2 alleles [144–146]. Furthermore, transient transfection assays suggested that the transcriptional induction capability of the A enhancer was over 100 times less than that of the B

enhancer [146]. The significance of this, in vivo, remains to be seen.

Many complexities of the ABO genes have been encountered. Most are relatively rare, but some are common in certain populations. About 80% of A^1 genes in Japanese (*A102) differ from the A^1 gene in Europeans (*A101) by encoding leucine instead of proline at position 156 [132,133]. This has no apparent affect on the phenotype. Some unusual ABO genes do affect activity of the gene products and these may result in subgroups of A and B (see Sections 2.7 and 2.8). A single nucleotide insertion in a string of seven guanosines at nucleotides 798–804 of an A^2 allele introduced a reading frameshift resulting in an enzymatically inactive product (O^3) [147]. Numerous genes have been identified that appear to be hybrids, comprising partly of sequences characteristic of one ABO allele and partly of sequences characteristic of another allele [139,141,148–150]. These fusion genes have probably arisen by meiotic crossing-over. In most of these hybrid genes the recombination has occurred within intron 6. Olsson and Chester [150] remark the presence of Chi or Chi-like sequences near the 3' end of intron 6, sequences associated with recombination hot-spots. Hybrid genes with exon 6 derived from O^1 or O^{1v} have a G261 deletion and are inactive, regardless of the origin of exon 7. Hybrid genes with exon 6 derived from A or B are generally active, with the origin of exon 7 determining specificity: exon 7 with A^1 or O^1 origin gives rise to A_1 activity; exon 7 with O^{1v} origin results in weakened A activity (A_2 or A_x).

Suzuki et al. [149] described a paternity case in which the mother was group B, the child group A, and the putative father group O; an apparent first-order exclusion of paternity. Many other polymorphic markers, however, failed to support this exclusion. Sequencing of the ABO genes of the family showed that the child had an ABO gene in which exon 6 (and, presumably, exons 1–5) had the sequence of a B allele and exon 7 the sequence of an O^1 allele. This hybrid gene had probably arisen in the germline of the mother as a result of crossing-over during meiosis (Fig. 2.5). This B-O^1 gene would encode an enzyme with A-transferase activity because O^1 and A^1 have an identical sequence in exon 7, the region encoding the catalytic site; the absense of the G261 deletion in exon 6 of B origin enables translation of this active enzyme. The child, therefore, had group A red cells, despite neither

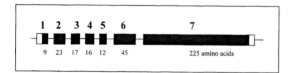

Fig. 2.4 Genomic organization of the ABO gene, showing the seven coding exons and number of amino acids encoded by each exon.

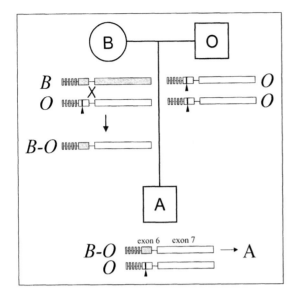

exon 6   exon 7

Fig. 2.5 A family with a group B mother, group O father, and group A child, an apparent first-order exclusion of paternity. Suzuki *et al.* [149] proposed that crossing-over between *B* and *O¹* alleles occurred in the germline of the mother, to create a *B-O* fusion gene that encodes a product with A-transferase activity, because exon 7 derived from an *O¹* gene has an identical sequence to exon 7 derived from an *A¹* gene. **X**, site of recombination; ▲, site of nucleotide deletion in *O¹* allele; open boxes represent exons derived from an *O¹* gene; shaded boxes represent exons derived from a *B* gene.

parent having an *A* gene. Such genetic events may be considered to be rare, yet Suzuki *et al* [149] estimate that similar recombinant alleles occur with a frequency of about 1% in the Japanese population.

The ABO genes have been well conserved during evolution [151–153]. Human *ABO* shares considerable sequence homology with non-primate α1,3-galactosyltransferase genes and with two human pseudogenes, one of which is localized, like *ABO*, to chromosome 9q33–34 [154,155]. A minimum of 95% homology in nucleotide and deduced amino acid sequences was detected in the *ABO* genes of primates [151]. Furthermore, the critical substitutions differentiating the *A* and *B* genes occurred before the divergence of the lineages leading to humans, chimpanzees, gorillas, and orang-utans [144]. This polymorphism is therefore at least 13 million years old and is most likely maintained by selection [144]. A labelled *ABO* gene probe hybridized with genomic DNA from marmoset, hamster, rat, mouse, sheep, cow, rabbit, cat, and dog [151]. The mouse *ABO* gene has a similar or-

ganization to human *ABO*, but has dual A- and B-transferase activity [156].

2.3.2.3 ABO genotyping from DNA

Numerous methods have been developed for *ABO* genotyping from genomic DNA. These mostly involve restriction enzyme analysis of PCR products [125,129,132,136,138,157–161] or PCR with allele specific primers [139–141,162]. Other methods involve analysis of PCR products by denaturing gradient gel electrophoresis [163,164], single-strand conformation [133,134], or sequence-specific oligonucleotide probing [130], and use of PCR with sequence-specific primers of different lengths [165]. Originally only *A*, *B*, and *O* could be identified, but later methods permitted the recognition of *A¹*, *A²*, *B*, *O¹* (including *O¹ᵛ*), and *O²* [129,130,134,138–141,160]. With the relatively common occurrence of so many variants, including fusion genes, results provided by these methods will not always be precise. However, providing the G261 deletion in exon 6 is detected and *A*, *B*, and *O²* are distinguished in exon 7, the tests will be reasonably reliable. Olsson *et al.* [166] devised a method for detecting recombinant hybrid *ABO* alleles by PCR with allele-specific primers that span intron 6.

Some gene frequencies, determined by PCR-based methods, are shown in Table 2.8.

2.3.3 Lewis antigens

In 1948 Grubb [167] made the observation that people with Le(a+) red cells were mostly non-secretors of ABH. Subsequently, the following general rule has been established for red cell Lewis phenotypes in adults:

Le(a+b–) red cells come from ABH non-secretors;
Le(a–b+) red cells come from ABH secretors;
Le(a–b–) red cells come from ABH secretors or non-secretors.

Grubb [168] later proposed a theory to explain the inheritance of the Lewis groups which, following family investigations, was confirmed and expanded by Ceppellini [169]. Basically, the theory of Grubb and Ceppellini states that the presence of Leᵃ in saliva is controlled by one locus (now called *LE* or *FUT3*) and thus Leᵇ might result from an interaction between the products of the Lewis and secretor genes. People with

Table 2.8 *ABO* allele frequencies determined by PCR-based analyses of genomic DNA.

Population	No. of alleles tested	Alleles					Reference
		A^1	A^2	B	O^1	O^2	
Europeans	600	0.215	0.062	0.112	0.583	0.028	[139]
English	172	0.198	0.075	0.105	0.605	0.017	[140]
Germans	234	0.214	0.068	0.051	0.650	0.017	[165]
Swedes	299	0.191	0.070	0.104	0.602	0.033	[138]
White Americans	240	0.188	0.017	0.108	0.671	0.017	[141]
Japanese	1040	0.287	ND	0.178	0.535	0	[132]
Japanese	208	0.288	0	0.178	0.534	0	[165]
Chinese	125	0.192	0	0.168	0.630	0	[134]

ND, not determined.

both Lewis and Secretor (*Se*) genes have Le^a and Le^b in their saliva and Le(a−b+) red cells, whereas those with a Lewis gene, but homozygous for the non-secretor allele (*se*), have only Le^a in their saliva and Le(a+b−) red cells. The Lewis and Secretor loci were shown by family studies to be genetically independent [170], although they are on the same chromosome (Chapter 32). The theories of Grubb and Ceppellini have now mostly been verified by biochemical evidence, although the situation is more complex in people from Eastern Asia and the Southern Pacific region, where a fourth red cell phenotype, Le(a+b+), is common.

The Lewis-related antigens, Le^c and Le^d, are described in Section 2.19.2.

2.3.3.1 Lewis biosynthesis

The Lewis (*Le*) gene product is an α1,4-L-fucosyltransferase [171,172], which catalyses the transfer of L-fucose from GDP-fucose to the *N*-acetylglucosamine of Type 1 acceptor substrates: to Type 1 precursor to form Le^a; to Type 1 H to form Le^b; to Type 1 A to form ALe^b; and to Type 1 B to form BLe^b. A pattern of interactions between genes at the *LE* (*FUT3*), *SE* (*FUT2*), and *ABO* loci determine whether Le^a or Le^b, or both, or neither, are present in secretions, plasma, and on red cells (Fig. 2.1).

At the simplest level, there are two alleles at the *LE* (*FUT3*) locus: *Le*, which encodes an α1,4-fucosyltransferase; and *le*, which is apparently silent. People homozygous for *le* secrete neither Le^a nor Le^b and have the Le(a−b−) red cell phenotype, regardless of their ABH and secretor phenotypes.

In ABH non-secretors (*se/se*), no α1,2-fucosyltransferase is present in secretions to convert Type 1 precursor to Type 1 H. Consequently, the Type 1 precursor is available as an acceptor substrate for the Le-transferase, resulting in production of the monofucosylated Le^a antigen; so the secretions contain Le^a and the red cells are Le(a+b−). People with an *Se* gene produce Type 1 H, which can then be converted by the Le-transferase to the difucosylated Le^b antigen. If they also have an *A* or *B* gene, much of the Type 1 H will be converted to A or B structures and so the Le-transferase will produce ALe^b or BLe^b. Although Le-transferase can utilize either Type 1 precursor or Type 1 H acceptor substrates to produce Le^a and Le^b, respectively, Le^a is a very poor substrate for the *Se* gene specified α1,2-fucosyltransferase [10,16]. Consequently, there is competition between these two enzymes for substrate [173,174]. If any Le^a is produced from Type 1 'precursor' by the Le-transferase it cannot be converted further to Le^b by Se-transferase, so secretions of a person with *Le* and *Se* genes contain Le^a and Le^b, although very little Le^a is detected in the plasma or on the red cells. Similarly, Le^b is not an acceptor substrate for A- or B-transferase [10,16], and secretions of an individual with *Le*, *Se*, and *A* genes contain Le^a, Le^b, and ALe^b (Fig. 2.1). The product of the weak secretor gene (*Se^w*), common in the Far East, competes with the Le-transferase less effectively than that of an *Se* allele, resulting in substantially greater production of Le^a than present in secretors. People homozygous for *Se^w*, or heterozygous *Se^w/se*, have Le^a and Le^b in their plasma and secretions and Le(a+b+) red cells [54,76,97,100,175,176].

Le-transferase has the exceptional ability to catalyse two distinct glycosidic linkages. In addition to α1,4-fucosyltransferase activity, it has some α1,3-fucosyltransferase activity and is usually referred to as an α1,3/4-L-fucosyltransferase [177–180], although it is almost 100 times more efficient on Type 1 H than Type 2 H acceptors [181]. Substitution of Trp111 to arginine by site-directed mutagenesis converted the acceptor specificity of the Le-transferase from Type 1 H to Type 2 H [182].

2.3.3.2 Molecular genetics

Kukowska-Latallo *et al.* [180] employed a gene transfer technique (like that described in Section 2.3.1.1 for isolation of the *H* gene) to clone and sequence cDNA encoding *Le*-gene-specified α1,3/4-fucosyltransferase. The gene contains an intronless coding region, which encodes a 361-amino acid protein with the three-domain structure typical of glyco-

syltransferases. There is a high level of sequence identity with some of the α1,2- and α1,3-fucosyltransferase genes.

The genetic basis for the Le(a–b–) red cell phenotype is heterogeneous, but is always associated with one or more missense mutations within the region of *FUT3* encoding the catalytic domain of the Lewis-transferase [183–193] (Table 2.9). No Lewis nonsense mutation has been found. Transfection experiments with cDNA or chimeric *FUT3* constructs showed that the following amino acid substitutions caused complete or almost complete inactivation of α1, 3/4-fucosyltransferase activity: Trp68Arg [194]; Gly170Ser [186]; Ile356Lys [185,186]. The enzyme is not inactivated by Thr105Met, which is always associated with Trp68Arg [194]. The mutation encoding Leu20Arg is common in Lewis-negative alleles (Table 2.9). This substitution occurs within the transmembrane domain of the enzyme and does not affect catalytic activity [183–185], but may affect anchoring

Table 2.9 *FUT3* alleles associated with inactivity of the Lewis-transferase and the encoded amino acid substitutions.

Symbol*	Amino acid position									Populations	References
	20	68	105	146	162	170	223	270	356		
†*Le*	Leu	Trp	Thr	Leu	Asp	Gly	Gly	Val	Ile		
‡*Le^{59}*	Arg	–	–	–	–	–	–	–	–	Indonesians, Europeans, Japanese, Chinese	[185,188,191–193]
le^{1067}	–	–	–	–	–	–	–	–	Lys	Indonesians, Europeans, Japanese, Chinese	[185,189,191,192]
le^{59,1067}	Arg	–	–	–	–	–	–	–	Lys	Europeans, Japanese, Indonesians, Africans, Chinese	[185,186,188–193]
le^{59,508}	Arg	–	–	–	–	Ser	–	–	–	Europeans, Japanese, Chinese, Africans	[183,184,186–188, 190–193]
le^{202,314}	–	Arg	Met	–	–	–	–	–	–	Europeans, Africans, Chinese	[188,190–192]
le^{59,68,1067}	Arg	Arg	–	–	–	–	–	–	Lys	Europeans	[188]
le^{59,445}	Arg	–	–	Met	–	–	–	–	–	Europeans	[188]
le^{202}	–	Arg	–	–	–	–	–	–	–	Europeans, Africans	[191]
le^{484,667}	–	–	–	–	Asn	–	Arg	–	–	Africans	[191]
le^{484,667,808}	–	–	–	–	Asn	–	Arg	Met	–	Africans	[191]
le^{202,314,484}	–	Arg	Met	–	Asn	–	–	–	–	Europeans	[191]

*Numbers represent nucleotide position of mutation.
†Common active allele.
‡Product enzymatically active, but may affect Golgi anchoring.

Table 2.10 Frequencies of *FUT3* alleles in three populations.

Allele	White South Africans (100)	Black South Africans (Xhosa) (100)	Japanese (808)
Le	0.675	0.500	0.643
Le⁵⁹	0	0.020	0
le¹⁰⁶⁷	0	0.005	0.001
le⁵⁹,¹⁰⁶⁷	0.130	0.025	0.082
le⁵⁹,⁵⁰⁸	0.010	0.310	0.274
le²⁰²,³¹⁴	0.140	0.080	0
le²⁰²	0.010	0.015	0
le⁴⁸⁴,⁶⁷	0	0.025	0
le⁴⁸⁴,⁶⁶⁷,⁸⁰⁸	0	0.020	0
le²⁰²,³¹⁴,⁴⁸⁴	0.005	0	0
Le³⁰⁴	0.005	0.020	0
Le³⁷⁰	0	0.005	0
References	[191]	[191]	[99,186,189]

of the enzyme in the Golgi membrane [185,193]. Leu20Arg in the absence of any other Lewis mutation is relatively common in Indonesians, and people homozygous for this allele have Le(a–b–) red cells but secrete Lewis antigens [185]. Two other missense mutations, *Le³⁰⁴* (Gln102Lys) and *Le³⁷⁰* (Ser124Ala), have no affect on enzyme activity [191].

In white populations, *le²⁰²,³¹⁴* and *le⁵⁹,¹⁰⁶⁷* are the two most frequent Lewis-negative alleles [190,191], whereas *le⁵⁹,⁵⁰⁸* is the most frequent in black Africans and in Japanese [99,186,189,191] (Table 2.10).

The positions of the inactivating mutations in *FUT3* suggest that the catalytic domain of the Lewis-transferase includes the region from amino acid residues 68–356. Expression of *FUT3* constructs that produce truncated proteins demonstrated that a protein consisting of amino acids 62–361 is enzymatically active, but shorter forms were inactive [195].

α1,4-fucosyltransferase activity has been identified in a number of tissues and secretions: kidney, gastric mucosa, submaxilliary glands, ovarian cyst linings, saliva, and milk (see [10]). α1,4-fucosyltransferase activity has not been detected in serum, red cells, lymphocytes, granulocytes, or platelets [178,196–198], suggesting that there is no haemopoietic origin for this enzyme. High levels of *FUT3* (*LE*) transcripts are present in colon, stomach, small intestine, lung, and kid-

ney; lesser amounts are present in salivary gland, bladder, uterus, and liver [199].

2.3.4 Le^x, Le^y, and sialyl-Le^x

Le^x (CD15) and Le^y represent the Type 2 isomers of Le^a and Le^b, respectively (Table 2.3). An α1,3-ʟ-fucosyltransferase catalyses the transfer of ʟ-fucose from a nucleotide donor to C-3 of the subterminal *N*-acetylglucosamine of Type 2 precursor, Type 2 H, Type 2 A, or Type 2 B to produce Le^x, Le^y, ALe^y, and BLe^y, respectively (Fig. 2.1). In analogy with the Lewis structures, Le^x antigen is not converted to Le^y antigen by H-transferase or Se-transferase, and Le^y antigen is not converted to ALe^y or BLe^y by A- or B-transferase. (The antigen described here as Le^x differs from the original Le^x antigen, called Le^abx in this chapter, see Section 2.19.1.)

In addition to *FUT3*, the Lewis gene, four other genes encoding enzymes with α1,3-fucosyltransferase activity have been cloned [200–206] (Table 2.6). *FUT3*, *FUT5*, and *FUT6* (plasma gene) have about 90% sequence homology and form a cluster on chromosome 19p13.3 (see Chapter 32). *FUT4* (myeloid gene) and *FUT7* (leucocyte gene) are located on chromosomes 11 and 19, respectively [205–207]. Fucosylation of a 2,3-sialylated acceptor produces sialyl-Le^x (sialyl-CD15) [203,204] (Table 2.3), a ligand for the selectin family of cell adhesion proteins [208–210] (Section 2.19.3). *FUT4* controls expression of Le^x on leucocytes and brain, whereas *FUT7* is responsible for synthesis of sialyl-Le^x on leucocytes. *FUT6* produces an α1,3-fucosyltransferase present in plasma, liver, kidney, colon, and salivary glands. The tissue distribution of the *FUT5* enzyme has not been determined (for review see [72]). In addition to Type 2 acceptors, the *FUT2* enzyme may be able utilize Type 1 acceptors [182,211] and so may be able to synthesize Lewis antigens.

The cluster of three homologous fucosyltransferase genes, *FUT3*, *FUT5*, and *FUT6*, and possibly the other fucosyltransferase genes (Table 2.6), probably arose by successive duplications followed by translocations and divergent evolution from a single ancestral gene. *FUT8*, which encodes an α1,6-fucosyltransferase, may represent the ancestral gene [181].

Homozygosity for *FUT6* alleles containing either a missense mutation (Glu247Lys) or a nonsense mutation (Tyr315Stop) is responsible for deficiency of plasma α1,3-fucosyltransferase in Indonesia [212], Polynesia and Sweden [213]. Nine per cent of Indonesians from Java have α1,3-fucosyltransferase deficiency, and 95% of these individuals have Le(a–b–) red cells, indicating linkage disequilibrium between the very closely linked *FUT3* (*LE*) and *FUT6* loci [212].

Part 3: ABO, Hh, and secretor systems

2.4 A$_1$ and A$_2$

The existence of subgroups of A, with red cells of one subgroup demonstrating weaker expression of A antigen than those of the other, was first recognized by von Dungern and Hirszfeld [214] in 1911. Landsteiner and Levine [215] named the two major subgroups A$_1$ and A$_2$.

The usual way of interpreting the A$_1$ and A$_2$ subgroups is as follows.

		Anti-A (group B serum)	
Group	Antigens	Anti-A	Anti-A$_1$
A$_1$	A A$_1$	+	+
A$_2$	A	+	–

Sera from group B individuals appear to contain two antibody components, anti-A and anti-A$_1$. A$_1$ cells react with both components, whereas A$_2$ cells react only with anti-A. Adsorption of some group B sera with A$_2$ cells removes anti-A leaving behind anti-A$_1$ [214]; continued adsorption of group B serum with A$_2$ cells, however, eventually removes all antibody [216]. Regrettably, the term anti-A has two meanings: the antiserum that reacts with A and AB cells; and one of the two antibody components present in group B serum. In this chapter, the precise meaning of 'anti-A' should be apparent from its context.

Anti-A$_1$ is present in the serum of some A$_2$ and A$_2$B people [217,218]. By agglutination of A$_1$ cells at room temperature, anti-A$_1$ was found in the serum of 1–2% of A$_2$ and 22–26% of A$_2$B individuals [219,220]. More sensitive techniques revealed anti-A$_1$ in higher proportions of A$_2$ and A$_2$B donors [221,222].

Probably the best and most widely used anti-A$_1$ reagent is *Dolichos biflorus* lectin [223]. Raw extract of *Dolichos* seeds agglutinates A$_1$ and A$_2$ red cells, but at a suitable dilution the lectin will easily distinguish

Table 2.11 A$_1$A$_2$BO genotypes and serologically determined phenotypes.

Genotype	Phenotype
A¹/A¹	
A¹/A²	A$_1$
A¹/O	
A²/A²	A$_2$
A²/O	
B/B	B
B/O	
A¹/B	A$_1$B
A²/B	A$_2$B
O/O	O

A$_1$ and A$_1$B from A$_2$ and A$_2$B. Red cells from group A babies usually react only weakly with *Dolichos* lectin and may not be agglutinated at all by human anti-A$_1$ [224]. It should be remembered that *Dolichos* lectin also agglutinates rare red cells with a very strong Sd^a antigen and Tn polyagglutinable red cells, regardless of ABO group (Chapters 29 and 31).

A$_2$ red cells have substantially higher expression of H antigen than A$_1$ cells.

When determined by serological means, the *A¹* gene appears dominant over *A²* and the genotypes *A¹/A¹* and *A¹/A²* cannot be discriminated by blood grouping techniques (Table 2.11). These genotypes may be determined by family studies, transferase assays, or molecular genetics.

2.4.1 A$_1$- and A$_2$-transferases, and the genes that produce them

The *A* gene product is an *N*-acetylgalactosaminyltransferase (Section 2.3.2.1). A-transferase isolated from sera or gastric mucosa of A$_1$ individuals is more effective at converting group O red cells to A-active cells than that from A$_2$ people [225–228]. When A$_2$ enzyme is used, the reaction is much slower and under normal conditions O cells are only converted to A$_2$ phenotype. However, after extended incubation with A$_2$ enzyme, O cells may be weakly agglutinated by A$_1$-specific reagents [228]. A$_1$ enzyme can convert A$_2$ cells to A$_1$ phenotype [226,227]. *N*-acetylgalactosaminyltransferases from

A_1 and A_2 sources have the same specificity for low molecular weight acceptors and both synthesize the same A determinant [10]. Yet at pH 5.5, activity of A-transferase from A_1 serum, with low molecular weight substrate, is 5–10 times higher than that from A_2 serum [229].

Schachter *et al.* [230] confirmed that A_1 and A_2 serum transferases are qualitatively different enzymes. They have different pH optima: 5.6 for A_1-transferase and between 7 and 8 for A_2-transferase. Sera from heterozygous A^1/A^2 individuals can be distinguished from sera from A^1/A^1 or A^1/O people by pH optima and by isoelectric point [231]. At pH 7.2, A_2-transferase, the less efficient enzyme, has a K_m value about 10 times higher than that for A_1-transferase [230]. *In vitro* conversion of O cells to A activity by A-transferase generally requires the presence of Mn^{2+} ions. If Mn^{2+} is substituted by Mg^{2+}, A_1-transferase remains active, but A_2-transferase does not [230].

The A^2 allele in people of European origin contains a deletion of one of the three cytosines at positions 1059–1061 (CCC to CC). This deletion is in the codon before the translation stop codon and causes a reading frameshift and loss of the stop codon, resulting in a gene product with an extra 21 amino acid residues at its C-terminus [128] (Figs 2.3 and 2.6). The A^2 allele also encodes Leu156, in place of Pro156 of the A^1 consensus sequence. A human cell line transfected with an A^1 cDNA construct with the C1059 deletion introduced artificially produced an A-transferase with drastically reduced activity. The Pro156Leu substitution had little effect on enzyme activity [128].

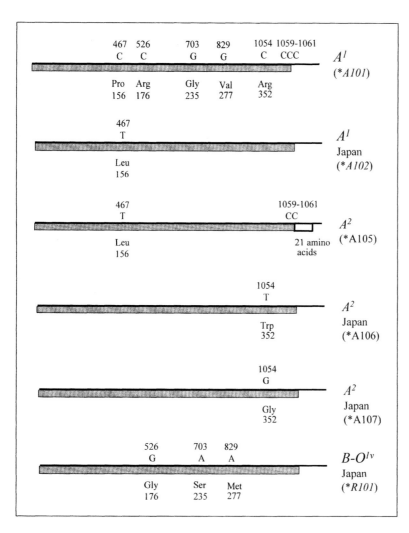

Fig. 2.6 Diagram representing cDNA and protein products of six ABO alleles. The top sequence is the consensus sequence (European A^1). The other sequences represent Japanese A^1 and four A^2 alleles, showing how they differ from the consensus sequence. Some silent nucleotide changes are not shown.

In Japan the situation is different [232,233]. The allele described above with a C1059 deletion (also called *A105) is rare. The two most common A^2 alleles do not have the C1059 deletion, but have different missense mutations within codon 352, only three codons before the normal stop codon: Arg352Trp (*A106) and Arg352Gly (*A107) (Fig. 2.6). A B-O^{1v} hybrid allele (*R101), also quite common in Japan, gives rise to an A_1 phenotype when paired with O, but an A_2B phenotype when paired with B, presumably because of competition for a common acceptor between the A-active hybrid transferase and the B-transferase [233]. This allele is responsible for an imbalance in A_2 and A_2B phenotype frequencies in Japan.

2.4.2 A_1 and A_2: do determinants differ qualitatively as well as quantitatively?

Since the A_1 and A_2 subgroups were first described there has been controversy as to whether A_1 and A_2 cells differ purely in the number of A determinants or whether these antigens actually show structural differences. Repeated adsorption of anti-A_1 from group B serum with A_2 cells will remove all antibody, suggesting a quantitative difference [216,234], but A_2 and A_2B individuals often make anti-A_1, suggesting that A_2 cells lack a determinant present on A_1 cells [217,218].

There is no doubt that a quantitative difference between A_1 and A_2 cells exists. A variety of techniques has been used to estimate the number of antigen sites on red cells. These include radioimmunoassay with labelled antibody or lectin [235–241], electron microscopy of red cells sensitized with ferritin-labelled lectin [242], conversion of H sites with radiolabelled UDP-N-acetylgalactosamine and A-transferase [27,238,239], and flow cytometry with monoclonal antibodies [243]. Estimated numbers of antigens sites per red cell can be summarized as follows:

A_1 $8-12\times10^5$
A_2 $1-4\times10^5$
A_1B $5-9\times10^5$
A_2B 1×10^5 [235–240,242,243].

Rochant et al. [244] found that the majority of red cells from A_2 individuals showed faint fluorescence with fluorescent Dolichos lectin, while a few cells demonstrated very strong fluorescence; conversely, in a population of A_1 cells, most had strong reactivity while around 10% exhibited only faint fluorescence. This may explain the 'mixed field' appearance of agglutination usually observed with anti-A_1 reagents.

A_1 and A_2 also differ qualitatively. Repetitive Type 3 A structures (see Section 2.2.2 and Table 2.3) are present on A_1 red cells, but not on A_2 cells [62,64,65]. Repetitive Type 3 chains are only present on group A cells because they are produced by the addition of a galactose residue to the terminal N-acetylgalactosamine of a Type 2 A chain followed by the fucosylation of that galactose to form Type 3 H (Fig. 2.7). A_1-transferase, but not A_2-transferase, is able to convert Type 3 H to Type 3 A by the addition of an N-acetylgalactosamine residue [65], so Type 3 H, but not Type 3 A, is detected on A_2 cells. Likewise, Type 4 H, but not Type 4 A, is detected on the glycolipids of A_2 cells [62,65]. It is probable that anti-A_1 is specific for, or shows a preference for, Type 3 A and/or Type 4 A structures. However, Dolichos lectin detects

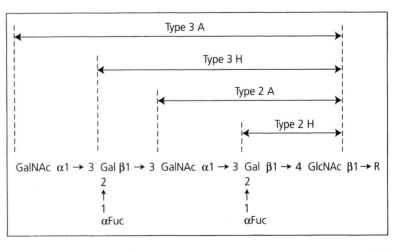

Fig. 2.7 Diagram showing how a repetitive Type 3 A chain is built up from a Type 2 H chain. From right to left, Type 2 H is converted to Type 2 A in group A people. Type 2 A may be converted to Type 3 H. Type 3 H is then further converted to Type 3 A in A_1, but not A_2 individuals.

N-acetylgalactosamine and, when present in sufficient concentration, agglutinates A_2 cells, so its use as a reagent for subtyping group A cells probably depends more on the quantitative than the qualitative difference between A_1 and A_2 phenotypes.

2.4.3 A_{int}

Landsteiner and Levine [215] recognized that the red cells of some group A individuals could not be defined as either A_1 or A_2, but fell into an intermediate category. A_{int} does not represent a true intermediate, however, as the level of H is as high as that found in A_2 and may be higher [224,245–248].

A_{int} is more common in black than white people. Of group A African Americans, 8.5% were found to be A_{int} compared with about 1% of group A white Americans [249]. Of group A black South Africans, 13.7% were A_{int} [245]. A_{int} appears to be inherited as an allele at the *ABO* locus [246,247].

Yoshida *et al.* [250] detected a unique form of A-transferase in A_{int} sera, which differed from A_2-transferase in having a high affinity for UDP-*N*-acetylgalactosamine and from A_1-transferase in having a low affinity for 2′-fucosyllactose, a soluble analogue for membrane-bound H-substance.

2.5 ABO phenotype and gene frequencies

Millions of people have been ABO grouped and the frequencies of the four phenotypes, A, B, AB, and O, differ substantially throughout the world, and often show marked variations even within quite small countries. In 1976, Mourant *et al.* [251] published the results of ABO tests on nearly 8 million people, together with previously published data on almost 7 million more. A supplement to this book included ABO data on about another million individuals [252]. Anyone requiring information on ABO frequencies of populations from virtually every country in the world is referred to these books.

As an example of ABO frequencies in britain, a study of unrelated individuals from the south of England is shown in Table 2.12. Red cells were tested with anti-A, -B, and -A_1, and sera were checked for reciprocal agglutinins. Methods for calculating *ABO* gene frequencies are given elsewhere [86] and computer programs also are available for this purpose. Detailed analyses of families tested for A_1A_2BO groups confirmed the accuracy of the genetical concepts of Bernstein [6,7] for ABO and of Thomsen *et al.* [8] for A_1A_2BO.

Populations with a high frequency of O (gene frequency greater than 0.7, i.e. 70%) are found in North and South America, and in parts of Africa and Australia, but not in most of Europe or Asia. Some native people of South and Central America are virtually all group O and probably were entirely so before the European invasion. The frequency of *A* is quite high (0.25–0.55) in Europe, especially in Scandinavia and

Table 2.12 A_1A_2BO phenotype, gene, and genotype frequencies in the south of England in 1939 [253].

Phenotype			Gene Calculated frequency		Genotype Calculated frequency	
	No.	Frequency				
O	1503	0.4345	*O*	0.6602	*O/O*	0.4349
A_1	1204	0.3481	*A¹*	0.2090	*A¹/A¹*	0.0437
					A¹/O	0.2760
					A¹/A²	0.0291
A_2	342	0.0989	*A²*	0.0696	*A²/A²*	0.0048
					A²/O	0.0919
B	297	0.0859	*B*	0.0612	*B/B*	0.0037
					B/O	0.0808
A_1B	91	0.0263			*A¹/B*	0.0256
A_2B	22	0.0063			*A²/B*	0.0085
Total	**3459**	**1.0000**		**1.0000**		**1.0000**

Table 2.13 Phenotype, gene, and genotype frequencies for secretor status of a random selection of people from Liverpool in 1960 [224].

Phenotype	No.	Frequency	Gene	Calculated frequency	Genotype	Calculated frequency
Secretors	864	0.7728	Se	0.5233	Se/Se	0.2739
					Se/se	0.4989
Non-secretors	254	0.2272	se	0.4767	se/se	0.2272

parts of Central Europe. High *A* frequency is also found in the Aborigines of South Australia (up to 0.45) and in certain Native American tribes, where the frequency reaches 0.35. A^2 is found mainly in Europe, the Near East, and Africa, but is either very rare or absent from indigenous populations throughout the rest of the world. The frequency of A^2 in Lapland reaches 0.37, but elsewhere in Europe it does not exceed 0.1. *B*, almost absent from Native Americans and most Australian Aborigines, probably was absent before the arrival of Europeans. High frequencies of *B* are found in Central Asia (0.2–0.3). In Europe, *B* frequency diminishes from about 0.15 in the east to less than 0.05 in the Netherlands, France, Spain, and Portugal (data compiled from Mourant *et al.* [251]). For a diagrammatic representation of some examples of gene frequencies in different populations see Fig. 2.8.

Some gene frequencies determined by molecular methods are provided in Table 2.8. The frequencies for English donors correlate remarkably well with those calculated from serological data (Table 2.12), considering changes in the ethnicity of the donor populations. It is important to remember that the serologically determined phenotypes—A_1, A_2, O, and to a lesser extent, B—are genetically heterogeneous (Sections 2.3.2.2 and 2.4.1).

2.6 Secretion of ABO and H antigens

By 1926 it was apparent that A and B antigens were not confined to red cells, but were present, in soluble form, in seminal fluid and saliva [255]. In 1930, Putkonen [256] noted that a proportion of A, B, and AB individuals lacked A or B antigens from their body fluids. The ability to secrete A, B, and 'O' was found to be inherited in a Mendelian manner, genetically inde-

pendent of ABO [85]. The locus controlling ABH secretion is called Secretor (*SE*, and subsequently *FUT2*): the ability to secrete (*Se*) is dominant over non-secretor (*se*) [85]. Although some other blood group antigens are also present in secretions, the terms 'secretor' and 'non-secretor' refer only to ABH secretion.

In secretor individuals of the appropriate ABO group, ABH antigens are detected in the secretions of the goblet cells and mucous glands of the gastrointestinal tract (saliva, gastric juice, bile, meconium), genitourinary tract (spermatic fluid, vaginal secretions, ovarian cyst fluid, urine), and respiratory tract, as well as in milk, sweat, tears, and amniotic fluid [35,254,257]. Secreted ABH antigens are mostly carried on glycoproteins of high molecular weight called mucins, but are also present in milk and urine as free oligosaccharides [10,36,37]. Secreted A, B, and H antigens are expressed on Type 1, 2, and 3 structures [10,14,44,61].

Se and *se* are alleles of the endodermal α1,2-fucosyltransferase gene, *FUT2*. The symbol *se* represents a number of alleles containing inactivating mutations (see Section 2.3.1.2 and Table 2.7). *Se* and *se* determine the presence or absence of H substance in secretions. A- and B-transferases are not under the control of the secretor gene, but are unable to catalyse the production of A and B substances in body fluids of non-secretors because of lack of H antigen, their acceptor substrate (see Section 2.3.2). The study of dispermic chimeras has shown that in order to secrete A, an *A* gene and an *Se* gene must be expressed in the same cell, and the corresponding situation applies to cells that secrete B substance [258,259].

The simplest method of determining secretor status is by inhibition of haemagglutination. Saliva is added to selected and appropriately diluted anti-A, -B, and

29

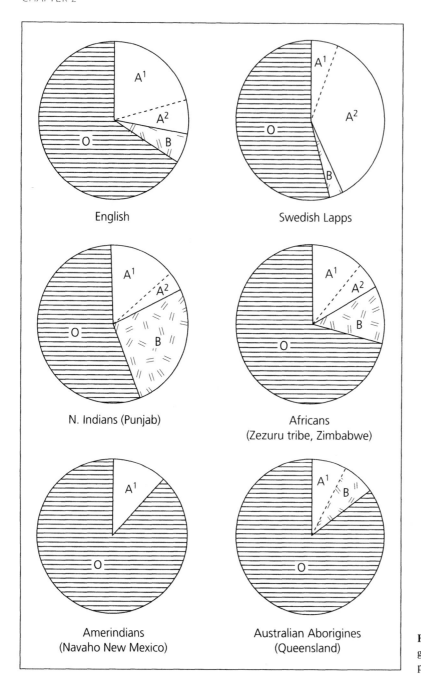

English

Swedish Lapps

N. Indians (Punjab)

Africans
(Zezuru tribe, Zimbabwe)

Amerindians
(Navaho New Mexico)

Australian Aborigines
(Queensland)

Fig. 2.8 Diagram showing A^1A^2BO gene frequencies in six selected populations.

-H (usually *Ulex europaeus* lectin), and inhibition determined by the failure of these mixtures to agglutinate A_2, B, and O cells, respectively.

2.6.1 Frequencies

In most European populations the frequency of secretors is about 80% [251]. Table 2.13 shows the results of secretor tests, with deduced gene and genotype frequencies, on over 1000 people from Liverpool [224]. *Ulex europaeus* lectin (anti-H) was used in agglutination inhibition tests and all A_1, A_1B, or B non-secretors were also checked for ability to inhibit agglutination by anti-A or -B.

The frequency of the *Se* gene does not differ greatly from 0.5 in most ethnic groups, although in Australian Aborigines, Inuits, some Native Americans, and some Melanesians, the frequency approaches 1.0 [251]. In India there is more variation with a high frequency of *Se* in the North (up to 0.75) and low frequency in the South (0.22).

2.6.2 Quantitative aspects

From a study of sibling pairs, Clarke *et al.* [260] report that individual quantitative variation of salivary A, B, or H antigens is, at least in part, inherited, and inherited in a polygenic manner. Sex and age, from 10 to 80 years, do not influence the concentration of ABH substances in saliva [261]. The primitive salivary glands of a human fetus produce secretion rich in ABH antigens from the gestational age of about nine weeks [262] and ABH antigens are well developed in neonatal saliva [263,264].

A variety of techniques, mostly employing human anti-A or *Dolichos biflorus* lectin, has provided substantial evidence that A_1 saliva contains more A antigen than A_2 saliva [173,261,265–269]. Clausen [14] has detected repetitive Type 3 A on A_1, but not A_2, ovarian cyst mucins. So, at least in part, the same basis for a qualitative difference between A_1 and A_2 determinants exists in secretions as on red cells (see Section 2.4.2).

Saliva from AB secretors contains less A and B substance than saliva from group A secretors and group B secretors, respectively [261,268,269] (Table 2.14), suggesting that in the saliva of AB secretors there is

competition between the A- and B-transferases for a common substrate.

The relative quantities of H antigen in secretor saliva of individuals of different ABO groups, shown in Table 2.14, has mostly been determined by inhibition of *Ulex europaeus* lectin [260,261,266,268,270], but extracts of seeds of *Cytisus sessilifolius* [270] and *Laburnum alpinum* [269] have also been used. The descending order of H quantity in saliva of different ABO groups differs from that found on red cells ($O > A_2 > B > A_1$), as determined by agglutination with *Ulex europaeus* lectin [266]. Three separate studies agreed that the quantity of secreted H substance is genetically determined and under the control of more genes than those at the secretor and *ABO* loci [260,271,272].

Small quantities of H, A, and B substances can be detected in the saliva of most non-secretors [174,254,273–275]. H-antigen production in non-secretor saliva is probably catalysed by the *H* (*FUT1*) gene-specified α1,2-fucosyltransferase and not the *Se* gene product. Betteridge and Watkins [75] detected a low level of α1,2-fucosyltransferase in submaxillary gland preparations from non-secretors, which showed the Type 2-acceptor preference typical of *H* gene-specified transferase.

2.6.3 Se^w

A weak secretor gene (Se^w or Se^{w385}), containing a missense mutation encoding an Ile129Phe substitution [76,97–100], is responsible for the Le(a+b+) red cell phenotype common in Orientals and Polynesians [54,175,176]. An α1,2-fucosyltransferase that is less efficient than the normal *Se* gene product would compete less effectively with the Lewis-transferase for the Type 1 precursor substrate. Consequently, a greater quantity of the substrate would be converted to Le^a antigen so that less would be available to be converted to Type 1 H and, subsequently, to Le^b (see Section 2.3.3.1).

2.6.4 A, B, and H antigens in plasma

A, B, and H antigens are found in the plasma of ABH secretors and non-secretors, although greater quantities are present in the former [90,276–278]. With anti-Type 1 H (serum from goats immunized with human saliva and adsorbed with immunoadsorbents coated

Table 2.14 Relative mean concentration of salivary blood group substances in secretions as determined by an automated quantitative inhibition method and approximate percentage relationships, according to red cell type [261].

Substance	Red cell type
A	$A_1 > A_1B > A_2 > A_2B$ 100 60 40 10
B	$B > A_2B > A_1B$ 100 75 25
H	$O > A_2 > A_1 > B \approx A_2B \approx A_1B$ 100 60 40 20 20 20

with Type 2 H trisaccharide) and anti-Type 2 H lectin (*Ulex europaeus*), Le Pendu *et al.* [90] showed that plasma from ABH secretors contains Type 1 H and Type 2 H, but plasma from non-secretors contains only Type 2 H. They estimated that all of the Type 1 H and about one-third of the Type 2 H in plasma is controlled by the secretor system, whereas most of the Type 2 H is independent of secretor and is presumably of haemopoietic origin. Plasma A, B, and H substances are carried on glycosphingolipids and glycoproteins [279,280]. Their quantity is greatly affected by Lewis phenotype: Le(a–b–) ABH secretors have substantially more ABH determinants in their plasma than do Le(a–b+) ABH secretors [90,278,279,281].

Over a period of about 2 weeks, group O transfused red cells adsorb A and B antigens from the plasma of an AB recipient and become agglutinable with some group O sera (anti-A,B) and with a few group A or group B sera [282]. A and B antigens adsorbed from plasma onto O red cells, *in vitro*, are glycosphingolipids and contain Type 1 chains [278].

2.7 Subgroups of A

In addition to the common phenotypes A_1 and A_2, numerous phenotypes with weak expression of A on the red cells have been found and a multitude of names have been adopted. Most of these phenotypes can be fitted into the following categories: A_3, A_x, A_{end}, A_m, A_y, and A_{el}. The serological characteristics of these phenotypes are shown in Table 2.15. All have normal or enhanced expression of H. In most cases the variant

phenotype results from inheritance of a rare allele at the *ABO* locus, which can be detected when paired with O or B, but not with A^1 or A^2. A_y probably results from germline mutation or from homozygosity for a rare gene at a locus independent of *ABO*. A_x, A_{end}, A_m, A_y, and A_{el} red cells are not agglutinated by most anti-A and are disclosed in routine testing because they resemble group O or B red cells, but no anti-A is present in the serum. A_x cells are agglutinated by group O (anti-A,B) serum. In A subgroups the A antigen is more easily detected if the cells are protease treated.

Cartron *et al.* [238,239] determined relative agglutinability by counting the number of cells agglutinated by anti-A in a Coulter counter, and site density by using a radiolabelled rabbit IgG anti-A (Table 2.16). These quantitative techniques demonstrate substantial individual variation within a subgroup, but do determine a hierarchy in respect to red cell A antigen expression.

Molecular techniques have confirmed that A subgroups are heterogeneous and have demonstrated that the phenotypic classification has little genetical basis (Table 2.17).

2.7.1 A_3

The least rare of the weak A phenotypes is A_3. The frequency has been estimated as 1 in 1000 group A Danes [265], 9 in 150 000 French donors (0.0136% of group A) [283], and 2 in about 180 000 Canadians [284]. The main serological feature of A_3 phenotype, first described by Friedenreich [285] in 1936, is a characteris-

Table 2.15 Serological and transferase characteristics of weak A subgroups.

Name	Reactions of cells with		Antibodies in serum		Antigens in saliva of secretors	A-transferase in serum
	Anti-A	Anti-A,B	Anti-A	Anti-A$_1$		
A_3	mf	mf	No	Sometimes	A H	Sometimes
A_{end}	mf	mf	No	Sometimes	H	No
A_x	–*/w	+	–/+	Usually	(A_x) H	Rarely
A_m	–*/w	–/+	No	No	A H	Yes
A_y	–*	–	No	No	A H	Trace
A_{el}	–*	–	Some	Yes	H	No

Red cells of none of the subgroups reacted with anti-A$_1$; all reacted with anti-H.
*Anti-A may be adsorbed onto and eluted from these cells.
(A_x), may require inhibition of agglutination of A_x cells for detection.
mf, mixed field agglutination; w, very weak agglutination.

Table 2.16 Relative agglutinability with anti-A and A site density per red cell [238].

Phenotype	No. of subjects	Agglutinability	Antigen site density (A sites per red cell $\times 10^5$)
A_1	4	100	10.5 (7.95–14.56)
A_2	10	96 ± 2	2.21 (1.29–3.53)
A_3	11	63 ± 10	0.35 (0.07–1.0)
A_{end}	7	10 ± 5	0.035 (0.011–0.044)
A_x	9	33 ± 10	0.048 (0.014–0.10)
A_m, A_y	4	0	0.012 (0.001–0.019)
A_{el}	4	0	0.007 (0.001–0.014)

Table 2.17 *ABO* alleles associated with weak A expression.

Phenotype	Allele	Nucleotide changes†	Amino acid changes†	Reference
A_3	A^3-1‡	G871A	Asp291Asn	[291]
A_3	A^3-2	G829A, del C1060	Val277Met, Pro354 FS	[292]
A_{finn}		5′ splice site intron 6		[293]
A_x	A^x-1	T646A	Phe216Ile	[150,232,290,294]
A_x	A^x-2, -4, -5§; A^1–O^{1v}	T646A, G681A, C771T, G829A	Phe216Ile, Val277Met	[150,290]
A_x	A^x-3; B/O^2–O^{1v}	A297G, T646A, G681A, C771T, G829A	Phe216Ile, Val277Met	[150,290]
A_x	A^x-6	G996A	Trp332Stop	[290]
A_{el}	A^{el}-1; $A*109$	+G G798–804	Phe269 frameshift	[232,290,295]
A_{el}	A^{el}-2; $A*110$	C467T, T646A, G681A	Pro156Leu, Phe216Ile	[232]
A_w	A^w-1	C407T, C467T, del C1060	Thr136Met, Pro156Leu	[290]
A_w	A^w-2	C350G, C467T, del C1060	Pro156Leu, Gly177Ala, Pro354 FS	[290]
A_w	A^w-3	G203C, C467T, del C1060	Arg68Thr, Pro156Leu, Pro354 FS	[290]
A_w	A^w-4	C712T	Arg241Trp	[290]
A_w	A^w-5	A965G	Glu322Gly	[290]

FS, reading frameshift; del, deletion.
†Changes from the A^1 consensus sequence.
‡See Olsson *et al.* [290].
§These alleles differ by the position of the cross-over site in intron 6 [290].

tic 'mixed field agglutination' when red cells are incubated with anti-A and with most anti-A,B. That is, small agglutinates are seen surrounded by a mass of unagglutinated, 'free' cells. On occasion, A_3 serum contains anti-A_1. Group A substance is detected in the saliva of secretors.

Unlike A_{mos} (described in Section 2.9), A_3 does not appear to be a mosaic of A_2 and O cells: in the A_3 phenotype anti-A can be eluted from the population of cells that was not agglutinated by it [284], and some anti-A,B agglutinate the whole population of cells [266]. When A_3 cells were stained with fluorescent anti-A, all the cells glowed, although there was vari-

ability in the degree of fluorescence [286]. It appears that only 3–4% of the cells have sufficient sites to permit agglutination with anti-A [286].

Investigation of serum transferases revealed heterogeneity within the A_3 phenotype. A_3 can be divided into the following three types on the basis of serum α-N-acetylgalactosaminyltransferases [287–289]:

1 the enzyme has a pH optimum of about 6, resembling A_1-transferase, but activity is about one-third of that found in A_1 serum;

2 the enzyme has a pH optimum of about 7 and thus resembles A_2-transferase, but has very low activity;

3 no A-transferase can be detected.

Under optimum conditions the enzyme in the first category can convert O cells to A-active cells, which do not display the characteristic A_3 agglutination pattern when incubated with anti-A and are agglutinated more strongly than are O cells converted with A_2 serum [287,289].

Surprisingly, in view of the high level of H antigen on the red cells, H-transferase levels in A_3 sera are generally considerably lower than H-transferase levels in A_1 or A_2 sera [289].

Sequencing of exons 6 and 7 of the A gene from two A_3B individuals revealed an A^1 sequence with a single base change encoding an Asp291Asn substitution [291] (Table 2.17). A single base change encoding Val277Met in a gene with the single nucleotide deletion characteristic of A^2, was present in two A_3 members of a Brazilian family, and another, unrelated, A_3 Brazilian was homozygous for this allele [292] (Table 2.17). Two other A_3 Brazilians had the Phe216Ile mutation characteristic of A_x phenotype [292]. Many other A_3 individuals had the normal A^1 or A^2 sequence in exons 6 and 7 [290–292,296], although they could have mutations in other exons, in a splice site, or in a promoter region.

2.7.2 A_{end} (A_{finn}, A_{bantu})

A_{end} was first described by Weiner et al. [297] in 1959 and named by Sturgeon et al. [298] 5 years later. A_{end} cells behave like weak A_3 cells: they give very weak 'mixed field' agglutination with some anti-A and -A,B. The saliva of A_{end} secretors, however, contains H, but no A substance. Anti-A_1 is present in some A_{end} sera.

Two examples of A_{end} were found in testing 150 000 French donors (0.003% of group A) [283]. A_{end} is inherited as an allele at the ABO locus [297]. No A-transferase has been detected in sera or red cell membranes of A_{end} individuals [287,288].

An A variant, which differs from A_{end} in only minor details, was found in Finns and named A_{finn} [299]. The frequency of A_{finn} in Finnish blood donors was estimated at about 1 in 6000 [299], but may be as high as 1 in 1000 in parts of Southern Finland [300]. Four A_{finn} individuals each had an A^1-like allele with an A to G transition in the 5′ donor splice site of intron 6 [293]. Although skipping of exon 6 would introduce a reading frameshift and no active enzyme product, the mutation is not in the invariable splice site sequence, so a minor fraction of the RNA might be spliced normally.

A_{bantu} is another variation of A_{end}, found in about 4% of group A black South Africans [245], and in up to 8% of Bushmen and Hottentots, the ethnic group in which the A_{bantu} gene may have originated [301]. Anti-A agglutinate A_{bantu} red cells more strongly than A_{end} cells.

2.7.3 A_x

The A_x phenotype was first described by Fischer and Hahn [302] in 1935. Its major serological characteristics are:

1 the red cells are not agglutinated by most anti-A (group B) sera, yet are agglutinated by the majority of anti-A,B (group O) sera; no mixed field pattern is observed;

2 the serum usually contains anti-A_1 and occasionally an antibody that agglutinates A_1 and A_2 cells [303];

3 in addition to H substance, the saliva of A_x secretors contains a trace of A, which is best detected when A_x cells are used as indicator cells for inhibition of anti-A [304].

A_x phenotype is very heterogeneous. Several other symbols—A_4, A_5, A_6, A_z, A_0—have been used to describe subgroups of A that differ from the original A_x by only fine serological details [265,305–307]. The term A_x will be used to describe all such variants. The subgroup called A_{pae} [308] may also be a variety of A_x.

Most sera from group B donors do not agglutinate A_x cells, although sera from group B volunteers immunized with A substance usually do [309]. Monoclonal anti-A reagents have been produced that are effective at detecting A_x cells although, under certain conditions, these antibodies may also agglutinate some group B cells [310–313] (Section 2.11). Anti-A can be readily adsorbed onto and eluted from A_x cells.

In two separate studies, the frequency of A_x in France has been estimated as 1 in 77 000 (0.003% of group A) [283] and as 1 in 40 000 [304].

A-transferase cannot usually be detected in A_x serum or red cell membranes [232,287–289]. H-transferase activity in A_x sera is low [289].

The molecular genetics of A_x reflects the heterogeneity of the serological phenotypes. The most common A^x allele has the A^1 consensus sequence with a missense mutation encoding a Phe216Ile substitution [150,232,290,294] (Table 2.17). Putative hybrid genes with crossover sites in intron 6 have been associated with A_x. In six Swedish families, exon 6 had the consensus (A^1) sequence and exon 7 the O^{1v} sequence [150,290]. In three Swedish families, one Pole, and one American, exon 6 had the B or O^2 sequence and exon 7 the O^{1v} sequence [150,290]. Three different crossover regions in intron 6 were detected [290]. It is no surprise that these hybrid alleles behave as A^x, because the O^{1v} exon 7 sequence encodes the amino acids important for A-specificity, but, like the typical A^x allele, also encodes Ile216. One A_x New Zealander had an A^1-like allele encoding a nonsense mutation (Trp332Stop), which predicts the loss of 23 amino acids from the C-terminus of the A-transferase [290].

Many families have shown that A_x is inherited in a regular fashion, as a rare allele at the ABO locus [265,303–307]. However, in a few families the genetic background is unclear: families with A_x children having group O parents [314,315] and a family in which three siblings with atypical A_x phenotypes had O and A^1/O parents [316]. In these families, if one of the group O parents were heterozygous O^2/O^{1v}, then crossing-over within intron 6 at meiosis to produce an O^2–O^{1v} hybrid gene could give rise to A_x children. Likewise, the A^1/O parent with A_x children might have been heterozygous A^1/O^{1v} and crossing-over could have produced an A^1–O^{1v} hybrid gene. These situations would resemble that proposed by Suzuki *et al.* [149] to explain abnormal ABO inheritance (Fig. 2.5), but the proposed explanations remain speculations until such families are studied at the molecular level.

A_x may be inherited through an A_2B parent [304,317–319] because the presence of a B gene sometimes enhances the expression of A^x to that expected of an A^2 gene (Section 2.10.2). Salmon and Cartron [319] detected weak A-transferase activity in the sera of people with an A_2B phenotype (genotype A^x/B) resulting from allelic enhancement; no enzyme was found in the serum of their A_x siblings who have the same A gene.

A very weak A-transferase, with higher activity at pH 8 than at pH 6 (A_2 type), was detected in the A_x mother of a baby who was A_2 at birth, but became A_x within 2 years [289,320].

2.7.4 A_m

A_m red cells are not agglutinated, or are agglutinated only very weakly, by anti-A and -A,B. Anti-A can be adsorbed onto and eluted from A_m cells. Saliva of A_m secretors contains normal quantities of A and H substances. A_m serum does not usually contain anti-A_1.

A_m is inherited as a rare allele at the ABO locus [321–326]. The name A_m was originally coined by Weiner *et al.* [327] for a new, weak-A phenotype assumed to arise from homozygosity for a recessive regulator gene at a locus independent of ABO, but this phenotype is now called A_y and is discussed below.

One example of A_m was found in 150 000 French donors (0.0015% of group A) [283] and one example was found in 400 000 Chinese in Taiwan [328].

Cartron *et al.* [287,288,324,329] distinguished two types of A_m from serum $\alpha 1,3$-N-acetylgalactosaminyltransferase analysis. In most samples the A-transferase had a pH optimum of 6 and the kinetic properties of an A_1-transferase, while in serum from one A_m person the enzyme had a pH optimum of 7 and resembled A_2-transferase. In all cases enzyme activity was between 30% and 50% of that found in A_1 or A_2 sera and probably originated from tissues other than the haemopoietic tissue [330].

An A gene in a Norwegian A_m mother and daughter had the A^1 consensus sequence in exons 6 and 7 [331]. A_m phenotype appears to result from a blocking of A^1 or A^2 genes in bone marrow cells, but not in mucus secreting cells, possibly by a mutation in the promoter region of the gene.

2.7.5 A_y

A_y phenotype is similar to A_m, but the most significant and definitive way in which A_y and A_m differ is by their mode of inheritance. A_y does not result from a rare allele at the ABO locus, but probably arises from a germline mutation of an A gene within a family. Weiner *et al.* [327] reported two families: one A_y (then called A_m) propositus had a group O parent and A_1 and O siblings; the other was A_yB and had A_1B and B parents. Other similar families have since been described [333–335], yet none of the A_y propositi had an A_y sibling. In one family the A_y son of A^1/O and B parents had an A_yB son who, in turn, had an A_y son [336].

A_y differs from A_m phenotypically in the following ways.

1 Substantially less anti-A is eluted from A_y cells than from A_m cells incubated with the same serum [332].
2 A_y secretor saliva contains considerably less A substance than A_m saliva [287,329].

35

3 A_y serum contains only a trace of A-transferase, whereas A_m serum contains readily detectable enzyme [288].

2.7.6 A_{el}

Under usual conditions A_{el} cells are not agglutinated by anti-A or -A,B, although they do bind these antibodies, as demonstrated by adsorption and elution [298,337–339]. Saliva from A_{el} secretors contains H, but no A substance. Serum from A_{el} individuals usually contains anti-A_1 and may also contain an antibody that agglutinates A_2 cells [337,339]. No A-transferase has been detected in A_{el} serum or red cell membranes [232,287–289]. Serum H-transferase is weaker than that found in A_1 or A_2 serum [289]. No example of A_{el} was found in testing 150 000 French blood donors [283], but five were found among 400 000 Chinese from Taiwan [328]. A_{el} appears to be inherited as a rare gene at the ABO locus [337–339]. As a result of allelic enhancement (Section 2.10.2), $A_{el}B$ cells may be weakly agglutinated by some monoclonal anti-A and may resemble B(A) phenotype [340] (Section 2.11).

The usual form of A^{el} has the A^1 consensus sequence except for a single G insert in a string of seven guanosines at nucleotides 798–804 [290,295] (Table 2.17). This insert creates a reading frameshift, altering the amino acid sequence after Gly268 and abolishing the translation stop codon, so that the gene product is 37 amino acids longer than the A_1-transferase and 16 amino acids longer than the A_2-transferase. Of four A_{el} Japanese, only one had the allele with the guanosine insert (*$A109$) [232]. One had an A allele with two missense mutations (*$A110$), encoding Pro156Leu and Phe216Ile substitutions (Table 2.17). The other two A_{el} Japanese and two A_{el} Norwegians had A^1 alleles with a normal sequence in exons 6 and 7 [232,331]. In one family, a guanosine insert at G798–804 was present in an otherwise normal A^2 allele [147]. The frameshift caused by the G insert was corrected by the C1059 deletion characteristic of A^2, but, despite encoding a product of normal length, this allele, called O^3, was associated with no A antigen expression.

Although most red cells of individuals with the A_{el} or A_m phenotypes have very little A antigen, 1–2% of cells were very strongly labelled with monoclonal anti-A as determined by scanning immunogold electron microscopy [331,341]. This provides a possible explanation of why red cells from these phenotypes may adsorb anti-A without being agglutinated by it.

2.7.7 A_w

Olsson et al. [290] sequenced exons, splice sites, and promoter regions of the ABO genes from other individuals with weak A antigens. As the phenotypes did not fit easily into any existing classification, the abnormal genes were called A^w (1–5) (Table 2.17). Three were A^2 alleles (Pro156Leu and the C1060 deletion) with additional missense mutations. In A^w-3 the mutation encoding Arg68Thr is in exon 4 and in A^w-2 the mutation encoding Gly177Ala is in exon 6. These are the only missense mutations associated with a weak subgroup outside exon 7. The other two (A^w-4 and -5) are A^1 alleles with an additional exon 7 missense mutation.

2.8 Subgroups of B

Weak variants of B are very rare. They appear to be much rarer than weak A subgroups, although this probably reflects the relatively low frequency of the B gene in many populations. In Japan, where the incidence of B is about half that of A, Yamaguchi et al. [342] analysed red cells from more than 700 000 donors and found that the frequencies of B_x and B_m are considerably higher than those of A_x and A_m.

Weak B subgroups have proved difficult to classify. Salmon [343] concluded that the best system for classifying B variants was by a loose analogy with the A variants: B_3, B_x, B_m, and B_{el}, plus B_w for those that do not fit any of the other four categories (Table 2.18).

Lopez et al. [344] defined three classes of B variants, B_{60}, B_{20}, and B_0, based on mean percentage agglutination with anti-B as measured in a Coulter counter. Although consistent within a family, substantial heterogeneity was found in each group, especially B_{60} [344–346].

2.8.1 B_3

First reported in 1972 by Wiener and Cioffi [347] in an ABH non-secretor, this phenotype is characterized by mixed field haemagglutination with anti-B and anti-A,B, by absence of anti-B in the serum, and by normal B antigen in the saliva. Despite being the least rare of the B variants [343], remarkably few examples of B_3

Table 2.18 Typical serological and transferase characteristics of weak B subgroups.

Name	Reactions of cells with			Anti-B in serum	Antigens in saliva of secretors	B-transferase in	
	Anti-B	Anti-A,B	Anti-H			Serum	Red cell membrane
B_3	mf	mf	+	No	B H	Yes	No
B_x	w	w	+	Yes	(B_x) H	No	No
B_m	–*/w	–/w	+	No	B H	Yes	Trace
B_{el}	–*	–	+	Sometimes	H	No	No

* Anti-B may be adsorbed onto and eluted from these cells.
(B_x), may require inhibition of agglutination of B_x cells for detection.
mf, mixed field agglutination; w, very weak agglutination.

Table 2.19 *ABO* alleles associated with weak B expression.

Phenotype	Allele		Nucleotide changes†	Amino acid changes†	References
B_3	B^3-1‡		C1054T	Arg352Trp	[291]
B_x	B^w-1	*B104	G871A	Asp291Asn	[232]
B_{el}	B^{el}-1	*B105	T641G	Met214Arg	[232]
B_{el}	B^{el}-2	*B106	G669T	Glu223Asp	[232]
B_w	B^w-2		C873G	Asp291Glu	[290]
B_w	B^w-3		C721T	Arg241Trp	[290]
B_w	B^w-4		A548G	Asp183Gly	[290]
B_w	B^w-5		G539A	Arg180His	[290]
B_w	B^w-6		A1036G	Lys346Glu	[290]
B_w	B^w-7		G1055A	Arg352Gln	[290]
B_w	B^w-8		T863G	Met288Arg	[290]

†Changes from the *B* sequence.
‡See Olsson *et al.* [290].

are reported. Three were in 350 000 (approximately 1 in 10 000 group B) French donors [348]. B_3 is less rare in Chinese: 1 in 900 group B donors was B_3 and 1 in 1800 A_1B donors was A_1B_3 [349].

B_3 generally results from inheritance of a rare gene at the *ABO* locus [343,345,347,348,350]. However, two A_1B_3 brothers with A_1 and *B/O* parents [348] and an $A_{int}B$ person with A_{int} and B_3 parents [351] are reported.

Badet *et al.* [352] were able to detect B-transferase in sera from B_3 individuals, but not in B_3 red cell membranes.

The *B* gene of one A_1B_3 individual had a single base change compared with a normal *B* gene, resulting in an Arg352Trp substitution [291] (Table 2.19). This substitution is also associated with a Japanese A^2 allele and with a variant O^1 allele [148,232]. No nucleotide

sequence change was detected in exons 6 and 7 of the B-transferase genes of two B_3 (B^3/O) individuals [291].

2.8.2 B_x

A heterogeneous group, but typical B_x red cells are weakly agglutinated by anti-B and anti-A,B. The serum contains weak anti-B and the saliva of B_x secretors contains some B substance, which is often only detected by inhibition of agglutination of B_x cells by anti-B. Studies of families with B variants, which can probably be classified as B_x, suggest that B^x is a rare allele at the *ABO* locus [342,343,345].

B-transferase was not detected in serum or red cell membranes of B_x individuals [232,352]. In the only example studied, an *ABO* allele from a person with B_x

red cells differed from a *B* allele by a single base change encoding Asp291Asn [232] (Table 2.19), a substitution also associated with A₃ [291] (Table 2.17).

2.8.3 B$_m$

B$_m$ cells are not agglutinated by anti-B or anti-A,B; the B antigen is only detected by sensitive techniques such as adsorption and elution of anti-B. The saliva of B$_m$ secretors contains about as much B substance as that of a normal B secretor. Characteristically, sera from B$_m$ individuals do not contain anti-B.

Generally, B$_m$ appears to be inherited as a variant gene at the *ABO* locus [112,353–358], but a couple of exceptions are described below.

Only very little B-transferase activity could be detected in B$_m$ red cell membranes [357]. B$_m$ sera demonstrated less than half of the B-transferase activity of B sera [112,356–359] and B$_m$ saliva had normal [112] or reduced [360] transferase activity compared with that of B secretor saliva. Yoshida *et al.* [358] found that serum B-transferase from a B$_m$ person differed from normal B-transferase in having a low affinity for UDP-galactose and in certain other physicochemical properties such as pH optimum; B-transferase in A₁B$_m$ members of another family appeared normal [361]. In families with B$_m$ and A₁B$_m$ members, much higher levels of B-transferase activity were apparent in the A₁B$_m$ sera than in the B$_m$ sera, presumably a result of allelic enhancement [356,357] (Section 2.10.2).

Homozygosity for a recessive gene that suppresses B in haemopoietic tissues has been proposed to explain abnormal inheritance of B$_m$-like phenotypes in a few families [362–364]. Red cells of the son of O and A₂B parents resembled B$_m$ phenotype and should probably be called B$_y$, in analogy with A$_y$ (Section 2.7.5). His serum contained normal H-transferase, but only about 70% of the normal level of B-transferase [364], the amount expected if all of it was non-haemopoietic in origin [330].

2.8.4 B$_{el}$

B$_{el}$ red cells are not agglutinated by anti-B or anti-A,B. They do bind anti-B, which can be detected in eluates. B is not present in the saliva of B$_{el}$ secretors; anti-B may be present in the serum.

B^{el} is inherited as a rare gene at the *ABO* locus [365,366]. No B-transferase was detected in B$_{el}$ sera or

red cell membranes [232,352,366]. In a family with B$_{el}$ and A₁B$_{el}$ members, the A₁B$_{el}$ red cells were weakly agglutinated by some anti-B [366]. In another family, B$_{el}$ was enhanced to B₃ in an *A/B* heterozygote [367] (see Section 2.10.2).

Two different abnormal alleles were found in two individuals with B$_{el}$ red cells. Each allele differed, in exons 6 and 7, from the normal *B* allele by a single nucleotide; one encoding Met214Arg, the other Glu223Asp [232] (Table 2.19).

2.8.5 B$_w$

Olsson *et al.* [290] identified seven novel *ABO* alleles, which differed from the common *B* sequence by single nucleotide changes, encoding a single amino acid substitution (*B^w*-2 to -8 in Table 2.19). All were associated with weak B expression, but were not classified further.

2.8.6 Other subgroups of B

An inherited variant B antigen called B$_v$ was characterized by the failure of B$_v$ red cells to react with human anti-B reagents that had been adsorbed with rabbit red cells [368,369]. B$_v$ red cells and secretions appear to lack normal human B antigen, but contain a B-like determinant, possibly the non-fucosylated B-like antigen on rabbit red cells (see [370]). B$_v$ also resembles serologically the B antigen characteristic of *cis*AB (Section 2.12.1). Sera of B$_v$ individuals contain a form of anti-B; no B-transferase activity could be detected. Among 567 210 Hong Kong Chinese blood donors, 46 examples of B$_v$ and eight examples of AB$_v$ were found [369].

A subgroup of B called B₂, analogous to A₂, was found in a Greek woman and her two children [371].

Based on a quantitative agglutination analysis, Gibbs *et al.* [372] divided 'normal B' into three types. Red cells of most group B white people fell into the middle strength category, whereas those of only about half of group B black people fitted the middle category, the other half having a stronger B antigen. Measuring relative B-transferase activity, Badet *et al.* [373] identified two types in white people: 84% (group I) had a relative enzyme activity of only about half that of the other 16% (group II). The majority of group B black people fitted neither of these groups, but a third group with an even higher relative transferase activity than group II. These strong *B* genes can result in depressed expression of A in some AB black people as a result of competition for acceptor substrate (Section 2.10.1).

2.9 A$_{mos}$ and B$_{mos}$

In 1975 Marsh *et al.* [374] applied the names A$_{mos}$ and B$_{mos}$ to remarkably similar variants of A and B. In A$_{mos}$, agglutination tests with anti-A and anti-A,B revealed two separable populations of cells, one A$_2$, the other O. A$_{mos}$ sera contained no anti-A, and the saliva contained H and possibly a trace of A. In addition to two A$_{mos}$ families, B$_{mos}$, A$_1$B$_{mos}$, and A$_{mos}$B phenotypes were described [374]. The inherited A+O and B+O mosaics previously reported in Japan probably represent earlier examples of A$_{mos}$ and B$_{mos}$ [375–377].

A$_{mos}$ is inherited, apparently at the *ABO* locus; a characteristic that distinguishes it from most other forms of red cell mosaicism. All A$_{mos}$ members within a family have about the same proportion of A and O cells, although these proportions vary substantially between different families. A$_{mos}$ differs from A$_3$ serologically as the cells left unagglutinated with anti-A do

not adsorb anti-A and the ratio of agglutinated : unagglutinated cells remains constant regardless of the strength of anti-A or anti-A,B used and whether or not the cells have been protease treated.

A family with B$_{mos}$ and A$_1$B$_{mos}$ members is shown in Fig. 2.9. In all members with the *B^{mos}* gene 12% of red cells expressed B antigen; the remaining red cells were O in B$_{mos}$ and A in AB$_{mos}$ [378]. All were ABH non-secretors. The level of serum B-transferase activity in the B$_{mos}$ members was only about 7–20% of that of normal B controls.

A healthy blood donor with 60% A$_1$B and 40% A$_1$ cells could not be A$_1$B$_{mos}$ as her parents had normal A$_1$ and A$_1$B red cells [379]. Somatic mutation involving the *B* gene in some erythropoietic cells is a possible cause of this mosaicism.

2.10 A and B gene interaction

2.10.1 Allelic competition

It is well established that A antigen is weaker on A$_2$B cells than on A$_2$ cells and that A$_1$ is weaker on A$_1$B than A$_1$ cells; the effect of two different glycosyltransferases

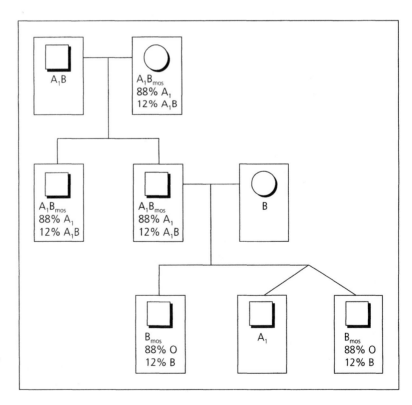

Fig. 2.9 Family with B$_{mos}$ and A$_1$B$_{mos}$ members, showing that all members inheriting a *B^{mos}* gene have 12% B cells, the other 88% being group O or A$_1$ [378].

competing for the same acceptor substrate. Although generally less obvious, B is often weaker in A_1B than in B [344,380–383].

In some cases A^1/B genotype may be expressed as an A_2B phenotype [247,367,382,384–386] and A^2/B may be expressed as A_3B phenotype [384,387]. In black populations the $A_2B:A_1B$ ratio is often significantly higher than would be expected from the $A_2:A_1$ ratio [367,385]. In a study of 5000 African Americans, 80% of group A individuals were A_1 and 20% were A_2, whereas 53% of the group AB individuals were A_1B and 47% were A_2B [385]. Similar discrepancies have been observed in white people [247,367], Chinese [349], and Japanese [233,386]. This imbalance in Japanese is caused, at least in part, by an ABO allele ($*R101$) that is expressed as A_1 in A^1/O genotype, but as A_2 in A^2/B genotype [233].

Sera from some A_2B black people contain A_1-transferase and no A_2-transferase, plus a B-transferase with activity considerably higher than that found in most group B sera [367,388,389]. Elevated B-transferase activity together with an A_1-transferase was found in the sera of 50% of the A_2B African Americans [385]. This superactive B-transferase utilizes the lion's share of available H sites, so that the A_1-transferase cannot produce sufficient A antigen to provide the high site density required for A_1 status.

2.10.2 Allelic enhancement

'Le renforcement allelique' is a gene interaction, the reverse of allelic competition described in the previous section [304,319]. It is an enhancement of expression of weak A or B genes in A/B heterozygotes. In a French family an A gene was expressed as A_x in A/O members, but as A_2 in A/B members [318]. The A_x cells had 11 200 A sites per red cell, whereas the A_2B cells had 96 000 A sites [319]. A-transferase activity was not apparent in the sera of the A_x members, but was detected in the sera of the A_2B individuals, although all had the same A gene [319]. In a Swedish family, an ABO allele with the A^2 sequence in exons 6 and 7 was expressed as A_2 in the A_2B mother, but as A_x in her A/O^{1v} children and grandchildren [150]. Other families have shown that a B gene responsible for B_x phenotype was expressed more strongly in A_1B members [390,391], and a B gene expressed as B_{el} in B/O members was represented by a B_3 phenotype in A/B members [392].

2.11 Overlapping specificities of A- and B-transferases: B(A) and A(B) phenotypes

The glycosyltransferase products of the A and B alleles differ in their donor substrate specificity, although they share a common acceptor substrate. This makes the ABO gene extremely unusual and at one time fuelled speculation that A and B may not be alleles. It has now been demonstrated that the A- and B-transferases are not precise in their choice of donor substrate and that there is a small degree of overlap between the A and B gene products [393–397].

Under the appropriate conditions, enzyme from group B serum can catalyse the transfer of N-acetylgalactosamine from UDP-N-acetylgalactosamine to 2′-fucosyllactose (a low molecular weight analogue of H) to form an A-active structure. Concentrated B-transferase could even make group O cells strongly agglutinable with anti-A. If equivalent quantities of UDP-galactose and UDP-N-acetylgalactosamine were present, only B activity could be detected; in the presence of UDP-galactose, thrice the quantity of UDP-N-acetylgalactosamine was required to produce A activity. As would be expected, when there is competition for substrate, the B-transferase is far more efficient at catalysing the transfer of galactose than of N-acetylgalactosamine [393,395,396]. Likewise, A-transferase can, under appropriate conditions, catalyse the synthesis of B-active structures [122,394].

The observation in several laboratories that highly potent monoclonal anti-A reagents capable of agglutinating A_x red cells also weakly agglutinated some group B cells led to the recognition that the phenomenon described above, the ability of B-transferase to produce A determinants in vitro, may also occur in vivo [311]. Red cells from 25 of 3458 group B donors were reactive with one example of monoclonal anti-A [398]. The reaction of these B(A) cells with some anti-A could be inhibited by group A secretor saliva [398] and the A-activity removed by treatment of the cells with α-N-acetylgalactosaminidase, but not α-galactosidase [399]. People with B(A) red cells were mostly black and were shown to have highly active serum B-transferase, in some cases 5–6 times more active than that from most other group B individuals [397,398]. In B(A), the hyperactive α1,3-galactosyltransferase catalyses the transfer of sufficient N-acetylgalactosamine to its acceptor sub-

Table 2.20 Enzymes with dual A- and B-transferase activity: amino acid substitutions at the four positions (176, 235, 266, 268) characteristic of *A* and *B* gene products and at position 234.

Phenotype	Amino acids					References
	176	234	235	266	268	
A	Arg	Pro	Gly	Leu	Gly	
*cis*AB	Arg	Pro	Gly	Leu	**Ala**	[400,401]
B	Gly	Pro	Ser	Met	Ala	
B(A)	Gly	Pro	**Gly**	Met	Ala	[294]
B(A)	Gly	**Ala**	Ser	Met	Ala	[402]
*cis*AB	Gly	Pro	Ser	**Leu**	Ala	[403]

strate to permit agglutination by certain anti-A. Furthermore, those anti-A capable of detecting B(A) will agglutinate all group B red cells that have been papain treated, suggesting some degree of *in vivo* A-transferase activity by most B-transferases [399].

Results of molecular genetical studies on three B(A) individuals, none of whom were of African origin, are not strictly concordant with the theory of a hyperactive B-transferase producing some A antigen. In two individuals the nucleotide sequence was identical to that of a normal *B* gene apart from one significant change encoding a Ser235Gly substitution, the A codon at the second site distinguishing *A* and *B* alleles [290,294] (Table 2.20). Two B(A) siblings had a *B*-like gene encoding a Pro234Ala substitution, the position before Ser235 [402] (Table 2.20). The siblings were *B(A)/O¹ᵛ* heterozygotes; their father was A₁B with an *A¹/B(A)* genotype. B expression in father and two siblings was slightly weaker than normal. With both mutations, B(A) phenotype is more likely to have resulted from a shift in substrate specificity of the enzyme rather than greatly enhanced B-transferase activity.

A monoclonal anti-B described by Voak *et al.* [404] brought about agglutination of 1.42% of group A red cell samples, all A₁, and this was considered to represent A(B) phenotype; B activity resulting from A₁-transferase activity. A(B) was not associated with elevated A-transferase activity, but A₁(B) cells did have elevated levels of H antigen and plasma H-transferase activity.

2.12 *Cis*AB

In 1964, Seyfried *et al.* [405] described a Polish family

in which inheritance of the ABO groups did not fit the single locus concept for ABO genetics. A and B appeared to have been inherited together in this family: an A₂B woman with a group O husband and a group O mother had two A₂B children. Numerous other similar families have been reported since [232,400,403,406–417]. Yamaguchi *et al.* [406] proposed the term *cis*AB for this phenotype. Fourteen *cis*AB samples were found from over 1 million Japanese blood donors, 0.012% of the 112 710 group AB bloods tested [410].

2.12.1 Serological characteristics

Although the main feature of *cis*AB is its unusual mode of inheritance, the *cis*AB phenotype almost always differs from '*trans*AB' serologically. Serological characteristics differ from family to family, but remain consistent within a family [411,418].

1 The A antigen is usually referred to as A₂, but *cis*AB cells generally express more A than A₂B and less than A₁B [411,413,414,417]. *Cis*A₁B phenotype is not unknown [408,409].

2 The B antigen is almost always expressed weakly, often being described as B₃ [410]. *Cis*AB cells react more strongly with A₂ sera than with A₁ sera [408,414]. Adsorption of immune anti-B with B cells removes all activity for *cis*AB cells, but anti-B adsorbed to exhaustion with *cis*AB cells will continue to agglutinate normal B cells [414]. The B antigen of *cis*AB may resemble B_v (Section 2.8.6), as rabbit anti-B did not react with *cis*AB cells and one adsorption of human immune anti-B with rabbit red cells removed all reactivity for *cis*AB cells [414]. The B antigen of

*cis*AB may not always be atypical; an A_2B mother of two group O children had an apparently normal B antigen [415].

3 *cis*AB cells have an unusually high level of H antigen, about the level found on A_2 cells, which is higher than that of normal A_2B cells [411].

4 Sera from *cis*AB people almost always contain weak anti-B. This antibody apparently recognizes that part of the B antigen lacking from *cis*AB cells [407,408]. Serum from the apparent *AB/O* woman with normal B antigen did not contain anti-B [415].

5 Salivas from *cis*AB secretors contain normal quantities of A substance and large quantities of H substance, plus a very little B substance that is only detectable by inhibition of agglutination of *cis*AB cells by anti-B [411,418].

2.12.2 Transferase studies and molecular genetics

There are two likely explanations for the *cis*AB phenomenon. One is unequal crossing-over, resulting in adjacent A and B genes and, presumably, separate gene products (transferase enzymes). The other involves mutation of an *A* or *B* gene to a gene producing an enzyme capable of transferring significant quantities of both *N*-acetylgalactosamine and galactose to the H acceptor substrate.

Transferase analyses of sera from *cis*AB individuals show heterogeneity between families and homogeneity within families [419]: generally *cis*AB sera have relatively low levels of A- and B-transferase activity [412–414,416,417,419,420]. In order to separate A- and B-transferases in serum, Yoshida *et al.* [416,420] exploited the fact that Sepharose 4B in a column binds A- but not B-transferase. In two *cis*AB sera no separation could be achieved because both A and B activity was adsorbed, support for a single mutant gene [420].

Sequencing of exons 6 and 7 of *ABO* from 21 unrelated individuals with *cis*AB (19 from Japan and two from the USA) revealed an A^1 sequence with a nucleotide change encoding a Gly268Ala substitution [232,400,420] (Table 2.20). This represents the *B* gene sequence at the fourth position of discrimination between *A* and *B* alleles and is probably responsible for the gene product having significant A- and B-transferase activity. In addition, all had the Pro156Leu mutation associated with A^2 and Japanese A^1, which is

not considered to affect A-transferase activity [128]. In one Vietnamese family *cis*AB resulted from a *B*-like gene with a single nucleotide change converting the methionine codon at position 266, the third position of discrimination between *A* and *B* alleles, to leucine, the codon characteristic of *A* [403] (Table 2.20).

In one *cis*AB individual Yoshida *et al.* [416] were able to separate two enzyme components from the serum, one similar to normal A_2-transferase and one similar to B-transferase, suggesting that two discrete genes are present on the same chromosome.

2.13 H-deficient phenotypes

The H-deficient phenotypes are those rare phenotypes in which the red cells are totally or partially deficient in H antigen. H may or may not be present in secretions; i.e. individuals with H-deficient red cell phenotypes may be ABH secretors or non-secretors. The various H-deficient phenotypes are summarized in Table 2.21.

2.13.1 Red cell H-deficient, non-secretor; the Bombay phenotype

In 1952, Bhende *et al.* [421] described the abnormal blood groups of three men from Bombay whose red cells were group O, but H-negative. All had anti-H in their serum. This rare phenotype later became known as the Bombay or O_h phenotype. Many other examples have been found since, all through the presence of anti-H in the serum.

2.13.1.1 Serological characteristics (Table 2.21)

O_h red cells are not agglutinated by anti-H, -A, -B, or -A,B. No H, A, or B antigen can be detected, by adsorption and elution techniques, on red cells with the 'typical O_h' phenotype [422,423]. Red cells of phenotypes that have been called 'atypical O_h', however, do bind anti-H, which can be detected in an eluate [424,425]. It may also be possible to adsorb and elute anti-A and/or anti-B from these cells [424,426,427].

As with most ABH non-secretors, O_h red cells are usually Le(a+b–), but may be Le(a–b–). O_h red cells never express Le^b.

No H, A, or B antigen is present in O_h saliva, which may contain Le^a, but never Le^b.

The serum of O_h individuals always contains anti-H, -A, and -B.

Table 2.21 H-deficient phenotypes.

Type	Notation	Antigens						Antibodies	Glycosyltransferases					
		Red cells*			Secretions				Serum			Red cells		
		A	B	H	A	B	H		A	B	H	A	B	H
H-deficient, non-secretor (Bombay)	O_h^O	–	–	–	–	–	–	Anti-H	–	–	–	–	–	–
	O_h^A	–	–	–	–	–	–	Anti-H	+	–	–	+	–	–
	O_h^B	–	–	–	–	–	–	Anti-H	–	+	–	–	+	–
H-partially deficient, non-secretor	$O_h^†$	–	–	–/w	–	–	–	Anti-H	+	–	–/+	–	–	–/+
	A_h	+/w	–	–/w	–	–	–	Anti-H	+	–	–/+	+	–	–/+
	B_h	–	+/w	–/w	–	–	–	Anti-H	–	+	–/+	–	+	–/+
H-deficient, secretor (para-Bombay)	O_h^O-secretor	–	–	–/w	–	–	+	Anti-HI	–	–	–/+	–	–	–/+
	O_h^A-secretor	+/w	–	–/w	+	–	+	Anti-HI	+	–	–/+	+	–	–/+
	O_h^B-secretor	–	+/w	–/w	–	+	+	Anti-HI	–	+	–/+	–	+	–/+
H_m (dominant)	OH_m	–	–	w	–	–	+	None	–	–	+	–	–	+
	AH_m	w	–	w	+	–	+	None	+	–	+	+	–	+
LADII		–	–	–	–	–	–	None	–	+	+	NT	NT	NT

*Tested by direct agglutination.
†Only distinguished from 'atypical' O_h-non-secretor by family studies.
NT, not tested; w, weak expression of antigen.

2.13.1.2 Inheritance

Ceppellini *et al.* [428] first proposed that an inhibitor gene might be responsible for the Bombay phenotype. In 1955, Watkins and Morgan [429] suggested that H expression may be controlled by a gene at a locus independent from *ABO*, and that the Bombay phenotype could arise from homozygosity for a rare allele, *h*, at this locus. This prediction has since been verified by biochemical and molecular genetical evidence. Individuals homozygous for *h* may have *A* and/or *B* genes, as demonstrated by the blood groups of their parents and children, but these genes are not expressed as antigens on red cells or in secretions [426,427,430,431]. When describing Bombay phenotypes the appropriate superscript may be added to the O_h notation when the *ABO* genotype is determined by family study, by glycosyltransferase analysis, or by molecular genetical tests—$O_h{}^O$, $O_h{}^A$, $O_h{}^B$, $O_h{}^{AB}$.

Like other phenotypes resulting from homozygosity of rare recessive genes, there is a high level of consanguinity among parents of O_h individuals [432].

2.13.1.3 Glycosyltransferases

H-transferase has not been detected in the serum or red cell membranes of O_h individuals [108,196,433,434]. O_h sera and red cells contain A- and B-transferases when *A* and *B* genes are present [108,225]. These enzymes are unable to act in the absence of their acceptor substrate (H antigen) and neither A nor B structure is produced. O_h red cells that have been made H-active *in vitro*, in the presence of H-transferase, can be converted to A- or B-active cells by the appropriate A- or B-transferase [93]. In families, sera from heterozygous *H/h* members have about half the H-transferase activity of sera from *H/H* homozygotes [435].

2.13.1.4 *In vivo* survival of O_h cells

Unlike Rh_{null} cells, there is no evidence to suggest that Bombay phenotype cells are haematologically abnormal. Autologous ^{51}Cr-labelled O_h red cells survive normally [436,437].

2.13.1.5 Frequency and distribution

The Bombay phenotype is very rare, but appears to be less rare in India than elsewhere. Bhatia and Sathe [438] tested 167 404 Indians in Bombay and obtained an O_h frequency of about 1 in 7600, an *h* gene frequency of 0.0115. Le Pendu *et al.* [439] discovered a rich source of two types of H-deficiency phenotype in Réunion Island in the Indian Ocean: typical O_h in the Tamoul Indian population and partial red cell H-deficiency, non-secretor in the population of European origin. O_h has also been found in the following ethnic groups: people of European origin [426,427,430,434, 436,440], where the 'atypical Oh' phenotype may predominate [423]; Japanese [441,442]; African Americans [443]; Thais [444]; and a Sudanese family of Arab and black African extraction [431].

2.13.2 Red cell H-partially deficient, non-secretor

Levine *et al.* [445] used the notation A_h to describe a phenotype in a non-secretor Czech woman whose red cells lacked H, but were weakly agglutinated by anti-A. The equivalent B phenotype, B_h, was found, also in a Czech, by Beranová *et al.* [446]. AB_h has also been described [439,447]. A_h, B_h, and AB_h have mainly been reported in people of European origin [439,445–449]. The term para-Bombay has been used for these red cell H-partially deficient, non-secretor phenotypes, but is better reserved for H-deficient and H-partially deficient secretors.

2.13.2.1 Serological characteristics (Table 2.21)

The strength of A expression on red cells of some A_h individuals resembles weak A_2 [445,448], whereas those of others are more like A_x, being agglutinated by only a minority of anti-A sera [449–451]. Likewise, B_h red cells have weak B antigen [446,452]. Little or no H antigen is detected on these cells. No H, A, or B antigen is present in the saliva and, like red cells of most non-secretors, A_h and B_h cells are usually Le(a+b−), but may be Le(a−b−) [435,447]. The serum contains anti-H. A_h serum contains anti-B, but no anti-A, although anti-A_1 is usually present [445,450,451]; in B_h, anti-A is always present and anti-B may also be detected [446,452].

Many examples of A_h, B_h, and AB_h, as well as O_h, have been identified in the people of French origin on the small island of Réunion, off the east coast of Africa [439,447]. O_h in this population arises from the same *H* genotype as the A_h, B_h, and AB_h phenotypes, because they are present in the same families and have the same *h* mutation [106]. This 'Réunion O_h phenotype' can be distinguished from Bombay phenotype by the quantity of H on the cells [439]. Purified *Ulex europaeus* lectin agglutinated papain-treated Réunion phenotype cells, but not Bombay phenotype cells, and high titred H antibodies found in the sera of Bombay phenotype Indians agglutinated Réunion phenotype cells. These same sera agglutinated red cells from some O_h Europeans [439]. The term O_h is ambiguous. It can represent homozygosity for an *h* allele that produces no active α1,2-fucosyltransferase (Bombay phenotype), or homozygosity for an *h* allele that produces weakly active α1,2-fucosyltransferase in people with no *A* or *B* gene and therefore no weak expression of A or B antigen. As predicted by Bhatia [423], there is a series of weak *H* alleles resulting in different degrees of red cell H-deficiency.

2.13.2.2 Glycosyltransferases

Mulet *et al.* [108,433] and Schenkel-Brunner *et al.* [196] were unable to detect H-transferase in sera or red cell membranes from A_h or B_h individuals. Le Pendu *et al.* [435] detected a very small amount of H-transferase activity in sera from red cell H-partially deficient, non-secretor individuals from Réunion Island. As with $O_h{}^A$ and $O_h{}^B$, A_h and B_h sera contain *A* and *B* gene-specified glycosyltransferases, respectively [108,433].

Red cell H-partially deficient phenotypes arise from homozygosity for a mutant gene at the *H* (*FUT1*) locus, which produces only a very weakly active H-transferase. Consequently, the small amount of H structure produced is completely converted to A or B (see Section 2.13.4). Mulet *et al.* [453] demonstrated ingeniously that H is the precursor of B on the cells of a B_h individual. B_h (B+H–) red cells treated with α-galactosidase extract of *Trichomonas foetus* lost their B antigen and became H-active. These B–H+ cells could then be converted to A_h (A+H–) by A-transferase. If the α-galactosidase-treated B_h red cells (B–H+) were treated with H-degrading α-fucosidase from *T. foetus*, they could no longer be converted to A activity.

2.13.3 Red cell H-deficient, secretor

Red cells of people with another type of H-deficiency

have little or no H, A, and B antigens, yet they are ABH secretors, with secretions containing normal quantities of H, A, and B substances. The first family showing that people lacking H from their red cells could secrete H was described by Solomon *et al.* [454] in 1965. Two brothers, whose red cells lacked H and bound anti-A, but were not agglutinated by it, secreted A and H; a third brother, with group O, H-negative red cells, secreted H alone. A secretor of B and H with H-deficient red cells was subsequently found [455]. In view of our current understanding of the genetical background of red cell H-deficient secretor phenotypes, the various symbols devised to describe these phenotypes — $A_m{}^h$, $B_m{}^h$ [454], O_{Hm} [456], Hz [457] — are no longer appropriate. The terms O_h-secretor, A_h-secretor, and B_h-secretor are recommended here (Table 2.21).

2.13.3.1 Serological characteristics (Table 2.21)

Red cells of O_h-secretors are not agglutinated by most H antibodies, but they may be agglutinated weakly by the potent anti-H in some O_h sera and by other strong anti-H reagents [423,458,459]. Adsorption and elution of anti-H may or may not reveal H antigen on red cells of O_h-secretors [91,440,455].

O_h-secretor red cells are not usually agglutinated by anti-A or -B, but some $O_h{}^A$-secretor cells behave like A_x cells and are agglutinated by anti-A,B and very potent anti-A [454,460]. Sometimes the A antigen can only be detected by adsorption and elution of anti-A [91,458]. A similar variation exists with B antigen strength in $O_h{}^B$-secretors [91,455,460,461].

Like those of most secretors, O_h-secretor red cells are usually Le(a–b+), but may be Le(a–b–). The Le(a+b+) phenotype, common in the Far East, was not found in 25 Taiwanese O_h-secretors [462], but was found in two of 51 Hong Kong Chinese O_h-secretors, about half the normal incidence [459].

H substance is present in saliva, in approximately normal quantities for an O secretor [91,454,455,459–461,463]. A and B substances are detected in normal quantities in the secretions when *A* and *B* genes are present.

The serum almost always contains an H-like antibody, which is generally weak and reacts only at low temperature. This antibody, called anti-HI, is not inhibited by secretor saliva and does not react with group O cord cells [224,458,460]. Two-thirds of O_h-

secretors from Hong Kong had anti-HI or anti-H active at 37°C [459].

2.13.3.2 Glycosyltransferases

Originally no H-transferase was detected in O_h-secretor sera or red cell membranes, although the appropriate A- and B-transferases were present [433,458,464]. In four O_h-secretor sera, Le Pendu *et al.* [91] found H-transferase activity representing about 5–10% of that found in sera of people with normal H phenotypes and suggested that this enzyme derived from secretory tissues.

2.13.3.3 Frequency and distribution

H-deficient secretors have been found in a diversity of ethnic groups and nationalities: Indian [423]; European [91,461,465]; Japanese [442,455,466]; Chinese [459,462,467–469]; South-East Asian [458,460]; Middle Eastern [91,458]; Native American [470]. Frequencies of 1 in 5000 Thais [460], 1 in 8000 Taiwanese [471], and 1 in 15 620 Hong Kong Chinese [459] have been estimated.

2.13.4 Genetics of red cell H-deficiency phenotypes

Before 1980, it was generally considered that a gene at the *H* locus was responsible for the production of H antigen both on red cells and in secretions, but that presence of H in secretions was further controlled by genes at a regulator locus called secretor. People with red cell H-deficient, non-secretor phenotypes were thought to be homozygous for rare *h* (or H^w) alleles at the *H* locus, preventing synthesis of H antigen in both red cells and secretions, regardless of secretor genotype. The discovery of secretors with H-deficient red cells introduced a further complexity and a third locus, named *Z*, a regulator for H-expression on red cells, but not in secretions, had to be invoked [454–456]. Red cell H-deficient, secretors would have normal *H* and secretor genes, but would be homozygous for a rare recessive gene, *z*, which would prevent synthesis of red cell H antigen, but permit secretion of H.

As described in Section 2.3.1, it is now known that the *H* (*FUT1*) locus controls α1,2-fucosyltransferase activity in haemopoietic tissue and consequently H antigen expression on red cells. The secretor (*FUT2*)

locus controls α1,2-fucosyltransferase activity in secretory tissue. Twenty-six *FUT1* alleles associated with red cell H-deficient phenotypes are listed in Table 2.22. They include 19 alleles containing missense mutations; 17 of these encoding single and two encoding double amino acid substitutions. There are also three nonsense mutations, converting the codon for an amino acid to a translation stop codon, and four frameshift mutations involving single or double nucleotide deletions. Most red cell H-deficient individuals were homozygous for a mutant allele, but some were found to be heterozygous for two different mutations [442,462,468,469,472,473]. One German with H-deficient red cells was heterozygous for an allele encoding an amino acid substitution and an allele with the normal sequence in the coding region of the gene [472].

The typical Bombay phenotype in people originating from India results from homozygosity for T725G in *FUT1*, encoding Leu242Arg, together with homozygosity for a deletion of *FUT2* [105,106]. The red cell H-partially deficient, non-secretor phenotype, relatively common in the European population of Réunion Island, results from homozygosity for an *FUT1* allele encoding a His117Tyr substitution in the stem region of the enzyme, together with the European non-secretor allele (*se^{428}*) in *FUT2* [106]. Bombay phenotype in an Austrian resulted from homozygosity for G785A and C786A mutations in *FUT1*, encoding Ser262Lys, and *se^{428}* in *FUT2* [434].

Expression of the mutant alleles by transfection of cultured cells has shown that some alleles give rise to no α1,2-fucosyltransferase activity and some produce low levels of enzyme activity [22,105,106,442,466,473]. This explains the different levels of H expression found in H-deficiency phenotypes. One Taiwanese allele (*h$^{35/980}$*) encoded two amino acid substitutions: one in the transmembrane domain, which probably does not affect enzyme activity, but could reduce stability of the enzyme in the Golgi membrane; and one in the catalytic domain [462]. Another H-deficiency allele, found in Japan, contained two missense mutations (*h^{460,1042}*) [442,466]. Wang *et al.* [466] found that expression of this allele in COS-7 cells resulted in no α1,2-fucosyltransferase activity, whereas chimeric alleles containing only the T460C mutation or only the G1042A mutation, yielded 1.0% and 9.3% of normal activity, respectively. The T460C mutation alone

Table 2.22 Mutations in *FUT1* associated with red cell H-deficient phenotypes.

Symbol	Mutation	Amino acid change	H-transferase expression	Secretor phenotype*	Population	References
$h^{35/980}$	C35T A980C	Ala12Val Asn327Thr	NT	Secretor	Taiwanese	[462]
h^{349}	C349T	His117Tyr	Low	Non-sec	Réunion	[106]
h^{442}	G442T	Asp148Tyr	Low	Non-sec†	Japanese	[442]
h^{460}	T460C	Tyr154His	NT	Secretor	Taiwanese	[462]
$h^{460,1042}$	T460C G1042A	Tyr154His Glu348Lys	Low/none	Secretor	Japanese	[442,466]
h^{461}	A461G‡	Tyr154Cys	NT	NR	European	[472]
h^{491}	T491A	Leu164His	None	Secretor	White US	[22,473]
h^{513}	G513C	Trp171Cys	NT	NR	European	[472]
h^{522}	C522A	Phe174Leu	NT	Secretor	Chinese	[469]
$h^{del\,547/548}$	del AG547–552	codon 183/184	NT	Secretor	Taiwanese, Chinese	[462,469]
h^{658}	C658T	Arg220Cys	NT	Secretor	Taiwanese	[462,468]
h^{659}	G659A	Arg220His	NT	Secretor	Taiwanese	[468]
h^{695}	G695A	Trp232stop	None	Non-sec†	Japanese	[442]
h^{721}	T721C	Tyr241His	Low	Secretor	Japanese	[442]
h^{725}	T725G	Leu242Arg	None	Non-sec	Indian	[105,106]
h^{776}	T776A	Val259Glu	NT	NR	European	[472]
$h^{785,786}$	G785A C786A	Ser262Lys	None	Non-sec	European	[434]
h^{801}	G801C or T	Trp267Cys	NT	NR	NR	[474]
h^{826}	C826T	Gln276stop	None	Secretor	White US	[22,473]
h^{832}	G832A	Asp278Asn	NT	NR	NR	[474]
$h^{del\,880/881}$	del TT880–882	codon 294	NT	Secretor	Taiwanese, Chinese	[462,469,474]
h^{944}	C944T	Ala315Val	NT	NR	European	[472]
h^{948}	C948G	Tyr316stop	None	Non-sec	White US	[473]
$h^{del\,969/970}$	del CT969,970	codon 323/324	NT	NR	European	[472]
$h^{del\,990}$	del G990	codon 330	Low	Secretor	Japanese	[442,474]
h^{1047}	G1047C	Trp349Cys	NT	NR	European	[472]
	None detected		NT	NR	European	[472]

* Secretor phenotypes of individuals with *FUT1* mutation shown.
† Homozygous for the weak secretor gene Se^{w385} [442] and would be expected to be weak secretors (Section 2.3.1.2).
‡ Silent mutations, A474G and T954A, also present.
NT, not tested; NR, not reported; del, deletion.

is responsible for a para-Bombay phenotype in Taiwanese [462].

The structural loci *FUT1* and *FUT2* are very closely linked (Chapter 32). In most cases, *FUT1* mutant alleles are associated with the same *FUT2* allele, even in unrelated individuals [106,442]. In six red cell H-deficient Japanese, nine h^{695} alleles were linked to Se^{w385}, whereas one h^{695} allele was linked to *Se*; the other two *H* alleles were h^{721} [442].

Two families are described in which recombination between the *FUT1* and *FUT2* loci may have occurred [89,440]. One family contains red cell H-deficient, secretor and non-secretor members [440]. In the other family it can be inferred that a father has passed *h* and *se* alleles to his five Bombay phenotype children, *H* and *Se* to his four group B, secretor children, and *H* and *se* to his group B, non-secretor daughter [89,475].

2.13.5 Other H-deficient phenotypes

2.13.5.1 H_m

The primary characteristic of the H_m phenotype (Table 2.21) is its dominant mode of inheritance, the rare phenotype appearing in several generations of the same family. Hrubisko [457] reported three Czech families with the H_m phenotype and several other families have been described since [433,465,476]. The H deficiency is not as dramatic as in Bombay or para-Bombay phenotypes: H_m red cells are weakly agglutinated by anti-H. The saliva contains normal quantities of H substance and H-transferase is present in serum and red cell membranes. AH_m cells show depression of the A antigen. In one family the propositus was A_2, but had very little H on his cells; the A-transferase was of the A_1 type, but presumably insufficient H was available for A_1 antigen expression [433,464]. Salmon *et al.* [477] suggest that the H deficiency in Hm must be caused by a dominant genetic defect unrelated to the *H* locus, because of the presence of normal H-transferase in serum and red cell membranes.

2.13.5.2 Leucocyte adhesion deficiency type II

Leucocyte adhesion deficiency type II (LADII) has been diagnosed in five patients: four Arab children [478,479] and boy of Turkish origin [480,481]. LADII is a generalized fucosylation defect associated with recurrent infections, short stature, mental retardation, and a distinctive facial appearance, but also with H-deficient (Bombay phenotype) red cells, ABH nonsecretion, and Le(a–b–) red cell phenotype (reviews in [482,483]). Transferase assays on one of the Arab patients revealed normal levels of serum H- and B-transferases and Le-transferase activity in his saliva [484]. The leucocyte adhesion defect results from a deficiency of sialyl-Le^x, a fucosylated ligand for E- and P-selectins (Section 2.19.3). The likely explanation for the generalized fucosylation deficiency in the Arab children is a defect in the biosynthesis of GDP-L-fucose, the donor substrate for fucosyltransferases, from GDP-D-mannose [482,483]. In the Turkish patient GDP-fucose biosynthesis was normal, so a defect of GDP-fucose import into the Golgi was proposed as a possible explanation for LADII in this patient [481].

A similar, but less complete, generalized fucosylation defect might explain the unusual phenotype of an English woman with weak expression of A and B antigens and no H antigen on her red cells, weak A and B, but no H in her saliva, and normal serum and red cell A-, B-, and H-glycosyltransferases [486]. Her saliva contained Le-transferase, but her red cells were Le(a–) and had very weak Le^b. A fucosylation defect could also explain the H_m phenotype [10].

2.13.6 I and i expression in H-deficient phenotypes

The I and i antigen structures represent carbohydrate chains that are precursors of H, A, B, Le^a, and Le^b substances, so it is not surprising that I and i expression is elevated in H-deficient red cells (see Chapter 25). This effect has been demonstrated on O_h cells by agglutination titrations with anti-I and anti-i [422–424,458]. Measurement of percentage agglutination by an electronic cell counter demonstrated significantly higher agglutination by anti-I with O_h, A_h, and B_h cells from non-secretors (90.2%), compared with control cells (73.5%) [487]. Despite a greater affinity of anti-I and anti-i for O_h cells than for O cells, Doinel [488] detected no increase in the number of I and i sites. Daniels [458] found elevated I expression on the red cells of red cell H-deficient, secretor members of two of three families tested.

2.14 Acquired alterations of A, B, and H antigens on red cells

Since the ABO blood groups were shown to be inherited characters, numerous rare variants have been recognized, many of which have been described in this chapter. Most of these variants are inherited, resulting from mutant genes at the *ABO*, *H*, and possibly other loci. Some ABO anomalies, however, are acquired, generally as a result of infection or malignancy and, occasionally, in the absence of any obvious disease.

2.14.1 Acquired B

Over a period of 4 years, Cameron *et al.* [489] identified seven patients with some kind of red cell B antigen, but with apparently normal anti-B in their sera. The anti-B did not react with the patients' own red cells. Cameron *et al.* [489] gradually came to appreciate that this B-like antigen was an acquired character, probably associated with disease. All seven patients were A_1; the secretors secreted A and H, but no B, and four had group O children and therefore had an A^1/O genotype.

Most individuals with acquired B are ill, although examples of acquired B in healthy subjects are recorded [490–492]. Gerbal and Ropars [493] estimated that 64% of reported cases had diseases of the digestive tract, most of those being carcinoma of the colon. In a survey of 200 patients (106 group O, 94 group A) with gastrointestinal disease, 10 cases of acquired B were found, all in group A patients [493,494]. Acquired B may be a transient phenomenon.

Sera from patients with acquired B antigen contain A-transferase, but no B-transferase [495]. No *B* gene was present in the genome of patients with acquired B red cell antigen [290,496,497].

2.14.1.1 Serological characteristics

Acquired B is only found on group A cells. These are nearly always A_1, although A expression may be depressed [493]. A few examples of A_2 with acquired B have been found: in one case the cells became A_1 as B expression diminished [498]; in another the patient had an A_2 serum transferase [499]; and in two cases the patients had A^2/O genotypes [290]. One example of acquired B was associated with weak expression of A and H antigens [500].

Acquired B antigen is usually weak, but varies in different individuals and with time. Often a proportion of cells remains unagglutinated with anti-B. Sera from A_2 donors are better at detecting acquired B than are sera from A_1 donors [495,498,501]; 10% of A_1 sera do not agglutinate acquired B cells [495]. Some group A and O sera contain a specific anti-acquired B, which does not react with normal B cells and can be separated from anti-B by adsorption and elution [491,502]. Herron *et al.* [491] produced anti-acquired B, which reacted with acquired B cells but not ordinary group B cells, by immunizing a rabbit with acquired B cells.

Some monoclonal anti-B react with acquired B cells [502–505] and monoclonal anti-acquired B has been produced by immunizing mice with acquired B red cells [506,507]. The introduction as a blood-grouping reagent of a monoclonal anti-B clone (ES4), which strongly agglutinates acquired B cells, greatly increased the rate of detection of this phenotype [505]. A group A patient with acquired B was grouped as AB with reagents containing ES4 and suffered a fatal haemolytic reaction following transfusion with four group AB units [508]. The patient's weak anti-B was not detected by abbreviated compatibility testing. Manufacturers of monoclonal anti-B have now lowered the pH of reagents containing ES4, so that they only detect the strongest examples of acquired B. This lowering of pH has caused problems, however, as the sera of about 1 in 500 blood donors have low pH-dependent autoagglutinins [509,510]. There are advantages in detecting acquired B, providing it is not mistaken for normal B. Detection of acquired B with a reagent containing ES4 in an apparently healthy blood donor led to the diagnosis of lymphoma and displacement of the small bowel [511].

Serum from acquired B individuals contains anti-B, which does not react with acquired B cells. Saliva of acquired B secretors contains A and H, but no B.

Acquired B red cells are often polyagglutinable (see below).

2.14.1.2 Cause of acquired B

Despite earlier suggestions that acquired B results from adsorption of B-like bacterial glycolipids [512,513], Marsh *et al.* [514,515] felt that acquired B resulted from enzyme action. Bacterial filtrates were used to simulate acquired B, *in vitro* [515]. A few sera from individuals with acquired B could convert group A cells to acquired B activity, *in vitro* [492,516,517]. Gerbal *et al.* [500] hypothesized that bacterial deacetylases convert N-acetylgalactosamine, the A immunodominant sugar, to galactosamine. This galactosamine is similar enough to galactose, the B immunodominant sugar, to react with some anti-B (Fig. 2.10). Gerbal *et al.* [495] suggest that acquired B is not

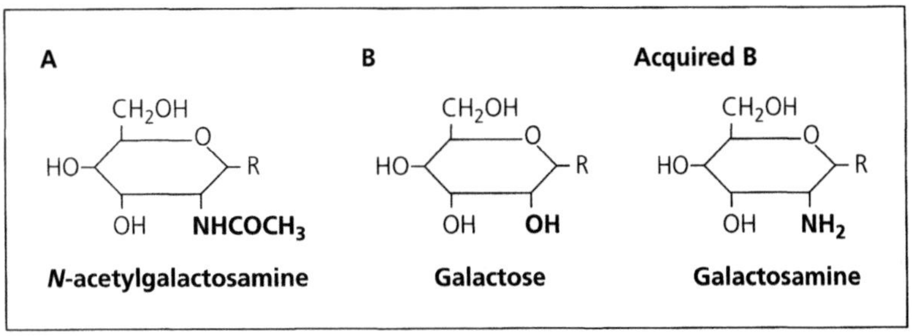

Fig. 2.10 Terminal immunodominant sugars for A, B, and acquired B, demonstrating the similarity between galactose and galactosamine (deacetylated *N*-acetylgalactosamine). R, remainder of molecule.

common because all A_2 people and 95% of A_1 people have anti-acquired B in their serum and because most bacteria do not produce the appropriate deacetylases. A wealth of evidence now exists confirming that deacetylation of N-acetylgalactosamine is the most common cause of acquired B [493–495,508,518].

2.14.1.3 Evidence for deacetylation of A as the cause of acquired B

1 Only group A cells acquire B antigen.

2 The strength of A antigen expression on acquired B cells is inversely related to the strength of the acquired B antigen [495] (Fig. 2.11). Gerbal and Ropars [493] used *Dolichos biflorus* lectin to separate two populations of red cells from a patient with acquired B. The A_1 cells agglutinated by the lectin had only weak acquired B, whereas the remaining A_2 cells had strong acquired B expression.

3 Deacetylases have been isolated from the bacteria *Clostridium tertium* A and *Escherichia coli* K12 [519,520]. Acquired B cells could be created, *in vitro*, by treating A_1 cells with culture filtrate from *C. tertium* or from one of six strains of *E. coli* [493,495]. Group O cells were not converted to B activity.

4 Chemical acetylation of acquired B cells with acetic anhydride destroyed the B activity and enhanced the A activity back to that of normal A_1 cells [518].

5 A-trisaccharide [GalNAcα1→3(Fucα1→2)Gal]

that has been chemically deacetylated inhibits the reaction of anti-B with acquired B, but not with normal B cells [521]. B-trisaccharide [Galα1→3(Fucα1→2)Gal], in which the hydroxyl group of carbon-2 of the α-galactose residue has been substituted by an amino group (see Fig. 2.10), had the same effect [522]. Agglutination of acquired B cells with anti-B is dispersed by the addition of galactosamine [523].

6 Suspension of acquired B red cells in an acid medium (pH 6) reduces reactivity with anti-B [495], presumably because the NH_2 group of the galactosamine residue is converted to NH_3^+.

2.14.1.4 Polyagglutination

Acquired B cells are usually polyagglutinable [493,524]; they are agglutinated, at least weakly, by most AB sera. This polyagglutination evolves in parallel with the acquired B phenomenon, but disappears before B activity during recovery; it is not apparent at pH 4.5 or below and it disappears after chemical acetylation of the cells [493,502,518]. Agglutination of acquired B cells by AB serum is inhibited by deacetylated A-trisaccharide, by amino-substituted B-trisaccharide, and by galactosamine [502,521,522].

It is possible that there are antibodies present in most human sera specific for the deacetylated A antigen that are responsible for the acquired B phenomenon. As polyagglutinable cells can be produced by deacetylation with *C. tertium* filtrate of O cells, as well as A cells [493], a different antigen from acquired B is probably involved, possibly involving glucosamine produced by deacetylation of N-acetylglucosamine [525].

Acquired B is a unique type of polyagglutination. Acquired B cells react with AB sera from which anti-T, -Tk, -Tn, -Cad, and anti-HEMPAS have been removed by adsorption [518,526] (see Chapter 31). However, other cryptantigens, responsible for other forms of polyagglutination, are often revealed on acquired B cells, especially Tk, but also T and Th [492,502,516,527,528].

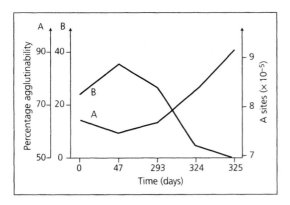

Fig. 2.11 Graph demonstrating the inverse relation between A and acquired B expression, as measured by percentage agglutination and number of A sites, in a patient studied over several months. As acquired B expression increased, A antigen expression decreased, and vice versa. Adapted from [495].

2.14.2 Alterations in leukaemia patients

2.14.2.1 Serology

In 1957, van Loghem *et al.* [529] suggested that very

weak A antigen expression on the red cells of a myeloblastic leukaemia patient, previously shown to have a normal A antigen, may have occurred as a result of his disease. A report of a similar case soon followed; a group A person whose red cells were no longer agglutinated by anti-A (although they did adsorb it) during the course of acute leukaemia [530,531].

The association of weak A antigen expression with acute leukaemia is now well documented (reviewed in [224,532–534]). In some cases all red cells show weakness of the A antigen, whereas in others two populations of red cells are clearly apparent [531,535–537]. Gold *et al.* [531] separated two populations of red cells from a patient with acute monoblastic leukaemia. Initially only 2% were agglutinated with anti-A, but in remission the proportion of agglutinable cells rose to 65% before falling again shortly before death. In a patient recorded by Renton *et al.* [538], 26% of the red cells were group AB, 12% A, 42% B, and 20% O. Presumably the patient was genetically *AB*; 62% of his cells had lost their A antigen and 32% their B antigen. Leukaemia-associated changes in B and H antigens are also recorded [537–539]. Between 17% and 37% of patients with leukaemia have significantly lower A, B, or H antigenic expression compared with healthy controls [539–542]. By flow cytometry 55% of A, B, or AB patients with myeloid malignancies had decreased expression of A or B compared with healthy controls of the same ABO genotype; 21% of group O patients had reduced H [543]. In almost all cases the changes represent a loss or diminution of antigen strength and not the expression of a new red cell antigen, although one case is reported of a group O (O^{1v}/O^{1v}) patient with myelodysplastic syndrome acquiring an A antigen [290].

Although modifications of ABH antigens are usually associated with acute leukaemia, they are also often manifested before diagnosis of malignancy and therefore indicate preleukaemic states [532]. Loss of an ABH antigen in a patient with a haematological disorder is generally prognostic of acute leukaemia [544]. For example, a four-year-old girl whose red cells gave mixed-field agglutination with anti-A initially had no sign of haematological disease, but was diagnosed as having acute myeloid leukaemia 18 months later [545].

Acute leukaemia has, on occasion, been associated with loss or weakening of Lewis antigens [531,544,546].

2.14.2.2 Transferases

Depression of A or B antigens in acute myeloid leukaemia (AML) and in preleukaemic states is generally associated with a severe reduction in red cell A- or B-transferase activity, but little or no reduction in red cell H-transferase activity [545,547,548]. In patients with separable populations of red cells, A- or B-transferase activity was greatly reduced in the membranes of those cells that had lost their A or B antigens, but were normal in those that had not [547]. No significant difference in H-transferase activity could be detected between the different cell populations. Furthermore, A or B antigen expression in those cells that had lost A or B activity could be converted to normal, *in vitro*. During clinical remission, the A antigen of one of the patients returned to normal, as did membrane A-transferase activity [547]. Thus, the loss of A or B expression in acute leukaemia results from a defect or deficiency of the *A* or *B* gene products and not a defect in enzyme substrates.

Serum H-transferase activity is generally reduced in patients with AML [547,549–551], but increased in those with chronic granulocytic leukaemia [551,552]. These changes appear to reflect the abnormal platelet counts often present in these conditions [551]. Serum A- and B-transferase activities may also be slightly reduced in AML patients [549].

In a patient with erythroleukaemia, about 50% of the red cells had lost their A antigen and those cells also showed a very low level of adenylate kinase-1 (AK_1), an enzyme encoded by a gene close to *ABO* on chromosome 9 [553] (Chapter 32). This was presumed to result from a chromosome lesion in the part of the chromosome containing both *ABO* and *AK1* loci. The *ABL1* oncogene locus maps between *ABO* and *AK1* on chromosome 9q34 [554]. *ABL1* is at the breakpoint of the Philadelphia-chromosome, a leukaemia-specific reciprocal translocation involving paternal chromosome 9 and maternal chromosome 22 [555]. In four informative cases of A or B antigen loss during AML, the allele that was lost could only have been maternally derived [556]. The significance of this is unclear, but the results suggest that imprinting affects other loci on chromosome 9q34 other than *ABL1*.

It is possible that down-regulation of *ABO* in haematological disorders involves methylation of the promoter region [143].

51

2.14.3 Other acquired changes in A, B, and H antigens

Acquired loss of A from a proportion of the red cells occasionally occurs in healthy, elderly individuals [557,558]. In one elderly woman, two red cell populations could be separated using anti-A$_1$ *Dolichos biflorus* lectin [557]. The A$_1$ cells, agglutinated by the lectin, were AK$_1$2-1, whereas the weak A (A$_x$-like) cells had lost the AK$_1$2 isozyme and only AK$_1$1 could be detected. In one clone, part of chromosome 9 appears to be partially inactivated.

An infant with congenital rubella infection lost her A antigen during the first few months of her life [559]. A healthy child who was A$_2$ at birth, but later became A$_x$, is described in Section 2.7.3 [320].

Following transplantation of a liver from a group AB donor, a proportion of the red cells of a group O child became transiently group AB, as did group O transfused red cells [560]. The cause of this phenomenon is unknown, but could have been caused by hepatic transferase activity. Weak A activity on red cells of group A recipients of group O bone marrow transplants may result from adsorption of A substance from the plasma of the recipient [561].

2.14.4 *In vitro* enzymatic degradation of A, B, and H antigens

A or B antigens on red cells can be converted to H antigen by removal of the immunodominant sugar with an appropriate exoglycosidase: α-N-acetylgalactosaminidase (A-zyme) or α-galactosidase (B-zyme). Such enzymes are derived from a variety of sources, especially bacteria (reviewed in [562]).

The enzyme that has brought most success in creating artificial group O cells from B cells is α-galactosidase from green coffee beans [562–564]. No B antigen could be detected on group B cells treated with this purified α-galactosidase and there was no apparent membrane damage. Phase I and II clinical trials, on healthy volunteers and patients, respectively, have shown that group B red cells treated with either native or recombinant α-galactosidase from coffee beans are safe and efficacious when transfused to group O or A subjects, once, in multiple-unit volumes, or on more than one occasion [565,566]. A minority of the recipients had increases in anti-B titres following transfusion, suggesting the presence of residual B antigens.

Furthermore, sera from 40% of group O and 20% of group A individuals weakly agglutinated the enzyme-modified group B red cells [566].

Attempts to find a suitable α-N-acetylgalactosaminidase have been less fruitful, probably because A antigens on A$_1$ cells are present at internal positions in addition to terminal positions of oligosaccharide chains and are not cleaved by exoglycosidases. A-zymes from chicken liver or from the enteric bacterium *Ruminococcus torques* IX-70 will convert A$_2$ red cells into O cells, but are less effective with A$_1$ cells [562,567].

An α-fucosidase isolated from *Aspergillus niger* abolished H activity on group O cells [568].

2.15 ABH antibodies and lectins

2.15.1 Anti-A and -B

Anti-A and -B are almost always present in sera of people who lack the corresponding antigen from their red cells (Table 2.2). With the exception of newborn infants, deviations from this rule are extremely rare. Dobson and Ikin [569] estimated that only about 1 in 12 000 adults lack expected anti-A or -B. Missing agglutinins may indicate a weak subgroup of A or B, a twin chimera, dispermy, hypogammaglobulinaemia, or old age. A few examples of missing agglutinins with no apparent explanation are recorded [570,571]. Springer and Tegtmeyer [571] showed that no immune response could be induced in a healthy group A woman lacking anti-B by injecting human blood group B glycoprotein. Van Loghem *et al.* [570] described three healthy group A individuals who, despite having no serologically detectable anti-B, demonstrated impaired *in vivo* survival of injected group B cells.

Antibodies detected in the serum of neonates are usually IgG and maternal in origin [572], but may, on occasion, be IgM and produced by the fetus [573]. Generally, ABO agglutinins are first detected at an age of about 3 months and continue to increase in titre, reaching adult levels between 5 and 10 years [573,574]. The low titres of anti-A and -B in elderly people detected in early studies [575,576] could not be confirmed [574].

Levels of A and B antibodies appear to be influenced mainly by environmental factors, genetics having no more than a minor role [577,578]. Anti-A and -B are often referred to as naturally occurring, but probably appear in children as a result of immunization by A and B substances present in the environment. Springer *et al.* [579,580] found that chickens, which normally develop an antibody to human group B red cells within a few months of hatching, fail to do so if kept in a germ-free environment. Feeding human infants with killed bacteria (*Escherichia coli* O_{86}) stimulated increased anti-B activity [581].

Changes in the characteristics of anti-A or -B occur as a result of further immunization by pregnancy or by artificial means, such as incompatible transfusion of red cells or other blood products. Typical changes, serologically detectable, are increase in titre and avidity of agglutinin, increase in haemolytic activity, and greater activity at 37°C. Such 'immune' sera are generally difficult to inhibit with saliva or with A or B substances.

Anti-A and -B molecules may be IgM, IgG or IgA; some sera may contain all three classes [573,582]. Anti-A and -B of non-stimulated individuals are predominantly IgM, although IgG and IgA may be present [583,584]. During a programme of immunizing donors with human A or B glycoproteins, with the purpose of producing potent blood grouping reagents, Contreras *et al.* [585] detected some IgG anti-A or -B in all donors prior to immunization. These donors, who had been selected for high titre antibodies, all showed

an increase in IgG after stimulation; IgA anti-A and -B, which could not be detected in any of the sera preimmunization, was present in all sera postimmunization. Table 2.23 shows some of the characteristics of IgM, IgG, and IgA ABO antibodies. IgG2 and IgG1 anti-A and/or -B were present in most sera from mothers of group A or B children; almost 40% of the sera also contained IgG3 and/or IgG4 anti-A/B [586]. IgG2 usually had a higher titre than antibodies of the other subclasses. A quantitative analysis of sera from 235 healthy blood donors again showed IgG1 and IgG2 anti-A/B predominant, with IgG3 and IgG4 having only a minor role [582].

ABO antibodies may be found in various body fluids including saliva, milk, cervical secretions, tears, and the contents of cysts [254,587–592]. They are primarily IgA [590] and generally most active in fluids from group O individuals.

Anti-A_1 is described in Section 2.4.

An interesting antibody described by Ikin *et al.* [593] in 1953 remains unique. In a saline medium this antibody agglutinated only group A Rh D+ cells; A_1 D+ cells gave stronger reactions than A_2 D+ cells. O D+ and A D– cells were not agglutinated. When the reactivity of the antibody was enhanced by addition of albumin it behaved as anti-D. The antibody could be completely adsorbed by O D+ cells, but it was not adsorbed by A_1 D– cells. Perhaps this anti-D-like anti-

Table 2.23 Some characteristics of IgM, IgG, and IgA anti-A and -B (compiled mostly from [573]).

Characteristic	IgM	IgG	IgA
Present in sera of:			
non-immunized donors	Yes	Sometimes	Rarely
immunized donors	Yes	Usually	Usually
Agglutinates red cells	Yes	Yes	Yes
Agglutination enhanced in serum medium	No	Yes	
Haemolytic	Yes	Yes	No
Binds complement	Yes	Yes	No
Titre increased in antiglobulin test	No	Yes	Yes
Inhibited by secretor saliva or purified glycoprotein	Yes, easily	Poorly	Yes, less easily than IgM
Thermal optimum	4°C	4–37°C	
Activity destroyed by 2-ME or DTT	Yes	No	Partially
Activity destroyed by heating to 56°C	Yes	No	No
Present in colostrum	Sometimes	No	Yes

DTT, dithiothreitol; 2-ME, 2-mercaptoethanol.

body recognized conformational changes in the Rh complex occurring with the presence or absence of an A determinant on the Rh-associated glycoprotein (see Section 5.5.7).

2.15.2 Anti-A,B of group O serum

Sera from group O people do not simply contain two separable antibodies, anti-A and -B, but a cross-reacting antibody called anti-A,B. If an eluate is made from group A cells incubated in group O serum the antibody in the eluate will agglutinate A and B cells [217]. The same effect is observed if group B cells are used. However, there is no such effect if artificial anti-A+B is made by mixing group A and group B sera [594,595].

The cross-reactivity of group O sera is often asymmetrical; some group O sera eluted from A cells react with B cells, yet when eluted from B cells will not react with A cells [595]. In group O people immunized with A cells or A substance the cross-reacting antibody usually shows a preference for A cells [585,596]; i.e. it has a higher binding constant for A cells than for B cells [597]. The reverse is true in group O individuals immunized with B antigen.

Although a number of theories have been put forward to explain the reactions of group O sera, the most feasible is that group O people make an antibody that detects a structure common to both A and B determinants [11,598–600]. Human monoclonal analysis by limiting-dilution methodology has confirmed that antibodies produced by group O donors bind to both A- and B-trisaccharide [601].

Anti-A,B are mostly IgG, but may be IgM or IgA [573].

2.15.3 Clinical significance of ABO antibodies

Transfusion of ABO incompatible red cells will almost always result in symptoms of haemolytic transfusion reaction and may cause disseminated intravascular coagulation, renal failure, and death. Signs of red cell destruction occasionally occurs following transfusion of group O blood to recipients of other ABO groups; the result of destruction of the patient's red cells by transfused ABO antibodies. (See [573] for details on transfusion reactions.)

Anti-A_1 is rarely clinically significant and most examples are not active above 25°C. However, there are

a few reports of haemolytic transfusion reactions caused by anti-A_1 [602–605].

Haemolytic disease of the fetus and newborn (HDN) caused by ABO antibodies usually occurs in A_1, B, or A_1B babies of group O mothers, yet IgG anti-A or -B is more often responsible than anti-A,B for HDN and tends to cause more severe symptoms [606,607]. Very rarely, group B babies of A_2 mothers may be affected. About 15% of pregnancies in women of European origin involve a group O mother with a group A or B fetus, yet ABO HDN requiring clinical intervention is rare, although minor symptoms involving a small degree of red cell destruction may be relatively common. Hydrops caused by ABO HDN is exceedingly rare, but very occasionally exchange transfusion for the prevention of kernicterus is indicated. Severe ABO HDN is relatively rare, despite the presence of IgG ABO antibodies in the serum of most group O women, because of the relatively low density of A and B antigens on fetal red cells and the presence of soluble A and B substances in the fetal plasma, which neutralize maternal antibodies. The complement deficiency of fetal plasma may also play a part in the rarity of ABO HDN as IgG anti-A that haemolyses red cells in the presence of complement will not lyse cord cells if neonatal serum is used as the source of complement [608].

Anti-A and -B will cause rejection of incompatible kidney, liver, and heart transplants. Transplantation of A_2 kidneys and livers into B and O patients may be satisfactory when patients are selected for low anti-A titre [609,610] and transplantation of incompatible hearts has been successful in newborn infants [611]. Anti-A and -B can usually be disregarded, however, for tissue transplants, including cornea, skin, and bone [612]. Although ABO is generally disregarded when selecting a bone marrow donor, ABO major incompatibility may reduce graft survival [613].

From the point of view of red cell transfusion, group O is generally considered the 'universal donor' and transfusion of O blood to an A or B recipient considered a compatible transfusion. There is now increasing evidence that infusion of relatively large quantities of ABO incompatible plasma, as frequently occurs when transfusing platelets, could cause impaired cellular immune function, infection, and multiorgan failure by a mechanism unrelated to haemolysis [614]. This might be a result of tissue damage caused by the presence of ABO antibodies in the transfused plasma or the presence of circulating immune complexes comprising soluble ABO substances in the transfused plasma and the recipient's antibodies. Heal and Blumberg [614] propose, 'That only ABO identical components, or those lacking incompatible antigen and antibody, be administered to patients with cancer, except when there are no alternatives.'

Some other effects of minor ABO incompatibility are described in Section 2.15.5.

2.15.4 ABO autoantibodies

ABO autoantibodies are apparently rare. In one English blood centre, of 4668 patients with autoantibodies studied over 32 years, only six had autoantibodies with ABO specificity [615]. Some apparent autoanti-A and -B do not react with group A or B cord cells and so their true specificity is anti-AI or -BI (Section 25.7.5). Several examples of autoanti-A and -B have caused autoimmune haemolytic anaemia [615], one resulting in fatal haemolysis and kidney failure [616]. Autoanti-A_1 has been reported, but not implicated in haemolytic anaemia [615].

Low affinity A and B autoantibodies are present in purified IgG and IgM fraction from sera of A and B individuals, respectively [617]. These autoantibodies are not detected in whole serum because of complementary interactions between V regions of the antibodies. This suggests that tolerance to autologous ABO antigens is dependent on peripheral control, rather than on clonal deletion or anergy at the B- or T-cell level [617].

2.15.5 Post-transplantation antibodies of graft origin

In 1971, Beck et al. [618] speculated that anti-A detected in the serum of a group A woman after transplantation of a lung from a group O donor may have been produced by lymphoreticular tissue transplanted with the lung. Since then there have been numerous accounts of apparent autoanti-A, -A_1, or -B, following transplantation of kidney, liver, heart, lung, pancreas, or spleen (review in [619]). Typically these ABO antibodies are IgG, appear 7–10 days after transplantation, and last for about 1 month. They are often responsible for haemolysis and have caused acute renal failure and, in one case, death [619,620]. The IgG allotype of anti-A eluted from the red cells of a group A_1 woman 14 days after receiving a group O kidney demonstrated that the antibody was of donor origin and could not have been produced by the patient [621].

Haemolysis induced by anti-A or -B produced by passenger lymphocytes of graft origin may also be a complication of minor ABO incompatibility in transplantation of bone marrow or peripheral blood progenitor cells [622–625]. This problem is more prevalent in patients treated with cyclosporin for prophylaxis against graft-vs.-host disease than in those receiving methotrexate [626]. Haemolysis may be severe and even fatal [625].

2.15.6 Monoclonal antibodies

Three years after Köhler and Milstein [627] described their method for in vitro production of monoclonal antibodies from hybridomas of murine myeloma cells and lymphocytes from immunized mice, Barnstable et al. [628] reported the first monoclonal blood group antibody, anti-A. This antibody resulted from immunizing a mouse with human tonsil lymphocyte preparations. Barnstable et al. [628] suggested that this anti-A might be of use in blood typing, but it was later shown to lack sufficient potency with A_2 and A_2B cells [629].

Numerous other monoclonal anti-A soon followed: some produced deliberately by immunizing mice with group A red cells or purified substance [630–633]; others accidentally by immunizing with cancer cell lines, other cells, or epidermal growth factor [629,634–637]. Some monoclonal antibodies behaving as anti-A_1 have also been reported [63,632,635].

Human anti-A and -A_1 monoclonal antibodies have been generated by Epstein–Barr virus (EBV) transformation of lymphocytes obtained either from hyperimmunized plasmapheresis donors [638] or from splenic tissue after in vitro stimulation with group A red cells [639]. Monoclonal anti-Type 2 A and anti-difucosylated A were produced by a heterohybridoma of EBV-transformed human lymphocytes and mouse myeloma cells [640].

Monoclonal antibodies have proved invaluable for studying the various types of carbohydrate chains determining A activity. Antibodies to Type 1 A, 2 A, 3 A, and 4 A have all been recognized [48,62,63,634,635,641], as have antibodies that show a preference for a difucosyl-A structure, either

Type 1 (ALe^b) or Type 2 (ALe^y) [636,642–645]. For reviews see [14,18,21,38,312,646]. Some monoclonal anti-A bind preferentially to the A-terminal trisaccharide, whereas others detect an epitope involving the oligosaccharide backbone. The former type of anti-A are more effective at agglutinating A$_2$B red cells with weak A expression than the latter type, and are more suitable for use as reagents [647,648].

Monoclonal anti-B have been produced following immunization of mice with B or AB red cells [503,632], purified B substance [383,504,632], or chemically synthesized B trisaccharide [649].

Several monoclonals that react with both A and B cells (anti-A,B) have been produced after immunizing mice with A substance, group A red cells, or AB red cells [310,632,633,650]. Some of these antibodies react more strongly with A cells than with B cells [310,650].

A Fab-phage was isolated, by panning with group B red cells, from a human IgG1 phage-display library derived from splenocytes from a group O donor. The 'antibody' agglutinated B, but not A or O red cells, but displayed interaction with A and B epitopes by inhibition techniques [651].

Details of numerous ABO monoclonal antibodies submitted to three international workshops are described in the workshop reports [652–654].

2.15.6.1 Monoclonal antibodies as blood grouping reagents

The advantage of monoclonal antibodies over polyclonal alloantibodies as ABO grouping reagents is not their monoclonality, which may even be a disadvantage, but the fact that they are manufactured *in vitro*. Vast quantities of specific antibody can be generated, containing no unwanted contaminating antibodies, and saving on human plasma and on the high cost of preparing and quality controlling conventional reagents made from pools of human serum. Furthermore, they remove the necessity to immunize human volunteers in order to make potent reagents. Monoclonal anti-A and -B have proved to be satisfactory reagents by both manual and automated techniques and are being used in most transfusion centres and hospital blood banks throughout the world [509,655].

Potent monoclonal anti-A reagents have been produced that agglutinate A$_x$ red cells [312,313]. This ob-

viates the requirement for anti-A,B. The complication of A(B) is discussed in Section 2.11. The hazard of using monoclonal anti-B reagents that detect acquired B antigen is described in Section 2.14.1.1.

Judson and Smythe [656] found that some monoclonal anti-B precipitate at 4°C. They deduced that this was because of B-like activity on the IgM molecules, a result of terminal α1,3-galactose on some *N*-glycans of mouse IgM. The suggested remedy for this cryoprecipitation is treatment of partially purified IgM with α-galactosidase or culturing the hybridoma in the presence of α-galactosidase or *N*-glycan processing inhibitors.

2.15.7 Anti-H

H antibodies detect the precursor of A and B antigens. They characteristically agglutinate group O and A$_2$ cells more strongly than A$_1$ and B cells.

Typically, H antibodies are inhibited by secretor saliva and react with group O cord cells, although often less strongly than with O adult cells. Morgan and Watkins [657] distinguished anti-H, which is inhibited by secretor saliva, from 'anti-O', which is not. The latter specificity is now generally called anti-HI (Section 2.15.8).

Antibodies specific for Type 1 H (Table 2.3) are often referred to as anti-Le^d or -Le^{dH} [281,658] (Section 2.19.2.1).

2.15.7.1 Anti-H in Bombay sera

Anti-H is generally present in the sera of people with H-deficient, non-secretor (Bombay, O$_h$, A$_h$, and B$_h$) phenotypes. These anti-H vary greatly in strength, ability to agglutinate cord cells, degree of inhibition by O saliva, and IgG content [458]. Sera with the greater IgG content show least difference in strength between O cord and O adult cells and are least readily inhibited by saliva. O$_h$ sera contain both anti-Type 1 H and anti-Type 2 H [659,660]. Réunion phenotype individuals (red cell H-partially deficient, non-secretors), however, produce a large quantity of anti-Type 1 H, but only little anti-Type 2 H, presumably because a small quantity of Type 2 H antigen is present on their red cells [660].

Anti-H in sera of red cell H-deficient and partially deficient, non-secretors is clinically significant and may cause severe HDN [661]. Only 2% of group O cells injected into an O_h patient survived 24 h [662]. In an A_h patient, 67% of A_1 cells were destroyed within 1 h of injection, despite being only weakly agglutinated at 37°C by the serum of the patient [663]. A transfusion reaction occurred in a B_h patient transfused with H-positive blood [452].

2.15.7.2 Other sources of human anti-H

Anti-H in the serum of people who do not have H-deficient red cell phenotypes are generally weak and only reactive at low temperatures. When present, they are usually found in ABH non-secretors [664].

An exceptionally potent anti-H from an A_1 Le(a–b+) person (Toml) was inhibited by secretor saliva, including the patient's own saliva, reacted with cord cells, and did not react with O_h cells [665]. Unlike sera from H-deficient, non-secretors, the anti-H of Toml and a high titred H autoagglutinin from a group B patient bound Type 2 H, but not Type 1 H, trisaccharides [659,666]. Monoclonal IgM autoanti-H in a patient with lymphoma was responsible for fatal autoimmune haemolytic anaemia [667]. Several autoanti-H (or -HI) have been reported that are only active in the presence of calcium chelators such as citrate or ethylenediaminetetraacetic acid (EDTA) [668,669].

2.15.7.3 Monoclonal anti-H

Numerous mouse monoclonal H antibodies have been produced, many unintentionally, following immunization by a variety of immunogens [60,64, 652–654,670–676]. Unlike human anti-H, murine monoclonal anti-H are often not inhibited by secretor salivas, or at least are inhibited by only a minority of secretor salivas [671,677]. Furukawa et al. [60] studied 11 H-like monoclonal antibodies: all reacted with either monofucosyl Type 2 H or difucosyl-Le^y, or with both structures; none reacted with the Type 1 structures. Those antibodies reactive with only Type 2 H reacted with red cells, but not with salivary substances, presumably because of a predominance of difucosylated structures in saliva; those specific for the difucosylated Le^y structure did react with salivary structures, but not with red cells; and those reactive with both monofucosylated and difucosylated structures reacted with red cells and with saliva. Mollicone et al. [675] subdivided 28 monoclonal anti-Type 2 H into seven

categories, based on their cross-reactivities with synthetic oligosaccharides.

2.15.7.4 Anti-H from other sources

Anti-H has been made in a number of animals by immunizing with O red cells or with purified H substance, and adsorbing with O_h cells. Bhatia [678] produced anti-H in chickens, cattle, buffalo, goats, and sheep. H-specific lectins are described in Section 2.15.9.4.

2.15.8 Anti-HI and -Hi

HI antibodies agglutinate red cells carrying both H and I determinants [679]; they do not agglutinate, or agglutinate only very weakly, H-deficient cells (non-secretor or secretor) or I-deficient cells (cord and adult i cells). Anti-HI are usually weak antibodies reacting only at low temperatures.

In line with the observation of Sanger [664] that anti-H is only made by ABH non-secretors, the H-like agglutinin found in the serum of H-deficient secretors is generally anti-HI [224,458,460]. Although anti-HI in the serum of H-deficient secretors was responsible for rapid destruction of small quantities of radiolabelled group O red cells, it was predicted that transfusion of whole units of blood would result in near normal survival [680].

Autoanti-HI is usually considered benign, but anti-HI of high titre and active at 37°C caused an acute haemolytic transfusion reaction in a group B woman with sickle cell disease, following transfusion of 100 mL of group O red cells [681]. Subsequent transfusion of group B cells through a blood warmer was satisfactory.

An autoagglutinin in the serum of an A_1 woman, which behaved like anti-H but was not inhibited by secretor saliva and reacted exceptionally strongly with group A_2 adult i cells, was called anti-Hi [682]. Three more examples have been reported since [683].

2.15.9 Lectins

The name lectin originally described plant extracts capable of agglutinating red cells [684]. In 1980, Goldstein et al. [685] broadened this definition to, 'A sugar-binding protein or glycoprotein of non-immune origin, which agglutinates cells and/or precipitates glycoconjugates'. Thus, the vast array of haemagglutinating substances found in plant (mostly seed) extracts and in some animals such as snails, fish, and snakes can all be termed lectins.

The agglutinating activity of lectins is inhibited by simple sugars, usually monosaccharides. It is assumed that these sugars represent the binding site for the lectin on the cell surface. Through the use of lectins, Morgan and Watkins [686] obtained some of the early information on the nature of the A, B, and H antigens. Some plant extracts contain more than one lectin, for example, seeds of *Ulex europaeus* and *Bandeiraea simplicifolia* (see below).

The variety of lectins with A, B, or H specificity are too numerous to itemize here. Most are seed extracts, predominantly from plants of the family Leguminosae, although many other sources exist. Lectins with anti-A, -B, and -H specificity are found in the fruiting bodies of many fungi [687]. A few lectins are listed in Table 2.24. For reviews see [688–691].

2.15.9.1 Anti-A

Renkonen [692] found anti-A activity in the seeds of *Vicia cracca*, the first blood group lectin to be recognized. Group A specificity has been found since in a number of seeds including *Dolichos biflorus*, an extremely useful blood grouping reagent because it agglutinates A_1 cells far more readily than A_2 cells and so, when appropriately diluted, distinguishes A_1 and A_1B from A_2 and A_2B [223]. *Dolichos* lectin is specific for terminal N-acetylgalactosamine [693] and so will also agglutinate Tn+ and Sd(a++) cells (see Chapters 29 and 31). Furukawa *et al.* [670] suggest that *Dolichos* lectin differentiates A_1 and A_2 red cells on the basis of quantitative rather than structural differences.

The eggs and albumin glands of several species of snails, mostly of the family Helicidae, contain anti-A (N-acetylgalactosamine) activity and have often been used in automated ABO grouping [689,694,695].

Table 2.24 Some lectins with A, B, A,B, or H activity.

Species	Source	Blood group activity	Monosaccharide specificity	Comments
Dolichos biflorus	Seed	Anti-A_1	GalNAc	Anti-Tn, -Cad also
Phaseolus limensis	Seed (lima bean)	Anti-A		
Phaseolus lunatus	Seed (lima bean)	Anti-A	GalNAc	
Helix pomatia	Snail	Anti-A	GalNAc	
Helix hortensis	Snail	Anti-A	GalNAc, NeuAc	
Fomes fometarius	Tree fungus	Anti-B		Anti-P^k also
Ptilota plumosa	Seaweed	Anti-B		
Salmo salar	Salmon roe	Anti-B	Gal	Anti-P also
Sophora japonica	Seed	Anti-A,B		Reacts strongly with En(a–) cells. Anti-B strongest
Phlomis fructosa	Seed (Jerusalem sage)	Anti-A,B	GalNAc, Gal	
Bandeiraea simplicifolia	Seed	Anti-A,B	GalNAc, Gal	BSI, one of 3 lectins. Anti-B strongest
Ulex europaeus	Seed (gorse)	Anti-H	I Fuc II GlcNAc*	Lectin most commonly used for detecting H secretion
Lotus tetragonolobus	Seed	Anti-H (-HI)	Fuc	
Anguilla anguilla	Eel serum	Anti-H (-HI)	Fuc	
Cystisus sessifolius	Seed	Anti-H	GlcNAc*	
Laburnum alpinum	Seed	Anti-H	GlcNAc*	

*Probably requires terminal Fuc residue.

2.15.9.2 Anti-B

B-specific lectins are less abundant than A-specific lectins. They are found, together with anti-H, in the arils (seed coats) of various species of *Evonymus* [696,697], in the fungus *Fomes fomentarius* [698], and in the seaweed *Ptilota plumosa*. Anti-B activity is also found in the roe of various species of fish, especially those of the salmon and herring families [699–701]. These lectins are D-galactose specific and may also show some P, P1, and P^k specificity as a result of the galactosyl determinants common to these antigens [701,702].

2.15.9.3 Anti-A,B

Several seed extracts agglutinate A and B cells but not O cells. In some cases this may be because of one lectin cross-reacting with both A and B structures. BSI, one of at least three lectins in *Bandeiraea simplicifolia* seeds, comprises five isolectins made up of different proportions of two subunits. Both subunits have a high affinity for galactose but one of the subunits also binds strongly to N-acetylgalactosamine [703]. Both A and B activity of *Phlomis fructicosa* lectin was inhibited by N-acetylgalactosamine, whereas galactose only inhibited B activity [704]. If separate A- and B-specific molecules are found in these lectins, the notation anti-A,B is inappropriate, anti-A+B being more suitable.

2.15.9.4 Anti-H

Lectins in the seeds of common gorse (*Ulex europaeus*) were shown to behave as anti-H by Cazal and Lalaurie [705]. This is the most widely used and probably the best reagent for identifying secretor status from salivas of group O individuals. At least two lectins are present in *U. europaeus* seed extracts [706]: Ulex I is inhibited by L-fucose; Ulex II is not inhibited by L-fucose, but is inhibited by di-N-acetylchitobiose, a sugar with an N-acetylglucosaminyl residue [707]. Both *Ulex* I and II are H specific and both fail to react with group O red cells treated with α-L-fucosidase [708]. It seems likely that *Ulex* II reacts with subterminal N-acetylglucosamine in the H structure, but only in the presence of terminal L-fucose.

Other H specific lectins fall into two classes [686,709]:

1 those, like *Ulex* I, that are inhibited by L-fucose, e.g. *Lotus tetragonolobus* seeds and eel serum; and

2 those, like *Ulex* II, that are inhibited by N-acetylglucosamine derivatives, e.g. seeds of *Cystisus sessilifolius* and *Laburnum alpinum*.

Ulex I is more readily inhibited by oligosaccharides with Type 2 chains, including those with difucosyl structures, than those with Type 1 chains [658, 659,710,711]. *Lotus tetragonolobus* lectin is strongly specific for Type 2 chains and does not react with Type 1 chains [712], which explains why it is not a useful reagent for inhibition tests. *Ulex europaeus* seed extract has a similar reaction strength with either I-positive or I-negative (adult i) cells, but *L. tetragonolobus* lectin and eel serum lectin behave like anti-HI, with little activity for adult i or cord cells [659,713]. *Cystisus sessilifolius* and *Laburnum alpinum* lectins occupy an intermediate position, reacting with adult i cells less strongly than with I-positive cells [713].

Part 4: Lewis system

2.16 Le^a and Le^b antigens and phenotypes

The structure and biosynthesis of the Lewis antigens is described in Part 2 of this chapter. The details discussed here are mainly related to the serological expression of Lewis antigens, although some structural matters are addressed.

2.16.1 Red cells

A general rule applies to red cell Lewis phenotypes of white and black people. Adults with an *Le* gene are Le(a–b+) or Le(a+b–); if they are secretors of ABH their red cells are Le(a–b+); if non-secretors they are Le(a+b–). People homozygous for *le* have Le(a–b–) red cells (Table 2.25). There are, as might be expected, a number of exceptions to this rule. Many anti-Le^b, often referred to as anti-Le^{bH}, fail to agglutinate A$_1$ Le(a–b+) cells (see Section 2.18.2.1) and A$_1$ Le(a–b+) cells may be falsely typed as Le(a–b–). Red cells from fetuses, cord samples, and neonates are generally Le(a–b–). Infants may be transiently Le(a+b+) before becoming Le(a+b–). Lewis-positive women may be-

Table 2.25 Interaction of Lewis and secretor genes and the resulting red cell and secreted phenotypes (in group O individuals).

Genotype		Red cell phenotype	Antigens in secretions	
Lewis	Secretor		Le^a	Le^b
Le/Le or Le/le	Se/Se or Se/se	Le(a–b+)	+	+
Le/Le or Le/le	Se^w/Se^w or Se^w/se	Le(a+b+)	+	+
Le/Le or Le/le	se/se	Le(a+b–)	+	–
le/le	Any	Le(a–b–)	–	–

come transiently Le(a–b–) during pregnancy (Section 2.16.6).

Flow cytometry appears to be a more reliable method for determining Lewis phenotypes of red cells than conventional serological techniques. The following results were obtained with commercial anti-Le^b reagents on red cells of Europeans genotyped for *FUT2* and *FUT3*: A$_1$ Le(a–b+), 71% positive; B Le(a–b+), 95%; O and A$_2$ Le(a–b+), 99%; Le(a–b–), and Le(a+b–), <10% [714].

The red cell phenotype Le(a+b+), with both Le^a and Le^b strongly expressed, is very rare in European adults, but is common in East and South-East Asia, and in the Pacific region [54,175,176,251,715]. The explanation for this is the presence of a weak *Se* gene and the rarity of *se* (explained in Section 2.6.3). Some anti-Le^b reagents do not detect the Le^b of Le(a+b+) red cells by some techniques, which may have led to failure to recognize Le(a+b+) in some studies [23].

Some Le^a expression may be detected with selected anti-Le^a on the red cells of O or A$_2$ Le(a–b+) adults if sensitive enough techniques are used, such as an indirect antiglobulin test with enzyme-treated cells [573]. Le(a–b+) red cells were destroyed, *in vivo*, in a patient with potent anti-Le^a [716].

2.16.2 Secretions

Lewis antigens are easily and conveniently detected in human saliva by haemagglutination inhibition. Anti-Le^a is inhibited by saliva of individuals with Le(a+b–) or Le(a–b+) red cells, the former inhibiting more strongly than the latter [167,168,717]. Le^b is present in saliva of individuals with Le(a–b+) red cells [168,718]. Le^a and Le^b is present in saliva of people with Le(a+b+) red cells [175,715] (Table 2.25).

Lewis antigens have also been detected in, and isolated from, human milk [41,42], gastrointestinal juices [719,720], urine [719,721,722], seminal fluid [719,723], ovarian cyst fluid [9,10], and amniotic fluid [724].

2.16.3 Plasma

Le^a is easily detected in plasma of individuals with Le(a+b–) red cells [717]. Unlike saliva, only a trace of Le^a may be detected in plasma of people with Le(a–b+) red cells [725]. Le^b is present in plasma of individuals with Le(a–b+) red cells [725–727].

The site of synthesis of plasma Lewis substances is unknown. Recipients of transplants of bone marrow [728,729], kidney [721], or liver grafts [730] maintain their own red cell Lewis phenotypes, even though Lewis antigens of donor origin are detected in the urine of kidney recipients and in the bile of liver recipients [721,730]. In view of the very high levels of intestinal Le^a active glycolipids, Hanfland and Graham [658] suggested that plasma Lewis substances might originate from the intestine. Non-secretor patients with coeliac disease have reduced quantities of urinary Le^a antigen [722]. Evans *et al.* [722] proposed that Le^a in urine and plasma derives from large Le^a-active molecules in the small intestine, which are digested to smaller molecules and absorbed into the bloodstream. Some of these small molecules are subsequently excreted via the kidney. In coeliac disease these molecules cannot be absorbed by the intestine, resulting in reduced levels of Le^a substance in the urine. Following regeneration of the intestinal mucosa, normal quantities of urinary Le^a are detected. Furthermore, all of eight patients with intestinal failure, seven of whom had resection of the ileum and 80% of the jejunum, had Le(a–b–) red cells [731]. This is statistically significant from the 6% expected and provides further evidence that plasma, and consequently red cell, Lewis glycolipids are intestinally derived. Henry *et al.* [23] consider that other exocrine organs, such as liver, kidney, and pancreas, may contribute to Lewis-active plasma glycolipids, explaining the differences in plasma and intestinal glycolipid profiles.

Trace amounts of glycolipids with the Le^b structure have been identified in plasma from individuals with Le(a–b–) red cells, suggesting some $\alpha1,4$-fucosyltransferase activity [732,733]. This probably occurs either because the Lewis-fucosyltransferase encoded by an *le* allele is not completely inactive or because one of the $\alpha1,3$-fucosyltransferases, possibly the product of *FUT5*, has low level $\alpha1,4$-fucosyltransferase activity [733].

Enhanced quantity of sialylated-Le^a (sLe^a or CA 19-9) in plasma is associated with cancer of the pancreas and colon, and has been used to support diagnosis (see Section 2.20.4).

2.16.4 Uptake of Lewis antigens by red cells

Red cells do not synthesize carbohydrate chains with a Type 1 backbone and consequently cannot synthesize Lewis antigens. Plasma lipids exchange slowly but freely with lipids in the red cell membrane; the composition of phospholipids and fatty acids in red cell membranes resembles that in plasma [734]. Consequently, plasma glycosphingolipids bearing Lewis structures become incorporated into the red cell membrane [52].

Sneath and Sneath [725] first recognized that Le(a–b–) red cells acquire Le^a and Le^b antigens during incubation in plasma from Le(a+b–) and Le(a–b+) individuals, respectively, and that Le(a+b–) and Le(a–b+) red cells lose their Lewis antigens during incubation in Le(a–b–) plasma. These experiments were carried out with one volume of packed red cells shaken continuously in 10 volumes of plasma at 35°C for at least 3 days, with the plasma being changed daily. Le^a antigen cannot be removed from Le(a+) red cells simply by repeated washing of the cells [716].

Group O red cells transfused into an A_1 Le(b+) recipient were not agglutinated by anti-A_1Le^b on the first and second days post-transfusion, but were weakly agglutinated on days 4 and 5, and were strongly agglutinated on day 6 [735]. Two days after transfusion of Le(b+) cells to an Le(a–b–) patient, the transfused cells still reacted strongly with anti-Le^b, but after 7 days the transfused cells gave a scarcely detectable reaction with anti-Le^b [736].

Marcus and Cass [52] isolated glycosphingolipids from plasma and found that this preparation was extremely effective at converting Le(b–) red cells to Le(b+); only 5-min incubation at 37°C made Le(b–) cells agglutinable with anti-Le^b. Group O Le(a–b–) red cells exposed to glycosphingolipid fractions prepared from plasma of A_1 Le(a–b+) donors were agglutinated by anti-A_1Le^b [278]. These glycosphingolipids, once adsorbed, could not be washed off with saline. About one-third of the total Le^b-active glycolipid in whole blood is associated with the red cells, the rest being found in the plasma [737]. Lewis antigens in saliva are glycoproteins and cannot be adsorbed onto red cells, despite being far more effective than plasma in inhibiting haemagglutination by Lewis antibodies [727].

Twin chimeras have permanent bone marrow grafts derived from their twin *in utero*. Their peripheral red cell population is often a mixture of their own cells and those of their twin, yet, unlike other blood groups, the chimera's own genes determine the Lewis phenotype of both populations of red cells, further proof that Lewis antigens are not haemopoietic in origin. In one chimeric twin, a secretor of H, all her red cells were Le(a–b+), despite half of her cells being derived from her non-secretor brother; all the red cells of her non-secretor brother were Le(a+b–), including those from his secretor sister [738].

A_1Le^b can only be produced by individuals with *Le*, *Se*, and *A^1* genes. Group A_1 red cells produced by grafted tissue in a group O secretor host are not agglutinated by anti-A_1Le^b, even though they carry both A_1 and Le^b antigens, because the A_1 originates from the graft and the Le^b originates from the host [330,735,739]. A chimeric twin reported by Crookston *et al.* [735] made anti-A_1Le^b even though 50% of her red cells were A_1 Le(b+). The antibody reacted with none of her own red cells, but did react with all of those of her chimeric twin brother, a secretor of A and H. Recipients of successful bone marrow transplants acquire the blood groups of the donor with the exception of Lewis, which remains that of the recipient [728,729].

2.16.5 Development of Lewis antigens

Le^a and Le^b cannot usually be detected on cord red cell samples by direct agglutination [13]. When more sensitive serological techniques are used, such as an indirect antiglobulin test or agglutination of enzyme-treated cells with potent antibodies, traces of Le^a and possibly Le^b may be detected on some cord or fetal red cells [716].

Lewis antigens start to appear on red cells soon after birth [740]. Le^a develops first; red cells of infants with an *Le* gene generally become Le(a+) during the first few months of life. In white people, at 3 months of age 80% of infants are Le(a+), this number dropping to the adult level of 20% by 2 years [741–743]. During this period the red cell phenotype Le(a+b+) is not uncommon [743,744]. By 6 years of age the proportion of Le(b+) reaches the adult level [743].

Appearance of Le^a and Le^b in the plasma of infants correlates with the appearance of those antigens on the red cells [744] and cord red cells can be made Le(b+) by incubation in plasma from an Le(b+) adult [727]. At the source of production of plasma Lewis substances in infants with an *Se* gene, the Le-fucosyltransferase becomes active before the *Se* gene specified fucosyltransferase, resulting in the appearance of Le^a in the plasma before Le^b.

In Chinese, 50% of cord samples were found to be Le(a–b+) and 50% Le(a–b–) [732]. The Le(a–b+) cells became Le(a+b+) before reverting to Le(a–b+); the Le(a–b–) cells either became Le(a+b+) and maintained that phenotype or remained Le(a–b–).

Lewis antigens in the saliva of neonates with an *Le* gene are the same as those detected in adult salivas: ABH secretors have Le^a and Le^b in their saliva; ABH non-secretors have only Le^a [744]. Lewis substances found in amniotic fluid obtained by amniocentesis corresponded to the Lewis and secretor phenotypes of the fetus and were present as early as 15 weeks' gestation [724].

2.16.6 Lewis antigens during pregnancy

Agglutinability of red cells with anti-Le^a or anti-Le^b may be reduced during pregnancy [745–748] and pregnant women with a transient Le(a–b–) phenotype may produce Lewis antibodies [607]. A woman in the seventh month of pregnancy had powerful anti-Le^b in her serum, yet 3 months after delivery no antibody was detectable and her red cells were Le(a–b+) [607].

Hammar *et al.* [748] found that the frequency of the Le(a–b–) red cell phenotype was 11% (8 of 73) in non-pregnant women, but 36% (27 of 74) in women at time of delivery. Those women who were A$_1$ most often became Le(b–) during pregnancy. The change in

Lewis phenotype occurred as early as the 24th week of the pregnancy and Le^b antigen was detectable again 6 weeks after delivery. The concentration of Le^b glycolipid in plasma decreased only slightly during pregnancy, so, unlike the situation in infants, changes in Le^b red cell expression during pregnancy do not appear to result directly from the quantity of Le^b in the plasma. Hammar *et al.* [748] suggest that, as a result of the increased concentration of plasma lipoprotein that occurs during pregnancy, more Lewis determinants become attached to plasma lipoproteins and consequently less are available to become bound to the red cell surface. Levels of Le^b-active oligosaccharides secreted in the urine of Le(a–b+) women increases during pregnancy and lactation [747].

2.17 Antigen, phenotype, and gene frequencies

2.17.1 Red cells

Based on 1796 tests on red cells, the frequency of Le^a in England was found to be 22.38% [749]. This frequency is very similar to that found in other European countries [251,749] and in white Americans [750,751]. Table 2.26 shows phenotype frequencies for Europeans and white Americans obtained from tests with anti-Le^a and -Le^b on O and A$_2$ cells. The frequency of the *Le* gene varies from 0.67 to 0.80 in white populations.

Two studies on African Americans revealed higher frequencies for the Le(a–b–) phenotype (Table 2.26) [726,751], giving a frequency of 0.46–0.53 for *Le*. The incidence of Le(a–b–) was as high as 35% in West

Table 2.26 Frequencies of Lewis phenotypes in three populations.

Phenotype	Europeans and white Americans	African Americans	Hong Kong Chinese
Le(a–b+)	70–72	52–55	62
Le(a+b–)	19–22	19–23	0
Le(a+b+)	0	0	27
Le(a–b–)	4–11	22–29	11
Reference	[168,750–752]	[726,751]	[753]

Africans ($Le=0.59$), with 15% Le(a+) (only O and A_2 tested [754]).

The Le(a+b+) red cell phenotype, rare in European and African people, is relatively common in East Asia, South-East Asia, the Pacific region, and Australasia [251]. Le(a+b+) has an incidence of 27% in Hong Kong Chinese [753] (Table 2.26), 16–25% Taiwan Chinese [715], 10–40% of Polynesians [755], and 10% in Australian Aborigines [756]. Le(a+b–) is rare or absent in Chinese [715,753,757].

Frequencies of Lewis genes derived from DNA analysis are shown in Table 2.10.

2.17.2 Secretions

Frequency of the *Le* gene can be determined by inhibition tests, using saliva to inhibit agglutination of Le(a+b–) red cells by anti-Le^a. Salivas of individuals with an *Le* gene contain Le^a; those of *le/le* individuals do not. From saliva tests the following estimates of *Le* gene frequency have been obtained: 0.82 in English; 0.69 in Swedes; about 0.45 in Africans; 0.70 in Australian Aborigines; and 0.36–0.57 in native South Americans [168,224,251,252]. These are similar frequencies to those determined by red cell testing.

2.18 Lewis antibodies

2.18.1 Anti-Le^a

2.18.1.1 Human anti-Le^a

Anti-Le^a is not uncommon; haemagglutination tests in Denmark [758] and France [759] revealed anti-Le^a in about 1 in every 300 sera. Agglutinating alloanti-Le^a is only found in people with Le(a–b–) red cells [224,726], possibly only those who are ABH secretors [726], and less often in group O individuals than in people of other ABO groups [758].

Le^a antibodies are usually 'naturally occurring' and predominantly IgM [573]. Very rarely is anti-Le^a purely IgG [573,760]. Most potent anti-Le^a sera contain an IgG component detectable by radioimmunoassay or enzyme-linked immunoadsorbent assay [760–762], but seldom detectable by an antiglobulin test with anti-IgG [573].

Anti-Le^a usually cross-react with Le^b oligosaccharide and will sometimes react with the Lewis disaccharide Fucα1→4GlcNAc or with Le^x, the Type 2 isomer

of Le^a (Table 2.3) [763]. IgM anti-Le^a have broader specificity for synthetic oligosaccharides than IgG anti-Le^a [764].

Despite the common occurrence of anti-Le^a, human antibodies potent enough to be useful as reagents are rare. As most sera containing anti-Le^a either contain weak anti-Le^b or cross-react with Le^b, methods of enhancing reactivity may lead to 'false positive' reactions with Le(a–b+) cells. Agglutination of red cells with anti-Le^a is generally strongest at low temperatures, often not occurring at all at 37°C. Anti-Le^a usually fix complement [765,766]; a two-stage complement-addition antiglobulin test is often a successful way of detecting anti-Le^a. Some Le^a antibodies lyse Le(a+) cells in the presence of complement. Another method for increasing the strength of reaction with anti-Le^a is to use protease-treated cells.

Some anti-Le^a are lymphocytotoxic [767,768].

2.18.1.2 Monoclonal anti-Le^a

Numerous murine monoclonal anti-Le^a have been produced [652–654,769–772]; some make excellent blood grouping reagents [771] and commercially produced monoclonal anti-Le^a are generally used.

Of the four monoclonal anti-Le^a described by Young *et al.* [769], one detected the Le^a trisaccharide Galβ1→3(Fucα1→4)GlcNAc, another the tetrasaccharide Galβ1→3(Fucα1→4)GlcNAcβ1→3Gal, and two were directed mainly towards the disaccharide Fucα1→4GlcNAc. All monoclonal anti-Le^a cross-react with the Type 1 precursor Galβ1→3GlcNAc (Le^c) [773]. Some monoclonal anti-Le^a cross-react with the T disaccharide Galβ1→3GalNAc and agglutinate Le(a–) T-activated red cells [774] (see Chapter 31).

2.18.2 Anti-Le^b

2.18.2.1 Human anti-Le^b

The original anti-Le^b, described by Andresen [13], only reacted specifically with group O Le(b+) or A_2 Le(b+) red cells, whereas the anti-Le^b reported by Brendemoen [718] reacted with all Le(b+) red cells. The two types of Le^b antibodies were named anti-Le^{bH} and anti-Le^{bL} by Ceppellini *et al.* [775].

Anti-Le^{bH}, which cross-reacts with H, can only be used reliably to type O or A_2 cells as it often fails to agglutinate A_1 or B, Le(a–b+) cells. Anti-Le^{bH} is inhibited by saliva from all ABH secretors regardless of whether their red cells are Le(a–b+) or Le(a–b–).

Anti-Le^{bL} agglutinates Le(b+) red cells regardless of ABO group. It is only inhibited by salivas of ABH secretors who also secrete Le^a; i.e. not those who have Le(a–b–) red cells. Only anti-Le^{bL} are suitable as anti-Le^b blood grouping reagents.

Like anti-Le^a, anti-Le^b are found most often in people with Le(a–b–) red cells; unlike anti-Le^a, these people are generally non-secretors of ABH [726]. However, there are reports of group A_1 or A_1B Le(a+b–) people who have made anti-Le^b of the anti-Le^{bH} type [718,776]. Compared with anti-Le^a, anti-Le^b is a relatively infrequent antibody. In tests on the sera of 72 000 Parisians, Salmon and Cartron [759] found 259 anti-Le^a, 29 anti-Le^{bH}, and only 2 anti-Le^{bL}.

Anti-Le^b show many of the serological characteristics described for anti-Le^a above. Anti-Le^b are generally IgM [573]. François et al. [763] tested 14 anti-Le^b sera with synthetic oligosaccharides: four cross-reacted with Le^a trisaccharide; seven cross-reacted with Le^y tetrasaccharide (the Type 2 isomer of Le^b), four of these also reacting with H trisaccharide (see Table 2.3).

Some anti-Le^b are lymphocytotoxic [718,777].

2.18.2.2 Animal anti-Le^b, polyclonal and monoclonal

Polyclonal anti-Le^b made in goats immunized with salivary blood group substances agglutinated Le(a–b+) cells of all ABO groups, but after adsorption with A_1 or B, Le(a–b+) cells only agglutinated O or A_2, Le(a–b+) cells [281]. The goat appeared to have made two separable antibodies: anti-Le^{bL} and anti-Le^{bH}.

Many monoclonal anti-Le^b have been produced, some anti-Le^{bL}, some anti-Le^{bH}, and some giving intermediate reactions (anti-Le^{bH,L}) [652–654,773,778, 779]. All anti-Le^{bL} and -Le^{bH,L} cross-react with Le^a; all anti-Le^{bH} and anti-Le^{bH,L} cross-react with Type 1 H (Le^d) and Le^y [773]. Despite these cross-reactivities, when the appropriate methods are adopted some monoclonal anti-Le^b make excellent blood grouping reagents.

2.18.3 Anti-ALe^b

Anti-A_1Le^b, an antibody that reacts only with the red cells of A_1 Lewis-positive secretors [A_1 Le(a–b+)], was first found in the serum of a group A_1B Le(a–b–) man [780]. Other examples have been described since [735,781]. Anti-ALe^b may be lymphocytotoxic [768]. Monoclonal anti-ALe^b may or may not cross-react with ALe^y, the Type 2 isomer [643,644].

Anti-BLe^b has not been reported.

2.18.4 Clinical significance of Lewis antibodies

Despite being relatively common antibodies, only a few examples of haemolytic transfusion reactions have been attributed to anti-Le^a [782–785], and even less to anti-Le^b [786–789]. This is probably because most Lewis antibodies are not active at 37°C, because Lewis antigens in the donor's plasma neutralize the recipient's Lewis antibodies, and because Le^a or Le^b antigens elute from red cells transfused into an Le(a–b–) recipient.

Lewis antibodies that are only active in vitro at temperatures below 37°C do not cause increased clearance of antigen-positive transfused red cells in vivo [573,607,790]. Consequently, patients with Lewis antibodies may be transfused with red cells that are crossmatch-compatible at 37°C. However, it is claimed that Lewis antibodies in South-East Asia are significantly more potent than in Europe and cause severe haemolytic transfusion reactions (D. Chandanayingyong, unpublished observations cited in [573]).

Lewis antibodies do not cause serious haemolytic disease of the newborn, presumably because Lewis antigens are present in fetal secretions, but generally not on fetal red cells. There are two recorded cases in which Lewis antibodies, one anti-Le^a [791] and one anti-Le^b [792], have been implicated in mild symptoms of HDN; in each the antibodies were IgG, active at 37°C, and could be eluted from the baby's direct antiglobulin test (DAT)-positive red cells.

2.18.5 Lewis antibodies and renal transplantation

Kidney cells biosynthesize Lewis antigens [721]. The role of cytotoxic Lewis antibodies in kidney graft survival is controversial. In 1978, from a retrospective study of 255 kidney transplant recipients, Oriol et al. [793] found that 2-year graft survival rates were significantly lower in Le(a–b–) recipients than in Le-positive recipients, leading to the proposal that antigens of the Lewis system represented histocompatability antigens in renal transplantation. This was supported by other retrospective studies [794–796] and by a prospective study [797] in which Lewis-identical donor–recipient pairs were shown to have better graft survival than Lewis-incompatible pairs. Further support came from individual cases in which Lewis antibodies were implicated as the possible cause of renal transplant rejection [798]. Spitalnik *et al.* [799], by their highly sensitive kinetic enzyme-linked immunosorbent assay, revealed the presence of anti-Le^a in all of eight Le(a–b–) patients with failed renal grafts, but not in the single Le(a–b–) recipient of an Le(a–b–) graft. Most of these antibodies could not be detected by haemagglutination. In two other prospective studies and one retrospective study [800–802], however, no significant difference in survival between Lewis-matched and Lewis-mismatched donor–recipient pairs was detected, although Le(a–b–) patients appeared to be at higher risk of graft failure when receiving HLA mismatched kidneys. These data led to the recommendation that kidneys should not be selected for engraftment on the basis of Lewis phenotype [801].

Anti-Le^a, presumably of graft origin, has been blamed for renal failure in bone marrow transplant recipients [729,803]. Autoanti-Le^{bH} in an Le(a–b+) patient who had received two kidney transplants that had both been rapidly rejected, agglutinated the patient's own red cells and was inhibited by his own saliva [798,804].

2.19 Other antigens associated with Lewis

2.19.1 Le^{abx}, the antigen originally called Le^x

An antigen named Le^x by Andresen and Jordal [743,805,806], present on Le(a+b–) and Le(a–b+) cells, but not Le(a–b–) cells, differs from inseparable anti-Le^{ab} because it reacts with 90% of umbilical cord red cell samples, despite cord red cells being Le(a–b–). These 90% are from infants with an *Le* gene, soon to develop red cell Le^a or Le^b [807]. As the symbol 'Le^x' is now commonly used for the monofucosyl Type 2 isomer of the Le^a trisaccharide CD15 (Section 2.19.3), the antigen originally called Le^x will be referred to as Le^{abx}.

Anti-Le^{abx} reacts equally strongly with A$_1$, A$_2$, and O, Le(abx+) cells [805,806]. Anti-Le^{abx} is inhibited by

saliva, amniotic fluid, and serum from Lewis-positive individuals [807].

Le^{abx} antibodies appear to be heterogeneous: some detect the Lewis disaccharide, Fucα1→4GlcNAc, and some detect larger determinants common to Le^a and Le^b [763,808,809]. These determinants must be more accessible on cord cells to anti-Le^{abx} than to anti-Le^a.

2.19.2 Le^c and Le^d

Le^c and Le^d are antigens on Le(a–b–) red cells from ABH non-secretor adults and ABH secretor adults, respectively. The symbols Le^c and Le^d are somewhat inappropriate as neither structure is produced by a Lewis gene-specified transferase, and Le^d is now known to be Type 1 H.

Like Le^a and Le^b, Le^c and Le^d are not intrinsic to the red cell but are incorporated into the red cell membrane from the plasma [810].

The phenotype Le(a–b–c–d–) is extremely rare and is associated with a deficiency of an α1,3-fucosyltransferase [811].

2.19.2.1 Le^d or Type 1 H (210002)

As a result of immunizing a goat with saliva from an Le(a–b+) person and adsorbing the serum with Le(a+b–) cells, Potapov [812] identified two antibodies: anti-Le^b and a new antibody, which agglutinated Le(a–b–) red cells from ABH secretors, but not those from non-secretors. He called this second antibody anti-Le^d, leaving anti-Le^c for the predicted antibody that would react with Le(a–b–) cells from non-secretors. Potapov proposed the following four Lewis phenotypes and corresponding genotypes:

Le(a+b–c–d–)	*Le/Le* or *Le/le*	*se/se*
Le(a–b+c–d–)	*Le/Le* or *Le/le*	*Se/Se* or *Se/se*
Le(a–b–c+d–)	*le/le*	*se/se*
Le(a–b–c–d+)	*le/le*	*Se/Se* or *Se/se*.

Two years later human anti-Le^c was identified [813].

Le^d and Type 1 H are synonymous. Anti-Le^d reacts with oligosaccharides containing the Type 1 H determinant, but not the Type 2 H determinant (Table 2.3) and Type 1 H active glycosphingolipids isolated from plasma of O Le(a–b–) secretors inhibited goat anti-Le^d [658]. Anti-Le^d, produced by immunizing rabbits with synthetic Type 1 H oligosaccharide, reacted with tissues of Le(a–b–) secretors [814].

Type 1 H in the plasma of Le(a–b–) ABH secretors

does not get converted to Le^b and so plenty is available to become adsorbed onto the red cell in detectable levels, giving rise to the Le(a–b–c–d+) red cell phenotype. Le^d in group A and B individuals is carried on Type 1 A (ALe^d) and Type 1 B (BLe^d), respectively (see Table 2.3).

Monoclonal anti-Type 1 A (anti-ALe^d) has been used in a biochemical analysis of red cell glycolipids [642]. Lymphocytotoxic murine monoclonal anti-A$_1$Le^d did not agglutinate red cells, but lysed A$_1$ Le(d+) red cells after addition of rabbit complement [641].

Antibodies that react with red cells of O and A$_2$ Le(a–b–) secretors, but not with those of A$_1$ Le(a–b–) secretors have been called anti-Le^{dH} [281].

2.19.2.2 Le^c (210001)

In 1957, Iseki et al. [815,816] produced a weak antibody by injecting a rabbit with Le(a–b–) secretor saliva. This antibody, which they called anti-Le^c, reacted with Le(a–b–) cells from secretors and non-secretors and so may have represented anti-Le^c+Le^d in the later notation [812]. Anti-Le^c of the type predicted by Potapov [812], an antibody that only reacts with red cells of Le(a–b–) non-secretors, was described by Gunson and Latham [813] in 1972. The antibody was found during the fourth pregnancy of an O Le(a–b+) woman (ARM), a secretor of H, Le^a, and Le^b. A second example of human anti-Le^c was found in a group A Le(a–b+) man who had never been transfused [817]. Other examples of anti-Le^c have subsequently been raised in goats by injection of Le(a–b–) non-secretor saliva and adsorption of the immune serum with Le(c–) red cells [281,818,819].

The structure of Le^c is less clearly defined than that of Le^d. Graham et al. [281] suggested that Le^c could represent the non-fucosylated Type 1 chain Galβ1→3GlcNAc, the precursor of Le^a and Type 1 H, unmodified by Le- or Se-fucosyltransferases. Further evidence that the Le^c determinant contains this disaccharide was provided when antibodies with anti-Le^c specificity were raised in rabbits immunized with Galβ1→3GlcNAc [819]. Furthermore, antibodies raised in goats immunized with Le(a–b–) non-secretor salivas and affinity-purified with Galβ1→3GlcNAc adsorbents behaved as anti-Le^c [819]. Hanfland et al. [820] found that the glycosphingolipid fractions isolated from O Le(a–b–) non-secretor plasma that were most effective at inhibiting anti-Le^c of either

human or goat origin carried a branched oligosaccharide chain, one branch containing Type 1 precursor Galβ1→3GlcNAc, the other a monofucosylated Type 2 structure. They concluded that unsubstituted Type 1 chain alone does not represent Le^c, although it does play a part. Further evidence that a monofucosylated Type 2 structure is an essential part of the Le^c determinant is provided by the very rare Le(a–b–c–d–) phenotype, which has only been found in two individuals, both with α1,3-fucosyltransferase-deficiency [811].

It is likely that anti-Le^c represents a heterogeneous group of antibodies that determine different structures abundant in the plasma of individuals who lack both Le and Se genes and which are incorporated into the red cell membrane.

2.19.3 Le^x, Le^y, and sialyl-Le^x

Le^x (CD15) and Le^y, the Type 2 isomers of Le^a and Le^b, are not really blood group antigens as they are not detectable on red cells [48]. Their structure and biosynthesis have been described in Part 2 of this chapter, and they are discussed briefly here because of their biochemical relationship to ABH and Lewis antigens (Table 2.3). Like Le^b and Le^d, the presence or absence of Le^y in secretions is principally dependent on genes at the secretor locus. Le^x differs from the Le^{abx} antigen discussed in Section 2.19.1.

Human alloantibodies to the Le^x and Le^y determinants have not been found, although some anti-Le^a cross-react with Le^x and some anti-Le^b cross-react with Le^y [763]. Murine monoclonal antibodies to the Le^x, Le^y, and ALe^y determinants have been described [47,59,642,643,821].

Sialyl-Le^x (sLe^x, CD15s), the sialylated derivative of Le^x antigen, and, to a lesser extent, sialyl-Le^a, function as ligands for the lectin-like N-terminal domains of selectins, a family of cell adhesion molecules on endothelium (E-selectin), leucocytes (L-selectin), and platelets (P-selectin) (reviews in [19,208–210]). Attachment of selectins to their carbohydrate ligands is important in the binding of leucocytes and platelets to endothelium, particularly at the region of inflammation.

Part 5 Tissue distribution, disease associations, and functional aspects

2.20 Expression of ABH and Lewis antigens on other blood cells and in other tissues

2.20.1 Leucocytes

A, B, and H antigens may be detected on lymphocytes, but they are acquired from the plasma and their expression is therefore under the control of the secretor (*FUT2*) locus [728,822–825]. Cytotoxic anti-A react with lymphocytes from A secretors, but not with lymphocytes from A non-secretors; the strongest reactors are lymphocytes from A Le(a–b–) secretors [823]. The same antibodies reacted with group O lymphocytes exposed to a glycosphingolipid fraction prepared from plasma of A Le(a–b–) secretors. Lymphocytes cultured in serum from A or B individuals acquired A or B antigens [768]. Following bone marrow transplantation, lymphocytes from group O donors may acquire A or B antigens from the recipient's plasma [728]. All the lymphocytes in a chimera with *A¹* and *Se* genes were equally susceptible to lysis by a lymphocytotoxic anti-A, yet half of them derived from the *O/O* twin brother [822]. Lymphocytes do not contain α1,2-fucosyltransferase [109,826] and previous reports [197,198] of α1,2-fucosyltransferase activity in lymphocytes was probably caused by platelet contamination. Like red cells, lymphocytes adsorb Lewis antigens from the plasma [768].

Granulocytes and monocytes do not express ABH or Lewis antigens regardless of secretor phenotype [825,827–829]. No α1,2-fucosyltransferase activity was detected in granulocytes or monocytes [109,198]. Granulocytes, monocytes, and lymphocytes do, however, have α1,3-fucosyltransferase activity [109] and express Le^x and sialyl-Le^x on their surface; determinants that function as ligands for selectins, a family of cell adhesion molecules [208–210].

2.20.2 Platelets

ABH antigens are present on platelets and megakaryocytes [826,830–832]. Type 1 ABH structures are adsorbed onto platelets from the plasma and are dependent on secretor phenotype; Type 2 structures are intrinsic and under control of the *H* (*FUT1*)

gene [826]. Platelet ABH antigens are expressed on glycolipids and on the platelet glycoproteins (GP) Ib, IIa, IIb, IIIa, IV, V, CD31 (PECAM), and CD109 [826,833–838]. Platelets from A_2 people carry very little A antigen [838]. Platelets contain H-, A-, and B-transferases [197] and release of α1,2-fucosyltransferase during clotting may represent a major source of this enzyme in plasma [109,551]. Unlike leucocytes, platelets do not contain α1,3-fucosyltransferase [109].

Le^a antigen, assimilated into the membrane from the plasma, can be detected on platelets [839].

ABO incompatibility may result in impaired efficacy of platelet transfusion in a minority of patients with high titred, IgG anti-A or -B, and in patients requiring long-term support [833,840–842]. Around 4–7% of A_1 and B Japanese and white Americans have high levels of expression of platelet A and B antigens [834, 843]; 2% of the A_1 Americans had seven times the normal level of platelet A antigen [843]. This inherited quantitative variation of platelet A and B antigens may affect platelet refractoriness caused by anti-A or -B.

2.20.3 Other tissues

ABH and Lewis antigens are widely distributed in the human body and should be called histo-blood group antigens [14]. There is a vast literature on this subject (reviews in [14,17,21,844]).

A scheme devised by Oriol [21] to summarize the genetic control of ABH and related antigens in various tissues is shown in Fig. 2.12. Although a few exceptions exist, the following general rules prevail.

1 In tissues derived from ectoderm and mesoderm, ABH antigens are under the control of the *H* (*FUT1*) locus. Type 2 ABH structures are expressed, often together with Le^x and/or Le^y antigens. In addition to haemopoietic tissue, these tissues include skin, primary sensory neurones, vascular endothelium, and renal glomeruli and convoluted tubules.

2 In tissues of endodermal origin—such as digestive and respiratory mucosae and renal urinary epithelium—ABH, Lewis, and Lewis-related structures may be Type 1 or 2 and are primarily controlled by the Secretor (*FUT2*) and Lewis (*FUT3*) loci.

Exceptions to these rules include some deep areas of digestive mucosa where, despite being of endodermal origin, histo-blood group antigens are independent of the secretor and Lewis genes; and parts of the mam-

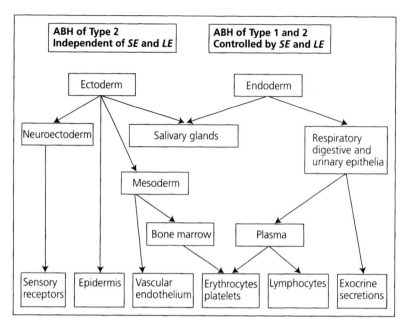

| ABH of Type 2 Independent of *SE* and *LE* | ABH of Type 1 and 2 Controlled by *SE* and *LE* |

Fig. 2.12 Scheme devised by Oriol [21] to demonstrate the genetic control of ABH and related antigens in human tissues derived from ectoderm, mesoderm, and endoderm. Some exceptions to this model are described in the text.

mary and sweat glands (tissues of ectodermal origin), where ABH and Lewis antigens are governed by the secretor and Lewis genes.

Ravn and Dabelsteen [844] have devised an alternative scheme, in which it is the process of differentiation of epithelial cells, rather than embryonic origin, that determines whether H antigens are controlled by *FUT1* or *FUT2*.

Le^a and Le^b have been detected, immunochemically and by structural analyses, in small intestine and colon of individuals with Le(a–b–) red cells and whose saliva contains no Le-transferase [845–847] (see Section 2.16.3 for a possible explanation).

2.20.4 Tumours

Kay and Wallace [848] first noticed that ABH antigens are sometimes absent from malignant tissue despite being present in the surrounding epithelium. Davidsohn [849] recognized the potential prognostic application of the loss of ABH antigen expression from some tumour cells. He became aware, from a study of many cases of carcinoma of the uterine cervix, lung, pancreas, and stomach, that, with very few exceptions, loss of ABH antigens preceded formation of distant metastases and hence a poor prognosis. In contrast, Nakagoe *et al.* [850] found that retention of tumour ABH antigens was associated with poor prog-

nosis in colorectal cancer. The changes in ABH and Lewis antigens associated with a variety of different cancers are reviewed by Le Pendu *et al.* [851].

The nature of altered ABH, Lewis, and related histo-blood group antigens has been studied by the use of monoclonal antibodies and by transferase analysis [14,17,18]. Loss of A or B antigens is generally caused by a disappearance of A- or B-transferase activity and results in an accumulation of H, Le^b, or Le^y. This may play a part in metastasis by affecting tumour cell interactions with cell adhesion molecules [18]. Loss of A and B antigens from malignant bladder tumours results from down-regulated transcription of the *ABO* gene, as neither *A* nor *B* mRNA can be detected in high-grade tumours [485]. Comparing A+ and A– clones derived from the same parental colonic cancer cells lines, in the clone that had lost A activity the enhancing activity of the 43 bp tandem repeat unit in the promoter region of *ABO* was reduced and there was enhanced CpG methylation of the promoter region [852] (see Section 2.3.2.2).

Type 1 and 2 ABH structures and Le^b, Le^x, and Le^y antigens are present on fetal distal colon; they are not present in healthy adult distal colon, but are often re-expressed in adults in carcinoma of the distal colon [853]. Ørntoft *et al.* [854] have shown that malignancy in the distal colon is associated with increased activity of α1,2-fucosyltransferase of H and Se types.

They conclude that α1,2-fucosyltransferases control, at least partially, oncodevelopmental expression of ABH and related antigens in colon.

Up-regulation of glycosyltransferases in tumours may result in increased levels of certain carbohydrate structures in the plasma [855]. The quantity of circulating sialylated-Le^a (sLe^a), otherwise known as the CA 19-9 antigen, is widely used as a marker to support diagnosis of colorectal, pancreatic, and gastric cancer, and as an aid to prognosis after potential curative surgery [49,856,857]. CA 19-9 levels vary according to Lewis and secretor genotypes, complicating cancer diagnosis; Le(a–b–) (le/le) individuals have no circulating CA 19-9 [857]. A marker for cancerous regions of colon of Le(a–b–) patients is sialyl-Le^c (DU-PAN-2), a precursor of sialyl-Le^a [857].

Another phenomenon associated with malignancy is the incompatible A antigen, occasionally expressed on tumours of group O or B people [858]. About 10% of colonic tumours from group O patients, shown to be homozygous for the O^1 allele, express A antigen and contain active A-transferase activity [859,860]. The molecular basis of this O to A conversion is not known, but Yamamoto et al. [124] pointed out that alternative splicing of ABO RNA, resulting in loss of exons 5 and 6, would introduce no frameshift or translation-termination codons. The putative gene product would be a truncated glycosyltransferase lacking the G261 nucleotide deletion, characteristic of the O^1 allele, and with a potential for A-transferase activity (see Section 2.3.2.2). It is feasible that the known higher incidence of gastric and ovarian adenocarcinomas in group A people [861] may be caused by a suppression of development of tumours bearing an A antigen by the anti-A naturally present in group O and B people.

2.21 Associations with disease

Some examples of associations between ABO group and disease have already been mentioned, notably haemolytic disease of the newborn (Section 2.15.3), leukaemia (Section 2.14.2), cancer (Section 2.20.4), acquired B resulting from bacterial infection (Section 2.14.1), and leucocyte adhesion deficiency type II (Section 2.13.5.2). A plethora of other associations between ABO and diseases has been reported, mostly based on observed ABO phenotype frequency discrepancies between patients with the disease and the healthy population (reviews in [24,861,862]). Susceptibility to infection by numerous pathogenic microorganisms is associated with ABO phenotype or secretor status [24]. In the concluding remarks of a very thorough review on ABO polymorphisms and their relationship with disease, Henry and Samuelsson [24] summarize as follows: 'There is tendency for bacterial infections to attack persons of group A, while virus infections tend, in a very general way, to be associated with group O. Cancers are mostly associated with group A, as are clotting diseases, while autoimmune diseases and bleeding are associated with O.'

Lewis antigens may act as receptors for several pathogenic bacteria [72,863]. Most attention has focused on *Helicobacter pylori*, a Gram-negative bacterium present in over 50% of the population and associated with development of gastritis, gastric and duodenal ulcers, and adenocarcinoma [864]. In 1993, Borén et al. [865] provided evidence that Le^b mediates attachment of certain strains of *H. pylori* to gastric mucosa cells. Bacterial binding to gastric mucosa cells was abolished by the presence of Le^b-active soluble glycoproteins and by Le^b-specific monoclonal antibodies. Gastric mucosa cells expressing Le^b bound *H. pylori* P466, whereas cells lacking Le^b did not. Type 1 H also mediated *H. pylori* attachment, but to a much lesser degree. As Le^a, ALe^b, and BLe^b did not bind the bacteria, this could explain why group O individuals have an increased probability of developing gastric and duodenal ulcers [866], but not why non-secretors run a substantially increased risk of developing duodenal ulcers [867]. Although some studies have shown no association of blood group and secretor status with occurrence of *H. pylori* or with the lymphomas closely associated with *H. pylori* infestation [868], Alkout et al. [869] found, by different techniques, that Type 2 H, Le^a, and Le^b bind *H. pylori*, and propose that Type 2 H is the key receptor. This would explain increased susceptibility to peptic ulcers in group O people. Furthermore, if Le^b in mucus competes more effectively than Le^a for the adhesin, this would reduce density of colonization among secretors and explain the increased risk of ulceration in non-secretors.

The O-antigen of lipopolysaccharides in most strains of *H. pylori* express Le^x, sialyl-Le^x, Le^y, Type 1 H, Le^a, Le^b, and A (review in [870]). These antigens undergo phase variation, the random, reversible high-frequency switching of phenotype. Le^x on *H. pylori* mediates adhesion to gastric epithelial cells and is essential for colonization. In contrast to previous suggestions, molecular mimicry between *H. pylori* and host glycoconjugates does not appear to play a significant part in host evasion or autoimmunity [870].

Fucosidosis is a rare lysosomal storage disease with an autosomally recessive mode of inheritance, often fatal within the first 5 years of life. It is characterized by an accumulation of fucosylated glycolipids and glycoproteins in neural and visceral tissues, as a result of an α-L-fucosidase deficiency resulting from inactivating mutations. Fucosidosis leads to mental and motor deterioration [871,872]. Fucosidosis patients may have enhanced expression of Lewis antigens on their red cells and in their saliva [873–875]. Two siblings with fucosidosis, described by Kousseff *et al.* [874], were both H secretors and yet had Le(a+b+) red cells, with very high levels of red cell and salivary Le^a and Le^b expression. Both patients had normal H activity, suggesting that the deficient fucosidase is specific for the α1→4 linkage to *N*-acetylglucosamine found in Lewis-active structures and not the α1→2 linkage to galactose of H-active structures (see Table 2.3). Furthermore, these results suggest that biosynthesis of fucosylated structures in healthy individuals depends on a balance of fucosyltransferase and fucosidase activities.

Loss of red cell Lewis antigen expression may occur in infectious mononucleosis complicated with immune haemolysis [876], in various forms of cancer (pancreatic, gastric, colorectal, bile duct, bladder) [877,878], and in alcoholic cirrhosis, alcoholic pancreatitis, and severe renal disease, but not in nonalcoholic liver disease [879].

2.22 Functional aspects

The part played by sialyl-Le^x and, to a lesser extent, sialyl-Le^a as ligands for lectin-like cell adhesion molecules, selectins, has been mentioned in Sections 2.3.4 and 2.19.3. Otherwise, almost nothing is known about the functions of ABO and Lewis antigens.

The red cell membrane has about 10^6 molecules of band 3 (anion transporter), 7×10^5 molecules of the glucose transporter, and about 10^6 molecules of polyglycosylated lipids [880]. All these molecules, plus some others of lower abundance, carry ABH antigens. The ABH-active oligosaccharides contribute to the glycocalyx or cell coat, an extracellular matrix of carbohydrate that protects the cell from mechanical damage and attack by pathogenic microorganisms [880,881].

Martinko *et al.* [152] propose that the A/B polymorphism is at least 13 million years old and probably maintained by selection. The nature of the selection pressures remains a mystery, but probably involved susceptibility to microbial infection throughout the body.

References

1 Landsteiner K. Zur Kenntnis der antifermentativen, lytischen und agglutinietenden Wirkungen des Blutserums und der Lymphe. *Zentralbl Bakt* 1900;27: 357–66.

2 Landsteiner K. Über Agglutinationserscheinungen normalen menschlichen Blutes. Agglutination phenomena in normal human blood. *Wien Klin Wochenschr* 1901;14:1132–4.

3 von Decastello A, Stürli A. Über die Isoagglutinie im Serum gesunder und kranker Menschen. *München Med Wochenschr* 1902;26:1090–5.

4 Epstein AA, Ottenberg R. A simple method of performing serum reactions. *Proc NY Path Soc* 1908;8:117–23.

5 von Dungern E, Hirschfeld L. Ueber Vererbung gruppenspezifischer Strukturen des Blutes. *Z Immun Forsch* 1910;6:284–92. [For translation see *Transfusion* 1962;2:70–4.]

6 Bernstein F. Ergebnisse einer biostatistischen zusammenfassenden Betrachtung über die erblichen Blutstrukturen des Menschen. *Klin Wochenschr* 1924;3:1495–7.

7 Bernstein F. Zussammenfassende Betrachttungen über die erblichen Blutstrukturen des Menschen. *Z Indukt Abstamm u VerebLehre* 1925;37:237–70.

8 Thomsen O, Friedenreich V, Worsaae E. Über die Möglichkeit der Existenz zweier neurer Blutgruppen; auch ein Beitrag zur Beleuchtung sogennanter Untergruppen. *Acta Path Microbiol Scand* 1930;7:157–90.

9 Morgan WTJ. A contribution to human biochemical genetics the chemical basis of blood-group specificity. *Proc R Soc Lond B* 1960;151:308–47.

10 Watkins WM. Biochemistry and genetics of the ABO, Lewis, and P blood group systems. In: Harris H, Hirschhorn K, eds. *Advances in Human Genetics* Vol. 10. New York: Plenum Press 1981:1–136.

11 Kabat EA. *Blood Group Substances: Their Chemistry and Immunochemistry.* New York: Academic Press 1956.

12 Mourant AE. A 'new' human blood group antigen of frequent occurrence. *Nature* 1946;158:237–8.

13 Andresen PH. The blood group system L: a new blood group L$_2$. A case of epistasy within the blood groups. *Acta Path Microbiol Scand* 1948;25:728–31.

14 Clausen H, Hakomori S. ABH and related histo-blood group antigens; immunochemical differences in carrier isotypes and their distribution. *Vox Sang* 1989;**56**:1–20.

15 Watkins WM, Greenwell P, Yates AD, Johnson PH. Regulation of expression of carbohydrate blood group antigens. *Biochimie* 1988;**70**:1597–611.

16 Hakomori S. Blood group ABH and Ii antigens of human erythrocytes: chemistry, polymorphism, and their developmental change. *Semin Hematol* 1981;**18**: 39–62.

17 Lloyd KO. Blood group antigens as markers for normal differentiation and malignant change in human tissues. *Am J Clin Pathol* 1987;**87**:129–39.

18 Hakomori S. Antigen structure and genetic basis of histo-blood groups A, B and O: their changes associated with human cancer. *Biochim Biophys Acta* 1999; **1473**:247–66.

19 Watkins WM, Skacel PO, Johnson PH. Human fucosyltransferases. In: Garegg PJ, Lindber AA, eds. *Carbohydrate Antigens. Amer Chem Soc Symp* Ser 1992:34–63.

20 Clausen H, Bennett EP, Grunnet N. Molecular genetics of the ABO histo-blood groups. *Transfus Clin Biol* 1994;**1**:79–89.

21 Oriol R. ABO, Hh, Lewis, and secretion: serology, genetics, and tissue distribution. In: Cartron J-P, Rouger P, eds. *Blood Cell Biochemistry* Vol. 6. New York: Plenum Press 1995:36–73.

22 Lowe JB. Biochemistry and biosynthesis of ABH and Lewis antigens: characterization of blood group-specific glycosyltransferases. In: Cartron J-P, Rouger P, eds. *Blood Cell Biochemistry* Vol. 6. New York: Plenum Press 1995:75–115.

23 Henry S, Oriol R, Samuelsson B. Lewis histo-blood group system and associated secretory phenotypes. *Vox Sang* 1995;**69**:166–82.

24 Henry S, Samuelsson B. ABO polymorphisms and their putative biological relationships with disease. In: King M-J, ed. *Human Blood Cells: Consequences of Genetic Polymorphism and Variations*. London: Imperial College Press 2000:1–103.

25 Finne J. Identification of the blood-group ABH-active glycoprotein components of human erythrocyte membrane. *Eur J Biochem* 1980;**104**:181–9.

26 Finne J, Krusius T, Rauvala H, Järnefelt J. Molecular nature of the blood-group ABH antigens of the human erythrocyte membrane. *Rev Franc Transfus Immuno-Hémat* 1980;**23**:545–52.

27 Schenkel-Brunner H. Blood-group-ABH antigens of human erythrocytes. *Eur J Biochem* 1980;**104**:529–34.

28 Wilczynska Z, Miller-Podraza H, Koscielak J. The contribution of different glycoconjugates to the total ABH blood group activity of human erythrocytes. *FEBS Lett* 1980;**112**:277–9.

29 Karhi KK, Gahmberg CG. Identification of blood group A-active glycoproteins in the human erythrocyte membrane. *Biochim Biophys Acta* 1980;**622**:344–54.

30 Fukuda M, Fukuda MN. Changes in cell surface glycoproteins and carbohydrate structures during the development and differentiation of human erythroid cells. *J Supramol Struct* 1981;**17**:313–24.

31 Anstee DJ. Blood group-active surface molecules of the human red blood cell. *Vox Sang* 1990;**58**:1–20.

32 Anstee DJ, Tanner MJA. Separation of ABH, I, Ss antigenic activity from the MN-active sialoglycoprotein of the human erythrocyte membrane. *Vox Sang* 1975; **29**:378–89.

33 Moore S, Green C. The identification of specific Rhesus polypeptide blood group ABH active glycoprotein complexes in the human red-cell membrane. *Biochem J* 1987;**244**:735–41.

34 Koscielak J, Miller-Podraza H, Krauze R, Piasek A. Isolation and characterization of poly (glycosyl) ceramides (megaloglycolipids) with A, H and I blood-group activities. *Eur J Biochem* 1976;**71**:9–18.

35 Morgan WTJ, Van Heyningen R. The occurrence of A, B and O blood group substances in pseudo-mucinous ovarian cyst fluids. *Br J Exp Path* 1944;**25**:5–15.

36 Kobata A. Isolation of oligosaccharides from human milk. *Methods Enzymol* 1972;**28**:262–71.

37 Lundblad A. Oligosaccharides from human urine. *Methods Enzymol* 1978;**50**:226–35.

38 Oriol R. Genetic control of the fucosylation of ABH precursor chains: evidence for new epistatic interactions in different cells and tissues. *J Immunogenet* 1990;**17**: 235–45.

39 Rege VP, Painter TJ, Watkins WM, Morgan WTJ. Isolation of serologically active fucose-containing oligosaccharides from human blood-group H substance. *Nature* 1964;**203**:360–3.

40 Lloyd KO, Kabat EA, Layug EJ, Gruezo F. Immunochemical studies on blood groups. XXXIV. Structures of some oligosaccharides produced by alkaline degradation of blood group A, B, and H substances. *Biochemistry* 1966;**5**:1489–501.

41 Watkins WM, Morgan WTJ. Specific inhibition studies relating to the Lewis blood-group system. *Nature* 1957;**180**:1038–40.

42 Watkins WM, Morgan WTJ. Further observations on the inhibition of blood-group specific serological reactions by simple sugars of known structure. *Vox Sang* 1962;**7**:129–50.

43 Rege VP, Painter TJ, Watkins WM, Morgan WTJ. Isolation of a serologically active, fucose-containing, trisaccharide from human blood-group Le^a substance. *Nature* 1964;**204**:740–2.

44 Lloyd KO, Kabat EA, Licerio E. Immunochemical studies on blood groups. XXXVIII. Structures and activities of oligosaccharides produced by alkaline degradation of blood-group Lewis^a substance: proposed structure of the carbohydrate chains of human blood-

group A, B, H, Le[a], and Le[b] substances. *Biochemistry* 1968;7:2967–90.

45 Marr AMS, Donald ASR, Watkins WM, Morgan WTJ. Molecular and genetic aspects of human blood-group Le[b] specificity. *Nature* 1967;215:1345–9.

46 Marr AMS, Donald ASR, Morgan WTJ. Two new oligosaccharides obtained from an Le[a]-active glycoprotein. *Biochem J* 1968;110:789–91.

47 Gooi HC, Feizi T, Kapadia A *et al.* Stage-specific embryonic antigen involves $\alpha 1 \rightarrow 3$ fucosylated type 2 blood group chains. *Nature* 1981;292:156–8.

48 Clausen H, Levery SB, Nudelman E, Baldwin M, Hakomori S. Further characterization of Type 2 and Type 3 chain blood group A glycosphingolipids from human erythrocyte membranes. *Biochemistry* 1986;25:7075–85.

49 Magnani JL, Nilsson B, Brockhaus M *et al.* A monoclonal antibody-defined antigen associated with gastrointestinal cancer is a ganglioside containing sialylated lacto-N-fucopentaose II. *J Biol Chem* 1982; 257:14365–9.

50 Picard JK, Loveday D, Feizi T. Evidence for sialylated Type 1 blood group chains on human erythrocyte membranes revealed by agglutination of neuraminidase-treated erythrocytes with Waldenström's macroglobulin IgM[WOO] and hybridoma antibody FC 10.2. *Vox Sang* 1985;48:26–33.

51 Fukushima K, Hirota M, Terasaki PI *et al.* Characterization of sialosylated Lewis[x] as a new tumor-associated antigen. *Cancer Res* 1984;44:5279–85.

52 Marcus DM, Cass LE. Glycosphingolipids with Lewis blood group activity: uptake by human erythrocytes. *Science* 1969;164:553–5.

53 Kannagi R, Levery SB, Hakomori S. Le[a]-active heptaglycosylceramide, a hybrid of Type 1 and Type 2 chain, and the pattern of glycolipids with Le[a], Le[b], X (Le[x]), and Y (Le[y]) determinants in human blood cell membranes (ghosts). *J Biol Chem* 1984;260:6410–5.

54 Henry SM, Woodfield DG, Samuelsson BE, Oriol R. Plasma and red-cell glycolipid patterns of Le (a+b+) and Le (a+b–) Polynesians as further evidence of the weak secretor gene Se[w]. *Vox Sang* 1993;65:62–9.

55 Henry SM, Oriol R, Samuelsson BE. Detection and characterization of Lewis antigens in plasma of Lewis-negative individuals: evidence of chain extension as a result of reduced fucosyltransferase competition. *Vox Sang* 1994;67:387–96.

56 Henry SM, Oriol R, Samuelsson BE. Expression of Lewis histo-blood group glycolipids in the plasma of individuals of Le (a+b+) and partial secretor phenotypes. *Glycocon J* 1994;11:593–9.

57 Stroud MR, Levery SB, Nudelman ED *et al.* Extended Type 1 chain glycosphingolipids: dimeric Le[a] (III[4]V[4]Fuc$_2$Lc$_6$) as human tumor-associated antigen. *J Biol Chem* 1991;266:8439–46.

58 Stroud MR, Levery SB, Salyan MEK, Roberts CE,

Hakomori S. Extended type-1 chain glycosphingolipid antigens: isolation and characterization of trifucosyl-Le[b] antigen (III[4]V[4]VI[2]Fuc$_3$Lc$_6$). *Eur J Biochem* 1992; 203:577–86.

59 Sakamoto J, Yin BWT, Lloyd KO. Analysis of the expression of H, Lewis, X, Y and precursor blood group determinants in saliva and red cells using a panel of mouse monoclonal antibodies. *Mol Immunol* 1984;21:1093–8.

60 Furukawa K, Welt S, Yin BWT *et al.* Analysis of the fine specificities of 11 mouse monoclonal antibodies reactive with Type 2 blood group determinants. *Mol Immunol* 1990;27:723–32.

61 Donald ASR. A-active trisaccharides isolated from A_1 and A_2 blood-group-specific glycoproteins. *Eur J Biochem* 1981;120:243–9.

62 Le Pendu J, Lambert F, Samuelsson B *et al.* Monoclonal antibodies specific for Type 3 and Type 4 chain-based blood group determinants: relationship to the A_1 and A_2 subgroups. *Glycocon J* 1986;3:255–71.

63 Clausen H, Levery SB, Nudelman E, Tsuchiya S, Hakomori S. Repetitive A epitope (type 3 chain A) defined by blood group A_1-specific monoclonal antibody TH-1: chemical basis of qualitative A_1 and A_2 distinction. *Proc Natl Acad Sci USA* 1985;82:1199–203.

64 Clausen H, Levery SB, Kannagi R, Hamomori S. Novel blood group H glycolipid antigens exclusively expressed in bood group A and AB erythrocytes (Type 3 chain H). I. Isolation and chemical characterization. *J Biol Chem* 1986;261:1380–7.

65 Clausen H, Holmes E, Hakomori S. Novel blood group H glycolipid antigens exclusively expressed in blood group A and AB erythrocytes (Type 3 chain H). II. Differential conversion of different H substrates by A_1 and A_2 enzymes, and Type 3 chain H expression in relation to secretor status. *J Biol Chem* 1986;261:1388–92.

66 Kannagi R, Levery SB, Hakomori S. Blood group H antigen with globo-series structure: isolation and characterization from human blood group O erythrocytes. *FEBS Lett* 1984;175:397–401.

67 Clausen H, Watanabe K, Kannagi R *et al.* Blood group A glycolipid (A[x]) with globo-series structure which is specific for blood group A_1 erythrocytes: one of the chemical bases for A_1 and A_2 distinction. *Biochem Biophys Res Commun* 1984;124:523–9.

68 Breimer ME, Jovall P-Å. Structural characterization of a blood group A heptaglycosylceramide with globo-series structure: the major glycolipid based blood group A antigen of human kidney. *FEBS Lett* 1985;179:165–72.

69 Holgersson J, Bäcker AE, Breimer ME *et al.* The blood group B type-4 heptaglycosylceramide is a minor blood group B structure in human B kidneys in contrast to the corresponding A type-4 compound in A kidneys: structural and *in vitro* biosynthetic studies. *Biochim Biophys Acta* 1992;1180:33–43.

70 Lindström K, Jovall P-Å, Ghardashkani S, Samuelsson

BE, Breimer ME. Blood group glycosphingolipid expression in kidney of an individual with the rare blood group A_1 Le (a–b+), p phenotype: absence of blood group structures based on the globoseries. *Glycocon J* 1996;13:307–13.

71 Paulson JC, Colley KJ. Glycosyltransferases: structure, localization, and control of cell type-specific glycosylation. *J Biol Chem* 1989;264:17615–18.

72 Costache M, Cailleau A, Fernandez-Mateos P, Oriol R, Mollicone R. Advances in molecular genetics of α-2- and α-3/4-fucosyltransferases. *Transfus Clin Biol* 1997;4:367–82.

73 Le Pendu J, Cartron JP, Lemieux RU, Oriol R. The presence of at least two different H-blood-group-related β-D-Gal α-2-L-fucosyltransferases in human serum and the genetics of blood group H substances. *Am J Hum Genet* 1985;37:749–60.

74 Kumazaki T, Yoshida A. Biochemical evidence that secretor gene, *Se*, is a structural gene encoding a specific fucosyltransferase. *Proc Natl Acad Sci USA* 1984;81:4193–7.

75 Betteridge A, Watkins WM. Variant forms of α-2-L-fucosyltransferase in human submaxillary glands from blood group ABH 'secretor' and 'non-secretor' individuals. *Glycocon J* 1985;2:61–78.

76 Henry S, Mollicone R, Fernandez P *et al.* Molecular basis for erythrocyte Le (a+b+) and salivary ABH partial-secretor phenotypes: expression of a FUT2 secretor allele with an A→T mutation at nucleotide 385 correlates with reduced α(1,2)fucosyltransferase activity. *Glycocon J* 1996;13:985–93.

77 Rouquier S, Lowe JB, Kelly RJ *et al.* Molecular cloning of a human genomic region containing the H blood group α(1,2)fucosyltransferase gene and two *H* locus-related DNA restriction fragments: isolation of a candidate gene for the human Secretor blood group locus. *J Biol Chem* 1995;270:4632–4639.

78 Kelly RJ, Rouquier S, Giorgi D, Lennon GG, Lowe JB. Sequence and expression of a candidate for the human Secretor blood group α(1,2)fucosyltransferase gene (*FUT2*): homozygosity for an enzyme-inactivating nonsense mutation commonly correlates with the non-secretor phenotype. *J Biol Chem* 1995;270:4640–4649.

79 Koda Y, Soejima M, Kimura H. Structure and expression of H-type GDP-L-fucose:β-D-galactoside 2-α-L-fucosyltransferase gene (*FUT1*). *J Biol Chem* 1997;272:7501–5.

80 Koda Y, Soejima M, Wang B, Kimura H. Structure and expression of the gene encoding 2-α-L-fucosyltransferase (*FUT2*). *Eur J Biochem* 1997;246:750–5.

81 Ernst LK, Rajan VP, Larsen RD, Ruff MM, Lowe JB. Stable expression of blood group H determinants and GDP-L-fucose:β-D-galactoside 2-α-L-fucosyltransferase in mouse cells after transfection with human DNA. *J Biol Chem* 1989;264:3436–47.

82 Rajan VP, Larsen RD, Aimera S, Ernst LK, Lowe JB. A cloned human DNA restriction fragment determines expression of a GDP-L-fucose:β-D-galactoside 2-α-L-fucosyltransferase in transfected cells: evidence for isolation and transfer of the human H blood group locus. *J Biol Chem* 1989;264:11158–67.

83 Larsen RD, Ernst LK, Nair RP, Lowe JB. Molecular cloning, sequence, and expression of a human GDP-L-fucose:β-D-galactoside 2-α-L-fucosyltransferase cDNA that can form the H blood group antigen. *Proc Natl Acad Sci USA* 1990;87:6674–8.

84 Prieto PA, Larsen RD, Cho M *et al.* Expression of human *H*-type α1,2-fucosyltransferase encoding for blood group H (O) antigen in Chinese hamster ovary cells. *J Biol Chem* 1997;272:2089–97.

85 Schiff F, Sasaki H. Der Ausscheidungstypus, ein auf serologischem Wege nachweisbares Mendelndes Merkmal. *Klin Wochenschr* 1932;11:1426–9.

86 Race RR, Sanger R. *Blood Groups in Man*, 5th edn. Oxford: Blackwell Scientific Publications 1968.

87 Lemieux RU. Human blood groups and carbohydrate chemistry. *Chem Soc Rev* 1978;7:423–52.

88 Oriol R. Interactions of ABO, Hh, secretor and Lewis systems. *Rev Franc Transfus Immuno-Hémat* 1980;23:517–26.

89 Oriol R, Danilovs J, Hawkins BR. A new genetic model proposing that the *Se* gene is a structural gene closely linked to the *H* gene. *Am J Hum Genet* 1981;33:421–31.

90 Le Pendu J, Lemieux RU, Lambert F, Dalix A-M, Oriol R. Distribution of H Type 1 and H Type 2 antigenic determinants in human sera and saliva. *Am J Hum Genet* 1982;34:402–15.

91 Le Pendu J, Oriol R, Juszozak G *et al.* α-2-L-fucosyltransferase activity in sera of individuals with H-deficient red cells and normal H antigen in secretions. *Vox Sang* 1983;44:360–5.

92 Sarnesto A, Köhlin T, Thurin J, Blaszczyk-Thurin M. Purification of H gene-encoded β-galactoside α1→2 fucosyltransferase from human serum. *J Biol Chem* 1990;265:15067–75.

93 Schenkel-Brunner H, Prohaska R, Tuppy H. Action of glycosyl transferases upon 'Bombay' (O_h) erythrocytes. *Eur J Biochem* 1975;56:591–4.

94 Henry S, Mollicone R, Lowe JB, Samuelsson B, Larson GA. A second nonsecretor allele of the blood group α (1,2)–fucosyltransferase gene (FUT2). *Vox Sang* 1996;70:21–25.

95 Yazawa S, Kishi K, Akamatsu S, Oh-kawara H, Seno T, Okubo Y. A search for the *Secretor* gene nonsense mutation (G428 to A428) in Japanese nonsecretors. *Transfusion* 1996;36:286 [letter].

96 Liu Y, Koda Y, Soejima M *et al.* Extensive polymorphism of the *FUT2* gene in an African (Xhosa) population of South Africa. *Hum Genet* 1998;103:204–10.

97 YuL-C, Yang Y-H, Broadberry RE, Chen Y-H, Chan

Y-S, Lin M. Correlation of a missense mutation in the human *Secretor* α1,2-fucosyltransferase gene with the Lewis (a+b+) phenotype: a potential molecular basis for the weak *Secretor* allele (*Se^w*). *Biochem J* 1995;**312**:329–32.

98 Koda Y, Soejima M, Liu Y, Kimura H. Molecular basis for secretor type α1,2-fucosyltransferase gene deficiency in a Japanese population: a fusion gene generated by unequal crossover responsible for the enzyme deficiency. *Am J Hum Genet* 1996;**59**:343–50.

99 Kudo T, Iwasaki H, Nishihara S *et al.* Molecular genetic analysis of the human Lewis histo-blood groups system. II. Secretor gene inactivation by a novel missense mutation A385T in Japanese nonsecretor individuals. *J Biol Chem* 1996;**271**:9830–7.

100 Henry S, Mollicone R, Fernandez P *et al.* Homozygous expression of a missense mutation at nucleotide 385 in the *FUT2* gene associates with the Le (a+b+) partial-secretor phenotype in an Indonesian family. *Biochem Biophys Res Commun* 1996;**219**:675–8.

101 Peng CT, Tsai CH, Lin TP *et al.* Molecular characterization of secretor type α (1,2)fucosyltransferase gene deficiency in the Philippine population. *Ann Hematol* 1999;**78**:463–7.

102 Yu L-C, Broadberry RE, Yang Y-H, Chen Y-H, Lin M. Heterogeneity of the human *Secretor* α(1,2)fucosyltransferase gene among Lewis(a+b–) non-secretors. *Biochem Biophys Res Commun* 1996;**222**:390–4.

103 Liu Y-H, Koda Y, Soejima M *et al.* The fusion gene at the ABO-secretor locus (*FUT2*): absence in Chinese populations. *J Hum Genet* 1999, 1996;**44**:181–4.

104 Yu L-C, Lee HL, Chu C-C, Broadberry RE, Lin MA. A newly identified nonsecretor allele of the human histo-blood group α (1,2) fucosyltransferase gene (*FUT2*). *Vox Sang* 1999;**76**:115–9.

105 Koda Y, Soejima M, Johnson PH, Smart E, Kimura H. Missense mutation of *FUT1* and deletion of *FUT2* are responsible for Indian Bombay phenotype of ABO blood group system. *Biochem Biophys Res Commun* 1997;**238**:21–5.

106 Fernandez-Mateos P, Cailleau A, Henry S *et al.* Point mutations and deletion responsible for the *Bombay* H null and the *Réunion* H weak blood groups. *Vox Sang* 1998;**75**:37–46.

107 Svensson L, Petersson A, Henry SM. Secretor genotyping for A385T, G428A, C571T, C628T, 685delTGG, G849A, and other mutations from a single PCR. *Transfusion* 2000;**40**:856–60.

108 Mulet C, Cartron JP, Badet J, Salmon C. Activity of 2-α-L-fucosyltransferase in human sera and red cell membranes. *FEBS Lett* 1977;**84**:74–8.

109 Skacel PO, Watkins WM. Fucosyltransferase expression in human platelets and leucocytes. *Glycocon J* 1987;**4**:267–72.

110 Schenkel-Brunner H, Tuppy H. Enzymes from human gastric mucosa conferring blood-group A and B specificities upon erythrocytes. *Eur J Biochem* 1970;**17**:218–22.

111 Race C, Watkins WM. The action of blood group B gene-specified α-galactosyltransferase from human serum and stomach mucosal extracts on group O and 'Bombay' O$_h$ erythrocytes. *Vox Sang* 1972;**23**: 385–401.

112 Kogure T, Furukawa K. Enzymatic conversion of human group O red cells into group B active cells by α-D-galactosyltransferases of sera and salivas from group B and its variant types. *J Immunogenet* 1976;**3**:147–54.

113 Pacuszka T, Koscielak J. The biosynthesis of blood-group-B character on human O-erythrocytes by a soluble α-galactosyltransferase from milk. *Eur J Biochem* 1972;**31**:574–7.

114 Barbolla L, Mojena M, Cienfuegos JA, Escartín P. Presence of an inhibitor of glycosyltransferase activity in a patient following an ABO incompatible liver transplant. *Br J Haematol* 1988;**69**:93–6.

115 Barbolla L, Mojena M, Boscá L. Presence of antibody to A- and B-transferases in minor incompatible bone marrow transplants. *Br J Haematol* 1988;**70**:471–6.

116 Kominato Y, Fujikura T, Shimada I *et al.* Monoclonal antibody to blood group glycosyltransferases, produced by hybrids constructed with Epstein–Barr-virus-transformed B lymphocytes from a patient with ABO-incompatible bone marrow transplant and mouse myeloma cells. *Vox Sang* 1990;**59**:116–8.

117 Rydberg L, Samuelsson BE. Presence of glycosyltransferase inhibitors in the sera of patients with long-term surviving ABO incompatible (A$_2$ to O) kidney grafts. *Transfus Med* 1991;**1**:177–82.

118 Amano J, Straehl P, Berger EG, Kochibe N, Kobata A. Structures of mucin-type sugar chains of the galactosyltransferase purified from human milk: occurrence of the ABO and Lewis blood group determinants. *J Biol Chem* 1991;**266**:11461–77.

119 Yoshida A, Yamaguchi YF, Dave V. Immunologic homology of human blood group glycosyltransferases and genetic background of blood group (ABO) determination. *Blood* 1979;**54**:344–50.

120 White T, Mandel U, Ørntoft TF *et al.* Murine monoclonal antibodies directed to the human histo-blood group A transferase (UDP-GalNAc: Fucα1→2Galα1→3-N-acetylgalactosaminyltransferase) and the presence therein of *N*-linked histo-blood group A determinant. *Biochemistry* 1990;**29**: 2740–7.

121 Clausen H, White T, Takio K *et al.* Isolation to homogeneity and partial characterization of a histo-blood group A defined Fucα1→2Galα1→3-N-acetylgalactosaminyltransferase from human lung tissue. *J Biol Chem* 1990;**265**:1139–45.

122 Navaratnam N, Findlay JBC, Keen JN, Watkins WM. Purification, properties and partial amino acid sequence of the blood-group-A-gene-associated α-3-N-

acetylgalactosaminyltransferase from human gut mucosal tissue. *Biochem J* 1990;**271**:93–8.

123 Yamamoto F, Marken J, Tsuji T *et al.* Cloning and characterisation of DNA complementary to human UDP-GalNAc:Fucα1→2Galα1→3GalNAc transferase (histo-blood group A transferase) mRNA. *J Biol Chem* 1990;**265**:1146–51.

124 Yamamoto F, McNeill PD, Hakomori S. Genomic organization of human histo-blood group ABO genes. *Glycobiology* 1995;**5**:51–8.

125 Yamamoto F, Clausen H, White T, Marken J, Hakomori S. Molecular genetic basis of the histo-blood group ABO system. *Nature* 1990;**345**:229–33.

126 Yamamoto F, Hakomori S. Sugar-nucleotide donor specificity of histo-blood group A and B transferases is based on amino acid substitutions. *J Biol Chem* 1990;**265**:19257–62.

127 O'Keefe DS, Dobrovic A. Decreased stability of the O allele mRNA transcript of the ABO gene. *Blood* 1996;**87**:3061–8 [letter].

128 Yamamoto F, McNeill PD, Hakomori S. Human histo-blood group A^2 transferase coded by A^2 allele, one of the A subtypes, is characterized by a single base deletion in the coding sequence, which results in an additional domain at the carboxyl terminal. *Biochem Biophys Res Commun* 1992;**187**:366–74.

129 Olsson ML, Chester MA. Frequent occurrence of a variant O^1 gene at the blood group ABO locus. *Vox Sang* 1996;**70**:26–30.

130 Mifsud NA, Haddad AP, Condon JA, Sparrow RL. ABO genotyping–identification of O^1, O^{1*}, and O^2 alleles using the polymerase chain reaction-sequence specific oligonucleotide (PCR-SSO) technique. *Immunohematology* 1996;**12**:149–53.

131 Olsson ML, Santos SEB, Guerreiro JF, Zago MA, Chester MA. Heterogeneity of the O alleles at the blood group *ABO* locus in Amerindians. *Vox Sang* 1998;**74**:46–50.

132 Fukumori Y, Ohnoki S, Shibata H, Nishimukai H. Sub-alleles of the ABO blood group system in a Japanese population. *Hum Hered* 1996;**46**:85–91.

133 Ogasawara K, Bannai M, Saitou N *et al.* Extensive polymorphism of ABO blood group gene: three major lineages of the alleles for the common ABO phenotypes. *Hum Genet* 1996;**97**:777–83.

134 Yip SP. Single-tube multiplex PCR-SSCP analysis distinguishes 7 common ABO alleles and readily identifies new alleles. *Blood* 2000;**95**:1487–92.

135 Yamamoto F, McNeill PD, Yamamoto M *et al.* Molecular genetic analysis of the ABO blood group system. IV. Another type of O allele. *Vox Sang* 1993;**64**:175–8.

136 Grunnet N, Steffensen R, Bennett EP, Clausen H. Evaluation of histo-blood group ABO genotyping in a Danish population: frequency of a novel O allele defined as O^2. *Vox Sang* 1994;**67**:210–5.

137 Yamamoto F, McNeill PD. Amino acid residue at codon 268 determines both activity and nucleotide-sugar donor substrate specificity of human histo-blood group A and B transferases: *in vitro* mutagenesis study. *J Biol Chem* 1996;**271**:10515–20.

138 Olsson ML, Chester MA. A rapid and simple ABO genotype screening method using a novel B/O^2 versus A/O^2 discriminating nucleotide substitution at the ABO locus. *Vox Sang* 1995;**69**:242–7.

139 Gassner C, Schmarda A, Nussbaumer W, Schönitzer D. ABO glycosyltransferase genotyping by polymerase chain reaction using sequence-specific primers. *Blood* 1996;**88**:1852–6.

140 Procter J, Crawford J, Bunce M, Welsh KIA. rapid molecular method (polymerase chain reaction with sequence-specific primers) to genotype for ABO blood group and secretor status and its potential for organ transplants. *Tissue Antigens* 1997;**50**:475–83 and *Tissue Antigens* 1998;**51**:319 [erratum].

141 Pearson SL, Hessner MJ. $A^{1,2}BO^{1,2}$ genotyping by multiplexed allele-specific PCR. *Br J Haematol* 1998;**100**:229–34.

142 Bennett EP, Steffensen R, Clausen H, Weghuis DO, van Kessel AG. Genomic cloning of the human histo-blood group ABO locus. *Biochem Biophys Res Commun* 1995;**206**:318–25.

143 Kominato Y, Hata Y, Takizawa H *et al.* Expression of human histo-blood group ABO genes is dependent upon DNA methylation of the promoter region. *J Biol Chem* 1999;**274**:37240–50.

144 Kominato Y, Tsuchiya T, Hata N, Takizawa H, Yamamoto F. Transcription of human ABO histo-blood group genes is dependent upon binding of transcription factor CBF/NF-Y to minisatellite sequence. *J Biol Chem* 1997;**41**:25890–8.

145 Irshaid NM, Chester MA, Olsson ML. Allele-related variation in minisatellite repeats involved in the transcription of the blood group *ABO* gene. *Transfus Med* 1999;**9**:219–26.

146 Yu L-C, Chang C-Y, Twu Y-C, Lin M. Human histo-blood group *ABO* glycosyltransferase genes: different enhancer structures with different transcriptional activities. *Biochem Biophys Res Commun* 2000;**273**:459–66.

147 Olsson ML, Chester MA. Evidence for a new type of O allele at the ABO locus, due to combination of the A^2 nucleotide deletion and the A^{el} nucleotide insertion. *Vox Sang* 1996;**71**:113–7.

148 Olsson ML, Guerreiro JF, Zago MA, Chester MA. Molecular analysis of the O alleles at the blood group ABO locus in populations of different ethnic origin reveals novel crossing-over events and point mutations. *Biochem Biophys Res Commun* 1997;**234**:779–82.

149 Suzuki K, Iwata M, Tsuji H *et al.* A de novo recombination in the ABO blood group gene and evidence for the occurrence of recombination products. *Hum Genet* 1997;**99**:454–61.

150 Olsson ML, Chester MA. Heterogeneity of the blood group A^x allele: genetic recombination of common alleles can result in the A_x phenotype. *Transfus Med* 1998;8:231–8.

151 Kominato Y, McNeill PD, Yamamoto M *et al.* Animal histo-blood group ABO genes. *Biochem Biophys Res Commun* 1992;189:154–64.

152 Martinko JM, Vincek V, Klein D, Klein J. Primate ABO glycosyltransferases: evidence for trans-species evolution. *Immunogenetics* 1993;37:274–8.

153 Saitou N, Yamamoto F. Evolution of primate ABO blood group genes and their homologous genes. *Mol Biol Evol* 1997;14:399–411.

154 Joziasse DH, Shaper JH, Jabs EW, Shaper NL. Characterization of an α1→3-galactosyltransferase homologue on human chromosome 12 that is organized as a processed pseudogene. *J Biol Chem* 1991;266: 6991–8.

155 Shaper NL, Lin S, Joziasse DH, Kim DY, Yang-Feng TL. Assignment of two human α-1,3-galactosyltransferase gene sequences (*GGTA1* and *GGTA1P*) to chromosomes 9q33-q34 and 12q14-q15. *Genomics* 1992;12: 613–15 and *Genomics* 1992;13:493 [erratum].

156 Yamamoto M, Lin X-H, Kominato Y *et al.* Murine equivalent of the human histo-blood group ABO gene is a *cis*AB gene and encodes a glycosyltransferase with both A and B transferase activity. *J Biol Chem* 2001;276:13701–8.

157 Chang J-G, Lee L-S, Chen P-H *et al.* Rapid genotyping of ABO blood group. *Blood* 1992;79:2176–7.

158 O'Keefe DS, Dobrovic A. A rapid and reliable PCR method for genotyping the ABO blood group. *Hum Mutat* 1993;2:67–70.

159 Stroncek DF, Konz R, Clay ME, Houchins JP, McCullough J. Determination of *ABO* glycosyltransferase genotypes by use of polymerase chain reaction and restriction enzymes. *Transfusion* 1995;35:231–40.

160 O'Keefe DS, Dobrovic A. A rapid and reliable PCR method for genotyping the ABO blood group. II. A^2 and O^2 alleles. *Hum Mutat* 1996;8:358–61.

161 Zago MA, Tavella MH, Simoes BP *et al.* Racial heterogeneity of DNA polymorphisms linked to the A and the O alleles of the ABO blood group gene. *Ann Hum Genet* 1996;60:67–72.

162 Ugozzoli L, Wallace RB. Application of an allele-specific polymerase chain reaction to the direct determination of the ABO blood group genotypes. *Genomics* 1992;12:670–4.

163 Johnson PH. Hopkinson DA. Detection of ABO blood group polymorphism by denaturing gradient gel electrophoresis. *Hum Mol Genet* 1992;1:341–4.

164 Yip SP, Yow CM, Lewis WHP. DNA polymorphism at the ABO locus in the Chinese population of Hong Kong. *Hum Hered* 1995;45:266–71.

165 Watanabe G, Umetsu K, Yuasa I, Suzuki T. Amplified product length polymorphism (APLP): a novel strategy for genotyping the ABO blood group. *Hum Genet* 1997;99:34–7.

166 Olsson ML, Hosseini-Maaf B, Hellberg Å, Chester MA. Allele-specific primer PCR across intron 6 resolves potential genotyping errors caused by recombinant hybrid alleles at the ABO locus [Abstract]. *Transfusion* 1998;38 (Suppl.):3S.

167 Grubb R. Correlation between Lewis blood group and secretor character in man. *Nature* 1948;162:933.

168 Grubb R. Observations on the human group system Lewis. *Acta Path Microbiol Scand* 1951;28:61–81.

169 Ceppellini R. On the genetics of secretor and Lewis characters: a family study. *Proc 5th Congr Int Soc Blood Transf*, 1955:207–11.

170 Sanger R, Race RR. The Lutheran-secretor linkage in man: support for Mohr's findings. *Heredity* 1958;12:513–20.

171 Grolman EF, Kobata A, Ginsburg V. An enzymatic basis for Lewis blood types in man. *J Clin Invest* 1969;48:1489–94.

172 Chester MA, Watkins WM. α-1-Fucosyltransferases in human submaxillary gland and stomach tissues associated with the H, Le^a and Le^b blood-group characters and ABH secretor status. *Biochem Biophys Res Commun* 1969;34:835–42.

173 Le Pendu J, Lemieux RU, Dalix AM, Lambert F, Oriol R. Competition between ABO and Le gene specified enzymes. I. A Lewis related difference in the amount of A antigen in saliva of A_1 and A_2 secretors. *Vox Sang* 1983;45:349–58.

174 Le Pendu J, Oriol R, Lambert F, Dalix AM, Lemieux RU. Competition between ABO and Le gene specified enzymes. II. Quantitative analysis of A and B antigens in saliva of ABH non-secretors. *Vox Sang* 1983;45:421–5.

175 Sturgeon P, Arcilla MB. Studies on the secretion of blood group substances. I. Observations on the red cell phenotype Le (a+b+x+). *Vox Sang* 1970;18:301–22.

176 Henry SM, Benny AG, Woodfield DG. Investigation of Lewis phenotypes in Polynesians: evidence of a weak secretor phenotype. *Vox Sang* 1990;58:61–6.

177 Prieels J-P, Monnom D, Dolmans M, Beyer TA, Hill RL. Co-purification of the Lewis blood group N-acetylglucosaminide α1→4 fucosyltransferase and an N-acetylglucosaminide α1→3 fucosyltransferase from human milk. *J Biol Chem* 1981;256:10456–63.

178 Clamagirand-Mulet C, Badet J, Cartron JP. Isoelectrofocusing pattern of 2-α-L, 3-α-L and 4-α-L-fucosyltransferases from human milk and serum. *FEBS Lett* 1981;126:123–6.

179 Johnson PH, Yates AD, Watkins WM. Human salivary fucosyltransferases: evidence for two distinct α-3-L-fucosyltransferase activities one of which is associated with the Lewis blood group *Le* gene. *Biochem Biophys Res Commun* 1981;100:1611–8.

180 Kukowska-Latallo JF, Larsen RD, Nair RP, Lowe JB. A cloned human cDNA determines expression of a mouse stage-specific embryonic antigen and the Lewis blood group α(1,3/1,4)fucosyltransferase. *Genes Dev* 1990;4:1288–303.

181 Costache M, Apoil P-A, Cailleau A *et al*. Evolution of fucosyltransferase genes in vertebrates. *J Biol Chem* 1997;272:29721–8.

182 Dupuy F, Petit J-M, Mollicone R *et al*. A single amino acid in the hypervariable stem domain of vertebrate α1,3/1,4–fucosyltransferases determines the Type 1/Type 2 transfer. *J Biol Chem* 1999;274:12257–62.

183 Koda Y, Kimura H, Mekada E. Analysis of Lewis fucosyltransferase genes from the human gastric mucosa of Lewis-positive and -negative individuals. *Blood* 1993;82:2915–9.

184 Nishihara S, Yazawa S, Iwasaki H *et al*. α(1,3/14)fucosyltransferase (FucT-III) gene is inactivated by a single amino acid substitution in Lewis histo-blood type negative individuals. *Biochem Biophys Res Commun* 1993;196:624–31.

185 Mollicone R, Reguigne I, Kelly RJ *et al*. Molecular basis for Lewis α(1,3/1,4)-fucosyltransferase gene deficiency (FUT3) found in Lewis-negative Indonesian pedigrees. *J Biol Chem* 1994;269:20987–94.

186 Nishihara S, Narimatsu H, Iwasaki H *et al*. Molecular genetic analysis of the human Lewis histo-blood group system. *J Biol Chem* 1994;269:29271–8.

187 Koda Y, Soejima M, Kimura H. Detection of G to A missense mutation of Lewis-negative gene by PCR on genomic DNA. *Vox Sang* 1994;67:327–8.

188 Ørntoft TF, Vestergaard EM, Holmes E *et al*. Influence of Lewis α1–3/4L-fucosyltransferase (*FUT3*) gene mutations on enzyme activity, erythrocyte phenotyping, and circulating tumor marker sialyl-Lewis a levels. *J Biol Chem* 1996;271:32260–8.

189 Liu Y, Koda Y, Soejima M, Uchida N, Kimura H. PCR analysis of Lewis-negative gene mutations and the distribution of Lewis alleles in a Japanese population. *J Forensic Sci* 1996;41:1018–21.

190 Elmgren A, Börjeson C, Svensson L, Rydberg L, Larson G. DNA sequencing and screening for point mutations in the human Lewis (FUT3) gene enables molecular genotyping of the human Lewis blood group system. *Vox Sang* 1996;70:97–103.

191 Pang H, Liu Y, Koda Y *et al*. Five novel missense mutations of the Lewis gene (*FUT3*) in African (Xhosa) and Caucasian populations in South Africa. *Hum Genet* 1998;102:675–80.

192 Liu Y-H, Koda Y, Soejima M, Pang H, Wang B, Kimura H. Lewis (*FUT3*) genotypes in two different Chinese populations. *J Forensic Med* 1999;44:82–6.

193 Nishihara S, Hiraga T, Ikehara Y *et al*. Molecular behavior of mutant Lewis enzymes *in vivo*. *Glycobiology* 1999;9:373–82.

194 Elmgren A, Mollicone R, Costache M *et al*. Significance of individual point mutations, T202C and C314T, in the human Lewis (*FUT3*) gene for expression of Lewis antigens by the human α(1,3/1,4)-fucosyltransferase, Fuc-TIII. *J Biol Chem* 1997;272:21994–8.

195 Xu Z, Vo L, Macher BA. Structure-function analysis of human α1,3-fucosyltransferase: amino acids involved in acceptor substrate specificity. *J Biol Chem* 1996; 271:8818–23.

196 Schenkel-Brunner H, Chester MA, Watkins WM. α-L-fusosyltransferases in human serum from donors of different ABO, secretor and Lewis blood-group phenotypes. *Eur J Biochem* 1972;30:269–77.

197 Cartron JP, Mulet C, Bauvois B, Rahuel C, Salmon C. ABH and Lewis glycosyltransferases in human red cells, lymphocytes and platelets. *Rev Franc Transfus Immuno-Hémat* 1980;23:271–82.

198 Greenwell P, Ball MG, Watkins WM. Fucosyltransferase activities in human lymphocytes and granulocytes: blood group *H*-gene-specified α-2-L-fucosyltransferase is a discriminatory marker of peripheral blood lymphocytes. *FEBS Lett* 1983;164: 314–17.

199 Cameron HS, Szczepaniak D, Weston BW. Expression of human chromosome 19p α(1,3)-fucosyltransferase genes in normal tissues: alternative splicing, polyadenylation, and isoforms. *J Biol Chem* 1995;270:20112–22.

200 Lowe JB, Stoolman LM, Nair RP *et al*. ELAM-1-dependent cell adhesion to vascular endothelium determined by a transfected human fucosyltransferase cDNA. *Cell* 1990;63:475–84.

201 Goelz SE, Hession C, Goff D *et al*. ELFT: a gene that directs the expression of an ELAM-1 ligand. *Cell* 1990;63:1349–56.

202 Weston BW, Nair RP, Larsen RD, Lowe JB. Isolation of a novel human α(1,3)fucosyltransferase gene and molecular comparison to the human Lewis blood group α(1,3/1,4)fucosyltransferase gene: syntenic, homologous, nonallelic genes encoding enzymes with distinct acceptor substrate specificities. *J Biol Chem* 1992; 267:4152–4160.

203 Koszdin KL, Bowen BR. The cloning and expression of a human α-1,3fucosyltransferase capable of forming the E-selectin ligand. *Biochem Biophys Res Commun* 1992;187:152–7.

204 Weston BW, Smith PL, Kelly RJ, Lowe JB. Molecular cloning of a fourth member of a human α(1,3)fucosyltransferase gene family: multiple homologous sequences that determine expression of the Lewis x, sialyl Lewis x, and difucosyl sialyl Lewis x epitopes. *J Biol Chem* 1992;267:24575–84.

205 Sasaki K, Kurata K, Funayama K *et al*. Expression cloning of a novel α1,3-fucosyltransferase that is involved in biosynthesis of the sialyl Lewis x carbohydrate

determinants in leukocytes. *J Biol Chem* 1994; **269**:14730–7.

206 Natsuka S, Gersten KM, Zenita K, Kannagi R, Lowe JB. Molecular cloning of a cDNA encoding a novel human leukocyte α-1,3-fucosyltransferase capable of synthesizing the sialyl Lewis x determinant. *J Biol Chem* 1994;**269**:16789–94; and *J Biol Chem* 1994;**269**: 20806.

207 Tetteroo PAT, de Heij HT, Van den Eijnden DH, Visser FJ, Schoenmaker E, van Kessel AHMG A GDP-fucose:[Galβ1→4]GlcNAcα1→3-fucosyltransferase activity is correlated with the presence of human chromosome 11 and the expression of the Le^x, Le^y, and sialyl-Le^x antigens in human-mouse cell hybrids. *J Biol Chem* 1987;**262**:15984–9.

208 Lasky LA. Selectin–carbohydrate interactions and the initiation of the inflammatory response. *Ann Rev Biochem* 1995;**64**:113–39.

209 McEver RP, Moore KL, Cummings RD. Leukocyte trafficking mediated by selectin–carbohydrate interactions. *J Biol Chem* 1995;**270**:11025–8.

210 Kansas GS. Selectins and their ligands: current concepts and contoversies. *Blood* 1996;**88**:3259–87.

211 de Vries T, Srnka CA, Paleic MM *et al.* Acceptor specificity of different length constructs of human recombinant α1,3/4-fucosyltransferases: replacement of the stem region and the transmembrane domain of fucosyltransferase V by protein A results in an enzyme with GDP-fucose hydrolyzing activity. *J Biol Chem* 1995; **270**:8712–22.

212 Mollicone R, Reguigne I, Fletcher A *et al.* Molecular basis for plasma α(1,3)-fucosyltransferase gene deficiency (FUT6). *J Biol Chem* 1994;**269**:12662–71.

213 Larson G, Börjeson C, Elmgren A *et al.* Identification of a new plasma α(1,3)-fucosyltransferase (FUT6) allele requires an extended genotyping strategy. *Vox Sang* 1996;**71**:233–41.

214 von Dungern E, Hirszfeld L. Über gruppenspezifische Strukturen des Blutes. III. *Z ImmunForsch* 1911; **8**:526–62.

215 Landsteiner K, Levine P. On the inheritance and racial distribution of agglutinable properties of human blood. *J Immunol* 1930;**18**:87–94.

216 Lattes L, Cavazzuti A. Sur l'existence d'un troisième élément d'isoagglutination. *J Immunol* 1924;**9**:407–25.

217 Landsteiner K, Witt DH. Observations on the human blood groups: irregular reactions. Isoagglutinins in sera of group IV. The factor A^1. *J Immunol* 1926;**11**:221–47.

218 Landsteiner K, Levine P. On the cold agglutinins in human serum. *J Immunol* 1926;**12**:441–60.

219 Taylor GL, Race RR, Prior AM, Ikin EW. Frequency of the iso-agglutinin α$_1$ in the serum of the subgroups A$_2$ and A$_2$B. *J Pathol Bacteriol* 1942;**54**:514–6.

220 Juel E. Anti-A agglutinins in sera from A$_2$B individuals. *Acta Path Microbiol Scand* 1959;**46**:91–5.

221 Juel E. Studies in the subgroups of the blood group A. *Acta Path Microbiol Scand* 1959;**46**:251–65.

222 Lenkiewicz B, Sarul B. Anti-A$_1$ antibodies in blood donors in the Warsaw region. *Arch Immunol Ther Exp* 1971;**19**:643–7.

223 Bird GWG. Relationship of the blood sub-groups A$_1$, A$_2$ and A$_1$B, A$_2$B to haemagglutinins present in the seeds of *Dolichos biflorus*. *Nature* 1952;**170**:674.

224 Race RR, Sanger R. *Blood Groups in Man*, 6th edn. Oxford: Blackwell Scientific Publications 1975.

225 Race C, Watkins WM. The enzymic products of the human *A* and *B* blood group genes in the serum of 'Bombay' O$_h$ donors. *FEBS Lett* 1972;**27**:125–30.

226 Schenkel-Brunner H, Tuppy H. Enzymatic conversion of human blood-group-O erythrocytes into A$_2$ and A$_1$ cells by a α-N-Acetyl-D-galactosaminyl transferases of blood-group-A individuals. *Eur J Biochem* 1973; **34**:125–8.

227 Fujii H, Yoshida A. Multiple components of blood group A and B antigens in human erythrocyte membranes and their difference between A$_1$ and A$_2$ status. *Proc Natl Acad Sci USA* 1980;**77**:2951–4.

228 Schenkel-Brunner H. Studies on blood-groups A$_1$ and A$_2$. *Eur J Biochem* 1982;**122**:511–4.

229 Schachter H, Michaels MA, Crookston MC, Tilley CA, Crookston JH. A quantitative difference in the activity of blood group A-specific *N*-acetylgalactosaminyltransferase in serum from A$_1$ and A$_2$ human subjects. *Biochem Biophys Res Commun* 1971;**45**:1011–8.

230 Schachter H, Michaels MA, Tilley CA, Crookston MC, Crookston JH. Qualitative differences in the *N*-acetyl-D-galactosaminyltransferases produced by human *A^1* and *A^2* genes. *Proc Natl Acad Sci USA* 1973;**70**:220–4.

231 Topping MD, Watkins WM. Isoelectric points of the human blood group *A^1*, *A^2* and *B* gene-associated glycosyltransferases in ovarian cyst fluids and serum. *Biochem Biophys Res Commun* 1975;**64**:89–96.

232 Ogasawara K, Yabe R, Uchikawa M *et al.* Molecular genetic analysis of variant phenotypes of the ABO blood group system. *Blood* 1996;**88**:2732–7.

233 Ogasawara K, Yabe R, Uchikawa M *et al.* Different alleles cause an imbalance in A$_2$ and A$_2$B phenotypes of the ABO blood group. *Vox Sang* 1998;**74**:242–7.

234 Mäkelä O, Ruoslahti E, Ehnholm C. Subtypes of human ABO blood groups and subtype-specific antibodies. *J Immunol* 1969;**102**:763–71.

235 Greenbury CL, Moore DH, Nunn LAC. Reaction of 7S and 19S components of immune rabbit antisera with human group A and AB red cells. *Immunology* 1963;**6**:421–33.

236 Economidou J, Hughes-Jones NC, Gardner B. Quantitative measurements concerning A and B antigen sites. *Vox Sang* 1967;**12**:321–8.

237 Lopez M, Benali J, Cartron JP, Salmon C. Some notes on

the specificity of anti-A$_1$ reagents. *Vox Sang* 1980; 39:271–6.

238 Cartron JP. Etude quantitative et thermodynamique des phénotypes érythrocytaires 'A faible'. *Rev Franc Transfus Immuno-Hémat* 1976;19:35–54.

239 Cartron JP, Gerbal A, Hughes-Jones NC, Salmon C. 'Weak A' phenotypes: relationship between red cell agglutinability and antigen site density. *Immunology* 1974;27:723–7.

240 Romano EL, Zabner-Oziel P, Soyano A, Linares J. Studies on the binding of IgG and F (ab) anti-A to adult and newborn group A red cells. *Vox Sang* 1983;45:378–83.

241 Matsumoto I, Osawa T. Specific purification of eel serum and *Cytisus sessilifolius* anti-H hemagglutinins by affinity chromatography and their binding to human erythrocytes. *Biochemistry* 1974;13:582–8.

242 Williams MA, Voak D. Studies with ferritin-labelled *Dolichos biflorus* lectin on the numbers and distribution of A sites on A$_1$ and A$_2$ erythrocytes, and on the nature of its specificity and enhancement by enzymes. *Br J Haematol* 1972;23:427–41.

243 Rouger P, Kornprobst M, Salmon C. Study of ABH red cell antigens by flow cytometry using monoclonal antigens [Abstract] *18th Congr International Soc Blood Transfus* 1984;32.

244 Rochant H, Tonthat H, Henri A, Titeux M, Dreyfus B. Abnormal distribution of erythrocytes A$_1$ antigens in preleukemia as demonstrated by an immunofluorescence technique. *Blood Cells* 1976;2:237–55.

245 Brain P. Subgroups of A in the South African Bantu. *Vox Sang* 1966;11:686–98.

246 Salmon C, De Grouchy J, Liberge G. Un nouvel antigène du système ABO: A$_{1(80)}$. *Nouv Rev Franc Hèmat* 1965;5:631–7.

247 Voak D, Lodge TW, Stapleton RR, Fogg H, Roberts HE. The incidence of H deficient A$_2$ and A$_2$B bloods and family studies on the AH/ABH status of an A$_{int}$ and some new variant blood types (A$_{intH\downarrow}$^{A1}, A$_{2\uparrow H}$w^{A1}, A$_{2\uparrow}$B$_H$w^{A1B} and A$_{2\downarrow}$B$_H$w^{A2B}). *Vox Sang* 1970;19:73–84.

248 Davey MG. Editorial note on paper 'Serology and genetics of the A$_1$ high H subgroup' by Malti Sathe and HM Bhatia. *Vox Sang* 1974;26:383–4.

249 Wiener AS. Heredity of the Rh blood types. IX. Observations in a series of 526 cases of disputed parentage. *Am J Hum Genet* 1950;2:177–97.

250 Yoshida A, Davé V, Branch DR, Yamaguchi H, Okubo Y. An enzyme basis for blood type A intermediate status. *Am J Hum Genet* 1982;34:919–24.

251 Mourant AE, Kopec AC, Domaniewska K. *The Distribution of Human Blood Groups and Other Polymorphisms*. London: Oxford University Press 1976.

252 Tills D, Kopec AC, Tills RE. *The Distribution of Human Blood Groups and Other Polymorphisms (Suppl. 1)*. Oxford: Oxford University Press 1983.

253 Ikin EW, Prior AM, Race RR, Taylor GL. The distribu-

tions in the A$_1$A$_2$BO blood groups in England. *Ann Eugen* 1939;9:409–11.

254 Wiener AS. *Blood Groups and Transfusion*, 3rd edn. Springfield: Thomas 1943.

255 Yamakami K. The individuality of semen, with reference to its property of inhibiting specifically isohemoagglutination. *J Immunol* 1926;12:185–9.

256 Putkonen T. Uber die gruppenspezifischen Eigenschaften Verschiedener Korperflussigkeiten. *Acta Soc Med Fenn Duodecim Ser A* 1930;14:113–53.

257 Buchanan DJ, Rapoport S. Composition of meconium: serological study of blood-group-specific substances found in individual meconiums. *Proc Soc Exp Biol NY* 1951;77:114–7.

258 Zuelzer WW, Beattie KM, Reisman LE. Generalized unbalanced mosaicism attributable to dispermy and probable fertilization of a polar body. *Am J Hum Genet* 1964;16:38–51.

259 Moores P. Blood group and tissue mosaicism in a Natal Indian woman. *Acta Haematol* 1973;50:299–304.

260 Clarke CA, McConnell RB, Sheppard PM. A genetical study of the variations in ABH secretion. *Ann Hum Genet* 1960;24:295–301.

261 Sturgeon P, McQuiston D, Van Camp S. Quantitative studies on salivary blood group substances. II. Normal values. *Vox Sang* 1973;24:114–25.

262 Szulman AE. The ABH antigens in human tissues and secretions during embryonal development. *J Histochem Cytochem* 1965;13:752–4.

263 Wiener AS, Belkin RB. Group-specific substances in the saliva of the new-born. *J Immunol* 1943;47:467–70.

264 Formaggio TG. Development and secretion of blood group factor O in the newborn. *Proc Soc Exp Biol NY* 1951;76:554–6.

265 Gammelgaard A. *Om Sjaeldne, Svage a-Receptorer (A$_3$, A$_4$, A$_5$ og A$_x$) Hos Mennesket.* Copenhagen: Busck 1942.

266 Boettcher B. Correlations between inhibition titres of blood group substances in salivas from A$_1$, A$_2$ and B secretors. *Aust J Exp Biol Med Sci* 1967;45:495–506.

267 Boettcher B. Precipitation of a substance in salivas from A$_1$ and A$_2$ secretors. *Aust J Exp Biol Med Sci* 1967;45:485–93.

268 Randeria KJ, Bhatia HM. Quantitative inhibition studies on the ABH and Lewis antigens in saliva. *Ind J Med Res* 1971;59:1737–53.

269 Prodanov P. Etude quantitative des antigènes ABH dans la salive des nouveau-nés et des adultes. *Rev Franc Transfus Immuno-Hémat* 1979;22:387–97.

270 Plato CC, Gershowitz H. Specific differences in the inhibition titers of the anti-H lectins from *Cytisus sessilifolius* and *Ulex europaeus*. *Vox Sang* 1961;6:336–47.

271 Plato CC, Gershowitz H. Differences between families in the amount of salivary H substances. *Ann Hum Genet* 1962;26:47–50.

272 Giusti GV, Panari G, Floris MT. Population and family

studies on the amount of salivary ABH blood group substances. *Vox Sang* 1972;**22**:54–63.

273 Fiori A, Giusti GV, Panari G. Gel filtration of ABH blood group substances. II. Individual gel chromatographic patterns of ABH substances in the saliva of secretors and non-secretors. *J Chromatogr A* 1971; **55**:351–63.

274 Kimberling WJ. The genetics of an expanded secretor system. *J Immunogenet* 1979;**6**:75–82.

275 Mohn JF, Owens NA, Plunkett RW. The inhibitory properties of group A and B non-secretor saliva. *Immunol Commun* 1981;**10**:101–26.

276 Hostrup H. A and B blood group substances in the serum of normal subjects. *Vox Sang* 1962;**7**:704–21.

277 Denborough MA, Downing HJ, Doig AG. Serum blood group substances and ABO haemolytic disease. *Br J Haematol* 1969;**16**:103–9.

278 Tilley CA, Crookston MC, Brown BL, Wherrett JR. A and B and A_1Le^b substances in glycosphingolipid fractions of human serum. *Vox Sang* 1975;**28**:25–33.

279 Holburn AM, Masters CA. The radioimmunoassay of serum and salivary blood group A and Le^a glycoproteins. *Br J Haematol* 1974;**28**:157–67.

280 Crookston MC. Antigens common to red blood cells and plasma. Plenary Sessions. *15th Congr Int Soc Blood Transfus.* Paris: Librairie Arnette 1978:51–61.

281 Graham HA, Hirsch HF, Davies DM Jr. Genetic and immunochemical relationships between soluble and cell-bound antigens of the Lewis system. *Human Blood Groups. 5th Int Convoc Immunol.* 1976. Basel: Karger 1977:257–67.

282 Renton PH, Hancock JA. Uptake of A and B antigens by transfused group O erythrocytes. *Vox Sang* 1962;**7**:33–8.

283 Garretta M, Muller A, Gener J, Matte C, Moullec J. Reliability in automatic determination of the ABO group by the groupamatic system. *Vox Sang* 1974;**27**:141–55.

284 Reed TE. The frequency and nature of blood group A_3. *Transfusion* 1964;**4**:457–60.

285 Friedenreich V. Eine bisher unbekannte Blutgruppeneigenschaft (A_3). *Z ImmunForsch* 1936;**89**:409–22.

286 Oguchi Y, Kawaguchi T, Suzuta T, Osawa T. The nature of human blood group A_3 erythrocytes. *Vox Sang* 1978;**34**:32–9.

287 Cartron JP. Etude des propriétés α-N-acétylgalactosaminyltransférasiques des sérums de sujets A et 'A faible'. *Rev Franc Transfus Immuno-Hémat* 1976;**19**:67–88.

288 Cartron JP, Badet J, Mulet C, Salmon C. Study of the α-N-acetylgalactosaminyltransferase in sera and red cell membranes of human A subgroups. *J Immunogenet* 1978;**5**:107–16.

289 Greenwell P, Watkins WM. Unpublished observations cited by Watkins WM, *Rev Franc Transfus Immuno-Hémat* 1978;**21**:201–28.

290 Olsson ML, Irshaid NM, Hosseini-Maaf B *et al.* Genomic analysis of clinical samples with serological ABO blood grouping discrepancies: identification of fifteen novel A and B subgroup alleles. *Blood* 2001;**98**:1585–1593.

291 Yamamoto F, McNeill PD, Yamamoto M *et al.* Molecular genetic analysis of the ABO blood group system. I. Weak subgroups: A_3 and B_3 Alleles. *Vox Sang* 1993; **64**:116–9.

292 Barjas-Castro ML, Carvalho MH, Locatelli MF, Bordin S, Saad STO. Molecular heterogeneity of the A_3 subgroup. *Clin Lab Haematol* 2000;**22**:73–8.

293 Olsson ML, Irshaid NM, Kuosmanen M, Pirkola A, Chester M. A splice-site mutation defines the A^{finn} allele at the blood group ABO locus. *Transfusion* 2000;**40** (Suppl.):13S [Abstract].

294 Yamamoto F, McNeill PD, Yamamoto M, Hakomori S, Harris T. Molecular genetic analysis of the ABO blood group system. A^x and $B^{(A)}$ alleles. *Vox Sang* 1993; **64**:171–4.

295 Olsson ML, Thuresson B, Chester MA. An A^{el} allele-specific nucleotide insertion at the blood group ABO locus and its detection using a sequence-specific polymerase chain reaction. *Biochem Biophys Res Commun* 1995;**216**:642–7.

296 Olsson ML, Chester MA. Polymorphisms at the *ABO* locus in subgroup A individuals. *Transfusion* 1996; **36**:309–13.

297 Weiner W, Sanger R, Race RRA. Weak form of the blood group antigen A: an inherited character. *Proc 7th Congr Int Soc Blood Transfus* 1959:720–5.

298 Sturgeon P, Moore BPL, Weiner W. Notations for two weak A variants: A_{end} A_{el}. *Vox Sang* 1964;**9**:214–5.

299 Mohn JF, Cunningham RK, Pirkola A, Furuhjelm U, Nevanlinna HR. An inherited blood group A variant in the Finnish population. I. Basic characteristics. *Vox Sang* 1973;**25**:193–211.

300 Nevanlinna HR, Pirkola A. An inherited blood group A variant in the Finnish population. II. Population studies. *Vox Sang* 1973;**24**:404–16.

301 Jenkins T. Blood group A_{bantu} population and family studies. *Vox Sang* 1974;**26**:537–50.

302 Fischer W, Hahn F. Ueber auffallende Schwäche der gruppenspezifischen Reaktionsfähigkeit bei einem Erwachsenen. *Z ImmunForsch* 1935;**84**:177–88.

303 Vos GH. Five examples of red cells with the A_x subgroup of blood group A. *Vox Sang* 1964;**9**:160–7.

304 Salmon C, Salmon D, Reviron J. Etude immunologique et génétique de la variabilité du phénotype A_x. *Nouv Rev Franc Hémat* 1965;**5**:275–90.

305 Jonsson B, Fast K. Ein eighartiger, familiärer typus von extrem schwachem A-faktor, 'A_6'. *Acta Path Microbiol Scand* 1948;**25**:649–55.

306 Estola E, Elo J. Occurence of an exceedingly weak 'A' blood group property in a family. *Ann Med Exp Fenn* 1952;30:79–87.

307 Grove-Rasmussen M, Soutter L, Levine P. A new blood subgroup (A₀) identifiable with group O serums. *Am J Clin Path* 1952;22:1157–63.

308 Stamps R, Sokol RJ, Leach M, Herron R, Smith G. A new variant of blood group A: A_{pae}. *Transfusion* 1987;27:315–8.

309 Mohn JF, Plunkett RW, Cunningham RK. Agglutination of group A_x erythrocytes by anti-A sera (group B). *Vox Sang* 1976;31:271–4.

310 Moore S, Chirnside A, Micklem LR, McClelland DBL, James K. A mouse monoclonal antibody with anti-A, (B) specificity which agglutinates A_x cells. *Vox Sang* 1984;47:427–34.

311 Beck ML, Hardman JT, Kowalski MA, Yates AD. Monoclonal anti-A reagents: correlation between reactivity with A_x and group B red blood cells. In: Rouger P, Salmon C, eds. *Monoclonal Antibodies Against Human Red Blood Cell and Related Antigens*. Paris: Arnette 1987:224–7.

312 Voak D. Monoclonal antibodies as blood grouping reagents. *Ballière's Best Pract Clin Haematol* 1990;3:219–42.

313 McDonald DF, Thompson JM. A new monoclonal anti-A antibody BIRMA-1: a potent culture supernatant which agglutinates A_x cells, but does not give undesirable reactions with B cells. *Vox Sang* 1991; 61:53–8.

314 van Loghem JJ, van der Hart M. The weak antigen A_4 occurring in the offspring of group O parents. *Vox Sang* 1954;4:69–75.

315 Beckers T, Dunsford I, van Loghem JJ. A second example of the weak antigen A_4 occurring in the offspring of group O parents. *Vox Sang* 1955;5:145–7.

316 Lanset S, Liberge G, Gerbal A, Ropartz C, Salmon C. Mise en évidence, dans une famille, d'une modification de l'expression des produits des locus ABO. *Rev Franc Transfus* 1970;13:431–4.

317 Cahan A, Jack JA, Scudder J et al. A family in which A_x is transmitted through a person of the blood group A_2B. *Vox Sang* 1957;2:8–15.

318 Ducos J, Marty Y, Ruffie J. A case of A_x phenotype transmitted by an A_2B parent. *Vox Sang* 1975;29: 390–3.

319 Salmon C, Carton JP. Le renforcement allèlique. *Rev Franc Transfus Immuno-Hémat* 1976;19:145–55.

320 Bird GWG, Roberts KD, Wingham J. Change of blood group from A_2 to A_x in a child with congenital abnormalities. *J Clin Path* 1975;28:962–3.

321 Salmon C, Borin P, André R. Le group sanguin A_m dans deux générations d'une mème famille. *Rev Hémat* 1958;13:529–37 and *Proc 7th Congr Int Soc Blood Transfus, Basel: Karger* 1959:709–15.

322 von Kindler M. Ein weiteres Beispiel einer schwachen A-Eigenschaft (A_m). *Blut* 1958, 1959;4:373–7.

323 Salmon C, Reviron J, Liberge G. Nouvel exemple d'une famille ou le phénotype A_m est observé dans 2 générations. *Nouv Rev Franc Hémat* 1964;4:359–64.

324 Cartron JP, Ropars C, Calkovská Z, Salmon C. Detection of A_1A_2 and $A_2A_m^{A1}$ heterozygotes among human A blood group phenotypes. *J Immunogenet* 1976; 3:155–61.

325 Ukita M, Yamada N, Seno T, Okubo Y, Yamaguchi H. An example of A_m due to a rare allele at the ABO locus with special reference to N-acetylgalactosaminyl-transferase assay in serum. *Proc Jpn Acad* 1980;56:534–7.

326 Wiener AS, Gordon EB. A hitherto undescribed human blood group, A_m. *Br J Haematol* 1956;2:305–7.

327 Weiner W, Lewis HBM, Moores P, Sanger R, Race RR. A gene, y, modifying the blood group antigen A. *Vox Sang* 1957;2:25–37.

328 Lin-Chu M, Broadberry RE, Tsai SJL. Incidence of ABO subgroups in Chinese in Taiwan. *Transfusion* 1987;27:114–5.

329 Cartron JP, Gerbal A, Badet J, Ropars C, Salmon C. Assay of α-N-acetylgalactosaminyltransferases in human sera: further evidence for several types of A_m individuals. *Vox Sang* 1975;28:347–65.

330 Wrobel DM, McDonald I, Race C, Watkins WM. 'True' genotype of chimeric twins revealed by bloodgroup gene products in plasma. *Vox Sang* 1974;27: 395–402.

331 Hansen T, Namork E, Olsson ML, Chester MA, Heier HE. Different genotypes causing indiscernible patterns of A expression on A_{el} red blood cells as visualized by scanning immunogold electron microscopy. *Vox Sang* 1998;75:47–51.

332 Gerbal A, Liberge G, Cartron J-P, Salmon C. Les phénotypes A_{end}: étude immunologique et génétique. *Rev Franc Transfus* 1970;13:243–50.

333 Darnborough J, Voak D, Pepper RM. Observations on a new example of the A_m phenotype which demonstrates reduced A secretion. *Vox Sang* 1973;24:216–27.

334 Ducos J, Marty Y, Ruffie J. A family with one child of phenotype A_m providing further evidence for the existence of the modifier genes Yy. *Vox Sang* 1975;28:456–9.

335 Drozda EA, Dean JD. Another example of the rare A_y phenotype. *Transfusion* 1985;25:280–1.

336 Koscielak J, Lenkiewicz B, Zielenski J, Seyfried H. Weak A phenotypes possibly caused by mutation. *Vox Sang* 1986;50:187–90.

337 Reed TE, Moore BPL. A new variant of blood group A. *Vox Sang* 1964;9:363–6.

338 Solomon JM, Sturgeon P. Quantitative studies of the phenotype A_{el}. *Vox Sang* 1964;9:476–86.

339 Lanset S, Liberge G, Gerbal A, Ropartz C, Salmon C. Le

phénotype Ael: étude immunologique et génétique. *Nouv Rev Franc Hémat* 1970;**10**:389–400.

340 Lau P, Sererat S, Beatty J, Oilschlager R, Kini J. Group A variants defined with a monoclonal anti-A reagent. *Transfusion* 1990;**30**:142–5.

341 Heier HE, Namork E, Calkovská Z, Sandin R, Kornstad L. Expression of A antigens on erythrocytes of weak blood group A subgroups. *Vox Sang* 1994;**66**:231–6.

342 Yamaguchi H, Okubo Y, Tanaka M. A rare blood B_x analogous to A_x in a Japanese family. *Proc Jpn Acad* 1970;**46**:446–9.

343 Salmon C. Les phénotypes B faibles B_3, B_x, B_{el} classification pratique proposée. *Rev Franc Transfus Immuno-Hémat* 1976;**19**:89–104.

344 Lopez M, Le Meud J, Gerbal A, Salmon C. Mesures d'agglutination quantitative des phénotypes B faibles. *Nouv Rev Franc Hémat* 1973;**13**:107–18.

345 Salmon C, Liberge G, Gerbal A, Lopez M. Heterogeneity of B_{60} phenotype including B_3 and some B_x. *Biomedicine* 1974;**21**:465–70.

346 Lopez M, Bouguerra A, Lemeud J, Badet J, Salmon C. Quantitative, kinetic and thermodynamic analysis of weak B_{60} erythrocyte phenotypes: heterogeneity among families—identity within a family. *Vox Sang* 1974; **27**:243–53.

347 Wiener AS, Cioffi AF. A group B analogue of subgroup A_3. *Am J Clin Path* 1972;**58**:693–7.

348 Garretta M, Muller A, Salmon C. Fréquence réelle des phénotypes B faible. *Rev Franc Transfus Immuno-Hémat* 1978;**21**:193–200.

349 Lin-Chu M, Broadberry RE, Chiou PW. The B_3 phenotype in Chinese. *Transfusion* 1986;**126**:428–30.

350 Chassaigne M, Lopez M, Krawczynska S, Saint-Paul B. Etude quantitative et thermodynamique de l'antigène B dans une famille comportant des sujets de phénotype B_3 et AB_3. *Rev Franc Transfus Immuno-Hémat* 1977;**20**:565–73.

351 Simie S. Weak B_3 antigen in a family. *Rev Franc Transfus Immuno-Hémat* 1983;**26**:625–6.

352 Badet J, Huet M, Mulet C et al. B-gene specified 3-α-D-galactosyltransferase activity in human blood group variants. *FEBS Lett* 1980;**122**:25–8.

353 Yokoyama M, Stacey SM, Dunsford I. B_x: a new subgroup of the blood group B. *Vox Sang* 1957;**2**:348–56.

354 Levine P, Celano M, Griset T. B_w: a new allele of the ABO locus. *Proc 6th Congr Int Soc Blood Transfus* 1958;132–5.

355 Ikemoto S, Furuhata T. Serology and genetics of a new blood type B_m. *Nature New Biol* 1971;**231**:184–5.

356 Simmons A, Twaitt J. Another example of a B variant. *Transfusion* 1975;**15**:359–62.

357 Koscielak J, Pacuszka T, Dzierzkowa-Borodej W. Activity of B-gene-specified galactosyltransferase in individuals with B_m phenotypes. *Vox Sang* 1976;**30**:58–67.

358 Yoshida A, Yamato K, Davé V, Yamaguchi H, Okubo Y. A case of weak blood group B expression (B_m) associated with abnormal blood group galactosyltransferase. *Blood* 1982;**59**:323–7.

359 Kogure T. The action of group B_m or CisAB sera on group O red cells in the presence of UDP-D-galactose. *Vox Sang* 1975;**29**:51–8.

360 Takizawa H, Kishi K, Iseki S. Biochemical and serological studies on α-galactosyltransferases in the sera and salivas from blood group B_m and A_1B_m individuals. *Proc Jpn Acad* 1978;**54**:402–7.

361 Yoshida A, Fujii H, Davé V, Cozant MJ, Morel PA. Membrane abnormality in red blood cells with weak type B expression. *Blood* 1980;**56**:881–5.

362 Kogure T, Iseki S. A family of B_m, due to a modifying gene. *Proc Jpn Acad* 1970;**46**:728–32.

363 Gundolf F, Andersen J. Variant of group B lacking the B antigen on the red cells. *Vox Sang* 1970;**18**:216–21.

364 Marsh WL, Ferrari M, Nichols ME, Fernandez G, Cooper K. $B_m{}^H$: a weak B antigen variant. *Vox Sang* 1973;**25**:341–6.

365 Yamaguchi H, Okazaki S, Hasegawa H et al. A weak B variant B_{el} occuring in a Japanese family. *Proc Jpn Acad* 1976;**52**:145–7.

366 Feng CS, Cook JL, Beattie KM et al. Variant type B blood in an El Salvador family: expression of a variant B gene enhanced by the presence of an A^2 gene. *Transfusion* 1984;**24**:264–6.

367 Yoshida A. The existence of atypical blood group galactosyltransferase which causes an expression of A_2 character in A_1B red blood cells. *Am J Hum Genet* 1983;**35**:1117–25.

368 Boorman KE, Zeitlin RA. B_v: a sub-group of B which lacks part of the normal human B antigen. *Vox Sang* 1964;**9**:278–88.

369 Mak KH, Voak D, Chu RW, Leong S, Chua KM. B_v: a distinct category of B sub-group among Chinese blood donors in Hong Kong. *Transfus Med* 1992;**2**:129–33.

370 Galili U. The two antibody specificities within human anti-blood group B antigens. *Transfus Med Rev* 1988;**2**:112–21.

371 Jakobowicz R, Simmons RT, Whittingham S. A sub-group of group B blood. *Vox Sang* 1961;**6**:706–9.

372 Gibbs MB, Akeroyd JH, Zapf JJ. Quantitative sub-groups of the B antigen in man and their occurrence in three racial groups. *Nature* 1961;**192**:1196–7.

373 Badet J, Ropars C, Cartron JP, Doinel C, Salmon C. Groups of α-D-galactosyltransferase activity in sera of individuals with normal B phenotype. *Vox Sang* 1976;**30**:105–13.

374 Marsh WL, Nichols ME, Øyen R et al. Inherited mocaicism affecting the ABO blood groups. *Transfusion* 1975;**15**:589–95.

375 Furuhata T, Kitahama M, Nozawa T. A family study of the so-called blood group chimera. *Proc Jpn Acad* 1959;**35**:55–7.

376 Kitahama M. Two families study of the erythrocyte antigen mosaicism. *Shinshu Med J* 1963;**12**:641–8.

377 Ogita Z, Kikkawa H, Yamamoto K, Murakami F. Erythrocyte antigen mosaicism in a Japanese family. *Jpn J Hum Genet* 1969;13:264–71.

378 Bird GWG, Wingham J, Watkins WM, Greenwell P, Cameron AH. Inherited 'mosaicism' within the ABO blood group system. *J Immunogenet* 1978;5:215–9.

379 Borley R, Hsu TCS, Sawitsky A, Johnson CL, Marsh WL. Mosaicism of red cell ABO type without reognizable cause. *Rev Franc Transfus Immuno-Hémat* 1980;23:299–304.

380 Gillespie EM, Gold ER. Weakening of the B-antigen by the presence of A_1 as shown by reactions with *Fomes fomentarius* (anti-B) extract. *Vox Sang* 1960;5:497–502.

381 Downie DM, Madin DF, Voak D. An evaluation of salmon anti-B reagent in manual and automated blood grouping. *Med Lab Sci* 1977;34:319–24.

382 Fernandez-Cabadi Y. Interaction entre allèles normaux A_1 ou A_2 et B chez l'hétérozygote AB. étude comparative portant sur des familles Européennes et Africaines. *Rev Franc Transfus Immuno-Hémat* 1980;23:661–74.

383 Sacks SH, Lennox ES. Monoclonal anti-B as a new blood-typing reagent. *Vox Sang* 1981;40:99–104.

384 Alter AA, Rosenfield RE. The nature of some subtypes of A. *Blood* 1964;23:605–20.

385 Morel PA, Watkins WM, Greenwell P. Genotype A^1B expressed as phenotype A^2B in a Black population. *Transfusion* 1984;24:426 [Abstract].

386 Yoshida A, Davè V, Hamilton HB. Imbalance of blood group A subtypes and the existence of superactive B^* gene in Japanese in Hiroshima and Nagasaki. *Am J Hum Genet* 1988;43:422–8.

387 Young LE, Witetsky E. Studies on the sub-groups of blood group A and AB. II. The agglutinogen A_3: its detection with potent B serum and an investigation of its inheritance. *J Immunol* 1945;51:111–6.

388 Watkins WM, Greenwell P. Molecular basis of human red cell antigens. *Proc 10th Int Congr Soc Forens Haemogenet* 1983:67–75.

389 Yoshida A. Identification of A_1B and A_2B blood types in paternity tests. *Transfusion* 1984;24:183–4.

390 Hrubriško M. Exemple d'une interaction allélique chez l'homme:interaction entre une variante du gène B (B_x ou B_{20}) et A_2. *Nouv Rev Franc Hémat* 1968;8:278–84.

391 Hrubisko M, Mergancová O, Prodanov P, Hammerová T, Racková M. Interallelic competition and complementation in the ABO blood group system. *Immunol Commun* 1980;9:139–53.

392 Salmon C, Cartron JP. Interactions in AB heterozygotes. In: Greenwalt TJ, Steane EA, eds. *CRC Handbook Series in Clinical Laboratory Science: Section D. Blood Banking* Vol. 1. Cleveland: CRC Press 1977:131–8.

393 Watkins WM, Greenwell P, Yates AD. The genetic and enzymic regulation of the synthesis of the A and B determinants in the ABO blood group system. *Immunol Commun* 1981;10:83–100.

394 Yates AD, Watkins WM. The biosynthesis of blood group B determinants by the blood group A gene-specified α-3-N-acetyl-D-galactosaminyltransferase. *Biochem Biophys Res Commun* 1982;109:958–65.

395 Yates AD, Feeney J, Donald ASR, Watkins WM. Characterisation of a blood-group A-active tetrasaccharide synthesised by a blood-group B gene-specified glycosyltransferase. *Carbohydr Res* 1984;130:251–60.

396 Greenwell P, Yates AD, Watkins WM. UDP-N-acetyl-D-galactosamine as a donor substrate for the glycosyltransferase encoded by the B gene at the human blood group *ABO* locus. *Carbohydr Res* 1986;149:149–70.

397 Yates AD. Overlapping functions of the glycosyltransferases encoded by the blood group A and B genes: biochemical basis and practical implications. In: Moore, SB, ed. *Progress in Immunohematology*. Arlington VA: American Association of Blood Banks 1988:65–91.

398 Beck ML, Yates AD, Hardman J, Kowalski MA. Identification of a subset of group B donors reactive with monoclonal anti-A reagent. *Am J Clin Pathol* 1989;92:625–9.

399 Goldstein J, Lenny L, Davies D, Voak D. Further evidence for the presence of A antigen on group B erythrocytes through the use of specific exoglycosidases. *Vox Sang* 1989;57:142–6.

400 Fukumori Y, Ohnoki S, Yoshimura K *et al*. Rapid detection of the cisAB allele consisting of a chimera of normal A and B alleles by PCR-RFLPs. *Transfus Med* 1996;6:337–44.

401 Yamamoto F, McNeill PD, Kominato Y *et al*. Molecular genetic analysis of the ABO blood group system. *cis*-AB alleles. *Vox Sang* 1993;64:120–3.

402 Yu L-C, Lee H-L, Chan Y-S, Lin M. The molecular basis for the *B(A)* allele: an amino acid alteration in the human histoblood group B α-(1,3)-galactosyltransferase increases its intrinsic α-(1,3)-N-acetylgalactosaminyltransferase activity. *Biochem Biophys Res Commun* 1999;262:487–93.

403 Mifsud NA, Watt JM, Condon JA, Haddad AP, Sparrow RL. A novel *cis*-AB variant allele arising from a nucleotide substitution A796C in the B transferase gene. *Transfusion* 2000;40:1276–7.

404 Voak D, Sonnerborn H, Yates A. The $A_1(B)$ phenomenon: a monoclonal anti-B (BS-85) demonstrates low level of B determinants on A_1 red cells. *Transfus Med* 1992;2:119–27.

405 Seyfried H, Walewska I, Werbilinska B. Unusual inheritance of ABO group in a family with weak B antigens. *Vox Sang* 1964;9:268–77.

406 Yamaguchi H, Okubo Y, Hazama F. Another Japanese A_2B_3 blood-group family with the propositus having O-group father. *Proc Jpn Acad* 1966;42:517–20.

407 Reviron J, Jacquet A, Delarue F *et al*. Interactions alléliques des gènes de groupes sanguines ABO: résultats préliminaires avec l'anti-B d'un sujet 'cis AB' et étude quantitative avec l'anti-B d'un sujet A_1O. *Nouv Rev Franc Hémat* 1967;7:425–33.

408 Reviron J, Jacquet A, Salmon C. Un exemple de chromosome 'cis A1': étude immunologique et génétique de phénotype induit. *Nouv Rev Franc Hémat* 1968;8:323–38.

409 Kogure T. A family with unusual inheritance of ABO blood groups. *Jpn J Hum Genet* 1971;16:69–87.

410 Yamaguchi H. A review of *cis*AB blood. *Jpn J Hum Genet* 1973;18:1–9.

411 Salmon C, Lopez M, Liberge G, Gerbal A. Le complexe CisAB du système ABO. *Rev Franc Transfus Immuno-Hémat* 1975;18:11–25.

412 Pacuszka T, Koscielak J, Seyfried H, Walewska I. Biochemical, serological and family studies in individuals with *CisAB* phenotypes. *Vox Sang* 1975;29:292–300.

413 Hummel K, Badet J, Bauermeister W *et al.* Inheritance of Cis-AB in three generations (family Lam). *Vox Sang* 1977;33:290–8.

414 Sabo BH, Bush M, German J, Carne LR, Yates AD, Watkins WM. The *cis*AB phenotype in three generations of one family: serological, enzymatic and cytogenetic studies. *J Immunogenet* 1978;5:87–106.

415 Valdes MD, Zoes C, Froker A. Unusual inheritance in the ABO blood group system: a group O child from a group A_2B mother. *Vox Sang* 1978;35:176–80.

416 Yoshida A, Yamaguchi H, Okubo Y. Genetic mechanism of *CisAB* inheritance. I. A case associated with unusual chromosomal crossing over. *Am J Hum Genet* 1980;32:332–8.

417 Bennett M, Levene C, Greenwell P. An Israeli family with six *cis*AB members: serologic and enzymatic studies. *Transfusion* 1998;38:441–8.

418 Lopez M. Le groupe sanguin *Cis* AB: étude quantitative et qualitative des antigènes ABH. *Rev Franc Transfus Immuno-Hémat* 1976;19:117–26.

419 Badet J, Ropars C, Salmon C. α-N-acetyl-D-galactosaminyl- and α-D-galactosyltransferase activities in sera of *cis* AB blood group individuals. *J Immunogenet* 1978;5:221–31.

420 Yoshida A, Yamaguchi H, Okubo Y. Genetic mechanism of Cis-AB inheritance. II. Cases associated with structural mutation of blood group glycosyltransferase. *Am J Hum Genet* 1980;32:645–50.

421 Bhende YM, Deshpande CK, Bhatia HM *et al.* A 'new' blood-group character related to the ABO system. *Lancet* 1952;i:903–4.

422 Moores PP, Issitt PD, Pavone BG, McKeever BG. Some observations on 'Bombay' bloods, with comments on evidence for the existence of two different O_h phenotypes. *Transfusion* 1975;15:237–43.

423 Bhatia HM. Serologic reactions of ABO and O_h (Bombay) phenotypes due to variations in H antigens. In: *Human Blood Groups. 5th Int Convoc Immunol, Buffalo NY.* Basel: Karger 1977:296–305.

424 Dzierzkowa-Borodej W, Meinhard W, Nestorowicz S,

425 Piróg J. Successful elution of anti-A and certain anti-H reagents from two 'Bombay' ($O_h{}^A$) blood samples and investigation of isoagglutinins in their sera. *Arch Immunol Ther Exp* 1972;20:841–9.

425 Rodier L, Lopez M, Liberge G *et al.* Anti-H absorbed by, and eluted from O_h (Bombay) red blood cells. *Biomedicine* 1974;21:312–6.

426 Levine P, Robinson E, Celano M, Briggs O, Falkinburg L. Gene interaction resulting in suppression of blood group substance B. *Blood* 1955;10:1100–8.

427 Lanset S, Ropartz C, Rousseau P-Y, Guerbet Y, Salmon C. Une famille comportant les phénotypes Bombay: $O_h{}^{AB}$ et $O_h{}^B$. *Transfusion (Paris)* 1966;9:255–63.

428 Ceppellini R, Nasso S, Tecilazich F. *La Malattia Emolitica de Neonato.* Istituto Sieroterapico Milanese Serafino Belfanti: Milano 1952;204.

429 Watkins WM, Morgan WTJ. Some observations on the O and H characters of human blood and secretions. *Vox Sang (Old Series)* 1955;5:1–14.

430 Aloysia M, Gelb AG, Fudenberg H *et al.* The expected 'Bombay' groups $O_h{}^{A1}$ and $O_h{}^{A2}$. *Transfusion* 1961;1:212–17.

431 Abu Sin AYH, Abdelrazig H, Ayoub M, Sabo BH. Bombay (O_h) blood in a Sudanese family. *Vox Sang* 1976;31:48–53.

432 Bhatia HM, Sanghvi LD. Rare blood groups and consanguinity: 'Bombay' Phenotype. *Vox Sang* 1962;7:245–8.

433 Cartron JP, Mulet C. Etude des activités 2-α-L fucosyltransférasiques des sérums et des membranes érythrocytaires de sujets 'Bombay' et 'Para-Bombay. *Rev Franc Transfus Immuno-Hémat* 1978;21:29–46.

434 Wagner T, Vadon M, Staudacher E *et al.* A new *h* allele detected in Europe has a missense mutation in a α (1,2)-fucosyltransferase motif II. *Transfusion* 2001;41:31–8.

435 Le Pendu J, Clamagirand-Mulet C, Cartron J-P *et al.* H-deficient blood groups of Réunion Island. III. α-2-L-fucosyltransferase activity in sera of homozygous and heterozygous individuals. *Am J Hum Genet* 1983;35:497–507.

436 Poschmann A, Fischer K, Seidl S, Spielmann W. ABH receptors and red cell survival in a 'Bombay' blood. *Vox Sang* 1974;27:338–46.

437 Bhatia HM, Sathe M, Gandhi S, Mehta BC, Levine P. Difference between Bombay and Rh$_{null}$ phenotypes. *Vox Sang* 1974;26:272–5.

438 Bhatia HM, Sathe MS. Incidence of 'Bombay' (O_h) phenotype and weaker variants of A and B antigen in Bombay (India). *Vox Sang* 1974;27:524–32.

439 Le Pendu J, Gerard G, Vitrac D *et al.* H deficient blood groups of Réunion Island. II. Differences between Indians (*Bombay phenotype*) Whites (*Réunion Phenotype*). *Am J Hum Genet* 1983;35:484–96.

440 Salmon C, Rouger P, Rodier L *et al.* Different H deficient

phenotypes present in one kindred. *Rev Franc Transfus Immuno-Hémat* 1980;23:251–8.

441 Iseki S, Takizawa H, Takizawa H. Immunological properties of 'Bombay' phenotype. *Proc Jpn Acad* 1970;46:803–7.

442 Kaneko M, Nishihara S, Shinya N *et al*. Wide variety of point mutations in the *H* gene of Bombay and para-Bombay individuals that inactivate H enzyme. *Blood* 1997;90:839–49.

443 Beattie KM, Saeed SM. Bombay phenotype. *Transfusion* 1976;16:290.

444 Sringarm S, Sombatpanich B, Chandanayingyong D. A case of O_h (Bombay) blood found in a Thai-Muslin patient. *Vox Sang* 1977;33:364–8.

445 Levine P, Uhlír M, White J. A_h, an incomplete suppression of A resembling O_h. *Vox Sang* 1961;6:561–7.

446 Beranová G, Prodanov P, Hrubisko M, Smálik S. A new variant in the ABO blood group system: B_h. *Vox Sang* 1969;16:449–56.

447 Gerard G, Vitrac D, Le Pendu J, Muller A, Oriol R. H-deficient blood groups (Bombay) of Réunion Island. *Am J Hum Genet* 1982;34:937–47.

448 Voak D, Stapleton RR, Bowley CC. $A_{2h}{}^{A1}$: a new variant of A_h, in two group A members of an English family. *Vox Sang* 1968;14:18–30.

449 Prodanov P, Drazhev G. $A_{xh}{}^{A1}$ variant of A_h in a Bulgarian family. *Vox Sang* 1978;34:162–3.

450 Gérard G, Guimbretière J, Guimbretière L. Difficultés de groupage chez un sujet vraisemblablement A_h. *Rev Franc Transfus* 1970;13:267–74.

451 Gerard G, Guimbretiere L, Lebot S, Guimbretiere J. Un nouveau cas de A_h. *Rev Franc Transfus Immuno-Hémat* 1975;18:321–3.

452 Liberge G, Salmon C, Gerbal A, Lopez M. Le phénotype B_h. *Rev Franc Transfus* 1970;13:357–63.

453 Mulet C, Cartron J-P, Schenkel-Brunner H *et al*. Probable biosynthetic pathway for the synthesis of the B antigen from B_h variants. *Vox Sang* 1979;37:272–80.

454 Solomon JM, Waggoner R, Leyshon WC. A quantitative immunogenetic study of gene suppression involving A_1 and H antigens of the erythrocyte without affecting secreted blood group substances: the ABH Phenotypes $A^h{}_m O^h{}_m$. *Blood* 1965;25:470–85.

455 Kitahama M, Yamaguchi H, Okubo Y, Hazama E. An apparently new B_h-like human blood-type. *Vox Sang* 1967;12:354–60.

456 Hrubisko M, Laluha J, Mergancová O, Zákovicova S. New variants in the ABOH blood group system due to interaction of recessive genes controlling the formation of H antigen in erythrocytes: the 'Bombay'-like phenotypes O_{Hm}, $O^B{}_{Hm}$ and $O^{AB}{}_{Hm}$. *Vox Sang* 1970; 19:113–22.

457 Hrubisko M. Deficient H phenotypes. *Rev Franc Transfus Immuno-Hémat* 1976;19:157–74.

458 Daniels GL. *Blood group antigens of high frequency: a serological and genetical study*. PhD thesis, University of London, 1980.

459 Mak KH, Lubenko A, Greenwell P *et al*. Serologic characteristics of H-deficient phenotypes among Chinese in Hong Kong. *Transfusion* 1996;36:994–9.

460 Sringarm S, Chupungart C, Giles CM. The use of *Ulex europaeus* and *Dolichos biflorus* extracts in routine ABO grouping of blood donors in Thailand: some unexpected findings. *Vox Sang* 1972;23:537–45.

461 Fawcett KJ, Eckstein EG, Innella F, Yokoyama M. Four examples of $B^h{}_m$ blood in one family. *Vox Sang* 1970;19:457–67.

462 Yu L-C, Yang Y-H, Broadberry RE, Chen Y-H, Lin M. Heterogeneity of the human *H* blood group $\alpha(1,2)$fucosyltransferase gene among para-Bombay individuals. *Vox Sang* 1997;72:36–40.

463 Rouger P, Juszczak G, Doinel C *et al*. Relationship between I and H antigens. II. Study of the H and I deficient phenotypes. *Immunol Commun* 1980;9:161–72.

464 Mulet C, Cartron JP, Lopez M, Salmon C. ABH glycosyltransferase levels in sera and red cell membranes from H_z and H_m variant bloods. *FEBS Lett* 1978;90:233–8.

465 Prodanov P. Etude des variantes H-déficitaires dans la population bulgare. *Rev Franc Transfus Immuno-Hémat* 1978;21:1093–101.

466 Wang B, Koda Y, Soejima M, Kimura H. Two missense mutations of H type $\alpha(1,2)$fucosyltransferase gene (*FUT1*) responsible for para-Bombay phenotype. *Vox Sang* 1997;72:31–5.

467 Lin-Chu M, Broadberry RE, Tsai SJL, Chiou PW. The para-Bombay phenotype in Chinese persons. *Transfusion* 1987;27:388–90.

468 Sun C-F, Lo M-D, Lee C-H, Chu D-C. Novel mutations, including a novel $G^{659}A$ missense mutation, of the *FUT1* gene are responsible for the para-Bombay phenotype. *Ann Clin Laboratory Sci* 2000;30:387–90.

469 Chee K, Yip S, Chan P, Chow EY, Wong H. Molecular genetic analysis of para-Bombay phenotypes in Hong Kong Chinese. *Transfusion* 2000;40 (Suppl.):118S [Abstract].

470 Salmon C, Schwartzenberg L, André R. Observations sérologiques et génétiques sur le groupe sanguin A_3. *Sang* 1959;30:227–36.

471 Lin M, Broadberry RE. Modification of standard Western pretransfusion testing procedures for Taiwan. *Vox Sang* 1994;67:199–202.

472 Wagner FF, Flegel WA. Polymorphism of the *h* allele and the population frequency of sporadic nonfunctional alleles. *Transfusion* 1997;37:284–90.

473 Kelly RJ, Ernst LK, Larsen RD *et al*. Molecular basis for H blood group deficiency in Bombay (O_h) and para-Bombay individuals. *Proc Natl Acad Sci USA* 1994;91:5843–7.

474 Johnson PH, Mak MK, Leong S *et al*. Analysis of muta-

tions in the blood-group H gene in donors with H-deficient phenotypes. *Vox Sang* 1994;67 (Suppl. 2):25 [Abstract].

475 Yunis EJ, Svardal JM, Bridges RA. Genetics of the Bombay phenotype. *Blood* 1969;33:124–32.

476 Salmon C, Juszczak G, Liberge G *et al*. Une famille où un phénotype 'Hm' est transmis à travers trois générations. *Rev Franc Transfus Immuno-Hémat* 1978;21:21–7.

477 Salmon C, Cartron JP, Rouger P *et al*. H deficient phenotypes: a proposed practical classification Bombay A_h, H_z, H_m. *Rev Franc Transfus Immuno-Hémat* 1980; 23:233–48.

478 Frydman M, Etzioni A, Eidlitz-Markus T *et al*. Rambam–Hasharon syndrome of psychomotor retardation, short stature, defective neutrophil motility, and Bombay phenotype. *Am J Med Genet* 1992;44:297–302.

479 Frydman M, Vardimon D, Shalev E, Orlin JB. Prenatal diagnosis of Rambam–Hasharon syndrome. *Prenat Diagn* 1996;16:266–9.

480 Marquardt T, Brune T, Lühn K *et al*. Leukocyte adhesion deficiency II syndrome: a generalized defect in fucose metabolism. *J Pediatr* 1999;134:681–8.

481 Körner C, Linnebank M, Koch HG *et al*. Decreased availability of GDP-L-fucose in a patient with LADII with normal GDP-D-mannose dehydratase and FX protein activities. *J Leukoc Biol* 1999;66:95–8.

482 Becker DJ, Lowe JB. Leukocyte adhesion deficiency type II. *Biochim Biophys Acta* 1999;1455:193–204.

483 Etziono A, Tonetti M. Leukocyte adhesion deficiency II: from A to almost Z. *Immunol Rev* 2000;178:138–47.

484 Schechter Y, Etzioni A, Levene C, Greenwell P. A Bombay individual lacking H and Le antigens but expressing normal levels of α-2- and α-4-fucosyltransferases. *Transfusion* 1995;35:773–6.

485 Ørntoft TF, Meldgaard P, Pedersen B, Wolf H. The blood group ABO gene transcript is down-regulated in human bladder tumors and growth-stimulated urothelial cell lines. *Cancer Res* 1996;56:1031–6.

486 Herron R, Greenwell P, Westwood MC, Race AC, Smith DS, Watkins WM. An H-deficient blood with normal *H* tranferase levels. *Vox Sang* 1980;39:186–94.

487 Lopez M, Gerbal A, Salmon C. Excès d'antigène I dans les érythrocytes de phénotypes O_h, A_h et B_h. *Rev Franc Transfus* 1972;15:187–94.

488 Doinel C. Antigénicité I des hématies Bombay. *Rev Franc Transfus Immuno-Hémat* 1976;19:185–91.

489 Cameron C, Graham F, Dunsford I *et al*. Acquisition of a B-like antigen by red blood cells. *Br Med J* 1959;ii:29–32.

490 Lanset S, Ropartz C. A second example of acquired B-like antigen in a healthy person. *Vox Sang* 1971;20:82–4.

491 Herron R, Young D, Clark M *et al*. A specific antibody for cells with acquired B antigen. *Transfusion* 1982; 22:525–7.

492 Kline WE, Sullivan CM, Bowman RJ, Linden M. Ac-

quired B antigen and polyagglutination in a apparently healthy blood donor. *Rev Franc Transfus Immuno-Hémat* 1982;25:119–26.

493 Gerbal A, Ropars C. L'antigène B acquis. *Rev Franc Transfus Immuno-Hémat* 1976;19:127–44.

494 Gerbal A, Salmon C, Lichtenstein H, Wagner JC. Acquisition d'un antigène B chez des sujets de groupe A: recherche chez 200 malades d'un service de gastro-entérologie. *Nouv Press Med* 1975;4:2884–5.

495 Gerbal A, Maslet C, Salmon C. Immunological aspects of the acquired B antigen. *Vox Sang* 1975;28:398–403.

496 Fisher GF, Faé I, Dub E, Pickl WF. Analysis of the gene polymorphism of ABO blood group specific transferases helps diagnosis of acquired B status. *Vox Sang* 1992;62:113–6.

497 Yip SP, Choy WL, Chan CW, Choi CH. The absence of a B allele in acquired B blood group phenotype confirmed by a DNA based genotyping method. *J Clin Pathol* 1996;49:180–1.

498 Reznikoff-Etievant MF, Garretta M, Sylvestre R *et al*. Trois observations de phénotype érythrocytaire 'B acquis'. *Rev Franc Transfus* 1974;17:15–39.

499 Andreu G, Mativet S, Simonneau M, Pierre J, Salmon C. Un antigène B acquis chez un sujet de groupe A_2. *Rev Franc Transfus Immuno-Hémat* 1978;21:185–92.

500 Gerbal A, Liberge G, Lopez M, Salmon C. Un antigène B acquis chez un sujet de phénotype érythrocytaire $A_h{}^m$. *Rev Franc Transfus* 1970;13:61–70.

501 Andersen J. Weak atypical B-like character in the blood cells of 7 group A persons. *Acta Path Microbiol Scand* 1960;48:289–304.

502 Janvier D, Reviron M, Biernat S, Saint Paul B, Reviron J. Etude immunohématologique de 7 transformations B acquis à l'aide d'anti-B et d'anti-B acquis sélectionnés. *Rev Franc Transfus Immuno-Hémat* 1983;26:467–80.

503 Rouger P, Edelman L, Doinel C *et al*. Study of blood group B antigen with a specific monoclonal antibody (anti-B, b-183). *Immunology* 1983;49:77–82.

504 Barrie EK, Fraser RH, Munro AC *et al*. Monoclonal anti-B produced by the immunization of mice with soluble salivary glycoproteins. *J Immunogenet* 1983; 10:41–4.

505 Beck ML, Kowalski MA, Kirkegaard JR, Korth JL. Unexpected activity with monoclonal anti-B reagents. *Immunohematology* 1992;8:22.

506 Janvier D, Veaux S, Reviron M, Guignier F, Benbunan M. Serological characterization of murine monoclonal antibodies directed against acquired B red cells. *Vox Sang* 1990;59:92–5.

507 Okubo Y, Seno T, Tanaka M *et al*. Conversion of group A red cells by deacetylation to ones that react with monoclonal antibodies specific for the acquired B phenotype. *Transfusion* 1994;34:456–7.

508 Garratty G, Arndt P, Co A, Rodberg K, Furmanski M. Fatal hemolytic transfusion reaction resulting from

ABO mistyping of a patient with acquired B antigen detectable only by some monoclonal anti-B reagents. *Transfusion* 1996;**36**:351–7.

509 Beck ML, Kirkegaard JR. Annotation–monoclonal ABO blood grouping reagents: a decade later. *Immunohematology* 1995;**11**:67.

510 Kennedy MS, Waheed A, Moore J. ABO discrepancy with monoclonal ABO reagents caused by a pH-dependent autoantibody. *Immunohematology* 1995; **11**:71–3.

511 Veneman SC, Mead JH, Boucock BP, Masterson KC. Acquired B antigen in a volunteer blood donor. *Transfusion* 1999;**39**:453–4.

512 Stratton F, Renton PH. Acquisition of B-like antigen. *Br Med J* 1959;ii:244.

513 Springer GF, Ansell Hahn NJ. Acquisition of blood-group B-like bacterial antigens by human A and O erythrocytes. *Proc 8th Congr Int Soc Blood Transfus* 1962:219–21.

514 Marsh WL, Jenkins WJ, Walther WW. Pseudo B: an acquired group antigen. *Br Med J* 1959;ii:63–6.

515 Marsh WL. The pseudo B antigen: a study of its development. *Vox Sang* 1960;**5**:387–97.

516 Stayboldt C, Rearden A, Lane TA. B antigen acquired by normal A_1 red cells exposed to a patient's serum. *Transfusion* 1987;**27**:41–4.

517 Herron R, Smith DS. *In vitro* conversion of group A_1 red cells to the acquired B state. *Transfusion* 1986;**26**:303.

518 Gerbal A, Ropars C, Gerbal R *et al.* Acquired B antigen disappearance by *in vitro* acetylation associated with A_1 activity restoration. *Vox Sang* 1976;**31**:64–6.

519 Yamamoto H, Iseki S. Development of H-specificity in A substance by A-decomposing enzyme from *Clostridum tertium* A. *Proc Jpn Acad* 1968;**44**:263–8.

520 Roseman S. Glucosamine metabolism. I. *N*-acetylglucosamine deacetylase. *J Biol Chem* 1957; **226**:115–23.

521 Salmon C, Gerbal A. The acquired B antigen. In: Greenwalt TJ, Steane EA, eds. *CRC Handbook Series in Clinical Laboratory Science: Section D. Blood Banking*, Vol. 1. Cleveland: CRC Press 1977:193–200.

522 Rahuel C, Lubineau A, David S, Salmon C, Cartron JP. Acquired B antigen: further studies using synthetic oligosaccharides. *Blood Transfus Immuno-Hémat* 1983;**26**:347–58.

523 Beck ML, Kirkegaard J, Korth J, Judd WJ. Monoclonal anti-B reagents and the acquired B phenotype. *Transfusion* 1993;**33**:623–4.

524 Judd WJ, Annesley TM. The acquired B phenomenon. *Transfus Med Rev* 1996;**10**:111–7.

525 Janvier D, Guignier F, Reviron M, Reviron JA. A new polyagglutination, specific for acquired B + Tk red blood cells [Abstracts]. *20th Congr Int Soc Blood Transfus* 1988;302.

526 Andreu G, Doinel C, Cartron JP, Mativet S. Induction of

527 Judd WJ, McGuire-Mallory D, Anderson KM *et al.* Comcommitant T- and Tk-activation associated with acquired-B antigens. *Transfusion* 1979;**19**:293–8.

528 Klarkowski DB, Ford DS. A case of polyagglutination with features of Th and Tk activation associated with an acquired B antigen. *Transfusion* 1983;**23**:59–61.

529 Van Loghem JJ, Dorfmeier H, Van Der Hart M. Two A antigens with abnormal serologic properties. *Vox Sang* 1957;**2**:16–24.

530 Stratton F, Renton PH, Hancock JA. Red cell agglutinability affected by disease. *Nature* 1958;**181**:62–3.

531 Gold ER, Tovey GH, Benney WE, Lewis FJW. Changes in the group A antigen in a case of leukæmia. *Nature* 1959;**183**:892–3.

532 Salmon C. Blood groups changes in preleukemic states. *Blood Cells* 1976;**2**:211–20.

533 Crookston MC. Anomalous ABO, H and Ii phenotypes in disease. In: Garratty, G, ed. *Blood Group Antigens and Disease*. Arlington VA: American Association of Blood Banks 1983:67–84.

534 Benson K. Decreased ABH blood group antigen expression associated with preleukemic conditions and acute leukemia: loss of detectable B, then A antigens in a group AB patient progressing from a myelodysplastic syndrome to leukemia. *Immunohematology* 1991; **7**:89–93.

535 Salmon C, Dreyfus B, André R. Double population de globules différent seulement par l'antigène de groupe ABO, observée chez un malade leucémique. *Rev Hémat* 1958;**13**:148–53.

536 Salmon C, André R, Dreyfus B. Existe-t-il des mutations somatiques du gène de groupe sanguin A au cours de certaines leucémies aiguës? *Rev Franc Étud Clin Biol* 1959;**4**:468–71.

537 Popp HJ, Nelson M, Forsyth C, Falson M, Kronenberg H. Quantifying the loss of ABO antigenicity in a patient with acute myeloid leukaemia by flow cytometric analysis. *Immunohematology* 1995;**11**:5–7.

538 Renton PH, Stratton F, Gunson HH, Hancock JA. Red cells of all four ABO groups in a case of leukaemia. *Br Med J* 1962;i:294–7.

539 Salmon C, Salmon D. Déficit en antigène H chez certains sujets de groupe O atteints de leucémie aiguë. *Rev Franc Étud Clin Biol* 1965;**10**:212–4.

540 Ayres M, Salzano FM, Ludwig OK. Blood group changes in leukaemia. *J Med Genet* 1966;**3**:180–5.

541 Starling KA, Fernbach DJ. Changes in strength of A antigen in children with acute leukaemia. *Transfusion* 1970;**10**:3–5.

542 Saichua S, Chiewsilp P. Red cell ABH antigens in leukaemias and lymphomas. *Vox Sang* 1978;**35**: 154–9.

543 Bianco T, Farmer BJ, Sage RE, Dobrovic A. Loss of red

Tk polyagglutination by bacteroides fragilis culture supernatants. *Rev Franc Transfus Immuno-Hémat* 1979;**22**:551–61.

cell A, B, and H antigens is frequent in myeloid malignancies. *Blood* 2001;97:3633–9.

544 Kolins J, Holland PV, McGinniss MH. Multiple red cell antigen loss in acute granulocytic leukemia. *Cancer* 1978;42:2248–53.

545 Lopez M, Bonnet-Gajdos M, Reviron M *et al.* An acute leukaemia augured before clinical signs by blood group antigen abnormalities and low levels of A and H blood group transferase activities in erythrocytes. *Br J Haematol* 1986;63:535–9.

546 Kolins J, Allgood JW, Burghardt DC, Klein HG, McGinniss MH. Modifications of B, I, i, and Lewis[b] antigens in a patient with DiGuglielmo's erythroleukemia. *Transfusion* 1980;20:574–7.

547 Salmon C, Cartron JP, Lopez M *et al.* Level of the A, B and H blood group glycosyltransferases in red cell membranes from patients with malignant hemopathies. *Rev Franc Transfus Immuno-Hémat* 1984;27:625–37.

548 Yoshida A, Kumazaki T, Davé V, Blank J, Dzik WH. Suppressed expression of blood group B antigen and blood group galactosyltransferase in a preleukemic subject. *Blood* 1985;66:990–2.

549 Kuhns WJ, Oliver RTD, Watkins WM, Greenwell P. Leukaemia-induced alterations of serum glycosyltransferase enzymes. *Cancer Res* 1980;40:268–75.

550 Kessel D, Ratanatharathorn V, Chou T-H. Electrofocusing patterns of fucosyltransferases in plasma of patients with neoplastic disease. *Cancer Res* 1979;39:3377–80.

551 Skacel PO, Watkins WM. Significance of altered α-2-L-fucosyltransferase levels in serum of leukemic patients. *Cancer Res* 1988;48:3998–4001.

552 Kessell D, Shah-Reddy I, Mirchandani I, Khilanani P, Chou T-H. Electrofocusing patterns of fucosyltransferase activity in plasma of patients with chronic granulocytic leukemia. *Cancer Res* 1980;40:3576–8.

553 Kahn A, Vroclans M, Hakim J, Boivin P. Differences in the two red-cell populations in erythroleukæmia. *Lancet* 1971;ii:933.

554 Ozelius LJ, Kwiatkowski DJ. Schuback DE *et al.* A genetic linkage map of human chromosome 9q. *Genomics* 1992;14:715–20.

555 Haas OA, Argyriou-Tirita A, Lion T. Parental origin of chromosomes involved in the translocation t(9;22). *Nature* 1992;359:414–416.

556 Dobrovic A, O'Keefe D, Sage RE, Batchelder E. Imprinting and loss of ABO antigens in leukemia. *Blood* 1993;82:1684–5.

557 Salmon C, Mannoni P, Séger J *et al.* Double population de globules rouges pour les antigènes ABH chez trois sujets âgés. *Nouv Rev Franc Hémat* 1970;10:303–12.

558 Race RR, Sanger R. Blood group mosaics. *Haematologia* 1972;6:63–71.

559 Sherman LA, Silberstein LE, Berkman EM. Altered blood group expression in a patient with congenital rubella infection. *Transfusion* 1984;24:267–9.

560 Comenzo RL, Malachowski ME, Rohrer RJ *et al.* Anomalous ABO phenotype in a child after an ABO-incompatible liver transplantation. *N Engl J Med* 1992;326:867–70.

561 Garratty G, Arndt PA, Noguerol P, Plaza E, Jiminez J. Differentiation of post-bone marrow transplant chimerism versus adsorption of A antigen onto transplanted group O RBCs. *Transfusion* 1999;39 (Suppl.):44S [Abstract].

562 Goldstein J. Conversion of ABO blood groups. *Transfus Med Rev* 1989;3:206–12.

563 Harpaz N, Flowers HM, Sharon N. Studies on B-antigenic sites of human erythrocytes by use of coffee bean α-galactosidase. *Arch Biochem Biophys* 1975;170:676–83.

564 Zhu A, Leng L, Monahan C *et al.* Characterization of recombinant α-galactosidase for use in seroconversion from blood group B to O of human erythrocytes. *Arch Biochem Biophys* 1996;327:324–9.

565 Lenny LL, Hurst R, Zhu A, Goldstein J, Galbraith RA. Multiple-unit and second transfusions of red cells enzymatically converted from group B to group O: report on the end of phase 1 trials. *Transfusion* 1995;35:899–902.

566 Kruskall MS, AuBuchon JP, Anthony KY *et al.* Transfusion to blood group A and O patients of group B RBCs that have been enzymatically converted to group O. *Transfusion* 2000;40:1290–8.

567 Hoskins LC, Larson G, Naff GB. Blood group A immunodeterminants on human red cells differ in biologic activity and sensitivity to α-N-acetylgalactosaminidase. *Transfusion* 1995;35:813–21

568 Doinel C, Ropars C, Rufin JM. I and H activities of human red blood cells treated with an 1,2-α-L-fucosidase from aspergillus niger. *Rev Franc Transfus Immuno-Hémat* 1980;23:259–69.

569 Dobson AM, Ikin EW. The ABO blood groups in the United Kingdom: frequencies based on a very large sample. *J Pathol Bacteriol* 1946;48:221–7.

570 van Loghem JJ, van der Hart M, von Moes M, dem Borne AEGK. Increased red cell destruction in the absence of demonstrable antibodies *in vitro*. *Transfusion* 1965;5:525–32.

571 Springer GF, Tegtmeyer H. Absence of B antibody in a blood group A₁ person. *Vox Sang* 1974;26:247–58.

572 Kochwa S, Rosenfield RE, Tallal L, Wasserman LR. Isoagglutinins associated with ABO erythroblastosis. *J Clin Invest* 1961;40:874–83.

573 Mollison PL, Engelfriet CP, Contreras M. *Blood Transfusion in Clinical Medicine*, 10th edn. Oxford: Blackwell Science 1997.

574 Auf der Maur C, Hodel M, Nydegger UE, Rieben R. Age dependency of ABO histo-blood antibodies: reexamination of an old dogma. *Transfusion* 1993;33:915–8.

575 Somers H, Kuhns WJ. Blood group antibodies in old age (36943). *Proc Soc Exp Biol Med NY* 1972;141:1104–7.

576 Baumgarten A, Kruchok AH, Weirich F. High frequency of IgG anti-A and -B antibody in old age. *Vox Sang* 1976;30:253–60.

577 Nijenhuis LE, Bratlie K. ABO antibodies in twins. *Vox Sang* 1962;7:236–8.

578 Grundbacher FJ. Genetics of anti-A and anti-B levels. *Transfusion* 1976;16:48–55.

579 Springer GF, Horton RE, Forbes M. Origin of anti-human blood group B agglutinins in white Leghorn chicks. *J Exp Med* 1959;110:221–44.

580 Springer GF, Horton RE, Forbes M. Origin of antihuman blood group agglutinins in germfree chicks. *Ann NY Acad Sci* 1959;78:272–5.

581 Springer GF, Horton RE. Blood group isoantibody stimulation in man by feeding blood group-active bacteria. *J Clin Invest* 1969;48:1280–91.

582 Rieben R, Buchs JP, Flückiger E, Nydegger UE. Antibodies to histo-blood group substances A and B: agglutination titers, Ig class, and IgG subclasses in healthy persons of different age categories. *Transfusion* 1991;31:607–15.

583 Kunkel HG, Rockey JH. β_{2A} and other immunoglobulins in isolated anti-A antibodies. *Proc Soc Exp Biol NY* 1963;113:278–81.

584 Filitti-Wurmser S. Natural antibodies to immune antibodies of human ABO blood group system. *Biochimie* 1976;58:1345–53.

585 Contreras M, Armitage SE, Hewitt PE. Response to immunization with A and B human glycoproteins for the procurement of blood grouping reagents. *Vox Sang* 1984;47:224–35.

586 Brouwers HAA, Overbeeke MAM, Gemke RJBJ *et al.* Sensitive methods for determining subclasses of IgG anti-A and anti-B in sera of blood-group-O women with a blood-group-A or -B child. *Br J Haematol* 1987;66:267–70.

587 Putkonen T. Ubie die gruppenspezifischen Eigenschaften Verschiedener Koperflussigkeiten. *Acta Soc Med Fenn Duodecim Ser A* 1930;14:113.

588 Boettcher B. ABO blood group agglutinins in saliva. *Acta Haematol* 1967;38:351–60.

589 Jakobowicz R, Ehrlich M, Graydon JJ. Crossreacting antibody and saliva agglutinins. *Vox Sang* 1967;12:340–53.

590 Bell CE, Fortwengler HP. Salivary anti-A and anti-B activity of group O males. *Vox Sang* 1971;21:493–508.

591 Gershowitz H, Behrman SJ, Neel JV. Hemagglutinins in uterine secretions. *Science* 1958;128:719–20.

592 Solish GI, Gershowitz H, Behrman SJ. Occurrence and titer of isohemagglutinins in secretions of the human uterine cervix. *Proc Soc Exp Biol NY* 1961;108:645–9.

593 Ikin EW, Mourant AE, Pugh VW. An anti-Rh serum reacting differently with O and A red cells. *Vox Sang (Old Series)* 1953;3:74–8.

594 Dodd BE. Linked anti-A and **anti-B** antibodies from group O sera. *Br J Exp Path* 1952;33:1–17.

595 Bird GWG. Observations on haemagglutinin 'linkage' in relation to iso-agglutinins and auto-agglutinins. *Br J Exp Path* 1953;34:131–7.

596 Dodd BE, Lincoln PJ. The effect of elution on the reactivity of antibodies of the ABO system, including cross-reacting antibodies, as demonstrated by use of red cells of various subgroups of A, and group B. *Br J Haematol* 1974;26:93–104.

597 Holburn AM. Radioimmunoassay studies of the cross-reacting antibody of human group O sera. *Br J Haematol* 1976;32:589–99.

598 Owen RD. Heterogeneity of antibodies to the human blood groups in normal and immune sera. *J Immunol* 1954;73:29–39.

599 Schiffman G, Howe C. The specificity of blood group A-B cross-reacting antibody. *J Immunol* 1965;94:197–204.

600 Franks D, Liske R. The specificity of the cross-reacting antibodies in blood group O sera which produce mixed agglutination. *Immunology* 1968;14:433–44.

601 Conger JD, Chan MM, DePalma L. Analysis of the repertoire of human B-lymphocytes specific for type A and type B blood group terminal trisaccharide epitopes. *Transfusion* 1993;33:200–7.

602 Salmon C, Schwartzenberg L, André R. Anémie hémolytique post-transfusionnelle chez un sujet A_2 à la suite d'une injection massive de sang A_1. *Sang* 1959;30:223–7.

603 Boorman KE, Dodd BE, Loutit JF, Mollison PL. Some results of transfusion of blood to recipients with 'cold' agglutinins. *Br Med J* 1946;i:751–4.

604 Lundberg WB, McGinniss MH. Hemolytic transfusion reaction due to anti-A_1. *Transfusion* 1975;15:1–9.

605 Pineda AA, Taswell HF, Brzica SM. Delayed hemolytic transfusion reaction: an immunologic hazard of blood transfusion. *Transfusion* 1978;18:1–7.

606 Voak D. The serological specificity of the sensitising antibodies in ABO heterospecific pregnancy of the group O mother. *Vox Sang* 1968;14:271–81.

607 Issitt PD, Anstee DJ. *Applied Blood Group Serology*, 4th edn. Miami: Montgomery Scientific Publications 1998.

608 Brouwers HAA, Overbeeke MAM, Huiskes E *et al.* Complement is not activated in ABO-haemolytic disease of the newborn. *Br J Haematol* 1988;68:363–6.

609 Nelson PW, Landreneau MD, Luger AM *et al.* Ten-year experience in transplantation of A_2 kidneys into B and O recipients. *Transplantation* 1998;65:256–60.

610 Fishbein TM, Emre S, Guy SR *et al.* Safe transplantation of blood group type A_2 livers to blood type O recipients. *Transplantation* 1999;67:1071–3.

611 West LJ, Pollock-Barziv SM, Dipchand AI *et al.* ABO-

incompatible heart transplantation in infants. *N Engl J Med* 2001;344:793–800.

612 Eastlund T. The histo-blood group ABO system and tissue transplantation. *Transfusion* 1998;38:975–88.

613 Benjamin RJ, McGurk S, Ralston MS, Churchill WH, Antin JH. ABO incompatibility as an adverse risk factor for survival after alloantigenic bone marrow transplantation. *Transfusion* 1998;39:179–87.

614 Heal JM, Blumberg N. The second century of ABO: and now for something completely different. *Transfusion* 1999;39:1155–9.

615 Sokol RJ, Booker DJ, Stamps R, Windle JA. Autoimmune haemolysis and red cell autoantibodies with ABO blood group specificity. *Haematologia* 1995; 26:121–9.

616 Szymanski IO, Roberts PL, Rosenfield RE. Anti-A autoantibody with severe intravascular hemolysis. *N Engl J Med* 1976;294:995–6.

617 Spalter SH, Kaveri AV, Bonnin E *et al.* Normal human serum contains natural antibodies reactive with autologous ABO blood group antigens. *Blood* 1999;93:4418–24.

618 Beck ML, Haines RF, Oberman HA. Unexpected serologic findings following lung homotransplantation. *Prog 24th Mtg Am Assoc Blood Banks* 1971;98 [Abstract].

619 Ramsey G. Red cell antibodies arising from solid organ transplants. *Transfusion* 1991;31:76–86.

620 Minakuchi J, Toma H, Takahashi K, Ota K. Autoanti-A and -B antibody induced by ABO unmatched blood group kidney allograft. *Transplant Proc* 1985;17:2297–300.

621 Ahmed KY, Nunn G, Brazier DM, Bird GWG, Crockett RE. Hemolytic anemia resulting from autoantibodies produced by the donor's lymphocytes after renal transplantation. *Transplantation* 1987;43:163–4.

622 Petz LD. Immunohematologic problems associated with bone marrow transplantation. *Transfus Med Rev* 1987;1:85–100.

623 Petz LD. The expanding boundaries of transfusion medicine. In: Nance SJ, ed. *Clinical and Basic Science Aspects of Immunohematology.* Arlington VA: American Association of Blood Banks 1991:73–113.

624 Toren A, Dacosta Y, Manny N, Varadi G, Or R, Nagler A. Passenger B-lymphocyte-induced severe hemolytic disease after allogeneic peripheral blood stem cell transplantation. *Blood* 1996;87:843–4.

625 Bolan CD, Childs RW, Procter JL, Barrett AJ, Leitman AJ. Massive immune haemolysis after allogeneic peripheral blood stem cell transplantation with minor ABO incompatibility. *Br J Haematol* 2001;112:787–95.

626 Hows J, Beddow K, Gordon-Smith E *et al.* Donor-derived red blood cell antibodies and immune hemolysis after allogeneic bone marrow transplantation. *Blood* 1986;67:177–81.

627 Köhler G, Milstein C. Continuous cultures of fused cells secreting antibody of predefined specificity. *Nature* 1975;256:495–7.

628 Barnstable CJ, Bodmer WF, Brown G *et al.* Production of monoclonal antibodies to group A erythrocytes, HLA and other human cell surface antigens: new tools for genetic analysis. *Cell* 1978;14:9–20.

629 Voak D, Sacks S, Alderson T *et al.* Monoclonal anti-A from a hybrid-myeloma: evaluation as a blood grouping reagent. *Vox Sang* 1980;39:134–40.

630 Edelman L, Rouger P, Doinel C *et al.* Thermodynamic and immunological properties of a monoclonal antibody to human blood group A. *Immunology* 1981; 44:549–54.

631 Lowe AD, Lennox ES, Voak D. A new monoclonal anti-A: culture supernatants with the performance of hyperimmune human reagents. *Vox Sang* 1984;46: 29–35.

632 Messeter L, Brodin T, Chester MA, Löw B, Lundblad A. Mouse monoclonal antibodies with anti-A, anti-B and anti-A,B specificities; some superior to human polyclonal ABO reagents. *Vox Sang* 1984;46:185–94.

633 Guest AR, Scott ML, Smythe J, Judson PA. Analysis of the structure and activity of A and A,B immunoglobulin A monoclonal antibodies. *Transfusion* 1992;32: 239–45.

634 Abe K, Levery SB, Hakomori S-I. The antibody specific to type 1 chain blood group A determinant. *J Immunol* 1984;132:1951–4.

635 Furukawa K, Clausen H, Hakomori S *et al.* Analysis of the specificity of five murine anti-blood group A monoclonal antibodies, including one that identifies Type 3 and Type 4 A determinants. *Biochemistry* 1985;24:7820–6.

636 Gooi HC, Hounsell EF, Picard JK *et al.* Differing reactions of monoclonal anti-A antibodies with oligosaccharides related to blood group A. *J Biol Chem* 1985;260:13218–24.

637 Telen MJ. An antibody to human thymic Hassall's body epithelium recognizes a subset of blood group A antigens. *J Immunogenet* 1985;12:3–15.

638 Goossens D, Champomier F, Rouger P, Salmon C. Human monoclonal antibodies against blood group antigens: preparation of a series of stable EBV immortalized B clones producing high levels of antibody of different isotypes and specificities. *J Immunol Methods* 1987;101:193–200.

639 Raubitschek A, Senyk G, Larrick J, Lizak G, Foung S. Human monoclonal antibodies against group A red blood cells. *Vox Sang* 1985;48:305–8.

640 Inoue H, Hirohasi S, Shimosato Y *et al.* Establishment of an anti-A human monoclonal antibody from a blood group A lung cancer patient: evidence for the occurrence of autoimmune response to difucosylated type-2 chain A. *Eur J Immunol* 1989;19:2197–203.

641 Iwaki Y, Kasai M, Terasaki PI *et al.* Monoclonal antibody against A$_1$ Lewis d antigen produced by the hy-

bridoma immunized with a pulmonary carcinoma. *Cancer Res* 1982;42:409–11.

642 Clausen H, Levery SB, McKibbin JM, Hakomori S. Blood group A determinants with mono- and difucosyl Type 1 chain in human erythrocyte membranes. *Biochemistry* 1985;24:3578–86.

643 Clausen H, McKibbin JM, Hakomori S. Monoclonal antibodies defining blood group A variants with difucosyl Type 1 chain (ALe^b) and difucosyl Type 2 chain (ALe^y). *Biochemistry* 1985;24:6190–4.

644 Gooi HC, Picard JK, Hounsell EF *et al*. Monoclonal antibody (EGR/G49) reactive with the epidermal growth factor receptor of A431 cells recognizes the blood group ALe^b and ALe^y structures. *Mol Immunol* 1985; 22:689–93.

645 Chen H-T, Kabat EA. Immunochemical studies on blood groups: the combining site specificities of mouse monoclonal hybridoma anti-A and anti-B. *J Biol Chem* 1985;260:13208–17.

646 Watkins WM. Monoclonal antibodies as tools in genetic studies on carbohydrate blood group antigens. *J Immunogenet* 1990;17:259–76.

647 Lubenko A, Ivanyi J. Epitope specificity of blood-group-A-reactive murine monoclonal antibodies. *Vox Sang* 1986;51:136–42.

648 Lubenko A, Savage J. Analysis of the heterogeneity of the binding site specificities of hyperimmune human anti-A and -A,B sera: the application of competition assays using murine monoclonal antibodies. *Vox Sang* 1989;57:254–60.

649 Bundle DR, Gidney MAJ, Kassam N, Rahman AFR. Hybridomas specific for carbohydrates: synthetic human blood group antigens for the production, selection, and characterization of monoclonal typing reagents. *J Immunol* 1982;129:678–82.

650 Voak D, Lowe AD, Lennox E. Monoclonal antibodies: ABO serology. *Biotest Bull* 1983;4:291–9.

651 Chang TY, Siegel DL. Isolation of an IgG anti-B from a human Fab-phage display library. *Transfusion* 2001; 41:6–12.

652 Rouger P, Anstee D, Salmon C, eds. First International Workshop on Monoclonal Antibodies Against Human Red Blood Cell and Related Antigens. *Rev Franc Transfus Immuno-Hémat* 1987;30:353–717.

653 Chester MA, Johnson U, Lundblad A *et al*. eds. Monoclonal Antibodies Against Human Red Blood Cell and Related Antigens. *Proceedings of the 2nd International Workshop and Symposium* 1990.

654 Beck ML, eds. Third International Workshop on Monoclonal Antibodies Against Human Red Blood Cell and Related Antigens. *Transfus Clin Biol* 1997;4:13–54.

655 McGowan A, Tod A, Chirnside A *et al*. Stability of murine monoclonal anti-A, anti-B and anti-A,B ABO grouping reagents and a multi-centre evaluation of their performance in routine use. *Vox Sang* 1989;56:122–30.

656 Judson PA, Smythe JS. Mechanism of cryoprecipitation of anti-blood group B murine monoclonal antibodies. *Transfus Med* 1991;1:97–102.

657 Morgan WTJ, Watkins WM. The detection of a product of the blood group O gene and the relationship of the so-called O-substance to the agglutinogens A and B. *Br J Exp Path* 1948;29:159–73.

658 Hanfland P, Graham HA. Immunochemistry of the Lewis-blood-group system: partial characterization of Le^{a-}, Le^{b-}, and H-Type 1 (Le^{dH})-blood-group active glycosphingolipids from human plasma. *Arch Biochem Biophys* 1981;210:383–95.

659 Daniels GL. Studies on anti-H reagents. *Rev Franc Transfus Immuno-Hémat* 1984;27:603–12.

660 Le Pendu J, Lambert F, Gérard G *et al*. On the specificity of human anti-H antibodies. *Vox Sang* 1986;50:223–6.

661 Moores PP, Smart E, Gabriel B. Hemolytic disease of the newborn in infants of an O$_h$ mother. *Transfusion* 1994;34:1015–6.

662 Davey RJ, Tourault MA, Holland PV. The clinical significance of anti-H in an individual with the O$_h$ (Bombay) phenotype. *Transfusion* 1978;18:738–42.

663 Whitsett CF, Cobb M, Pierce JA, Parvin M. Immunological characteristics and clinical significance of anti-H in the A$_h$ phenotype. *Transfusion* 1984;24:164–5.

664 Sanger R. A relationship between the secretion of the blood group antigens and the presence of anti-O or anti-H in human serum. *Nature* 1952;170:78.

665 Watkins WM, Morgan WTJ. A potent group-O cell-agglutinin of human origin with H-specific character. *Lancet* 1954;i:959–61.

666 Uchikawa M, Tohyama H. A potent cold autoagglutinin that recognizes Type 2H determinant on red cells. *Transfusion* 1986;26:240–2.

667 Kuipers EJ, van Imhoff GW, Hazenberg CAM, Smit J. Anti-H IgM (kappa) autoantibody mediated severe intravascular haemolysis associated with malignant lymphoma. *Br J Haematol* 1991;78:283–5.

668 Joshi SR. Citrate-dependent auto-antibody causing an error in blood grouping. *Vox Sang* 1997;72:229–32.

669 Janvier D, Reviron M, Maury J. Relationship between antibodies dependent on calcium chelators and the H antigen. *Vox Sang* 1998;75:79–80.

670 Furukawa K, Mattes MJ, Lloyd KO. A$_1$ and A$_2$ erythrocytes can be distinguished by reagents that do not detect structural differences between the two cell types. *J Immunol* 1985;135:4090–4.

671 Knowles RW, Bai Y, Daniels GL, Watkins WM. Monoclonal anti-Type 2 H: an antibody detecting a precursor of the A and B blood group antigen. *J Immunogenet* 1982;9:69–76.

672 Anger BR, Lloyd KO, Oettgen HF, Old LO. Mouse monoclonal IgM antibody against human lung cancer line SK-LC-3 with specificity for H (O) blood group antigen. *Hybridoma* 1982;1:139–47.

673 Doinel C, Edelman L, Rouger P et al. A murine monoclonal antibody against blood group H type-1 and -2 structures. Immunology 1983;50:215–21.

674 Fredman P, Richert ND, Magnani JL et al. A monoclonal antibody that precipitates the glycoprotein receptor for epidermal growth factor is directed against the human blood group H Type 1 antigen. J Biol Chem 1983;258:11206–10.

675 Mollicone R, Cailleau A, Imberty A et al. Recognition of the blood group H type 2 trisaccharide epitope by 28 monoclonal antibodies and three lectins. Glycocon J 1996;13:263–71.

676 Kudryashov V, Ragupathi G, Kim IJ et al. Characterization of a mouse monoclonal IgG3 antibody to the tumor-associated globo H structure produced by immunization with a synthetic glycoconjugate. Glycocon J 1998;15:243–9.

677 Daniels GL. Unpublished observations.

678 Bhatia HM. Serological specificity of anti-H blood group antibodies. Ind J Med Res 1964;52:5–14.

679 Rosenfield RE, Schroeder R, Ballard R et al. Erythrocytic antigenic determinants characteristic of H, I in the presence of H [IH], or H in the absence of i [H(-i)]. Vox Sang 1964;9:415–9.

680 Lin-Chu M, Broadberry RE. Blood transfusion in the para-Bombay phenotype. Br J Haematol 1990; 75:568–72.

681 Campbell SA, Shirey RS, King KE, Ness PM. An acute hemolytic transfusion reaction due to anti-IH in a patient with sickle cell disease. Transfusion 2000;40:828–31.

682 Bird GWG, Wingham J. Erythrocyte autoantibody with unusual specificity. Vox Sang 1977;32:280–2.

683 Pierce SR, Kowalski MA, Hardman JT, Beck ML. Anti-Hi: more common than previously thought? [Abstracts]. Joint Congr Int Soc Blood Transfus and Am Assoc Blood Banks 1990:79.

684 Boyd WC, Shapleigh E. Antigenic relations of blood group antigens as suggested by tests with lectins. J Immunol 1954;73:226–31.

685 Goldstein IJ, Hughes RC, Monsigny M, Osawa T, Sharon N. What should be called a lectin? Nature 1980;285:66.

686 Morgan WTJ, Watkins WM. The inhibitions of the haemagglutinins in plant seeds by human blood group substances and simple sugars. Br J Exp Path 1953; 34:94–103.

687 Furukawa K, Ying R, Nakajima T, Matsuki T. Hemagglutinins in fungus extracts and their blood group specificity. Exp Clin Immunogenet 1995;12:223–31.

688 Boyd WC. The lectins: their present status. Vox Sang 1963;8:1–32.

689 Prokop O, Uhlenbruck G, Köhler W. A new source of antibody-like substances having anti-blood group specificity: discussion on the specificity of Helix agglutinins. Vox Sang 1968;14:321–33.

690 Sharon N, Lis H. Lectins: cell-agglutinating and sugar-specific proteins. Science 1972;177:949–59.

691 Bird GWG. Lectins in immunohematology. Transfus Med Rev 1989;3:55–62.

692 Renkonen KO. Studies on hemagglutinins present in seeds of some representatives of the family Leguminoseae. Ann Med Exp Fenn 1948;26:66–72.

693 Etzler ME, Kabat EA. Purification and characterization of a lectin (plant hemagglutinin) with blood group A specificity from Dolichos biflorus. Biochemistry 1970;9:869–77.

694 Boyd WC, Brown R. A specific agglutinin in the snail Otala (Helix) lactea. Nature 1965;208:593–4.

695 Hammarström S, Kabat EA. Studies on specificity and binding properties of the blood group A reactive hemagglutinin from Helix pomatia. Biochemistry 1971;10:1684–92.

696 Potapov MI. Untersuchung von Blutflecken und menschlichen Ausscheidungsprodukten mit dem Gruppenlektin Anti-B$_1$ (Evonymus alata). Folia Haemat 1970; 93:458–64.

697 Ottensooser F, Sato R, Sato M. A new anti-B lectin. Transfusion 1968;8:44–6.

698 Mäkelä O, Mäkelä P, Krüpe M. Zur spezifität der Anti-B-Phythamagglutine. Z ImmunForsch 1959;117: 220–9.

699 Prokop O, Schlesinger D, Geserick G. Thermostabiles B-agglutinin aus Konserven von Lachskaviar. Z Immun-Forsch 1967;132:491–4.

700 Todd GM. Blood group antibodies in Salmonidae roe. Vox Sang 1971;21:451–4.

701 Anstee DJ, Holt PDJ, Pardoe GI. Agglutinins from fish ova defining blood groups B and P. Vox Sang 1973;25:347–60.

702 Voak D, Todd GM, Pardoe GI. A study of the serological behaviour and nature of the anti-B/P/Pk activity of Salmonidae roe protectins. Vox Sang 1974;26:176–88.

703 Goldstein IJ, Blake DA, Ebisu S, Williams TJ, Murphy LA. Carbohydrate binding studies on the Bandeiraea simplicifolia I isolectins. J Biol Chem 1981;256:3890–3.

704 Bird GWG, Wingham J. Agglutinins from Jerusalem sage (Phlomis fruticosa). Experientia 1970;26:1257–8.

705 Cazal P, Lalaurie M. Recherches sur quelques phyto-agglutinines spécifiques des groups sanguins ABO. Acta Haemat 1952;8:73–80.

706 Flory LL. Differences in H antigen on human buccal cells from secretor and non-secretor individuals. Vox Sang 1966;11:137–56.

707 Matsumoto I, Osawa T. Purification and characterization of an anti-H (O) phytohemagglutinin of Ulex europeus. Biochim Biophys Acta 1969;194:180–9.

708 Matsumoto I, Osawa T. Purification and characterization of a Cytisus-type anti-H (O) phytohemagglutinin

from *Ulex europeus* seeds. *Arch Biochem Biophys* 1970;**140**:484–91.

709 Bird GWG. Heterogeneity of anti-H lectin. *Rev Franc Transfus Immuno-Hémat* 1976;**19**:175–83.

710 Pereira MEA, Kisailus EC, Gruezo F, Kabat EA. Immunochemical studies on the combining site of the blood group H-specific lectin 1 from *Ulex europeus* seeds. *Arch Biochem Biophys* 1978;**185**:108–15.

711 Hindsgaul O, Norberg T, Le Pendu J, Lemieux RU. Synthesis of Type 2 human blood-group antigenic determinants: the H, X, and Y haptens and variations of the H Type 2 determinant as probes for the combining site of the lectin I of *Ulex europaeus*. *Carbohydr Res* 1982;**109**:109–42.

712 Pereira MEA, Kabat EA. Specificity of purified hemagglutinin (lectin) from *Lotus tetragonolobus*. *Biochemistry* 1974;**13**:3184–92.

713 Voak D, Lodge TW. The demonstration of anti-HI/HI-H activity in seed anti-H reagents. *Vox Sang* 1971;**20**:36–45.

714 Larson G, Svensson L, Hynsjö L, Elmgren A, Rydberg L. Typing of the human Lewis blood group system by quantitative fluorescence-activated flow cytometry: large differences in antigen presentation between A_1, A_2, B, O phenotypes. *Vox Sang* 1999;**77**:227–36.

715 Broadberry RE, Lin-Chu M. The Lewis blood group system among Chinese in Taiwan. *Hum Hered* 1991;**41**:290–4.

716 Cutbush M, Giblett ER, Mollison PL. Demonstration of the phenotype Le(a+b+) in infants and in adults. *Br J Haematol* 1956;**2**:210–20.

717 Brendemoen OJ. Studies of agglutination and inhibition in two Lewis antibodies. *J Lab Clin Pathol* 1949;**34**:538–42.

718 Brendemoen OJ. Further studies of agglutination and inhibition in the Le^a-Le^b system. *J Lab Clin Med* 1950;**36**:335–41.

719 McConnell RB. Lewis blood group substances in body fluids. *Proc 2nd Congr Hum Genet* 1961:858–861.

720 Hounsell EF, Feizi T. Gastrointestinal mucins: structures and antigenicities of their carbohydrate chains in health and disease. *Med Biol* 1982;**60**:227–36.

721 Oriol R, Cartron JP, Cartron J, Mulet C. Biosynthesis of ABH and Lewis antigens in normal and transplanted kidneys. *Transplantation* 1980;**29**:184–8.

722 Evans DAP, Donohoe WTA, Hewitt S, Linaker BD. Le^a blood group substance degradation in the human alimentary tract and urinary Le^a in coeliac disease. *Vox Sang* 1982;**43**:177–87.

723 Lodge TW, Usher A. Lewis blood group substances in seminal fluid. *Vox Sang* 1962;**7**:329–33.

724 Arcilla MB, Sturgeon P. Lewis and ABH substances in amniotic fluid obtained by amniocentesis. *Pediatr Res* 1972;**6**:853–8.

725 Sneath JS, Sneath PHA. Transformation of the Lewis groups of human red cells. *Nature* 1955;**176**:172.

726 Miller EB, Rosenfield RE, Vogel P, Haber G, Gibbel N. The Lewis blood factors in American Negroes. *Am J Phys Anthropol* 1954;**12**:427–44.

727 Mäkelä O, Mäkelä P. Le^b antigen: studies on its occurrence in red cells, plasma and saliva. *Ann Med Exp Fenn* 1956;**34**:157–62.

728 Oriol R, Le Pendu J, Sparkes RS *et al.* Insights into the expression of ABH and Lewis antigens through human bone marrow transplantation. *Am J Hum Genet* 1981;**33**:551–60.

729 Blajchman MA, King DJ, Heddle NM *et al.* Association of renal failure with Lewis incompatibility after allogenic bone marrow transplantation. *Am J Med* 1985;**79**:143–6.

730 Dzik WH, Mondor LA, Maillet SM, Jenkins RL. ABO and Lewis blood group antigens of donor origin in the bile of patients after liver transplantation. *Transfusion* 1987;**27**:384–7.

731 Ramsey G, Fryer JP, Teruya J, Sherman LA. Lewis (a–b–) red blood cell phenotype in patients undergoing evaluation for small intestinal transplantation. *Transfusion* 2000;**40** (Suppl.):114S [Abstract].

732 Lin M, Shieh S-H. Postnatal development of red cell Le^a and Le^b antigens in Chinese infants. *Vox Sang* 1994;**66**:137–40.

733 Henry SM, Jovall P-E, Ghardashkani S, Gustavsson ML, Samuelsson BO. Structural and immunochemical identification of Le^b glycolipids in the plasma of a group O Le(a–b–) secretor. *Glycocon J* 1995;**12**:309–17.

734 Cooper RA. Abnormalities of cell-membrane fluidity in the pathogenesis of disease. *N Engl J Med* 1977;**297**:371–7.

735 Crookston MC, Tilley CA, Crookston JH. Human blood chimaera with seeming breakdown of immune tolerance. *Lancet* 1970;**ii**:1110–2.

736 Mollison PL, Polley MJ, Crome P. Temporary suppression of Lewis blood-group antibodies to permit incomplete transfusion. *Lancet* 1963;**i**:909–12.

737 Rohr TE, Smith DF, Zopf DA, Ginsburg V. Le^b-active glycolipid in human plasma: measurement by radioimmunoassay. *Arch Biochem Biophys* 1980;**199**:265–9.

738 Nicholas JW, Jenkins WJ, Marsh WL. Human blood chimeras: a study of surviving twins. *Br Med J* 1957;**i**:1458–60.

739 Swanson J, Crookston MC, Yunis E *et al.* Lewis substances in a human marrow-transplantation chimaera. *Lancet* 1971;**i**:396.

740 Brendemoen OJ. Development of the Lewis blood group in the newborn. *Acta Path Microbiol Scand* 1961;**52**:55–8.

741 Andresen PH. Blood group with characteristic phenotypical aspects. *Acta Path Microbiol Scand* 1948;**24**:616–8.

742 Jordal K, Lyndrup S. The distribution of C-D and Le^a in 1000 mother–child combinations. *Acta Path Microbiol Scand* 1952;31:476–80.

743 Jordal K. The Lewis blood groups in children. *Acta Path Microbiol Scand* 1956;39:399–406.

744 Lawler SD, Marshall R. Lewis and secretor characters in infancy. *Vox Sang* 1961;6:541–54.

745 Brendemoen OJ. Some factors influencing Rh immunization during pregnancy. *Acta Path Microbiol Scand* 1952;31:579–83.

746 Rosenfield RE, Haber GV, Kissmeyer-Nielsen F *et al.* Ge, a very common red-cell antigen. *Br J Haematol* 1960;6:344–9.

747 Zopf DA, Ginsburg V, Hallgren P *et al.* Determination of Le^b-active oligosaccharides in urine of pregnant and lactating women by radioimmunoassay. *Eur J Biochem* 1979;93:431–5.

748 Hammar L, Månsson S, Rohr T *et al.* Lewis phenotype of erythrocytes and Le^b-active glycolipid in serum of pregnant women. *Vox Sang* 1981;40:27–33.

749 Race RR, Sanger R. *Blood Groups in Man*, 2nd edn. Oxford: Blackwell Scientific Publications 1954:233–43.

750 Miller EB, Rosenfield RE, Vogel P. On the incidence of some of the new blood agglutinogens in Chinese and Negroes. *Am J Phys Anthropol* 1951;9:115–26.

751 Molthan L. Lewis phenotypes of American Caucasians, American Negroes and their children. *Vox Sang* 1980;39:327–30.

752 Salmon C, Malassenet R. Considérations sur les anticorps anti-Lewis et pourcentage des différents phénotypes Lewis chez les donneurs de sang de Paris. *Rev Hémat* 1953;8:183–8.

753 Mak KH, Cheng S, Yuen C *et al.* Survey of blood group distribution among Chinese blood donors in Hong Kong. *Vox Sang* 1994;67 (Suppl. 2):50 [Abstract].

754 Barnicot NA, Lawler SD. A study of the Lewis, Kell, Lutheran and P blood group systems and the ABH secretion in West African Negroes. *Am J Phys Anthropol* 1953;11:83–90.

755 Henry SM, Simpson LA, Woodfield DG. The Le(a+b+) phenotype in Polynesians. *Hum Hered* 1988;38:111–16.

756 Boettcher B, Kenny R. A quantitative study of Le^a, A and H antigens in salivas of Australian Caucasians and Aborigines. *Hum Hered* 1971;21:334–45.

757 Broadberry RE, Lin M. Comparison of the Lewis phenotypes among the different population groups of Taiwan. *Transfus Med* 1996;6:255–60.

758 Kissmeyer-Nielsen F. Irregular blood group antibodies in 200000 individuals. *Scand J Haematol* 1965;2:331–42.

759 Salmon C, Cartron JP. The Lewis blood group system. In: Greenwalt TJ, Steane EA, eds. *CRC Handbook Series in Clinical Laboratory Science: Section D. Blood Banking*, Vol. 1. Cleveland: CRC Press 1977:309–40.

760 Spitalnik S, Cowles J, Cox MT *et al.* A new technique in quantitative immunohematology: solid-phase kinetic enzyme-linked immunoadsorbent assay. *Vox Sang* 1983;45:440–8.

761 Holburn AM. IgG anti-Le^a. *Br J Haematol* 1974;27:489–500.

762 Spitalnik S, Cowles J, Cox MT, Blumberg N. Detection of IgG anti-Lewis (a) antibodies in cord sera by kinetic elisa. *Vox Sang* 1985;48:235–8.

763 François A, Sansonetti N, Mollicone R *et al.* Heterogeneity of Lewis antibodies: a comparison of the reaction of human and animal reagents with synthetic oligosaccharides. *Vox Sang* 1986;50:227–34.

764 Cowles JW, Spitalnik SL, Blumberg N. The fine specificity of Lewis blood group antibodies: evidence for maturation of the immune response. *Vox Sang* 1989;56:107–11.

765 Polley MJ, Mollison PL. The role of complement in the detection of blood group antibodies: special reference to the antiglobulin test. *Transfusion* 1961;1:9–22.

766 Stratton F. Complement-fixing blood group antibodies with special reference to the nature of anti-Le^a. *Nature* 1961;190:240–1.

767 Dorf ME, Eguro SY, Cabrera G *et al.* Detection of cytotoxic non-HL-A antisera. I. Relationship to anti-Le^a. *Vox Sang* 1972;22:447–56.

768 Oriol R, Danilovs J, Lemieux R, Terasaki P, Bernoco D. Lymphocytoxic definition of combined ABH and Lewis antigens and their transfer from sera to lymphocytes. *Hum Immunol* 1980;3:195–205.

769 Young WW, Johnson HJ, Tamura Y *et al.* Characterization of monoclonal antibodies specific for the Lewis a human blood group determinant. *J Biol Chem* 1983;258:4890–4.

770 Fraser RH, Allan EK, Inglis G *et al.* Production and immunochemical characterization of mouse monoclonal antibodies to human Lewis^a blood group structures. *Expl Clin Immunogenet* 1984;1:145–51.

771 Cowles JW, Cox MT, McMican A, Blumberg N. Comparison of monoclonal antisera with conventional antisera for Lewis blood group antigen determination. *Vox Sang* 1987;52:83–4.

772 Dickson L, Richman PI, Shaw M-A, Donald ASR, Swallow DM. Three antibodies to human intestinal brush border membrane are characterized as anti-Le^a. *J Immunogenet* 1989;16:193–202.

773 Good AH, Yau O, Lamontagne LR, Oriol R. Serological and chemical specificities of twelve monoclonal anti-Le^a and anti-Le^b antibodies. *Vox Sang* 1992;62:180–9.

774 Písacka M, Stambergová M. Activation of Thomsen–Friedenreich antigen on red cells: a possible source of errors in antigen typing with some monoclonal antibodies. *Vox Sang* 1994;66:300.

775 Ceppellini R, Dunn LC, Filomena I. Immunogenetica II. Analisi genetica formale de caratteri Lewis con particolare riguardo alla natura epistatica della speci-

ficita' serologica Le^b. *Fol Hered Path* 1959;8:261–96.

776 Garratty G, Kleinschmidt G. Two examples of anti-Le^b detected in the sera of patients with the Lewis phenotype Le(a+b–). *Vox Sang* 1965;10:567–71.

777 Hudelson B, Liu J, Ocariz J, Martin D, Slater LM. Lymphocytotoxic anti-Lewis^{bH} antibody. *Transplantation* 1981;31:449–51.

778 Messeter L, Brodin T, Chester MA *et al*. Immunochemical characterization of a monoclonal anti-Le^b blood grouping reagent. *Vox Sang* 1984;46:66–74.

779 Brockhaus M, Magnani JL, Blaszczyk M *et al*. Monoclonal antibodies directed against the human Le^b blood group antigen. *J Biol Chem* 1981;256:13223–5.

780 Seaman MJ, Chalmers DG, Franks D. Siedler: an antibody which reacts with A$_1$Le(a–b+) red cells. *Vox Sang* 1968;15:25–30.

781 Gundolf F. Anti-A$_1$Le^b in serum of a person of a blood group A$_1$h. *Vox Sang* 1973;25:411–9.

782 de Vries SI, Smitskamp HS. Haemolytic transfusion reaction due to anti-Lewis^a agglutinin. *Br Med J* 1951;i:280–1.

783 Brendemoen OJ, Aas K. Hemolytic transfusion reaction probably caused by anti-Le^a. *Acta Med Scand* 1952;141:458–60.

784 Mollison PL, Cutbush M. Use of isotope-labelled red cells to demonstrate incompatibility in vivo. *Lancet* 1955;i:1290–5.

785 Roy RB, Wesley RH, Fitzgerald JDL. Haemolytic transfusion reaction caused by anti-Le^a. *Vox Sang* 1960;5:545–50.

786 Weir AB, Woods LL, Chesney C, Neitzer G. Delayed hemolytic transfusion reaction caused by anti-Le^{bH} antibody. *Vox Sang* 1987;53:105–7.

787 Contreras M, Mollison PL. Delayed haemolytic transfusion reaction caused by anti-Le^{bH} antibody. *Vox Sang* 1989;56:290.

788 Quiroga H, Leite A, Baía F *et al*. Clinically significant anti-Le^b. *Vox Sang* 2000;78 (Suppl. 1) [Abstract P125].

789 Jesse JK, Sheek KJ. Anti-Le^b implicated in acute hemolytic transfusion reaction: a rare occurrence. *Transfusion* 2000;40 (Suppl.):115S [Abstract].

790 Waheed A, Kennedy MS, Gerhan S, Senhauser DA. Transfusion significance of Lewis system antibodies: success in transfusion with crossmatch-compatible blood. *Am J Clin Pathol* 1981;76:294–8.

791 Carreras Vescio LA, Torres OW, Virgilio OS, Pizzolato M. Mild hemolytic disease of the newborn due to anti-Lewis^a. *Vox Sang* 1993;64:194–5.

792 Bharucha ZS, Joshi SR, Bhatia HM. Hemolytic disease of the newborn due to anti-Le^b. *Vox Sang* 1981; 41:36–9.

793 Oriol R, Cartron J, Yvart J *et al*. The Lewis sytem: new histocompatibility antigens in renal transplantation. *Lancet* 1978;i:574–5.

794 Fischer E, Lenhard V, Römer W *et al*. The Lewis antigen system and its relevance for clinical transplantation. *Z Immun Forsch* 1979;155:420–3.

795 Oriol R, Opelz G, Chun C, Terasaki PI. The Lewis system and kidney transplantation. *Transplantation* 1980;29:397–400.

796 Pfaff WW, Howard RJ, Ireland J, Scornik J. The effect of Lewis antigen and race on kidney graft survival. *Transplant Proc* 1983;15:1139–41.

797 Lenhard V, Roelcke D, Dreikorn K *et al*. Significance of Lewis and HLA system in kidney transplantation: a multicenter study in Germany. *Transplant Proc* 1981;13:930–3.

798 Williams G, Pegrum GD, Evans CA. Lewis antigens in renal transplantation. *Lancet* 1978;i:878.

799 Spitalnik S, Pfaff W, Cowles J *et al*. Relation of humoral immunity to Lewis blood group antigens with renal transplant rejection. *Transplantation* 1984;37:265–8.

800 Rydberg L, Samuelsson BE, Brynger H. Influence of Lewis incompatibility in living donor kidney transplantation. *Transplant Proc* 1985;17:2292–3.

801 Posner MP, McGeorge MB, Mendez-Picon G, Mohanakumar T, Lee HM. The importance of the Lewis system in cadaver renal transplantation. *Transplantation* 1986;41:474–7.

802 Gratama JWC, Hendriks GFJ, Persijn GG *et al*. The interaction between the Lewis blood group system and HLA-matching in renal transplantation. *Transplantation* 1988;45:926–9.

803 Myser T, Steedman M, Hunt K *et al*. A bone marrow transplant with an acquired anti-Le^a: a case study. *Hum Immunol* 1986;17:102–6.

804 Giles CM, Poole J. Auto-anti-Le^b in the serum of a renal dialysis patient. *Clin Lab Haematol* 1979;1:239–42.

805 Andresen PH, Jordal K. An incomplete agglutinin related to the L-(Lewis) system. *Acta Path Microbiol Scand* 1949;26:636–8.

806 Jordal K. The Lewis factors Le^b and Le^X and a family series tested by anti-Le^a, anti-Le^b, and anti-Le^X. *Acta Path Microbiol Scand* 1958;42:269–84.

807 Arcilla MB, Sturgeon P. Le^x, the spurned antigen of the Lewis blood group system. *Vox Sang* 1974; 26:425–38.

808 Schenkel-Brunner H, Hanfland P. Immunochemistry of the Lewis blood-group system. III. Studies on the molecular basis of the Le^x property. *Vox Sang* 1981;40:358–66.

809 AuBuchon JP, Davey RJ, Anderson HJ *et al*. Specificity and clinical significance of anti-Le^x. *Transfusion* 1986;26:302–3.

810 Hirsch HF, Graham HA. Adsorption of Le^c and Le^d from plasma onto red blood cells. *Transfusion* 1980;20:474–5.

811 Greenwell P, Johnson PH, Edwards JM *et al*. Association of the human Lewis blood group Le(a–b–c–d–) with the failure of expression of α-3-L fucosyltrans-

ferase. *Rev Franc Transfus Immuno-Hémat* 1986; **24**:233–49.

812 Potapov MI. Detection of the antigen of the Lewis system, characteristic of the erythrocytes of the secretory group Le(a–b–). *Probl Haemathol (Moscow)* 1970; **11**:45–9 [in Russian with English summary].

813 Gunson HH, Latham V. An agglutinin in human serum reacting with cells from Le(a–b–) non-secretor individuals. *Vox Sang* 1972;**22**:344–53.

814 Lemieux RU. Baker DA, Weinstein WM, Switzer CM. Artifical antigens: antibody preparations for the localization of Lewis determinants in tissues. *Biochemistry* 1981;**20**:199–205.

815 Iseki S, Masaki S, Shibasaki K. Studies on Lewis blood group system. I. Le^c blood group factor. *Proc Jpn Acad* 1957;**33**:492–7.

816 Iseki S, Masaki S, Shinasaki K. Studies on Lewis blood group system. II. Distribution and heredity of Le^c blood group factor. *Proc Jpn Acad* 1957;**33**:686–91.

817 Sistonen P, Nevanlinna HRA. Second example of human anti-Le^c [Abstract]. *19th Congr Int Soc Blood Transfus* 1986:652.

818 Potapov MI. Production of immune anti-Lewis sera in goats. *Vox Sang* 1976;**30**:211–13.

819 Le Pendu J, Lemieux RU, Oriol R. Purification of anti-Le^c antibodies with specificity for βDGal(1→3)βDGlc-NAcO- using a synthetic immunoadsorbent. *Vox Sang* 1982;**43**:188–95.

820 Hanfland P, Kordowicz M, Peter-Katalinic J *et al.* Immunochemistry of the Lewis blood-group system: isolation and structures of Lewis-c active and related glycosphingolipids from the plasma of blood-group O Le(a–b–) nonsecretors. *Arch Biochem Biophys* 1986; **246**:655–72.

821 Solter D, Knowles BB. Monoclonal antibody defining a stage-specific mouse embryonic antigen (SSEA-1). *Proc Natl Acad Sci USA* 1978;**75**:5565–9.

822 Mayr WR, Pausch VP. RB, a determinant defined by lymphocytotoxicity being associated with ABO blood groups and ABH secretor status. *J Immunogenet* 1976;**3**:367–72.

823 Rachkewich RA, Crookston MC, Tilley CA, Wherrett JR. Evidence that blood group A antigen on lymphocytes is derived from the plasma. *J Immunogenet* 1978;**5**:25–9.

824 Bernoco M, Danilovs J, Terasaki PI *et al.* Detection of combined ABH and Lewis glycosphingolipids in sera of H-deficient donors. *Vox Sang* 1985;**49**:58–66.

825 Dunstan RA. Status of major red cell blood group antigens on neutrophils, lymphocytes and monocytes. *Br J Haematol* 1986;**62**:301–9.

826 Mollicone R, Caillard T, Le Pendu J *et al.* Expression of ABH and X (Le^x) antigens on platelets and lymphocytes. *Blood* 1988;**71**:1113–9.

827 Kelton JG, Bebenek G. Granulocytes do not have surface ABO antigens. *Transfusion* 1985;**25**:567–9.

828 Dunstan RA, Simpson MB, Borowitz M. Absence of ABH antigens on neutrophils. *Br J Haematol* 1985;**60**:651–7.

829 Gaidulis L, Branch DR, Lazar GS, Petz LD, Blume KG. The red cell antigens A, B, D, U, Ge, Jk3 and Yt^a are not detected on human granulocytes. *Br J Haematol* 1985;**60**:659–68.

830 Gurevitch J, Nelken D. ABO groups in platelets. *Nature* 1954;**173**:356.

831 Dunstan RA, Simpson MB, Knowles RW, Rosse WF. The origin of ABH antigens on human platelets. *Blood* 1985;**65**:615–19.

832 Dunstan RA. The expression of ABH antigens during *in vitro* megakaryocyte maturation: origin of heterogeneity of antigen density. *Br J Haematol* 1986;**62**:587–93.

833 Santoso S, Kiefel V, Mueller-Eckhardt C. Blood group A and B determinants are expressed on platelet glycoproteins IIa IIIa, and Ib. *Thromb Haemost* 1991;**65**:196–201.

834 Ogasawara K, Ueki J, Takenaka M, Furihata K. Study on the expression of ABH antigens on platelets. *Blood* 1993;**82**:993–9.

835 Hou M, Stockelberg D, Rydberg L, Kutti J, Wadenvik H. Blood group A antigen expression in platelets is prominently associated with glycoprotein Ib and IIb: evidence for A$_1$/A$_2$ difference. *Transfus Med* 1996;**6**:51–9.

836 Stockelberg D, Hou M, Rydberg L, Kutti J, Wadenvik H. Evidence for expression of blood group A antigen on platelet glycoproteins IV and V. *Transfus Med* 1996;**6**:243–8.

837 Kelton JG, Smith JW, Horsewood P *et al.* ABH antigens on human platelets: expression on the glycosyl phosphatidylinositol-anchored protein CD109. *J Lab Clin Med* 1998;**132**:142–8.

838 Skogen B, Hansen B, Husebekk A, Havnes T, Hannestad K. Minimal expression of blood group A antigen on thrombocytes from A$_2$ individuals. *Transfusion* 1988;**28**:456–9.

839 Dunstan RA, Simpson MB, Rosse WF. Le^a blood group antigen on human platelets. *Am J Clin Path* 1985; **83**:90–4.

840 Murphy S. ABO blood groups and platelet transfusion. *Transfusion* 1988;**28**:401–2.

841 Lee EJ, Schiffer CA. ABO compatibility can influence the results of platelet transfusion: results of a randomized trial. *Transfusion* 1989;**29**:384–9.

842 Heal JM, Rowe JM, McMican A *et al.* The role of ABO matching in platelet transfusion. *Eur J Haematol* 1993;**50**:110–7.

843 Curtis BR, Edwards JT, Hessner MJ, Klein JP, Aster RH. Blood group A and B antigens are strongly expressed on platelets of some individuals. *Blood* 2000;**96**:1574–81.

844 Ravn V, Dabelsteen E. Tissue distribution of histo-blood group antigens. *APMIS* 2000;**108**:1–28.

845 Ørntoft TF, Holmes EH, Johnson P, Hakomori S, Clausen H. Differential tissue expression of the Lewis

blood group antigens: enzymatic, immunohistologic, and immunochemical evidence for Lewis a and b antigen expression in Le(a–b–) individuals. *Blood* 1991;77:1389–96.

846 Henry SM, Samuelsson BO, Oriol R. Immunochemical and immunohistological expression of Lewis histoblood group antigens in small intestine including individuals of the Le(a+b+) and Le(a–b–) nonsecretor phenotypes. *Glycoconj J* 1994;11:600–7.

847 Henry S, Jovall P-A, Ghardashkani S *et al.* Structural and immunochemical identification of Le[a], Le[b], H type 1, and related glycolipids in small intestinal mucosa of a group O Le(a–b–) nonsecretor. *Glycoconj J* 1997;14: 209–23.

848 Kay HEM, Wallace DM. A and B antigens in tumors arising from urinary epithelium. *J Natl Cancer Inst* 1961;26:1349–65.

849 Davidsohn I. Early immunologic diagnosis and prognosis of carcinoma. *Am J Clin Path* 1972;57:715–30.

850 Nakagoe T, Nanshima A, Sawai T *et al.* Expression of blood group antigens A, B and H in carcinoma tissue correlates with a poor prognosis for colorectal cancer patients. *J Cancer Res Clin Oncol* 2000;126:375–82.

851 Le Pendu J, Marionneau S, Cailleau-Thomas A *et al.* ABH and Lewis histo-blood group antigens in cancer. *APMIS* 2001;109:9–31.

852 Iwamoto S, Withers DA, Handa K, Hakomori S. Deletion of A-antigen in a human cancer cell line is associated with reduced promoter activity of CBF/NF-Y binding region, and possibly with enhanced DNA methylation of A transferase promoter. *Glycoconj J* 1999;16:659–66.

853 Yuan M, Itzkowitz SH, Palekar A *et al.* Distribution of blood group antigens A, B, H, Lewis[a], and Lewis[b] in human normal, fetal, and malignant colonic tissue. *Cancer Res* 1985;45:4499–511.

854 Ørntoft TF, Greenwell P, Clausen H, Watkins WM. Regulation of the oncodevelopmental expression of type 1 chain ABH and Lewis[b] blood group antigens in human colon by α-2-L-fucosylation. *Gut* 1991;32:287–93.

855 Ørntoft TF, Bech E. Circulating blood group related carbohydrate antigens as tumour markers. *Glycoconj J* 1995;12:200–5.

856 Steinberg W. The clinical utility of the CA 19-9 tumor-associated antigen. *Am J Gastroenterol* 1990; 85:350–5.

857 Narimatsu H, Iwasaki H, Nakayama F *et al.* Lewis and *Secretor* gene dosages affect CA19-9 and DU-PAN-2 serum levels in normal individuals and colorectal cancer patients. *Cancer Res* 1998;58:512–8.

858 Häkkinen I. A-like blood group antigen in gastric cancer cells of patients in blood groups O or B. *J Natl Cancer Inst* 1970;44:1183–93.

859 Clausen H, Hakomori S, Graem N, Dabelsteen E. Incompatible A antigen expressed in tumors of blood group O individuals: immunochemical, immunohisto-

logic, and enzymatic characterization. *J Immunol* 1986;136:326–30.

860 David L, Leitao D, Sobrinho-Simoes M *et al.* Biosynthetic basis of incompatible histo-blood group A antigen expression: anti-A transferase antibodies reactive with gastric cancer tissue of type O individuals. *Cancer Res* 1993;53:5494–500.

861 Mourant AE, Kopec AC, Domaniewska-Sobczak K. *Blood Groups and Diseases: A Study of Associations of Diseases with Blood Groups and Other Polymorphisms.* Oxford: Oxford Universty Press 1978.

862 Garratty G. Blood groups and disease: a historical perspective. *Transfus Med Rev* 2000;14:291–301.

863 Essery SD, Weir DM, James VS *et al.* Detection of microbial surface antigens that bind Lewis[a] antigen. *FEMS Immunol Med Microbiol* 1994;9:15–22.

864 Goodwin CS, Mendall MM, Northfield TC. *Helicobacter pylori* infection. *Lancet* 1997;349:265–9.

865 Borén T, Falk P, Roth KA, Larson G, Normark S. Attachment of *Helicobacter pylori* to human gastric epithelium mediated by blood group antigens. *Science* 1993;262:1892–5.

866 Clarke CA, Cowan WK, Wyn Edwards J *et al.* The relationship of the ABO blood groups to duodenal and gastric ulceration. *Br Med J* 1955;ii:643–6.

867 Clarke CA, Edwards JW, Haddock DRW *et al.* ABO blood groups and secretor character in duodenal ulcer: population and sibship studies. *Br Med J* 1956; ii:725–31.

868 Oberhuber G, Kranz A, Dejaco C *et al.* Blood group Lewis[b] and ABH expression in gastric mucosa: lack of inter-relation with *Helicobacter pylori* colonisation and occurrence of gastric MALT lymphoma. *Gut* 1997;41:37–42.

869 Alkout AM, Blackwell CC, Weir DM *et al.* Isolation of a cell surface component of *Helicobacter pylori* that binds H Type 2, Lewis[a], and Lewis[b] antigens. *Gastroenterology* 1997;112:1179–87.

870 Appelmelk BJ, Monteiro MA, Martin SL, Moran AP, Vandenbroucke-Grauls MJE. Why *Helicobacter pylori* has Lewis antigens. *Trends Microbiol* 2000;8: 565–570.

871 Durand P, Borrone C, Cella GD. Fucosidosis. *J Pediatr* 1969;75:665–74.

872 Tiberio G, Filocamo M, Gatti R, Durand P. Mutations in fucosidosis gene: a review. *Acta Genet Med Gemellol* 1995;44:223–32.

873 Gatti R, Borrone C, Trias X, Durand P. Genetic heterogeneity in fucosidosis. *Lancet* 1973;ii:1024.

874 Kousseff BG, Beratis NG, Strauss L *et al.* Fucosidosis type 2. *Pediatrics* 1976;57:205–13.

875 Romeo G, Borrone C, Gatti R, Durand P. Fucosidosis in Calabria: founder effect or high gene frequency. *Lancet* 1977;i:368–9.

876 Lee CH, Hagen MA, Chong BH, Grace CS, Rozenberg MC. The Lewis system and secretor status in autoim-

mune hemolytic anemia complicating infectious mononucleosis. *Transfusion* 1980;20:585–8.

877 Hirano K, Kawa S, Oguchi H *et al.* Loss of Lewis antigen expression on erythrocytes in some cancer patients with high serum CA-19-9 levels. *J Natl Cancer Inst* 1987;79:1261–8.

878 Langkilde NC, Wolf H, Meldgård P, Ørntoft TF. Frequency and mechanism of Lewis antigen expression in human urinary bladder and colon carcinoma patients. *Br J Cancer* 1991;63:583–6.

879 Stigendal L, Olsson R, Rydberg L, Samuelsson BE. Blood group Lewis phenotype on erythrocytes and in saliva in alcoholic pancreatitis and chronic liver disease. *J Clin Pathol* 1984;37:778–82.

880 Viitala J, Järnefelt J. The red cell surface revisited. *Trends Biol Sci* 1985;14:392–5.

881 Koscielak J. A hypothesis on the biological role of ABH, Lewis and P blood group determinant structures in glycosphingolipids and glycoproteins. *Glycocon J* 1986;3:95–108.

3.1 History and introduction

MNS, the second blood group system discovered, is probably second only to Rh in its complexity. Many of the serological intricacies of MNS are now understood at the molecular level. The 43 antigens of the MNS system are listed in Table 3.1.

The first antibodies to the M and N red cell antigens were found in rabbits immunized with human red cells. This was the result of a deliberate search by Landsteiner and Levine [1–4] in 1927 for more human blood groups, at a time when A and B were the only red cell antigens known. Although human alloanti-M and -N exist, they are relatively uncommon antibodies and generally not clinically significant. Landsteiner and Levine [3,4] showed that M and N are inherited as the products of alleles, and this was soon confirmed by further family studies [5,6]. MN is polymorphic in all populations tested: the frequencies of the common phenotypes in white people are M+N– 28%, M+N+ 50%, and M–N+ 22%.

In 1947, Walsh and Montgomery [7] found an alloantibody, anti-S, detecting an antigen related to M and N. As a result of testing 190 English blood samples, Sanger *et al.* [8,9] found that 86% of S+ samples were M+, whereas only 63% of S– samples were M+, a highly significant difference. The relationship between M, N, and *S* was clearly not allelic, but could result from very closely linked loci as had been proposed to explain the relationship between Cc, D, and Ee of the Rh system. Anti-*s*, an alloantibody detecting the product of an allele of *S*, was reported in 1951 by Levine *et al.* [10]. Very close linkage between *MN* and *Ss* was subsequently confirmed by family studies [11,12]; very few examples of recombination between these loci are documented. Ss is polymorphic in most populations.

Table 3.1 Antigens of the MNS system (system 002).

Number	Name	Characteristics
MNS1	M	Polymorphic; GPA 1–5 Ser-Ser*-Thr*-Thr*-Gly-
MNS2	N	Polymorphic; GPA 1–5 Leu-Ser*-Thr*-Thr*-Glu-
MNS3	S	Polymorphic; GPB Met29
MNS4	s	Polymorphic; GPB Thr29
MNS5	U	HFA associated with presence of S or s
MNS6	He	LFA; GPB 1–5 Trp-Ser*-Thr*-Thr*-Gly-
MNS7	Mi^a	LFA; probably product of junction of A2 and BΨ3 (or altered A3)
MNS8	M^c	GPA 1–5 Ser-Ser*-Thr*-Thr*-Glu-
MNS9	Vw	LFA; GPA Thr28Met, Asn26 not glycosylated
MNS10	Mur	LFA associated with expression of *GYPB* pseudoexon
MNS11	M^g	LFA; GPA 1–5 Leu-Ser-Thr-Asn-Glu-
MNS12	Vr	LFA; GPA Ser47Tyr
MNS13	M^e	Determinant common to M on GPA and He on GPB
MNS14	Mt^a	LFA; GPA Thr58Ile
MNS15	St^a	LFA; product of junction of exons B2 or A2 and A4
MNS16	Ri^a	LFA; GPA Glu55Lys
MNS17	Cl^a	LFA; inherited with *Ms*
MNS18	Ny^a	LFA; GPA Asp27Glu
MNS19	Hut	LFA; GPA Thr28Lys, Asn26 not glycosylated
MNS20	Hil	LFA; product of junction of exons A3 and B4 with s
MNS21	M^v	LFA; GPB Thr3Ser
MNS22	Far	LFA; possibly inherited with *MS* or *Ns*
MNS23	s^D	LFA; GPB Pro39Arg
MNS24	Mit	LFA; GPB Arg35His
MNS25	Dantu	LFA; probably product of junction of exons B4 and A5
MNS26	Hop	LFA; GPA Arg49Thr*
MNS27	Nob	LFA; GPA Arg49Thr* + GPA Tyr52Ser
MNS28	En^a	Heterogeneous: HFAs on GPA
MNS29	ENKT	HFA; GPA, antithetical to Nob (MNS27)
MNS30	'N'	HFA; GPB 1–5 Leu-Ser*-Thr*-Thr*-Glu-
MNS31	Or	LFA; GPA Arg31Trp
MNS32	DANE	LFA; possibly Asn45 of GP(A-B-A)Dane (normal = Ile46)
MNS33	TSEN	LFA; product of junction of exons A3 and B4 with S
MNS34	MINY	LFA; product of junction of exons A3 and B4 with S or s
MNS35	MUT	LFA; generally behaves as anti-Mur + Hut
MNS36	SAT	LFA; probably product of junction of exons A4 and B5
MNS37	ERIK	LFA; GPA Gly59Arg
MNS38	Os^a	LFA; GPA Pro54Ser
MNS39	ENEP	HFA; GPA, antithetical to HAG (MNS41)
MNS40	ENEH	HFA; GPA, antithetical to Vw (MNS9)
MNS41	HAG	LFA; GPA Ala65Pro
MNS42	ENAV	HFA; GPA, antithetical to MARS (MNS43)
MNS43	MARS	LFA; GPA Glu63Lys

*O-glycosylated.
HFA and LFA, high and low frequency antigens.

Phenotype frequencies in white people are as follows: S+s– 11%, S+s+ 44%, and S–s+ 45%. Greenwalt *et al.* [13] found that about 1% of African Americans are S–s– and lack the high frequency antigen named U by Wiener *et al.* [14,15]; S–s– is extremely rare in Europeans. Complexities involving S–s– associated with weak expression of U soon became apparent [16]. Table 3.2 shows the common MNSs phenotypes and genotypes, and their frequencies in white English and African American populations.

M and N determinants are carried on glycophorin A (GPA), the major red cell sialic acid-rich glycoprotein (sialoglycoprotein, SGP). M differs from N in the amino acid composition of the extracellular tip of GPA: M has serine at position 1 and glycine at position 5; N has leucine at position 1 and glutamic acid at position 5. Carbohydrate, especially sialic acid, also plays a part in the expression of M and N antigens.

S and s are carried on another red cell SGP called glycophorin B (GPB). The S/s distinction arises from a single amino acid substitution at position 29 of GPB: S has methionine and s has threonine at position 29. The first 26 amino acid residues from the extracellular terminus of GPB are identical to those of N-active GPA (GPA^N). Consequently, GPB also demonstrates N activity (often referred to as 'N'), which is detected on the red cells of homozygous *M/M* individuals by some anti-N.

Red cells of individuals homozygous for the very rare MNS-null gene M^K lack all MNS antigens and have no GPA or GPB. Cells of another very rare phenotype, called En(a–), lack GPA and, consequently, MN antigen expression (apart from the 'N' antigen carried on GPB). En(a–) cells express normal Ss antigens but lack a variety of GPA-borne high frequency antigens collectively named En^a. En(a–) cells also lack Wr^b, expression of which results from an interaction between GPA and the red cell glycoprotein band 3 (Chapter 10). S–s–U– cells are deficient in GPB, but express normal MN antigens. GPA- and GPB-deficient phenotypes mostly result from gene deletions.

Numerous low frequency red cell antigens associated with the MNS system have been identified (Table 3.1). Some are known to result from amino acid substitutions and/or glycosylation changes in GPA or GPB, but many are associated with abnormal hybrid glycophorin molecules comprising partly GPA and partly of GPB. These hybrid glycophorins are presumed to have arisen as a result of chromosome misalignment followed by unequal crossing-over or gene conversion involving the GPA and GPB genes.

GYPA and *GYPB*, the genes encoding GPA and GPB, are homologous and, together with a third homologous gene, *GYPE*, which may produce glycophorin E, they constitute a gene cluster on chromosome 4 at 4q28→q31 (Chapter 32).

Table 3.2 Common MNSs phenotypes and genotypes and their frequencies in white European and African American populations.

| Phenotype | Europeans* | | African Americans† | |
	Genotype	%	Genotype	%
M+N–S+s–	*MS/MS*	5.7	*MS/MS* or *MS/Mu*	2.1
M+N–S+s+	*MS/Ms*	14.0	*MS/Ms*	7.0
M+N–S–s+	*Ms/Ms*	10.1	*Ms/Ms* or *Ms/Mu*	15.5
M+N–S–s–		0	*Mu/Mu*	0.4
M+N+S+s–	*MS/NS*	3.9	*MS/NS, MS/Nu, Mu/NS*	2.2
M+N+S+s+	*MS/Ns* or *Ms/NS*	22.4	*MS/Ns* or *Ms/NS*	13.0
M+N+S–s+	*Ms/Ns*	22.6	*Ms/Ns, Ms/Nu, Mu/Ns*	33.4
M+N+S–s–		0	*Mu/Nu*	0.4
M–N+S+s–	*NS/NS*	0.3	*NS/NS* or *NS/Nu*	1.6
M–N+S+s+	*NS/Ns*	5.4	*NS/Ns*	4.5
M–N+S–s+	*Ns/Ns*	15.6	*Ns/Ns* or *Ns/Nu*	19.2
M–N+S–s–		0	*Nu/Nu*	0.7

*Frequencies from tests on 1000 white English people [17].

†Frequencies compiled by Race and Sanger [18] from tests on 1322 African Americans.

u represents all genes that result in no expression of S or s.

3.2 Antigen, gene, and phenotype frequencies

3.2.1 M and N

All the early frequency studies, and very many others since, were performed with anti-M and -N alone [19,20]. MN frequencies vary less between different populations than do those of the ABO and Rh antigens. In most populations, including most of Europe, Africa, and East Asia, the frequency of the M allele is between 50% and 60% and, consequently, the frequency of N is between 40% and 50%. A higher frequency of M is found in east Baltic countries, including European Russia, and in most of South Asia and western Indonesia. Highest M frequencies, over 90%, are found among the Inuit and some Native Americans. Lowest M frequencies are in the Pacific area and among Australian Aborigines. In regions of Papua New Guinea incidence of M drops below 2%.

3.2.2 M, N, S, and s

The different S antigen frequencies between people of the three MN phenotypes (Table 3.3) led Sanger et al. [8,9] to recognize the association between MN and S; if there were no association the frequency of S+ would be the same in M+N−, M+N+, and M−N+ individuals. Family analyses (Section 3.3) and molecular genetics (Section 3.4.5) have demonstrated conclusively that the MN and Ss polymorphisms are controlled by very closely linked loci.

There are four common haplotypes in white people, MS, Ms, NS, and Ns. Anti-s has often been considered too scarce to be used in large population studies but, because u, a silent allele at the Ss locus, is extremely rare in white people, the S− phenotype can be considered to result from homozygosity for s in white populations and haplotype frequencies can be deduced. Fisher [21,22] used the maximum likelihood method devised for Rh, but now computer programs are available for this purpose. In Europeans, MS and Ms have similar frequencies, but Ns is about five or six times more common than NS. In white British donors the following haplotype frequencies were calculated: MS, 25%; Ms 29%; NS 7%; Ns 39% [17,18].

S is less common in the Far East than it is in Europe [19]: 52 624 Taiwanese were all s-positive [23]. S is virtually absent from Australian Aborigines [19].

Although Ss antigens are almost always present in white people, the phenotype S−s− is not uncommon in people of African origin (see Table 3.2). The presence of S and/or s is associated with a high frequency antigen, U. S−s− cells are either U− or have a variant form of U (Section 3.7). Wiener et al. [15] proposed that a pair of alleles controlled U expression: U which determines the presence of the antigen and u, recessive to U, which determines its absence. When the association with Ss expression was recognized, the name S^u was proposed [13] for the silent allele of S and s that produces no U antigen. For the purposes of describing gene frequencies u will be used here to represent a silent gene at the Ss locus (Table 3.2). Table 3.4 shows frequencies for the six most common haplotypes in three different populations of African Americans and in two regions of Africa.

3.3 Inheritance

A wealth of family evidence has proven that MN and Ss behave as two very closely linked loci with virtually

Table 3.3 Some approximate phenotype frequencies in the MNS system for people of northern European extraction (after [18]).

MN phenotype	Ss phenotype		
	All (%)	S+ (%)	s+ (%)
All	100	55	89
M+N−	28	72	78
M+N+	50	56	92
M−N+	22	31	97

Table 3.4 Frequencies of MNSs haplotypes in black populations.

Haplotype	USA (1000) [18–20,24]	Senegal (459) [19,25]
MS	0.1001	0.0244
Ms	0.3496	0.0492
Mu	0.0454	0.0747
NS	0.0614	0.0640
Ns	0.3744	0.2940
Nu	0.0691	0.1137

All tested with anti-M, -N, -S, and -s; u represents all genes that result in no expression of S or s.

no recombination occurring between them. Analyses are reported of 882 white families, with a total of 2354 children, tested for M, N, S, and s [11,12,26,27]. The inheritance of MNSs in black families is complicated by *u* (Section 3.7), but, from the point of view of analysing families, *u* (elsewhere called S^u) can be considered an allele at the *Ss* locus, recessive to *S* and *s*. No large series of black families has been analysed for MNSs, but a few pedigrees are described [28–30].

With the knowledge that *MN* and *Ss* represent two discreet gene loci encoding different proteins, it should be no surprise that recombination, presumably as a result of crossing-over, occurs between them. However, documented examples of such recombination are rare. In one family an M−N+S−s+ father and M+N+S+s+ mother had three M−N+S−s+, three M+N+S+s+, and one M+N+S−s+ children [31]. The mother must be *MS/Ns* because she has three presumed *Ns/Ns* children and three presumed *MS/Ns* children (because the father is probably *Ns/Ns*); yet the other child appears to be *Ms/Ns*. Thus the mother appears to have passed *Ns* to three children, *MS* to three children, and *Ms* to another. This anomaly of inheritance may be explained by any one of several genetic mechanisms—suppression, deletion, mutation, or recombination—but Chown *et al.* [31] favour recombination between *MS* and *Ns* producing an *Ms* oocyte in the mother. Gedde-Dahl *et al.* [32] describe six families in which MNSs inheritance anomalies may be a result of recombination.

3.4 Biochemistry and molecular genetics

3.4.1 Glycophorins

Numerous intrinsic membrane proteins and glycoproteins are anchored within the phospholipid bilayer of the red cell membrane. Some of the glycoproteins are heavily glycosylated and rich in sialic acid (*N*-acetylneuraminic acid) and are called sialoglycoproteins or glycophorins. Two of these glycophorins carry the MN and Ss determinants. A variety of different terminologies has been used to describe the glycophorins and these are shown in Table 3.5. The major sialoglycoprotein, which carries M or N determinants, is called glycophorin A (GPA) and the minor sialoglycoprotein, which carries the S or s determinants, glycophorin B (GPB) (reviewed in [33–38]). Glycophorin C and D, which carry the Gerbich antigens, are genetically unrelated to the MNS system and are described in Chapter 18.

Glycophorins traverse the red cell membrane and consist of a polypeptide backbone with its carboxy-terminus (C-terminus) inside the cell, possibly interacting with the membrane skeleton, and its amino-terminus (N-terminus) outside the membrane (Fig. 3.1). Attached to the polypeptide chain are two types of carbohydrate structures, *N*-linked oligosaccharides and O-linked oligosaccharides, often referred to as *N*-glycans and O-glycans. *N*-glycans are generally complex carbohydrate chains attached to the amide-nitrogen of asparagine, usually through *N*-

Table 3.5 Red cell glycophorins and some notations used in early publications.

Glycophorin	Gene		M_r	Blood group antigens	Other notations		
Glycophorin A	GPA	*GYPA*	43 000	M/N Enª	CD235A MN glycoprotein	α	PAS-2
Glycophorin B	GPB	*GYPB*	25 000	S/s 'N'	CD235B Ss glycoprotein	δ	PAS-3
Glycophorin E*	GPE	*GYPE*					
Glycophorin A dimer	GPA₂		86 000	M/N Enª		α	PAS-1
Glycophorin B dimer	GPB₂		50 000	S/s 'N'		δ	
Glycophorin AB heterodimer	GPAB		68 000	M/N S/s Enª 'N'		αδ	PAS-4
Glycophorin C	GPC	*GYPC*	40 000	Ge3 Ge4	CD236C	β	PAS-2′
Glycophorin D	GPD	*GYPC*	30 000	Ge2 Ge3		γ	

*Existence of a product of *GYPE* in the red cell membrane has not been confirmed.

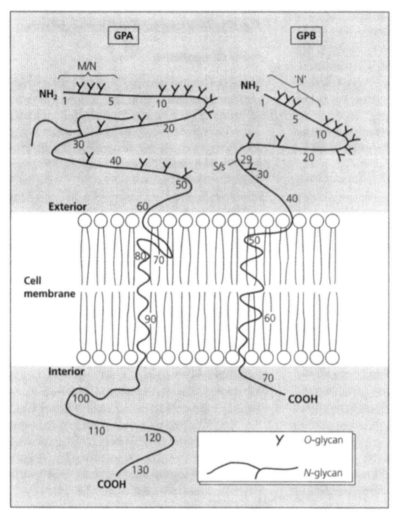

Fig. 3.1 Diagrammatic representation of glycophorin A (GPA) and glycophorin B (GPB), and their situation in the red cell membrane (GPA after [39]).

acetylglucosamine. The tripeptide Asn-Xaa-Thr/Ser (where Xaa is any amino acid except proline) is a prerequisite for N-glycosylation. GPA has one N-glycan; GPB is not N-glycosylated. On glycophorins, the O-glycans are smaller molecules than N-glycans and are attached to the hydroxyl-oxygen of serine or threonine. In glycophorins it is the O-glycans that carry most of the sialic acid. They typically have the disialotetrasaccharide structure shown in Fig. 3.4, although other structures have been identified [34]. All carbohydrate chains are attached to the extracellular domain of the polypeptide backbone (Fig. 3.1). Transfection of *GYPA* cDNA into Chinese hamster ovary cells, including mutant cells with glycosylation defects, demonstrated that O-glycosylation is required for insertion of GPA into the plasma membrane [41],

but in the absence of O-glycosylation, an N-glycan can support some expression of GPA at the cell surface [42].

Glycophorins, especially GPA and GPB, probably exist in the membrane in their monomeric (GPA and GPB) and dimeric (GPA$_2$ and GPB$_2$) forms, and as a heterodimer (GPAB) (Table 3.5).

3.4.2 Identification of glycophorins

Separation and identification of the intrinsic glycoproteins of the red cell membrane was facilitated by the procedure of sodium dodecyl sulphate polyacrylamide gel electrophoresis (SDS PAGE) [43,44]. Washed ghosts from haemolysed red cells are solubilized in the ionic detergent SDS, which releases the glycoproteins

$$NeuNac\alpha2 \rightarrow 3Gal\beta1 \rightarrow 3GalNAc\alpha1 \rightarrow O - Ser/Thr$$
$$6$$
$$\downarrow$$
$$NeuNAc\alpha2$$

Fig. 3.2 Disialotetrasaccharide: the predominant O-glycan of glycophorins [40]. For abbreviations see Table 2.4.

from the phospholipid bilayer and gives them a negative charge. During the process of electrophoresis, the charged glycoproteins are drawn by an electric current through a polyacrylamide gel, which acts as a molecular sieve. Larger molecules tend to move through the gel more slowly than smaller molecules and the glycoproteins become sorted throughout the gel roughly according to their molecular weight. The glycoproteins can then be visualized by a variety of methods.

Coomassie brilliant blue staining of gels following SDS PAGE of red cell membranes reveals several proteins including band 3 (anion exchanger, AE1), band 4.5 (glucose transport protein), and components of the membrane skeleton, spectrin, actin, ankyrin, and protein 4.1. Coomassie blue does not readily stain the glycophorins, probably because of their high degree of glycosylation. Periodic acid–Schiff (PAS) stains glycoproteins rich in sialic acid, which makes it ideal for staining the red cell glycophorins. When the gels are stained with PAS at least seven bands are seen, representing GPA, GPB, GPC, and GPD, dimers of GPA and of GPB, and a heterodimer of GPA and GPB (Fig. 3.3, Table 3.5). More sensitive methods of visualizing glycophorins in a polyacrylamide gel involve autoradiography and fluorography. The association of MN and Ss antigens with GPA and GPB, respectively, was originally demonstrated by SDS PAGE and PAS staining of butanol extracted components from red cell membranes. These components were shown to have M, N, S, or s activity by haemagglutination inhibition [45,46]. Further evidence came from the absence of GPA from cells of individuals with the rare M–N–En(a–) phenotype and the absence of GPB from S–s–U– cells (Sections 3.6 and 3.7, and Fig. 3.3).

The technique of immunoblotting (Western blotting), originally developed by Towbin *et al.* [47], has proved to be a very effective method of identifying glycophorins and other blood group-active glycoproteins. After SDS PAGE, a filter of nitrocellulose, nylon, or similar substance is laid onto the surface of the slab

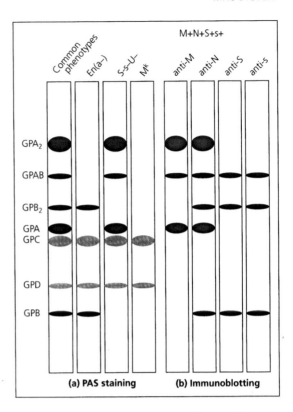

Fig. 3.3 Diagrammatic representation of the red cell membrane glycophorins after sodium dodecyl sulphate polyacrylamide slab gel electrophoresis. (a) Gel stained with periodic acid–Schiff (PAS); cells of common and 'null' phenotypes used. (b) Gel electroblotted onto nitrocellulose filters and immunostained with anti-M, -N, -S, and -s; M+N+S+s+ cells used. Anti-M detects GPA and its complexes, anti-S and -s detect GPB and its complexes, and anti-N detects GPA and GPB and their complexes.

gel and the proteins are transferred electrophoretically onto the filter, where they are immobilized. The filter can then be incubated with an antibody of known blood group specificity. Immunostaining is visualized by the use of labelled antiglobulin reagent. After electrophoresis and electroblotting of membranes from M+N+S+s+ cells, anti-M immunostains GPA, GPA$_2$ and GPAB, anti-N immunostains GPA, GPB, GPA$_2$, GPB$_2$ and GPAB, and anti-S and -s immunostain GPB, GPB$_2$ and GPAB (Fig. 3.3) [48–50].

3.4.3 Glycophorin A (CD235A)

GPA is the most abundant red cell sialoglycoprotein and, together with band 3, with which it is associated [51], the most abundant red cell membrane glycopro-

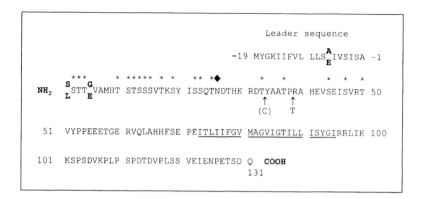

Fig. 3.4 Amino acid sequence of glycophorin A (see Table 3.6 for code). Sequences for GPA^M (above line) and GPA^N (below line) are distinguished at positions –7, 1, and 5. * represents probable sites of O-glycosylation. ◆ represents site of N-glycosylation. The membrane spanning domain is underlined. T, major trypsin cleavage site on intact cells. (C), partial chymotrypsin cleavage site. The leader sequence is cleaved after insertion of the protein into the membrane.

Table 3.6 The 20 common amino acids: one and three letter codes.

A	Ala	Alanine
C	Cys	Cysteine
D	Asp	Aspartic acid
E	Glu	Glutamic acid
F	Phe	Phenylalanine
G	Gly	Glycine
H	His	Histidine
I	Ile	Isoleucine
K	Lys	Lysine
L	Leu	Leucine
M	Met	Methionine
N	Asn	Asparagine
P	Pro	Proline
Q	Gln	Glutamine
R	Arg	Arginine
S	Ser	Serine
T	Thr	Threonine
V	Val	Valine
W	Trp	Tryptophan
Y	Tyr	Tyrosine

tein. The number of copies of GPA per red cell has been estimated to be about 1×10^6 [52]. For more details on the nature of the association between GPA and band 3, see Sections 3.6.1.3, 3.16, and 3.25 and Chapter 10.

GPA consists of 131 amino acids, organized into three domains:

1 an extracellular N-terminal domain of 72 amino acids;

2 a hydrophobic membrane-spanning domain of 23 amino acids; and

3 a C-terminal cytoplasmic domain of 36 amino acids.

The extracellular domain contains a high proportion of serine and threonine residues and is heavily glycosylated with about 15 O-glycans and a single N-glycan. GPA is generally present in the membrane in dimeric form, with the polypeptides associated at the hydrophobic membrane-spanning domain [39,53]. The prevalence of glycines and β-branched amino acids in the GPA transmembrane domain and, in particular the Gly79-x-x-x-Gly83 motif, is responsible for GPA dimerization [54,55]. The molecular organization of GPA is described in detail by Welsh *et al.* [39].

The amino acid sequence of GPA is shown in Fig. 3.4 and a diagrammatic representation of how it may appear in relation to the red cell membrane in Fig. 3.1. Most of the amino acid sequence for GPA was resolved by degradation amino acid sequencing techniques [34,56,57]. The complete sequence in Fig. 3.4 was deciphered from the nucleotide sequence of *GYPA* cDNA isolated by Siebert and Fukuda [58]. The amino acids numbered –1 to –19 represent a leader sequence, which ensures correct insertion of the whole molecule into the cell membrane. Translation of mRNA is initiated at the methionine codon at position –19 and amino acid residues –19 to –1, presumed to be present at the N-terminus when the protein is synthesized, are cleaved after membrane insertion [58].

The predominant O-glycan of glycophorins is the branched tetrasaccharide shown in Fig. 3.2, comprising two molecules of sialic acid, one galactose, and one N-acetylgalactosamine [40]. Several variations of this molecule have been recognized, including mono-sialotrisaccharides and trisialopentasaccharides [34,59]. Glycosylation of GPA is incomplete and variable; only about 15 of the 21 extracellular serine or threonine amino acid residues are glycosylated [57,60] and variation in O-glycosylation of different GPA molecules occurs within the same individual [52,61]. The asparagine residue at position 26 bears an N-linked oligosaccharide, a branched structure of about 11–13 sugar residues and approximate molecular weight of 3000 [62,63].

3.4.3.1 M and N antigens

The amino acid sequence of GPA demonstrates polymorphic variation at positions 1 and 5, represented serologically as the MN blood groups. GPA isolated from M+N– individuals has serine at position 1 and glycine at position 5; GPA from M–N+ individuals has leucine at position 1 and glutamic acid at position 5 (Table 3.7) [60,64,65]. Both forms of GPA can be isolated from M+N+ individuals. The terminal serine of M-active GPA is not glycosylated; amino acid residues 2, 3, and 4 of GPA^M and GPA^N are O-glycosylated. The Ser/Leu polymorphism at position 1 results from a single base change (TCA/TTA) that creates a *Sfa*NI restriction site in the *M* allele and an *Mse*I site in the *N* allele; the Gly/Glu change at position 5 results from two nucleotide changes (GGT/GAG), creating a *Bsr*I site in *M* and a *Dde*I site in *N* [66]. In addition, nucleotide sequencing has predicted that glutamic acid and alanine are present at residue –7 of the leader peptide of GPA^N and GPA^M, respectively (Fig. 3.4) [67]. A total of 17 nucleotide differences in exons 1, 2, and 7 and introns 1–4 distinguish the standard *M* allele and

N [68]. Another *M* allele, common in Asians, shares characteristics of both standard *M* and *N* [68].

Although the amino acid residues at positions 1 and 5 of GPA are primarily responsible for the MN polymorphism, glycosylation is also important in the serological expression of the M and N antigens. Many anti-M and -N do not bind sialidase-treated red cells [48,69–72]. This could be because of an alteration in steric presentation of receptors dependent on an interaction between sialic acid and amino groups [73,74]. GPA contains a small number of non-galactosylated N-acetylgalactosamine residues, which may be partially sialylated. The number of these residues on Ser2, Thr3, and Thr4 is substantially higher in GPA^N than in GPA^M [75]. The role of sialic acid in M and N specificity is discussed further in Section 3.5.2.

PCR techniques with allele-specific primers have been developed for MN genotyping from genomic DNA [76–79] and reticulocyte-derived cDNA [66]. Most methods utilize primers that are specific for either the M- or N-associated sequence paired with a common primer specific for *GYPA*. Unfortunately, internal controls for successful amplification have not always been included. If the *M*- and *N*-specific primers are designed to recognize different allele-specific sites (codons 1 and 5), the products representing the alleles are of slightly different lengths [78].

3.4.4 Glycophorin B (CD235B)

GPB, another sialic acid-rich red cell membrane glycoprotein, is closely related in structure to GPA. It consists of 72 amino acids which, like GPA, fit into three domains:

Table 3.7 Some N-terminal pentapeptides of GPA and GPB.

Glycophorin A	Human M	Ser–Ser*–Thr*–Thr*–Gly–
	Human N	Leu–Ser*–Thr*–Thr*–Glu–
	Human M^g	Leu–Ser–Thr–Asn–Glu–
	Human M^c	Ser–Ser*–Thr*–Thr*–Glu–
	Chimpanzee	Ser–Ser–Thr*–Thr*–Glu–
Glycophorin B	Human 'N'	Leu–Ser*–Thr*–Thr*–Glu–
	Human He	Trp–Ser*–Thr*–Ser*–Gly–

*O-glycosylated.

```
                                          Leader sequence
                               -19 MYGKIIFVL LLSEIVSISA -1

           ***      *  * ***** * *    ** *
     NH2  LSTTEVAMHT STSSSVTKSY ISSQTNGE M G QLVHRFTVPA PVVIILIILC 50
                                        T    ↑
                                     29      C

     51  VMAGIIGTIL LISYSIRRLI KA  COOH
                                72
```

Fig. 3.5 Amino acid sequence of glycophorin B (see Table 3.6 for code). Amino acid characteristic of GPB[S] at position 29 is above the line, that for GPB[s] is below the line. * Represents probable sites of O-glycosylation. The membrane spanning domain is underlined. C, chymotrypsin cleavage site. The leader sequence is cleaved after insertion of the protein into the membrane.

1 an N-terminal glycosylated extracellular domain of 44 amino acids;

2 a hydrophobic membrane-spanning domain of 20 amino acids; and

3 a very short C-terminal cytoplasmic tail of eight amino acids.

The amino acid sequence shown in Fig. 3.5 was deduced from the nucleotide sequence of *GYPB* cDNA [67,80] and differs only slightly from that obtained by peptide sequencing techniques [81]. Figure 3.1 shows a diagrammatic representation of GPB in the membrane. GPB has about 11 O-glycans and is devoid of N-glycosylation [34].

The first 26 amino acids from the N-terminus of GPB are identical to those of the N form of GPA (GPA[N]). This accounts for the N activity of GPB, usually denoted 'N' to distinguish it from the N activity of GPA[N]. Unlike GPA, the N-terminal amino acids of GPB are not cleaved by trypsin treatment of intact red cells, so 'N' is a trypsin-resistant N antigen. The only difference between amino acid residues 1–26 of GPA[N] and GPB is that Asn26 is N-glycosylated in GPA, but not in GPB [82]. This is because, unlike GPA, GPB does not have the requisite serine or threonine residue at position 28. GPA and GPB show other homologies. Amino acid residues 59–67 and 75–100 of GPA closely resemble residues 27–35 and 46–71 of GPB [34,81]. Also, the leader sequences of GPA and GPB, deduced from cDNA analysis, are almost identical, and sequencing of genomic DNA has revealed more close homologies (see Section 3.4.5).

There are an estimated $1.7–2.5 \times 10^5$ molecules of GPB per red cell [52]. S+s– red cells have about 1.5 times as much GPB as S–s+ cells, with S+s+ cells having an intermediate quantity [34,83].

3.4.4.1 S and s antigens

The S/s polymorphism is represented by a single amino acid substitution in GPB at position 29; S-active GPB has Met29 and the s-active molecule has Thr29 [83]. Dahr *et al.* [84] found that a synthetic peptide representing residues 25–33 of S-specific GPB inhibited anti-S poorly and the equivalent s-specific peptide did not inhibit anti-s at all. This suggests that the S/s antigen sites are more complex than just the amino acid residue at position 29 and there is evidence that residues 34 and 35 and possibly the glycosylation of Thr25 are all involved in S and s activity [85]. Anti-S sera are heterogeneous; a synthetic peptide representing residues 25–43 of GPB[S] inhibited six of 16 anti-S [86] and two human monoclonal anti-S demonstrated different serological characteristics [87] (Section 3.20.9).

S/s genotyping on genomic DNA can be carried out by PCR-based techniques with an allele-specific primer [77].

3.4.5 Cloning and organization of the genes for glycophorins A, B, and E

Siebert and Fukuda [58] synthesized mixed oligonucleotides corresponding to amino acid sequences in the C-terminal region of GPA and used them to prime the synthesis of *GYPA* cDNA from a K562 cell line cDNA library. *GYPA* cDNA from this library was then isolat-

Table 3.8 Structural organization of *GYPA*, *GYPB*, and *GYPE*. Amino acid residues encoded by each exon are numbered from the N-terminal residue of the mature protein (assuming that *GYPE* is translated). The exons are numbered according to the system used by Huang *et al.* [36] in which pseudoexons are numbered so that homologous exons maintain the same number in all three genes.

GYPA		GYPB		GYPE	
A1	5′ UT, −19 to −8	B1	5′ UT, −19 to −8	E1	5′ UT, −19 to −8
A2	−7 to 26	B2	−7 to 26	E2	−7 to 26
A3	27–58	B3	Pseudoexon	E3	Pseudoexon
A4	59–71	B4	27–39	E4	Pseudoexon
A5	72–100	B5	40–71	E5	27–58
A6	101–126	B6	72, 3′ UT	E6	59, 3′ UT
A7	127–131, 3′ UT				

ed with mixed oligonucleotides representing the central region of GPA. Siebert and Fukuda [80] then proceeded to isolate *GYPB* cDNA from a K562 cDNA library by the use of two oligonucleotide probes, one specific for a *GYPA* sequence and the other representing a sequence common to *GYPA* and *GYPB* cDNA. Subsequently full-length *GYPA* and *GYPB* cDNA clones were isolated from human reticulocyte cDNA libraries [67] and from *GYPA* cDNA from a human fetal liver library [88].

GPA and GPB are encoded by discrete, single-copy genes specific to each polypeptide [89]. *GYPA* is about 40 kb and contains seven exons [90,91] (Fig. 3.6, Table 3.8). Exon A1 codes for most of the leader peptide and is separated by a large intron of about 30 kb from exon A2, which codes for the remainder of the leader peptide and the first 26 amino acids of the extracellular domain. Exons A3 and A4 encode the remainder of the extracellular domain, exon A5 the transmembrane portion, and exon A6 and part of exon A7 the cytoplasmic portion of the polypeptide. Most of the seventh exon is not translated. Three *GYPA* mRNA transcripts, of 2.8, 1.7, and 1.0 kb differing from each other in the lengths of their 3′ untranslated regions, have been identified in erythroleukaemic cell lines [58,66,92], fetal liver [88], and reticulocytes [58,67].

Figure 3.6 shows that *GYPB* has only five exons [90,91]. Exons B1 and B2 are almost identical to exons A1 and A2 of *GYPA*. The third exon, numbered B4 to demonstrate homology with exon A4, encodes the S/s polymorphism. Exon B5 codes for most of the C-terminal part of the polypeptide and exon B6 encodes the C-terminal amino acid residue, the remainder of exon B6 being untranslated (Table 3.8). A sequence within the second intron of *GYPB* is homologous to

exon 3 of GYPA. This 'pseudoexon' is not translated because the gt (gu in RNA) consensus splice site at the 5′ end of intron 3 is mutated to tt (uu) [90], and other changes in intron 2 may also affect splicing. So the 'pseudoexon' is spliced out of *GYPB* mRNA, together with the regions homologous to the second and third introns of *GYPA* [93]. GPB therefore lacks a segment homologous to amino acid residues 27–58 of GPA. The *GYPB* pseudoexon may be translated in rare phenotypes where a functional acceptor splice site is transplanted into *GYPB* from *GYPA* by gene conversion [36] (see Section 3.10).

During isolation of *GYPA* and *GYPB*, a closely associated gene, *GYPE*, was discovered [91,94,95]. The three genes show 90% nucleotide sequence homology, the coding regions demonstrating more diversity than the non-coding introns [36,90]. *GYPE* is present in all human DNA investigated including that from En(a−), S−s−U−, homozygous M^K, and homozygous *GYP(A–B)Hil* (Mi.V) individuals [91,94,96–98]. *GYPE* has a similar genomic structure to that of *GYPB*, but contains four exons and two pseudoexons [95,98] (Fig. 3.6, Table 3.8). The predicted polypeptide has 78 amino acids including a 19 residue leader peptide. The mature cell surface glycoprotein protein would be 59 amino acid residues long, carry 11 O-glycans and no N-glycan, have an M_r of 17 000, and express M antigen. Anstee [99] speculated that a red cell membrane component of approximate molecular weight 20 000, revealed on immunoblots of membranes from red cells of all MN groups by monoclonal anti-M, might be GPE. GPE may also express S or s antigen [100].

The three genes are situated on chromosome 4q31 in the order 5′–*GYPA*–*GYPB*–*GYPE*–3′ [97,98] and

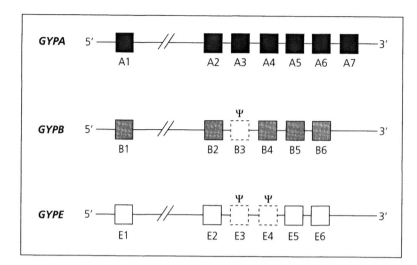

Fig. 3.6 Genomic organization of *GYPA*, *GYPB*, and *GYPE*. Boxes represent exons and pseudoexons (ψ). The exons are numbered according to the system used by Huang *et al.* [36] in which pseudoexons are numbered so that homologous exons maintain the same number in all three genes.

are over 95% identical to each other from the 5' flanking region to an *Alu* repeat sequence 1 kb downstream of the exon encoding the transmembrane domain [95]. Isolation of a yeast artificial chromosome (YAC) encoding the entire region demonstrated that the glycophorin gene family occupies 330 kb of genomic DNA and that the three genes are about an equal distance apart [101]. These genes appear to have evolved from a common ancestral gene through homologous recombination events involving *Alu* sequences [95] (see Fig. 3.13). A putative precursor fragment downstream from *GYPA* has been isolated [102].

Like other genes active predominantly in erythroid tissue, promoters for the three glycophorin genes are driven mainly by GATA-1 and SP1 binding to well-characterized *cis*-acting elements [103]. The proximal promoters for the three glycophorin genes had very similar sequences and the three genes exhibited similar transcriptional activities [103,104]. *GYPB* mRNA transcript was less stable than *GYPA* transcript, however, and *GYPE* transcript was very unstable [104]. Post-transcriptional regulation therefore may be responsible for the very different quantities of the three protein products at the cell surface. Regulatory factors controlling transcription of *GYPB* have been analysed in detail and at least two factors (Ku70 and factor U) that appear to be involved in the repression of *GYPB* transcription in non-erythroid cells, have been identified [105–107].

For reviews on the molecular genetics of glycophorins see [36–38,108].

3.5 Effects of enzyme treatment on the MNSs antigens

3.5.1 Proteases

Various proteolytic enzymes have proved very useful in the serological identification, analysis, and definition of antigens belonging to the MNS system. The effects on isolated sialoglycoproteins of proteases, glycanases, and various peptide bond-splitting chemicals, such as cyanogen bromide, have been extremely valuable in elucidating the biochemical structure of these glycoproteins and of some of the antigens associated with them. Certain proteases, such as trypsin and chymotrypsin, are highly specific for the peptide bonds they cleave, although access of enzymes may be blocked by the presence of neighbouring oligosaccharides or, when intact cells are treated, by the red cell membrane or other membrane-bound components.

3.5.1.1 Trypsin

Trypsin catalyses the hydrolysis of peptide bonds on the carboxyl side of lysine and arginine residues. There are at least seven trypsin cleavage sites on GPA, at amino acid residues 30, 31, 39, 61, 97, 101, and 102; desialylation of the molecule is required before cleavage can occur at some of these sites [57,61]. The sites at residues 30 and 31 are partial cleavage sites; 50% of native GPA molecules are cleaved at residue 31 and 10% at residue 30 [61]. When intact cells are treated with trypsin the N-terminal 39 amino acid residues of

GPA are severed, resulting in loss of M antigen and GPA-borne N antigens, as well as any other determinants located on this portion of the glycoprotein. Purified GPB may be cleaved by trypsin at amino acid residue 35 [83], but trypsin treatment of intact cells does not denature GPB. The blood group antigens S and s, and the 'N' antigen located at the N-terminus of GPB are therefore trypsin-resistant [109,110].

3.5.1.2 Chymotrypsin

Chymotrypsin, or more accurately α-chymotrypsin, normally hydrolyses the peptide bond on the carboxyl side of the aromatic amino acids phenylalanine, tryptophan, and tyrosine, as well as leucine, methionine, asparagine, and glutamine. Isolated GPA may be cleaved at residues 34, 64, 98, and 118 [57,61]. M and N antigens on intact cells are partially resistant to chymotrypsin treatment [109,110]; red cell membrane-bound GPA may be cut by chymotrypsin behind residue 34, but only in those molecules devoid of an O-glycan on Thr33 [61]. Treatment of red cells with sialidase followed by chymotrypsin results in abolition of all M and N activity. Treatment of red cells with chymotrypsin cleaves the N-terminal region of GPB at amino acid residue 34 [83,85], destroying S, s, and 'N' activity [109,110]. S-active GPB is denatured by a lower concentration of chymotrypsin than s-active GPB [110].

3.5.1.3 Papain, ficin, bromelin, pronase

The enzymes papain, ficin, and bromelin have a rather broad specificity and the preparations available are often crude compared with trypsin and chymotrypsin. Most GPA- and GPB-borne antigens are destroyed by treatment of red cells with these enzymes, only those situated close to the red cell membrane survive. Pronase, a bacterial enzyme, behaves in a similar way [110]. Whereas papain or ficin treatment of cells readily destroys M, N, 'N', and s antigens, S activity is less easily abolished [109–111].

3.5.2 Sialidase

GPA and GPB carry about 15 and 11 O-linked oligosaccharides, respectively, most of which contain two molecules of sialic acid. In addition, GPA has one N-glycan, which may also be sialylated. Sialidase (neu-raminidase) treatment of red cells removes at least some of these sialic acid residues, altering the charge and possibly the shape of the molecules. Most human sera contain an antibody, anti-T, which recognizes desialylated O-linked oligosaccharides and consequently agglutinates sialidase-treated red cells (Section 3.17.2). High concentrations of sialidase are required to remove most of the sialic acid from GPA; α2→3 linked sialic acid is more easily removed from GPA by sialidase than α2→6 linked sialic acid [112].

M and N antibodies vary in their requirements for sialic acid in order to agglutinate red cells. Judd et al. [71] obtained the following results from testing human MN sera (adsorbed to remove anti-T) with sialidase-treated cells: 27 anti-M, reaction abolished with nine, unaffected with 16, and enhanced with two; seven anti-N, reaction abolished with three, weakened with two, and unaffected with two. Specific M and N antibodies produced by immunizing rabbits with desialylated red cell glycoproteins only agglutinated sialidase-treated cells [113]. Most monoclonal anti-M and -N do not react, or react comparatively weakly, with desialylated red cells or isolated glycophorins (see Section 3.20.7). The effect of sialidase applies equally to N on GPA and 'N' on GPB. M and N activity may be restored to sialidase-treated red cells by resialylation catalysed by sialyltransferases [114].

S, s, and most other MNS system antibodies are not sialic acid-dependent.

3.6 The rare glycophorin A-deficient phenotypes En(a–) and M^K

The following section describes unusual MNS phenotypes caused by two very rare gene deletions. En, a deletion of the coding region of GYPA, causes a deficiency of GPA, but not GPB. M^K, a deletion of the coding regions of GYPA and GYPB, is responsible for deficiency of GPA and GPB. The multifarious antibodies detecting non-polymorphic determinants on GPA, collectively called anti-En^a, will also be described here. There are many other variant MNS genes that do not produce normal GPA, and many rare phenotypes in which part of GPA is missing and consequently anti-En^a (and/or anti-Wr^b) may be made. These are described in other sections, especially those on hybrid glycophorins.

3.6.1 En(a–)

When Darnborough *et al.* [115] described a 'new' antibody to a high-frequency red cell antigen, they noted that the red cells of the antibody maker, a pregnant English woman (MEP), and of several members of her family, gave a variety of unusual blood grouping reactions. These effects were deduced as being 'due to some factor affecting the red cell structure possibly by modifying the cell envelope'. The antibody was named anti-En^a (for envelope) and the rare red cell phenotype En(a–). A second En(a–) propositus (VB) with anti-En^a was found in Finland by Furuhjelm *et al.* [116] and two subsequent En(a–) propositi with anti-En^a, one found in Finland (GW) [117] and the other in the USA (ERP) [118], are part of the same extended family. Two other En(a–) propositi with anti-En^a, a French-Canadian (RL) [119] and a Pakistani (SD) [120], have been identified. Two En(a–) Japanese blood donors without anti-En^a were found by screening red cells from Japanese blood donors with monoclonal anti-En^a [121,122].

Anti-En^a represents an umbrella term, which describes antibodies to determinants on various parts of GPA. The En(a–) phenotype can arise in a number of ways. Typically, En(a–) represents homozygosity for a rare gene deletion (called *En* for convenience) at the *GYPA* locus, resulting in no production of GPA, but normal production of GPB. The original En(a–) phenotype in an English family [115], however, did not arise in this way and probably represents heterozygosity for a complex *GYP(A–B)* hybrid gene [often called *En(UK)*] and an *M^K* gene [123–125]; this En(a–)UK phenotype will be discussed in more detail in Section 3.11.4. The Finnish [116–118], French-Canadian [119], Pakistani [120], and Japanese [121,122] En(a–) phenotypes [En(a–)Fin] appear to result from homozygosity for *En* [often called *En(Fin)*].

Nine En(a–) individuals presumed to have the *En/En* genotype are known; five come from the three branches of the Finnish family [116–118]. This family strongly suggests that *En* is inherited as a recessive character and behaves as a silent allele of *M* and *N*. The parents of two of the Finnish propositi and of the Canadian propositus were cousins [116,117,119]. In the family shown in Fig. 3.8, in which there was no En(a–) member, presence of *En* explained an apparent exclusion of paternity; the M+N– father had three M–N+ children (M. Izatt, cited in [126]).

3.6.1.1 Serological characteristics of En(a–) cells

En(a–) cells do not react with the anti-En^a in the sera of En(a–) propositi, with autoanti-En^a, or with monoclonal antibodies to epitopes restricted to GPA.

En(a–)Fin cells lack any M antigen or trypsin-sensitive N antigen; they do express trypsin-resistant N because of the 'N' antigen of GPB. En(a–)UK cells lack N and 'N', but have a trypsin-resistant 'M' antigen [123,127,128], for reasons that will be described in Section 3.11.4.

En(a–) cells have normal or enhanced expression of S and/or s.

En(a–) cells are Wr(a–b–). The significance of this is discussed below (Section 3.6.3.2) and in Chapter 10.

En(a–) cells have a number of other unusual serological characteristics, probably because of their reduced sialic acid content, which results from absence of the major red cell surface sialic acid-rich glycoprotein. Most of these characteristics are seen, to a lesser extent, in red cells of individuals heterozygous for *En* and are also apparent in other MNS variants that result in a reduction of red cell membrane sialic acid content. En(a–) cells are not aggregated, or at least are aggregated only very weakly, by polybrene and protamine sulphate [118,119,129]. En(a–) cells are agglutinated more strongly than En(a+) cells by non-immune animal sera [116]. Consequently, En(a–) cells may be nonspecifically agglutinated by rabbit anti-M or -N sera as a result of residual anti-human antibodies. Saline suspensions of En(a–) cells are directly agglutinated by 'incomplete' anti-D and other Rh antibodies when the appropriate Rh antigens are present on the cell; these antibodies do not agglutinate En(a+) cells of the same Rh phenotype. En(a–) cells react more strongly than En(a+) cells with certain lectins [116,130]. Particularly useful for this purpose are extracts from the seeds of *Sophora japonica* (adsorbed with group AB cells to remove anti-A+B activity) and *Glycine soja*, although extracts from seeds of *Bauhinia purpurea* (anti-N), *Dolichos biflorus* (anti-A$_1$), *Phaseolus lunatus* (anti-A), and *Arachis hypogea* (anti-T) can all distinguish En(a–) cells from En(a+) cells. *Maclura aurantiaca* lectin, which binds to red cell sialoglycoproteins [127], reacts only weakly with En(a–) cells [130].

En heterozygotes can generally be recognized because their red cells show some of the serological characteristics associated with reduced sialic acid described above. Parents or offspring of an En(a–) individual, and those people presumed to be

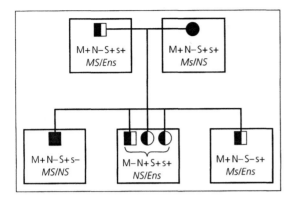

Fig. 3.7 Family demonstrating how the presence of *En* can explain an M+N− father with three M−N+ children and associated red cell membrane modifications. Red cells of all family members are En(a+). The genotype of the mother is deduced from her parents and sibs (not shown). ■● no modification of red cell membrane; ▯◖ modified red cell membrane, single dose of M or N. Redrawn from [126].

heterozygous for *En* because of the unusual serological characteristics of their red cells or because of abnormal inheritance of M or N antigens (Fig. 3.7), are M+N− or M−N+ ; none is M+N+.

3.6.1.2 Frequency of *En*

En is very rare; only five unrelated *En/En* individuals are known. Tests with anti-En[a] on 12 500 English, 8800 Finnish, and 200 Estonian donors revealed no En(a−) individual [115,116]; tests on 250 000 Japanese donors revealed one [121,122]. As mentioned above, saline suspensions of En(a−) cells are directly agglutinated by 'incomplete' Rh antibodies. Three possible *En* heterozygotes were found by screening 6202 donors with 'incomplete' anti-D and anti-c [131]. An investigation of red cells from 1300 Scottish donors for aggregation in protamine sulphate revealed two probable *En* heterozygotes, one with *En(UK)* and the other with *En(Fin)* [129].

3.6.1.3 Biochemistry

Typical En(a−) red cells lack GPA; no GPA, or its dimer (GPA$_2$) and heterodimer (GPAB), is detected by SDS PAGE of En(a−) cells (see Fig. 3.3) [48,49,60,118–120,122,127,128,132]. GPB of En(a−) cells has normal mobility on SDS PAGE. Band 3, the anion transport protein, has an elevated molecular weight in En(a−) cells, resulting from an increase in the length of its N-glycan [119,120,122,127,128,132,133]. If GPA facilitates the movement of band 3 from internal membranes to the cell surface, as suggested from its effect in *Xenopus* oocytes, then in GPA-deficient cells band 3 protein may remain longer in the Golgi network providing greater opportunity for elongation of the N-glycan [134] (see Section 3.25).

Furuhjelm *et al.* [116], in their study of the first Finnish En(a−) propositus, observed reduced red cell electrophoretic mobility resulting from a low level of sialic acid. En(a−) cells have about 40% of the sialic acid of normal cells and cells from *En* heterozygotes, about 70% of normal levels [116,119,132]. This reduction in sialic acid appears to increase the agglutinability of red cells, explaining many of the unusual serological characteristics of GPA-deficient red cells.

3.6.1.4 Molecular genetics

Results of Southern blotting of genomic DNA from two individuals with the En(a−)Fin phenotype initially suggested a complete deletion of *GYPA* and normal *GYPB* [88,94,96]. Vignal *et al.* [98,103] subsequently showed that exon A1 and the upstream untranslated region of *GYPA* is not deleted in *En*, and that the deletion encompasses exons A2–7 of *GYPA* and exon B1 of *GYPB* (Fig. 3.8). As exon 1 of both genes codes for most of the leader sequence, but not for any of the mature protein, this would result in production of no GPA. However, it would permit normal expression of GPB, which would be produced by a *GYP(A–B)* hybrid gene comprising the promoter sequences and exon A1 of *GYPA* and exons B2–6 of *GYPB*.

3.6.2 *M^K*

The name *M^K* was coined by Metaxas and Metaxas-Bühler [135] for a new allele of *M* and *N* that appeared to produce neither M nor N. A second family showed that not only did *M^K* appear to be a silent allele at the *MN* locus, it was also silent at the *Ss* locus [136]. The effect of the *M^K* gene was highlighted in this family by apparent maternal exclusions in three generations: an M+N−S−s+ woman (presumed genotype *Ms/M^K*) had an M−N+S−s+(*Ns/M^K*) daughter, who married an M+N−S+s+(*MS/Ms*) man and had one M+N−S+s− (*MS/M^K*) and two M+N−S−s+(*Ms/M^K*) daughters, one of whom had an M−N+S−s+(*Ns/M^K*) child.

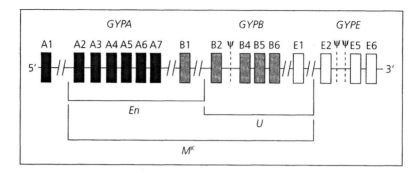

Fig. 3.8 Diagram to show the extent of deletions of *GYPA*, *GYPB*, and *GYPE* responsible for En(a–) (*En*), U– (*u*), and M^K phenotypes [98,103]. In each case the deletion breakpoints occur within the very long first introns (–//–) of these genes. *En* represents a deletion of exons A2–A7 and B1; *u*, a deletion of exons B2–B6 and E1; and M^K, a deletion of exons A2–A7, B1–B6, and E1. Other mechanisms may also be responsible for S–s–U– phenotypes (see Section 3.7.4).

Red cells of individuals with one M^K gene resemble cells of *En* heterozygotes regarding the unusual serological characteristics associated with reduced sialic acid levels [131,137–140] (see Section 3.6.1.1). Eight heterozygous M^K individuals were found in 10 097 Swiss donors, either by testing with 'incomplete' anti-D and anti-c by direct agglutination of untreated cells or by M and N dosage determination [131,141]. Apart from the Swiss examples, at least six other M^K heterozygous propositi have been reported: one Dane [136]; one Swede [142]; two English [115,143]; one white American [144]; one Chilean [145]; and one Chinese [138]. The Chinese family also contains the rare gene for GP.Mur (Mi.III) [138] (Section 3.12.1). The American [144] and Chilean [145] are heterozygous for M^K and the gene for GP.Hil (Mi.V) (Section 3.11.1). One of the English propositi [115] is heterozygous for M^K and *En(UK)* [123,124] (Section 3.11.4).

A dysmorphic, mentally deficient child with part of the long arm of chromosome 2 translocated onto the long arm of chromosome 4 appeared to have the genotype *MS/M^K* [146,147]. His father was M–N+S–s+, with a double dose of N antigen, and his mother was M+N+S+s+. The child, whose red cells had a single dose of M antigen, had probably not inherited M^K from either parent, the rare gene resulting *de novo* from the effect of his chromosomal translocation. *MNS* is on the long arm of chromosome 4 (Chapter 32).

The first *M^K/M^K* homozygotes were a Japanese blood donor and his brother, reported by Tokunaga *et al.* [148] in 1979. Their red cells were M–N–S–s–U–En(a–) Wr(a–b–) and showed all the reactions charac-

teristic of reduced sialic acid. This M^K phenotype has subsequently been found in two Japanese sisters [149], in an African American child [150], and in a Turkish woman and her brother [151]. Parents of each of the Japanese propositi were consanguineous.

3.6.2.1 Biochemistry

M^K produces neither GPA nor GPB; red cells from *M^K/M^K* homozygotes are devoid of GPA and GPB [148–150]. Red cells of people heterozygous for M^K have about half the normal quantity of GPA and GPB [40,152–154].

Band 3 of M^K cells, like that of En(a–) cells, shows an increase in molecular weight resulting from increased glycosylation (Section 3.6.1.3). This amounted to an increase of about 3000 in the M_r of band 3 in M^K homozygotes [148,149] and heterozygotes [152]. M^K red cells have reduced sulphate transport activity because of a lowered binding affinity of band 3 for sulphate ions [155]. M^k red cells also appear to have a reduction in size of the glucose transporter GLUT1 [155] and an M_r 2000 increase in the cytoskeletal glycoprotein, band 4.1 [148]. Red cell sialic acid content is reduced by about 30% in cells of M^K heterozygotes [137,140,144,152] and 70% in cells from *M^K/M^K* homozygotes [148].

The *M^K/M^K* genotype had no obvious adverse effect on the health of five M^K individuals and no abnormal haematological effects were apparent [148]. The *M^K/M^K* genotype therefore has not been very informative about the functions of GPA and GPB (see Section 3.25).

3.6.2.2 Molecular genetics

From Southern blot analysis, Tate *et al*. [94] showed that genomic DNA from one of the Japanese M^K/M^K individuals lacked all fragments of *GYPA* and *GYPB* that encode mature GPA and GPB, suggesting a single deletion spanning both genes. This agrees with the conclusions of Rahuel *et al*. [96] from their studies on an *En(UK)/M^K* individual. *GYPE* is not deleted in M^K [94,98]. As shown in Fig. 3.8, the deletion does not include exon A1 and the upstream promoter region of *GYPA*, but does include exon E1 of *GYPE*, to leave a hybrid *GYP(A–E)* gene [98,103].

3.6.3 Anti-En^a, anti-Wr^b, and the determinants they define

3.6.3.1 Alloanti-En^a

The first three examples of anti-En^a, those from the English En(a–) propositus (MEP) and the first two Finnish En(a–) propositi (VB, GW), appeared to be antibodies of identical specificity, which reacted with all red cells save those of the En(a–) phenotype [115–117]. All three propositi had been transfused. None of the four En(a–) siblings of the three propositi had made anti-En^a; none had been transfused, but one had been pregnant five times. These three anti-En^a sera were later shown to contain at least two antibodies to high frequency antigens, anti-En^a and -Wr^b [116,156–158]. Neither antibody reacted with cells of the En(a–) Wr(a–b–) phenotype, but anti-En^a, unlike anti-Wr^b, did react with En(a+) Wr(a+b–) cells (described below). The other En(a–) propositus from the Finnish family (ERP), who had never been transfused but had been pregnant twice, made a similar mixture of antibodies [118]. The French-Canadian En(a–) propositus (RL), a man with no transfusion history, made anti-En^a and no anti-Wr^b; his anti-En^a differed from the other examples in that it defined a trypsin-sensitive antigen and could be inhibited by extracted M and N substances [119].

Adsorption and elution studies with red cells treated with different proteases (trypsin, papain, ficin) and with red cells of rare MNS phenotypes in which only part of GPA is present, have shown that anti-En^a is a collective term for antibodies to determinants at a variety of sites on the extracellular domain of GPA [116,158–161]. For convenience, Issitt *et al*. [162] de-fined three broad categories of anti-En^a according to the effect of proteases on the antigenic determinants they detect.

Anti-En^aTS recognizes a trypsin-sensitive determinant and is typified by the antibody of the French-Canadian En(a–) propositus (RL) [119]. It does not react with En(a+) red cells treated with trypsin, ficin, or papain and can be inhibited by isolated GPA. GPA on intact cells is cleaved by trypsin at amino acid residue 39. Dahr *et al*. [61] found that three anti-En^aTS (two alloantibodies and one autoantibody) had different binding sites on the N-terminus of GPA. The antibody of RL reacts with a determinant around amino acid residues 31–39, but only on those GPA molecules that are not glycosylated at Thr33 [61].

Anti-En^aFS represents those En^a antibodies that recognize a ficin-sensitive (papain-sensitive), trypsin-resistant determinant. Anti-En^aFS is found as a separable component in the sera of the En(a–) propositi MEP, VB, GW, and ERP and may also be an autoantibody [163]. Anti-En^aFS is inhibited by isolated GPA [158–160]. Six anti-En^aFS analysed by Dahr *et al*. [61] were very similar; all six were directed at a determinant around residues 46–56 of GPA and five of the sera required glycosylation at Thr50 for binding.

Anti-En^aFR represents those antibodies that react with a ficin-resistant (papain-resistant), trypsin-resistant determinant. They differ from anti-Wr^b by reacting with En(a+) Wr(a+b–) cells. Anti-En^aFR can also be isolated from the sera of MEP, VB, and GW. Anti-En^aFR is not easily inhibited with isolated GPA. En^aFR appears to represent a labile structure within amino acid residues 62–72 of GPA, requiring lipid for complete antigenic expression [164].

3.6.3.2 Anti-Wr^b and the Wr^b antigen

The name anti-Wr^b was tentatively used by Adams *et al*. [165] in 1971 for an antibody detecting a public antigen in the serum of a woman whose Wr(a+) red cells appeared to have a double dose of Wr^a. The antibody reacted more strongly with Wr(a–) cells than with Wr(a+) cells. The association between Wr^b and MNS first became apparent when Issitt *et al*. [156,166] found that En(a–) cells were Wr(a–b–) and subsequent immunochemical studies suggested that the Wr^b determinant is located on GPA [164,167]. This presented an enigma, as it had long been known that Wr^a is genetically independent of MNS [18].

Details of the nature of the relationship of Wr^b to the MNS system are provided in Chapter 10. The Wr^a/Wr^b dimorphism results from an amino acid substitution within band 3 [168], but Wr^b can only be detected when band 3 is associated with GPA in the membrane. Hence, GPA-deficient red cells are Wr(b–). Whether Wr^a expression also requires GPA presence is unclear as no GPA-deficient individual with a *Wr^a* allele has been found.

3.6.3.3 Clinical significance of anti-En^a

The clinical outcome of transfusing En(a+) red cells to patients with anti-En^a is varied. A patient with anti-En^{a}TS and depressed red cell GPA expression died of a post-transfusion haemolytic reaction [169] and an En(a–) patient (GW) with anti-En^a and anti-Wr^b suffered a mild delayed haemolytic transfusion reaction after receiving 6 units of En(a+) blood [117]. Predominantly IgG1 anti-En^a with a lesser IgG3 component in an *M^K/M^K* patient was responsible for severe haemolytic disease of the newborn (HDN) [151]. Functional assays with anti-En^{a}FR/Wr^b provided further evidence that these antibodies are of clinical importance [170].

3.6.3.4 Autoanti-En^a

Autoantibodies with En^a specificity have been identified [171], some in patients with severe and fatal autoimmune haemolytic anaemia [163,172,173]. These are usually of the anti-En^{a}FS type, though some may be anti-En^{a}FR [173]. Moulds *et al.* [174] found that pure anti-En^{a}FS occurs in 1.6% of warm autoantibody cases. Anti-Wr^b is not an uncommon autoantibody specificity (Chapter 10).

3.6.3.5 Antibodies produced by *M^K/M^K* individuals

Neither of two Japanese men with *M^K/M^K* genotype had been transfused, yet both produced an antibody to a public antigen [148]. These antibodies did not react directly with En(a–) cells, but their reactivity with En(a+) cells was reduced by adsorption with En(a–) cells. The antibodies, which did not react with sialidase or pronase-treated cells and could be inhibited by sialoglycoprotein preparations, probably detect a Pr-like determinant common to GPA and GPB (see Section 3.6.4). The other Japanese propositus [149]

and the Turkish woman [151] made anti-En^a; both had been pregnant several times, but had not been transfused.

3.6.3.6 Monoclonal antibodies to non-polymorphic determinants on GPA

In 1982, Anstee and Edwards [175] described three monoclonal antibodies, produced by immunization of mice with human red cells, which detected different epitopes on GPA. None was anti-M or anti-N. Many more monoclonal antibodies to non-polymorphic epitopes on GPA have been described since [48,52,87,176–178]. These antibodies can be loosely divided into four categories.

1 Antibodies to trypsin-, ficin-, and papain-sensitive epitopes on GPA, but not GPB (anti-En^{a}TS). These epitopes are either on the N-terminal side of the trypsin cleavage site at Arg39 or overlap Arg39. They are mostly within the region of amino acid residues 30–45.

2 Antibodies to trypsin-resistant, but ficin- and papain-sensitive epitopes on GPA (anti-En^{a}FS). These epitopes are mostly in the region of amino acid residues 49–58.

3 Antibodies that detect epitopes, usually sialic acid-dependent, common to GPA and GPB. This epitope is generally situated within the N-terminal 26 amino acid acids, which are identical in GPA^N and GPB. Antibodies of this type react with En(a–) and S–s–U– cells, which lack either GPA or GPB, respectively; they do not react with M^K cells, which lack both GPA and GPB, or with trypsin-treated S–s–U– cells, which lack GPB plus the N-terminal 39 amino acids of GPA.

4 Antibodies to epitopes on the cytoplasmic C-terminal domain of GPA. These antibodies do not react with intact red cells and are usually detected by immunoblotting.

One murine monoclonal antibody bound to [53]Pro-Pro-Glu-Glu-Glu[57] of GPA (anti-En^{a}FS), but also reacted with [395]Pro-Pro-Glu-Gln[398] of the cytoskeletal component, protein 4.1 [179]. Monoclonal antibodies directed at different epitopes on GPA have proved extremely valuable in the analysis of the many rare MNS variants described later in this chapter.

3.6.4 Pr and Sa antigens

The protease labile Pr antigens [180,181] were originally named Sp$_1$ by Marsh and Jenkins [182] and HD by Roelcke [183] (Chapter 25). They are generally detected by cold-active IgM human monoclonal autoantibodies in cold haemagglutinin disease or postinfection [184], but on rare occasions may be associated with warm autoimmune haemolytic anaemia [172,173]. Pr antigens have been subdivided into a number of subspecificities; Pr_1, Pr_2, and Pr_3 are distinguished by chemical modification of sialic acid residues with periodate oxidation and carbodiimide treatment (reviewed in [181]). Anti-Sa cold agglutinins are similar to anti-Pr in detecting a sialic acid-dependent antigen, but anti-Sa react, albeit only weakly, with papain-treated cells [185].

Anti-Pr_1, -Pr_2, -Pr_3, and -Sa react with O-linked oligosaccharides on sialoglycoproteins [34,186–188]. Most anti-Pr and all anti-Sa recognize immunodominant $\alpha2,3$-N-neuraminic acid groups linked to galactose, but a minority of anti-Pr may recognize $\alpha2,6$-N-neuraminic acid groups [189]. It is probable that anti-Pr_{1-3} detect the predominant form of O-glycan, the disialotetrasaccharide shown in Fig. 3.2, and that anti-Sa detects incompletely sialylated glycoconjugates (monosialotetrasaccharides) found on the more internal parts of GPA [181]. GPA and GPB express Pr_{1-3} [34,186,187]; GPA is also Sa-active [185,187]. Pr_2 and Sa are also detected on red cell gangliosides [188]. Pr antibodies agglutinate En(a–) cells very weakly and do not agglutinate M^K cells at all [18,119,190]. Unfortunately, no adsorption–elution studies were performed with M^K cells, which would be expected to carry some Pr determinants on other membrane components such as GPC and GPD.

3.7 U antigen and the GPB-deficient phenotypes S–s–U– and S–s–U+^{var}

3.7.1 U and anti-U

U was the name given by Wiener et al. [15,191] in 1953 to a new high-frequency blood group antigen present on the red cells of 977 of 989 African Americans and all of 1100 white Americans. When, in the following year, Greenwalt et al. [13] found a second example of anti-U, it became apparent that U was associated with the MNS system; both U– samples available were also S–s–, a phenotype not previously encountered. Adsorption and elution studies showed that anti-U was not a separable mixture of anti-S and -s [13,192]. Greenwalt et al. [13] proposed that the gene that did

not produce any S, s, or U antigen be called S^u. As we now know that this gene cannot strictly be considered an allele of S and s, the original notation of Wiener et al. [191] will be used here; U for the gene producing U antigen, u for that not producing U antigen.

U– red cells are almost always S–s–, but S–s– cells are often U+ [16,30,193,194]. S–s–U+ is often referred to as S–s–U+^{var} [195]. Strength of U antigen expression on S–s–U+ red cells is variable; adsorption–elution tests or sensitive agglutination tests with a particularly potent antibody may be required for its detection [16,196]. Like S–s–U–, the S–s–U+^{var} phenotype is virtually exclusive to people of African origin. About 50% of S–s– red cell samples are U+^{var} [194,197].

The precise serological definition of anti-U is unclear, but the term is traditionally used to describe antibodies produced by S–s– individuals to high-frequency determinants on GPB. In a study of 17 'anti-U', Storry and Reid [194] found that five failed to react with all S–s– red cells. They called these antibodies anti-U. The other 12, which reacted with S–s–U+^{var} cells, but not S–s–U– cells, they called anti-U/GPB. By these definitions, S–s–U– cells are U–, U/GPB–, whereas S–s–U+^{var} cells are U–, U/GPB+. In this respect, anti-U and -U/GPB could be considered analogous to anti-En^a [194]. S–s–U– cells are totally GPB-deficient, whereas S–s–U+^{var} cells have a variant GPB molecule that expresses neither S nor s. Following transfusion or pregnancy, anti-U may broaden in specificity to become anti-U/GPB and react with S–s–U+^{var} red cells that had previously been non-reactive with serum from the same patient [198,199].

S–s–U– and S–s–U+^{var} cells usually lack the trypsin-resistant N antigen carried on GPB ('N') [18,30,195,200,201], although Dahr et al. [202] detected weak 'N' activity on isolated sialoglycoprotein from two M+N–S–s–U+^{var} individuals. Consequently, apart from cells of certain very rare MNS variant phenotypes, M+N–S–s– cells are the only cells with no obvious expression of N antigen. Immunized N– U– people are likely to make anti-U and/or potent anti-N, which reacts strongly with the N antigen on both GPA and GPB [195].

The low-frequency antigen He is expressed at the N-terminus of a GPB molecule that does not express 'N' (see Section 3.8.3). There is a strong correlation between expression of variant U antigen and He. Reid et al. [197,203] found that 54 (51%) of 106 S–s– red cell samples reacted with anti-U/GPB, but not anti-U;

of these 54 S–s–U+^{var} samples, 37 (68.5%) were He+. None of the S–s–U– red cells that were non-reactive with anti-U/GPB was He+. PCR with allele-specific primers revealed that 90% of people with the S–s–U+^{var} phenotype have a *He* allele of *GYPB*; the remainder have an 'N' allele of *GYPB* [203]. This confirms that S–s–U+^{var} results from the presence of a variant GPB molecule (see Sections 3.7.3 and 3.7.4). Storry and Reid [194] considered that anti-U/GPB could be categorized as either inseparable anti-U,N,He or -U,He.

U antigen is generally resistant to denaturation by sialidase, trypsin, chymotrypsin, papain, and ficin. However, unusual examples of anti-U do not react with papain-treated cells and an antibody component to a papain-sensitive determinant was identified in about 50% of anti-U sera [204]. An antibody component to a papain-sensitive determinant was present in 21 of 40 sera containing anti-U.

S–s–U– red cells do not show most of the unusual serological reactions associated with reduced sialic acid that are characteristic of red cells deficient in GPA (Section 3.6.1.1), though *Glycine soja* lectin may agglutinate U-deficient cells [205].

Other rare phenotypes in which the red cells may be S–s–U– are the Rh-deficiency phenotypes (Section 5.16.5) and phenotypes arising from homozygosity for hybrid genes encoding the rare SAT and St^a antigens (Sections 3.11.3 and 3.15.2).

Further details of anti-U, including clinical significance and autoanti-U, can be found in Section 3.20.11. Anti-U^Z and anti-U^X are described in Section 3.20.12.

3.7.2 Frequency and inheritance of U

Results of screening donors with anti-U are unreliable, because they vary according to the proportion of S–s–U+^{var} samples that give positive or negative results with the antibody reagent used. Issitt and Anstee [195] draw attention to six series of tests on red cells from African Americans. In three series the frequency of U– is between 0.2% and 0.3%. This probably represents the true figure for U–. In the other three series, the frequency is between 1.2% and 1.4%, probably representing not only U–, but also those with a weak variant U antigen.

Table 3.2 shows M, N, S, and s phenotype frequencies in African Americans, together with genotypes in which the S–s– phenotype is assumed to have resulted

from homozygosity for *u* at the *Ss* locus. The *MN* and *Ss* haplotype frequencies derived from studies of African American and African populations shown in Table 3.4 reflect a similar approach. Of 126 Pygmies from Zaire, 35% were U– [206]. No S–s–U– individual was found among 1000 Bantu-speaking people of Natal [207], whereas three were found among 1000 black antenatal patients from the eastern Cape [208].

No large series of black families has been studied for MNSs, but a few are described in references [28–30]. In black people it is not uncommon for a S+s– (genotype *S/u*) parent to have a S–s+(*s/u*) child, or for a S–s+(*s/u*) parent to have a S+s– (*S/u*) child.

Although extremely rare, *u* and the U– phenotype have been identified in people of non-African descent. Four S–s–U– members were found in a white family from France [209] and four S–s–U– individuals were found in a family originating from India [210]. Six of 324 Finnish Lapps [19] and two of 63 Central American Indians from Honduras [20] were S–s–. Presence of a *u* gene in white families has often been used to explain otherwise unlikely parentage exclusion through Ss groups [18,211–214]. Although this proposal is usually backed-up with serological evidence from dosage studies with anti-S, -s, and even anti-U, dosage effects with anti-U are generally very difficult to detect [215].

3.7.3 Biochemistry

S–s–U– red cells are deficient in GPB. This has been demonstrated by failure to inhibit anti-S, -s, or -U with sialoglycoproteins isolated from S–s–U– cells [216], by SDS PAGE of red cell membranes or isolated sialoglycoproteins [200,202,209,216–218], and by immunoblotting with antibodies and lectins directed at determinants on GPB [49,50,209,217]. Red cells of individuals heterozygous for *u* have roughly half of the normal quantity of GPB [200,201,216].

By heavy loading of gels, Dahr *et al.* [202] were able to detect small quantities of GPB, about 2–3% of normal, on S–s–U+^{var} cells. GPB normally carries about 11 O-glycans, and S–s–U– and S–s–U+^{var} red cells demonstrate a reduction in sialic acid by about 15% compared with normal cells [216,219]. Cells of individuals heterozygous for *u* have about a 9% sialic acid reduction [216]. Unlike En(a–) and M^K, the GPA-deficiency phenotypes, S–s–U– is not associated with any apparent alteration of band 3 [216].

U appears to be a labile structure requiring lipid for full expression [220]. In this respect it resembles En^{a}FR, which is located close to the membrane on GPA (Section 3.6.3). From the results of anti-U haemagglutination inhibition tests with GPB extracts, in the presence of lipids, Dahr and Moulds [220] proposed that amino acid residues 33–39 of GPB are essential for U antigen expression. Unlike S and s, U escapes denaturation by chymotrypsin treatment of intact cells, because the cleavage site for chymotrypsin is between residues 32 and 33.

3.7.4 Molecular genetics

The S–s– phenotype has two major molecular backgrounds. In about 53% of S–s– African Americans there is a substantial deletion of *GYPB*, encompassing exons B2–6 of *GYPB* and also including exon E1 of *GYPE* [94,98,217,221,222] (see Fig. 3.8). Homozygosity for this deletion is probably responsible for the S–s–U– phenotype.

The molecular basis for S–s–U+^{var} is less clear. S–s–U+^{var} phenotypes probably arise from the presence of abnormal *GYPB*-like genes that usually express an He-specific sequence within exon B2 [203], the most common of which is a phenotype called GP.He(P$_2$) [223] present in about 42% of S–s– African Americans [222]. In addition to a *GYPA* insert within exon 2 responsible for He expression (see Section 3.12.2), splice site mutations at the 3′ end of exon B5 and near to the 5′ end of the adjacent intron (position +5) result in complete skipping of exon B5 and a reading frameshift within exon B6. The skipping of exon B5 leads to the loss of the region that usually constitutes the membrane-spanning domain of GPB. The reading frameshift abolishes the translation stop codon close to the 5′ end of exon B6 so that the C-terminus of the glycoprotein is elongated by a novel sequence of 41 amino acids. Expression of He antigen on intact red cells and immunoblotting experiments demonstrated that this abnormal GPB was present in the membrane. The novel amino acid sequence encoded by exon B6 is highly hydrophobic and is, presumably, utilized as a membrane-spanning domain (Fig. 3.9). Furthermore, fusion of the extracellular domain to an abnormal hydrophobic sequence must be responsible for the failure of the structure to express S or U (although U/GPB is expressed), despite the presence of a linear sequence for these antigens. This demon-

strates the conformational importance of the region around the insertion of GPB into the membrane for expression of S, s, and U antigens.

3.8 M and N variants representing amino acid substitutions within the N-terminal region of GPA and GPB

M and N antigens are determined by the sequence and glycosylation of the N-terminal five amino acids of GPA and GPB (Table 3.7). Amino acid substitutions within this pentapeptide may affect expression of M or N and may create a new antigen. Three such variants are described in this section: M^g and M^c on GPA; He on GPB.

3.8.1 M^g (MNS11)

M^g, a very rare antigen first described by Allen *et al.* [224] in 1958, is encoded by a gene that produces virtually no M or N antigen. Undetected, an *M^g* allele in a family could result in apparent exclusion of parentage as an M+N– (*M/M^g*) parent can have a M–N+ (*N/M^g*) child.

Tests with anti-M^g on over 100 000 English and American blood donors revealed no M^g+ sample [225]. In Swiss and Sicilians a much higher incidence of about one in 600 was found [225–227] (Table 3.9). Analysis of 21 Swiss families with the mating type M^g+ ×M^g– and a total of 51 children confirmed that *M^g* behaves as an allele of *M* and *N* [225,226]. In two Bostonian families [224,270], a family from mainland Italy [227], and all of the Swiss families [225,226], M^g was aligned with *s*; in four families of Sicilian origin [227,271], the alignment was *M^{g}S*. The M^g+ daughter of one of the Swiss propositi was found to have an M^g+ husband and an M–N–M^g+ child [225], the only known person homozygous for *M^g* and the source of much of our serological and biochemical knowledge of M^g.

Red cells from the *M^g* homozygote have a reduction in sialic acid level of about 12% from normal; heterozygotes have a 7% reduction [152]. They demonstrate many of the serological and physicochemical features characteristic of cells with reduced membrane sialic acid levels [137] (described in Section 3.6.1.1). Like M and N, M^g is denatured by treatment of the cells with trypsin, but not chymotrypsin [153,272,273]; unlike most anti-M and -N, anti-M^g

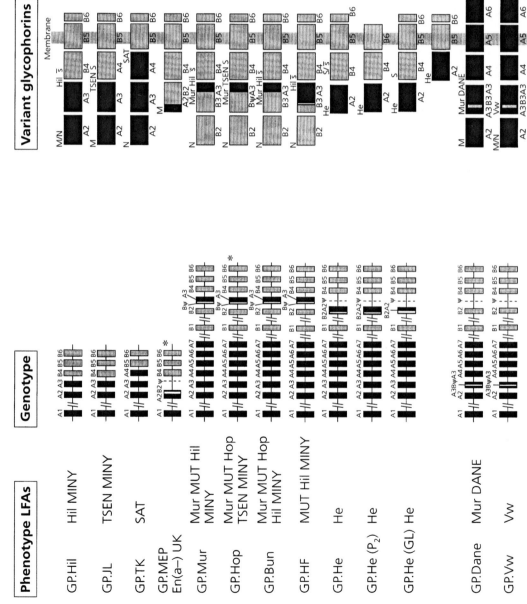

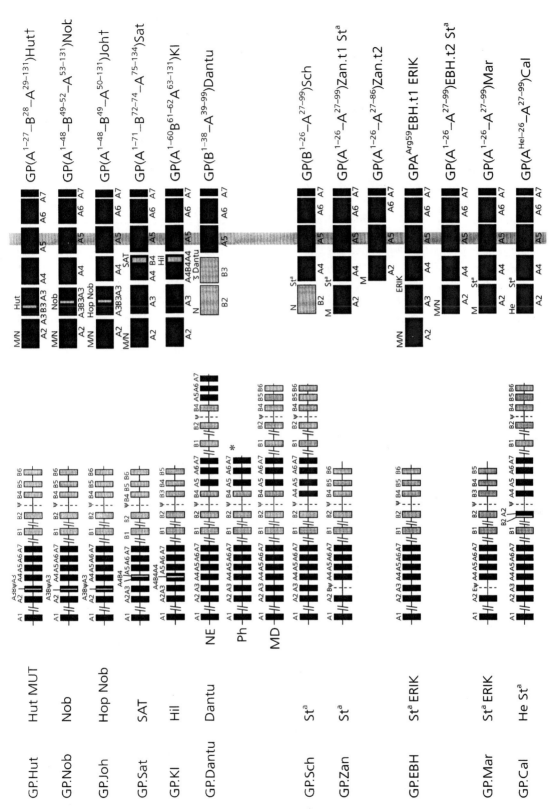

Fig. 3.9 Rare MNS phenotypes associated with hybrid glycophorins. * Possible genotypes deduced from serological and biochemical evidence. † Alternatively could result from a point mutation.

121

generally react with sialidase-treated M^g+ cells [71,274,275].

In 1981, three research teams showed that the M^g phenotype results from a threonine to asparagine substitution at position 4 of GPA^N [272,275–277], the result of a point mutation in an N allele of $GYPA$ [66]. This asparagine residue is not glycosylated and the amino acid substitution also prevents, or at least grossly reduces, glycosylation of the serine and threonine residues at positions 2 and 3, a total reduction of three O-glycans responsible for a degree of sialic acid deficiency (Table 3.7).

Although Furthmayr et al. [275] detected no glycosylation of residues 2 and 3 of $GPAM^g$, Dahr et al. [276] found them to be glycosylated in up to 25% of $GPAM^g$ molecules. Furthermore, 30% of $GPAM^g$ molecules lack the N-terminal leucine residue and up to 10% lack N-terminal leucine and serine residues, probably because of in vivo action of amino-peptidase [84].

Anti-M^g is easily inhibited by the glycosylated N-terminal octapeptide cleaved from $GPAM^g$, but not by that from GPA^N [275]. Haemagglutination inhibition studies with various synthetic peptides and glycopeptides representing the N-terminal region of GPA showed that most anti-M^g primarily recognize a non-glycosylated structure with N-terminal leucine; only a minority are dependent on Asn4 [278,279]. Glycosylation of M^g-active peptides at positions 2, 3, or 4 abolishes M^g activity [278]. Two murine monoclonal anti-M^g have been produced [280]: for one the epitope is dependent on Glu5, but not Asn4; for the other, Leu1 and Asn4 were the most essential components of the epitope.

Judd et al. [71] found that one of six M^g antibodies reacted with a sialic acid-dependent antigen. Perhaps this antibody detects a determinant on the minority glycosylated form of $GPAM^g$ [34]. A variant of M^g, in which the cells reacted with only two of six anti-M^g, had the same N-terminal amino acid sequence as normal $GPAM^g$, but up to 75% of these aberrant $GPAM^g$ molecules were glycosylated at residues 2 and 3 [281].

Roughly half of the monoclonal anti-M tested reacted with cells of M^g/N or M^g/M^g individuals and, on immunoblots, bound to GPA of reduced molecular weight characteristic of M^g [48,176,282–284]. The epitope detected by monoclonal anti-M that agglutinate M–M^g+ red cells is dependent on Val6 and Met8

of deglycosylated GPA (as occurs in $GPAM^g$), but also requires Gly5 when the GPA is normally glycosylated [285]. Monoclonal anti-N may agglutinate cells from M^g/M or M^g/M^g individuals [48,239], but bind to GPB and not $GPAM^g$ on immunoblots [286]. Immunoblotting of M^g+ cells with anti-M^g, polyclonal or monoclonal, revealed only the GPA molecule of reduced molecular weight ($GPAM^g$) [239,284].

M^g+ red cells reacted with anti-DANE (-MNS32) and with the original anti-Mur (Murrell), but not with 14 other examples of anti-Mur [284]. Immunoblotting showed that the Murrell anti-Mur was binding $GPAM^g$. A possible explanation for these reactions is provided in Section 3.14.2.

3.8.1.1 Anti-M^g

M^g is extremely rare, yet anti-M^g is possibly the most common MNS antibody [18]. In four separate searches for anti-M^g in sera of normal people the following frequencies were obtained: four from 500 sera (0.8%) in the USA [224]; 23 from 703 (3.3%) [18] and six from 340 (1.8%) [153] in England; 12 from 1614 (0.7%) in India [238]. In order to explain the high incidence of anti-M^g, Dahr et al. [276,279] speculated that people might be exposed to M^g-like structures by removal of carbohydrate from normal glycophorin during natural red cell destruction. Anti-M^g in 17.6% of sera from Liberia was attributed to the high level of parasitic infection [287].

Anti-M^g has been produced in rabbits [288] and as murine monoclonal antibodies [280].

3.8.2 M^c (MNS8)

Despite having an International Society of Blood Transfusion (ISBT) red cell antigen number, M^c cannot strictly be regarded as a blood group antigen as no anti-M^c exists. M^c is often considered to represent an intermediate between M and N.

M^c, a rare allele of M and N found by Dunsford et al. [289] in an English family, produces a determinant that reacts with the majority of anti-M (as demonstrated by the red cells of the N/M^c member of the family) and with the minority of rabbit anti-N (as demonstrated by the two M/M^c members). M^c has subsequently been defined by a pattern of reactions with known anti-M and -N reagents. Several more examples of M^c have been reported, all in people of European origin

Table 3.9 Incidence of MNS-associated low frequency antigens (in ISBT number order).

Antigen	Population	No. tested	No. positive	Antigen frequency (%)	References
He (MNS6)	African Americans	6 997	207	2.958	[24,228–230]
	West Africans	1 428	38	2.661	[231]
	Congolese	70	10	14.286	[230]
	South African Bantu	4 000	247	6.175	[232]
	Pygmy Bush people	428	32	7.477	[233]
	African Bushmen	188	4	2.128	[234]
	Hottentots	201	21	10.448	[234]
	Papuans	33	3	9.091	[235]
	Europeans	1 500	0		[231]
	White New Yorkers	5 00	4	0.800	[24]
	White South Africans	1 000	0		[232]
Vw (MNS9)	White people	52 635	30	0.057	[18]
	Grisons, SE Switzerland	1 541	22	1.428	[18]
	Thais	2 500	1	0.040	[236]
Mur (MNS10)	Thais	2 500	1	9.640	[236]
	Minnan Chinese (Taiwan)	400	18	4.500	[237]
	Hakka Chinese (Taiwan)	100	3	3.000	[237]
	Ami Taiwanese	138	122	88.406	[237]
	Bunun Taiwanese	100	0		[237]
	White people	50 101	6	0.012	[18]
M^g (MNS11)	Boston, USA	44 000	0		[225]
	English	61 128	0		[225]
	Swiss	6 530	10	0.153	[225,226]
	Sicilians (in Belgium)	1 889	3	0.159	[227]
	Italians (in Belgium, non-Sicilians)	4 408	1	0.023	[227]
	Belgians	36 683	0		[227]
	Bombay	9 000	2	0.022	[238]
	African Americans	4 254	0		[239]
Vr (MNS12)	Dutch	1 200	3	0.250	[240]
Mt^a (MNS14)	White Americans	11 907	28	0.235	[241]
	Swiss (Zürich)	1 435	5	0.348	[18]
	Irish	1 000	0		[242]
	African Americans	1 007	1	0.099	[241]
	Thais	318	3	0.943	[243]
St^a (MNS15)	Chinese	490	8	1.633	[244,245]
	Japanese	220	14	6.364	[245]
	English	17 013	20	0.118	[246]
Ri^a (MNS16)	Londoners	70 501	1	0.001	[246,247]
Cl^a (MNS17)	Europeans	12 541	0		[18,248]
Ny^a (MNS18)	Norwegians	9 687	18	0.186	[249–251]
	Swiss	9 395	1	0.010	[18]
	Germans	20 000	0		[252]
	Americans	7 400	0		[253]
	African Americans	350	0		[254]
	Japanese	3 281	0		[254]
	Chinese	1 032	0		[254]

Continued

Table 3.9 *Continued*

Antigen	Population	No. tested	No. positive	Antigen frequency (%)	References
Hut (MNS19)	White people	32 591	21	0.064	[18]
	Thais	2 500	1	0.040	[236]
Mᵛ (MNS21)	English	2 372	14	0.590	[255]
Far (MNS22)	Europeans	15 373	0		[256,257]
sᴰ (MNS23)	White South Africans	1 000	1*	0.100	[258]
	Black South Africans	1 000	0		[258]
	Indian South Africans	500	0		[258]
	'Coloured' South Africans	1 000	1	0.100	[258]
Mit (MNS24)	Canadians	3 311	4	0.121	[259]
	North Londoners	8 278	7	0.085	[260]
	Africans	662	0		[259]
	African East Indians	500	0		[259]
	Manitoba Cree	555	0		[259]
Dantu (MNS25)	African Americans	3 200	16	0.500	[261]
	N London (mostly white)	44 112	1†	0.002	[262]
Hop (MNS26)	Thais	2 500	17	0.680	[236]
Nob (MNS27)	English	4 929	3	0.061	[263]
	Mixed race Americans	1 766	0		[264]
Or (MNS31)	English	887	0		[265]
	African Americans	163	1	0.613	[265]
	Japanese	17 200	2	0.012	[266]
DANE (MNS32)	Danes	467‡	2	0.428	[267]
SAT (MNS36)	Japanese	10 480	1	0.010	[268]
Osᵃ (MNS38)	Japanese	50 000	0		[269]

*Member of original family [258].
†Black/Indian/English/French donor from Maurutius.
‡Trypsin-treated cells screened with anti-M.

[18,290]. M^c exists as $M^c s$ and $M^c S$ [18,289,290]. Because anti-M^c does not exist, there is very little information on the frequency of M^c. Metaxas *et al.* [290] screened red cells of 3895 Swiss with anti-M and -N reagents designed to disclose MN variants and found one M^c/M individual.

The serological behaviour of M^c cells was explained in 1981 when the N-terminal amino acid sequence of GPAM^c was determined [275,291]. At position 1 is serine, characteristic of M, and at position 5 is glutamic acid, characteristic of N (Table 3.7). Residues 2, 3, and 4 have normal glycosylation. If M^c represents an evolutionary link between M and N, the rarity of M^c suggests that it might have been at some selective disadvantage to M and N.

The reactivity of the majority of anti-M and minority of anti-N with M^c cells shows that, for most antibodies, it is the N-terminal amino acid residue that is recognized, although the residue at position 5 is important for some. This applies not only to polyclonal rabbit and human reagents [18,289], but also to monoclonal antibodies [48,176,282,292].

3.8.3 He (MNS6) and Mᵉ (MNS13)

3.8.3.1 He

The original anti-He was found by Ikin and Mourant [293] in a rabbit serum containing anti-M. Another example was made deliberately by immunizing a rabbit with He+ red cells, the cells of Mr Henshaw from whom the antigen derived its name [231]. Human alloanti-He have been identified since [18,294,295]. Monoclonal anti-He were produced by immunizing mice with He+ red cells [87,228].

He antigen is found in about 3% of African Americans and in various African populations with a similar or higher incidence (Table 3.9). He is very rare in white people; no example was found in 1500 Europeans [231] or 1000 white South Africans [232], but four He-positives were found among 500 white New Yorkers [24]. He may be associated with MS, Ms, NS or Ns, predominantly with NS in black New Yorkers [229] and West Africans [231], with MS in Congolese [235], and with Ns in Papuans [235].

Judd et al. [296] suggested that an He+ woman who had made potent anti-N and whose red cells lacked all expression of N antigen, including the 'N' antigen associated with GPB, had the genotype MsHe/Mu. The gene complex encoding He was producing no 'N', suggesting that He is located on GPB. Biochemical analysis of GPB from He+ red cells confirmed the association with GPB and explained the absence of 'N'. Three of the five N-terminal amino acid residues of GPBHe differ from those of normal N-active GPB: tryptophan replaces leucine at position 1; serine replaces threonine at position 4; glycine replaces glutamic acid at position 5 [297]. Glycosylation of this region is unchanged as the serine residue at position 4 of GPBHe is O-glycosylated (Table 3.7). Immunoblotting with human and mouse anti-He confirmed the location of He antigen on GPB [228,298]. As would be expected of a determinant on GPB, He is resistant to trypsin treatment of the red cells, but weakened or abolished by chymotrypsin treatment [273,296,297]. The requirement for sialic acid is variable [71,297].

DNA analysis has shown that He is associated with GYPB in which a small segment, including part of exon B2 and intron B2, have been replaced by the homologous segment from GYPA [298]. Huang et al. [298] propose that a gene conversion event was responsible for creating this GYP(B–A–B) gene (see Section 3.10). A number of untemplated nucleotide changes would have occurred during the gene conversion, some of which produced the amino acid sequence characteristic of the He antigen. He-active glycophorins are produced by several other hybrid genes (Fig. 3.9) discussed elsewhere in this chapter: GYP(B–A–B)He(P$_2$) (Section 3.7.4);

GYP(B–A–B)He(GL) (Section 3.12.2); and GYP(B–A–B–A)Cal (Section 3.15.2.5).

Serological and immunochemical studies with monoclonal anti-He revealed a marked variation in He antigen strength [197,228]. Reid et al. [197] divided He expression into strong (He^s), moderate (He^{mod}), and weak (He^w). He^s is associated with S/s+U+ phenotypes, He^w with S–s– phenotypes, and He^{mod} with either S/s+ or S–s– phenotypes (see Section 3.7). He^w only reacted serologically with undiluted monoclonal and rabbit anti-He, and not at all with human anti-He. Ninety per cent of S–s– red cell samples that reacted with anti-U/GPB had the nucleotide sequence characteristic of He [203].

Of 38 He+ donors of African origin, all with the normal (strong) He antigen, 35 (92%) were S+ [228]. As about 30% S+ would be expected for the whole population, the GYP(B–A–B) gene encoding He usually produces S.

3.8.3.2 M^e

Wiener and Rosenfield [299] described a rabbit anti-M that unexpectedly reacted with M–N+He+ cells. Anti-M and -He activity could not be separated by adsorption and elution tests and the determinant shared by M and He was named M^e. Twenty years later the first human anti-M^e was found [295]. Whereas the rabbit anti-M^e had reacted preferentially with M, the human antibody reacted equally strongly with M+He– cells and M–He+ cells. Anti-M^e was found to be present in nine of 14 anti-M sera from M–N+ Israeli blood donors [300] and five of nine monoclonal 'anti-M' had anti-M^e activity [301]. Reactivity of anti-M^e with M+He– cells is trypsin-sensitive; reactivity of anti-M^e with M–He+ cells is trypsin-resistant [300]. On immunoblots, monoclonal anti-M^e stains GPA on M+He– membranes, GPB on M–He+ membranes, and both GPA and GPB on M+He+ membranes.

The existence of anti-M^e is no surprise. Anti-M that are dependent on the presence of terminal leucine will not react with an He determinant on GPB, but anti-M that recognizes glycine at position 5 of GPA would be expected to react with GPA^M and GPBHe (Table 3.7).

3.9 The Miltenberger series

Miltenberger is a series of relatively rare phenotypes associated with the MNS system, related to each other through the overlapping specificities of a number of low frequency alloantigens. The characteristics that place an MNS variant phenotype into the Miltenberger series, rather than just being considered as one of the many MNS variants, are purely serological and some of these serological connections between the categories are tenuous. It is no longer feasible to expand the Miltenberger series to accommodate new phenotypes, or to incorporate some existing MNS variant phenotypes, such as M^g, which would become candidates for inclusion on the grounds of serological findings. Although the Miltenberger classification is now obsolete, it is mentioned here because it has appeared in the literature for many years and still continues to do so. Described below is a brief history of the Miltenberger series followed by an outline of an alternative notation proposed by Tippett et al. [302] and designed to encompass all variant MNS phenotypes. The Miltenberger classes, together with the new terminology, are listed in Table 3.10. A review by Dahr [307] puts an alternative point of view by asserting that the Miltenberger subsystem should be expanded to incorporate new findings.

Cleghorn [308] initiated the Miltenberger series in 1966 in an attempt to bring some order to a complex pattern of reactions with several different antibodies to low incidence antigens. These antibodies were categorized into four type sera:

1 Verweyst (Vw), also called Graydon (Gr) [305,309];
2 Miltenberger (Mi^a) [310];
3 Murrell (Mur) [311];
4 Hill (Hil) [18].

These four type sera defined four phenotypes:
Class I in which the cells are Mi(a+) Vw+;
Class II initially [312,313] Mi(a+) Vw−, but later found also to react with anti-Hut [308,313];
Class III Mi(a+), Mur+, Hil+, and Hut+; and
Class IV Mi(a+), Mur+, Hut+.

The original association with the MNS system originated from the observation that Vw appeared to be inherited with MNS [314]. Cleghorn [308] named the series Miltenberger after the type serum that reacted with red cells of all four classes. Six more classes have been added since (Table 3.10). The original meaning of anti-Hut has been changed. Giles [273,304] has suggested that Hut is specific for Class II, the original reactivity with cells of other classes being a result of a mixture of anti-Hut and -Mur. As these two specifici-

ties cannot always be separated, Giles's revised definition of anti-Hut (specific for Class II cells) is used in Table 3.10 and the term anti-MUT is used for the inseparable anti-Mur+Hut originally called anti-Hut by Cleghorn [308].

A fifth class was added to the series in 1970 [255]. Mi.V cells do not react with any of the antibodies found in Miltenberger type sera, but were included because, like Mi.III cells, they reacted with anti-Hil.

Miltenberger became even more complex with the addition of three more classes—Mi.VI, Mi.VII, and Mi.VIII [273,315,316]—following the identification of three more type sera, Anek, Raddon, and Lane [263,304]. Giles [273] proposed that Miltenberger could be simplified by considering determinants rather than type sera and by dismissing some weak reactions as cross-reactivity. Anek serum, which subdivided Mi.III into Mi.III (Anek−) and Mi.VI (Anek+), and also reacts with Mi.IV cells, became anti-Hop. Raddon and Lane type sera became anti-Nob. Mi.VII cells react with anti-Nob, but not anti-Hop; Mi.VIII cells react with both anti-Hop and anti-Nob (Table 3.10). Even this explanation is an oversimplification; some of the further complexities of Hop and Nob specificity are described by Tippett et al. [302].

Miltenberger class IX was introduced by Skov et al. [267] in 1991 when they found four propositi with Mur+ cells that also reacted with anti-DANE, a new antibody specific for Mi.IX. Despite being Mur+, Mi.IX cells are MUT−. Mi.X, added in 1992, is represented by red cells that are Hil+ and MUT+, yet Mur− and Hut− [317]. Mi.XI was added [307] for the phenotypes of two propositi, JR and JL, on the basis of the reactions of their red cells with anti-TSEN and -MINY [318,378].

The notation proposed by Tippett et al. [302] replaces the Miltenberger classes with a symbol comprising GP (for glycophorin) followed, after a full stop, by the abbreviated name of the first propositus (with the exception of Mi.V where the familiar name Hil is used). So, for example, for Mi.III, Mur is the abbreviated name of the first propositus, GP.Mur is the phenotype, GP(B–A–B)Mur the variant glycophorin, and GYP(B–A–B)Mur the gene that produces it. This notation can also be used for other abnormal MNS phenotypes, thus abolishing the concept of the Miltenberger subsystem. The new terminology will be used for the rest of this chapter, and the 'Miltenberger phenotypes'

Table 3.10 Serological definition of the Miltenberger phenotypes and a replacement notation proposed by Tippett *et al.* [302] (and slightly modified [303]).

Mi class	New notation	Antigens										
		Mi[a]	Vw	Mur	Hil	Hut*	MUT†	Hop	Nob	DANE	TSEN	MINY
I	GP.Vw	+	+	−	−	−	−	−	−	−	−	−
II	GP.Hut	+	−	−	−	+	+	−	−	−	−	−
III	GP.Mur	+	−	+	+	−	+	−	−	−	−	+
IV	GP.Hop	+	−	+	−	−	+	+	−	−	+	+
V	GP.Hil	−	−	−	+	−	−	−	−	−	−	+
VI	GP.Bun	+	−	+	+	−	+	+	−	−	−	+
VII	GP.Nob	−	−	−	−	−	−	−	+	−	−	−
VIII	GP.Joh	−	−	−	−	−	−	+	+	−	NT	−
IX	GP.Dane	−	−	+	−	−	−	−	−	+	−	−
X	GP.HF‡	+	−	−	+	−	+	−	−	−	−	+
XI	GP.JL	−	−	−	−	−	NT	−	−	−	+	+

*As defined by Giles *et al.* [273,304].
†Originally called Hut [18,305,306].
‡GP.HF previously named GP.Mor [302].
NT, not tested.

will be described more fully in various sections according to their biochemical basis. For the convenience of readers more accustomed to Miltenberger classes, these will be provided in parentheses at regular intervals.

3.10 Hybrid glycophorins and the low frequency antigens associated with them

In 1979, Anstee *et al.* [218] looked to haemoglobin to provide an explanation for the unusual serological and biochemical characteristics observed with red cells of the GP.Hil (Mi.V) phenotype. The model illustrated in Fig. 3.10 predicts that misalignment between *GYPA* and *GYPB*, followed by unequal crossing-over, results in the production of two new haplotypes. In one there is a loss of *GYPA* and *GYPB* and the formation of a novel fusion gene that produces a GP(A–B) hybrid molecule made up of the N-terminal region of GPA and the C-terminal region of GPB. This is often referred to as the Lepore type of hybrid glycophorin, after the analogous rare haemoglobin variant Lepore in which the non-α chain is a hybrid comprising a fusion of part δ-chain and part β-chain [319]. In the opposite haplotype, formed at the same event (anti-Lepore), not only is a hybrid gene predicted that produces a GP(B–A) glycoprotein consisting of the N-terminus of GPB and the

C-terminus of GPA, but also normal *GYPA* and *GYPB* flanking the hybrid gene.

There is now substantial evidence confirming the validity of Anstee *et al.*'s [218] proposal. Lepore type hybrids may explain the unusual MNS phenotypes associated not only with GP.Hil, but also with several other variants including En(UK) and GP.Sat. Anti-Lepore haplotypes are responsible for the unusual phenotypes associated with expression of Dantu and St[a] antigens. It is likely that chromosomal misalignment, involving *GYPA* and *GYPB*, occurs as a result of the homology that occurs between some regions of those genes. Intron 3 of *GYPA* and the homologous intron of *GYPB* appear to be particular hotspots for recombination (reviews in [36,320]).

More complex GP(B–A–B) and GP(A–B–A) hybrids also exist, the former being a GPB molecule with a small GPA insert and the latter a GPA molecule with a GPB insert. The likelihood of two crossing-over events occurring in such close proximity is small, so gene conversion provides a more likely explanation for these aberrant glycophorins [36]. The mechanism of gene conversion is poorly understood, but it is a non-reciprocal exchange of genetic material from one homologous gene to another resulting in a small segment of one gene being replaced by the equivalent segment of its homologue. A model for gene conversion is

127

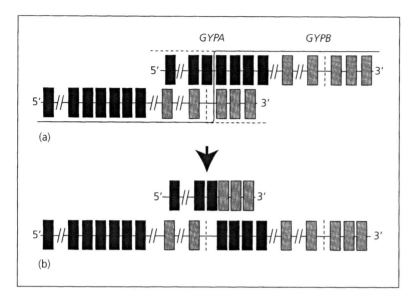

Fig. 3.10 Model demonstrating development of hybrid genes involving *GYPA* and *GYPB* by chromosomal misalignment and unequal crossing-over. (a) The two homologous genes become misaligned at meiosis and intergenic crossing-over occurs. (b) Result: one haplotype containing a *GYP(A–B)* fusion gene and another haplotype containing a *GYP(B–A)* fusion gene flanked by normal *GYPA* and *GYPB*. The two hybrid genes produced are typical of those encoding GP(A–B)Hil and GP(B–A)Sch.

illustrated in Fig. 3.11. In some cases, the insertion of a functional splice-site consensus sequence from *GYPA* into *GYPB* has led to the expression of the *GYPB*-pseudoexon [36].

The creation of novel amino acid sequences by the production of hybrid glycophorins often results in the expression of low frequency antigens. Some of these amino acid sequences and their associated antigenic determinants may arise by more than one genetic mechanism. The various hybrid glycophorin molecules and their associated low frequency antigens will be described in Sections 3.11–3.15.

Figure 3.9 shows the rare phenotypes resulting from hybrid glycophorins, the haplotypes that produce them, and a diagrammatic representation of the hybrid glycophorins. Often it is not possible to determine the precise location of recombination sites. In Fig. 3.9 the smallest possible insert is assumed.

3.11 GP(A–B)-associated variants (Lepore type)

3.11.1 GP.Hil (Mi.V) and the Hil (MNS20) antigen

Red cells of a new phenotype identified by Crossland *et al.* [255] reacted with anti-Hil, which also reacted with GP.Mur (Mi.III) cells, but they did not react with anti-Mur (Table 3.10). Family studies have shown that the gene for GP.Hil may be inherited with weakened N or M and elevated expression of s [144,145,159, 255,322].

Owing to the shortage of anti-Hil, no frequency studies have been reported. All the recorded GP.Hil individuals are probably of European origin.

Since Anstee *et al.* [218] suggested that the unusual glycophorins associated with GP.Hil (Mi.V) represented a Lepore type of hybrid glycophorin, its dimer, and its heterodimers with GPA and GPB, substantial serological and biochemical supportive evidence has followed [49,91,144,145,159,323,324]. This was facilitated by the finding of an M–N+S–s+ Spanish-American woman homozygous for the GP.Hil gene [159] and of two individuals heterozygous for the GP.Hil gene and M^K [144,145]. Immunochemical studies revealed only two structures, the putative hybrid (apparent M_r 40 000) and its dimer. Antibodies to the N-terminal region of GPA bound to the putative hybrid molecule; those to the C-terminal domain did not. The final proof that GP.Hil is a hybrid glycophorin molecule came from an analysis of the genomic DNA [91,97,103,325]. *GYP(A–B)Hil* comprises exons A1–A3 of *GYPA* fused to exons B4–6 of *GYPB* (Fig. 3.9). The crossing-over point is located within intron 3 of *GYPA* and *GYPB* [97,325]. The primary structure of the polypeptide encoded by *GYP(A–B)Hil* therefore comprises amino acid residues 1–58 of GPA fused to residues 27–72 of GPB.

It is now possible to provide biochemical explanations for many of the unusual serological characte-

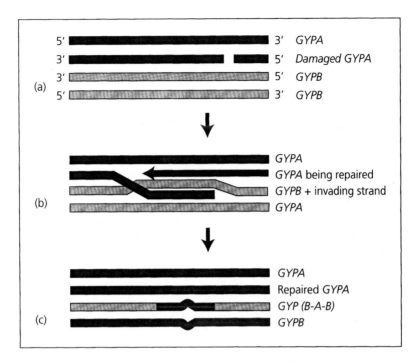

Fig. 3.11 A model for gene conversion occurring as the result of damage repair to *GYPA* and involving homologous regions of *GYPA* and *GYPB*. (a) *GYPA/GYPB* heteroduplex, resulting from chromosomal misalignment, with a nick in one *GYPA* strand. (b) An extra copy of one strand of the *GYPA* DNA is synthesized, displacing the original copy, which pairs with one strand of the homologous region of the *GYPB* DNA. The unpaired region of *GYPB* is then degraded. (c) Result: one *GYPB* gene contains a short segment of *GYPA* DNA. After [321].

ristics of GP.Hil red cells, especially those of *GYP(A–B)Hil* homozygotes (and heterozygotes with M^K).

1 Reduced M or N expression; no 'N'. The N-terminus of the hybrid glycophorin carries M or N, although the gene produces less GP(A–B) than GPA produced by a normal gene [91,218,326]. These M or N antigens are trypsin-sensitive because of an intact trypsin cleavage site at amino acid residue 39 of GPA. There is no trypsin-resistant 'N' because no GPB is produced.

2 Elevated s expression. The hybrid contains Thr29 of GPB responsible for s expression. Although there is less GP(A–B) than normal GPA, there is substantially more than normal GPB. U antigen is also produced.

3 Presence of En[a]TS and En[a]FS; very weak expression of En[a]FR; absence of Wr[b]. The part of GPA associated with trypsin- and ficin-sensitive determinants is retained in the hybrid, that associated with Wr[b] and most of En[a]FR are lost. En[a]FR is detectable only by adsorption experiments [159]. The homozygous *GYP(A–B)Hil* woman and those women heterozy-

gous for *GYP(A–B)Hil* and M^K were found because they had produced anti-Wr[b] (and/or anti-En[a]FR) [144,145,159].

4 Serological characteristics associated with reduced red cell surface sialic acid [131,144,159] (described for En(a–) in Section 3.6.1.1). Red cells of *GYP(A–B)Hil* homozygotes and heterozygotes have about 53% and 80% of normal sialic acid, respectively [140,159].

5 Hil antigen. Hil, which is trypsin-resistant, represents the unique amino acid sequence present at the point of fusion of GPA and GPB, but only when the third amino acid residue of the GPB derived sequence is threonine (representing s). More details on the Hil antigen are provided in Section 3.14.1.

3.11.2 GP(A–B) hybrids associated with S antigen

Johe *et al.* [327] described an M+N+S+s+ individual (JL) heterozygous for *Ns* and a gene producing a hybrid glycophorin. The red cells were Hil– and had

129

unusual S; they reacted with only 14 of 19 anti-S. The hybrid glycophorin is identical to GP(A–B)Hil apart from having methionine instead of threonine at position 61 (equivalent to position 29 of GPB), explaining the S activity (Fig. 3.9). Genomic sequencing has shown that *GYP(A–B)Hil* and *GYP(A–B)JL* differ in the location of the crossing-over sites within intron 3 [325]. A purine-rich sequence, AAAGT, orientated in either forward or reverse direction, was identified within the crossing-over region of both hybrid genes. A single nucleotide substitution in exon 4 of *GYP(A–B)Hil* and *GYP(A–B)JL*, responsible for the Thr/Met and S/s differences, showed that different *GYPB* alleles had participated in the recombination events responsible for the generation of these two hybrid genes [325]. GP.JL has also been referred to as Mi.XI [307].

Other examples of GP(A–B)JL have been described in people of European origin and in Chinese [160,161,170,318,328,329]. A similar phenotype was found in a Spanish-American woman (AG) who appeared to be homozygous for genes producing GP(A–B) hybrid glycophorins carrying M and S, but whose red cells were weakly Hil+ [330]. Most of the propositi had produced anti-En^a and/or anti-Wr^b.

All these S-active GP(A–B) hybrids express TSEN antigen, whereas the s-active GP(A–B)Hil molecule does not [318] (see Section 3.14.1).

3.11.3 SAT (MNS36)

A new low incidence antigen called SAT, found in two Japanese families, is described here because it is associated with a novel Lepore type of hybrid glycophorin in one of the families [268]. The second SAT+ propositus was found as a result of screening 10 480 Japanese blood donors (Table 3.9). Four examples of anti-SAT are known.

The red cells of one of the SAT+ propositi (TK), who had produced anti-Wr^b and/or anti-En^aFR, were M–N+S–s–U– En^aTS+ En^aFS+ En^aFR– Wr(b–). The results of SDS PAGE and immunoblotting were consistent with the propositus being homozygous for a gene producing a GP(A–B) hybrid. All SAT+ members of his family had the same variant glycophorin; the SAT– members did not. Unlike all other GP(A–B) molecules described, GP(A–B)TK did not express S, s, or U [268]. Analysis of cDNA demonstrated that GP(A–B)TK is

encoded by a gene comprising exons A1–4 of *GYPA* and B5 and B6 of *GYPB*, with a crossover point within intron 4 [331] (Fig. 3.9). This represents the reverse arrangement to that seen in GP(B–A)Dantu (Section 3.15.1). GP(A–B)TK is a 104 amino acid glycoprotein with the novel sequence Ser-Glu-Pro-Ala-Pro-Val produced by the junctions of exons A4 and B5 [331]. This sequence may represent the SAT antigen.

In the only other family with SAT+ members there was no sign of a hybrid molecule and SAT appeared to be associated with normal GPA and GPB, except that the GPA carried a very weak M antigen [268]. Uchikawa *et al.* [332] found six more SAT+ propositi in Japan, three with the GP(A–B) hybrid glycophorin and three with apparently normal GPA and GPB. Analysis of *GYPA* cDNA from the latter type revealed an insert, between exons A4 and A5, of nine nucleotide bases derived from the 5′ end of exon B5 of *GYPB*. This predicted an insert of Ala-Pro-Val in a GPA molecule, creating the SAT specific sequence of Ser-Glu-Pro-Ala-Pro-Val.

3.11.4 En(UK)

En(UK) is one of the genes responsible for the aberrant phenotype of the original En(a–) proposita (MEP) [115], who is heterozygous for *En(UK)* and *M^K* [123–125]. Unlike *En(Fin)* (a deletion of *GYPA* with normal *GYPB*), *En(UK)* probably produces a Lepore type of hybrid glycophorin of the same molecular weight as GPB [125]. En(a–)UK cells lack the En^a, Wr^b, and C-terminal determinants associated with GPA. They have a weak trypsin-resistant M antigen, and no trypsin-resistant 'N' [17,60,123–125,128,326]. They also have enhanced expression of S. It is probable that En(UK) arose from the misalignment and unequal crossing-over between an *M* allele of *GYPA* and an *S* allele of *GYPB*, with the crossing-over occurring either within the homologous region encoding the first 26 amino acid residues of both molecules or within intron 1. Preliminary DNA analysis supported the hypothesis of a gene encoding a GP(A–B) hybrid [96].

Screening of red cells from 1300 British blood donors for reduced sialic acid by protamine sulphate aggregation revealed one donor who appeared to have *En(UK)* producing S and trypsin-resistant M [129]. Two individuals with *En(UK)* producing M and s [333], presumably represent a separate recombination event from that responsible for *En(UK)* in the other families studied [115,129]. Anti-M reagents that depend on Ser1 reacted with the M produced by *En(UK)*, whereas those that require Gly5 did not. This suggests that the original recombination may have occurred between the codons for amino acid residues 1 and 5, producing a molecule identical to GPB apart from a Leu1Ser substitution.

3.12 GP(B–A–B)-associated variants

3.12.1 GP.Mur (Mi.III), GP.Hop (Mi.IV), GP.Bun (Mi.VI), and GP.HF (Mi.X)

3.12.1.1 Serology, frequency, and inheritance

GP.Mur and GP.Bun are similar phenotypes. The red cells are Mur+, Hil+, MUT+, and MINY+, but GP.Bun cells are Hop+ whereas GP.Mur cells are Hop– (Table 3.10). GP.Mur and GP.Bun are always inherited with s. In people of European origin GP.Mur may be inherited with *Ns* or with *Ms*, the former being more frequent than the latter [308]. In Thais [236] and Chinese [244], GP.Mur is usually inherited with *Ms*. GP.Bun is generally inherited with *Ms* [315]. For examples of GP.Mur families see [138,236,308,311,334,335] and for GP.Bun families see [315]. GP.Mur and GP.Bun phenotypes are associated with an elevated expression of 'N', the trypsin-resistant N antigen carried on GPB [138,244,308,315,334,336]. The s antigen produced by the GP.Mur gene differs qualitatively from normal s. GP.Mur red cells may fail to react with some potent anti-s sera [308] and one s+ woman with GP.Mur red cells made an anti-s, which did not react with her own cells (M. Moulds, C. Lomas and E. Holbrook, unpublished observations, 1981).

Only two GP.Hop propositi are known [308,337]. Like GP.Bun, GP.Hop red cells are also Mur+, MUT+, Hop+, and MINY+, but are Hil– and TSEN+ (Table 3.10). In the only family studied, GP.Hop is inherited with *NS* [308]. Cells from individuals heterozygous for *Ms* and the GP.Hop gene reacted with only some anti-S sera [308,337] and failed to react with a monoclonal anti-GPB (MAb148), which usually reacts preferentially with S+ cells [338].

Tests on over 50 000 white people revealed only six Mur-positives [18]; five were GP.Mur (or possibly GP.Bun as anti-Hop was not used) and one was GP.Hop (Table 3.9). Mur is much more common in people of East Asia. About 10% of Thai blood donors were Mur+; of these, 93% were Hop– (GP.Mur) and 7% were Hop+ (GP.Bun) [236,315] (Table 3.9). GP.Mur has a frequency of around 6% in Hong Kong Chinese [335] and a mean frequency of about 7% in Taiwan Chinese, although there is substantial regional variation [237]. The frequency of GP.Mur reaches 88% in the Ami mountain people of Taiwan, but was not found in some other Taiwanese indigenous groups [237].

GP.HF (Mi.X) cells are unique in being MUT+, yet Mur– and Hut–; they are also Hil+, Hop–, TSEN–, and MINY+ (Table 3.10), and are M+ with elevated 'N' and S– with elevated s [302,317]. Several GP.HF propositi are known, all of Japanese ancestry (M. Uchikawa, unpublished observations 1993).

Another phenotype, named GP.Kip, found in German and Australian propositi, is very similar to GP.Mur[339]. The red cells were Mur+, Hil+, MINY+, and MUT+, but despite being non-reactive with anti-Hop and -Nob, they did react with sera containing Hop+Nob specificities (Anek and Raddon sera).

3.12.1.2 Biochemistry and molecular genetics

In contrast to many other MNS variants, GP.Mur cells have an increased level of sialic acid [140,154,218]. Red cells from heterozygotes have about 13%, and those from homozygotes about 21% more sialic acid than normal cells [218].

GP.Mur, GP.Hop, and GP.Bun are associated with replacement of normal GPB by a component resembling GPB, but of increased apparent M_r (31 000–38 000) [50,154,218,324,340,341]. This abnormal component, which also exists in dimeric form and as heterodimers with GPA and GPB, has the same molecular weight in all three phenotypes and carries about twice as much sialic acid as normal GPB [218,324]. In addition to the abnormal GPB molecule, the GP.Mur haplotype produces normal GPA, but no normal GPB [154,218]. King *et al.* [324] showed that R18, a monoclonal antibody to an epitope on GPA between amino acid residues 46 and 56, bound to the abnormal GPB of GP.Mur cells. This supported a previous suggestion that GP.Mur, GP.Hop, and GP.Bun phenotypes may result from the production of GPB molecules with GPA inserts [342].

DNA analysis has demonstrated that GP.Mur, GP.Hop, GP.Bun, and GP.HF arise from the replacement of a small segment of *GYPB* with a homologous segment from the 5′ end of exon A3 and the 3′ end of intron 3 of *GYPA*, probably the result of gene conversion [317,337,343–345] (see Section 3.10). This piece of *GYPA* replaces the non-functional donor splice-site for the *GYPB* pseudoexon with the functional splice-site sequence from *GYPA*, hence a new composite exon is now expressed consisting of the 5′ end of the pseudoexon of *GYPB* and the 3′ end of exon A3 of *GYPA*, resulting in an enlarged GPB molecule (Fig. 3.12). This GP(B–A–B) molecule consists of the products of exons B1 and B2 of *GYPB* as its N-terminal domain (although exon 1 product is cleaved from the mature protein), followed by the composite exon comprising most of the activated *GYPB* pseudoexon and part of *GYPA* exon A3, followed by exons B4–6 as its C-terminal domain (although most of exon B6 is untranslated) (Fig. 3.9).

GYP(B–A–B)Mur, *GYP(B–A–B)Bun*, and *GYP(B–A–B)HF* have *GYPA* inserts of 55, 131, and 98 bp, respectively. The precise size of the *GYP(B–A–B)Hop* insert is not known. Only minimal differences exist between the glycophorins these genes encode. GP(B–A–B)Mur and GP(B–A–B)Bun differ only at amino acid residue 48, arginine in the former and threonine in the latter. GP(B–A–B)Hop and GP(B–A–B)Bun have the same insert and differ only by Met60Thr (equivalent to position 29 in GPB), responsible for S and s expression. GP(B–A–B)Mur and GP(B–A–B)HF differ by five amino acid residues.

3.12.1.3 Anti-Mur and other antibodies to GP.Mur red cells

Anti-Mur is a fairly common separable component of 'anti-Mi^a' sera [336,346,347], although it also occurs alone [308,334,336,346]. Antibodies to GP.Mur red cells (probably mainly anti-Mur, but often called 'anti-Mi^a') have been responsible for immediate and delayed haemolytic transfusion reactions [348,349] and severe HDN [349,350]. GP.Mur phenotype and antibodies to GP.Mur cells are relatively common in South-East Asia [236,237,335]. Antibodies to GP.Mur cells in Hong Kong are present in 0.34% and 0.46% of patients and pregnant women, respectively; the most common atypical alloantibody. It is important that in South-East Asia GP.Mur red cells are included in antibody screening panels, particularly where abbreviated crossmatch procedures are employed. Complex PCR-based techniques make it possible to predict whether the fetus of a mother with anti-Mur or -Mi^a has GP.Mur or a related phenotype [351].

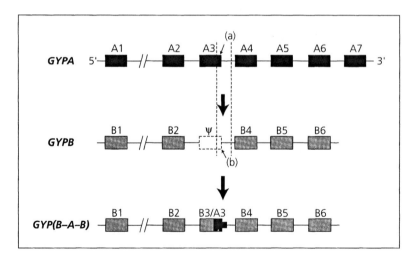

Fig. 3.12 Diagram demonstrating the replacement of a small segment of *GYPB* by the homologous region from *GYPA*, including part of exon A3 and part of intron 3, to generate a novel *GYP(B–A–B)* gene; the result of non-reciprocal recombination by gene conversion. The mutated, non-functional splice-site (b) responsible for the *GYPB* pseudoexon (ψ) is replaced by a functional splice-site from intron 3 of *GYPA* (a), and a composite exon comprising part of the *GYPB* pseudoexon and part of exon A3 is expressed. The resultant *GYP(B–A–B)* gene produces a GP(B–A–B) hybrid glycophorin typical of those present in GP.Mur, GP.Hop, GP.Bun, and GP.HF phenotypes.

Human IgM monoclonal anti-Mur was produced by fusion of Epstein–Barr virus-transformed lymphoblastoid cells with myeloma cells [352].

3.12.2 He (MNS6)

As mentioned in Section 3.8.3.1, a hybrid glycophorin is responsible for the He antigen. The gene encoding He is *GYPB* in which a segment near the 5′ end is replaced by the homologous segment from *GYPA* [298]. A number of untemplated nucleotide changes, probably introduced during a gene conversion event, encode the abnormal amino acid sequence within the N-terminal pentapeptide of the hybrid glycophorin responsible for He antigen expression (Table 3.7). Although the gene is a *GYP(B–A–B)* hybrid, the *B–A* recombination site probably lies in the region of exon 2 encoding the leader peptide and the *A–B* site in intron 2, so the mature protein, after cleavage of the leader peptide, is a GP(A–B) hybrid (Fig. 3.9).

Variants of *GYP(B–A–B)He*, involving splice-site mutations, have been reported. In one [GP.He(P$_2$)], splicing-out of exon B5 and utilization of a novel sequence as a membrane-spanning domain gives rise to a S–s–U+^{var} phenotype [223] and is described in Section 3.7.4. In another variant [GP.He(GL)] there is a point mutation in exon B5 of the gene encoding the He-active glycophorin, which creates a new acceptor splice-site, and another mutation in the exon B6 acceptor site in intron B5 [353]. These mutations affect splicing of exon B4 in a proportion of the mRNA transcripts, so that two glycoprotein isoforms are produced from the same gene: one virtually identical to GP(A–B)He; the other, with an apparent M$_r$ reduced by about 3000 as a result of the absence of the product of exon B4, expresses He, but no S, s, or U (Fig. 3.9). These two glycoproteins were easily detected by immunoblotting with anti-He, but the serological phenotype is not readily distinguished from common He+ phenotypes.

3.13 GP(A–B–A)-associated variants

3.13.1 GP.Dane (Mi.IX)

DANE (MNS32) was identified by Skov *et al.* [267] in four Danish families. In each family DANE was inherited with *MS*; the M was trypsin-resistant. Two of the four propositi were found by screening trypsin-treated red cells from 467 Danish blood donors with monoclonal anti-M (Table 3.9). DANE is trypsin-sensitive. All DANE+ cells are also positive for the Mur antigen, but are MUT– (Table 3.10).

Immunoblotting of M+N+ DANE+ cells with anti-M and with other antibodies to epitopes on the N- and C-terminal domains of GPA showed that DANE is associated with a GPA-like molecule with an apparent M$_r$ about 1000 less than that of normal GPA. This GPA-like molecule appeared to lack the trypsin cleavage site at amino acid residue 39 and also the determinants recognized by alloanti-En^{a}TS and by a number of monoclonal antibodies that detect epitopes between residues 26 and 39 of GPA. Skov *et al.* [267] suggested that DANE is associated with an aberrant GPA molecule with an alteration in the region between amino acid residues 35 and 39, and possibly the loss of one O-glycan.

DNA analysis revealed that the abnormal glycophorin associated with DANE is a GPA molecule with a small segment replaced by GPB, probably as the result of gene conversion [354]. The whole *GYPB* insert is derived from the pseudoexon and replaces an internal segment of exon A3 of *GYPA*, creating two hybrid junctions within the exon. The minimal amount of DNA transferred is 16 nucleotides. Amino acid residues 35–41 of GPA (-Ala-Ala-Thr-Pro-Arg-Ala-His-) are replaced by six residues from GPB (-Pro-Ala-His-Thr-Ala-Asn-). This results in the loss of the trypsin cleavage site at Arg39 of GPA and also the loss of one O-glycan. The sequence derived from the *GYPB*-pseudoexon may represent the Mur determinant, although adjacent amino acid residues may also be involved (see Section 3.14.2). There is an additional untemplated point mutation, Ile46 of GPA to Asn45 of GP(A–B–A)Dane. This amino acid substitution may be responsible for DANE antigen expression and the presence of asparagine may explain the reactions of anti-DANE with M^g cells (see Section 3.8.1).

Only one example of anti-DANE has been identified [267], made by a non-transfused man who is now dead. Very little of the antibody remains.

3.13.2 GP.Vw and GP.Hut, and the Vw (MNS9) and Hut (MNS19) antigens

3.13.2.1 Serology, frequency, and inheritance of Vw

Anti-Vw defines the phenotype GP.Vw (Mi.I)

(Table 3.10). No aberrant expression of M or N antigens has been associated with Vw.

The frequency of Vw in white people is about 0.06%, although in south-east Switzerland a frequency of 1.43% was found [18] (Table 3.9). Family studies have shown Vw to be associated with Ns, NS, Ms, and MS, in decreasing order of frequency [308]; Vw associated with M is very rare [302]. Family analyses are described in references [308,309,311,313,314, 355,356]. One person assumed to be homozygous for the gene producing Vw has been described, an M–N+ S–s+ multiparous woman with an antibody of the anti-En^{a}TS type, named anti-ENEH (–MNS40) [357].

3.13.2.2 Serology, frequency, and inheritance of Hut

Anti-Hut (as defined by Giles [273,304]) determines the GP.Hut (Mi.II) phenotype. GP.Hut cells also react with anti-MUT (originally called anti-Hut [18]), which reacts with most Hut+ or Mur+ cells. Hut is not associated with aberrant expression of M or N antigens.

Hut has a frequency in white people of about 0.06% [18], similar to that of Vw (Table 3.9). Hut has been shown to be aligned with MS, Ns, and Ms in decreasing order of frequency [308], but not with NS. Examples of family studies are given in references [311,313, 358,359].

3.13.2.3 Biochemistry and molecular genetics of Vw and Hut

Vw and Hut are associated with the presence of abnormal GPA molecules, each with a decrease in apparent M_r of about 3000 compared with normal GPA [49,190,324,360–362]. Sialic acid levels of Vw+ and Hut+ red cells appear normal [361]. Manual amino acid sequencing revealed that the unusual GPA molecules contain amino acid substitutions at residue 28; threonine was replaced by methionine in GPAVw and by lysine in GPAHut [361]. Asn26 of GPA normally carries an N-glycan. The required amino acid sequence for N-glycosylation is Asn-Xaa-Thr/Ser (where Xaa represents any amino acid except proline). In normal GPA, which has Asn26 and Thr28, these criteria are fulfilled; in GPAVw and GPAHut Thr28 is substituted, so Asn26 is not N-glycosylated. This lack of N-glycosylation was demonstrated by the failure of the molecule to bind Phaseolus vulgaris lectin [361]

and accounts for the 3000 decrease in M_r compared with normal GPA. Treatment of GPA with N-glycanase reduces the M_r to that of GPAVw; similar treatment of GPAVw has no effect [363].

Vw and Hut are trypsin-sensitive and anti-Vw and -Hut could be inhibited by tryptic peptides comprising the N-terminal 30 or 39 amino acids of GPA from Vw+ and Hut+ cells, respectively [361]. GPA expressed by Chinese hamster ovary cells transfected with GYPA cDNA that has been altered, by site-directed mutagenesis, to encode GPAVw or GPAHut, lacked N-glycosylation and bound anti-Vw and -Hut, respectively [42]. Anti-Vw bound the abnormal GPA of Vw+ cells on immunoblots [364]. It is probable that anti-ENEH, the En^{a}TS antibody produced by a woman homozygous for GYPAVw [357], is specific for Thr28 of GPA, for GPA N-glycosylated at Asn26, or for both.

The codon for amino acid residue 28 of GYPA is ACG (Thr), that for GYPAVw is ATG (Met) [363], an apparent point mutation. One of the codons for lysine is AAG, so point mutation could also account for GYPAHut. Huang et al. [36,363] point out that AAG at the codon for amino acid residue 28 is identical to the equivalent codon within the unexpressed pseudoexon of GYPB. GYPAHut could have arisen by gene conversion with the replacement of a small segment of GYPA with the homologous segment from GYPB (Fig. 3.9). As the nucleotide substitution in GYPAVw is at the same position as that for GYPAHut, GYPAVw could have arisen as a result of gene conversion during which an untemplated replacement of the mismatched nucleotide has occurred because of a failure in heteroduplex repair [363]. The changed nucleotides lie between the two half sites of a direct repeat sequence that has been implicated in recombination events responsible for the production of other hybrid glycophorins. It should be pointed out, however, that creation of the two rare genes by straightforward point mutations has not been ruled out.

3.13.2.4 Anti-Vw

Anti-Vw occurs in mixtures of antibodies to low frequency MNS antigens (as a component of 'anti-Mi^a') [336] or by itself [305,314], where it has been responsible for severe HDN [362,365–367] and, possibly, for a fatal transfusion reaction [368] (although this is disputed [369]). Molecular genotyping can be used to predict fetal Vw phenotype when the mother has anti-

Vw [351]. Anti-Vw is not uncommon in the sera of healthy individuals, with about 1% of normal sera containing anti-Vw [18,309,311,355,356]. It can be found regularly in sera of patients with autoimmune haemolytic anaemia [308]. Of eight anti-Vw sera, seven were IgG alone and one was IgG+IgM [370].

3.13.2.5 Anti-Hut and -MUT

Anti-Hut, an antibody specific for GP.Hut (Mi.II) cells, was first defined by Giles [273,304]. The original Hut antibodies, which would now be called anti-MUT, were isolated from 'anti-Miᵃ' sera [308,313], but independent examples have also been identified and are reported to have caused HDN [18]. Anti-MUT is not simply an antibody that cross-reacts with Mur and Hut antigens. GP.Dane cells are Mur+, but MUT– [267]; GP.HF cells are Mur–Hut–, but MUT+ [302,317] (Table 3.10).

3.13.3 GP.Nob (Mi.VII) and GP.Joh (Mi.VIII), and the Hop (MNS26) and Nob (MNS27) antigens

3.13.3.1 Serology, frequency, and inheritance

Anti-Nob defines two phenotypes, called GP.Nob and GP.Joh [263,273,304,316] (Table 3.10). These phenotypes are distinguished by anti-Hop, which reacts with GP.Joh, but not with GP.Nob cells. Anti-Hop also reacts weakly with GP.Hop (Mi.IV) and GP.Bun (Mi.VI) phenotype cells (Section 3.12.1). This serological description is an oversimplification; anti-Hop sera may contain weak anti-Nob and vice versa, and these specificities may be inseparable. Some of the complexities are mentioned in Sections 3.13.3.3 and 3.13.3.4.

Hop and Nob antigens are trypsin-resistant, but papain- and ficin-sensitive [263,264,273,316].

Unusual expression of M, N, S, s, U, or 'N' antigens has not been reported for GP.Nob or GP.Joh phenotype cells. Red cells of a woman homozygous for the gene responsible for the GP.Nob phenotype lacked ENKT, a form of EnᵃFS antigen [342].

Few families with GP.Nob or GP.Joh members have been identified. In three families, the GP.Nob gene was aligned with *MS* and in one family with *Ms* [263,316]. In two families the GP.Joh gene was aligned with *Ns* [316,371]. Nob has a frequency

of about one in 1643 English blood donors [263] (Table 3.9).

3.13.3.2 Biochemistry and molecular genetics

GP.Nob and GP.Joh phenotypes result from amino acid substitutions within GPA. Both have O-glycosylated Thr49 instead of arginine, but GPANob also has serine (which may be O-glycosylated) instead of Tyr52 [372–374]. Both substitutions could be accounted for by point mutations or by the product of gene conversion [36]. Codons for Thr49 and Ser52, peculiar to GPANob, occur in the corresponding codons of the pseudoexon of a normal *GYPB*. Consequently, a process of gene conversion between *GYPA* and *GYPB* could account for both amino acid substitutions in GPANob, and a similar process involving a smaller segment of *GYPB*, could account for the single amino acid substitution in GPAJoh (Fig. 3.9).

Inhibition assays showed that Hop and Nob antigens on GP(A–B–A)Nob and GP(A–B–A)Joh are located within amino acid residues 40–61 [372–374]. As Hop and Nob are both sialidase-sensitive determinants [373], it seems likely that they are dependent on the glycosylation of Thr49 for binding to native GP(A–B–A)Nob and GP(A–B–A)Joh, yet binding of anti-Hop also appears to require Tyr52. The B–A junction in GP(B–A–B)Bun, but not GP(B–A–B)Mur, creates a Thr-Thr-Val-Tyr (TTVY) sequence that is also present in GP(A–B–A)Joh. It is probable that this sequence is required for the Hop determinant. In the GP.Nob phenotype, the Tyr residue is substituted by Ser and these cells are Hop–. A synthetic decapeptide (EISVTTVYPP), representing amino acid residues 44–53 of GP(B–A–B)Bun and 45–54 of GP(A–B–A)Joh and containing the Thr-Thr-Val-Tyr (TTVY) sequence, inhibited anti-Hop [375].

3.13.3.3 Anti-Hop

The original anti-Hop, found in the serum of a Thai man (Anek) who had never been transfused and whose red cells were of the GP.Mur (Mi.III) phenotype [315], is now considered to be anti-Hop+(Nob) [302]. Other anti-Hop found since [273,316,371] can more accurately be called anti-Hop as, unlike Anek serum, they do not react with GP.Nob (Mi.VII) cells [302] (Table 3.10).

135

3.13.3.4 Anti-Nob

Of the original two anti-Nob sera [263], only one (Lane) is now considered anti-Nob (Table 3.10); the other serum (Raddon) behaves as anti-Nob+(Hop) as it reacts weakly with GP.Hop (Mi.IV) and GP.Bun (Mi.VI) cells [302]. Another antibody reported as anti-Nob [264] behaves as anti-Nob+Hop. This apparently 'naturally occurring' antibody caused minor symptoms of a haemolytic reaction after transfusion of 1 unit of GP.Nob (Mi.VII) blood.

3.13.4 GP(A–B–A)KI

Red cells of a Czech blood donor (KI) and her sister had a novel phenotype. They were Hil+, yet they were MINY– and no abnormal structure was detected by immunoblotting with monoclonal antibodies to GPA and GPB [376]. Genomic sequencing revealed *GYPA* with two nucleotide changes encoding Arg61Thr and Val62Gly substitutions [377] (Fig. 3.9). This creates the sequence PEEETGETGQL, a sequence recognized by anti-Hil (see Section 3.14.1 and Table 3.11). The abnormal GPA molecule is probably the product of a gene conversion event, with Thr61 and Gly62 encoded by a small *GYPB*-derived segment.

3.13.5 GP(A–B–A)Sat

Phenotypes in which the red cells react with anti-SAT occur as the result of at least two backgrounds. One involves a GP(A–B) hybrid and the other a GP(A–B–A) molecule with a small GPB insert [332]. Both are discussed in Section 3.11.3.

Table 3.11 Results of inhibition experiments with synthetic peptides representing amino acids encoded by the 3′ end of *GYPA* exon A3 and the 5′ end of *GYPB* exon B4 [318,375,378].

Peptides GPA-GPB	Antibodies			
	Hil	TSEN	MINY	S^JL
PEEET-GETGQLVHR s	+	–	+	–
PEEET-GEMGQLVHR s	–	+	+	+

+Inhibition; – no inhibition.

3.14 Further details on Hil, TSEN, MINY, Mur, and Mi^a; antigens associated with GP(A–B), GP(B–A–B), and GP(A–B–A) hybrid glycophorins

These antigens are considered together here because they are common to hybrid glycophorins of the GP(A–B) and GP(B–A–B) types, and Hil and Mur are also associated with a GP(A–B–A) molecule.

3.14.1 Hil (MNS20), TSEN (MNS33), and MINY (MNS34)

Hil, TSEN, and MINY are low frequency antigens that react with GP(A–B) and GP(B–A–B) hybrid glycophorins produced by genes with A–B junctions within intron 3; Hil is expressed when s is present, TSEN when S is present, and MINY when either s or S is present [318,375,378]. These hybrid glycophorins have the product of the 3′ end of exon A3 of *GYPA* (or of a *B–A* fusion exon) fused to the product of the 5′ end of exon B4 of *GYPB* (Fig. 3.9, Table 3.11). GP(A–B)Hil, GP(B–A–B)Mur, GP(B–A–B)Bun, and GP(B–A–B)HF all have Thr29 of normal GPB and express an unusual s antigen; they are all Hil+TSEN–MINY+. GP(A–B)JL, similar GP(A–B) hybrids, and GP(B–A–B)Hop express an unusual S antigen and presumably have the Met29 of normal GPB; they are Hil– TSEN+ MINY+.

A 14 amino acid synthetic peptide representing amino acid residues 54–67 of GP(A–B)Hil, including the Thr-Gly A–B junction and the threonine residue responsible for s activity, inhibited anti-Hil [375], but did not inhibit anti-TSEN [318] (Table 3.11). Another peptide, identical apart from the threonine residue replaced by methionine, inhibited anti-TSEN and those anti-S sera (S^JL) that react with red cells with the GP(A–B)JL hybrid glycophorin, but did not inhibit anti-Hil [318,375]. Both peptides inhibited anti-MINY [378]. The Hil determinant is probably smaller than that shown in Table 3.11, as the sequence of PEEETGETGQL is present in GP(A–B–A)KI (Section 3.13.4), which expresses Hil [377].

3.14.1.1 Anti-Hil, -TSEN, and -MINY

The original anti-Hil caused HDN [18,308]. One other example has been reported [379] and a few more examples are now known. Five examples of anti-TSEN have been found, four of them by screening sera from 80 000 donors [318,329]. Only a single example anti-MINY is reported [378].

3.14.2 Mur (MNS10)

GP(B–A–B)Mur, GP(B–A–B)Hop, and GP(B–A–B) Bun include the product of the *GYPB*-pseudoexon activated by a *GYPA* insert, and all express the Mur antigen. Anti-Mur was inhibited by a 13 amino acid synthetic peptide (DTYPAHTANEVSE), representing a sequence encoded by this pseudoexon and amino acid residues 32–44 of GP(B–A–B)Mur and GP(B–A–B)Bun [375]. Location of Mur on GP(B–A–B)Mur was confirmed by immunoblotting [364].

GP(A–B–A)Dane contains the sequence Pro-Ala-His-Thr-Ala-Asn (PAHTAN) originating from the *GYPB*-pseudoexon. DANE+ cells react with anti-Mur, so presumably this sequence represents at least part of the Mur determinant [354]. The original anti-Mur (Murrell) does not contain anti-M^g but reacts with M^g+ cells. The tripeptide Asn-Glu-Val (NEV) could represent the epitope of this atypical form of anti-Mur as it is present in the product of the *GYPB*-pseudoexon (Table 3.11), in GP(B–A–B)Dane (last residue of GPB insert and following two residues), and in GPAM^g (residues 4–6).

Clinical significance of anti-Mur is discussed in Section 3.12.1.3.

3.14.3 Mi^a (MNS7)

Although anti-Mi^a was the antibody that originally defined the phenotypes of the Miltenberger subsystem, it was subsequently considered to represent mixtures of antibodies to low frequency antigens, especially anti-Vw, -Mur, -Hut, and -MUT [133,302,336]. However, production of two murine monoclonal anti-Mi^a demonstrated that anti-Mi^a could exist as a separate entity [352,380]. Dahr [307] speculated that anti-Mi^a might detect the amino acid sequence QTND(M or K)HKRDTY. This sequence represents the junction of the 3′ end of *GYPA* exon 2 and the *GYPB*-pseudoexon, present in GP(B–A–B)Mur, GP(B–A–B)Hop, GP(B–A–B)Bun, and GP(B–A–B)HF, but is also present in the putative GP(B–A–B) molecules associated with GP.Vw and GP.Hut.

3.15 GP(B–A)-associated variants (anti-Lepore type)

3.15.1 Dantu (MNS25)

When Anstee *et al.* [218] postulated a GP(A–B) type of hybrid to account for the GP.Hil (Mi.V) MNS variant phenotype, the genetic mechanism proposed for the creation of the GP(A–B) molecule included the simultaneous production of a haplotype encoding a GP(B–A) type of hybrid glycophorin together with normal GPA and GPB (Fig. 3.10). In 1980, Tanner *et al.* [381] described a new MNS variant in an M+N+S–s+ black Zimbabwean (Ph) and his M+N+S–s– father, in which a novel glycoprotein of M_r 32 000, its dimer, and its heterodimers with GPA and GPB, were identified. Tanner *et al.* [381] proposed that this novel glycoprotein, which carried a trypsin-resistant N antigen, was a GP(B–A) type of glycophorin. The gene producing this GP(B–A) molecule appeared to be inherited with a gene encoding a normal M-active GPA molecule, but no *GYPB* (Fig. 3.9). So it seemed that the initial recombination producing the unusual haplotype must have involved a *u* gene, not uncommon in Africans, which produces no GPB. The putative GP(B–A) molecule was precipitated by a rabbit antibody to a determinant on the cytoplasmic (C-terminal) domain of GPA, but not by a monoclonal antibody to an epitope on the extracellular (N-terminal) domain of GPA [323]; the opposite result to that obtained with GP(A–B)Hil.

In 1984, Contreras *et al.* [262] described Dantu, a new MNS-associated low frequency red cell antigen, found in seven black propositi including the Zimbabwean blood donor (Ph) [381] and an American woman (NE), who also appeared to have a GP(B–A) hybrid glycophorin [382]. In addition to the protease-resistant Dantu antigen, Dantu+ cells carry protease-resistant N and weak s (not denatured by trypsin, chymotrypsin, papain, ficin, or pronase). At first site the family appeared to demonstrate segregation of Dantu from MNS, until it was appreciated that the Dantu haplotype produces both M and N antigens.

The Dantu+ phenotype of Ph differs from that of NE, the latter having a substantially higher ratio of GP(B–A) molecules to GPA than the former [262,326,383]. NE is the usual variety of Dantu+ phenotype [261]; a second Dantu+ propositus of the Ph variety is yet to be found. One white Dantu+ propositus has been identified [384] and her phenotype represents a third variety.

The Dantu haplotype generally produces a normal M-active GPA and a variant glycophorin consisting of the N-terminal 39 amino acid residues of a s-active GPB fused to residues 72–131 of GPA [343,385,386]. The GYP(B–A) breakpoint resides in intron 4 [344] and therefore GP(B–A)Dantu is the reciprocal of GP(A–B)TK described in Section 3.11.3 [331]. GP(B–A)Dantu is protease-resistant [385,387], explaining the trypsin- and papain-resistant N and s antigens [262,381,383]. The s antigen differs qualitatively from normal s. The Dantu haplotype produces little or no U [262,382,383] and GP(B–A)Dantu expresses no Wr^b [388]. The reason why a molecule containing the 39 N-terminal amino acid residues of GPB should have altered s and little or no U is not obvious, but may be because of a conformational change in the molecule.

Dantu+ cells of the NE type have substantially more GP(B–A)Dantu (315 000 sites) than those of Ph (200 000) [326]. The molar ratio of GP(B–A) to GPA in NE type cells is about 2.4:1 [385–387], compared with about 1:1 in Ph [381]. Heterozygotes for the NE type of Dantu have only about 43% the quantity of normal GPA found in cells of common MNS phenotypes despite having two active GYPA genes. This is reflected serologically in weak expression of M and some En^a antigens [262,382]. Huang and Blumenfeld [343] showed that the gene producing GP(B–A)Dantu is duplicated and arranged in tandem (Fig. 3.9), providing an explanation for the high level of GP(B–A) in Dantu+ cells of the NE type. Presumably, the gene producing the Ph type of GP(B–A)Dantu is not duplicated. In contrast to En(a–), M^K, and other phenotypes with reduced GPA (Section 3.6.1.3), the apparent M_r of band 3 is reduced by about 3000, because of shortening of the N-glycan [387].

Dahr *et al.* [385] showed that purified GP(B–A)Dantu inhibited activity of anti-N and -s, but only inhibited anti-Dantu in the presence of lipid. They concluded that Dantu was probably a labile structure, like En^{a}FR and U, and might be located within residues 28–40 of GP(B–A)Dantu.

Dantu+ cells are unusual in having a ficin-resistant N antigen. A simple way of searching for Dantu+ is to screen ficin-treated cells with *Vicia graminea* lectin [261,389]. Sixteen Dantu+ individuals were found by this method, from testing 3200 African American

blood donors (Table 3.9); all were of the NE type [261]. In South Africa, Dantu is rare in the black, white, and Asian populations, but relatively common (1.1%) in the people of mixed race ('Coloureds'), who have Khoi, Asian, black, and European ethnic origin [390]. This suggests that the Dantu gene originated from the Khoi people, an indigenous group of southern Africa.

Red cells of the only known Dantu+ white person (MD) contained a GP(B–A) hybrid, which expressed N and s and could not be distinguished from that of the NE and Ph types [384]. The molar ratio of hybrid to GPA was only about 0.6:1, suggesting that there was no duplication of the hybrid gene in this individual [384,386]. The Dantu haplotype, in addition to producing GP(B–A)Dantu and normal GPA^M, also contained normal *GYPB*. Unlike the two types of Dantu found in Africans, Dantu of the MD type appears to have originated from an unequal crossing-over event involving active *GYPA* and *GYPB*—no surprise considering that the *GYPB* deletion gene (*u*) is extremely rare in white people.

In summary, three types of Dantu phenotype are known. In each type the Dantu haplotype probably produces an identical N- and s-active GP(B–A) hybrid glycophorin plus GPA^M. In the NE type the gene producing GP(B–A) is duplicated, in the Ph and MD types it is not. In the white MD type, the gene encoding GP(B–A) is flanked by *GYPA* and *GYPB*; in the African NE and Ph types *GYPA* and *GYP(B–A)* are in tandem, but there is no *GYPB*.

3.15.1.1 Anti-Dantu

Several examples of anti-Dantu are known. All are in sera containing other specificities, especially sera containing numerous antibodies to private antigens, but also in some anti-S and -s reagents [262]. Most anti-Dantu are non-immune, although one immune IgG anti-Dantu was responsible for a positive direct antiglobulin reaction on neonatal red cells [262]. Screening of 1348 donor sera with Dantu+ red cells produced no anti-Dantu [262].

3.15.2 St^a (Stones, MNS15) and ERIK (MNS37)

The low incidence antigen St^a, first described by Cleghorn [246] in 1962, is described in this section because it is usually associated with a GP(B–A) molecule. However, in a few individuals St^a is encoded by *GYP(A–B–A)*, *GYP(A–E–A)*, and *GYP(B–A–B–A)* genes.

St^a is far more frequent in Oriental people than in people of European origin, with a frequency of over 6% in Japanese [245] compared with only about 0.1% in Europeans [131,246] (Table 3.9). Screening with anti-N *Vicia graminea* lectin against ficin-treated cells revealed St^a frequencies of between 1.0% and 5.2% in different populations of Chinese in Taiwan [391], but no St^a-positive in 100 African Americans [389]. Homozygosity for the St^a gene has been identified in a Japanese family [392].

3.15.2.1 GP.Sch (M^r)

Anstee *et al.* [393] first recognized the association of St^a with a GP(B–A) type of hybrid glycophorin. This hybrid molecule, now called GP(B–A)Sch, binds antibodies directed at the cytoplasmic domain of GPA, but not antibodies to the extracellular domain of GPA [49,388,393,394]. GP(B–A)Sch usually carries N, St^a, and Wr^b antigens, but neither S nor s [388,392,394–396]. GP(B–A)Sch is resistant to cleavage by trypsin and low concentrations of ficin [389,393–395,397], but is less protease-resistant than GP(B–A)Dantu [326].

DNA analysis has confirmed that GP(B–A)Sch is a hybrid molecule comprising amino acid residues 1–26 of GPB at its N-terminal region and residues 59–131 of GPA it its C-terminal region [325,398,399] (Fig. 3.9); the result of intergenic crossing-over between intron 3 of *GYPA* and the third intron of *GYPB* on the 3′ side of the pseudoexon. The pseudoexon of *GYPB* is spliced out of *GYP(B–A)Sch* mRNA, as it is with *GYPB* mRNA. Asn26 is not glycosylated [395]. The product of the 3′ end of exon B2 of *GYPB* fused to the product of the 5′ end of exon A4 of GYPA results in a novel amino acid sequence, -Gln-Thr-Asn-Gly-Glu-Arg-Val-, which probably represents the St^a antigen.

Huang and Blumenfeld [400] have identified three types of *GYP(B–A)Sch*, all producing identical hybrid glycophorins, but differing in their intronic recombination sites. Two types were found in African Americans, the third in Japanese. Clearly, the St^a phenotype has arisen from different events involving unequal crossing-over within the recombination 'hot-spot' of intron 3 of *GYPA* and the homologous region of

GYPB. One type of *GYP(B–A)Sch* has the same crossing-over site as *GYP(A-B)Hil* (Mi.V), but in a reciprocal arrangement; these two variant genes may be derived from a single recombination event [325,400]. *GYP(B–A)Sch* is flanked by *GYPA* and *GYPB* [392–394,398,399] (Fig. 3.9). The molar ratio of variant glycophorin to normal GPA^M is 1:1 in an individual homozygous for *GYP(B–A)Sch* and 0.5:1 in a typical heterozygote [392,401]. Screening of 264 Taiwanese by a PCR-based test designed to recognize *GYP(B–A)Sch* revealed eight positives, one of whom was homozygous; a gene frequency of 0.017 [351].

3.15.2.2 GP.Zan (M^z)

Metaxas *et al.* [290] found that St(a+) red cells from members of one family reacted with an M-like antibody called anti-M′. This antibody, which is no longer available, did not react with other St(a+) samples. Unlike the usual St^a phenotype red cells (originally called M^r, but now GP.Sch), these variant St(a+) cells (originally M^z, but now GP.Zan) have trypsin-resistant M [396,401]. A variant glycophorin with the same amino acid sequence as that found in GP.Sch cells, except that the N-terminal pentapeptide had the M sequence, was isolated from the red cells of the only known GP.Zan propositus and his daughter [401].

The suggestion by Dahr *et al.* [401] that the M-active variant glycophorin in GP.Zan cells is not a GP(B–A) hybrid, but a GPA molecule lacking amino acid residues 27–58 because of a deletion of exon A3 of *GYPA*, was confirmed by DNA analysis [402]. A GPA^M molecule lacking residues 27–58 would be identical to GP(B–A)Sch, apart from expressing M instead of N, because amino acid residues 1–26 of GPA^M and GPB differ only at positions 1 and 5. GP(A–A)Zan is the product of a *GYP(A–B–A)* hybrid gene, the result of gene conversion, in which the whole of exon A3 and the 5′ end of intron 3 of *GYPA* is replaced by the homologous segment from *GYPB*. This *GYPB* segment includes the pseudoexon and the defective splice site. Consequently, no product of exon 3 is expressed in the mature protein (Fig. 3.9). Analysis of cDNA confirmed the skipping of exon 3, but also showed the presence of a minor transcript, a mRNA species in which both exons 3 and 4 are skipped. Immunoblotting revealed that both transcripts are represented as aberrant glycophorins at the red cell surface, one expressing M and St^a, the other only expressing M [402].

3.15.2.3 GP.EBH and the ERIK antigen

Another St^a variant is associated with the low frequency antigen ERIK [396]. In St(a+) ERIK+ red cells a variant glycophorin was detected with an apparent M_r identical to that of GP(B–A)Sch. In two families (one of Italian origin, one Australian), St(a+) ERIK+ red cells had trypsin-resistant M and the variant glycophorin expressed St^a and M; in another two families (one Danish, one South African of mixed race) no M antigen was detected and the variant glycophorin expressed St^a and N. Immunoblotting of red cell membranes from the Italian and Danish propositi revealed that ERIK was carried, not on the St^a-active variant glycophorin molecule, but on an apparently normal GPA.

The GP.EBH phenotype in the Danish and Italian families is caused by a G to A mutation in the 3′ terminal nucleotide of exon A3 of GYPA [403] (Fig. 3.9). This creates a Gly59Arg substitution in an otherwise normal GPA molecule, presumably responsible for the ERIK antigen. As the mutation resides in the exonic part of the donor splice-site consensus sequence for intron 3, partial disruption of RNA splicing occurs. At least four transcripts are produced from this mutated GYPA: t1, a normally spliced transcript, which produces the ERIK-active GPA molecule; t2, a transcript lacking exon A3, which produces a GPA molecule lacking amino acid residues 27–59 and therefore with the amino acid sequence characteristic of the St^a determinant, but no ERIK antigen; t3 and t4, two abnormally spliced transcripts in which exons A2 and A3 (t3), and A2, A3, and A4 (t4) have been removed [403]. Protein products of transcripts t3 and t4 have not been detected, probably because of the loss of exon A2, which encodes part of the leader sequence involved in the incorporation of the glycoprotein into the red cell membrane.

3.15.2.4 A molecule expressing St^a and ERIK derived from a GYP(A–E–A) gene

In the Australian family with St(a+) ERIK+ members, yet another genetic mechanism is involved [404]. Loss of the product of exon A3 to produce an St^a-active GP(A–A) molecule (like that in GP.Zan) resulted from the replacement of exon A3 and the active 5′ splice site of intron 3 with pseudoexon E3 and its inactive splice site in intron 3 from GYPE. Thus GP(A–A)TF is encoded by a GYP(A–E–A) hybrid gene (Fig. 3.9). No explanation has been provided for ERIK expression on these cells.

3.15.2.5 A molecule expressing St^a and He derived from a GYP(B–A–B–A) gene

Immunoblotting of membranes from red cells expressing St^a and He demonstrated that both antigens resided on the same molecule, an aberrant glycophorin resembling GP(B–A)Sch. DNA analysis showed that this unusual glycophorin molecule was encoded by a GYP(B–A–B–A) gene, which probably arose from unequal crossing-over between GYP(B–A–B)He and GYPA [298]. The first (5′) GYPB segment encodes the 5′ untranslated region and part of the leader sequence, the second GYPB segment is intronic and includes the GYPB pseudoexon; neither is expressed in the mature protein. The first GYPA segment represents exon A2 and encodes the N-terminal 26 amino acid residues of the mature protein including the sequence associated with He expression (see Section 3.8.3); the second GYPA segment represents exons A4–A7 of GYPA (Fig. 3.9). The junction of the products of GYPA exons A2 and A4 creates the St^a antigen.

3.15.2.6 Anti-St^a and -ERIK

The original anti-St^a was found in a serum together with separable anti-Ri^a, -Wr^a, and -Sw^a [246]. Although other examples have been found since [245], anti-St^a is not a common specificity.

Anti-ERIK is present in the serum of the wife of the Danish St(a+) ERIK+ propositus and caused a positive DAT on the red cells of their baby [396]. Anti-ERIK is also present in two multispecific sera containing numerous antibodies to low frequency antigens [396].

3.16 Antigens associated with abnormal expression of Wr^b

GPA appears to be associated in the membrane with band 3, the red cell anion exchanger and Diego blood group antigen. This association is described further in Section 3.25 and in Chapter 10. The Wr^a/Wr^b

(DI3/DI4) dimorphism is determined by a single amino acid substitution in band 3 [168]. As mentioned in Section 3.6.3, Wr^b is not expressed if GPA is not present or, more specifically, if the region around the junction of the extracellular and membrane-spanning domains of GPA is not present (Section 10.4.2). Described below are amino acid substitutions at positions 63 and 65 of GPA that create low frequency MNS antigens and affect Wr^b expression.

3.16.1 HAG (MNS41) and ENEP (MNS39)

A previously transfused man with an antibody to a high frequency determinant on GPA (anti-ENEP) was found to be homozygous for a G250C change in exon A4 of *GYPA*, encoding an Ala654Pro substitution in GPA [405]. This substitution, which appears to have created a new low frequency antigen HAG and abolished the high frequency antigen ENEP, also affected expression of Wr^b. Only eight of 15 monoclonal and polyclonal anti-Wr^b reacted with the red cells. The band 3 genes were apparently normal and had the sequence for Wr^b homozygosity. Pro65 may disrupt the putative α-helix between GPA residues 56 and 70, and this may be responsible for the aberrant Wr^b expression. An unrelated HAG+ person, heterozygous for the Ala65Pro mutation, has been identified.

Anti-HAG was present in several sera containing multiple antibodies to low frequency antigens and in one monospecific serum.

3.16.2 MARS (MNS43) and ENAV (MNS42)

Concurrent absence of the high frequency MNS antigen ENAV (initially AVIS) and presence of the low frequency antigen MARS in a Native American woman results from homozygosity for a single nucleotide change in *GYPA* exon 4, encoding a Glu63Lys substitution in GPA. Her red cells also had weak expression of Wr^b, yet no abnormality was detected in her band 3 gene [406,407]. MARS appears to be unique to the Choctaw tribe of Native Americans, where it is aligned with *Ms*, with an incidence of about 15% [408]. No MARS+ individual was found among 2000 white people, 200 Japanese, 155 Thais, 128 Mexican Americans, 96 Cree, 75 Peruvians, 38 Inuits, or 81 African Americans [408]. Anti-MARS was found in sera containing multiple antibodies to low frequency red cell antigens.

3.17 Other low incidence antigens of the MNS system

The ISBT Working Party on blood group terminology recognizes 29 low frequency antigens belonging to the MNS system. Many of these have been described already; this section includes the remainder. All are inherited and some also accompany aberrant expression of MNSs antigens. Six are associated with single amino changes in GPA and three with single amino changes in GPB. They will be mentioned in numerical order according to the ISBT nomenclature. Frequencies are shown in Table 3.9.

3.17.1 Vr (MNS12)

Aligned with *Ms* in three Dutch families and one Orcadian family (with a Dutch name) [240,409]; no unusual expression of MNSs antigens. Vr results from a Ser47Tyr substitution in GPA, encoded by a C197A transversion in exon 3 of *GYPA* [410]. Tyr47 introduces an α-chymotrypsin cleavage site, explaining the chymotrypsin sensitivity of Vr despite being located on GPA [409].

The original anti-Vr was apparently immune; the antibody producer had three Vr+ children, but none had HDN [240]. Other examples of anti-Vr have been identified in anti-S sera and in multispecific sera; no example of anti-Vr was found in sera from 202 blood donors [240].

3.17.2 Mt^a (Martin, MNS14)

Aligned with *Ns* in the four families reported [241,242,411]. Mt^a has been found in white and black people, and in Thais (Table 3.9). Mt^a is destroyed by papain and ficin, but not by trypsin [242,273]. Eleven Mt(a+) individuals were heterozygous for C230T at the 3' end of exon A3 of *GYPA*, encoding a Thr58Ile substitution [410]. This mutation destroys an *Msp*I restriction site.

The original anti-Mt^a was identified in a serum containing antibodies to other low frequency antigens, as were two subsequent examples [411]. No anti-Mt^a was found in 3500 donor sera [411]. In a case of HDN caused by anti-Mt^a, the baby was jaundiced and required exchange transfusion [242].

141

3.17.3 Riᵃ (Ridley, MNS16)

Riᵃ is extremely rare. The original Ri(a+) propositus [246] is the only one known, despite the testing of 70 501 London blood donors [246,247]. The family of the propositus shows that Riᵃ is inherited with *MS* and M and S antigens are expressed normally [247]. Riᵃ is trypsin-sensitive, but resistant to treatment of the cells with chymotrypsin, papain, or pronase [247], a pattern not usually associated with MNS antigens. Riᵃ is associated with G220A in *GYPA* exon 3, encoding a Glu55Lys substitution in GPA [412]. This amino acid change introduces a trypsin cleavage site and ablates a papain cleavage site.

Screening of 42 886 sera for anti-Riᵃ revealed one example, in a woman with no history of transfusion or pregnancy [247]. Twelve other anti-Riᵃ are known, all in sera containing other antibodies to low incidence antigens [247]. Twelve of the 13 anti-Riᵃ are IgM.

3.17.4 Clᵃ (Caldwell, MNS17)

Aligned with *Ms* in two Scottish families (one originating from Ireland) [248]. Apparently normal expression of M and s. Antigen destroyed by trypsin and by papain.

Anti-Clᵃ was found in 24 of 5326 (0.45%) donor sera. No anti-Clᵃ was found in sera of five Cl(a–) women with Cl(a+) children [248].

3.17.5 Nyᵃ (Nyberg, MNS18)

Nyᵃ is present on the red cells of almost 0.2% of Norwegians [249–251], yet only one Ny(a+) person (a Swiss [18]) was found from screening many thousands of European, white American, and Oriental blood donors (Table 3.9). In 19 Norwegian families and one Swiss family Nyᵃ was inherited with *Ns* [18,249–251]. The N and s antigens of Ny(a+) cells appear normal [250]. Nyᵃ is denatured by trypsin, papain, and pronase treatment [250,252,273]. Two unrelated Ny(a+) individuals were heterozygous for a T138A change in exon 3 of *GYPA*, encoding a GPA Asp27Glu substitution [413]. Amino acid 27 of GPA represents the Xaa residue in the Asn-Xaa-Ser/Thr consensus sequence for N-glycosylation of Asn26. SDS PAGE and immunoblotting with antibodies to GPA revealed no abnormality of GPA from Ny(a+) cells, so the Asp27Glu substitution does not appear to affect N-glycosylation [190,413].

Anti-Nyᵃ was found in about 0.1% of Norwegian and German blood donors [250,252]. Anti-Nyᵃ is generally not immune; anti-Nyᵃ was not found in the sera of seven Ny(a–) women with Ny(a+) babies [250].

3.17.6 Mᵛ (MNS21)

Mᵛ is a low incidence antigen associated with a variant form of GPB. The original 'anti-Mᵛ', which reacted with all N+ cells and with cells of about one in 400 M+N– white Americans [414], was later considered to be inseparable anti-NMᵛ [255]. A second example of anti-Mᵛ, which lacked the anti-N activity, reacted with cells of about 0.6% of English blood donors [255] (Table 3.9). Mᵛ was inherited with *Ms* in 14 families and with *MS* in two families [255,414]. Weakened expression of s antigen was noticed when Mᵛ was associated with *Ms*, but no similar effect on S expression was apparent when Mᵛ was associated with *MS* [255,414,415]. Mᵛ is resistant to trypsin cleavage, but is destroyed by chymotrypsin, papain, ficin, and sialidase treatment [273,416,417].

Red cells of a woman heterozygous for GP.Hil (Mi.V) and Mᵛ genes have no trypsin-resistant 'N' antigen and only about 25% of the normal quantity of GPB [125,154,417]. *GYP(A–B)Hil* produces no 'N' or GPB (Section 3.11.1). Expression of Mᵛ and loss of 'N' from GPB is associated with a C65G change in *GYPB* exon 2, encoding a Thr3Ser substitution [418]. It is not clear whether this amino acid change is also responsible for reduced GPB expression as other mutations, possibly in the promoter region of *GYPB*, might also be present. An analogy can be drawn between anti-NMᵛ (the original anti-Mᵛ) and anti-Mᶜ; the former cross-reacting with Mᵛ on GPB and N on GPA, and the latter cross-reacting with He on GPB and M on GPA.

Anti-Mᵛ may be red cell immune [414,416] or 'naturally occurring' [255]. IgG anti-Mᵛ caused HDN in two of the five Mᵛ+ children of an Mᵛ– woman with an Mᵛ+ husband [416].

3.17.7 Far (MNS22)

In the Far family the gene producing the Far antigen appeared to be aligned with an *Ns* complex [256,419]. Far was subsequently shown to be the same as the

Kamhuber antigen [257,420]. In the Kamhuber family Far may be associated with *MS*, although neither family proves close linkage with *MNS*. Far is resistant to trypsin, papain, and ficin [257,273].

Anti-Far has been responsible for severe HDN [419] and for a haemolytic transfusion reaction [257]. Both Far antibodies are probably red cell immune, one arising from fetal–maternal immunization [256,419], the other from transfusion of Far+ blood [257]. No example of anti-Far was found in 541 sera from normal donors [256].

3.17.8 s^D (Dreyer, MNS23)

Aligned with *Ms* in a white South African family with 41 s^D+ members in four generations [258]. Screening of red cells from 1000 white South Africans revealed one s^D-positive, subsequently shown to belong to the original family [258]. One of 1000 donors of mixed race was also s^D+ (Table 3.9). *GYPB* exon 4 from two s^D+ individuals contained a C173G transversion, encoding Pro39Arg in GPB^s [418]. Red cells of S+s+s^D+ individuals reacted weakly, or not at all, with several anti-s sera [258]. This altered expression of s may be caused by conformational changes in GPB resulting from the Pro39Arg substitution [418].

Anti-s^D caused HDN [258].

3.17.9 Mit (Mitchell, MNS24)

Of 15 reported families, Mit was inherited with *MS* in 13, with *NS* in one, and with *Ms* in one [259,260,421]. With anti-Mit of low titre, Lubenko *et al.* [260] found four Mit+ individuals from 17 951 North London donors, but with a high-titred anti-Mit, they identified seven Mit-positives from a further 8278 donors. In S+s+ Mit+ individuals, S expression is often depressed [418,421], as is s antigen expression in one informative family [260]. The extent of the S depression is variable and very dependent on the anti-S reagents used. A G161A transition encoding an Arg35His substitution was present in exon 4 of *GYPB^S* of three Mit+ individuals [418]. This is consistent with Arg35 of GPB being part of the S and s epitopes [85] (Section 3.4.4.1). Immunochemical techniques revealed no obvious reduction in GPB quantity in Mit+ red cells [260,418,421], although immunoblotting with anti-S clearly demonstrated a reduction in staining intensity of GPB with S+s+ Mit+

cells [50]. Mit expression is reduced by pronase treatment of the cells, but not by trypsin or chymotrypsin treatment [260].

No example of anti-Mit was found in 500 antenatal sera or 660 donor sera [259]. The original anti-Mit was responsible for slight neonatal jaundice [259].

3.17.10 Or (Orriss, MNS31)

Or was transmitted with *Ms* in a white Australian family with seven Or+ members in three generations [422]. Or+ has also been found in two Japanese [266], an African American [265], and a Jamaican [423] (Table 3.9). Anti-Or was inhibited by sialoglycoproteins isolated from Or+ red cells and gave a positive result in a monoclonal antibody-specific immobilization of erythrocyte antigens (MAIEA) analysis with monoclonal antibodies to GPA [266,422]. Or+ cells give normal PAS staining patterns after SDS PAGE [422]. A C148T base change in exon 3 of *GYPA*, encoding a GPA Arg31Trp substitution, was detected in cDNA from three unrelated Or+ individuals [266,423]. The M antigen of the Or+ individuals is more resistant to trypsin denaturation than normal M antigen. Or antigen is destroyed by pronase, ficin, and sialidase treatment of cells, is chymotrypsin-resistant, and shows the same partial resistance to trypsin treatment as the M antigen on Or+ cells [422,423]. Fifty per cent of native GPA molecules are cleaved by trypsin at Arg31 [61]. Sialidase sensitivity suggests that glycosylation of Thr33 and Thr37 are involved in the Or epitope [423].

The original anti-Or was found in the serum of an autoimmune haemolytic anaemia patient [265]. Anti-Or has caused HDN of moderate severity [423]. Twenty examples of anti-Or have been found in about 17 000 normal sera, and five in 50 sera containing antibodies to other low frequency antigens [265,266,422].

3.17.11 Os^a (MNS38)

Os^a has been found in one Japanese family where it was associated with *Ms* [269]. No further Os(a+) was detected among 50 000 Japanese donors. Os^a is trypsin-resistant, but destroyed by papain, ficin, and pronase. Immunoblotting with anti-Os^a showed that Os^a resides on a GPA molecule of normal electrophoretic mobility and the location of Os^a on GPA was confirmed by a MAIEA test [413]. Sequencing *GYPA* exon 3 of an Os(a+) individual from the only family with Os^a revealed heterozygosity for a C217T base change, encoding a Pro54Ser substitution [413]. A synthetic peptide representing part of GPA with the Os^a mutation (VRTVYPSEEETGE) inhibited anti-Os^a, whereas the control peptide (VRTVYPPEEETGE) did not.

Anti-Os^a is present in several sera containing multispecific antibodies to low frequency antigens, but no example was found in testing 100 000 sera from Japanese donors [269].

3.18 Antigens associated with atypical glycophorin glycosylation

3.18.1 Hu, M$_1$, Tm, Sj, and Can

Several antibodies have been identified that show a distinct preference for either M+ or N+ cells, but are not anti-M or -N. They react with red cells from a greater proportion of black than white people and demonstrate a great deal of individual variation in antigen strength. These antibodies are not simply showing variation in the strength of M or N antigen; the M-related antibodies will often react more strongly with M+N+ cells (with a single dose of M antigen) than with M+N− cells (with a double dose). The same applies to the N-related antibodies with M+N+ and M−N+ cells. Table 3.12 shows the frequencies of antigens detected by these antibodies in black and white populations.

Binding of many examples of anti-M and -N is partially dependent on oligosaccharide moieties located on GPA and GPB. However, the polymorphism they detect is determined primarily by the nucleotide sequence of the genes responsible for the amino acid sequence of the polypeptide chain of GPA and GPB. The antibodies described in this section appear to be recognizing differences in the structures of the oligosaccharides around the N-terminus of GPA and possibly GPB, arising from inherited glycosyltransferase variation. Such heterogeneity in transferase specificity presumably derives from polymorphism at a gene locus separate from the *MNS* complex locus.

3.18.1.1 Serology and genetics

Hu (Hunter) Hu is the oldest MNS antigen after M and N. In 1934 Landsteiner *et al.* [427] injected rabbits

with the red cells of an African American, Mr Hunter, and the resulting antibody agglutinated the red cells of about 7% of African Americans [24,427]. Twenty-two per cent of West Africans were later found to be Hu+ [231]. Hu is relatively rare in white people [24] (Table 3.12). All Hu+ samples, giving 'distinct, positive reactions' with anti-Hu, are N+ , although many N+ red cells are Hu−. Anti-Hu has only been produced by immunizing rabbits with Mr Hunter's red cells [427,428]; because these cells are no longer available, Hu specificity is close to extinction. Limited family data suggested that Hu is inherited in a Mendelian manner [231].

Wright *et al.* [424] described an antibody, provisionally named anti-Sext, which may represent alloanti-Hu. The antibody reacted with red cells of 24% of African Americans and no white people; all reactive cells were N+. Few red cells of known Hu type were available, but all 13 Hu+ samples reacted with anti-Sext; 3 Hu− samples did not.

M$_1$ M$_1$ is only present on M+ red cells [429]. Early examples of anti-M$_1$ were found associated with anti-M in the sera of M−N+ individuals [18,193,362,429]. At the appropriate pH and dilution these sera behaved as anti-M$_1$ and, with these sera, 24% of African Americans were found to be M$_1$+ [24,193]. Later, two examples of anti-M$_1$ from M+N+ individuals provided somewhat lower frequencies for M$_1$ antigen; 17% of black people and <1% of white people were M$_1$+ [425,430] (Table 3.12).

Tm and Sj Anti-Tm reacts preferentially with N+ cells [431]. Most M+N+ Tm+ cells are also M$_1$+ [432]. Anti-Sj was identified as a second antibody in the serum containing the original anti-Tm [24]. Like Tm, Sj has a slightly higher incidence in black than white people. Sj has only been detected on N+ cells.

Can (Canner) The only example of anti-Can reacted with the red cells of 60% and 27% of black and white people, respectively, and showed a preference for M+ cells [426]. Results of tests with anti-Can against desialylated red cells provided the first suggestion that carbohydrate structures played an important part in the specificity of anti-Can and similar antibodies [426]. Most M$_1$+ cells are also Can+ [432].

Table 3.12 Relative frequencies of antigens partially determined by *N*-acetylgalactosamine content of *O*-glycans on GPA, shown as a percentage of antigen-positive individuals in the whole ethnic group and in people of each MN phenotype.

| Antigen | African Americans | | | | | White people | | | | | References |
| | No. tested | Percentage antigen positive | | | | No. tested | Percentage antigen positive | | | | |
		Whole pop.	M+N−	M+N+	M−N+		Whole pop.	M+N−	M+N+	M−N+	
Hu	500	7	1	8	12	500	1	0	2	3	[24]
Sext	335	24	0	28	33	167	0	0	0	0	[424]
$M_1{}^a$	822	24	46	26	0	500	4	10	1	0	[24,193]
$M_1{}^b$	230	13	32	10	0	218	1*	1	0	0	[425]
Tm	500	31	3	27	64	900	25	2	24	61	[24]
Sj	500	4	0	3	9	500	2	0	3	3	[24]
Can	447	60	74	67	37	541	27	44	24	5	[426]

*One sample positive.
[a]Anti-M+M_1 used by condition in which only anti-M_1 reacts; [b]anti-M_1 used.

3.18.1.2 Biochemistry

When tested with desialylated red cells, anti-Can and -Tm behaved as anti-M and -N, respectively [426,433]. The sera had to be adsorbed free of anti-T with sialidase-treated red cells of the appropriate phenotype. One of the major factors determining Hu, Sext, M_1, Tm, Sj, and Can activity appears to be the *N*-acetylglucosamine content of the *O*-glycans attached to amino acid residues 2–4 of GPA and GPB [432]. The predominant *O*-glycan on GPA is the disialotetrasaccharide shown in Fig. 3.2. An alternative oligosaccharide, in which one of the sialic acid residues is replaced by *N*-acetylglucosamine, also occurs, more commonly in black than white people [277,434]. Dahr *et al.* [432] have suggested that anti-Hu, -Sext, -M_1, -Tm, -Sj, and -Can react with GPA molecules with these variant *O*-glycans when present on the appropriate M or N peptide backbone. If a high enough level of the variant *O*-glycan is present, then some of these antibodies will react with the red cell regardless of MN type. Race and Sanger [18] noted a weakening of N antigen on M_1+M+N+ cells compared with M_1−M+N+ cells. This could be caused by anti-N binding less effectively to GPA^N with a high proportion of oligosaccharides containing *N*-acetylglucosamine.

There can be little doubt that the series of antibodies described in this section are distinguishing not only a polymorphism at the *MN* (*GYPA*) locus, but also polymorphism of genes producing the glycosyltransferases responsible for the biosynthesis of the *O*-glycans of the N-terminal region of GPA. Limited family studies have implied that Hu, M_1, and Tm have a regular mode of inheritance [231,435], although one family study suggests anomalous inheritance of M_1 [436].

3.18.2 T, Tn, and Cad

T, Tn and Cad antigens represent alterations of the *O*-linked oligosaccharides of glycophorins. Although studied predominantly on GPA, these determinants are not found exclusively on red cell sialoglycoproteins and may be detected on other red cell components as well as on other cells. Consequently, they will be considered only briefly here.

T and Tn are cryptantigens; they are not normally detectable. Most human sera contain anti-T and -Tn, so red cells expressing these antigens are polyagglutinable (agglutinated by most human sera) and are described in detail in Chapter 31. Red cells become T-active when they are desialylated, either by sialidase treatment *in vitro* or by the action of bacterial sialidase *in vivo*. This results in the cleavage of the sialic acid residues from the *O*-linked tetrasaccharides, revealing the T-active structure Galβ1→3GalNAc. T expression is depressed in desialylated En(a−) cells [115,116,119].

The Tn determinant is *N*-acetylgalactosamine linked to serine or threonine; the *O*-glycans of Tn-active cells consist of this monosaccharide or of a sialylated disaccharide. Tn-active red cells lack β1,3-D-galactosyltransferase (T-transferase), probably as a result of somatic mutation. Consequently, galactose cannot be added to the *O*-linked *N*-acetylgalactosamine of glycophorins and other structures. T- and Tn-active red cells have depressed expression of M and N.

In the Sd(a++) phenotype (described in Chapter 29) some of the *O*-linked oligosaccharides of glycophorins have an additional *N*-acetylgalactosamine residue linked to galactose, producing a disialopentasaccharide (reviewed in [35]).

3.19 Quantitative variants

The symbols N_2 and S_2 have been used to describe weakened expression of N and S (for references see [437]). In the absence of any biochemical analysis or testing with modern serological reagents, these phenotypes are no longer of any significance.

Four families are described in which a positive direct antiglobulin test (DAT), with no signs of haemolytic anaemia, was inherited as a dominant character. In one family [438] the positive DAT is inherited with a weak expression of M antigen (called M_2). In two families [439,440], including one with 11 members with DAT-positive red cells, it was inherited with weak N (N_2, but different from that mentioned above). In the fourth family [18] no aberrant expression of MN antigens was detected. Anti-IgG, -IgA, and -C3 in the antiglobulin reagent were not involved in the reaction, but the presence of anti-IgM did seem to be important [439,440].

3.20 MNSsU antibodies

3.20.1 Human anti-M

Anti-M is a relatively common 'naturally occurring' antibody. Thousands of examples have been identified since the original description by Wolff and Jonsson [441] in 1933. With a low ionic-strength polybrene Auto-Analyser and M+N+ screening cells, Perrault [442] identified 64 anti-M in 22 500 (0.3%) donor sera, 62 from M– and two from M+ donors. Most anti-M are only reactive at temperatures below 37°C, with

an optimum temperature of 4°C, but occasional examples will agglutinate red cells at body temperature [443]. Although generally considered to be 'naturally occurring', there is evidence that anti-M may be stimulated by transfusion [444,445] or by bacterial infection in children [446]. Many examples of anti-M show a pronounced dosage effect, reacting more strongly with M+N– than with M+N+ cells [18]; weaker examples of anti-M are often not detected in tests with M+N+ cells. By an agglutination technique at room temperature with M+N– cells, A. Lubenko (cited in [443]) found an incidence of anti-M of 1 in 2500 donor sera, but only of 1 in 5000 sera when M+N+ cells were used for screening. Anti-M is more common in infants than in adults [447], particularly in patients with burns [448].

Most human anti-M contain an IgM component [443], although 78% were found to be at least partially IgG and these IgG antibodies could agglutinate saline suspensions of M+ red cells [449]. Anti-M bind very little or no complement [443,445,450].

MN antibodies are often pH dependent and this topic will be discussed in more detail in Section 3.20.7 on monoclonal antibodies. By acidifying sera from 1000 M–N+ donors, Beattie and Zuelzer [451] found 21 examples of anti-M dependent on low pH. These IgM anti-M had a pH optimum of 6.5 and were mostly inactive at pH 7.5; below pH 6.5 they became non-specific.

M-like alloantibodies, which do not react with the antibody maker's own cells, have occasionally been identified in the sera of M+ individuals [452–454]. In one case, the patient's M-like alloantibody did not react with the cells of his four M+N+ children who had inherited his M [452]. In another example, the M-like antibody did not react with the M+N+ red cells of the patient's sister [454].

3.20.2 Human anti-N

Any discussion on anti-N and the N antigen is complicated by the presence of N determinant, not only on GPA of individuals with an *N* allele, but also on GPB of most people. Consequently, most *M/M* people (often denoted M+N–) do have N on their red cells (usually designated 'N') and only very rarely make anti-N. When they do it is generally weakly reactive. These antibodies, which will often agglutinate M+N– cells at low temperatures and can be removed from the serum by adsorption with M+N– cells [30,455,456], are not strictly alloantibodies.

Red cells of individuals with the rare M+N–S–s–(U– or U+^{var}) phenotypes lack 'N' and may produce a potent alloanti-N, which will agglutinate all cells carrying an N determinant, whether on GPA or GPB [193,456–458]. These antibodies have been referred to as anti'N', -N'N', or -NU; misleading terminologies that suggest they differ in specificity from the anti-N produced by M+N–S+/s+ people.

Anti-N is relatively rare compared with anti-M [18,442]. Most anti-N are 'naturally occurring', IgM, and inactive above 25°C [443]. Immune anti-N resulting from multiple transfusions do occur [458], usually in people of African origin with M+N–S–s–U– red cells. A pH-dependent anti-N in the serum of an M+N–S–s+ man demonstrated optimum reactivity at a pH below 7 [460]. Anti-N often show a pronounced dosage effect [18].

A few healthy M+N+ people have produced N-like antibodies, which did not agglutinate autologous cells [461–465].

3.20.3 Clinical significance of anti-M and -N

3.20.3.1 Alloantibodies

Most anti-M and anti-N are not active at 37°C and are not clinically significant. They can generally be ignored in transfusion practice and, if room temperature incubation is eliminated from compatibility testing and screening for antibodies, they will not be detected. When M or N antibodies active at 37°C are encountered, crossmatch-compatible blood should be provided.

Anti-M and -N have been implicated as the cause of immediate and delayed haemolytic transfusion reactions [447,458,466–469], although Issitt and Anstee [195] cast doubt on the validity of some of these claims. The suggestion that anti-M and -N can have haemolytic activity was supported by the results of ^{51}Cr survival tests and monocyte phagocytosis assays [458,468].

HDN caused by anti-M is rare. There are reports of anti-M HDN leading to fetal death or requiring treatment by exchange transfusion [459,470–475]. One high titre IgG plus IgM anti-M was responsible for neonatal pure red cell aplasia and caused a substantial reduction in proliferation of erythroid cells in culture [475]. Therefore, like anti-K (Section 7.3.5.2), anti-M may cause HDN primarily by destroying erythroid progenitors rather than mature erythrocytes. No serious case of HDN caused by anti-N is recorded, but anti-N in a woman of phenotype M+N–S–s–U+^{var} caused mild HDN in her M+N+ baby [457].

3.20.3.2 Autoantibodies

At least 15 cases of patients with autoanti-M have been reported and these are reviewed by Sacher et al. [476]. Of these 15 autoantibodies, 11 were considered innocuous, whereas the other four gave some symptoms of cold haemagglutinin disease. Where anaemia was reported, it was mild and easily controlled [477,478]. A Pr-like antibody with a binding preference for M+ cells caused chronic cold haemagglutinin disease and autoimmune haemolytic anaemia in an M+N+ patient [479]. A few cases of warm AIHA caused by autoanti-N have been described [173], one of which had a fatal outcome [480]. Autoanti-M responsible for warm AIHA has not been found [173].

3.20.4 Anti-N and renal dialysis

In 1972, Howell and Perkins [481] identified 12 examples of apparent anti-N from the sera of 416 prospective kidney transplant patients maintained on chronic haemodialysis. The antibodies disappeared after transplantation. Production of these N-like antibodies (anti-Nf) arises from immunization of the patients by small numbers of residual red cells on which N determinants have been altered by the formaldehyde used in sterilization of the dialysis membranes [481–491]. Between 21% and 27% of dialysis patients using formaldehyde-sterilized membranes have anti-Nf, regardless of their MN phenotype [487,488,491].

When tested with red cells treated with formaldehyde solution, anti-Nf show greatly increased reactivity and will often agglutinate red cells of all MN groups, including M+N–S–s– cells [483,485–488,492]. Furthermore, many sera from dialysis patients that do not contain anti-Nf have this 'antiformaldehyde' specificity. Antibodies to formaldehyde-treated cells are both IgM and IgG, whereas antibodies to untreated N+ cells (anti-Nf) are IgM and can be considered as separate antibodies appearing at a late stage of immunization [489].

Dahr and Moulds [492] showed that formaldehyde treatment greatly increased the ability of glycophorin to inhibit haemagglutination by anti-Nf, but only if there had been no prior blocking of N-terminal amino groups. They concluded that anti-Nf recognizes N determinants on GPA and GPB in which the free amino group of N-terminal leucine is modified by reacting with formaldehyde. Sialic acid residues on the second, third, and fourth amino acids may also be involved in the binding site. Presumably, the antiformaldehyde antibodies are stimulated by other formaldehyde modified proteins, as the reaction with M+N−S−s− red cells could not be inhibited by formaldehyde-treated GPA N-terminal octapeptides.

3.20.5 Glucose dependent antibodies

Some antibodies that only react with red cells previously exposed to glucose have M or N specificity [494–496]. They were identified because of the presence of glucose in red cell preservative solutions used for antibody identification panels. Incubation in 1–2% glucose solutions at neutral or alkaline pH, for a few hours at 37°C or days at 4°C, rendered red cells agglutinable by these glucose-dependent antibodies. With some of the antibodies other sugars, such as galactose, mannose, or N-acetylglucosamine, had the same effect [494,496]. One glucose specific anti-M, produced in an M−N+ diabetic, agglutinated M+ red cells from six of seven patients with diabetes mellitus without prior incubation of the cells in glucose, presumably as a result of non-enzymatic glycosylation of proteins because of elevated serum glucose levels [495].

It is probable that glucose binds to the amino group of the N-terminal amino acid residues of GPA and GPB, altering the steric configuration of the M or N determinant [494–496].

3.20.6 Anti-M and -N produced in animals

Before the advent of monoclonal antibodies (see below), anti-M and -N reagents were generally produced by injecting rabbits with human red cells of the appropriate MN phenotype. The original M and N antibodies of Landsteiner and Levine [1–4], which led to the discovery of the MN system, were hetero-agglutinins produced in rabbits.

3.20.7 Monoclonal anti-M and -N

Numerous monoclonal antibodies to M and N antigens have been produced and many examples have been analysed in three international workshops [48,87,176]. They have been made by the murine hybridoma technique employing spleen cells from mice immunized with either human red cells or with glycophorin isolated from human red cells. Most were IgG, although some IgM anti-M and -N have been generated.

Fraser et al. [497,498] produced two monoclonal anti-N by immunizing mice with M+N−S−s+ red cells, the immunogen presumably being the 'N' determinant on GPB. Both antibodies reacted with GPA^N and GPB. Two monoclonal anti-N differed in their affinity for N and 'N', one antibody having a much higher avidity for the N determinant on GPA and the other having a higher avidity for 'N' on GPB [499]. Although the primary structures of N and 'N' are identical, these monoclonal antibodies may be able to distinguish differences in their tertiary structures [499].

Monoclonal antibodies are usually more sensitive to variations in pH than are the polyclonal antibodies in human and animal sera, which are cocktails of antibody molecules to different epitopes on the same antigenic determinant, all with different pH optima. A number of charged groups exist in the region of the M and N determinants, including the free amino group of the terminal amino acid residue, the carboxyl groups of sialic acid on amino acid residues 2, 3, and 4, and the glutamic acid at position 5 in N. Variations in pH affect the charge on these groups leading to conformational changes in the region of the M and N determinants, altering the binding affinity with various monoclonal antibodies [500]. At pH, temperature, and concentration optimal for reaction strength, many monoclonal anti-M (or, more accurately, anti-M-like) will agglutinate M−N+ cells [282,283,501]. From the point of view of reagent production this problem can usually be overcome by dilution or by pH adjustment.

Most MN monoclonal antibodies do not react with, or show greatly reduced avidity for, sialic acid-depleted red cells or glycophorins. However, there are a few monoclonal anti-M and -N that detect sialic acid-independent epitopes [48,87,176].

M and N antigens differ at the first and fifth amino acids of the N-terminus of GPA (see Table 3.7); anti-M detect either Ser1 or Gly5; anti-N either Leu1 or Glu5. Other factors, especially the presence of oligosaccharides, are usually also important to epitope integrity. Red cells with the rare M^c and He phenotypes (see Table 3.7) have been very useful in the elucidation of some of these fine specificities, as have techniques for modification of the terminal amino acid residue by acetylation of the free amino group or by removal of the N-terminal amino acid by Edman degradation [48,87,176,502]. As a rough guide, anti-M that detect the presence of Ser1 react with M^c/N cells but not with acetylated cells [282,503], whereas those that detect Gly5 do not react with M^c cells, but do react with acetylated cells and may bind to He active GPB, which has glycine at position 5 [501]. Some anti-M that react with a Gly5-dependent epitope cross-react with M^g [285]. The fine specificity of N antibodies is more difficult to determine. Anti-N recognizing Leu1 rather than Glu5 should not react with GPA from M^c/M cells [503,504].

The fine specificity of MN antibodies has also been analysed by haemagglutination inhibition tests with acetone powders prepared from Chinese hamster ovary cells transfected with *GYPA* cDNA [505,506]. The cDNA either encoded GPA^M or GPA^N, or was modified by site directed mutagenesis to encode the M^c sequence or a novel NM N-terminal sequence, Leu-Ser-Thr-Thr-Gly (see Table 3.7). One monoclonal anti-M required Gly5 and sialic acid for binding, three human alloanti-M required Ser1 and not Gly5, and two monoclonal anti-N and *Vicia graminea* lectin required Leu1, but not Glu5.

Fab fragments of murine monoclonal anti-M and -N displayed on the surface of bacteriophages transformed with cDNA representing light-chain variable region had similar immunological properties to those of their parental hybridoma antibodies [493,507]. The affinity of soluble, recombinant, anti-N Fab-fragment, derived from murine cDNA, was enhanced 100-fold by shuffling of Fd fragments with library-derived light-chains. These mutant Fab fragments had similar affinity to the parental immunoglobulin molecules and agglutinated N+ red cells in the presence of antiglobulin [508].

3.20.8 Lectins

A seed extract from *Iberis amara* was found to have M specificity [509], but no seed lectin has proved satisfactory as an anti-M blood grouping reagent [510].

One of the most useful lectins in blood group serology was identified by Ottensooser and Silberschmidt [511] in the seeds of a Brazilian plant, *Vicia graminea*. At the appropriate dilution, this lectin behaves as anti-N and is a useful blood grouping reagent. M–N+ cells bind approximately 20 times more molecules of *V. graminea* lectin than M+N– cells [512,513]. *V. graminea* lectin binds to GPA and GPB from M–N+ and M+N+ cells, but only to GPB from M+N– cells [513,514].

Trypsin treatment enhances the ability of *V. graminea* lectin to bind to 'N'. The lectin agglutinates all trypsin-treated red cells apart from those of the S–s–U– and S–s–U+^{var} phenotypes, and those of other rare phenotypes in which 'N' is not present [515]. *V. graminea* lectin binds sialidase-treated cells more strongly than untreated cells and agglutinates sialidase-treated M+N– red cells as strongly as sialidase-treated M–N+ cells; after desialylation, M+N– and M–N+ cells have a similar number of binding sites [513]. The determinant recognized by *V. graminea* lectin is often referred to as N_{Vg} to distinguish it from N.

The minimum binding requirement for *V. graminea* lectin is the disaccharide Galβ1→3GalNAc [109,516], present in the O-glycosidically linked tetrasaccharides located around the N-terminus of GPA and GPB. For most efficient binding, N-terminal leucine, which probably affects the steric arrangement of neighbouring O-glycans, is required, hence the binding preference for N-active glycophorins. The lectin does not bind GPAM^c [517] which, like N, has glutamic acid at position 5 but, unlike N, has serine at position 1 (see Table 3.7). Edman degradation of GPA^N, which removes the N-terminal amino acid residue, results in failure of the molecule to combine with *V. graminea* lectin [518].

Some other lectins are potentially useful as anti-N reagents, especially seed extracts from *Bauhinia purpurea* [519] and *B. variegata* [520], and the extract from leaves of *Vicia unijuga* [521]. Lectins prepared from the seeds of *Mollucella laevis* [522] and *Bandeiraea simplicifolia* [523] have A+N activity; they agglutinate all group A cells and also N+ group O and B cells.

A number of other lectins that have proved useful are those that signpost rare variants of the MNS system by detecting deficiency of normal GPA and/or GPB. Lectin from the seeds of *Maclura aurantiaca* is specific for the disaccharide Galβ1→3GalNAc but, unlike *V. graminea* lectin, does not distinguish between M and N [524]. Haemagglutination by this lectin is depressed in En(a–) cells compared with En(a+) cells [130]. *Phaseolus vulgaris* lectin binds to the N-linked oligosaccharide present on GPA [127]. Like *M. aurantiaca* lectin, radioiodinated *P. vulgaris* lectin has been useful for visualizing GPA in gels after electrophoresis [127]. Some lectins, such as *Sophora japonica* (after adsorption with A_1B cells) and *Glycine soja*, preferentially agglutinate sialic acid-deficient red cells [116,130]. These lectins have been utilized in screening for MNS variants with deficiency or alteration of GPA and/or GPB.

3.20.9 Anti-S

Since the discovery of anti-S in 1947 [7,8], many more examples have been found [525,526]. Anti-S are usually immune [443,525], although 'naturally occurring' examples are known [525,527]. Anti-S, -s, and -U are generally non-complement binding IgG antibodies [195,443], although IgM anti-S has been reported [528]. S, s, and U antibodies usually react at 37°C, but most are optimally reactive at temperatures between 10 and 22°C by manual antiglobulin tests under normal ionic conditions [529,530].

Anti-S reagents are notorious for containing antibodies to private antigens. Lubenko [531] found that of nine single donor anti-S sera tested, four contained one antibody to a low frequency antigen, one contained two such antibodies, and two were polyspecific with 15 antibodies to low frequency antigen detected in each serum.

Anti-S has been implicated in haemolytic transfusion reactions [532,533] and has caused severe and fatal HDN [526,534].

Autoanti-S has been responsible for AIHA [535,536]. An autoanti-S appeared in the serum of an S+ patient 2 months after treatment for AIHA caused by an apparently 'non-specific' autoantibody [537]. Autoantibodies that are probably detecting non-polymorphic determinants on GPB may 'mimic' anti-

S because of the greater quantity of GPB molecules on S+ cells than on S– cells [538,539] (see Section 3.4.4).

Two human IgM monoclonal anti-S submitted to the third monoclonal antibody workshop were considered suitable as blood grouping reagents [87]. Both directly agglutinated S+ red cells, but they had different serological characteristics. MS94 detected a sialidase-sensitive epitope and did not react with the abnormal S antigen associated with TSEN (see Section 3.14.1); MS95 detected a sialidase-resistant epitope and did react with TSEN+ cells [87].

A murine monoclonal antibody, MAb148, behaved as anti-S by agglutination or indirect antiglobulin tests, but when more sensitive tests or a pH of 6.5 was employed, the antibody reacted with all red cells with GPB [338]. MAb148 gave some unexpected results. It reacted strongly with S–St(a+) and S–Dantu+ cells, but did not react with S+GP.Hop (Mi.IV) cells. Hemming and Reid [338] deduced that MAb148 detects the tetrapeptide Thr-Asn-Gly-Glu at positions 25–28 of GPB, but binds more efficiently when methionine (S), rather than threonine (s), is at position 29.

Some human alloanti-S behave as anti-GPB when tested with ficin-treated cells, agglutinating all such cells save those of S–s–U– and S–s–U+^{var} phenotypes [111].

3.20.10 Anti-s

Anti-s was discovered 4 years after anti-S [10]. Although anti-s is rare, many examples have been found. Anti-s may be IgM or IgG and four of five anti-s consisted of IgG3 alone [540]. No 'naturally occurring' anti-s is reported. Anti-s are usually optimally reactive at 22°C or below [529,530].

Anti-s has been responsible for severe and fatal HDN [10,541,542] and for a delayed haemolytic transfusion reaction [533,543].

3.20.11 Anti-U

Many of the serological complexities of anti-U are given in Section 3.7.1. Described here are details about the antibodies themselves and their clinical significance.

The original anti-U was reported by Wiener *et al.* [191] in 1953. Many examples have been found since and, because the U– phenotype is relatively rare, anti-

U creates a far greater transfusion problem than anti-S or -s. Anti-U are generally non-complement-binding IgG antibodies [195] containing an IgG1 component [540]; no 'naturally occurring' anti-U has been reported. Like anti-S and -s, U antibodies may have greater reactivity at temperatures below 22°C than at body temperature [529,530].

The first anti-U was responsible for a fatal haemolytic transfusion reaction [191] and several examples of delayed haemolytic transfusion reaction caused by anti-U are documented [198,544–547]. In one case the transfused cells responsible for the reaction were S–s–U+^{var}, the U antigen being too weak to be detected during compatibility testing [198]. Several examples of anti-U causing HDN are reported, including one resulting in stillbirth [548]. However, in one case maternal anti-U had a titre of 1024 and gave a very high score (> 100%) in an antibody-dependent cellular cytotoxicity (ADCC) assay yet, despite IgG1 and IgG3 anti-U being eluted from the baby's red cells, cord haemoglobin and bilirubin levels were almost normal and no treatment was required [549]. No monocyte-blocking antibody was detected.

Autoanti-U, either alone or associated with other autoantibodies, has been implicated in AIHA [550–555]. An IgG2 autoanti-U was responsible for severe AIHA with apparent intravascular haemolysis and bone marrow dyserythropoiesis [555]. Autoanti-U has also been involved in alpha-methyldopa-induced haemolytic anaemia [556]. Nine of 28 (32%) hospitalized patients with AIDS had autoanti-U, detectable in their serum by enzyme tests only [557]. Some autoanti-U only react at low pH and low temperature [551,558] and one case of LISS-dependent autoanti-U is described [559]. Whereas makers of alloanti-U are almost invariably black, most patients with autoanti-U are white.

3.20.12 Anti-U^Z and -U^X

Anti-U^Z and -U^X were detected by Booth [560,561] in the sera of Melanesians. Anti-U^Z reacts with the red cells of 36% of Melanesians and 61% of white people. U^Z is associated with S. Most S+ samples are U^Z+, although the phenotypes S+U^Z– and S–U^Z+ do exist. Anti-U^X is a similar antibody. It is likely that U^Z and U^X represent determinants on GPB, the apparent association with S resulting from greater quantity of GPB on S+ cells than S– cells (Section 3.4.4).

An antibody closely resembling anti-U^Z was detected in the serum of a S–s+U+He+(weak) Hispanic woman and in an eluate from the red cells of her newborn fourth child [562]. Despite causing a strongly positive DAT on the baby's red cells, HDN was not diagnosed.

3.21 GYPA mutation assay

The proportion of a small minority of M–N+ or M+N– red cells in M+N+ individuals can be determined by flow cytometry with monoclonal anti-M and -N. This has been exploited to estimate the frequency of somatic mutation in erythroid precursor cells [563,564]. Significant increases in apparent mutation were found in cancer patients after exposure to mutagenic chemotherapy drugs [563], in Hiroshima atomic bomb survivors [565], and in Chernobyl accident victims exposed to ionizing radiation [566]. The technique has also been used to monitor the mutagenic effects of radioiodine therapy for thyroid cancer [567,568]. In M+N+ Chinese chemical industry workers exposed to benzene, the presence of M–N+ red cells with a double dose of N (*NN*), but not with a single dose of N (*NØ*), suggested that benzene is responsible for gene-duplicating mutations rather than gene-inactivating mutations [569].

3.22 Association with Rh

The first signs of an association between antigens of the MNS and Rh systems came with the recognition that Rh$_{null}$ cells, which lack all Rh antigens, often have reduced expression of S, s, and U antigens [18,570]. Depression of U expression is generally more manifest than that of S or s. Rh$_{null}$ (regulator and amorph type) and Rh$_{mod}$ cells have between 60% and 70% reduction in GPB compared with normal cells [571,572]. Red cells of individuals heterozygous for the regulator alleles have about a 30% decrease in GPB content. Dahr *et al.* [571] propose that Rh proteins form a complex with GPB, which might facilitate the incorporation of GPB into the membrane and contribute to complete expression of the U antigen.

Anti-Duclos, an alloantibody to a high frequency antigen, reacted with red cells expressing either Rh antigens or U antigen, but not with Rh$_{null}$ U– cells [573]. Red cells of the antibody maker had normal Rh antigens and slightly depressed U. Inhibition of anti-

Duclos with various GPB fractions suggested that Duclos represents a lipid-dependent labile structure in the region of amino acid residues 35–40 of GPB [220]. A mouse monoclonal antibody, MB-2D10, behaved serologically in a very similar way to anti-Duclos, except that the former reacted with red cells of the maker of anti-Duclos. Immunoblotting revealed that the monoclonal antibody bound to the Rh-associated glycoprotein (RhAG) [574]. U, Duclos, and MB-2D10 determinants appear to require an association between GPB and various Rh-related structures for optimum expression [574,575] (see also Sections 5.5.7 and 5.5.8).

An antibody in a multiply transfused Rh D+ S–s+ heart surgery patient reacted only with cells bearing both D and S antigens [576]. This combined specificity was confirmed by adsorption studies and provides serological evidence for an association between Rh protein and GPB in the red cell membrane.

3.23 Glycophorins as receptors for pathogens

3.23.1 Glycophorins and malaria

Of the four species of malarial protozoa that parasitize humans, *Plasmodium falciparum* is responsible for the most severe and prevalent form of malaria. An essential stage in the life cycle of malarial parasites is the invasion of host red cells by merozoites. This invasion involves an interaction between receptors on the parasite and ligands on the surface of the red cell. The first suggestion that human glycophorin may be involved in this interaction came from the observation by Miller *et al.* [577] that GPA-deficient, En(a–), red cells are more resistant to invasion than normal cells. This was confirmed by Pasvol *et al.* [578] (Table 3.13), who showed that the minority of merozoites that do succeed in entering the En(a–) cells develop normally (reviewed in [581,582]). S–s– cells, which lack GPB, were less susceptible to invasion than S+/s+ cells, but substantially less resistant than En(a–) cells [579,583]. GPC- and GPD-deficient red cells of the rare Gerbich-negative Leach phenotype demonstrated a degree of resistance to invasion [580], but this could be a result of their elliptocytic morphology [584] (see Chapter 18). Trypsin treatment of red cells, which removes N-terminal segments of GPA, GPC, and GPD, makes

them relatively resistant to invasion [577,579, 583,585]. The degree of resistance is greater in trypsin-treated S–s– cells, suggesting that GPA, GPB, and possibly GPC and GPD act as receptors for *P. falciparum* attachment. The results shown in Table 3.13 are those of Pasvol *et al.* Other workers, sometimes using different strains of the parasite, have often obtained different data, but the trends are much the same. An observed inhibition of parasite invasion by monoclonal antibodies to GPA, including anti-Wr[b], is probably the result of increased red cell rigidity [586]. Epitopes on GPA responsible for antibody and parasite binding are concealed by coating red cells with polyethylene glycol, rendering the cells relatively resistant to *P. falciparum* invasion [587].

Sialic acid clustered on the O-linked oligosaccharides of sialoglycoproteins is critical to the invasion process of *P. falciparum*. As GPA carries about 70% of total red cell sialic acid, it is difficult to determine the relative importance of GPA and sialic acid as receptors for parasite adhesion and invasion. Sialidase treatment of red cells reduced invasion by about 50% [577]. Furthermore, Tn red cells, which lack sialic acid and galactose from their O-linked oligosaccharides, are virtually refractory to invasion by some strains of *P. falciparum* [579,588,589] (Table 3.13). Sd(a++) (Cad) cells, which have a normal level of sialic acid but have an additional N-acetylgalactosamine residue at-

Table 3.13 Invasion of red cells of various phenotypes with *Plasmodium falciparum* merozoites [578–580].

Phenotype	Deficient structure	Invasion (percentage of normal)
Normal		100
En(a–) GW	GPA	8
En(a–) RL	GPA	14
S–s–U–	GPB	72
Ge:–2,–3,–4 Leach	GPC	57
Tn*	Gal+ sialic acid	8
Trypsin-treated normal	GPA-T1, GPC-T1	38
Trypsin-treated S–s–U–	GPA-T1, GPC-T1, GPB	5

*Approximately 90% Tn and 10% normal cells.
GPA-T1 and GPC-T1, N-terminal glycopeptides of GPA and GPB.

tached to most of their *O*-glycans (Chapter 29) are relatively resistant to *P. falciparum* invasion, possibly because the additional *N*-acetylgalactosamine residue prevents access of the parasite to its sialic acid ligand [588]. Adherence of *P. falciparum* microgametes to red cells during exflagellation also appears to be dependent on GPA, or at least on sialic acid [590].

EBA-175, a *P. falciparum* protein that acts as a ligand for red cell binding, bound specifically to GPA and to a glycopeptide comprising the N-terminal 64 amino acids of GPA, but did not bind GPB [591]. Both sialic acid and the peptide backbone of GPA were essential for binding EBA-175. This contrasts evidence suggesting that GPA acts as a receptor for *P. falciparum* purely on the basis of being a carrier of sialic acid. The degree of dependence on sialic acid, however, varies with the strain of parasite.

3.23.2 Other pathogens

GPA, especially GPA^M, acts as a receptor for some bacteria. The uropathogenic *Escherichia coli* strain 1H11165 specifically agglutinates red cells carrying an M antigen [592]. This agglutination is not affected by sialidase treatment of the cells. GPA^M, but not GPA^N, binds the bacteria. This binding could be inhibited by the glycosylated N-terminal octapeptide of GPA^M. A haemagglutinating adhesin isolated from *E. coli* F41 agglutinated M+ red cells more effectively than M− cells [593]. Glycophorins appear to act as receptors for bacterial toxins that lyse red cells. Coating of red cells with antibodies to GPA and GPB protects the cells from lysis by haemolysins from *E. coli* and *Vibrio cholerae*, respectively [594,595].

GPA acts as a receptor for influenza virus [596] and certain other viruses [597,598]. Purified GPA, GPB, GPC, and GPD inhibited haemagglutination by influenza viruses A and B [599].

3.24 Development and distribution of MNS antigens

M, N, S, s, U, and most of the other MNS system antigens are well developed at birth, and some have been shown to be present on red cells quite early in fetal life [18]. The biosynthesis of GPA has been well studied and is reviewed by Gahmberg *et al.* [600]. GPA is present on proerythroblasts, the earliest morphologically recognizable red cell precursor [601–603], appearing after the Rh-associated glycoprotein and slightly before band 3 during *in vitro* erythropoiesis [604–606]. The degree of O-glycosylation increases as the erythroid precursor cells differentiate [603], hence M and N antigens are only detectable at a later stage in erythroid development [607].

GPA is restricted to blood cells of erythroid lineage [608] and is often used as an erythroid marker. It is not present on lymphocytes, granulocytes, megakaryocytes, or platelets [34,601,609]. Sialoglycoproteins resembling GPA and GPB are present on the erythroleukaemia cell line K562 [601,609,610], which has been used as a source of *GYPA* and *GYPB* cDNA [58,80]. M and N antigens have been detected on K562 cells [609]; M antigen is more readily detected after induction of haemoglobin synthesis by hemin [611].

GPA, or at least a closely related molecule, has been detected on renal endothelium [612]. Immunocytochemical studies have shown that M, N, and certain other GPA-borne antigens are expressed on endothelial cells of human kidney, but only those anti-M and -N detecting sialic acid-independent determinants reacted with kidney tissue, suggesting that the GPA in renal endothelium is incompletely sialylated [613].

3.25 Function and evolution of glycophorins

The main characteristic that the glycophorins have in common is a long heavily glycosylated extracellular domain. The function of this domain is not known. Glycophorins carry a lot of sialic acid and therefore a substantial negative charge. Consequently, their prime function may be to keep red cells apart and prevent spontaneous aggregation. They also contribute to the glycocalyx or cell coat, an extracellular matrix of carbohydrate that protects the cell from mechanical damage and microbial attack [614]. Phenotypes in which red cells are totally deficient in GPA and GPB (M^K) or GPC and GPD (Leach) are rare and are not associated with ill health. In GPA-deficiency phenotypes, in which the most abundant glycophorin is absent, sialic acid deficiency is partially compensated by increased glycosylation of band 3 glycoprotein. M^K red cells have only a 20% reduction in sialic acid content, compared with a predicted 60% reduction if there were no increased glycosylation of band 3 [615].

153

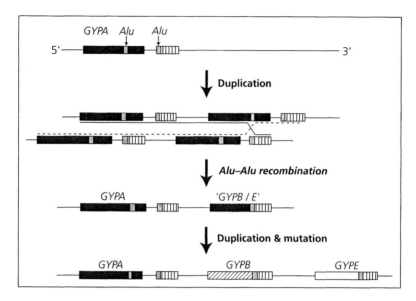

Fig. 3.13 Model to explain the evolution of the three glycophorin genes on chromosome 4. Duplication of an ancestral *GYPA* was followed by chromosomal misalignment and unequal crossing-over occurring at an *Alu* sequence within intron A5 of the duplicated *GYPA* ancestral gene and another *Alu* sequence downstream of that gene. Duplication of the resulting hybrid *GYPB/E* progenitor then produced ancestral *GYPB* and *GYPE*. All three genes have been further modified by insertion and deletion. Redrawn from [102].

GPA is associated with the anion transporter band 3 in the membrane (see Section 10.4.2). *Xenopus* oocytes in which human band 3 and *GYPA* cDNAs were coexpressed had higher levels of chloride transport and higher level of band 3 in their plasma membrane than oocytes expressing band 3 alone [134]. Furthermore, band 3 with a Gly701Asp mutation is unstable in the membrane of oocytes unless *GYPA* cDNA is coexpressed with the mutant band 3 cDNA [616]. Young *et al.* [617] propose that a role of GPA in the red cell is to enhance the rate of folding and maturation of band 3 during band 3 biosynthesis in the maturing erythroid cell. In En(a–) phenotypes, band 3 may remain in the Golgi complex longer, resulting in increased extension of the oligosaccharide chains of the *N*-glycan on band 3. Band 3-deficient red cells of mice with targeted inactivation of the band 3 gene did not express GPA at their cell surface despite the presence of *GYPA* mRNA, prompting the suggestion that band 3 may act as a chaperone for GPA, facilitating its translocation to the plasma membrane [618]. However, in human cells GPA can be expressed in the absence of band 3; GPA appears before band 3 on erythroid progenitors during *ex vivo* erythropoiesis [604,606] and K562 cells express GPA, but not band 3 [619].

GPA may have a role in ligand-induced signal transduction. In its native state, GPA has little or no direct interaction with the membrane skeleton, a network of proteins beneath the lipid bilayer (see Chapter 18). Binding of antibodies, monovalent Fab fragments, or lectins to GPA resulted in decreased red cell membrane deformability and reduced lateral movement of GPA [615]. If a transmembrane signal can be induced by the binding of ligands to the extracellular domain of GPA, it probably passes to the membrane skeleton *via* band 3 [620].

GPA may function as a complement regulator, providing limited protection to red cells from complement-induced reactive lysis by inhibiting the formation or binding of C5b–7 [621]. GPA inserted into K562 cells by electropulsation increased their resistance to natural killer cell attack, an effect that appeared to be dependent on *N*-glycosylation of the GPA, but not on sialic acid or *O*-glycosylation [622].

GPA is an important factor for the invasion of red cells by malarial parasites (Section 3.23.1). GPA-deficiency phenotypes should therefore have a strong selective advantage in areas where *P. falciparum* is endemic, particularly as no pathology has been associated with these phenotypes. Yet GPA-deficiency phenotypes are extremely rare. This suggests that GPA does have an important function, or had one until recent evolutionary history.

The three glycophorin genes on human chromosome 4 show marked homology from their 5′ flanking sequences to an *Alu* sequence approximately 1 kb downstream of exon 5, the exon encoding the transmembrane domains [90,95]. Figure 3.13 outlines the probable series of events that led to the formation of the three-gene cluster [102]. Duplication of an ancestral *GYPA*[N] gene was followed by unequal crossing-over between the *Alu* sequence within intron A5 of the duplicated *GYPA* gene and another *Alu* sequence downstream of that gene. This produced a precursor *GYPB/E* gene lacking the 3′ exons of *GYPA*, but acquiring a new sequence from the region downstream of the ancestral *GYPA*. Duplication of this *GYPB/E* gene, followed by divergence, produced ancestral *GYPB* and *GYPE*. *GYPE* subsequently appeared to acquire a segment of *GYPA*[M], including exon 2, by gene conversion [623,624]. This would explain why GPB has the N sequence, but GPE has the M sequence.

A *GYPA* gene has been detected in all primate species tested; a *GYPB* gene is present in chimpanzee, pygmy chimpanzee, and gorilla, but absent from orang-utan and gibbon; and a *GYPE* gene is present in all species with *GYPB*, but only seven of 16 gorillas had *GYPE* [625]. *GYPB* and *GYPE* probably arose from the ancestral *GYPA* prior to gorilla divergence [625,626]. Chimpanzee and gorilla GPB is larger than human GPB, because of expression of the exon B3, which has become the *GYPB*-pseudoexon in humans. *GYPE* has acquired mutation much more rapidly than *GYPB* or *GYPA*, suggesting that *GYPE* is non-functional, or less functional than the other glycophorin genes [625,626]. Two allelic forms of *GYPA* are found in gorillas: one in which exon A3 is represented in the mRNA transcript and one in which exon A3 is a pseudoexon [626].

Chimpanzee red cells express an M-like antigen. This is probably because of terminal serine on chimpanzee GPA, which has an N-terminal pentapeptide sequence identical to that of the human M[c] sequence (see Table 3.7) [627]. N-like activity in red cells of some chimpanzees probably derives from chimpanzee GPB [625,627]. He activity in some gorillas may arise from N-terminal Trp-Ser-Trp on GPA, GPB, and, possibly, GPE [626]. For a review on the expression of MNS antigens on the red cells of non-human primates see [628].

References

1 Landsteiner K, Levine P. A new agglutinable factor differentiating individual human bloods. *Proc Soc Exp Biol NY* 1927;**24**:600–2.

2 Landsteiner K, Levine P. Further observations on individual differences of human blood. *Proc Soc Exp Biol NY* 1927;**24**:941–2.

3 Landsteiner K, Levine P. On individual differences in human blood. *J Exp Med* 1928;**47**:757–75.

4 Landsteiner K, Levine P. On the inheritance of agglutinogens of human blood demonstrable by immune agglutinins. *J Exp Med* 1928;**48**:731–49.

5 Schiff F. Die Vererbungsweise der Faktoren M und N von Landsteiner und Levine. *Klin Wochnschr* 1930;**2**:1956–9.

6 Wiener AS, Vaisberg M. Heredity of the agglutinogens M and N of Landsteiner and Levine. *J Immunol* 1931;**20**:371–88.

7 Walsh RJ, Montgomery CM. A new human iso-agglutinin subdividing the MN blood groups. *Nature* 1947;**160**:504–6.

8 Sanger R, Race RR. Subdivisions of the MN blood groups in man. *Nature* 1947;**160**:505.

9 Sanger R, Race RR, Walsh RJ, Mongomery C. An antibody which subdivides the human MN blood groups. *Heredity* 1948;**2**:131–9.

10 Levine P, Kuhmichel AB, Wigod M, Koch E. A new blood factor, s, allelic to S. *Proc Soc Exp Biol NY* 1951;**78**:218–20.

11 Sanger R, Race RR. The MNSs blood group system. *Am J Hum Genet* 1951;**3**:332–43.

12 Race RR, Sanger R. *Blood Groups in Man*, 2nd edn. Oxford: Blackwell Scientific Publications, 1954.

13 Greenwalt TJ, Sasaki T, Sanger R, Sneath J, Race RR. An allele of the S(s) blood group genes. *Proc Natl Acad Sci USA* 1954;**40**:1126–9.

14 Wiener AS, Unger LJ, Gordon EB. Fatal hemolytic transfusion reaction caused by sensitization to a new blood factor U. *J Am Med Assoc* 1953;**153**:1444–6.

15 Wiener AS, Unger LJ, Cohen L. Distribution and heredity of blood factor U. *Science* 1954;**119**:734–5.

16 Race RR, Sanger R. *Blood Groups in Man*, 4th edn. Oxford: Blackwell Scientific Publications, 1962:88–93.

17 Cleghorn TE. MNSs gene frequencies in English blood donors. *Nature* 1960; **187**: 701.

18 Race RR, Sanger R. *Blood Groups in Man*, 6th edn. Oxford: Blackwell Scientific Publications, 1975.

19 Mourant AE, Kopec AC, Domaniewska-Sobczak K. *The Distribution of the Human Blood Groups and Other Polymorphisms*, 2nd edn. London: Oxford University Press, 1976.

20 Tills D, Kopec AC, Tills RE. *The Distribution of the Human Blood Groups and Other Polymorphisms* (Suppl. 1). Oxford: Oxford University Press, 1983.

21 Fisher RA. The fitting of gene frequencies to data on Rhesus reactions. *Ann Eugen* 1946;**13**:150–5.

22 Fisher RA. Note on the calculation of the frequencies of Rhesus allelomorphs. *Ann Eugen* 1947;**13**:223–4.

23 Lin-Chu M, Broadberry RE, Chang FJ. The distribution of blood group antigens and alloantibodies among Chinese in Taiwan. *Transfusion* 1988;**28**:350–2.

24 Issitt PD, Haber JM, Allen FH. Sj, a new antigen in the MN system, and further studies on Tm. *Vox Sang* 1968;**15**:1–14.

25 Bouloux C, Gamila J, Langaney. Hemotypology of the Bedik. *Hum Biol* 1972;**44**:289–302.

26 Chown B, Lewis M, Kaita H. The inheritance of the MNSs blood groups in a Caucasian population sample. *Am J Hum Genet* 1967;**19**:86–93.

27 Heiken A. A genetic study of the MNSs blood group system. *Hereditas* 1965;**53**:187–211.

28 Morton NE, Mi MP, Yasuda N. A study of the S^u alleles in Northeastern Brazil. *Vox Sang* 1966;**11**:194–208.

29 Sanger R, Race RR, Greenwalt TJ, Sasaki T. The S, s and S^u blood group genes in American negroes. *Vox Sang* 1955;**5**:73–81.

30 Allen FH, Madden HJ, King RW. The MN gene *MU*, which produces M and U but no N, S, or s. *Vox Sang* 1963;**8**:549–56.

31 Chown B, Lewis M, Kaita H. An anomaly of inheritance in the MNSs blood groups. *Am J Hum Genet* 1965;**17**:9–13.

32 Gedde-Dahl T, Grimstad AL, Gundersen S, Vogt E. A probable crossing over or mutation in the MNSs blood group system. *Acta Genet* 1967;**17**:193–210.

33 Steck TL. The organization of proteins in the human red blood cell membrane: a review. *J Cell Biol* 1974;**62**:1–19.

34 Dahr W. Immunochemistry of sialoglycoproteins in human red blood cell membranes. In: V Vengelen-Tyler, WJ Judd, eds. *Recent Advances in Blood Group Biochemistry*. Arlington, VA: American Association of Blood Banks, 1986:23–65.

35 Blanchard D. Human red cell glycophorins: biochemical and antigenic properties. *Transfus Med Rev* 1990;**4**:170–86.

36 Huang C-H, Blumenfeld OO. MNS blood groups and major glycophorins: molecular basis for allelic variation. In: J-P Cartron, P Rouger, eds. *Blood Cell Biochemistry*, Vol. 6. New York: Plenum, 1995: 153–88.

37 Cartron J-P, Rahuel C. Human erythrocyte glycophorins: protein and gene structure analyses. *Transfus Med Rev* 1992;**6**:63–92.

38 Chasis JA, Mohandas N. Red blood cell glycophorins. *Blood* 1992;**80**:1869–79.

39 Welsh EJ, Thom D, Morris ER, Rees DA. Molecular organization of glycophorin A: implications for membrane interactions. *Biopolymers* 1985;**24**:2301–32.

40 Thomas DB, Winzler RJ. Structural studies on human erythrocyte glycoproteins. *J Biol Chem* 1969;**244**: 5943–6.

41 Remaley AT, Ugorski M, Wu N *et al.* Expression of human glycophorin A in wild type and glycosylation-deficient Chinese hamster ovary cells: role of *N*- and *O*-linked glycosylation in cell surface expression. *J Biol Chem* 1991;**266**:24176–83.

42 Ugorski M, Blackall DP, Påhlsson P *et al.* Recombinant Miltenberger I and II human blood group antigens: the role of glycosylation in cell surface expression and antigenicity of glycophorin A. *Blood* 1993;**82**:1913–20.

43 Laemmli UK. Cleavage of structural proteins during the assembly of the head of bacteriophage T4. *Nature* 1970;**227**:680–5.

44 Fairbanks G, Steck TL, Wallach DFH. Electrophoretic analysis of the major polypeptides of the human erythrocyte membrane. *Biochemistry* 1971;**10**:2606–17.

45 Fujita S, Cleve H. Isolation and partial characterization of two minor glycoproteins from human erythrocyte membranes. *Biochim Biophys Acta* 1975;**382**:172–80.

46 Hamaguchi H, Cleve H. Solubilization of human erythrocyte membrane glycoproteins and separation of the MN glycoprotein from a glycoprotein with I, S, and A activity. *Biochim Biophys Acta* 1972;**278**:271–80.

47 Towbin H, Staehelin T, Gordon J. Electrophoretic transfer of proteins from polyacrlyamide gels to nitrocellulose sheets: procedure and some applications. *Proc Natl Acad Sci USA* 1979;**76**:4350–4.

48 Rouger P, Anstee D, Salmon C, eds. First International Workshop on Monoclonal Antibodies Against Human Red Blood Cell and Related Antigens. *Rev Franc Transfus Immuno-Hémat* 1988;**31**:261–364 (11 papers).

49 Lu Y-Q, Nichols ME, Bigbee WL, Nagel RL, Blumenfeld OO. Structural polymorphisms of glycophorins demonstrated by immunoblotting techniques. *Blood* 1987;**69**:618–24.

50 Khalid G, Green CA. Immunoblotting of human red cell membranes: detection of glycophorin B with anti-S and anti-s antibodies. *Vox Sang* 1990;**59**:48–54.

51 Nigg EA, Bron C, Giradet M, Cherry RJ. Band 3–glycophorin A association in erythrocyte membranes demonstrated by combining protein diffusion measurements with antibody-induced cross-linking. *Biochemistry* 1980;**19**:1887–93.

52 Gardner B, Parsons SF, Merry AH, Anstee DJ. Epitopes on sialoglycoprotein α: evidence for heterogeneity in the molecule. *Immunology* 1989;**68**:283–9.

53 Marchesi VT. Functional proteins of the human red blood cell membrane. *Semin Hematol* 1979;**16**:3–20.

54 MacKenzie KR, Prestegard JH, Engelman DM. A transmembrane helix dimer: structure and implications. *Science* 1997;**276**:131–3.

55 Brosig B, Langosch D. The dimerization motif of the glycophorin A transmembrane segment in membranes: importance of glycine residues. *Protein Sci* 1998;**7**:1052–6.

56 Tomita M, Marchesi VT. Amino-acid sequence and oligosaccharide attachment sites of human erythrocyte glycophorin. *Proc Natl Acad Sci USA* 1975;72:2964–8.

57 Tomita M, Furthmayr H, Marchesi VT. Primary structure of human erythrocyte glycophorin A: isolation and characterization of peptides and complete amino acid sequence. *Biochemistry* 1978;17:4756–70.

58 Siebert PD, Fukuda M. Isolation and characterization of human glycophorin A cDNA clones by a synthetic oligonucleotide approach: nucleotide sequence and mRNA structure. *Proc Natl Acad Sci USA* 1986;83:1665–9.

59 Fukuda M, Lauffenburger M, Sasaki H, Rogers ME, Dell A. Structures of novel sialylated O-linked oligosaccharides isolated from human erythrocyte glycophorins. *J Biol Chem* 1987;262:11952–7.

60 Furthmayr H. Structural comparison of glycophorins and immunochemical analysis of genetic variants. *Nature* 1978;271:519–24.

61 Dahr W, Müller T, Moulds J et al. High frequency antigens of human erythrocyte membrane sialoglycoproteins. I. En^a receptors in the glycosylated domain of the MN sialoglycoprotein. *Biol Chem Hoppe-Seyler* 1985;366:41–51.

62 Yoshima H, Furthmayr H, Kobata A. Structures of the asparagine-linked sugar chains of glycophorin A. *J Biol Chem* 1980;255:9713–8.

63 Irimura T, Tsuji T, Tagami S, Yamamoto K, Osawa T. Structure of a complex-type sugar chain of human glycophorin A. *Biochemistry* 1981;20:560–6.

64 Blumenfeld OO, Adamany AM. Structural polymorphism within the amino-terminal region of MM, NN, and MN glycoproteins (glycophorins) of the human erythrocyte membrane. *Proc Natl Acad Sci USA* 1978;75:2727–31.

65 Wasniowska K, Drzeniek Z, Lisowska E. The amino acids of M and N blood group glycopeptides are different. *Biochem Biophys Res Commun* 1977;76:385–90.

66 DuPont BR, Grant SG, Oto SH et al. Molecular characterization of glycophorin A transcripts in human erythroid cells using RT-PCR, allele-specific restriction, and sequencing. *Vox Sang* 1995;68:121–9.

67 Tate CG, Tanner MJA. Isolation of cDNA clones for human erythrocyte membrane sialoglycoproteins α and δ. *Biochem J* 1988;254:743–50.

68 Akane A, Mizukame H, Shiono H. Classification of standard alleles of the MN blood group system. *Vox Sang* 2000;79:183–7.

69 Springer GF, Ansell NJ. Inactivation of human erythrocyte agglutinogens M and N by influenza viruses and receptor-destroying enzyme. *Proc Natl Acad Sci USA* 1958;44:182–9.

70 Mäkelä O, Cantell K. Destruction of M and N blood group receptors of human red cells by some influenza viruses. *Ann Med Exp Fenn* 1958;36:366–74.

71 Judd WJ, Issitt PD, Pavone BG, Anderson J, Aminoff D. Antibodies that define NANA-independent MN-system antigens. *Transfusion* 1979;19:12–18.

72 Issitt PD, Wilkinson SL. Further studies on the dependence of some examples of anti-M and anti-N on the presence of red-cell-borne sialic acid. *Transfusion* 1983;23:117–19.

73 Lisowska E, Duk M. Modification of amino groups of human-erythrocyte glycoproteins and the new concept on the structural basis of M and N blood-group specificity. *Eur J Biochem* 1975;54:469–74.

74 Lisowska E, Duk M. Effect of modification of amino groups of human erythrocytes on M, N and N_{Vg} blood group specificities. *Vox Sang* 1975;28:392–7.

75 Krotkiewski H, Duk M, Syper D et al. Blood group MN-dependent difference in degree of galactosylation of O-glycans of glycophorin A is restricted to the GalNAc residues located on amino acid residues 2–4 of the glycophorin polypeptide chain. *FEBS Lett* 1997;406:296–300.

76 Corfield VA, Moolman JC, Martell R, Brink PA. Polymerase chain reaction-based detection of MN blood group-specific sequences in the human genome. *Transfusion* 1993;33:119–24.

77 Eshleman JR, Shakin-Eshleman SH, Church A, Kant JA, Spitalnik SL. DNA typing of the human MN and Ss blood group antigens in amniotic fluid and following massive transfusion. *Am J Clin Pathol* 1995;103:353–7.

78 Nakayashiki N, Sasaki Y. An improved method for MN genotyping by the polymerase chain reaction. *Int J Legal Med* 1996;109:216–7.

79 Li Z-X, Yoshimura S, Kobayashi T, Akane A. Allele-specific, inverse-PCR amplification for genotyping MN blood group. *Biotechniques* 1998;25:358–62.

80 Siebert PD, Fukuda M. Molecular cloning of a human glycophorin B cDNA: nucleotide sequence and genomic relationship to glycophorin A. *Proc Natl Acad Sci USA* 1987;84:6735–9.

81 Blanchard D, Dahr W, Hummel M et al. Glycophorins B and C from human erythrocyte membranes: purification and sequence analysis. *J Biol Chem* 1987;262:5808–11.

82 Furthmayr H. Glycophorins A, B, and C: a family of sialoglycoproteins. Isolation and preliminary characterization of trypsin derived peptides. *J Supramol Struct* 1978;9:79–95.

83 Dahr W, Beyreuther K, Steinbach H, Gielen W, Krüger J. Structure of the Ss blood group antigens. II. A methionine/threonine polymorphism within the N-terminal sequence of the Ss glycoprotein. *Hoppe-Seyler Z Physiol Chem* 1980;361:895–906.

84 Dahr W, Beyreuther K, Bause E, Kordowicz M. Structures and antigenic properties of human erythrocyte membrane sialoglycoproteins. *Prot Biol Fluids* 1982;29:57–62.

85 Dahr W, Gielen W, Beyreuther K, Krüger J. Structure of the Ss blood group antigens. I. Isolation of Ss-active

glycopeptides and differentiation of the antigens by modification of methionine. *Hoppe-Seyler Z Physiol Chem* 1980;**361**:145–52.

86 Storry JR, Reid ME. Synthetic peptide inhibition of anti-S [Abstract]. *Transfusion* 1996;**36**:55S.

87 Reid ME, Lisowska E, Blanchard D, eds. Third International Workshop on Monoclonal Antibodies Against Human Red Blood Cell and Related Antigens. *Transfus Clin Biol* 1997;**4**:57–96 (9 papers).

88 Rahuel C, London J, d'Auriol L *et al.* Characterization of cDNA clones for human glycophorin A: use for gene localization and for analysis of normal of glycophorin-A-deficient (Finnish type) genomic DNA. *Eur J Biochem* 1988;**172**:147–53.

89 Siebert PD, Fukuda M. Human glycophorin A and B are encoded by separate, single copy genes coordinately regulated by a tumor-promoting phorbol ester. *J Biol Chem* 1986;**261**:12433–6.

90 Kudo S, Fukuda M. Structural organization of glycophorin A and B genes: glycophorin B gene evolved by homologous recombination at *Alu* repeat sequences. *Proc Natl Acad Sci USA* 1989;**86**:4619–23.

91 Vignal A, Rahuel C, El Maliki B *et al.* Molecular analysis of glycophorin A and B gene structure and expression in homozygous Miltenberger class V (Mi. V) human erythrocytes. *Eur J Biochem* 1989;**184**:337–44.

92 Hamid J, Burness ATH. The mechanism of production of multiple mRNAs for human glycophorin A. *Nucl Acid Res* 1990;**18**:5829–36.

93 Reid ME. Some concepts relating to the molecular genetic basis of certain MNS blood group antigens. *Transfus Med* 1994;**4**:99–111.

94 Tate CG, Tanner MJA, Judson PA, Anstee DJ. Studies on human red-cell membrane glycophorin A and glycophorin B genes in glycophorin-deficient individuals. *Biochem J* 1989;**263**:993–6.

95 Kudo S, Fukuda M. Identification of a novel human glycophorin, glycophorin E, by isolation of genomic clones and complementary DNA clones utilizing polymerase chain reaction. *J Biol Chem* 1990;**265**:1102–10.

96 Rahuel C, London J, Vignal A *et al.* Alteration of the genes for glycophorin A and B in glycophorin-A-deficient individuals. *Eur J Biochem* 1988;**177**:605–14.

97 Kudo S, Chagnovich D, Rearden A, Mattei M-G, Fukuda M. Molecular analysis of a hybrid gene encoding human glycophorin variant Miltenberger V-like molecule. *J Biol Chem* 1990;**265**:13285–89.

98 Vignal A, Rahuel C, London J *et al.* A novel gene member of the human glycophorin A and B gene family: molecular cloning and expression. *Eur J Biochem* 1990;**191**:619–25.

99 Anstee DJ. The nature and abundance of human red cell surface glycoproteins. *J Immunogenet* 1990;**17**:219–25.

100 Huang C-H, Guizzo ML, McCreary J, Leigh EM, Blumenfeld OO. Typing of MNSs blood group specific sequences in the human genome and characterization of a restriction fragment tightly linked to S–s– alleles. *Blood* 1991;**77**:381–6.

101 Onda M, Kudo S, Fukuda M. Genomic organization of glycophorin A gene family revealed by yeast artificial chromosomes containing human genomic DNA. *J Biol Chem* 1994;**269**:13013–20.

102 Onda M, Kudo S, Rearden A, Mattei M-G, Fukuda M. Identification of a precursor genomic segment that provided a sequence unique to glycophorin B and E genes. *Proc Natl Acad Sci USA* 1993;**90**:7220–4.

103 Vignal A, London J, Rahuel C, Cartron J-P. Promoter sequence and chromosomal organization of the genes encoding glycophorins A, B and E. *Gene* 1990;**95**:289–93.

104 Rahuel C, Elouet J-F, Cartron J-P. Post-transcriptional regulation of the cell surface expression of glycophorins A, B, and E. *J Biol Chem* 1994;**269**:32752–8.

105 Rahuel C, Vinit M-A, Lemarchandel V, Cartron J-P, Romeo P-H. Erythroid-specific activity of the glycophorin B promoter requires GATA-1 mediated displacement of a repressor. *EMBO J* 1992;**11**:4095–102.

106 Camara-Clayette V, Thomas D, Rahuel C *et al.* The repressor which binds the –75 GATA motif of the GPB promoter contains Ku70 as the DNA binding subunit. *Nucl Acid Res* 1999;**27**:1656–63.

107 Camara-Clayette V, Rahuel C, Bertrand O, Cartron J-P. The E-box of the human glycophorin B promoter is involved in the erythroid-specific expression of the GPB gene. *Biochem Biophys Res Commun* 1999;**265**:170–6.

108 Fukuda M. Molecular genetics of the glycophorin A gene cluster. *Semin Hematol* 1993;**30**:138–51.

109 Dahr W, Uhlenbruck G, Knott H. Immunochemical aspects of the MNSs-blood group system. *J Immunogenet* 1975;**2**:87–100.

110 Judson PA, Anstee DJ. Comparative effect of trypsin and chymotrypsin on blood group antigens. *Med Lab Sci* 1977;**34**:1–6.

111 Case J. The behaviour of anti-S antibodies with ficin treated human red cells [Abstract]. *Transfusion* 1978;**18**:392–3.

112 Herron B, Smith GA. The effect of increasing concentration of neuraminidase on the removal of α2,3– and α2,6–linked sialic acids from intact red cells [Abstract]. *Transfus Med* 1992;**2**(Suppl.1):70.

113 Lisowska E, Kordowicz M. Specific antibodies for desialized M and N blood group antigens. *Vox Sang* 1977;**33**:164–9.

114 Sadler JE, Paulson JC, Hill RL. The role of sialic acid in the expression of human MN blood group antigens. *J Biol Chem* 1979;**254**:2112–9.

115 Darnborough J, Dunsford I, Wallace JA. The En^a antigen and antibody: a genetical modification of human red cells affecting their blood grouping reactions. *Vox Sang* 1969;**17**:241–55.

116 Furuhjelm U, Myllylä G, Nevanlinna HR *et al.* The red

cell phenotype En(a–) and anti-En^a: serological and physicochemical aspects. *Vox Sang* 1969;17:256–78.

117 Furuhjelm U, Nevanlinna HR, Pirkola A. A second Finnish En(a–) propositus with anti-En^a. *Vox Sang* 1973;24:545–9.

118 Walker PS, Bergren MO, Busch MP, Carmody AM, Perkins HA. Finnish En(a–) propositus with anti-En^{a}FS and anti-En^{a}FR: *in vitro* and *in vivo* characteristics. *Vox Sang* 1987;52:103–6.

119 Taliano V, Guévin R-M, Hébert D *et al.* The rare phenotype En(a–) in a French-Canadian family. *Vox Sang* 1980;38:87–93.

120 Rapini J, Batts R, Yacob M *et al.* En(a–) FIN phenotype in a Pakistani. *Immunohematology* 1995;11:51–3.

121 Shinozuka T, Miyata Y, Kuroda N *et al.* Serological and biochemical studies on En(a–) human erythrocytes in a Japanese family. *Jpn J Legal Med* 1992;46:301–9.

122 Okubo Y, Seno T, Yamaguchi H *et al.* En(a–) phenotype in a Japanese blood donor. *Imunohemat* 1993;9:105–8.

123 Dahr W, Uhlenbruck G, Wagstaff W, Leikola J. Studies on the membrane glycoprotein defect of En(a–) erythrocytes. II. MN antigenic properties of En(a–) erythrocytes. *J Immunogenet* 1976;3:383–93.

124 Anstee DJ, Barker DM, Judson PA, Tanner MJA. Inherited sialoglycoprotein deficiencies in human erythrocytes of type En(a–). *Br J Haematol* 1977;35:309–20.

125 Dahr W, Uhlenbruck G, Leikola J, Wagstaff W. Studies on the membrane glycoprotein defect of En(a–) erythrocytes. III. N-terminal amino acids of sialoglycoproteins from normal and En(a–) red cells. *J Immunogenet* 1978;5:117–27.

126 Metaxas MN, Metaxas-Bühler M. *Human Blood Groups, 5th Int Convoc Immunol, Buffalo, NY.* Basel: Karger, 1977:344–52.

127 Tanner MJA, Anstee DJ. The membrane change in En(a–) human erythrocytes: absence of the major erythrocyte sialoglycoprotein. *Biochem J* 1976;153:271–7.

128 Dahr W, Uhlenbruck G, Leikola J, Wagstaff W, Landeried K. Studies on the membrane glycoprotein defect of En(a–) erythrocytes. I. Biochemical aspects. *J Immunogenet* 1976;3:329–46.

129 Inglis G, Anstee DJ, Giles CM, Tanner MJA, Mitchell R. Probable *En^{a}En* heterozygotes in two British families. *J Immunogenet* 1979;6:145–54.

130 Bird GWG, Wingham J. The action of seed and other reagents on En(a–) erythrocytes. *Vox Sang* 1973;24:48–57.

131 Metaxas MN, Metaxas-Bühler M. The detection of MNSs 'variants' in serial tests with incomplete Rh antisera in saline. *Vox Sang* 1972;22:474–7.

132 Gahmberg CG, Myllyla G, Leikola J, Pirkola A, Nordling S. Absence of the major sialoglycoprotein in the membrane of human En(a–) erythrocytes and increased glycosylation of Band 3. *J Biol Chem* 1976;251:6108–16.

133 Tanner MJA, Jenkins RE, Anstee DJ, Clamp JR. Abnormal carbohydrate composition of the major penetrating membrane protein of En(a–) human erythrocytes. *Biochem J* 1976;155:701–3.

134 Groves JD, Tanner MJA. Glycophorin A facilitates the expression of human band 3-mediated anion transport in *Xenopus* oocytes. *J Biol Chem* 1992;267:22163–70.

135 Metaxas MN, Metaxas-Buehler M. M^k: an apparently silent allele at the MN locus. *Nature* 1964;202:1123.

136 Henningsen K. Exceptional MNSs- and Gm-types within a Danish family: causal relationship or coincidence? *Acta Genet* 1966;16:239–41.

137 Nordling S, Sanger R, Gavin J *et al.* M^k and M^g: some serological and physicochemical observations. *Vox Sang* 1969;17:300–2.

138 Sturgeon P, Metaxas-Bühler M, Metaxas MN, Tippett P, Ikin EW. An erroneous exclusion of paternity in a Chinese family exhibiting the rare MNSs gene complexes M^k and Ms^{III}. *Vox Sang* 1970;18:395–406.

139 Metaxas MN, Metaxas-Bühler M, Romanski Y. The inheritance of the blood group gene *M^k* and some considerations on its possible nature. *Vox Sang* 1971;20:509–18.

140 Luner SJ, Sturgeon P, Szklarek D, McQuiston DT. Cell electrophoretic, membrane sialic acid and quantitative hemagglutination studies on some MN variants. *Vox Sang* 1975;29:440–9.

141 Metaxas MN, Metaxas-Bühler M, Edwards JH. MNSs frequencies in 3895 Swiss blood donors. *Vox Sang* 1970;18:385–94.

142 Heiken A, Ikin EW, Mårtensson L. On the M^k allele of the MNSs system. *Acta Genet* 1967;17:328–37.

143 Hodson C, Lee D, Cooper DG *et al.* M^k in three generations of an English family. *J Immunogenet* 1979;6:391–401.

144 Judd WJ, Geisland JR, Issitt PD *et al.* Studies on the blood of an *Mi^v/M^k* proposita and her family. *Transfusion* 1983;23:33–6.

145 Habash J, Lubenko A, Pizzaro I *et al.* Studies on a Chilean *Mi^V/M^k* proposita and her family [Abstract]. *Joint Congr Int Soc Blood Transfus and Am Assoc Blood Banks* 1990:155.

146 German JL, Walker ME, Stiefel FH, Allen FH. Autoradiographic studies of human chromosomes. II. Data concerning the position of the *MN* locus. *Vox Sang* 1969;16:130–45.

147 German J, Metaxas MN, Metaxas-Buhler M, Louie E, Chaganti RSK. Further evaluation of a child with the M^k phenotype and a translocation affecting the long arms of chromosomes 2 and 4 [Abstract]. *Cytogenet Cell Genet* 1979;25:160.

148 Tokunaga E, Sasakawa S, Tamaka K *et al.* Two apparently healthy Japanese individuals of type *M^{k}M^k* have erythrocytes which lack both the blood group MN and Ss-active sialoglycoproteins. *J Immunogenet* 1979;6:383–90.

149 Okubo Y, Daniels GL, Parsons SF et al. A Japanese family with two sisters apparently homozygous for M^k. Vox Sang 1988;54:107–11.

150 Gutendorf R, Lacey P, Moulds J, Dahr W. Recognition of an M^kM^k Black child during paternity testing [Abstract]. Transfusion 1985;25:481.

151 Leak M, Poole J, Kaye T et al. The rare M^kM^k phenotype in a Turkish antenatal patient and evidence for clinical significance of anti-En^a [Abstract]. Joint Congr Int Soc Blood Transfus and Am Assoc Blood Banks 1990:57.

152 Dahr W, Uhlenbruck G, Knott H. The defect of M^k erythrocytes as revealed by sodium dodecylsulphate-polyacrylamide gel electrophoresis. J Immunogenet 1977;4:191–200.

153 Anstee DJ, Tanner MJA. Genetic variants involving the major membrane sialoglycoprotein of human erythrocytes. Biochem J 1978;175:149–57.

154 Dahr W, Longster G, Uhlenbruck G, Schumacher K. Studies on Miltenberger class III, V, M^v and M^k red cells. I. Sodium–dodecylsulfate polyacrylamide gel electrophoretic investigations. Blut 1978;37:129–138.

155 Bruce LJ, Groves JD, Okubo Y, Thilaganathan B, Tanner MJA. Altered band 3 structure and function in glycophorin A- and B-deficient (M^kM^k) red blood cells. Blood 1994;84:916–22.

156 Issitt PD, Pavone BG, Wagstaff W, Goldfinger D. The phenotypes En(a−), Wr(a−b−), and En(a+), Wr(a+b−), and further studies on the Wright and En blood group systems. Transfusion 1976;16:396–407.

157 Pavone BG, Pirkola A, Nevanlinna HR, Issitt PD. Demonstration of anti-Wr^b in a second serum containing anti-En^a. Transfusion 1978;18:155–9.

158 Daniels GL. Blood group antigens of high frequency: a serological and genetical study. PhD thesis, University of London, 1980.

159 Vengelen-Tyler V, Anstee DJ, Issitt PD et al. Studies on the blood of an Mi^V homozygote. Transfusion 1981;21:1–14.

160 Langley JW, Issitt PD, Anstee DJ et al. Another individual (J.R.) whose red blood cells appear to carry a hybrid MNSs sialoglycoprotein. Transfusion 1981;21:15–24.

161 Issitt PD, Wilkinson-Kroovand S, Langley JW, Smith N. Production of allo-anti-En^a by an individual whose red blood cells carry some En^a antigen. Transfusion 1981;21:211–14.

162 Issitt PD, Daniels G, Tippett P. Proposed new terminology for En^a. Transfusion 1981;21:473–4.

163 Pavone BG, Billman R, Bryant J, Sniecinski I, Issitt PD. An auto-anti-En^a, inhibitable by MN sialoglycoprotein. Transfusion 1981;21:25–31.

164 Dahr W, Wilkinson S, Issitt PD et al. High frequency antigens of human erythrocyte membrane sialoglycoproteins III. Studies on the En^{a}FR, Wr^b and Wr^a antigens. Biol Chem Hoppe-Seyler 1986;367:1033–45.

165 Adams J, Broviac M, Brooks W, Johnson NR, Issitt PD. An antibody, in the serum of a Wr(a+) individual, reacting with an antigen of very high frequency. Transfusion 1971;11:290–1.

166 Issitt PD, Pavone BG, Goldfinger D, Zwicker H. An En(a−) red cell sample that types as Wr(a−b−). Transfusion 1975;15:353–5.

167 Ridgwell K, Tanner MJA, Anstee DJ. The Wr^b antigen, a receptor for Plasmodium falciparum malaria, is located on a helical region of the major membrane sialoglycoprotein of human red blood cells. Biochem J 1983;209:273–6.

168 Bruce LJ, Ring SM, Anstee DJ et al. Changes in the blood group Wright antigens are associated with a mutation at amino acid 658 in human erythrocyte band 3: a site of interaction between band 3 and glycophorin A in the red cell membrane under certain conditions. Blood 1994;85:541–7.

169 Postoway N, Anstee DJ, Wortman M, Garratty G. A severe transfusion reaction associated with anti-En^{a}TS in a patient with an abnormal alpha-like red cell sialoglycoprotein. Transfusion 1988;28:77–80.

170 Banks J, Malde R, King M-J, Poole J. An individual of phenotype GP.JL with anti-Wr^b/En^{a}FR: a case study [Abstract]. Transfus Med 1998;8(Suppl.1):28.

171 Bell CA, Zwicker H. Further studies on the relationship of anti-En^a and anti-Wr^b in warm autoimmune hemolytic anemia. Transfusion 1978;18:572–5.

172 Garratty G, Arndt P, Domen R et al. Severe autoimmune hemolytic anemia associated with IgM warm autoantibodies directed against determinants on or associated with glycophorin A. Vox Sang 1997;72:124–30.

173 Garratty G. Specificity of autoantibodies reacting optimally at 37°C. Immunohematology 1999;15:24–40.

174 Moulds MK, Lacey P, Bradford MF et al. An in vitro phenomenon unique to auto anti-En^{a}FS in eight patients [Abstract]. 19th Congr Int Soc Blood Transfus 1986:653.

175 Anstee DJ, Edwards PAW. Monoclonal antibodies to human erythrocytes. Eur J Immunol 1982;12:228–32.

176 Chester MA, Johnson U, Lundblad A et al. eds. Monoclonal Antibodies Against Human Red Blood Cell and Related Antigens. Proceedings of the 2nd International Workshop and Symposium 1990.

177 Wasniowska K, Duk M, Czerwinski M et al. Analysis of peptidic epitopes recognized by the three monoclonal antibodies specific for the same region of glycophorin A but showing different properties. Mol Immunol 1992;29:783–91.

178 Rasamoelisolo M, Czerwinski M, Bruneau V, Lisowska E, Blanchard D. Fine characterization of a series of new monoclonal antibodies directed against glycophorin A. Vox Sang 1997;72:185–91.

179 Rasamoelisolo M, Czerwinski M, Willem C, Blanchard D. Shared epitopes of glycoprotein A and protein 4.1 defined by antibody NaM10–3C10. Hybridoma 1998;17:283–8.

180 Roelcke D, Uhlenbruck G. Letter to the editor. *Vox Sang* 1970;**18**:478–9.

181 Roelcke D. Cold agglutination. *Transfus Med Rev* 1989;**3**:140–66.

182 Marsh WL, Jenkins WJ. Anti-Sp₁: the recognition of a new cold auto-antibody. *Vox Sang* 1968;**15**:177–86.

183 Roelcke D. A new serological specificity in cold antibodies of high titre: anti-HD. *Vox Sang* 1969;**16**:76–9.

184 Roelcke D, Kreft H. Characterization of various anti-Pr cold agglutinins. *Transfusion* 1984;**24**:210–13.

185 Roelcke D, Pruzanski W, Ebert W *et al*. A new human monoclonal cold agglutinin Sa recognizing terminal N-acetylneuraminyl groups on the cell surface. *Blood* 1980;**55**:677–81.

186 Ebert W, Fey J, Gärtner C *et al*. Isolation and partial charaterization of the Pr autoantigen determinants. *Molec Immunol* 1979;**16**:413–19.

187 Dahr W, Lichthardt D, Roelcke D. Studies on the receptor sites of the monoclonal anti-Pr and -Sa cold agglutinins. *Prot Biol Fluids* 1982;**29**:365–8.

188 Uemura K, Roelcke D, Nagai Y, Feizi T. The reactivities of human erythrocyte autoantibodies anti-Pr₂, anti-Gd, Fl and Sa with gangliosides in a chromatogram binding assay. *Biochem J* 1984;**219**:865–74.

189 Kewitz S, Groß HJ, Kosa R, Roelcke D. Anti-Pr cold agglutinins recognize immunodominant α2,3- or α2,6-sialyl groups on glycophorins. *Glycocon J* 1995;**12**:714–20.

190 Anstee DJ. Blood group MNSs-active sialoglycoproteins of the human erythrocyte membrane. In: SG Sandler, J Nusbacher, MS Schanfield, eds. *Immunobiology of the Erythrocyte*. New York: Liss, 1980: 67–98.

191 Wiener AS, Unger LJ, Gordon EB. Fatal hemolytic transfusion reaction caused by sensitization to a new blood factor U: report of a case. *J Am Med Assoc* 1953;**153**:1444–6.

192 Hackel E. Elution of anti-U from SS and ss cells. *Vox Sang* 1958;**3**:92–3.

193 Francis BJ, Hatcher DE. MN blood types. The S–s– U+ and the M₁ phenotypes. *Vox Sang* 1966;**11**:213–16.

194 Storry JR, Reid ME. Characterization of antibodies produced by S–s– individuals. *Transfusion* 1996;**36**: 512–16.

195 Issitt PD, Anstee DJ. *Applied Blood Group Serology*, 4th edn. Durham, NC: Montgomery Scientific Publications, 1998.

196 Reid ME, Storry JR, Maurer J, Nance ST. Practical method for determination of the U status of S–s– erythrocytes. *Immunohematology* 1997;**13**:111–14.

197 Reid ME, Storry JR, Ralph H, Blumenfeld OO, Huang C-H. Expression and quantitative variation of the low-incidence blood group antigen He on some S–s– red cells. *Transfusion* 1996;**36**:719–24.

198 Beattie KM, Sigmund KE, McGraw J, Shurafa M. U-variant blood in sickle cell patients. *Transfusion* 1982;**22**:257.

199 Mentor J, Richards HS. Anti-U recognizing a variant of the U-blood group. *Vox Sang* 1989;**56**:62.

200 Dahr W, Uhlenbruck G, Issitt PD, Allen FH. SDS-polyacrylamide gel electrophoretic analysis of the membrane glycoprotein from S–s–U– erythrocytes. *J Immunogenet* 1975;**2**:249–51.

201 Tanner MJA, Anstee DJ, Judson PA. A carbohydrate-deficient membrane glycoprotein in human erythrocytes of phenotype S–s–. *Biochem J* 1977;**165**:157–61.

202 Dahr W, Issitt P, Moulds J, Pavone B. Further studies on the membrane glycoprotein defects of S–s– and En(a–) erythrocytes. *Hoppe-Seyler Z Physiol Chem* 1978;**359**:1217–24.

203 Storry JR, Reid ME. Serological and molecular characteristics of S–s– glycophorin B variants [Abstract]. *Transfusion* 1997;**7**(Suppl.1):18.

204 Issitt PD, Marsh WL, Wren MR, Theuriere M, Mueller K. Heterogeneity of anti-U demonstrable by the use of papain-treated red cells. *Transfusion* 1989;**29**:508–13.

205 McKeever BG, Pochedley M, Meyer JD. Reactivity of U negative cell samples with Glycine lectin [Abstract]. *Transfusion* 1980;**20**:634.

206 Fraser GR, Giblett ER, Motulsky AG. Population genetic studies in the Congo. III. Blood groups (ABO, MNSs, Rh, Jsᵃ). *Am J Hum Genet* 1966;**18**:546–52.

207 Lowe RF, Moores PP. S–s–U– red cell factor in Africans of Rhodesia, Malawi, Mozambique and Natal. *Hum Hered* 1972;**22**:344–50.

208 Hoekstra A, Albert AP, Newell GAI, Moores P. S–s–U– phenotype in South African Negroes. *Vox Sang* 1975;**29**:214–16.

209 Sondag-Thull D, Girard M, Blanchard D, Bloy C, Cartron J-P. S–s–U– phenotype in a Caucasian family. *Exp Clin Immunogenet* 1986;**3**:181–6.

210 Moores P. Four examples of the S–s–U– phenotype in an Indian family. *Vox Sang* 1972;**23**:452–4.

211 Giblett ER, Gartler SM, Waxman SH. Blood group studies on the family of an XX/XY hermaphrodite with generalized tissue mosaicism. *Am J Hum Genet* 1963;**15**:62–8.

212 Polesky HF, Moulds J. Anomalous inheritance of Ss in a Caucasian family. *Am J Hum Genet* 1975;**27**:543–6.

213 Austin RJ, Riches G. Inherited lack of Ss antigens with weak expression of U in a Caucasian family. *Vox Sang* 1978;**34**:343–6.

214 Mauff G, Pulverer G, Hummel K, Spielmann W, Bender K. Occurrence of Sᵘ in a German family. *Blut* 1977;**34**:357–62.

215 Issitt PD, Pavone BG, Rolih SD. Failure to demonstrate dosage of U antigen. *Vox Sang* 1976;**31**:25–31.

216 Dahr W, Issitt PD, Uhlenbruck G. New concepts of the MNSs blood group system. In: *Human Blood Groups, 5th Int Convoc Immunol, Buffalo, NY*. Basel: Karger, 1977:197–205.

217 Huang C-H, Johe K, Moulds JJ *et al*. δ glycophorin (glycophorin B) gene deletion in two individuals

homozygous for the S–s–U– blood group phenotype. *Blood* 1987;**70**:1830–5.

218 Anstee DJ, Mawby WJ, Tanner MJA. Abnormal blood-group-Ss-active sialoglycoproteins in the membrane of Miltenberger class III, IV and V human erythrocytes. *Biochem J* 1979;**183**:193–203.

219 Ballas SK, Reilly PA, Murphy DL. The blood group U antigen is not located on glycophorin B. *Biochim Biophys Acta* 1986;**884**:337–43.

220 Dahr W, Moulds JJ. High-frequency antigens of human erythrocyte membrane sialoglycoproteins. IV. Molecular properties of the U antigen. *Biol Chem Hoppe-Seyler* 1987;**368**:659–67.

221 Rahuel C, London J, Vignal A, Ballas SK, Cartron J-P. Erythrocyte glycophorin B deficiency may occur by two distinct gene alterations. *Am J Hematol* 1991;**37**:57–8.

222 Storry JR, Reid ME. Analysis of silenced glycophorin B alleles by PCR-RFLP of exon 5 of the glycophorin B gene [Abstract]. *Transfusion* 2000;**40**:13S.

223 Huang C-H, Reid ME, Blumenfeld OO. Remodelling of the transmembrane segment in human glycophorin by aberrant RNA splicing. *J Biol Chem* 1994;**269**:10804–12.

224 Allen FH, Corcoran PA, Kenton HB, Breare N. M^g, a new blood group antigen in the MNS system. *Vox Sang* 1958;**3**:81–91.

225 Metaxas MN, Metaxas-Bühler M, Romanski J. Studies on the blood group antigen M^g. I. Frequency of M^g in Switzerland and family studies. *Vox Sang* 1966;**11**:157–69.

226 Metaxas MN, Matter M, Metaxas-Bühler M, Romanski Y, Hässig A. Frequency of the M^g blood group antigen in Swiss blood donors and its inheritance in several independent families. *Proc 9th Congr Int Soc Blood Transfus* 1964:206–9.

227 Brocteur J. Confirmation of the M^gS gene complex found in 3 new Sicilian families [Abstract]. *Joint Mtg Int Soc Haematol and Am Assoc Blood Banks* 1972:12.

228 Reid ME, Lomas-Francis C, Daniels GL *et al.* Expression of the erythrocyte antigen Henshaw (He; MNS6): serological and immunochemical studies. *Vox Sang* 1995;**68**:183–6.

229 Pollitzer WS. The Henshaw blood factor in New York City Negroes. *Am J Phys Anthrop* 1956;**14**:445–7.

230 Greenwalt TJ. Practical applications of recent advances in the red cell blood groups with emphasis on the rarer types. In: LM Tocantins, ed. *Progress in Hematology.* New York: Grune & Stratton, 1962:71–91.

231 Chalmers JNM, Ikin EW, Mourant AE. A study of two unusual blood-group antigens in West Africans. *Br Med J* 1953;**ii**:175–7.

232 Shapiro M. Inheritance of the Henshaw (He) blood factor. *J Forensic Med* 1956;**3**:152–60.

233 Nijenhuis LE, Wortel L. Weak examples of the Henshaw antigen. *Vox Sang* 1968;**14**:462–4.

234 Zoutendyk A. The blood groups of South African na-

tives with particular reference to a recent investigation of the Hottentots. *Proceedings of the 5th Congr International Soc Blood Transfus* 1955:247–9.

235 Nijenhuis LE. The Henshaw bloodgroup (He) in Papuans and Congo negroes. *Vox Sang* 1953;**3**:112–14.

236 Chandanyingyong D, Pejrachandra S. Studies on the Miltenberger complex frequency in Thailand and family studies. *Vox Sang* 1975;**28**:152–5.

237 Broadberry RE, Lin M. The distribution of the MiIII (GP.Mur) phenotype among the population of Taiwan. *Transfus Med* 1996;**6**:145–8.

238 Joshi SR, Bharucha ZS, Sharma RS, Bhatia HM. The M^g blood group antigen in two Indian families. *Vox Sang* 1972;**22**:478–80.

239 Reid ME, Halverson GR. Characterization of monoclonal antibodies in section 2B using enzymes and variant red blood cells. *Transfus Clin Biol* 1997;**4**:65–8.

240 van der Hart M, van der Veer M, van Loghem JJ, Sanger R, Race RR. Vr, an antigen belonging to the MNSs blood group system. *Vox Sang* 1958;**3**:261–5.

241 Konugres AA, Fitzgerald H, Dresser R. Distribution and development of the blood factor Mt^a. *Vox Sang* 1965;**10**:206–7.

242 Field TE, Wilson TE, Dawes BJ, Giles CM. Haemolytic disease of the newborn due to anti-Mt^a. *Vox Sang* 1972;**22**:432–7.

243 Chandanayingyong D, Sasaki TT, Greenwalt TJ. Blood groups of the Thais. *Transfusion* 1967;**7**:269–76.

244 Metaxas-Buehler M, Metaxas MN, Sturgeon P. MNSs and Miltenberger frequencies in 211 Chinese. *Vox Sang* 1975;**29**:394–9.

245 Madden JH, Cleghorn TE, Allen FH, Rosenfield RE, Mackeprang M. A note on the relatively high frequency of St^a on the red blood cells of Orientals, and report of a third example of anti-St^a. *Vox Sang* 1964;**9**:502–4.

246 Cleghorn TE. Two human blood group antigens, St^a (Stones) and Ri^a (Ridley), closely related to the MNSs system. *Nature* 1962;**195**:297–8.

247 Contreras M, Armitage SE, Stebbing B. The MNSs antigen Ridley (Ri^a). *Vox Sang* 1984;**46**:360–5.

248 Wallace J, Izatt MM. The Cl^a (Caldwell) antigen: a new and rare human blood group antigen related to the MNSs system. *Nature* 1963;**200**:689–90.

249 Örjasaeter H, Kornstad L, Heier AM *et al.* A human blood group antigen, Ny^a (Nyberg), segregating with the Ns gene complex of the MNSs system. *Nature* 1964;**201**:832.

250 Örjasaeter H, Kornstad L, Heier A-M. Studies on the Ny^a blood group antigen and antibodies. *Vox Sang* 1964;**9**:673–83.

251 Kornstad L, Heier Larsen AM, Weisert O. Further observations on the frequency of the Ny^a blood-group antigen and its genetics. *Am J Hum Genet* 1971;**23**:612–13.

252 Schimmack L, Müller I, Kornstad L. A contribution to the Ny^a problem. *Hum Hered* 1971;**21**:346–50.

253 Pineda AA, Taswell HF. First example of Ny^a blood group antigen in American population. *Vox Sang* 1969;17:459–61.

254 Nakajima H, Ohkura K, Orjasaeter H, Kornstad L. The Ny^a blood group antigen among Japanese, Ryukyuan, and Chinese and the Mountainous Aborigines in Taiwan. *Jpn J Hum Genet* 1967;11:263–5.

255 Crossland JD, Pepper MD, Giles CM, Ikin EW. A British family possessing two variants of the MNSs blood group system, M^v and a new class within the Miltenberger complex. *Vox Sang* 1970;18:407–13.

256 Cregut R, Liberge G, Yvart J, Brocteur J, Salmon C. A new rare blood group antigen, 'FAR', probably linked to the MNSs system. *Vox Sang* 1974;26:194–8.

257 Speiser P, Kühböck Mickerts D et al. 'Kamhuber' a new human blood group antigen of familial occurrence, revealed by a severe transfusion reaction. *Vox Sang* 1966;11:113–15.

258 Shapiro M, Le Roux ME. Serology and genetics of a 'new' red cell antigen: s^D [Abstract]. *Transfusion* 1981;21:614.

259 Battista N, Stout TD, Lewis M, Kaita H. A new rare blood group antigen: 'Mit'. Probable genetic relationship with the MNSs blood group system. *Vox Sang* 1980;39:331–4.

260 Lubenko A, Savage JL, Gee SW, Cullen EM, Burslem SJ. Serology and genetics of the Mit antigen in North London blood donors [Abstract]. *Proc 20th Congr Int Soc Blood Transfus* 1988:116.

261 Unger P, Procter JL, Moulds JJ et al. The Dantu erythrocyte phenotype of the NE variety. II. Serology, immunochemistry, genetics, and frequency. *Blut* 1987; 55:33–43.

262 Contreras M, Green C, Humphreys J et al. Serology and genetics of an MNSs-associated antigen Dantu. *Vox Sang* 1984;46:377–86.

263 Webb AJ, Giles CM. Three antibodies of the MNSs system and their association with the Miltenberger complex of antigens. II. Raddon and Lane Sera. *Vox Sang* 1977; 32:274–6.

264 Baldwin ML, Barrasso C, Gavin J. The first example of a Raddon-like antibody as a cause of a transfusion reaction. *Transfusion* 1981;21:86–9.

265 Cleghorn TE. Cited in [18].

266 Tsuneyama H, Uchikawa M, Matsubara M et al. Molecular basis of Or in the MNS blood group system. *Vox Sang* 1998;74(Suppl.1):abstract 1446.

267 Skov F, Green C, Daniels G, Khalid G, Tippett P. Miltenberger class IX of the MNS blood group system. *Vox Sang* 1991;61:130–6.

268 Daniels GL, Green CA, Okubo Y et al. SAT, a 'new' low frequency blood group antigen, which may be associated with two different MNS variants. *Transfus Med* 1991;1:39–45.

269 Seno T, Yamaguchi H, Okubo Y et al. Os^a, a 'new' low-frequency red cell antigen. *Vox Sang* 1983;45:60–1.

270 Winter NM, Antonelli G, Walsh EA, Konugres AA. A second example of blood group antigen M^g in the American population. *Vox Sang* 1966;11:209–12.

271 Brocteur J. The M^{g}S gene complex of the MNSs blood group system, evidenced in a Sicilian family. *Hum Hered* 1969;19:77–85.

272 Dahr W, Metaxas-Bühler M, Metaxas MN, Gallasch E. Immunochemical properties of M^g erythrocytes. *J Immunogenet* 1981;8:79–87.

273 Giles CM. Serological activity of low frequency antigens of the MNSs system and reappraisal of the Miltenberger complex. *Vox Sang* 1982;42:256–61.

274 Springer GF, Stalder K. Action of influenza viruses, receptor-destroying enzyme and proteases on blood group agglutinogen M^g. *Nature* 1961;191:187–8.

275 Furthmayr H, Metaxas MN, Metaxas-Bühler M. M^g and M^c: mutations within the amino-terminal region of glycophorin A. *Proc Natl Acad Sci USA* 1981;78:631–5.

276 Dahr W, Beyreuther K, Gallasch E, Krüger J, Morel P. Amino acid sequence of the blood group M^g-specific major human erythrocyte membrane sialoglycoprotein. *Hoppe-Seyler Z Physiol Chem* 1981;362:81–5.

277 Blumenfeld OO, Adamany AM, Puglia KV. Amino acid and carbohydrate structural variants of glycoprotein products (M-N glycoproteins) of the *M-N* allelic locus. *Proc Natl Acad Sci USA* 1981;78:747–51.

278 Cartron JP, Ferrari B, Huet M, Pavia AA. Specificity of anti-M^g antibody: a study with synthetic peptides and glycopeptides. *Expl Clin Immunogenet* 1984;1: 112–16.

279 Dahr W, Weinberg R, Roelcke D, Bunke D, Beyreuther K. Studies of the specificity of anti-M^g [Abstract]. *Transfusion* 1992;32:54S.

280 Jaskiewicz E, Blanchard D, Rasamoelisolo M et al. Fine specificities of murine anti-M^g monoclonal antibodies. *Transfus Med* 1999;9:161–6.

281 Dahr W, Collins P, Shin C, Schanfield MS. Studies on the structure of a variant of the M^g blood group [Abstract]. *Transfusion* 1983;23:422.

282 Fraser RH, Inglis G, Mackie A et al. Mouse monoclonal antibodies reacting with M blood group-related antigens. *Transfusion* 1985;25:261–6.

283 Nichols ME, Rosenfield RE, Rubinstein P. Two blood group M epitopes disclosed by monoclonal antibodies. *Vox Sang* 1985;49:138–48.

284 Green C, Daniels G, Skov F, Tippett P. The M^g+ MNS blood group phenotype: further observations. *Vox Sang* 1994;66:237–41.

285 Jáskiewicz E, Czerwinski M, Syper D, Lisowska E. Anti-M monoclonal antibodies cross reacting with variant M^g antigen: an example of modulation of antigenic properties of peptide by its glycosylation. *Blood* 1994;84:2340–5.

286 Edelman L, Blanchard D, Rouger P et al. A monoclonal antibody directed against the homologous N-terminal

domain of glycophorin A and B. *Expl Clin Immunogenet* 1984;**1**:129–39.

287 Neppert J. Blood group antibody anti-M^g and isoagglutinin frequency in the Republic of Liberia, West Africa. *Transfusion* 1980;**20**:448–9.

288 Ikin EW. The production of anti-M^g in rabbits. *Vox Sang* 1966;**11**:217–18.

289 Dunsford I, Ikin EW, Mourant AE. A human blood group gene intermediate between M and N. *Nature* 1953;**172**:688–9.

290 Metaxas MN, Metaxas-Bühler M, Ikin EW. Complexities of the *MN* locus. *Vox Sang* 1968;**15**:102–17.

291 Dahr W, Kordowicz M, Beyreuther K, Krüger J. The amino acid sequence of the M^c-specific major red cell membrane sialoglycoprotein: an intermediate of the blood group M- and N-active molecules. *Hoppe Seyler Z Physiol Chem* 1981;**362**:363–6.

292 Bigbee WL, Langlois RG, Vanderlaan M, Jensen RH. Binding specificities of eight monoclonal antibodies to human glycophorin A: studies with M^{c}M, and M^{k}En(UK) variant human erythrocytes and M- and MN^v-type chimpanzee erythrocytes. *J Immunol* 1984;**133**:3149–54.

293 Ikin EW, Mourant AE. A rare blood group antigen occurring in Negroes. *Br Med J* 1951;**i**:456–7.

294 MacDonald KA, Nichols ME, Marsh WL, Jenkins WJ. The first example of anti-Henshaw in human-serum. *Vox Sang* 1967;**13**:346–8.

295 McDougall DCJ, Jenkins WJ. The first human example of anti-M^c. *Vox Sang* 1981;**40**:412–15.

296 Judd WJ, Rolih SD, Dahr W *et al.* Studies on the blood of an *MsHe/MS^u* proposita and her family: serological evidence that Henshaw-producing genes do not code for the 'N' antigen. *Transfusion* 1983;**23**:382–6.

297 Dahr W, Kordowicz M, Judd WJ *et al.* Structural analysis of the Ss sialoglycoprotein specific for Henshaw blood group from human erythrocyte membranes. *Eur J Biochem* 1984;**141**:51–5.

298 Huang CH, Lomas C, Daniels G, Blumenfeld OO. Glycophorin He(St^a) of the human red cell membrane is encoded by a complex hybrid gene resulting from two recombinational events. *Blood* 1994;**83**:3369–76.

299 Wiener AS, Rosenfield RE. M^e, a blood factor common to the antigenic properties of M and He. *J Immunol* 1961;**87**:376–8.

300 Levene C, Sela R, Lacser M *et al.* Further examples of human anti-M^e found in sera of Israeli donors. *Vox Sang* 1984;**46**:207–10.

301 Zelinski T, Coghlan G, Belcher E *et al.* Preliminary serological studies on 31 samples of monoclonal antibodies directed against red cell glycophorins. *Rev Franc Transfus Immuno-Hémat* 1988;**31**:273–9.

302 Tippett P, Reid ME, Poole J *et al.* The Miltenberger subsystem: is it obsolescent? *Transfus Med Rev* 1992; **6**:170–82.

303 Reid ME, Tippett P. Review of a terminology proposed

to supersede Miltenberger. *Immunohematology* 1993;**9**:91–5.

304 Giles CM, Chandanayingyong D, Webb AJ. Three antibodies of the MNSs system and their association with the Miltenberger complex of antigens. III. Anek, Raddon and Lane antisera in relation to each other and the Miltenberger complex. *Vox Sang* 1977;**32**:277–9.

305 Graydon JJ. A rare iso-hæmagglutinogen. *Med J Aust* 1946;**ii**:9–10.

306 Chandanayingyong D, Pejrachandra S. Separable anti-Hut which is specific for class II of the Miltenberger complex. *Vox Sang* 1975; **28**:149–51.

307 Dahr W. Miltenberger subsystem of the MNSs blood group system: review and outlook. *Vox Sang* 1992;**62**: 129–35.

308 Cleghorn TE. A memorandum on the Miltenberger blood groups. *Vox Sang* 1966;**11**:219–22.

309 Simmons RT, Albrey JA, McCulloch WJ. The duplication of the Gr (Graydon) blood group by Vw (Verweyst). *Vox Sang* 1959;**4**:132–7.

310 Levine P, Stock AH, Kuhmichel AB, Bronikovsky N. A new human blood factor of rare incidence in the general population. *Proc Soc Exp Biol* 1951;**77**:402–3.

311 Cleghorn TE. *The occurrence of certain rare blood group factors in Britain.* MD thesis, University of Sheffield, 1961.

312 Wallace J, Milne GR, Mohn J *et al.* Blood group antigens Mi^a and Vw and their relation to the MNSs system. *Nature* 1957;**179**:478.

313 Mohn JF, Lambert RM, Rosamilia HG *et al.* On the relationship of the blood group antigens Mi^a and Vw to the MNSs system. *Am J Hum Genet* 1958;**10**:276–86.

314 van der Hart M, Bosman H, van Loghem JJ. Two rare human blood group antigens. (Preliminarily designed as Vw and Rm). *Vox Sang* 1954;**4**:108–16.

315 Chandanayingyong D, Pejrachandra S, Poole J. Three antibodies of the MNSs system and their association with the Miltenberger complex of antigens. I. Anek serum. *Vox Sang* 1977;**32**:272–3.

316 Dybkjaer E, Poole J, Giles CM. A new Miltenberger class detected by a second example of Anek type serum. *Vox Sang* 1981;**41**:302–5.

317 Huang C-H, Kikuchi M, McCreary J, Blumenfeld OO. Gene conversion confined to a direct repeat of the acceptor splice site generates allelic diversity at human glycophorin (*GYP*) locus. *J Biol Chem* 1992;**267**:3336–42.

318 Reid ME, Moore BPL, Poole J *et al.* TSEN: a novel MNS-related blood group antigen. *Vox Sang* 1992; **63**:122–8.

319 Weatherall DJ, Clegg JB. Recent developments in the molecular genetics of human hemoglobin. *Cell* 1979; **16**:467–79.

320 Reid ME. Hybrid sialoglycoproteins, Gerbich, Webb and Cad blood group determinants. In: Vengelen-Tyler, V, Judd, WJ, eds. *Recent Advances in Blood Group Bio-*

chemistry. Arlington: American Association of Blood Banks, 1986:67–104.

321 Alberts B, Bray D, Lewis J, Raff M, Roberts K, Watson JD. *Molecular Biology of the Cell*, 3rd edn. New York: Garland, 1994.

322 Metaxas MN, Metaxas-Bühler M, Heiken A, Vamosi M, Ikin EW, Bull W. Further examples of Miltenberger cell class V, one of them inherited with a depressed M antigen. *Vox Sang* 1972;23:420–8.

323 Mawby WJ, Anstee DJ, Tanner MJA. Immunochemical evidence for hybrid sialoglycoproteins of human erythrocytes. *Nature* 1981;291:161–2.

324 King MJ, Poole J, Anstee DJ. An application of immunoblotting in the classification of the Miltenberger series of blood group antigens. *Transfusion* 1989; 29:106–12.

325 Huang C-H, Blumenfeld OO. Identification of recombination events resulting in three hybrid genes encoding human MiV, MiV(J.L.), and St^a glycophorins. *Blood* 1991;77:1813–20.

326 Merry AH, Hodson C, Thomson E, Mallinson G, Anstee DJ. The use of monoclonal antibodies to quantify the levels of sialoglycoproteins α and δ and variant sialoglycoproteins in human erythrocyte membranes. *Biochem J* 1986;233:93–8.

327 Johe KK, Smith AJ, Vengelen-Tyler V, Blumenfeld OO. Amino acid sequence of an α-δ-glycophorin hybrid: a structure reciprocal to St^a α-glycophorin hybrid. *J Biol Chem* 1989;264:17486–93.

328 Lin F, Lu Y-Q, Liu J-F. Three types of Miltenberger glycophorin found in families of Chinese minorities in a malaria hyperendemic area [Abstract]. *Blood* 1994;84(Suppl.1):544a.

329 Storry J, Lindsay G, Rolih S *et al*. Four examples of anti-TSEN and three of TSEN-positive erythrocytes. *Transfusion* 2000;79:175–9.

330 Morel PA, Vengelen-Tyler V, Williams EA *et al*. Another MNSs variant producing a hybrid MNSs sialoglycoprotein. *Rev Franc Transfus Immuno-Hémat* 1982;25: 597–610.

331 Huang C-H, Reid ME, Blumenfeld OO, Okubo Y, Daniels GL. Glycophorin SAT of the human erythrocyte membrane is specified by a hybrid gene reciprocal to glycophorin Dantu gene. *Blood* 1995;85:2222–7.

332 Uchikawa M, Tsuneyama H, Wang L *et al*. A novel amino acid sequence result in the expression of the MNS related private antigen, SAT [Abstract]. *Vox Sang* 1994;67(Suppl.2):116.

333 Hodson C, Lee D. A new MNSs S.G.P. (α-δ) hybrid of the En(UK) type [Abstract]. *2nd Mtg Br Blood Transfus Soc* 1984:G50.

334 Cornwall S, Wright J, Moore BPL. Studies on Mur (Murrell), a rare antigen associated with the MNSs ststem. *Vox Sang* 1968;14:295–8.

335 Poole J, King M-J, Mak KH *et al*. The Mi^{III} phenotype among Chinese donors in Hong Kong: immunochemi-

cal and serological studies. *Transfus Med* 1991;1: 169–75.

336 Chandanayingyong D, Pejrachandra S. Studies on anti-Mi^a and the Mi^{III} complex. *Vox Sang* 1975;29:311–15.

337 Storry JR, Poole J, Condon J, Reid ME. Identification of a novel hybrid glycophorin gene encoding GP.Hop. *Transfusion* 2000;40:560–5.

338 Hemming NJ, Reid ME. Evaulation of monoclonal anti-glycophorin B as an unusual anti-S. *Transfusion* 1994;34:333–6.

339 Green C, Poole J, Ford D, Glameyer T. A postulated glycophorin B-A-B hybrid demonstrating heterogeneity of anti-Hop and anti-Nob sera [Abstract]. *Transfus Med* 1992;2(Suppl.1):67.

340 Huang C-H, Puglia KV, Bigbee WL *et al*. A family study of multiple mutations of alpha and delta glycophorins (glycophorins A and B). *Hum Genet* 1988;81:26–30.

341 Wu AM, Duk M, Lin M, Broadberry RE, Lisowska E. Identification of variant glycophorins of human red cells by lectinoblotting: application to the Mi.III variant that is relatively frequent in the Taiwanese population. *Transfusion* 1995;35:571–6.

342 Laird-Fryer B, Moulds JJ, Dahr W, Min YO, Chandanayingyong D. Anti-En^{a}FS detected in the serum of an Mi^{VII} homozygote. *Transfusion* 1986;26:51–6.

343 Huang C-H, Blumenfeld OO. Characterization of a genomic hybrid specifying the human erythrocyte antigen Dantu: Dantu gene is duplicated and linked to a δ glycophorin gene deletion. *Proc Natl Acad Sci USA* 1988;85:9640–4.

344 Huang C-H, Blumenfeld OO. Molecular genetics of human erythrocyte Mi^{III} and Mi^{VI} glycophorins: use of a pseudoexon in construction of two δ-α-δ hybrid genes resulting in antigenic diversification. *J Biol Chem* 1991;266:7248–55.

345 Johe KK, Smith AJ, Blumenfeld OO. Amino acid sequence of Mi^{III} glycophorin: demonstration of δ-α and α-δ junction regions and expression of δ pseudoexon by direct protein sequencing. *J Biol Chem* 1991;266:7256.

346 Mak KH, Banks JA, Lubenko A *et al*. A survey of the incidence of Miltenberger antibodies among Hong Kong Chinese blood donors. *Transfusion* 1994;34:238–41.

347 Broadberry RE, Lin M. The incidence and significance of anti-'Mi^a' in Taiwan. *Transfusion* 1994;34:349–52.

348 Lin M, Broadberry RE. An intravascular transfusion reaction due to anti-'Mi^a' in Taiwan. *Vox Sang* 1994;67:320.

349 Lin CK, Mak KH, Cheng G *et al*. Serologic characteristics and clinical significance of Miltenberger antibodies among Chinese patients in Hong Kong. *Vox Sang* 1998;74:59–60.

350 Lin CK, Mak KH, Yuen CMY *et al*. A case of hydrops fetalis, probably due to antibodies directed against antigenic determinants of GP.Mur (Miltenberger class III) cells. *Immunohematology* 1996;12:115–18.

351 Shih MC, Yang LH, Wang NM, Chang JG. Genomic

typing of human red cell Miltenberger glycophorins in a Taiwanese population. *Transfusion* 2000;**40**:54–61.

352 Uchikawa M, Suzuki Y, Onodera Y *et al.* Monoclonal anti-Miª and anti-Mur. *Vox Sang* 2000;**78**(Suppl.1):Abstract P021.

353 Huang C-H, Blumenfeld OO, Reid ME *et al.* Alternative splicing of a novel glycophorin allele GPHe(GL) generates two protein isoforms in the human erythrocyte membrane. *Blood* 1997;**90**:391–7.

354 Huang C-H, Skov F, Daniels G, Tippett P, Blumenfeld OO. Molecular analysis of human glycophorin MiIX gene shows a silent segment transfer and untemplated mutation resulting from gene conversion via sequence repeats. *J Biol Chem* 1992;**80**:2379–87.

355 Darnborough J. Further observations on the Verweyst blood group antigen and antibodies. *Vox Sang* 1957;**2**: 362–7.

356 Kornstad L, Orjasæter H, Heier Larsen AM. The blood group antigen Vw and anti-Vw antibodies: some observations in the Norwegian population. *Acta Genet* 1966;**16**:355–61.

357 Spruell P, Moulds JJ, Martin M *et al.* An anti-EnªTS detected in the serum of an *Mi^I* homozygote. *Transfusion* 1993;**33**:848–51.

358 Lewis M, Kaita H, Uchida I. Segregation of *Miª* with *Ms.* *Vox Sang* 1963;**8**:245.

359 Mohn JF, Lambert RM, Iseki S, Masaki S, Furukawa K. The blood group antigen Miª in Japanese. *Vox Sang* 1963;**8**:430–7.

360 Blanchard D, Asseraf A, Prigent M-J, Cartron J-P. Miltenberger class I and II erythrocytes carry a variant of glycophorin A. *Biochem J* 1983;**213**:399–404.

361 Dahr W, Newman RA, Contreras M *et al.* Structure of Miltenberger class I and II specific major human erythrocyte membrane sialoglycoproteins. *Eur J Biochem* 1984;**138**:259–65.

362 Rearden A, Frandson S, Carry JB. Severe hemolytic disease of the newborn due to anti-Vw and detection of glycophorin A antigens on the Miltenberger I sialoglycoprotein by western blotting. *Vox Sang* 1987; **52**:318–21.

363 Huang C-H, Spruell P, Moulds JJ, Blumenfeld OO. Molecular basis for the human erythrocyte glycophorin specifying the Miltenberger class I (MiI) phenotype. *Blood* 1992;**80**:257–63.

364 Herron R, Smith GA. Identification by immunoblotting of the erythrocyte membrane sialoglycoproteins that carry the Vw and Mur antigens. *Vox Sang* 1991; **60**:118–22.

365 Alcalay D, Tanzer J. Maladie hémolytique du nouveau-né par anticorps anti-Miltenberger. *Rev Franc Transfus Immuno-Hémat* 1977;**20**:623–5.

366 Taylor AM, Knighton GJ. A case of severe hemolytic disease of the newborn due to anti-Verweyst (Vw). *Transfusion* 1982;**22**:165–6.

367 Gorlin JB, Beaton M, Poortenga M, Davidson S,

368 Molthan L. Intravascular hemolytic transfusion reaction due to anti-Vw+Miª with fatal outcome. *Vox Sang* 1981;**40**:105–8.

369 Avoy DR. Letter. *Vox Sang* 1982;**42**:54–5.

370 Smith L, Hsi R, McQuiston D, Goldfinger D. IgG subclassing of antibodies reactive with the MiI (Miltenberger) class of red blood cells [Abstract]. *Transfusion* 1985;**25**:447.

371 Vengelen-Tyler V, Goya K, Green CA, Poole J. The second example of Mi: VIII phenotype [Abstract]. *Transfusion* 1985;**25**:464.

372 Dahr W, Beyreuther K, Moulds JJ. Structural analysis of the major human erythrocyte membrane sialoglycoprotein from Miltenberger class VII cells. *Eur J Biochem* 1987;**166**:27–30.

373 Dahr W, Beyreuther K, Dybkjaer E, Moulds J, Vengelen-Tyler V. Biochemical characterization of class VII and VIII cells within the Miltenberger system. In: WR Mayr, ed. *Advances in Forensic Haemogenetics*, Vol. 2. Berlin: Springer-Verlag, 1988:22–5.

374 Dahr W, Vengelen-Tyler V, Dybkjaer E, Beyreuther K. Structural analysis of glycophorin A from Miltenberger class VIII erythrocytes. *Biol Chem Hoppe-Seyler* 1989;**370**:855–9.

375 Johe KK, Vengelen-Tyler V, Leger R, Blumenfeld OO. Synthetic peptides homologous to human glycophorins of the Miltenberger complex of variants of MNSs blood group system specify the epitopes for Hil, S^{JL}, Hop, and Mur antisera. *Blood* 1991;**78**:2456–61.

376 Pisacka M, Poole J, Rodrigues M, King M-J. Serological basis of a new variant glycophorin [Abstract]. *24th Congr Int Soc Blood Transfus* 1996:147.

377 Poole J, Bruce LJ, Tanner MJA, Pisacka M. Novel molecular basis for the Hil (MNS20) antigen [Abstract]. *Transfusion* 1998;**38**:103S.

378 Reid ME, Poole J, Green C, Neill G, Banks J. MINY: a novel MNS-related blood group antigen. *Vox Sang* 1992;**63**:129–32.

379 Ellisor SS, Zelski D, Sugasawara E, Dean WD, Bradburn S. A second example of anti-Hil. *Transfusion* 1982; **22**:402.

380 Moulds M, Moulds J, Halverson GR, Reid ME, Chen V. The first example of monoclonal anti-Miª [Abstract]. *Transfusion* 1999;**39**:42S.

381 Tanner MJA, Anstee DJ, Mawby WJ. A new human erythrocyte variant (Ph) containing an abnormal membrane sialoglycoprotein. *Biochem J* 1980;**187**: 493–500.

382 Unger P, Orlina A, Dahr W *et al.* Two new gene complexes in the MNSs blood group system [Abstract]. *Forensic Sci Int* 1981;**18**:258.

383 Dahr W, Moulds J, Unger P, Blanchard D, Cartron JP. Serological and biochemical investigations on the

N.E. variety of the Dantu red cell phenotype. In: B Brinkmann, K Henningsen, eds. *Advances in Forensic Haemogenetics* 1. Berlin: Springer-Verlag, 1986:3–7.

384 Dahr W, Pilkington PM, Reinke H, Blanchard D, Beyreuther K. A novel variety of the Dantu gene complex (*Dantu^{MD}*) detected in a Caucasian. *Blut* 1989;58:247–53.

385 Dahr W, Beyreuther K, Moulds J, Unger P. Hybrid glycophorins from human erythrocyte membranes. I. Isolation and complete structural analysis of the hybrid sialoglycoprotein from Dantu-positive red cells of the N.E. variety. *Eur J Biochem* 1987;166:31–6.

386 Blumenfeld OO, Smith AJ, Moulds JJ. Membrane glycophorins of Dantu blood group erythrocytes. *J Biol Chem* 1987;262:11864–70.

387 Dahr W, Moulds J, Unger P, Kordowicz M. The Dantu erythrocyte phenotype of the NE variety. I. Dodecylsulfate polyacrylamide gel electophoretic studies. *Blut* 1987;55:19–31.

388 Ridgwell K, Tanner MJA, Anstee DJ. The Wr^b antigen in St^a-positive and Dantu-positive human erythrocytes. *J Immunogenet* 1984;11:365–70.

389 Vengelen-Tyler V, Mogck N. A new test useful in identifying red cells with a (δ-α) hybrid sialoglycoprotein. *Transfusion* 1986;26:231–3.

390 Moores P, Smart E, Marais I. The Dantu phenotype in southern Africa [Abstract]. *Transfus Med* 1992; 2(Suppl.1):68.

391 Broadberry RE, Chang FC, Jan YS, Lin M. The distribution of the red-cell St^a (Stones) antigen among the population of Taiwan. *Transfus Med* 1998;8:57–8.

392 Blumenfeld OO, Adamany AM, Kikuchi M, Sabo B, McCreary J. Membrane glycophorins in St^a blood group erythrocytes. *J Biol Chem* 1986;261:5544–52.

393 Anstee DJ, Mawby WJ, Parsons SF, Tanner MJA, Giles CM. A novel hybrid sialoglycoprotein in St^a positive human erythrocytes. *J Immunogenet* 1982;9:51–5.

394 Blanchard D, Cartron J-P, Rouger P, Salmon C. Pj variant, a new hybrid MNSs glycoprotein of the human red-cell membrane. *Biochem J* 1982;203:419–26.

395 Blanchard D, Dahr W, Beyreuther K, Moulds J, Cartron J-P. Hybrid glophorins from human erythrocyte membranes: isolation and complete structural analysis of the novel sialoglycoprotein from St(a+) red cells. *Eur J Biochem* 1987;167:361–6.

396 Daniels GL, Green CA, Poole J et al. ERIK, a low frequency red cell antigen of the MNS blood group system associated with St^a. *Transfus Med* 1993;3:129–35.

397 Rearden A. Hybrid sialoglycoprotein content of St(a+) red cells. *Transfusion* 1988;28:119–22.

398 Huang C-H, Guizzo ML, Kikuchi M, Blumenfeld OO. Molecular genetic analysis of a hybrid gene encoding St^a glycophorin of the human erythrocyte membrane. *Blood* 1989;74:836–43.

399 Rearden A, Phan H, Dubnicoff T, Kudo S, Fukuda M. Identification of the crossing-over point of a hybrid gene

encoding human glycophorin variant St^a. *J Biol Chem* 1990;265:9259–63.

400 Huang C-H, Blumenfeld OO. Multiple origins of the human glycophorin St^a gene: identification of hot spots for independent unequal homologous recombinations. *J Biol Chem* 1991;266:23306–14.

401 Dahr W, Blanchard D, Chevalier C et al. The M^z variety of the St(a+) phenotype: a variant of glycophorin A exhibiting a deletion. *Biol Chem Hoppe-Seyler* 1990;371:403–10.

402 Huang C-H, Reid ME, Blumenfeld OO. Exon skipping caused by DNA recombination that introduces a defective donor splice site into the human glycophorin A gene. *J Biol Chem* 1993;268:4945–52.

403 Huang C-H, Reid M, Daniels G, Blumenfeld OO. Alteration of splice site selection by an exon mutation in the human glycophorin A gene. *J Biol Chem* 1993;268:25902–8.

404 Huang C-H, Chen Y, Blumenfeld OO. A novel St^a glycophorin produced via gene conversion of pseudoexon III from glycophorin E to glycophorin A gene. *Hum Mutat* 2000;15:533–40.

405 Poole J, Banks J, Bruce LJ et al. Glycophorin A mutation Ala65→Pro gives rise to a novel pair of MNS alleles ENEP (MNS39) and HAG (MNS41) and altered Wr^b expression: direct evidence for GPA/band 3 interaction necessary for normal Wr^b expression. *Transfus Med* 1999;9:167–74.

406 Moulds JJ, Moulds MK, Lacey B et al. Two antigens showing a relation to the MNS and Wright blood groups [Abstract]. *Transfusion* 1992;32:55S.

407 Jarolim P, Moulds JM, Moulds JJ, Rubin HL, Dahr W. MARS and AVIS blood group antigens: polymorphism of glycophorin A affects band 3–glycophorin A interaction [Abstract]. *Blood* 1996;88(Suppl.1):182A.

408 Moulds JM, Reveille JD, Arnett FC et al. MARS: a glycophorin A determinant unique to the Choctaw Indians [Abstract]. *Transfusion* 1997;37:32S.

409 Poole J, Banks J, Hemming N, Sheffield E. The rare MNS-related antigen Vr: a family study [Abstract]. *Transfus Med* 1993;3(Suppl.1):98.

410 Storry JR, Coghlan G, Poole J, Figueroa D, Reid ME. The MNS blood group antigens, Vr (MNS12) and Mt^a (MNS14), each arise from an amino acid substitution on glycophorin A. *Vox Sang* 2000;78:52–6.

411 Swanson J, Matson GA. Mt^a, a 'new' antigen in the MNSs system. *Vox Sang* 1962;7:585–90.

412 Storry JR, Reid ME. A point mutation in *GYPA* exon 3 encodes the low incidence antigen, MNS16. *Vox Sang* 2000;78(Suppl.1):Abstract P025.

413 Daniels GL, Bruce LJ, Mawby WJ et al. The low frequency MNS blood group antigens Ny^a (MNS18) and Os^a (MNS38) are associated with GPA amino acid substitutions. *Transfusion* 2000;40:555–9.

414 Gershowitz H, Fried K. Anti-M^v, a new antibody of the MNSs blood group system. I. M^v, a new inherited vari-

ant of the *M* gene. *Am J Hum Genet* 1966;18:264–81.

415 Beck ML, Hardman JT. Anti-s reagents. *Transfusion* 1980;20:479.

416 Walsh TJ, Giles CM, Poole J. Anti-M^v causing haemolytic disease of the newborn and serological considerations of the M^v red cell determinant. *Clin Lab Haematol* 1981;3:137–42.

417 Dahr W, Longster G. Studies of M^v red cells. II. Immunochemical investigations. *Blut* 1984;49:299–306.

418 Storry JR, Reid ME, MacLennan S, Lubenko A, Nortman P. The low incidence MNS antigens, M^v, s^D, and Mit arise from single amino acid substitutions on GPB. *Transfusion* 2001;41:269–75.

419 Cregut R, Lewin D, Lacomme M, Michot O. Un cas d'anasarque fœto-placentaire par iso-immunisation contre un antigène 'privé'. *Rev Franc Transfus* 1968;11:139–43.

420 Giles CM. The identity of Kamhuber and Far antigens. *Vox Sang* 1977;32:269–71.

421 Skradski KJ, McCreary J, Zweber M, Sabo B. Further investigation of the effect of Mitchell (Mit) antigen on S antigen expression [Abstract]. *Transfusion* 1983;23:409.

422 Bacon JM, Macdonald EB, Young SG, Connell T. Evidence that the low frequency antigen Orriss is part of the MN blood group system. *Vox Sang* 1987;52:330–4.

423 Reid ME, Sausais L, Øyen R *et al.* First example of hemolytic disease of the newborn caused by anti-Or and confirmation of the molecular basis of Or. *Vox Sang* 2000;79:180–2.

424 Wright J, Lim FC, Freeman J, Giles CM. An unusual antibody related to the MN blood group system. *Transfusion* 1983;23:120–3.

425 Moltham L. The second example of anti-M$_1$ antibodies produced by a group MN person. *Vox Sang* 1980;38:210–12.

426 Judd WJ, Issitt PD, Pavone BG. The Can serum: demonstrating further polymorphism of M and N blood group antigens. *Transfusion* 1979;19:7–11.

427 Landsteiner K, Strutton WR, Chase MW. An agglutination reaction observed with some human bloods, chiefly among Negroes. *J Immunol* 1934;27:469–72.

428 Rosenfield RE, Haber GV, Schroeder R, Ballard R, Driscoll J. A Negro family revealing Hunter–Henshaw information, and independence of the genes for Js and Lewis. *Am J Hum Genet* 1960;12:143–6.

429 Jack JA, Tippett P, Noades J, Sanger R, Race RR. M$_1$, a subdivision of the human blood-group antigen M. *Nature* 1960;186:642.

430 Giles CM, Howell P. An antibody in the serum of an MN patient which reacts with M$_1$ antigen. *Vox Sang* 1974;27:43–51.

431 Issitt PD, Haber JM, Allen FH. Anti-Tm, an antibody defining a new antigenic determinant within the MN blood-group system. *Vox Sang* 1965;10:742–3.

432 Dahr W, Knuppertz G, Beyreuther K *et al.* Studies on structures of the Tm, Sj, M$_1$, Can, Sext and Hu blood group antigens. *Biol Chem Hoppe-Seyler* 1991;372:573–84.

433 Issitt PD, Wilkinson SL. Anti-Tm is anti-N polypeptide. *Transfusion* 1981;21:493–7.

434 Adamany AM, Blumenfeld OO, Sabo B, McCreary J. A carbohydrate structural variant of MM glycoprotein (glycophorin A). *J Biol Chem* 1983;258:11537–45.

435 Issitt PD, Wren MR, Moore RE, Roy RB. The M$_1$ and Tm antigens require M and N gene-specified amino acids for expression. *Transfusion* 1986;26:413–18.

436 Richmond RS, Innella F. Anomalous expression of the M$_1$ antigen of the MN system in an American Negro family. *Vox Sang* 1968;15:463–6.

437 Daniels G. *Human Blood Groups.* Oxford: Blackwell Science, 1995.

438 Jakobowicz R, Bryce LM, Simmons RT. Occurrence of unusual positive Coombs reactions and M factors in the blood of a mother and her first baby. *Nature* 1950;165:158–9.

439 Jensen KG, Freiesleben E. Inherited positive Coombs' reaction connected with a weak N-receptor (N$_2$). *Vox Sang* 1962;7:696–703.

440 Jeannet M, Metaxas-Bühler M, Tobler R. Anomalie héréditaire de la membrane érythrocytaire avec test de Coombs direct positif et modification de l'antigène de groupe N. *Vox Sang* 1964;9:52–5.

441 Wolff E, Jonsson B. Studien uber die Untergruppen A$_1$ und A$_2$ mit besonderer Berucksichtigung der Paternitätsuntersuchungen. *Dtsch Ztschr Gerichtl Med* 1933;22:65–85.

442 Perrault R. Naturally-occurring anti-M and anti-N with special case: IgG anti-N in a NN donor. *Vox Sang* 1973;24:134–49.

443 Mollison PL, Engelfriet CP, Contreras M. *Blood Transfusion in Clinical Medicine*, 10th edn. Oxford: Blackwell Science, 1997.

444 Freiesleben E, Knudsen EE. A human incomplete immune anti-M. In: *P.H. Andresen, Papers in Dedication of His Sixtieth Birthday.* Copenhagen: Munksgaard, 1957: 26–31.

445 Branch DR, McBroom R, Jones GL. Discrepant *in vitro* versus *in vivo* interaction of M-positive donor red cells with IgG1 anti-M. *Rev Franc Transfus Immuno-Hémat* 1983;26:565–72.

446 Kao YS, Frank S, de Jongh DS. Anti-M in children with acute bacterial infections. *Transfusion* 1978;18:320–2.

447 Strahl M, Pettenkofer HJ, Hasse W. A haemolytic transfusion reaction due to anti-M. *Vox Sang* (old series) 1955;5:34–37.

448 Reid ME, Lomas-Francis C. *The Blood Group Antigen Facts Book.* San Diego: Academic Press, 1997.

449 Smith ML, Beck ML. The immunoglobulin structure of human anti-M agglutinins. *Transfusion* 1979;19:472–4.

450 Freedman J, Massey A, Chaplin H, Monroe MC. Assessment of complement binding by anti-D and anti-M antibodies employing labelled antiglobulin antibodies. *Br J Haematol* 1980;45:309–18.

451 Beattie KM, Zuelzer WW. The frequency and properties of pH-dependent anti-M. *Transfusion* 1965;5:322–6.

452 Schmidt AP, Taswell HF. Coexistence of MN erythrocytes and apparent anti-M antibody. *Transfusion* 1969;9:203–4.

453 Howard PL, Picoff RC. Another example of anti-M in an M-positive patient. *Transfusion* 1972;12:59–61.

454 Lawe JE, LaRoche LL. Study of a family with a variant M antigen. *Vox Sang* 1983;44:92–7.

455 Hirsch W, Moores P, Sanger R, Race RR. Notes on some reactions of human anti-M and anti-N sera. *Br J Haematol* 1957;3:134–42.

456 Allen FH, Corcoran PA, Ellis FR. Some new observations on the MN system. *Vox Sang* 1960;5:224–31.

457 Telischi M, Behzad O, Issitt PD, Pavone BG. Hemolytic disease of the newborn due to anti-N. *Vox Sang* 1976;31:109–16.

458 Ballas SK, Dignam C, Harris M, Marcolina MJ. A clinically significant anti-N in a patient whose red cells were negative for N and U antigens. *Transfusion* 1985;25:377–80.

459 Yoshida Y, Yoshida H, Tatsumi K et al. Successful antibody elimination in severe M-incompatible pregnancy. *N Engl J Med* 1981;305:460–1.

460 Reid ME, Ellisor SS, Barker JM. A human alloanti-N enhanced by acid media. *Transfusion* 1984;24:222–3.

461 Metaxas-Bühler M, Ikin EW, Romanski J. Anti-N in the serum of a healthy blood donor of group MN. *Vox Sang* 1961;6:574–82.

462 Greenwalt TJ, Sasaki T, Steane EA. Second example of anti-N in a blood donor of group MN. *Vox Sang* 1966;11:184–8.

463 Moores P, Botha MC, Brink S. Anti-N in the serum of a healthy type MN person: a further example. *Am J Clin Pathol* 1970;54:90–3.

464 Lahmann N. Ein weiterer Fall von anti-N im Serum einer Person der Blutgruppe MN. *Haematologia* 1970;4:79–84.

465 Booth PB, Anti N^A. An antibody sub-dividing Melanesian N. *Vox Sang* 1971;21:522–30.

466 Wiener AS. Réaction transfusionnelle hémolytique due a une sensibilisation anti-M. *Rev Hémat* 1950;5:3–6.

467 Furlong MB, Monaghan WP. Delayed hemolytic episodes due to anti-M. *Transfusion* 1981;21:45–9.

468 Alperin JH, Riglin H, Branch DR, Gallagher MT, Petz LD. Anti-M causing delayed hemolytic transfusion reaction. *Transfusion* 1983;23:322–4.

469 Sancho JM, Pujol M, Fernández F et al. Delayed haemolytic transfusion reaction due to anti-M antibody. *Br J Haematol* 1998;103:268–9.

470 Stone B, Marsh WL. Haemolytic disease of the newborn caused by anti-M. *Br J Haematol* 1959;5:344–7.

471 Macpherson CR, Zartman ER. Anti-M antibody as a cause of intrauterine death: a follow-up. *Am J Clin Pathol* 1965;43:544–7.

472 Duguid JKM, Bromilow IM, Entwistle GD, Wilkinson R. Haemolytic disease of the newborn due to anti-M. *Vox Sang* 1995;68:195–6.

473 Furukawa K, Nakajima T, Kogure T et al. Example of a woman with multiple intrauterine deaths due to anti-M who delivered a live child after plasmapheresis. *Exp Clin Immunogenet* 1993;10:161–7.

474 Kanra T, Yüce K, Özcebe OI. Hydrops fetalis and intrauterine deaths due to anti-M. *Acta Obstet Gynecol Scand* 1996;75:415–17.

475 Nolan B, Hinchliffe R, Vora A. Neonatal pure red cell aplasia due to maternal anti-M [Abstract]. *Blood* 2000;96:8A.

476 Sacher RA, Abbondanzo SL, Miller DK, Womack B. Auto anti-M: clinical and serological findings of seven patients from one hospital and review of the literature. *Am J Clin Pathol* 1989;91:305–9.

477 Sangster JM, Kenwright MG, Walker MP, Pembroke AC. Anti blood group-M autoantibodies with livedo reticularis, Raynaud's phenomenon, and anaemia. *J Clin Pathol* 1979;32:154–7.

478 Chapman J, Murphy MF, Waters AH. Chronic cold haemagglutinin disease due to an anti-M-like autoantibody. *Vox Sang* 1982;42:272–7.

479 Roelcke D, Dahr W, Kalden JR. A human monoclonal IgMκ cold agglutinin recognizing oligosaccharides with immunodominant sialyl groups preferentially at the blood group M-specific peptide backbone of glycophorins: anti-Pr^M. *Vox Sang* 1986;51:207–11.

480 Garratty G, Arndt P, Tsuneta R, Kanter M. Fatal hemolytic anemia associated with autoanti-N. *Transfusion* 1994;34:20S.

481 Howell ED, Perkins HA. Anti-N-like antibodies in the sera of patients undergoing chronic hemodialysis. *Vox Sang* 1972;23:291–9.

482 McLeish WA, Brathwaite AF, Peterson PM. Anti-N antibodies in hemodialysis patients. *Transfusion* 1975;15:43–5.

483 Boettcher B, Nanra RS, Roberts TK, Mallan M, Watterson CA. Specificity and possible origin of anti-N antibodies developed by patients undergoing chronic haemodialysis. *Vox Sang* 1976;31:408–15.

484 Crosson JT, Moulds J, Comty CM, Polesky HF. A clinical study of anti-N$_{DP}$ in the sera of patients in a large repetitive hemodialysis program. *Kidney Int* 1976;10:463–70.

485 Bird GWG, Wingham J. Anti-N antibodies in renaldialysis patients. *Lancet* 1977;i:1218.

486 White WL, Miller GE, Kaehny WD. Formaldehyde in the pathogenesis of hemodialysis-related anti-N antibodies. *Transfusion* 1977;17:443–7.

487 Fassbinder W, Seidl S, Koch KM. The role of formalde-hyde in the formation of haemodialysis-associated anti-N-like antibodies. *Vox Sang* 1978;**35**:41–8.

488 Sandler SG, Sharon R, Bush M, Stroup M, Sabo B. Formaldehyde-related antibodies in hemodialysis patients. *Transfusion* 1979;**19**:682–7.

489 Lynen R, Rothe M, Gallasch E. Characterization of formaldehyde-related antibodies encountered in hemodialysis patients at different stages of immunization. *Vox Sang* 1983;**44**:81–9.

490 Dzik WH, Darling CA. Positive direct antiglobulin test result in dialysis patients resulting from antiformalde-hyde antibodies. *Am J Clin Pathol* 1989;**92**:214–17.

491 Ng Y-Y, Chow M-P, Wu S-C *et al.* Anti-N_{form} antibody in hemodialysis patients. *Am J Nephrol* 1995;**15**:374–8.

492 Dahr W, Moulds J. An immunochemical study on anti-N antibodies from dialysis patients. *Immunol Commun* 1981;**10**:173–83.

493 Czerwinski M, Siegel DL, Moore JS, Spitalnik PF, Spitalnik SL. Construction of bacteriophage expressing mouse monoclonal Fab fragments directed against the human MN glycophorin blood group antigens. *Transfusion* 1995;**35**:137–44.

494 Morel PA, Bergren MO, Hill V, Garratty G, Perkins HA. M and N specific hemagglutinins of human erythrocytes stored in glucose solutions. *Transfusion* 1981;**21**:652–62.

495 Reid ME, Ellisor SS, Barker JM, Lewis T, Avoy DR. Characteristics of an antibody causing agglutination of M-positive non-enzymatically glycosylated human red cells. *Vox Sang* 1981;**41**:85–90.

496 Drzeniek Z, Kusnierz G, Lisowska E. A human antiserum reacting with modified blood group M determinants. *Immunol Commun* 1981;**10**:185–97.

497 Fraser RH, Munro AC, Williamson AR *et al.* Mouse monoclonal anti-N. I. Production and serological characterization. *J Immunogenet* 1982;**9**:295–301.

498 Fraser RH, Munro AC, Williamson AR *et al.* Mouse monoclonal anti-N. II. Physicochemical characterization and assessment for routine blood grouping. *J Immunogenet* 1982;**9**:303–9.

499 Rubocki R, Milgrom F. Reactions of murine monoclonal antibodies to blood group MN antigens. *Vox Sang* 1986;**51**:217–25.

500 Fraser RH, Inglis G, Mitchell R. pH effect on anti-M and anti-N reactivity. *Transfusion* 1986;**26**:118.

501 Lisowska E, Messeter L, Duk M, Czerwinski M, Lundblad A. A monoclonal anti-glycophorin A antibody recognizing the blood group M determinant: studies on the subspecificity. *Mol Immunol* 1987;**24**:605–13.

502 Lisowska E. MN monoclonal antibodies as blood group reagents. In: P Rouger, C Salmon, eds. *Monoclonal Antibodies Against Human Red Blood Cell and Related Antigens.* Paris: Arnette, 1987: 181–91.

503 Jaskiewicz E, Moulds JJ, Kraemer K, Goldstein AS, Lisowska E. Charaterization of the epitope recognized by a monoclonal antibody highly specific for blood group M antigen. *Transfusion* 1990;**30**:230–5.

504 Wasniowska K, Duk M, Steuden I *et al.* Two monoclonal antibodies recognizing different epitopes of blood group N antigen. *Arch Immunol Ther Exp* 1988;**36**:623–32.

505 Blackall DP, Ugorski M, Smith ME, Påhlsson P, Spitalnik SL. The binding of human alloantibodies to recombinant glycophorin A. *Transfusion* 1992;**32**:629–32.

506 Blackall DP, Ugorski M, Påhlsson P, Shakin-Eshleman SH, Spitalnik SL. A molecular biologic approach to study the fine specificity of antibodies directed to the MN human blood group antigens. *J Immunol* 1994;**152**:2241–7.

507 Czerwinski M, Blackall DP, Abrams WR, Rubocki RJ, Spitalnik SL. Restricted V_H gene usage by murine hybridomas directed against human N, but not M, blood group antigen. *Mol Immunol* 1994;**31**:279–88.

508 Czerwinski M, Krop-Watorek A, Siegel DL, Spitalnik SL. A molecular approach for isolating high-affinity Fab fragments that are useful in blood group serology. *Transfusion* 1999;**39**:364–71.

509 Allen NK, Brilliantine L. A survey of hemagglutinins in various seeds. *J Immunol* 1969;**102**:1295–9.

510 Bird GWG. Lectins in immunohematology. *Transfus Med Rev* 1989;**3**:55–62.

511 Ottensooser F, Silberschmidt K. Haemagglutinin anti-N in plant seeds. *Nature* 1953;**172**:914.

512 Duk M, Lisowska E. *Vicia graminea* anti-N lectin: partial characterization of the purified lectin and its binding to erythrocytes. *Eur J Biochem* 1981;**118**:131–6.

513 Prigent MJ, Blanchard D, Cartron J-P. Membrane receptors for *Vicia graminea* anti-N lectin and its binding to native and neuraminidase-treated human erythrocytes. *Arch Biochem Biophys* 1983;**222**:231–44.

514 Duk M, Lisowska E, Kordowicz M, Wasniowska K. Studies on the specificity of the binding site of *Vicia graminea* anti-N lectin. *Eur J Biochem* 1982;**123**:105–12.

515 Rolih SD, Issitt PD. Effects of trypsin on the *Vicia graminea* receptors of glycophorin A and B [Abstract]. *Transfusion* 1978;**18**:637.

516 Lisowska E. The degradation of M and N blood group glycoproteins and glycopeptides with alkaline borohydride. *Eur J Biochem* 1969;**10**:574–9.

517 Prigent MJ. Erythrocyte receptors for *Vicia graminea* anti-N lectin. In: J-P Cartron, P Rouger, C Salmon, eds. *Red Cell Membrane Glycoconjugates and Related Genetic Markers.* Paris: Arnette, 1983:43–50.

518 Dahr W, Uhlenbruck G. Structural properties of the human MN blood group antigen receptor sites. *Hoppe Seyler Z Physiol Chem* 1978;**359**:835–43.

519 Boyd WC, Everhart DL, McMaster MH. The anti-N lectin of *Bauhinia purpurea.* *J Immunol* 1958;**81**:414–18.

520 Fletcher G. The anti-N phytagglutinin of *Bauhinia variegata*. *Aust J Sci* 1959;**22**:167.

521 Moon GJ, Wiener AS. A new source of anti-N lectin: leaves of the Korean *Vicia unijuga*. *Vox Sang* 1974;**26**:167–70.

522 Bird GWG, Wingham J. Agglutinins for antigens of two different human blood group systems in the seeds of *Moluccella laevis*. *Vox Sang* 1970;**18**:235–9.

523 Judd WJ, Murphy LA, Goldstein IJ, Campbell L, Nichols ME. An anti-B reagent prepared from the α-D-galactopyranosyl-binding isolectins from *Bandeiraea simplicifolia* seeds. *Transfusion* 1978;**18**:274–80.

524 Dahr W, Uhlenbruck G, Bird GWG. Further characterization of some heterophile agglutinins reacting with alkali-labile carbohydrate chains of human erythrocyte glycoproteins. *Vox Sang* 1975;**28**:133–48.

525 Coombs HI, Ikin EW, Mourant AE, Plaut G. Agglutinin anti-S in human serum. *Br Med J* 1951;**i**:109–11.

526 Levine P, Ferraro LR, Koch E. Hemolytic disease of the newborn due to anti-S: a case report with a review of 12 anti-S sera cited in the literature. *Blood* 1952;**7**:1030–7.

527 Constantoulis NC, Paidoussis M, Dunsford I. A naturally occurring anti-S agglutinin. *Vox Sang* (old series) 1955;**5**:143–4.

528 Adinolfi M, Polley MJ, Hunter DA, Mollison PL. Classification of blood-group antibodies as β₂M or gamma globulin. *Immunology* 1962;**5**:566–79.

529 Lalezari P, Malamut DC, Dreisiger ME, Sanders C. Anti-s and anti-U cold-reacting antibodies. *Vox Sang* 1973;**25**:390–7.

530 Arndt P, Garratty G. Evaluation of the optimal incubation temperature for detecting certain IgG antibodies with potential clinical significance. *Transfusion* 1988;**28**:210–13.

531 Lubenko A. Anti-S sera and their co-existing 'private antibodies [Abstract]. *5th Mtg Br Blood Transfus Soc* 1987: 01/17.

532 Cutbush M, Mollison PL. Haemolytic transfusion reaction due to anti-S. *Lancet* 1949;**ii**:102–3.

533 Moore SB, Taswell HF, Pineda AA, Sonnenberg CL. Delayed hemolytic transfusion reactions. *Am J Clin Pathol* 1980;**74**:94–7.

534 Mayne KM, Bowell PJ, Green SJ, Entwistle CC. The significance of anti-S sensitization in pregnancy. *Clin Lab Haematol* 1990;**12**:105–7.

535 Johnson MH, Plett MJ, Conant CN, Worthington M. Autoimmune hemolytic anemia with anti-S specificity [Abstract]. *Transfusion* 1978;**18**:389.

536 Fabijanska-Mitek J, Kopec J, Seyfried H. Autoimmune haemolytic anaemia with autoantibody of anti-S specificity [Abstract]. *Vox Sang* 1994;**67**(Suppl.2):123.

537 Alessandrino EP, Costamagna L, Pagani A, Coronelli M. Late appearance of autoantibody-anti S in autoimmune hemolytic anemia. *Transfusion* 1984;**24**:369–70.

538 Issitt PD, Tregellas WM, Lee C, Wilkinson SL. An antibody that recognizes a determinant common to S and s-bearing sialoglycoproteins. *Transfusion* 1982;**22**:174–9.

539 Puig N, Carbonell F, Soler MA *et al*. Mimicking anti-S simulating a delayed transfusion reaction. *Vox Sang* 1987;**53**:173–4.

540 Hardman JT, Beck ML. Hemagglutination in capillaries: correlation with blood group specificity and IgG subclass. *Transfusion* 1981;**21**:343–6.

541 Giblett E, Chase J, Crealock FW. Hemolytic disease of the newborn resulting from anti-s antibody: report of a fatal case resulting from the fourth example of anti-s antibody. *Am J Clin Pathol* 1958;**29**:254–6.

542 Drachmann O, Hansen KB. Haemolytic disease of the newborn due to anti-s. *Scand J Haematol* 1969;**6**:93–8.

543 Kalyanaraman M, Heidemann SM, Sarnaik AP, Meert KL, Sarnaik SA. Anti-s antibody-associated delayed hemolytic transfusion reaction in patients with sickle cell anemia. *J Pediatr Hematol Oncol* 1999;**21**:70–3.

544 Meltz DJ, Bertles JF, David DS, deCiuths AC. Delayed haemolytic transfusion reaction with renal failure. *Lancet* 1971;**ii**:1348–9.

545 Rothman IK, Alter HJ, Stewler GJ. Delayed overt hemolytic transfusion reaction due to anti-U antibody. *Transfusion* 1976;**16**:357–60.

546 Taliano V, Fleury M, Pichette R, Lamothe M, Décary F. Réaction transfusionnelle hémolytique retardée due à un anti-U. *Rev Franc Transfus Hémobiol* 1989;**32**:17–26.

547 Pillay GS, Womack B, Sandler SG. Immune-mediated hemolysis in a postoperative patient. Case report: anti-U and differential diagnosis. *Immunohematology* 1993;**9**:41–6.

548 Smith G, Knott Rissik J, de la Fuente J, Win N. Anti-U and haemolytic disease of the fetus and newborn. *Br J Obstet Gynaecol* 1998;**105**:1318–21.

549 Garner SF, Devenish A. Do monocyte ADCC assays accurately predict the severity of hemolytic disease of the newborn caused by antibodies to high-frequency antigens? *Immunohematology* 1996;**12**:20–6.

550 Nugent ME, Colledge KI, Marsh WL. Auto-immune hemolytic anemia caused by anti-U. *Vox Sang* 1971;**20**:519–25.

551 Bell CA, Zwicker H. pH-dependent anti-U in autoimmune hemolytic anemia. *Transfusion* 1980;**20**:86–9.

552 Sacher RA, McGinniss MM, Shashat GG, Jacobson RJ, Rath CE. The occurrence of an auto-immune hemolytic anemia with anti-U specificity in a patient with myelodysplastic syndrome. *Am J Clin Pathol* 1982;**77**:356–9.

553 Marsh WL, Reid ME, Scott EP. Autoantibodies of U blood group specificity in autoimmune haemolytic anaemia. *Br J Haematol* 1972;**22**:625–9.

554 Vos GH, Petz LD, Garratty G, Fudenberg HH. Autoantibodies in acquired hemolytic anemia with special reference to the LW system. *Blood* 1973;**42**:445–53.

555 Roush GR, Rosenthal NS, Gerson SL *et al*. An unusual

case of autoimmune hemolytic anemia with reticulocytopenia, erythroid dysplasia, and an IgG2 autoanti-U. *Transfusion* 1996;36:575–80.

556 Kessey EC, Pierce S, Beck ML, Bayer WL. Alphamethyldopa induced hemolytic anemia involving autoantibody with U specificity [Abstract]. *Transfusion* 1973;13:360.

557 McGinniss MH, Macher AM, Rook AH, Alter HJ. Red cell autoantibodies in patients with acquired immune deficiency syndrome. *Transfusion* 1986;26:405–9.

558 Wojcicki RE, Hardman JT, Beck ML *et al.* pH, temperature and ionic strength: significant variables in detection of auto anti-U [Abstract]. *Transfusion* 1980;20:628.

559 Chiofolo JT, Reid ME, Charles-Pierre D. LISS-dependent autoantibody with apparent anti-U specificity. *Immunohematology* 1995;11:18–19.

560 Booth PB. A 'new' blood group antigen associated with S and s. *Vox Sang* 1972;22:524–8.

561 Booth PB. Two Melanesian antisera reacting with SsU components. *Vox Sang* 1978;34:212–20.

562 Read SM, Taylor MM, Reid ME, Popovsky MA. Anti-U^z found in mother's serum and child's eluate. *Immunohematology* 1993;9:47–9.

563 Langlois RG, Bigbee WL, Jensen RH. Measurements of the frequency of human erythrocytes with gene expression loss phenotypes at the glycophorin A locus. *Hum Genet* 1986;74:353–62.

564 Grant SG, Jensen RH. Use of hematopoietic cells and markers for the detection and quantitation of human *in vivo* somatic mutation. In: G Garratty, ed. *Immunobiology of Transfusion Medicine.* New York: Dekker, 1994: 299–323.

565 Langlois RG, Bigbee WL, Kyoizumi S *et al.* Evidence of increased somatic cell mutations at the glycophorin A locus in atomic bomb survivors. *Science* 1987;236:445–8.

566 Jensen RH, Langlois RG, Bigbee WL *et al.* Elevated frequency of glycophorin A mutations in erythrocytes from Chernobyl accident victims. *Radiat Res* 1995;141:129–35.

567 Schiweitz J, Lorenz R, Scheubeck M, Börner W, Hempel K. Improved determination of variant erythrocytes at the glycophorin A (GPA) locus and variant frequency in patients treated with radioiodine for thyroid cancer. *Int J Radiat Biol* 1996;70:131–43.

568 Jensen RH, Reynolds JC, Robbins J *et al.* Glycophorin A as a biological dosimeter for radiation dose to the bone marrow from iodine-131. *Radiat Res* 1997; 147:747–52.

569 Rothman N, Haas R, Hayes RB *et al.* Benzene induces gene-duplicating but not gene-inactivating mutations at the glycophorin A locus in exposed humans. *Proc Natl Acad Sci USA* 1995;92:4069–73.

570 Schmidt PJ, Lostumbo MM, English CT, Hunter OB. Aberrant U blood group accompanying Rh$_{null}$. *Transfusion* 1967;7:33–4.

571 Dahr W, Kordowicz M, Moulds J *et al.* Characterization of the Ss sialoglycoprotein and its antigens in Rh$_{null}$ erythrocytes. *Blut* 1987;54:13–24.

572 Dahr W, Issitt PD, Wren MR. The Ss SGP in an X^Q homozygote and heterozygotes [Abstract]. *Transfusion* 1986;26:560.

573 Habibi B, Fouillade MT, Duedari N *et al.* The antigen Duclos: a new high frequency red cell antigen related to Rh and U. *Vox Sang* 1978;34:302–9.

574 Mallinson G, Anstee DJ, Avent ND *et al.* Murine monoclonal antibody MB-2D10 recognizes Rh-related glycoproteins in the human red cell membrane. *Transfusion* 1990;30:222–5.

575 von dem Borne AEGK, Bos MJE, Lomas C *et al.* Murine monoclonal antibodies against a unique determinant of erythrocytes, related to Rh and U antigens: expression on normal and malignant erythrocyte precursors and Rh$_{null}$ red cells. *Br J Haematol* 1990;75:254–61.

576 Le Pennec PV, Rouger P, Klein MT, Le Basnerais M, Salmon C. An antibody supporting the evidence of an association between the Rh polypeptides and glycophorin B on the red cell membrane [Abstract]. *Joint Congr Int Soc Blood Transfus Am Assoc Blood Banks* 1990:29.

577 Miller LH, Haynes JD, McAuliffe FM *et al.* Evidence for differences in erythrocyte surface receptors for the malarial parasites *Plasmodium falciparum* and *Plasmodium knowlesi. J Exp Med* 1977;146:277–81.

578 Pasvol G, Wainscoat JS, Weatherall DJ. Erythrocytes deficient in glycophorin resist invasion by the malarial parasite *Plasmodium falciparum. Nature* 1982;297: 64–6.

579 Pasvol G, Jungery M, Weatherall DJ *et al.* Glycophorin as a possible receptor for *Plasmodium falciparum. Lancet* 1982;ii:947–51.

580 Pasvol G, Anstee D, Tanner MJA. Glycophorin C and the invasion of red cells by *Plasmodium falciparum. Lancet* 1984;i:907–8.

581 Pasvol G. Receptors on red cells for *Plasmodium falciparum* and their interaction with merozoites. *Phil Trans R Soc Lond B* 1984;307:189–200.

582 Hadley TJ, McGinniss MH, Klotz FW, Miller LH. Blood group antigens and invasion of erythrocytes by malaria parasites. In: G Garratty, ed. *Red Cell Antigens and Antibodies.* Arlington VA: American Association of Blood Banks, 1986:17–33.

583 Facer CA. Erythrocyte sialoglycoproteins and *Plasmodium falciparum* invasion. *R Soc Trop Med Hyg* 1983;77:524–30.

584 Chisti AH, Palek J, Fisher D, Maalouf GJ, Liu S-C. Reduced invasion and growth of *Plasmodium falciparum* into elliptocytic red blood cells with a combined deficiency of protein 4.1, glycophorin C, and p55. *Blood* 1996;87:3462–9.

585 Perkins M. Inhibitory effects of erythrocyte membrane proteins on the *in vitro* invasion of the human malarial

parasite (*Plasmodium falciparum*) into its host cell. *J Cell Biol* 1981;**90**:563–7.

586 Pasvol G, Chasis JA, Mohandas N *et al.* Inhibition of malarial parasite invasion by monoclonal antibodies against glycophorin A correlates with reduction in red cell membrane deformability. *Blood* 1989;**74**:1836–43.

587 Blackall DP, Armstrong JK, Meiselman HJ, Fisher TC. Polyethylene glycol-coated red blood cells fail to bind glycophorin A-specific antibodies and are impervious to invasion by the *Plasmodium falciparum* malaria parasite. *Blood* 2001;**97**:551–6.

588 Cartron JP, Prou O, Luilier M, Soulier JP. Susceptibility to invasion by *Plasmodium falciparum* of some human erythrocytes carrying rare blood group antigens. *Br J Haematol* 1983;**55**:639–47.

589 Mitchell GH, Hadley TJ, McGinniss MH, Klotz FW, Miller LH. Invasion of erythrocytes by *Plasmodium falciparum* malaria parasites: evidence for receptor heterogeneity and two receptors. *Blood* 1986;**67**:1519–21.

590 Templeton TJ, Keister DB, Muratova O, Procter JL, Kaslow DC. Adherence of erythrocytes during exflagellation of *Plasmodium falciparum* microgametes is dependent on erythrocyte surface sialic acid and glycophorins. *J Exp Med* 1998;**187**:1599–609.

591 Sim BKL, Chitnis CE, Wasniowska K, Hadley TJ, Miller LH. Receptor and ligand domains for invasion of erythrocytes by *Plasmodium falciparum*. *Science* 1994; **264**:1941–4.

592 Jokinen M, Ehnholm C, Väisänen-Rhen V *et al.* Identification of the major human sialoglycoprotein from red cells, glycophorin A^M, as the receptor for *Escherichia coli* IH 11165 and characterization of the receptor site. *Eur J Biochem* 1985;**147**:47–52.

593 Brooks DE, Cavanagh J, Jayroe D *et al.* Involvement of the MN blood group antigen in shear-enhanced hemagglutination induced by the *Escherichia coli* F41 adhesin. *Infect Immun* 1989;**57**:377–83.

594 Cortajarena AL, Goñi FM, Ostolaza H. Glycophorin as a receptor for *Escherichia coli* α-haemolysin in erythrocytes. *J Biol Chem* 2001;**276**:12513–9.

595 Zhang D, Takahashi J, Seno T, Tani Y, Honda T. Analysis of receptor for *Vibrio cholerae* E1 Tor hemolysin with a monoclonal antibody that recognizes glycophorin B of human erythrocyte membrane. *Infect Immun* 1999;**67**:5332–7.

596 Kathan RH, Winzler RJ, Johnson CA. Preparation of an inhibitor of viral hemagglutination from human erythrocytes. *J Exp Med* 1961;**113**:37–45.

597 Allaway GP, Burness ATH. Site of attachment of encephalomyocarditis virus on human erythrocytes. *J Virol* 1986;**59**:768–70.

598 Paul RW, Lee PWK. Glycophorin is the reovirus receptor on human erythrocytes. *Virology* 1987; **159**:94–101.

599 Ohyama K, Endo T, Ohkuma S, Yamakawa T. Isolation and influenza virus receptor activity of glycophorins B,

C and D from human erythrocyte membranes. *Biochim Biophys Acta* 1993;**1148**:133–8.

600 Gahmberg CG, Jokinen M, Karhi KK *et al.* Biosynthesis of the major human red cell sialoglycoprotein, glycophorin A: a review. *Rev Franc Transfus Immuno-Hémat* 1981;**24**:53–73.

601 Yurchenco PD, Furthmayr H. Expression of red cell membrane proteins in erythroid precursor cells. *J Supramol Struct* 1980;**13**:255–69.

602 Robinson J, Sieff C, Delia D, Edwards PAW, Greaves M. Expression of cell-surface HLA-DR, HLA-ABC and glycophorin during erythroid differentiation. *Nature* 1981;**289**:68–71.

603 Gahmberg CG, Ekblom M, Andersson LC. Differentiation of human erythroid cells is associated with increased O-glycosylation of the major sialoglycoprotein, glycophorin A. *Proc Natl Acad Sci USA* 1984;**81**:6752–6.

604 Southcott MJG, Tanner MJA, Anstee DJ. The expression of human blood group antigens during erythropoiesis in a cell culture system. *Blood* 1999; **93**:4425–35.

605 Bony V, Gane P, Bailly P, Cartron J-P. Time–course expression of polypeptides carrying blood group antigens during human erythroid differentiation. *Br J Haematol* 1999;**107**:263–74.

606 Daniels G, Green C. Expression of red cell surface antigens during erythropoiesis. *Vox Sang* 2000; **78**(Suppl.1):149–53.

607 Ekblom M, Gahmberg CG, Andersson LC. Late expression of M and N antigens on glycophorin A during erythroid differentiation. *Blood* 1985;**66**:233–6.

608 Gahmberg CG, Jokinen M, Andersson LC. Expression of the major sialoglycoprotein (glycophorin) on erythroid cells in human bone marrow. *Blood* 1978; **52**:379–87.

609 Gahmberg CG, Jokinen M, Andersson LC. Expression of the major red cell sialoglycoprotein, glycophorin A, in the human leukemic cell line K562. *J Biol Chem* 1979;**254**:7442–8.

610 Silver RE, Adamany AM, Blumenfeld OO. Glycophorins of human erythroleukemic K562 cells. *Arch Biochem Biophys* 1987;**256**:285–94.

611 McGinniss MH, Dean A. Expression of red cell antigens by K562 human leukemia cells before and after induction of hemoglobin synthesis by hemin. *Transfusion* 1985;**25**:105–9.

612 Hawkins P, Anderson SE, McKenzie JL *et al.* Localization of MN blood group in kidney. *Transplant Proc* 1985;**2**:1697–700.

613 Harvey J, Parsons SF, Anstee DJ, Bradley BA. Evidence for the occurrence of human erythrocyte membrane sialoglycoproteins in human kidney endothelial cells. *Vox Sang* 1988;**55**:104–8.

614 Jentoft N. Why are proteins O-glycosylated? *Trends Biochem Sci* 1990;**15**:291–4.

615 Chasis JA, Mohandas N. The role of red cell gly-cophorins in regulating membrane function. In: PC Agre, J-P Cartron, eds. *Protein Blood Group Antigens of the Human Red Cell: Structure, Function and Clinical Significance.* Baltimore: Johns Hopkins, 1992:152–69.

616 Tanphaichitr VS, Sumboonnanonda A, Ideguchi H *et al.* Novel AE1 mutations in recessive distal renal tubular acidosis: loss-of-function is rescued by glycophorin A. *J Clin Invest* 1998;102:2173–9.

617 Young MT, Beckmann R, Toye AM, Tanner MJA. Red-cell glycophorin A–band 3 interactions associated with the movement of band 3 to the cell surface. *Biochem J* 2000;350:53–60.

618 Hassoun H, Hanada T, Lutchman M *et al.* Complete deficiency of glycophorin A in red blood cells from mice with targeted inactivation of the band 3 (AE1) gene. *Blood* 1998;91:2146–51.

619 Beckman R, Smythe JS, Anstee DJ, Tanner MJA. Func-tional cell surface expression of band 3, the human red blood cell anion exchange protein (AE1), in K562 erythroleukemia cells: band 3 enhances the cell surface reactivity of Rh antigens. *Blood* 1998;92:4428–38.

620 Paulitschke M, Nash GB, Anstee DJ, Tanner MJA, Gratzer WB. Perturbation of red blood cell membrane rigidity by extracellular ligands. *Blood* 1995;86:342–8.

621 Tomita A, Radike EL, Parker CJ. Isolation of erythro-cyte membrane inhibitor of reactive lysis type II: identi-fication as glycophorin A. *J Immunol* 1993;151:3308–23.

622 El Ouagari K, Teissié J, Benoist H. Glycophorin A protects K562 cells from natural killer cell attack: role of oligosaccharides. *J Biol Chem* 1995;270:26970–5.

623 Kudo S, Fukuda M. Contribution of gene conversion to the retention of the sequence for M blood group type determinant in glycophorin E gene. *J Biol Chem* 1994;269:22969–74.

624 Onda M, Fukuda M. Detailed physical mapping of the genes encoding glycophorins A, B and E, as revealed by P1 plasmids containing human genomic DNA. *Gene* 1995;159:225–230.

625 Rearden A, Magnet A, Kudo S, Fukuda M. Glycophorin B and glycophorin E genes arose from the glycophorin A ancestral gene via two duplications during primate evolution. *J Biol Chem* 1993;268:2260–7.

626 Xie S-S, Huang C-H, Reid ME, Blancher A, Blumenfeld OO. The glycophorin A gene family in gorillas: structure, expression, and comparison with the human and chimpanzee homologues. *Biochem Genet* 1997;35:59–76.

627 Blumenfeld OO, Adamany AM, Puglia KV, Socha WW. The chimpanzee M blood-group antigen is a variant of the human M-N glycoproteins. *Biochem Genet* 1983;21:333–48.

628 Blancher A, Reid ME, Socha WW. Cross-reactivity of antibodies to human and primate red cell antigens. *Transfus Med Rev* 2000;14:161–79.

4 P blood groups

4.1 Introduction

While looking for new polymorphisms by injecting rabbits with human red cells, Landsteiner and Levine [1] discovered the P blood group system in a series of experiments that also revealed the MN groups. To remove anti-species agglutinins, the immune sera were adsorbed with red cells from subjects other than those used to immunize the rabbits. The sera were then tested for antibodies that reacted differently with red cells from different people. One such antibody, which could not be explained by the ABO or MN groups, defined two types of blood called P+ and P–. Human alloantibodies of the same specificity were found soon after.

The P system was expanded in 1955 by Sanger [2], who observed that all red cells of the very rare phenotype Tj(a–) were P–. The notation was altered to accommodate the new phenotype: P+ became P_1, P– became P_2, and Tj(a–) was renamed p; the original P antigen has now become P1. Recognition in 1959 of another rare phenotype, P^k (CD77), created further complexity [3]. P^k red cells have strong expression of P^k antigen, and lack a high frequency antigen, now called P, which is strongly expressed on all other red cells except those of the p phenotype (Table 4.1). P^k red cells may be P_1 or P_2. The Luke antigen (LKE), another associated antigen of relatively high incidence lacking from p cells, was found in 1965 [4]. The reactions of antibodies defining these phenotypes are shown in Table 4.1.

The first biochemical steps were taken by Morgan and Watkins [5], who isolated a P1-active glycoprotein from hydatid cyst fluid (HCF). The P1 determinant was identified as a trisaccharide [6]. The identification of the P1, P, and P^k red cell antigens as glycosphingolipids followed the exciting work of Naiki and Marcus [7] in identifying the P antigen as the most abundant red cell glycosphingolipid, globoside. Elucidation of the structures of P1, P, and P^k demonstrated that two biosynthetic pathways were involved in the production of these antigens. The genes encoding the glycosyltransferases that catalyse the synthesis of P^k and P have been cloned (see Section 4.3.3), but the genetics of P1 biosynthesis remains unresolved. As more than one gene locus is involved, the P blood groups cannot be considered a single blood group system.

4.2 Notation

The International Society of Blood Transfusion (ISBT) Terminology Working Party has awarded the number 003 to the P system. This system has the symbol P1 and contains only one antigen, P1 (003001). P, P^k, and LKE are not included in the P system, because P and LKE are not controlled by genes at the same locus as that governing P1 and the position of P^k is unclear. As there are obvious serological and biochemical relationships between P, P^k, and LKE, they have been assembled into collection 209, the globoside collection: P is GLOB1; P^k is GLOB2; and LKE is GLOB3.

Phenotype names are shown in Table 4.1. P_1 is used for P1+ P+ cells and P_2 for P1– P+ cells; P_1^k and P_2^k are used for P1+ P– P^k+ and P1– P– P^k+ cells, respectively. The symbol p is used for the 'null' phenotype. Symbols for the genes are not straightforward because P^2 has been used in two ways:

1 originally as the allele of P^1; and
2 later as the gene responsible for the β-N-

Table 4.1 P blood groups: phenotypes and antibodies.

Phenotype	Frequency in white people (%)	Anti-P1	Anti-P	Anti-Pk	Anti-LKE	Anti-PP1Pk
P_1	75	+	+	−*	+	+
P_2	25	−	+	−*	+	+
p	Very rare	−	−/w	−	−	−
P_1^k	Very rare	+	−	+	−	+
P_2^k	Very rare	−	−	+	−	+
LKE+	98	+ or −	+	−	+	+
LKE−	2	+ or −	+	+†	−	+
Source of antibody		P_2 people; animals; MAbs	P^k people; MAbs	Anti-PP1P^k adsorbed with P_1 cells; MAbs	LKE−people; MAbs	p people

*Very weak P^k on these cells cannot be detected by agglutination tests with anti-P^k separated from anti-PP1P^k by adsorption with P$_1$ cells.
†P^k expression on LKE− cells less strong than P^k expression on P$_1^k$ and P$_2^k$ cells.
MAbs, monoclonal antibodies; w, weak positive reaction.

acetylgalactosaminyltransferase that catalyses the conversion of ceramide trihexose (Gb3, P^k antigen) to globoside (P).

These are conflicting definitions so, to avoid confusion, $P2$ will not be used. The symbols $P1^+$ and $P1^-$, P^{k+} and P^{k-}, and P^+ and P^- will be used for the genes that control the production of P1 from paragloboside, of P^k from lactosylceramide, and of P from P^k, respectively (see Section 4.3). A better notation should be devised when the genetics are fully understood.

4.3 Biochemistry

P antigenic determinants on red cells reside in the carbohydrate residues of glycosphingolipids, oligonucleotide chains attached to ceramide. Identification of the chemical structures of P1, P, and P^k showed that neither P nor P^k could be the precursor of P1. Two biosynthetic pathways are involved in production of these antigens (Table 4.2 and Fig. 4.1). Reviews on P biochemistry include [8–10].

4.3.1 Paragloboside series of antigens

Paragloboside (lacto-N-neotetraosylceramide, Table 4.2) is a precursor of Type 2 ABH antigens, of some gangliosides, and of P1 (Fig. 4.1).

4.3.1.1 P1 antigen

The first information on the biochemical nature of the P antigens was derived from inhibition tests. From studies on the effect of many monosaccharides, disaccharides, and trisaccharides on the agglutination of P_1 cells by anti-P1, Watkins and Morgan [11] indicated the involvement of α-D-galactose in P1 specificity. They applied techniques previously used for extracting A, B, and H substances from body fluids to isolate a P1-active glycoprotein from HCF of sheep, which inhibits anti-P1 [5]. The products of partial acid hydrolysis of this glycoprotein led to characterization of a trisaccharide, Galα1→4Galβ1→4GlcNAc as the P1 determinant [6].

P1 on red cells is a glycosphingolipid [12–14]. After extensive purification, the structure of the active glycolipid was identified as the ceramide pentasaccharide shown in Table 4.2 [15,16], with the terminal trisaccharide identical to that isolated from the sheep P1 glycoprotein [6]. This structure is paragloboside with an additional non-reducing α-galactosyl residue.

P1-trisaccharide is very efficient at inhibiting monoclonal anti-P1 [17,18]. Synthetic glycoproteins containing the P1-trisaccharide have been used to immunize mice in the production of monoclonal anti-P1 [19] (Section 4.4.5.3). P1-trisaccharide bound to an insoluble immunoadsorbent removed alloanti-P1 from human sera [20].

4.3.1.2 Sialosylparagloboside

An antibody reacting preferentially with p cells was specifically inhibited by sialosylparagloboside [21,22]

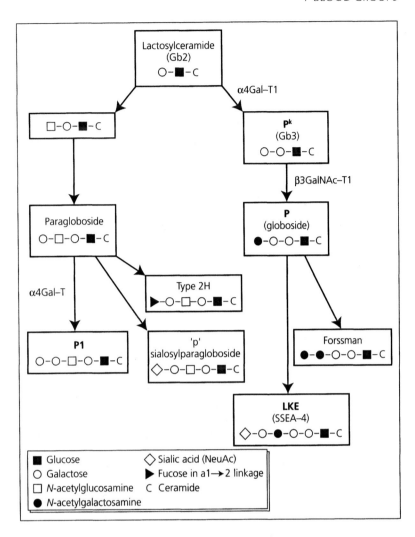

Fig. 4.1 Possible biosynthetic pathways for formation of P antigens from a common precursor, lactosylceramide. Glycosyltransferases responsible for production of P1, P^k, and P antigens are shown.

(Section 4.10.1), paraglioboside with a terminal sialic acid residue (Table 4.2). Sialosylparagloboside levels may be increased in p cells because a blockage in the synthesis of P^k (Gb3) results in increased quantities of precursor glycolipids for other biosynthetic pathways [22] (Fig. 4.1).

4.3.2 Globoside series of antigens

The early biochemical studies showed a close relationship between P1 and P^k antigens, but gave no clue to the structure of P antigen. Using purified glycolipids to inhibit anti-PP1P^k, Naiki and Marcus [7] made the observation that globoside and ceramide trihexoside (Gb3), two very well-characterized glycolipids, constituted red cell P and P^k antigens, respectively (Table 4.2). Characterization of the P and P^k antigens demonstrated that P^k was the direct precursor of P and that P1 arises from a different biosynthetic pathway (Fig. 4.1).

The sugar sequences that determine P1, P^k, and P occur as glycolipids on red cells; P1 and P^k occur as glycoproteins in HCF.

4.3.2.1 P^k antigen

The involvement of α-D-galactose in P^k specificity, first postulated by Voak *et al.* [23], was subsequently confirmed [24,25]. Anti-P^k, like anti-P1, is inhibited by HCF [3]. Partial acid hydrolysis of the P1P^k glycoprotein, isolated from HCF, yielded the P1-trisaccharide, which inhibited anti-P^k and -P1, and a disaccharide Galα1→4Gal, which inhibited anti-P^k, but not anti-P1 [25]. Other α-galactosyl-terminal oligosaccharides

Table 4.2 Structures of some glycosphingolipids associated with P antigens.

Antigen	Structure	
	Lactosylceramide (Gb2)	Galβ1→4Glc-Cer
P1	*Paragloboside series* Paragloboside Galactosylparagloboside Sialosylparagloboside	Galβ1→4GlcNAcβ1→3Galβ1→4Glc-Cer Galα1→4Galβ1→4GlcNAcβ1→3Galβ1→4Glc-Cer NeuAcα2→3Galβ1→4GlcNAcβ1→3Galβ1→4Glc-Cer
P^k P	*Globoside series* Globotriosylceramide (Gb3) Globoside (globotetraosylceramide, Gb4)	Galα1→4Galβ1→4Glc-Cer GalNAcβ1→3Galα1→4Galβ1→4Glc-Cer
LKE, SSEA-4	Sialosylgalactosylgloboside (SGG)	NeuAcα2→3Galβ1→3GalNAcβ1→3Galα1→4Galβ1→4Glc-Cer
	Disialosylgalactosylgloboside (DSGG)	NeuAcα2→3Galβ1→3(NeuAcα2→6)GalNAcβ1→3Galα1→4 Galβ1→4Glc-Cer
H	Globo-H (Type 4 H)	Fucα1→2Galβ1→3GalNAcβ1→3Galα1→4Galβ1→4Glc-Cer
Forssman	Forssman (Gb5)	GalNAcα1→3GalNAcβ1→3Galα1→4Galβ1→4Glc-Cer

also inhibited anti-P^k [25], confirming the immunodominance of α-galactose in P^k expression.

Using glycosphingolipids of known structure, Naiki and Marcus [7] identified the P^k antigen as Gb3, which has the expected terminal galactose residue (Table 4.2). Glycosphingolipid analysis demonstrated that Gb3 was absent from p red cells and increased in P^k red cells [26,27]. Monoclonal anti-P^k (Section 4.6.4.3) react with Gb3 [28]. Several monoclonal anti-P^k were derived from mice immunized with synthetic glycoproteins containing the P^k-trisaccharide (Galα1→4Galβ1→4Glc) [19].

Study of glycosphingolipids from P₁ and P₂ red cells showed that Gb3 is a common component of their membranes [7,16]. Thus, contrary to expectation from early serology, P^k is not a rare antigen, but an antigen of very high incidence (Section 4.6.3).

4.3.2.2 P antigen (globoside)

The glycoproteins that inhibited anti-P1 and -P^k did not cross-react with anti-P and nothing was known of the structure of P until, in the same inhibition studies as those that revealed that P^k is Gb3, Naiki and Marcus [7] identified P as globoside (Gb4). Subsequently, globoside was shown to be lacking from P^k red cells and present in only trace amounts in p red cells [26,27].

Globoside is the most abundant red cell membrane glycolipid, with about 14×10^6 molecules per cell [29,30]. Globoside represents Gb3 (P^k) with an additional non-reducing N-acetylgalactosamine residue (Table 4.2).

Monoclonal anti-P (Section 4.5.2.3) was inhibited by the terminal trisaccharide of globoside (GalNAcβ1→3Galα1→4Gal) and by Galβ1→3GalNAcβ1→3Gal [31]. Another monoclonal antibody that behaved serologically as anti-P was completely inhibited by T-specific immunoadsorbent (Galβ1→3GalNAc-R) [32]. Human anti-P were not inhibited by this disaccharide.

Despite the lack of two abundant glycosphingolipids, Gb3 and globoside (Gb4), p red cells appear normal in behaviour and in morphology. Red cells with p phenotype have increased quantities of lactosylceramide and other complex glycolipids [26,33,34]. Kidney contains high levels of extended globoseries compounds. Kidney, obtained at autopsy, from a group A, p phenotype individual, had enhanced levels of lactosylceramide, no Gb3 or globoside, and no Type 4 A (globo-A) chain structure [35] (Section 2.2.2).

4.3.2.3 LKE antigen

Recognition that a monoclonal antibody detecting

the murine stage-specific embryonic antigen (SSEA-4) [31] defined the red cell antigen LKE, implied that LKE is a globoseries antigen [36]. SSEA-4 represents a globoside molecule with additional galactose and sialic acid residues (Table 4.2). Confirmation that LKE has the same dependence on sialic acid as SSEA-4 is awaited.

4.3.3 Transferases and the genes that encode them

Biosynthesis of the P antigens, like the ABH antigens, occurs by the sequential addition of monosaccharides to a precursor substrate, catalysed by glycosyltransferases. Although the biochemical pathway is now established (Fig. 4.1), the genetical background is still not clear. Indirect evidence for active transferases was first presented by Fellous *et al.* [37] from complementation experiments; P was found to be re-expressed on polykaryon cells obtained by fusion of P^k and p fibroblasts, providing further evidence that two independent genes were responsible for P^k and p phenotypes.

4.3.3.1 P^k (Gb3) synthase

As the gene governing the P_1/P_2 polymorphism has been mapped to chromosome 22q13.2 (Chapter 32), Steffenson *et al.* [38] carried out a database search within this region for a sequence homologous to that encoding an α-N-acetylglucosaminyltransferase in the hope of finding the gene for the P1 α1,4-galactosyltransferase. They identified a cDNA that encodes an α1,4-galactosyltransferase (named α4Gal-T1), which catalyses the transfer of galactose from UDP-galactose to lactosylceramide (Gb2) to produce globotriosylceramide (Gb3), the P^k antigen (Fig. 4.1). However, it did not convert paragloboside to P1 antigen. When transfected with an α4Gal-T1 cDNA construct, Namalawa human lymphoblastoid cells, which have no endogenous α1,4-galactosyltransferase activity, strongly expressed P^k. The α4Gal-T1 gene has two exons, but only one of them contains coding sequence [39]. α4Gal-T1 belongs to a family of glycosyltransferases that are conserved in mammals, insects, and plants, and possibly throughout evolution [40].

4.3.3.2 P (globoside) synthase

Okajima *et al.* [41] used an eukaryotic cell expression cloning system to isolate the cDNA encoding globoside synthase, a β1,3-N-acetylgalactosaminyltransferase (β3GalNAc-T1). In order to achieve this, mouse fibroblast cells were transfected with Gb3 synthase cDNA, to produce P^k, a human kidney cDNA library, and Forssman synthase cDNA to produce Forssman antigen from any globoside that may be synthesized (Fig. 4.1). Cells isolated by panning with anti-Forssman therefore must have incorporated cDNA for globoside synthase. The cloned cDNA encodes β3GalNAc-T1, an enzyme that was previously considered to be a galactosyltransferase (β3Gal-T3) [42]. β3GalNAc-T1 synthesizes P antigen from P^k by catalysing the transfer of N-acetylgalactosamine from UDP-N-acetylgalactosamine to Gb3 (P^k). The gene is located at chromosome 3q25 [42] and contains a single coding exon [41]. It is widely expressed, with strong expression in brain and heart, moderate expression in lung, placenta, and testis, and low expression in kidney liver, spleen, and stomach [41,42]. Cultured fibroblasts from individuals with P^k phenotype lack globoside synthase, confirming that P^k phenotype is caused by a deficient synthase and not to degradation by an α-galactosidase [43].

4.3.3.3 P1 synthase

The putative α1,4-galactosyltransferase responsible for the synthesis of P1 from paragloboside (Fig. 4.1) has not been identified.

Red cells of the p phenotype lack P^k (Gb3), P (globoside), and P1 (Table 4.1). The p phenotype is associated with homozygosity for inactivating mutations in the Gb3 synthase (α4Gal-T1) gene, explaining the absence of P^k [38,39] (Section 4.8.1). Globoside synthase was present in cultured fibroblasts and B-lymphocytes from p individuals [34,43], but could not synthesize globoside in the absence of its acceptor substrate, Gb3.

Any genetic model for biosynthesis of the P antigens must explain why red cells of p people lack P1 (a paragloboside series glycosphingolipid) as well as Gb3 and globoside (globoseries glycosphingolipids), yet P_2 (P1–) red cells have Gb3 and globoside. The possibility that P_2 might reflect the lack of the precursor of P1 was eliminated by the observation that normal amounts of paragloboside were found in P_2 cells [29,33].

A genetic model proposed by Graham and Williams [44] predicts three alleles at the *P1* locus:
1 $P_1{}^k$ coding for an α1,4-galactosyltransferase, which

can utilize both paragloboside and lactosylceramide as acceptor substrates and synthesizes P1 and P^k;

2 *P^k* coding for an α1,4-galactosyltransferase, which can only use lactosylceramide and only synthesizes P^k; and

3 *p*, an amorph, which synthesizes neither P1 nor P^k (Table 4.3).

At the second locus there are two alleles: *P$^+$* encoding globoside synthase and *P$^-$*, which is an amorph. In this model, no P$_1$ children would be expected from p×P$_2$ matings. Ten such matings produced 37 children, none of whom was P$_1$.

P^k synthase (α4Gal-T1), however, did not catalyse the synthesis of P1 from paragloboside [38]. Furthermore, no polymorphism correlating to P$_1$/P$_2$ phenotypes was detected in the coding region of the α4Gal-T1 gene [38,39].

An alternative model has three loci, *P1*, *P^k*, and *P*, with the *P1$^+$* allele altering the acceptor specificity requirements of P^k synthase so that it could utilize paragloboside as well as lactosylceramide [16]. A precedent for this form of interaction exists in the β4Gal-T family, where binding of α-lactalbumin to two enzymes changes the acceptor substrate specificity from *N*-acetylglucosamine to glucose [45]. If three independent loci were involved, P$_1$ children would be expected from the mating type p×P$_2$. This has not been observed, so if three loci were involved, *P1* and *P^k* must be closely linked. This might be expected as the *P1* locus and the gene for P^k synthase are both on chromosome 22q13.2, but searches of the available chromosome 22 sequence did not reveal additional homologous genes [38].

In contrast, Iizuka *et al.* [46] found that extracts from p and P$_1$ lymphoblastoid cells were equally effective at transferring galactose from a UDP-galactose donor to lactosylceramide to produce P^k-active Gb3. Yet, *in vivo*, no P^k is produced and lactosylceramide accumulates in p cells. The reason for these unexpected results is not known.

4.4 P1 antigen and anti-P1

4.4.1 Frequency and inheritance

The frequency of P1 varies in different populations. About 80% of white people are P$_1$. The frequency of P1 is much higher in some African and South American people and very much lower in some Asian populations, as low as 30% in Japanese. For details of frequencies for many populations see [47].

Some of the early estimates in white people are inaccurate because of the anti-P1 reagents used; if a weak anti-P1 were used the frequency of P1 was low. Race and Sanger [48] considered the work of Henningsen [49,50] to be the most reliable and used it for calculation of the phenotype, gene, and genotype frequencies. In a survey of 2345 Scandinavians, 78.85% were P$_1$ and 21.15% were P$_2$. These figures provided the following gene and genotype frequencies:

P1$^+$ 0.5401 *P1$^+$/P1$^+$* 0.2917
P1$^-$ 0.4599 *P1$^+$/P1$^-$* 0.4968
          P1$^-$/P1$^-$ 0.2115.

Landsteiner and Levine [1] showed that P1 was inherited and behaved as a Mendelian dominant character. This is supported by all subsequent work. In many family studies, too many P$_2$ children were observed from P$_1$×P$_1$ and P$_1$×P$_2$ matings compared with the expected values calculated from the gene frequencies. These discrepancies are attributed to the difficulty in detecting weak P1 (Section 4.4.2), especially in young children (Section 4.5.3) [48]. Henningsen's [51] results

Table 4.3 Two gene locus genetical model proposed to explain production of the P1, P, and P^k antigens and their expression in the five P phenotypes [44].

P1 locus	P locus	PG→P1	Gb2→P^k	P^k→P	Phenotype
$P_1{}^k/P_1{}^k$, $P_1{}^k/P^k$, or $P_1{}^k/p$	P^+/P^+ or P^+/P^-	+	+	+	P$_1$
P^k/P^k or P^k/p	P^+/P^+ or P^+/P^-	−	+	+	P$_2$
p/p	P^+/P^+ or P^+/P^-	−	−	No P^k	p
$P_1{}^k/P_1{}^k$, $P_1{}^k/P^k$, or $P_1{}^k/p$	P^-/P^-	+	+	−	$P_1{}^k$
P^k/P^k or P^k/p	P^-/P^-	−	+	−	$P_2{}^k$
p/p	P^-/P^-	−	−	No P^k	p

Gb2, lactosylceramide; PG, paragloboside.

of family studies using his rigorous criteria for P_1 and P_2 agreed very well with the expected values.

4.4.2 Variation in strength

The strength of P1 on red cells shows individual variation and appears to be under genetic control [49–51]. Dosage contributes to this variation in strength. Fisher [52] analysed Henningsen's data and calculated that 66% of individuals with strong P1 were homozygous $P1^+/P1^+$ and all individuals with weak P1 were heterozygous $P1^+/P1^-$.

In(Lu), the rare dominant inhibitor of Lutheran and other red cell antigens, inhibits P1 expression [53,54] and has been responsible for P_2 parents having a P_1 child [54,55]. *In(Lu)*, which is not closely linked to the *P1* locus [54], is discussed in Chapter 6.

4.4.3 Development and distribution

P1 is considerably weaker in children than in adults and the frequency of P_2 is substantially higher in newborn babies than in adults [49]. Complete development of P1 is not reached until 7 years of age or older [56]. Despite this weak expression at birth, P1 is strongly expressed on fetal red cells. Fetal P1 expression is weaker than adult P1, but the strength of P1 decreases with increasing age of the fetus; P1 was more strongly, and more frequently, expressed by 12-week fetuses than by 28-week fetuses [57].

Flow cytometry with alloanti-P1 revealed that P1 is expressed on lymphocytes, granulocytes, and monocytes [58].

4.4.4 Other sources of P1 substance

Helminths (tapeworms and flukes) are sources of P1-active substances. Fluid from hydatid cysts of sheep livers inhibits anti-P1, but only if the fluid contains scolices [59]. The frequency and avidity of anti-P1 is increased in P_2 patients infested with certain tapeworms (hydatid disease) and liver flukes [59–62]. Annelid and nematode worms are also sources of P1 substance; extracts of *Lumbricus terrestris* (earthworm) and *Ascaris suum* inhibit anti-P1 [63].

Some other sources of P1 substance are avian in origin. Red cells, plasma, and excrement of pigeons and turtle doves, and ovomucoid of turtle dove egg white, all contain P1 substance [64–66]. Anti-P1 is more commonly found in P_2 pigeon-fanciers (34%) than in P_2 donors (6%) [64]. Substances like turtle dove ovomucoid and the hydatid cyst wall and protoscoleces of helminths, which inhibit anti-P1 and can be used to stimulate anti-P1 production, have branching structures with the P1-trisaccharide, Galα1→4Galβ1→4GlcNAc [67,68].

4.4.5 Anti-P1

4.4.5.1 Alloanti-P1

Alloanti-P1 is a common specificity, usually as a weak agglutinin active only at low temperature. Rarely has anti-P1 been attributed to stimulation by transfusion of red cells [69–72].

Most examples of anti-P1 do not agglutinate red cells at 25°C or above and these cold-reactive antibodies should not be considered clinically significant [73]. There are two reports of immediate haemolytic transfusion reactions (IHTR), one with a fatal outcome, caused by anti-P1 that agglutinate red cells at 37°C [74,75]. Some examples have been reported to have caused delayed transfusion reactions, although no anti-P1 was detected in the pretransfusion sample and, in one case, the antibody had disappeared within 4 months of the reaction [71,76]. Anti-P1 active at 37°C rapidly eliminated 50% of radiolabelled P1 cells; the rest were eliminated slowly [77]. Anti-P1 responsible for an IHTR gave results of up to 22% (normal ≤ 3%) in an indirect monocyte monolayer assay with P1 red cells [75].

Anti-P1 has been found as a separable specificity in the serum of some p people by adsorption with P_2 cells [48]. Anti-P1 has not been reported in any P_2^k individual. Alloanti-P1 in a P_1 pigeon breeder led to the suggestion that the antibody might be directed at a determinant absent from the patient's own P1 antigen [78].

4.4.5.2 Animal anti-P1

The first anti-P1 resulted from immunization of rabbits with human red cells [1]. Since then, anti-P1 has been found as a 'naturally occurring' antibody in rabbits and other animals. Anti-P1 reagents have been made by injecting rabbits or goats with tanned P_2 cells, which had been exposed to HCF [79], with partially purified P1 substance from sheep HCF coupled with a

181

protein from *Shigella shigae* [11], with extracts of earthworms [63], or with soluble ovomucoid from turtle dove eggs [66].

4.4.5.3 Monoclonal anti-P1

Monoclonal antibodies with P1 specificity have been produced by immunizing mice with turtle dove ovomucoid [17], with synthetic glycoproteins containing the P1-trisaccharide (Galα1$\rightarrow$4Galβ1$\rightarrow$4GlcNAc) [19], or with human red cells expressing strong P1 [80]. Agglutination of P1 red cells by monoclonal anti-P1 was inhibited by the P1 trisaccharide and by the disaccharide (Galα1$\rightarrow$4Gal), the former being 200 times more efficient than the latter [17,18]. P1 monoclonal antibodies produced by immunization with P1-trisaccharide bound equally well to the P1-trisaccharide and the P^k-trisaccharide (Galα1$\rightarrow$4Galβ1$\rightarrow$4Glc) [19]. P1 monoclonal antibodies have been analysed at three International Workshops [18,81,82]. One monoclonal antibody, produced by immunizing mice with synthetic glycoprotein containing the P^k-trisaccharide, behaved as anti-P1P^k; it agglutinated P$_1$, P$_1^k$, and P$_2^k$ cells, but not P$_2$ or p cells [19].

4.5 P antigen and anti-P

4.5.1 P antigen

P antigen, the glycolipid globoside (Section 4.3.2.2), is found on all red cells except those of the rare phenotypes p and P^k (Table 4.1 and Sections 4.6 and 4.8). P antigen is expressed equally on cells from P$_1$ and P$_2$ adults [3]. P is well developed at birth, but P$_2$ cord cells have a weaker expression of P than P$_1$ cord cells [83].

Expression of P on other blood cells is controversial. P was detected, by flow cytometry with human alloanti-P, on lymphocytes, granulocytes, and monocytes [58]. With monoclonal anti-P, however, von dem Borne *et al.* [84] could not detect P on granulocytes and most peripheral blood lymphocytes, although they did detect it on endothelial cells and on subsets of platelets, megakaryocytes, and fibroblasts. With a different monoclonal antibody, Shevinsky *et al.* [85] failed to demonstrate P on lymphocytes or fibroblasts. P antigen is found on malignant cells and cell lines derived from them [84–87]. P has also been detected on fetal liver, fetal heart, and on placenta [10].

4.5.2 Anti-P

4.5.2.1 Alloanti-P

Anti-P is found in the serum of all P^k individuals and can be separated from serum of p individuals by adsorption with P$_1^k$ or P$_2^k$ cells [3,88], or by inhibition with HCF [25]. When complement is present, anti-P will haemolyse P$_1$ or P$_2$ cells. Anti-P in the serum of p individuals may be solely IgM [89], but most anti-P sera are IgG and IgM [90–92], and may also contain IgA anti-P [93].

4.5.2.2 Autoanti-P and paroxysmal cold haemoglobinuria

Paroxysmal cold haemoglobinuria (PCH) is a rare form of autoimmune haemolytic anaemia (AIHA), occurring predominantly in young children following viral infections. Sera from patients with PCH usually give a positive Donath–Landsteiner test; i.e. the antibody binds in the presence of complement at 0°C and haemolyses the cells when subsequently warmed (reviewed in [94]). These biphasic haemolysins, or Donath–Landsteiner (DL) antibodies, generally have P specificity [95–97]. Sera from PCH patients react with P$_1$ and P$_2$ red cells, but not with p or P^k cells. Anti-P DL antibody is always IgG [89]. Often the DL test is very weak in PCH and papain-treated red cells [94,98] or acidified sera [99] may be required before a positive result is obtained. Very rarely the specificity of DL antibodies may anti-I, -i, -Pr [98] or 'anti-p' [83, 100] (Section 4.10.1). A few cases of AIHA, one with fatal consequences, were caused by IgG monophasic anti-P, haemolytic at temperatures between 20 and 32°C [101–103]. P autoantibodies only detected in low ionic-strength solution (LISS) at room temperature did not give a positive DL reaction [104,105].

4.5.2.3 Monoclonal anti-P

A rat monoclonal antibody (MC631), raised against mouse embryo, was shown to define a murine stage-specific embryonic antigen, SSEA-3, related to globoside [85]. MC631 was inhibited by the terminal trisaccharide of globoside (GalNAcβ1$\rightarrow$3Galα1$\rightarrow$4Gal) and reacted with P$_1$ and P$_2$ red cells, but not with p or P^k cells [31,36].

An IgM murine monoclonal anti-P, which reacted

with purified globoside, was a relatively weak cold agglutinin, but a strong haemolysin [18,84]. Another murine monoclonal antibody, raised against an *Escherichia coli* immunogen, behaved serologically as anti-P, but was completely inhibited by T-specific immunoadsorbent (Galβ1→3GalNAc-R) [18,32].

4.5.2.4 Lectins

Extracts of salmon, trout, and herring roes react with red cells that have B, P, P1, or P^k antigen; they do not agglutinate O p or A p cells [23,106,107]. These specificities cannot be separated so the extracts are not useful as reagents.

4.6 P^k phenotype, P^k antigen, and anti-P^k

4.6.1 P^k phenotype

Further expansion, increasing the complexity of the P blood groups, occurred with the recognition of another rare phenotype, P^k. Matson *et al.* [3] investigated an anti-Tj^a-like agglutinin in the serum of a woman whose red cells reacted with the serum of p people. Adsorption tests showed that this reaction was caused by a third antibody in serum of p individuals, which they called anti-P^k. The red cell antigen P^k was of particular interest because, unlike most other red cell antigens, it did not appear to be inherited in a dominant manner.

Red cells of all P^k individuals express P^k and lack P. The expression of P^k on red cells of P^k people is uniformly strong regardless of P_1 or P_2 status; the variation in strength of P1 antigen is similar to that of P+ people. All P^k individuals have 'naturally occurring' anti-P in their serum, which reacts equally strongly with P_1 and P_2 cells (Section 4.5.2). Most sera from P^k people react weakly with p cells [88,108], an unexpected observation which has not been explained.

4.6.2 Frequency and inheritance of P^k phenotype

All P^k propositi have been ascertained through anti-P in their sera. No random P^k individual has been reported despite the testing of 28 677 Finnish and 39 939 English donors [48]. This suggests that P^k is even rarer than p. P^k appears less uncommon in Finland and Japan.

The red cells of parents of P^k propositi are not agglutinated by anti-P^k separated from anti-PP1P^k by adsorption with P1 cells, suggestive of recessive inheritance for the P^k phenotype. In family studies, 33 P^k propositi have 21 P^k and 56 not-P^k siblings; good agreement with expectations for a recessive character [48,109,110; personal communications from many colleagues]. The parents of at least seven of the propositi were consanguineous. P^k phenotype has a recessive mode of inheritance because P^k is the precursor for P antigen and is only detected, by conventional serological methods, on red cells of individuals homozygous for the gene responsible for inactive globoside (P) synthase (Section 4.3 and Fig. 4.1).

The normal distribution of $P_1:P_2$ phenotypes for children of P^k propositi had shown that a recessive gene at the *P1* locus was unlikely to be responsible for expression of P^k on red cells. Any possibility of a recessive gene at the *P1* locus was eliminated by a family in which a P_1^k mother and P_2 father had one P_1 and three P_2 children [88].

4.6.3 P^k antigen (CD77)

Initially, red cells of all people other than those with the rare P^k phenotype were thought to lack P^k antigen. Red cells of parents and children of P^k propositi were not agglutinated by anti-P^k (separated from anti-P1PP^k by adsorption with P_1 cells) and adsorption tests appeared to confirm this lack of P^k. Kortekangas *et al.* [111] adsorbed anti-P1PP^k serum with red cells from each of the 18 family members of the second P^k propositus. The strength of anti-P^k left after adsorption with the cells from the parents, both P_1, was similar to that left by adsorption by cells of other P_1 members.

P^k is, however, a public antigen and not, as originally thought, a private antigen. Fellous *et al.* [112] made the surprising observation that P^k was present on the fibroblasts of all P_1 and P_2 individuals, and only absent from those of p people. Then Naiki and Marcus [7] showed that ceramide trihexoside (Gb3), a common glycolipid component of red cell membranes, inhibited anti-P^k (Section 4.3). Naiki and Kato [113] considered that P^k was expressed on P_1 and P_2 red cells and was not a cryptantigen because anti-P1P^k, made by addition of globoside to anti-P1PP^k (to inhibit anti-P), agglutinated P_2 cells. They suggested that this P^k expression on P_2 cells had not been detected before because anti-P^k reagents had been prepared previously by adsorption of anti-PP1P^k with P$_1$ cells, which contain Gb3. Monoclonal anti-P^k, an antibody of high titre, reacts very weakly with P$_1$ and P$_2$ cells [M. Fellous, J-P. Catron, J. Wiels, T. Tursz, unpublished observations], confirming that P^k is present on P+ red cells. Weak expression of P^k on P$_1$ and P$_2$ cells is probably explained by incomplete conversion of Gb3 to globoside (P).

Red cells of P$_1$ LKE– and P$_2$ LKE– people have stronger expression of P^k antigen than those of individuals with the common P$_1$ LKE+ and P$_2$ LKE+ phenotypes, but weaker P^k expression than cells of P$_1^k$ and P$_2^k$ phenotypes, which are always LKE– [114] (Section 4.7).

P^k (also known as CD77) has been detected on lymphocytes, granulocytes, monocytes, platelets, smooth muscle of the digestive track and urogenital system, and in other tissues [115]. P^k is also expressed on malignant cells and cell lines derived from them [28,87,116] and is a useful marker for Burkitt's lymphoma [116]. P^k in B lymphocytes is largely restricted to germinal centre cells and may have a role in B cell differentiation. Ligation of P^k (CD77) to CD19, a B cell-restricted antigen, and their subsequent internalization, appears to be involved in germinal centre B cell apoptosis [117]. There is evidence that P^k is involved in B cell receptor-mediated apoptosis by regulating Lyn kinase activity in B cells and thus participates in the negative selection of germinal centre B cells [118].

4.6.4 Anti-P^k

4.6.4.1 Alloanti-P^k

Alloanti-P^k is found, together with anti-P and -P1, in sera of p people. It can be separated from some of these sera by adsorption with P$_1$ cells [48,108]. These anti-P^k react equally strongly with P$_1^k$ and P$_2^k$ cells [48,88].

The reaction of anti-P^k is completely inhibited by HCF [3,111]. By inhibition of anti-P^k with fractions of HCF prepared by partial acid hydrolysis, and with oligosaccharides of known structure, Watkins and Morgan [25] concluded that anti-P^k was less demanding in its specificity than anti-P1. They found that the disaccharide Galα1$\rightarrow$4Gal purified from the P$_1^k$ glycoprotein of HCF inhibited anti-P^k, as did the P1 trisaccharide (Galα1$\rightarrow$4Galβ1$\rightarrow$4GlcNAc) and other oligosaccharides with terminal Galα1$\rightarrow$4Gal. Anti-

P1P^k, isolated by addition of globoside to anti-PP1P^k, was completely inhibited by P^k glycosphingolipid (Gb3) [113].

4.6.4.2 Autoanti-P^k

Four examples of autoanti-P^k are recorded [48]. One was found in the serum of a P$_1$ woman with AIHA. The other three were found by screening sera of patients, one from 55 patients with AIHA and two from 60 patients with biliary cirrhosis.

4.6.4.3 Monoclonal anti-P^k

A monoclonal antibody (38.13), raised in a rat to a human Burkitt's lymphoma cell line (Daudi) [116], was shown to define the neutral glycolipid Gb3 [28]. Tests against red cells demonstrated the expected anti-P^k specificity: the antibody agglutinated P$_1^k$ and P$_2^k$ cells to a very high titre, reacted very weakly with papain treated P$_1$ and P$_2$ cells, and did not react with p cells. Other monoclonal anti-P^k resulted from immunizing mice with synthetic glycoproteins containing the P^k trisaccharide (Galα1$\rightarrow$4Galβ1$\rightarrow$4Glc) [19], with Gb3 isolated from pig red cells [119], or with an oesophageal squamous cell carcinoma line [115]. One anti-P^k (OSK7) was investigated at an international workshop [81].

4.7 LKE and anti-LKE

The P story was made more complex in 1965 by Tippett et al. [4] when they reported an agglutinating system called Luke. An agglutinin to a high frequency antigen in the serum of Mr Luke P behaved like anti-P because it did not react with p and P^k cells but, unlike anti-P, it also failed to react with the cells of about 2% of P$_1$ and P$_2$ people. In 1985, the monoclonal antibody 813-70, which defined the murine stage-specific embryonic antigen, SSEA-4 [31], was shown to recognize the same red cell antigen as that detected by the antibody in the Luke serum [36]. The red cell antigen was given the symbol LKE [36].

SSEA-4 had been identified as the terminal trisaccharide of a unique globoseries ganglioside NeuAcα2$\rightarrow$3Galβ1$\rightarrow$2GalNAc [31]. This structure is equivalent to the addition to globoside of two sugars, galactose and sialic acid, and thus offers an explanation for the serological specificity of anti-LKE.

4.7.1 Frequency and inheritance of LKE

The frequency of LKE– was about 2% in tests with the original Luke serum [4]. A total of 950 English donors were tested with 813-70 and gave the phenotype frequencies LKE+ 98.84% and LKE– 1.16% [36]. From these the following gene and genotype frequencies were calculated:

LKE^+	0.8923	LKE^+/LKE^+	0.7962
LKE^-	0.1077	LKE^+/LKE^-	0.1922
		LKE^-/LKE^-	0.0116.

Applying these frequencies to the 454 donors tested with the Luke serum [4], the observed figures of 445 LKE+ and nine LKE– do not differ significantly from those expected. Only four LKE– individuals were found among 2400 Scottish blood donors [120], an incidence for LKE– of 0.0017, much lower than in England.

LKE– individuals have been found in various populations: black, English, Italian, French, Scottish, Algerian, Jewish, and Turkish.

LKE appears to be inherited as a Mendelian dominant character. Data from family studies are consistent with dominant inheritance, but are too few to be conclusive. LKE is not controlled by the loci for MNS, P1, Rh, Lu, Kell, Fy, Xg, or Secretor.

4.7.2 Variation in strength of LKE

Variation in strength of reaction of LKE+ cells was observed with the Luke serum [4]. The reactions were classified as LKE+, LKEw, and LKE–. LKEw was more common in P_2 than in P_1, and more common in A_1 and A_1B than in O, A_2, A_2B, and B. Variation in the strength of LKE+ cells was also observed with the monoclonal antibody 813-70, but no effect of P_1 or A_1 was demonstrated [36]. With the monoclonal antibody, LKEw was more common in groups B and AB than in O, A_1, and A_2. These results suggest that LKEw, which had been defined by the Luke serum in 1965, differed from that defined by 813-70 in 1985. It was unfortunate that the two antibodies could not be tested in parallel. The second human anti-LKE did not show any effect of P_1 or ABO groups on the strength of LKE+ reactions.

4.7.3 Development and distribution

Cord red cell samples react well with anti-LKE [36,120]. LKE antigen is not passively acquired from the mother; the child of a P^k LKE– mother was LKE+ [36] as was the child of a P_1 LKE– mother [120]. Monoclonal antibody 813-70 defines a mouse embryonic antigen, SSEA-4, which is also found on human teratoma cell lines [31], signalling the possibility that LKE may be expressed on human embryos.

LKE-active structures were detected in gangliosides isolated from platelets [121].

4.7.4 Involvement of other P antigens

LKE– individuals may be P_1 or P_2. The strength of P1 on P_1 LKE– cells can be very strong or weak depending on the $P1^+$ allele governing it [4]. Parallel testing with anti-P from P^k people and with monoclonal anti-P demonstrated that the strength of P on LKE– cells is the same as that on LKE+ cells [4].

P^k is more strongly expressed on P+ LKE– red cells than on P+ LKE+ red cells [114]. Unlike P_1^k and P_2^k cells, which express P^k equally strongly, P_1 LKE– red cells have stronger P^k expression than P_2 LKE– red cells [120].

4.7.5 Anti-LKE

Five examples of human alloanti-LKE are known. The first was found in the serum of a black patient with a lymphomatous tumour [4]. He had never been transfused. The antibody was an agglutinin; the strength of reaction was increased by incubation at low temperature and by enzyme (trypsin, papain, or ficin) treatment of cells. When fresh, the Luke serum lysed papain-treated LKE+ red cells. The agglutinin was not inhibited by saliva or HCF. Four other examples of alloanti-LKE have been found [120,122], one present together with anti-P1 [122]. LKE+ babies of mothers with anti-LKE had no symptoms of HDN [120,122].

4.8 p Phenotype and anti-PP1P^k

In 1951, Levine *et al.* [123] described an antibody in the serum of a woman with gastric carcinoma, which reacted with all cells except for her own and those of her sister. The antibody was called anti-Tj^a (T for tumour, j for the patient's name). The involvement of Tj^a with the P blood group resulted from Sanger's [2] observation that six unrelated Tj (a–) individuals were P_2. Sanger [2] proposed that Tj(a–) be called p and considered the result of homozygosity for a recessive allele at the *P1* locus.

4.8.1 Frequency and inheritance of p phenotype

The p phenotype is very rare. Race and Sanger [48] calculated a frequency of 0.0024 for the *p* gene, giving a p phenotype frequency of 5.8 per million people of European origin. The p phenotype is more common in Japan [73], but screening of over 1 million Hong Kong Chinese revealed no example of p [124]. In the Vasterbotten country of northern Sweden, eight p individuals were found from screening 40 149 donors with anti-PP1P^k [125]. Allowing for inbreeding, the calculated *p* gene frequency for this part of Sweden is 0.0119 and the p phenotype frequency is about 141 per million.

Information from many families with p propositi supports recessive inheritance of *p* [48,126–129]. The high consanguinity rate of the parents of p propositi also support recessive inheritance. The rare p phenotype has been reported in two generations in some families, all in inbred communities or small isolates [129–132].

4.8.2 Molecular genetics of p phenotype

The p phenotype is associated with homozygosity for mutations in the gene that encodes Gb3 synthase, the enzyme responsible for converting lactosylceramide to P^k (Gb3) [38,39] (Fig. 4.1). In seven p Swedes, the mutation encodes a Met183Lys substitution, though a mutation encoding Gly187Asp was found in one p Swede [38,39]. A Pro251Leu mutation was found in three p Japanese; one other p Japanese was homozygous for a mutation converting the codon for Trp261 to a translation stop codon [39]. Transfection experiments showed that all these mutations resulted in either no enzymatic activity or only marginal activity *in vitro* [39]. Inactivity of Gb3 synthase explains the absence of P^k and P in p phenotype, but not the absence of P1. Possible explanations are provided in Section 4.3.3.

4.8.3 Antibodies in serum of p individuals

All p people have antibody in their serum; this antibody agglutinates and/or haemolyses all red cells except p cells. Sanger [2] showed that anti-P1 was a component in serum of p people; adsorption with P$_2$ cells to remove anti-P left activity against P1 cells.

Later it was realized a third component, anti-P^k, was present, so the antibody in serum of p people is now generally called anti-PP1P^k.

Adsorption of anti-PP1P^k with P$_1$^{k} cells removes anti-P1 and -P^k leaving anti-P [3]; surprisingly, adsorption with P$_2$^{k} cells has the same effect [88]. Specific anti-P^k can be made from only some anti-PP1P^k sera. Tippett [108] adsorbed sera from 47 p people with P$_1$ cells, but only succeeded in making anti-P^k from less than half of these sera, and even with those sera continued adsorption with P$_1$ cells removed or weakened the anti-P^k. Naiki and Kato [113] used complement fixation and haemagglutination tests to investigate the effect of inhibition of four p sera with various glycosphingolipids and concluded that, after inhibition of anti-P with globoside, most of the remaining antibody is cross-reacting anti-P1P^k. This offers an explanation for the inability to isolate anti-P1 from anti-PP1P^k by adsorption with P$_2$^{k} cells. Anti-P1P^k was mostly IgG [113], in contrast to the anti-P1 of P$_2$ people, which is usually IgM. By similar techniques, Kato *et al.* [133] found that most of the anti-P component in the sera of two p individuals was IgM and cross-reacted with Forssman antigen; the rest was IgG and specific for globoside. Most of the anti-P^k in these sera was IgG [133].

IgG and IgA activity to P, P1, and P^k carbohydrate structures, but IgM activity to only P1 and P^k structures, was detected in p sera by radioimmunoassay [134]. All but one of 13 p sera contained IgG3 antibodies to P, P1, and P^k oligosaccharides; some also contained IgG1 and/or IgG2 antibodies, but none contained IgG4 [134]. IgG1 antibodies also bound strongly to A- and H-active globoseries glycosphingolipids (Type 4 A and Type 4 H), probably because of recognition of internal sequences within the carbohydrate chain [134].

Anti-PP1P^k is capable of causing rapid removal of transfused cells; injection of the original p individual with 25 mL of incompatible red cells resulted in a severe haemolytic reaction [123]. Anti-PP1P^k as a potential cause of early abortion and HDN is discussed in Section 4.12.

4.8.4 p Phenotype and cancer

The original p phenotype was in a woman with gastric carcinoma [123]. She was treated by subtotal gastrectomy, which was a complete success and in the 22 years until her death from unrelated causes there was no evidence of tumour recurrence or metastasis [135]. Unlike her red cells, the tumour expressed P system antigens [136], which led Levine [135] to propose his theory of 'illegitimate' antigens, antigens present on tumours contrary to the genetic constitution of the patient. Moreover, Levine suggested that her anti-PP1P^k had prevented further growth of the tumour.

4.9 Some unusual phenotypes

The unexpected presence of an apparent anti-PP1P^k in the serum of a P$_2$ patient, O.H., started a more rigorous investigation of the patient's cells with P antisera [48]. O.H.'s cells were P1– P^k– LKE–, yet they reacted with all of nine anti-P from P^k donors, but with only eight of 12 anti-PP1P^k from p donors, and did not react with anti-P from a PCH patient. The antibody of O.H., which was not an autoantibody, reacted strongly with P$_1$, P$_2$, and P^k cells, but did not react with any of 16 p samples. A similar phenotype was found in a patient who made anti-IP1 and -IP (Section 4.10.2) [137]. The patient's cells were P1– P^k– and had a weaker P antigen than that of control P$_2$ cells. Her I phenotype was also unusual; I^F was normal, I^D was weakened, and i was enhanced (see Chapter 25).

The P$_2$ red cells of a Chinese propositus had much reduced expression of P and reacted weakly with anti-PP1P^k [138]. His serum did not contain a P-related antibody. The globoside and Gb3 content of his red cells was less than 25% of normal and 30–40% of normal, respectively. Kundu et al. [138] suggested this 'new' P phenotype could reflect homozygosity of a defective P^k allele or could be due to a gene at another locus, which inhibits the normal expression of the P^k gene.

An agglutinin, reacting strongly with P$_1$ and P$_2$ red cells and weakly with p cells, revealed an unusual P^k phenotype [139]. The red cells were P1+ P^k+ P–, but biochemical analysis of the red cell membranes revealed that there was only about 50% of the normal quantity of globoside and about 4–6 times the normal quantity of Gb3. The serological phenotype is similar to that of P$_1$ LKE– individuals, but the cells were not tested with anti-LKE. The antibody is P-like and not anti-LKE, because it was inhibited by globoside and reacted weakly with p cells.

4.10 Other P antibodies

4.10.1 'Anti-p'

Three alloantibodies have been described that react strongly with p cells and much more weakly, or not at all, with P$_1$, P$_2$, and P^k cells [21,83,100]. All three antibodies differed slightly in their serological characteristics. One of the antibodies (Fol) [21] was an agglutinin and biphasic haemolysin, which reacted very strongly with p cells, less strongly with P$_2$ and P$_2$^{k} cells, and much less strongly with P$_1$ and P$_1$^{k} cells. The red cell antigen recognized by the Fol antibody was destroyed by sialidase treatment and was identified as sialosylparagloboside [22] (Table 4.2). Schwarting et al. [22] suggested that p red cells accumulate paragloboside and lactosylceramide, which are available for sialylation. Anti-Gd agglutinins that also react with sialic acid dependent antigens do not have the same specificity, although one anti-Gd showed a slight preference for p cells [140]. Anti-Gd is discussed with other cold agglutinins in Chapter 25. Marcus et al. [8] mention two glycolipids with terminal sialosylparagloboside, which inhibit both Fol and anti-Gd. A murine monoclonal antibody (BIRMA-2G4) gave very similar reactions to those of the Fol antibody, but showed enhanced reactivity with sialidase-treated p cells [141].

4.10.2 Anti-IP1, -I^{T}P1, -I^{T}P, and -IP

Issitt et al. [142] described four antibodies, called anti-IP1, which behaved as anti-P1, except they were non-reactive with P1 cord or P1 adult i cells. Booth [143] identified an antibody in a Melanesian as anti-I^{T}P1. Bithermic anti-I^{T}P, identified in a non-Melanesian, behaved as anti-I^T, apart from its failure to agglutinate p cells [144]. Anti-IP, together with anti-IP1, was found in a patient with unusual P and I antigens [137] (see Section 4.9).

4.11 P antigens as receptors for pathogenic microorganisms

4.11.1 Pathogenic bacteria and their toxins

Escherichia coli is responsible for most recurrent urinary tract infections. Uropathogenic *E. coli* attach to uroepithelial cells before they invade them. Adherence is achieved by lectin-like structures called adhesins, encoded by *pap* genes and located on P fimbriae on the bacterial surface. Isolates of uropathogenic *E. coli* expressing *pap*-encoded adhesins bind to globo-series glycoconjugates containing the disaccharide Galα1→4Gal, including P^k, P1, P, LKE (sialosylgalactosylgloboside, SGG), disialosylgalactosylgloboside (DSGG), and globo-A (Type 4 A) (Table 4.2) (reviewed in [145,146]). Red cells of the p phenotype are not agglutinated by pyelonephritogenic *E. coli* fimbriae and the bacteria have impaired adhesion to uroepithelial cells from p individuals [147]. It is possible therefore that women of the p phenotype have enhanced resistance to urinary tract infection and pyelonephritis. Several population studies examining the effect of P1 phenotype on urinary tract infections have produced conflicting results [146].

ABH non-secretor phenotype may also be associated with increased occurrence of recurrent urinary tract infections, although this is not supported by all population studies [146]. Stapleton *et al.* [148] found that uroepithelial cells from non-secretor women showed enhanced adherence to uropathogenic *E. coli* compared to those from secretors. *E. coli* R45 bound to SGG (LKE antigen) and the disialylated form of this antigen (DSGG). These structures are selectively expressed by epithelial cells of non-secretors, presumably as a result of sialylation of the galactosylgloboside precursor, which is fucosylated to globo-H (Type 4 H) in secretors [148].

Some strains of enterohaemorrhagic *E. coli* produce enterotoxins, called verotoxins, which are highly homologous to the Shiga toxin produced by *Shigella dysenteriae*. These verotoxins are associated with diarrhoeal illness and other diseases including haemolytic uraemic syndrome [146]. Terminal Galα1→4Gal disaccharides on P^k and P1 antigens are ligands for verotoxin [149]. Chinese hamster ovary cells that do not express Gb3 (P^k) and are resistant to Shiga verotoxin become susceptible to the toxin following transfection with Gb3 synthase cDNA [40]. A meta-analysis of five separate studies failed to show any protective effect of P1 phenotype on haemolytic uraemic syndrome [150]. Verotoxin may induce apoptosis in Burkitt's lymphoma cells through binding to P^k (CD77) [151] (see Section 4.6.3).

Streptococcus suis, an important pathogen in pigs and a cause of meningitis in humans, binds the Galα1→4Galβ1→4Glc trisaccharide of P^k, although Galα1→4Galβ1→4GlcNAc (P1) is also recognized by

the adhesin [152]. *S. suis* bacteria are more affective at agglutinating P_1^k and P_2^k cells than P_1 and P_2 cells, and do not agglutinate p cells [152].

4.11.2 Viruses

P antigen (globoside) is a cellular receptor for parvovirus B19 [153], a human pathogen that is highly tropic to bone marrow and replicates in erythroid progenitor cells, the only nucleated cells expressing P. B19 is the cause of fifth disease, a common childhood illness, and occasionally more severe disorders of erythropoiesis, particularly in immunocompromised patients [154]. B19 empty capsids agglutinate P_1 and P_2 red cells, but not P^k or p cells. The cytotoxic effect of B19 parvovirus on erythroid colony formation in culture is prevented by sensitizing the cells with monoclonal anti-P (but not with anti-P1 or -P^k); there is no cytotoxicity when cells are derived from a p marrow [153,155]. Dual immunostaining of cells derived from B19-infected bone marrow showed that only cells expressing P antigen also expressed B19 antigen [156]. Individuals with the p phenotype appear to be naturally resistant to parvovirus B19 infection [155].

There is evidence that Gb3 (P^k) may act as a fusion cofactor involved in the entry of human immunodeficiency virus type 1 (HIV-1) [157,158].

4.12 The association of P antibodies with early abortion

The incidence of habitual spontaneous abortion is significantly higher in women with the p phenotype than in the normal population. Many women with the p phenotype have been ascertained because of habitual abortion, although other p women have several live children. Abortions occur characteristically in the first trimester; embryos that survive this critical period usually develop to healthy babies. Most P_1 or P_2 babies of p mothers have no sign of HDN [131,159], although there are a few reports of mild HDN [126,160].

It is almost certain that anti-$PP1P^k$ in the sera of p women is the cause of the abortions [161], but which of the specificities is the causative agent is unknown. Because P1 is strongly expressed on red cells of the early fetus [57], Levine [162] considered anti-P1 the culprit antibody and proposed that p women regularly abort if the fetus receives the father's P1 antigen. Sanger and Tippett [163] pointed out that this hypothesis was unconvincing because of the existence of P_1 children of p mothers. Moreover, the observed ratio of $P_1 : P_2$ children was close to that expected.

Because P^k is present on growing tissues and fetal organs, Kato et al. [133] suggested that anti-P^k might be culpable. They found that 75% of the anti-P^k in the sera of p women were IgG and results from antibody-dependent cell-mediated cytotoxicity assays provided further evidence that anti-P^k may be the responsible antibody [90].

Enzyme-linked and radioimmune assays revealed that sera from almost all p people contain IgG3 antibodies to P, P1, and P^k oligosaccharides and glycosphingolipids [92,134]. IgG3 is known to pass the placenta.

Glycosphingolipid fractions prepared from 12- and 17-week-old fetuses obtained following spontaneous abortions by two p women, had only trace amounts of P and P^k antigen activity, whereas the placental fractions had high P and P^k activity [164]. IgG3 antibodies from the serum of one of the p mothers bound strongly to placental glycolipids, but not to glycolipid fractions from the fetus. The primary target for antibodies in p aborters appears therefore to be the placenta and not the fetus [164].

Initially anti-P did not appear to cause early abortion in P^k women. Children born to P^k mothers were reported to have no sign of HDN or only suffered from mild HDN [109,131]. A P_2^k Japanese woman and a P_1^k Kuwaiti woman, who had suffered four and 13 early abortions, respectively, demonstrated that anti-P can be responsible for abortion [91,165]. Neither had any live children, but in both a procedure of therapeutic plasmapheresis begun at the fifth or sixth week of pregnancy was rewarded by a live birth. Neither baby required any treatment other than phototherapy. IgM, IgG (mostly IgG3), and IgA antibodies, strongly reactive with globoside (P antigen) isolated from placenta, were present in the serum of the Kuwaiti woman [93]. In the Japanese case, autologous plasma was returned to the mother after ex vivo removal of anti-P by adsorption with donor red cells [91]. These plasmapheresis procedures have subsequently been used successfully for p women with a history of multiple abortions and no live children [134,166–168].

An unusual antibody was reported in the serum of 'habitual aborters' (pregnant women who threatened to abort for at least a second time) in Perth, Western Australia [169]. This antibody haemolysed, but did not agglutinate, all P_1 and P_2 red cells, but did not haemolyse or agglutinate p cells. (There is no report of tests with P^k cells.) The patients were of normal P1 groups. The haemolysin was only present at the time of the threatened abortion; it was not found in other pregnant or non-pregnant women [169]. The haemolytic activity did not appear to be complement dependent [170]. The haemolysin was not found in sera of similar patients in Canada, USA, or Hungary [169,171]. Vos [169,170,172,173] exhaustively studied these puzzling patients, looking for an environmental or immunological cause for the phenomenon, but no explanation was forthcoming.

References

1 Landsteiner K, Levine P. Further observations on individual differences of human blood. Proc Soc Exp Biol NY 1927;24:941–2.

2 Sanger R. An association between the P and Jay systems of blood groups. Nature 1955;176:1163–4.

3 Matson GA, Swanson J, Noades J, Sanger R, Race RR. A 'new' antigen and antibody belonging to the P blood group system. Am J Hum Genet 1959;11:26–34.

4 Tippett P, Sanger R, Race RR, Swanson J, Busch S. An agglutinin associated with the P and the ABO blood groups system. Vox Sang 1965;10:269–80.

5 Morgan WTJ, Watkins WM. Blood group P_1 substance. I. Chemical properties. Proc 9th Congr Int Soc Blood Transfus 1962: 225–9.

6 Cory HT, Yates AD, Donald ASR, Watkins WM, Morgan WTJ. The nature of the human blood group P_1 determinant. Biochem Biophys Res Commun 1974;61:1289–96.

7 Naiki M, Marcus DM. Human erythrocyte P and P^k blood group antigens: identification as glycosphingolipids. Biochem Biophys Res Commun 1974; 60:1105–11.

8 Marcus DM, Kundu SK, Suzuki A. The P blood group system: recent progress in immunochemistry and genetics. Semin Hematol 1981;18:63–71.

9 Bailly P, Bouhours J-F. P blood group and related antigens. In: Cartron J-P, Rouger P, eds. Blood Cell Biochemistry, Vol. 6. New York: Plenum Press, 1995:299–329.

10 Spitalnik PF, Spitalnik SL. The P blood group system: biochemical, serological, and clinical aspects. Tranfus Med Rev 1995;9:110–22.

11 Watkins WM, Morgan WTJ. Blood-group P_1 substance. II. Immunological properties. Proc 9th Congr Int Soc Blood Transfus 1962:230–4.

12 Marcus DM. Isolation of a substance with blood-group P_1 activity from human erythrocyte stroma. Transfusion 1971;11:16–18.

13 Anstee DJ, Tanner MJA. The distribution of blood-

group antigens on butanol extraction of human erythrocyte 'ghosts'. *Biochem J* 1974;138:381–6.

14 Yang Z, Bergström J, Karlsson K-A. Glycoproteins with Galα4Gal are absent from human erythrocyte membranes, indicating that glycolipids are the sole carriers of blood group P activities. *J Biol Chem* 1994;269: 14620–4.

15 Naiki M, Fong J, Ledeen R, Marcus DM. Structure of the human erythrocyte blood group P_1 glycosphingolipid. *Biochemistry* 1975;14:4831–7.

16 Naiki M, Marcus DM. An immunochemical study of the human blood group P_1, P, and P^k glycosphingolipid antigens. *Biochemistry* 1975;14:4837–41.

17 Bailly P, Chevaleyre J, Sondag D *et al.* Characterization of a murine monoclonal antibody specific for the human P1 blood group antigen. *Mol Immunol* 1987;24:171–6.

18 Rouger P, Anstee D, Salmon C, eds. First International Workshop on Monoclonal Antibodies Against Human Red Blood Cell and Related Antigens. *Rev Franc Transfus Immuno-Hémat* 1987;30:627–708.

19 Brodin NT, Dahmén J, Nilsson B *et al.* Monoclonal antibodies produced by immunization with neoglycoproteins containing Galα1–4Galβ1–4Glcβ-O and Galα1–4Galβ1–4GlcNAcβ-O residues: useful immunochemical and cytochemical reagents for blood group P antigens and a differentiation marker in Burkitt lymphoma and other B-cell malignancies. *Int J Cancer* 1988;42:185–94.

20 Cowles JW, Blumberg N. Neutralization of P blood group antibodies by synthetic solid-phase antigens. *Transfusion* 1987;27:272–5.

21 Metaxas MN, Metaxas-Buehler M, Tippett P. A 'new' antibody in the P blood group system [Abstract]. *14th Congr International Soc Blood Transfus* 1975:95.

22 Schwarting GA, Marcus DM, Metaxas M. Identification of sialosylparagloboside as the erythrocyte receptor for an 'anti-p' antibody. *Vox Sang* 1977;32:257–61.

23 Voak D, Anstee D, Pardoe G. The α-galactose specificity of anti-P^k. *Vox Sang* 1973;25:263–70.

24 Furukawa K. Properties of P blood group antigen and antibodies. *Jpn J Hum Genet* 1975;20:32–3.

25 Watkins WM, Morgan WTJ. Immunochemical observations on the human blood group P system. *J Immunogenet* 1976;3:15–27.

26 Marcus DM, Naiki M, Kundu SK. Abnormalities in the glycosphingolipid content of human P^k and p erythrocytes. *Proc Natl Acad Sci USA* 1976;73:3263–7.

27 Koscielak J, Miller-Prodraza H, Krauze R, Cedergren B. Glycolipid composition of blood group P erythrocytes. *FEBS Lett* 1976;66:250–3.

28 Nudelman E, Kannagi R, Hakomori S *et al.* A glycolipid antigen associated with Burkitt lymphoma defined by a monoclonal antibody. *Science* 1983;220:509–11.

29 Fletcher KS, Bremer EG, Schwarting GA. P blood group regulation of glycosphingolipid levels in human erythrocytes. *J Biol Chem* 1979;254:11196–8.

30 Anstee DJ. Blood group-active surface molecules of the human red blood cell. *Vox Sang* 1990;58:1–20.

31 Kannagi R, Cochran NA, Ishigami F *et al.* Stage-specific embryonic antigens (SSEA-3 and -4) are epitopes of a unique globo-series ganglioside isolated from human teratocarcinoma cells. *EMBO J* 1983;2:2355–61.

32 Inglis G, Fraser RH, Mitchell AAB *et al.* Serological characterisation of a mouse monoclonal anti-P-like antibody. *Vox Sang* 1987;52:79–82.

33 Kundu SK, Suzuki A, Sabo B *et al.* Erythrocyte glycosphingolipids of four siblings with the rare blood group, p phenotype and their parents. *J Immunogenet* 1981;8:357–65.

34 Wiels J, Taga S, Tétaud C *et al.* Histo-blood group p: biosynthesis of globoseries glycolipids in EBV-transformed B cell lines. *Glycocon J* 1996;13:529–35.

35 Lindström K, Jovall P-Å, Ghardashkani S, Samuelsson BE, Breimer ME. Blood group glycosphingolipid expression in kidney of an individual with the rare blood group A_1 Le(a–b+) p phenotype: absence of blood group structures based on the globoseries. *Glycocon J* 1996;13:307–13.

36 Tippett P, Andrews PW, Knowles BB, Solter D, Goodfellow PN. Red cell antigens P (globoside) and Luke: identification by monoclonal antibodies defining the murine stage-specific embryonic antigens -3 and -4 (SSEA-3 and SSEA-4). *Vox Sang* 1986;51:53–6.

37 Fellous M, Gerbal A, Nobillot G, Weils J. Studies on the biosynthetic pathway of human P erythrocyte antigen using genetic complementation tests between fibroblasts from rare, p and P^k phenotype donors. *Vox Sang* 1977;32:262–8.

38 Steffenson R, Carlier K, Wiels J *et al.* Cloning and expression of the histo-blood group P^k UDP-galactose: Galβ1–4Glcβ1-Cer α1,4-Galactosyltransferase—molecular basis of the p phenotype. *J Biol Chem* 2000;275:16723–9.

39 Furukawa K, Iwamura K, Uchikawa M *et al.* Molecular basis for the p phenotype: identification of distinct and multiple mutations in the α1,4-Galactosyltransferase gene in Swedish and Japanese individuals. *J Biol Chem* 2000;275:37752–6.

40 Keusch JJ, Manzella SM, Nyame KA, Cummings RD, Baenziger JU. Cloning of Gb3 synthase, the key enzyme in globo-series glycosphingolipid synthesis, predicts a family of α1,4-glycosyltransferases conserved in plants, insects and mammals. *J Biol Chem* 2000; 275:25315–21.

41 Okajima T, Nakamura Y, Uchikawa M *et al.* Expression cloning of human globoside synthase cDNAs: identification of β3Gal-T3 as UDP-N-acetylgalactosamine: globotriosylceramide β1,3-N-acetylgalactosaminyltransferase. *J Biol Chem* 2000;275:40498–503.

42 Amado M, Almeida R, Carneiro F *et al.* A family of human β3-galactosyltransferases. Characterization of four members of a UDP-galactose:β-N-acetyl-

glucosamine/β-N-acetyl-galactosamine β-1,3-galacto-syltransferase family. *J Biol Chem* 1998;**273**:12770–8.

43 Kijimoto-Ochiai S, Naiki M, Makita A. Defects of glycosyltransferase activities in human fibroblasts of P^k and, p blood group phenotypes. *Proc Natl Acad Sci USA* 1977;**74**:5407–10.

44 Graham HA, Williams AN. A genetic model for the inheritance of the P, P$_1$ and P^k antigens. *Immunol Commun* 1980;**9**:191–201.

45 Almeida R, Amado M, David L *et al*. A family of human β4-galactosyltransferases: cloning and expression of two novel UDP-galactose:β-N-acetylglucosamine β1, 4-galactosyltransferases, β4Gal-T2 and β4Gal-T3. *J Biol Chem* 1997;**272**:31979–91.

46 Iizuka S, Chen S-H, Yoshida A. Studies on the human blood group P system: an existence of UDP-Gal:Lacto-sylceramide α1→4 galactosyltransferase in the small p type cells. *Biochem Biophys Res Commun* 1986;**137**:1187–95.

47 Mourant AE, Kopec AC, Domaniewska-Sobczak K. *The Distribution of Human Blood Groups and Other Polymorphisms*, 2nd edn. London: Oxford University Press, 1976.

48 Race RR, Sanger R. *Blood Groups in Man*, 6th edn. Oxford: Blackwell Scientific Publications, 1975.

49 Henningsen K. Investigations on the blood factor P. *Acta Path Microbiol Scand* 1949;**26**:639–54.

50 Henningsen K. On the heredity of blood factor P. *Acta Path Microbiol Scand* 1949;**26**:769–85.

51 Henningsen K. Etude d'ensemble du facteur sanguin P. *Rev Hémat* 1950;**5**:276–84.

52 Fisher R. The variation in strength of the human blood group P. *Heredity* 1953;**7**:81–9.

53 Crawford MN, Tippett P, Sanger R. Antigens Au^a, i and P$_1$ of cells of the dominant type of Lu(a–b–). *Vox Sang* 1974;**26**:283–7.

54 Shaw MA, Leak MR, Daniels GL, Tippett P. The rare Lutheran blood group phenotype Lu(a–b–): a genetic study. *Ann Hum Genet* 1984;**48**:229–37.

55 Contreras M, Tippett P. The Lu (a–b–) syndrome and an apparent upset of P$_1$ inheritance. *Vox Sang* 1974;**27**:369–71.

56 Heiken A. Observations on the blood group receptor P$_1$ and its development in children. *Hereditas* 1966; **56**:83–98.

57 Ikin EW, Kay HEM, Playfair JHL, Mourant AE. P$_1$ antigen in the human foetus. *Nature* 1961;**192**:883.

58 Dunstan RA. Status of major red cell blood group antigens on neutrophils, lymphocytes and monocytes. *Br J Haematol* 1986;**62**:301–9.

59 Cameron GL, Staveley JM. Blood group P substance in hydatid cyst fluids. *Nature* 1957;**179**:147–8.

60 Ben-Ismail R, Rouger P, Carme B, Gentilini M, Salmon C. Comparative automated assay of anti-P$_1$ antibodies in acute hepatic distomiasis (fascioliasis) and in hydatidosis. *Vox Sang* 1980;**38**:165–8.

61 Bevan B, Hammond W, Clarke RL. Anti-P$_1$ associated with liver-fluke infection. *Vox Sang* 1970;**18**:188–9.

62 Petit A, Duong TH, Bremond JL *et al*. Allo-anticorps irréguliers anti-P$_1$ et Clonorchiase à clonorchis sinensis. *Rev Franc Transfus Immuno-Hémat* 1981;**24**:197–208.

63 Prokop O, Schlesinger D. P$_1$ blood group substance in *Lumbricus terrestris* (earthworm) and *Ascaris suum*. *Nature* 1966;**209**:1255.

64 Radermecker M, Bruwier M, François C *et al*. Anti-P$_1$ activity in pigeon breeders' serum. *Clin Exp Immunol* 1975;**22**:546–9.

65 François-Gerard C, Gerday C, Beeley JG. Turtledove ovomucoid, a glycoprotein proteinase inhibitor with P$_1$-blood-group antigen activity. *Biochem J* 1979;**177**:679–85.

66 François-Gérard C, Brocteur J, André A. Turtledove: a new source of P$_1$-like material cross-reacting with the human erythrocyte antigen. *Vox Sang* 1980;**39**: 141–8.

67 François-Gerard C, Brocteur J, Andre A *et al*. Demonstration of the existence of a specific blood-group P$_1$ antigenic determinant in turtle-dove ovomucoid. *Rev Franc Transfus Immuno-Hémat* 1980;**23**:579–88.

68 Khoo K-H, Nieto A, Morris HR, Dell A. Structural characterization of the N-glycans from *Echinococcus granulosus* hydatid cyst membrane and protoscoleces. *Mol Biochem Parasitol* 1997;**86**:237–48.

69 Wiener AS, Unger LJ. Isoimmunization to factor P by blood transfusion. *Am J Clin Pathol* 1944;**14**:616–8.

70 Cheng MS. Potent anti-P$_1$ following blood transfusion. *Transfusion* 1984;**24**:183.

71 Chandeysson PL, Flye MW, Simpkins SM, Holland PV. Delayed hemolytic transfusion reaction caused by anti-P$_1$ antibody. *Transfusion* 1981;**21**:77–82.

72 Cox MT, Roberts M, LaJoie J *et al*. An apparent primary immune response involving anti-Jk^a and anti-P$_1$ detected 10 days after transfusion. *Transfusion* 1992;**32**:874.

73 Issitt PD, Anstee DJ. *Applied Blood Group Serology*, 4th edn. Durham, NC: Montgomery Scientific Publications, 1998.

74 Moureau P. Les réactions post-transfusionnelles. *Rev Belge Sci Med* 1945;**16**:258–300.

75 Arndt PA, Garratty G, Marfoe RA, Zeger GD. An acute hemolytic transfusion reaction caused by an anti-P$_1$ that reacted at 37°C. *Transfusion* 1998;**38**:373–7.

76 DiNapoli JB, Nichols ME, Marsh WL, Warren D, Mayer K. Hemolytic transfusion reaction caused by IgG anti-P$_1$ [Abstract]. *Transfusion* 1978;**18**:383.

77 Mollison PL, Cutbush M. The use of isotope-labelled red cells to demonstrate incompatibility *in vivo*. *Lancet* 1955;**i**:1290–5.

78 Norman P, MacIntyre D, Poole J, Mallan M. Allo-anti-P1 in a P1-positive person. *Vox Sang* 1985;**49**:211–14.

79 Levine P, Celano M, Staveley JM. The antigenicity of P

substance in *Echinococcus* cyst fluid coated on to tanned red cells. *Vox Sang* 1958;**3**:434–8.

80 Bouhours D, Bouhours JF, Willem C, Planus E, Blanchard D. Over expression of the P1 blood group antigen on red cells from a CDAII patient [Abstract]. *Vox Sang* 1994;**67**(Suppl. 2):118.

81 Chester MA, Johnson U, Lundblad A *et al.*, eds. *Proc 2nd Int Workshop and Symposium on Monoclonal Antibodies Against Human Red Blood Cells and Related Antigens* 1990, 86–92.

82 Beck ML, ed. Third International Workshop on Monoclonal Antibodies Against Human Red Blood Cell and Related Antigens. *Transfus Clin Biol* 1997;**4**:13–54 (8 papers).

83 Issitt CH, Duckett JB, Osborne BM, Gut JB, Beasley J. Another example of an antibody reacting optimally with p red cells. *Br J Haematol* 1976;**34**:19–23.

84 von dem Borne AEGK, Bos MJE, Joustra-Maas N *et al.* A murine monoclonal IgM antibody specific for blood group P antigen (globoside). *Br J Haematol* 1986;**63**:35–46.

85 Shevinsky LH, Knowles BB, Damjanov I, Solter D. Monoclonal antibody to murine embryos defines a stage-specific embryonic antigen expressed on mouse embryos and human teratocarcinoma cells. *Cell* 1982;**30**:697–705.

86 Kelus A, Gurner BW, Coombs RRA. Blood group antigens on HeLa cells shown by mixed agglutination. *Immunology* 1959;**2**:262–7.

87 Bono R, Cartron JP, Mulet C, Avner P, Fellous M. Selective expression of blood group antigens on human teratocarcinoma cell lines. *Rev Franc Transfus Immuno-Hémat* 1981;**24**:97–107.

88 Kortekangas AE, Kaarsalo E, Melartin L *et al.* The red cell antigen P^k and its relationship to the P system: the evidence of three more P^k families. *Vox Sang* 1965;**10**:385–404.

89 Adinolfi M, Polley MJ, Hunter DA, Mollison PL. Classification of blood-group antibodies as β2M or gamma globulin. *Immunology* 1962;**5**:566–79.

90 Lopez M, Cartron J, Cartron JP *et al.* Cytotoxicity of anti-PP_1P^k antibodies and possible relationship with early abortions of p mothers. *Clin Immunol Immunopath* 1983;**28**:296–303.

91 Yoshida H, Ito K, Emi N, Kanzaki H, Matsuura S. A new therapeutic antibody removal method using antigen-positive red cells. II. Application to a P-incompatible pregnant woman. *Vox Sang* 1984;**47**:216–23.

92 Söderström T, Enskog A, Samuelsson BE, Cedergren B. Immunoglobulin subclass (IgG3) restriction of anti-P and anti-P^k antibodies in patients of the rare p blood group. *J Immunol* 1985;**134**:1–3.

93 Hansson GC, Wazniowska K, Rock JA *et al.* The glycosphingolipid composition of the placenta of a blood group P fetus delivered by a blood group P_1^k woman and analysis of the anti-globoside antibodies found in maternal serum. *Arch Biochem Biophys* 1988;**260**: 168–76.

94 Heddle NM. Acute paroxysmal cold hemoglobinuria. *Transfus Med Rev* 1989;**3**:219–29.

95 Levine P, Celano MJ, Falkowski F. The specificity of the antibody in paroxysmal cold hemoglobinuria (PCH). *Transfusion* 1963;**3**:278–80.

96 van der Hart M, van der Giessen M, van der Veer M, Peetoom F, van Loghem JJ. Immunochemical and serological properties of biphasic haemolysins. *Vox Sang* 1964;**9**:36–9.

97 Worlledge SM, Rousso C. Studies on the serology of paroxysmal cold haemoglobinuria (PCH), with special reference to its relationship with the P blood group system. *Vox Sang* 1965;**10**:293–8.

98 Sokol RJ, Booker DJ, Stamps R. Paroxysmal cold hemoglobinuria and the elusive Donath–Landsteiner antibody. *Immunohematology* 1998;**14**:109–12.

99 Judd WJ. A pH-dependent auto-agglutinin with anti-P specificity. *Transfusion* 1975;**15**:373–6.

100 Engelfriet CP, von Beckers D, dem Borne AEGK, Reynierse E, van Loghem JJ. Haemolysins probably recognizing the antigen p. *Vox Sang* 1971;**23**:176–81.

101 Ries CA, Garratty G, Petz LD, Fudenberg HH. Paroxysmal cold hemoglobinuria: report of a case with an exceptionally high thermal range Donath–Landsteiner antibody. *Blood* 1971;**38**:491–9.

102 Lindgren S, Zimmerman S, Gibbs F, Garratty G. An unusual Donath–Landsteiner antibody detectable at 37°C by the antiglobulin test. *Transfusion* 1985;**25**:142–4.

103 Mensinger E, Lerner W, Leger R *et al.* Serological profile associated with a fatal case of paroxysmal cold hemoglobinuria [Abstract]. *Transfusion* 1995;**35**:21S.

104 Judd WJ, Steiner EA, Capps RD. Autoagglutinins with apparent anti-P specificity reactive only by low-ionic-strength salt techniques. *Transfusion* 1982;**22**: 185–8.

105 Cohen DW, Nelson L. Auto-anti-P reacting only by low-ionic-strength solutions in a patient with hemolysis. *Transfusion* 1983;**23**:79–80.

106 Anstee DJ, Holt PDJ, Pardoe GJ. Agglutinins from fish ova defining blood groups B and P. *Vox Sang* 1973;**25**:347–60.

107 Voak D, Todd GM, Pardoe GI. A study of the serological behaviour and nature of the anti-B/P/P^k activity of *Salmonidae* roe protectins. *Vox Sang* 1974;**26**:176–88.

108 Tippett P. Antibodies in the sera of p and P^k people. *Abstracts from 14th Congr Int Soc Blood Transfus* 1975: 94.

109 Nakagima H, Yokota T. Two Japanese families with P^k members. *Vox Sang* 1977;**32**:56–8.

110 Moullec J, Muller A, Garretta M, Kerouanton F, Bare J. L'antigène P^k chez trois membres d'une même fratrie. *Ann Génét* 1974;**2**:95–8.

111 Kortekangas AE, Noades J, Tippett P, Sanger R, Race RR. A second family with the red cell antigen P^k. *Vox Sang* 1959;**4**:337–49.

112 Fellous M, Gerbal A, Tessier C *et al*. Studies on the biosynthetic pathway of human P erythrocyte antigens using somatic cells in culture. *Vox Sang* 1974;26:518–36.

113 Naiki M, Kato M. Immunological identification of blood group Pk antigen on normal human erythrocytes and isolation of anti-Pk with different affinity. *Vox Sang* 1979;37:30–8.

114 Tippett P. Contributions of monoclonal antibodies to understanding one new and some old blood group systems. In: Garratty G, ed. *Red Cell Antigens and Antibodies*. Arlington: American Association of Blood Banks, 1986, 83–98.

115 Kasai K, Galton J, Terasaki PI *et al*. Tissue distribution of the P^k antigen as determined by a monoclonal antibody. *J Immunogenet* 1985;12:213–20.

116 Wiels J, Fellous M, Tursz T. Monoclonal antibody against a Burkitt lymphoma-associated antigen. *Proc Natl Acad Sci USA* 1981;78:6485–8.

117 Khine A-A, Firtel M, Lingwood CA. CD77-dependent retrograde transport of CD19 to the nuclear membrane: functional relationship between CD77 and CD19 during germinal center B-cell apoptosis. *J Cell Physiol* 1998;176:281–92.

118 Mori T, Kiyokawa N, Katagiri YU *et al*. Globotriaosyl ceramide (CD77/Gb$_3$) in the glycolipid-enriched membrane domain participates in B-cell receptor-mediated apoptosis by regulating Lyn kinase activity in human B cells. *Exp Hematol* 2000;28:1260–8.

119 Miyamoto D, Ueno T, Takashima S *et al*. Establishment of a monoclonal antibody directed against Gb$_3$Cer/CD77: a useful immunochemical reagent for a differentiation marker in Burkitt's lymphoma and germinal centre B cells. *Glycocon J* 1997;14:379–88.

120 Bruce M, Watt A, Gabra GS *et al*. LKE red cell antigen and its relationship to P$_1$ and P^k: serological study of a large family. *Vox Sang* 1988;55:237–40.

121 Cooling LLW, Zhang D, Koerner TAW. Human platelets express gangliosides with LKE activity and ABH blood group activity. *Transfusion* 2001;41:504–16.

122 Møller B, Jørgensen J. Anti-LKE in a pregnant woman. *Transfusion* 1988;28:88.

123 Levine P, Bobbitt OB, Waller RK, Kuhmichel A. Isoimmunization by a new blood factor in tumor cells. *Proc Soc Exp Biol NY* 1951;77:403–5.

124 Lin CK, Mak KH, Cheng CK, Yang CP. The first case of the p phenotype in a Ghurka Nepalese. *Immunohematology* 1998;14:30–2.

125 Cedergren B. Population studies in northern Sweden. IV. Frequency of the blood type P. *Hereditas* 1973;73:27–30.

126 Levene C, Sela R, Rudolphson Y *et al*. Hemolytic disease of the newborn due to anti-PP$_1$P^k (anti-Tj^a). *Transfusion* 1977;17:569–72.

127 Cantin G, Lyonnais J. Anti-PP$_1$P^k and early abortion. *Transfusion* 1983;23:350–1.

128 Weiss DB, Levene C, Aboulafia Y, Isacsohn M. Anti-PP$_1$P^k (anti-Tj^a) and habitual abortion. *Fertil Steril* 1975;26:901–4.

129 Salmon D, Bouchmel S, Hafsia A *et al*. p phenotypes observed in two generations of tunisian family with a high rate of inbreeding. *Rev Franc Transfus Immuno-Hémat* 1979;22:563–70.

130 Catino ML, Busch S, Huestis DW, Stern K. Transmission of the blood group genotype *pp* (Tj^a-negative) in a kinship with multiple consanguineous marriages. *Am J Hum Genet* 1965;17:36–41.

131 Yamaguchi H, Okubo Y, Tanaka M, Murakami W, Honkawa T. Rare blood type p and P^k in Japanese families. *Proc Jpn Acad* 1974;50:764–7.

132 Miwa S, Matuhasi T, Yasuda J. The p phenotype in two successive generations of a Japanese family. *Vox Sang* 1974;26:565–7.

133 Kato M, Kubo S, Naiki M. Complement fixation antibodies to glycosphingolipids in sera of rare blood group p and P^k phenotypes. *J Immunogenet* 1978;5:31–40.

134 Rydberg L, Cedergren B, Breimer ME *et al*. Serological and immunochemical characterization of anti-PP$_1$P^k (anti-Tj^a) antibodies in blood group p individuals: blood group A Type 4 recognition due to internal binding. *Mol Immunol* 1992;29:1273–86.

135 Levine P. Illegitimate blood group antigens P$_1$, A, and MN (T) in malignancy: a possible therapeutic approach with anti-Tj^a, anti-A, and anti-T. *Ann NY Acad Sci* 1976;277:428–35.

136 Kannagi R, Levine P, Watanabe K, Hakomori S. Recent studies of glycolipid and glycoprotein profiles and characterization of the major glycolipid antigen in gastric cancer of a patient of blood group phenotype (Tj^a–) first studied in 1951. *Cancer Res* 1982;42:5249–54.

137 Allen FH, Marsh WL, Jensen L, Fink J. Anti IP: an antibody defining another product of interaction between the genes of the I and P blood group systems. *Vox Sang* 1974;27:442–6.

138 Kundu SK, Steane SM, Bloom JEC, Marcus DM. Abnormal glycolipid composition of erythrocytes with a weak P antigen. *Vox Sang* 1978;35:160–7.

139 Kundu SK, Evans A, Rizvi J, Glidden H, Marcus DM. A new P^k phenotype in the P blood group system. *J Immunogenet* 1980;7:431–9.

140 Roelcke D, Riesen W, Geisen HP, Ebert W. Serological identification of the new cold agglutinin specificity anti-Gd. *Vox Sang* 1977;33:304–6;372.

141 McDonald DF, Thompson JM, Lowe JA. A murine monoclonal antibody agglutinates P$_1$–ve cord blood red cells and detects an antigen expressed preferentially by adult red cells of pp phenotype [Abstract]. *Transfus Med* 1996;6(Suppl. 2):25.

142 Issitt PD, Tegoli J, Jackson V, Sanders CW, Allen FH. Anti IP$_1$: antibodies that show an association between the I and P blood group systems. *Vox Sang* 1968;14:1–8.

143 Booth PB. Anti I^{T}P$_1$: an antibody showing a further as-

sociation between the I and P blood group systems. *Vox Sang* 1970;19:85–90.

144 Ramos RR, Curtis BR, Eby CS, Ratkin GA, Chaplin H. Fatal outcome in a patient with autoimmune hemolytic anemia associated with an IgM bithermic anti-I^{T}P. *Transfusion* 1994;34:427–31.

145 Moulds JM, Nowicki S, Moulds JJ, Nowicki BJ. Human blood groups: incidental receptors for viruses and bacteria. *Transfusion* 1996;36:362–4.

146 Eder AF, Spitalnik SL. Blood group antigens as receptors for pathogens. In: A Blancher, J Klein, WW Socha, eds. *Molecular Biology and Evolution of Blood Group and MHC Antigens in Primates.* Berlin: Springer-Verlag 1997, 268–304.

147 Källenius G, Svenson SB, Möllby R et al. Structure of carbohydrate part of receptor on human uroepithelial cells for pyelonephritogenic *Escherichia coli. Lancet* 1981;ii:604–6.

148 Stapleton A, Nudelman E, Clausen H, Hakomori S, Stamm WE. Binding of uropathogenic *Escherichia coli* R45 to glycolipids extracted from vaginal epithelial cells is dependent on histo-blood group secretor status. *J Clin Invest* 1992;90:965–72.

149 Lingwood CA, Law H, Richardson S et al. Glycolipid binding of purified and recombinant *Escherichia coli* produced verotoxin *in vitro. J Biol Chem* 1987;262:8834–9.

150 Green DA. P1 blood group and haemolytic uraemic syndrome. *Clin Lab Haematol* 2000;22:55.

151 Mangeney M, Lingwood CA, Taga S et al. Apoptosis induced in Burkitt's lymphoma cells via Gb3/CD77, a glycolipid antigen. *Cancer Res* 1993;53:5314–9.

152 Haataja S, Tikkanen K, Liukkonen J, François-Gerard C, Finne J. Characterization of a novel bacterial adhesin specificity of *Streptococcus suis* recognizing blood group P receptor oligosaccharides. *J Biol Chem* 1993;268:4311–7.

153 Brown KE, Anderson SM, Young NS. Erythrocyte P antigen: cellular receptor for B19 parvovirus. *Science* 1993;262:114–17.

154 Brown KE. Haematological consequences of parvovirus B19 infection. *Baillière's Best Pract Res Clin Haematol* 2000;13:245–59.

155 Brown KE, Hibbs JR, Gallinella G et al. Resistance to parvovirus B19 infection due to lack of virus receptor (erythrocyte P antigen). *N Engl J Med* 1994; 330:1192–6.

156 Kerr JR, McQuaid S, Coyle PV. Expression of P antigen in parvovirus B19-infected bone marrow. *N Engl J Med* 1995;332:128.

157 Puri A, Hug P, Jernigan K et al. The neutral glycosphingolipid globotriaosylceramide promotes fusion mediated by a CD4-dependent CXCR4-utilizing HIV type 1 envelope glycoprotein. *Proc Natl Acad Sci USA* 1998;95:14435–40.

158 Hammache D, Yahi N, Maresca M, Piéroni G, Fantini J. Human erythrocytes glycosphingolipids as alternative cofactors for human immunodeficiency virus type 1 (HIV-1) gp120 and reconstituted membrane microdomains of glycosphingolipids (Gb3 and GM3). *J Virol* 1999;73:5244–8.

159 Sheehan J, Pochedley M, Toy E. A retrospective study of cord blood samples from infants born to p phenotype mothers [Abstracts]. *Joint Congr Int Soc Blood Transfus and Am Assoc Blood Banks*, 1990: 84.

160 Hayashida Y, Watanabe A. A case of p Taiwanese woman delivered of an infant with hemolytic disease of the newborn. *Jpn J Legal Med* 1968;22:10–15.

161 Levine P, Koch EA. The rare human isoagglutinin anti-Tj^a and habitual abortion. *Science* 1954;120:239–41.

162 Levine P. Comments on hemolytic disease of newborn due to anti-PP$_1$P^k (anti-Tj^a). *Transfusion* 1977; 17:573–8.

163 Sanger R, Tippett P. Live children and abortions of p mothers. *Transfusion* 1979;19:222–3.

164 Lindström K, dem Borne AEGK, Breimer ME et al. Glycosphingolipid expression in spontaneously aborted fetuses and placenta from blood group p women: evidence for placenta being the primary target for anti-Tj^a-antibodies. *Glycocon J* 1992;9:325–9.

165 Shirey RS, Ness PM, Kickler TS et al. The association of anti-P and early abortion. *Transfusion* 1987;27: 189–91.

166 Shechter Y, Timor-Tritsch IE, Lewit N, Sela R, Levene C. Early treatment by plasmapheresis in a woman with multiple abortions and the rare blood group p. *Vox Sang* 1987;53:135–8.

167 Yoshida H, Ito K, Kusakari T et al. Removal of maternal antibodies from a woman with fetal loss due to P blood group incompatability. *Transfusion* 1994;34:702–5.

168 Fernández-Jiménez MC, Jiménez-Marco MT, Hernández D et al. Treatment with plasmapheresis and intravenous immunoglobulin in pregnancies complicated with anti-PP$_1$P^k or anti-K immunization: a report of two patients. *Vox Sang* 2001;80:117–20.

169 Vos GH, Celano MJ, Falkowski F, Levine P. Relationship of a hemolysin resembling anti-Tj^a to threatened abortion in Western Australia. *Transfusion* 1964;4:87–91.

170 Vos GH. The serology of anti-Tj^a-like hemolysins observed in the serum of threatened aborters in Western Australia. *Acta Haematol* 1966;35:272–83.

171 Horváth E, Paisz I. Absence of anti-Tj^a-like hemolysin in pregnant aborters in Budapest. *Transfusion* 1966;6:499–500.

172 Vos GH. A comparative observation of the presence of anti-Tj^a-like hemolysins in relation to obstetric history, distribution of the various blood groups and the occurrence of immune anti-A or anti-B hemolysins among aborters and nonaborters. *Transfusion* 1965;5:327–35.

173 Vos GH. A study related to the significance of hemolysins observed among aborters, nonaborters and infertility patients. *Transfusion* 1967;7:40–7.

5 Rh blood group system

5.1 Introduction

Rh is the most complex of the blood group systems, comprising 46 antigens numbered RH1 to RH53 with seven numbers obsolete (Table 5.1). The Rh antigens are encoded by two homologous, closely linked, genes on the short arm of chromosome 1 (Chapter 32): *RHD*, producing the D antigen, and *RHCE*, producing the Cc and Ee antigens. *RHD* and *RHCE* encode RhD (CD240D) and RhCcEe (CD240CE), highly hydrophobic, non-glycosylated proteins, which span the red cell membrane 12 times. Rh antigens are very dependent on the conformation of the Rh proteins in the membrane and may involve interactions between two or more extracellular loops.

The first discovered and clinically most important antigen is D (RH1). D is often referred to as the Rh or rhesus antigen, because it was initially thought to be the same as the antigen, now called LW, defined by antibodies produced in rabbits immunized with rhesus monkey red cells (Section 5.2). D is present on red cells of about 85% of white people and is more frequent in Africans and Asians. Before the introduction of the anti-D immunoglobulin prophylaxis programme, anti-D was a common cause of severe haemolytic disease of the newborn (HDN) (Section 5.18.1.3).

Although most people are either D+ or D–, variants of D exist, some resulting in weak expression of the D antigen, others representing a variety of qualitative differences in which D+ people may make a D-like antibody (Section 5.6). D– phenotype occurs from the absence of the RhD protein from the red cell membrane. In white people, D– is usually a result of homozygosity for a deletion of *RHD*, but in D– Africans inactive *RHD* is common.

C and c, and E and e, represent two pairs of antithetical antigens; polymorphisms controlled by *RHCE*. As no recombination between D, Cc, and Ee has been disclosed, the alleles are inherited as haplotypes denoted *DCe*, *DcE*, *dce*, etc. (where *d* represents an *RHD* deletion or any inactive *RHD* gene). From serological results it is often impossible to determine the true genotype of an individual and phenotypes are often symbolized as the most probable genotype deduced from known haplotype frequencies. It is important to remember that DCe/dce, for example, is a phenotype; although *DCe/dce* is the most common genotype responsible for the DCe/dce phenotype in a white population, *DCe/DCe* and *dce/DCe* also produce the DCe/dce serological phenotype (Section 5.4).

The term 'haplotype' is used throughout this chapter to represent the haploid complement of Rh genes,

195

Table 5.1 Antigens of the Rh system.

No.	Names CDE	Names Rh-Hr	Names Other	Comments
RH1	D	Rh_o		Polymorphic; no antithetical antigen
RH2	C	rh′		Polymorphic; antithetical to c
RH3	E	rh″		Polymorphic; antithetical to e
RH4	c	hr′		Polymorphic; antithetical to C
RH5	e	hr″		Polymorphic; antithetical to E
RH6	ce	hr	f	Polymorphic; c and e encoded by the same gene
RH7	Ce	rh_1		Polymorphic; C and e encoded by the same gene
RH8	C^w	$rh_1^{\,w}$		Polymorphic; antithetical to C^x and MAR
RH9	C^x	$rh_1^{\,x}$		LFA; antithetical to C^w and MAR
RH10		hr^v	V	Associated with ce^s VS+, but not (C)ce^s VS+
RH11	E^w	$rh_2^{\,w}$		LFA associated with weak E
RH12	G	rh^G		Polymorphic; when either C or D present
RH17		Hr_o		HFA; absent from Rh_{null}, D−−
RH18		Hr		HFA; absent from E−e+hr^S−, D−−, Rh_{null}
RH19		hr^S		e variant in black people
RH20			VS	Associated with ce^s V+ and (C)ce^s V−
RH21	C^G			C-like antigen of r^G
RH22	CE			LFA; C and E encoded by the same gene
RH23	D^w			LFA; associated with DV
RH26	c-like			Variant of c
RH27	cE			Polymorphic; c and E encoded by the same gene
RH28		hr^H		Variant of VS
RH29			Total Rh	HFA; only absent from Rh_{null}
RH30			Go^a	LFA; associated with DIVa
RH31		hr^B		e variant in black people
RH32		R^N		LFA; associated with D(C)(e) R^N and DBT
RH33			Har	LFA; associated with DHAR
RH34		Hr^B		HFA; anti-RH34 may be anti-hr^B+-Hr^B
RH35				LFA; associated with D(C)(e)
RH36			Be^a	LFA; associated with d(c)(e)
RH37			Evans	LFA; associated with D·· and DIVb
RH39				Anti-C-like autoantibody
RH40			Tar	LFA; associated with DVII
RH41				Ce-like
RH42	Cce^s			Associated with (C)ce^s VS+ V−
RH43			Crawford	
RH44			Nou	HFA; on DIV(C)− and common phenotypes
RH45			Riv	LFA; associated with DIV(C)−
RH46			Sec	HFA; absent from R^N, D −−, Rh_{null} cells
RH47			Dav	HFA; on D·· and common phenotypes
RH48			JAL	LFA; associated with D(C)(e) and D(c)(e)
RH49			STEM	LFA; associated with some hr^S− and hr^B−
RH50			FPTT	LFA; associated with DFR and DHAR
RH51			MAR	HFA; antithetical to C^w and C^x
RH52			BARC	LFA; associated with DVI type II
RH53			JAHK	LFA; associated with r^G

LFA and HFA, low and high frequency antigens.
Obsolete: RH13 (Rh^A), RH14 (Rh^B), RH15 (Rh^C), RH16 (Rh^D), RH24 (E^T), RH25 (LW, now system 16), RH38 (Duclos, now 901013).

even though most D– 'haplotypes' will comprise a single Rh gene.

Numerous variants exist that involve aberrant expression of one or more Rh antigens. These rare haplotypes often produce one or more characteristic low frequency antigens (Section 5.17) and, in the homozygous state, may result in absence of high frequency antigens.

Abnormal expression of D or CcEe antigens may be caused by missense mutations in *RHD* or *RHCE*, but often involve exchange of genetic material between the two Rh genes.

Red cells of the Rh deficiency phenotype Rh_{null} express none of the Rh system antigens (Section 5.16). Rh_{null} has two genetic backgrounds:

1 homozygosity for an *RHD* deletion together with an inactive *RHCE* gene; and

2 homozygosity for inactivating mutations in the gene encoding the Rh-associated glycoprotein, which is essential for the expression of Rh antigens.

Rh_{null} red cells also have abnormal expression of a variety of antigens that do not belong to the Rh system.

Functions of the Rh proteins remain a mystery, although there is a suggestion that they could be involved in ammonium transport.

5.2 History

In 1939, Levine and Stetson [1] investigated a haemolytic reaction, which resulted from the transfusion of a woman with blood from her husband. She had recently given birth to a stillborn baby. An antibody in the mother's serum agglutinated her husband's red cells and those of 80% of ABO compatible blood donors. Levine and Stetson [1] showed that this new antigen, which they did not name, was independent of the known blood groups, ABO, MN, and P. They suggested that the mother had been immunized by a fetal antigen of paternal origin and that the haemolytic episode was caused by maternal antibody reacting with that antigen on the transfused husband's red cells.

In 1940, Landsteiner and Wiener [2] made an antibody by injecting rhesus monkey red cells into rabbits (and later guinea pigs [3]). The antibody, called anti-Rh, agglutinated rhesus monkey red cells, but also agglutinated the red cells from 85% of white New Yorkers. Studies of 60 families showed that Rh-positive was inherited as a dominant character [3]. In the same year Wiener and Peters [4] identified antibod-

ies of apparently identical specificity in the sera of patients who had transfusion reactions after receiving ABO compatible blood. Levine and Stetson's antibody also appeared to be the same as anti-Rh [5].

As early as 1942 Fisk and Foord [6] demonstrated a difference between animal and human anti-Rh: red cells from all newborn babies, whether Rh+ or Rh– as defined by human anti-Rh, were positive with animal anti-Rh. It took another 20 years to prove that human and animal Rh antibodies did not react with the same antigen. The name Rh for antigens recognized by human antibodies could not be changed because it appeared in thousands of publications and so Levine *et al.* [7] proposed that the antigen defined by animal anti-rhesus be called LW in honour of Landsteiner and Wiener. The accumulated information illustrating the differences between LW and Rh (D), and the genetic independence of Rh and LW, is described in Chapter 16.

Meanwhile, the complexity of the Rh groups had increased. By 1943 Race *et al.* [8] had four antisera of different Rh specificities, which defined seven alleles; in New York, Wiener [9] with three different antisera could define six alleles.

When Levine *et al.* [5,10,11] confirmed that incompatibility between mother and fetus was the cause of erythroblastosis fetalis or haemolytic disease of the newborn (HDN), one of the success stories of prophylactic medicine began. The story culminated in the 1960s with the discovery that primary D immunization caused by an incompatible pregnancy can be prevented by the passive administration of anti-D immunoglobulin shortly after delivery. Only a quarter of a century had elapsed between the identification of the cause and the introduction of an effective preventive measure for the disease.

5.3 Notation and genetic models

Two symbolic notations were developed to explain the increasing complexity of the Rh groups. These notations were based on different genetic theories: the Fisher–Race theory postulated three closely linked loci, *C*, *D*, and *E*, whereas Wiener's Rh–Hr theory predicted multiple alleles of a single gene.

5.3.1 Fisher's synthesis

In 1943, when Fisher [cited in 12] noticed that the reactions of two of the four antibodies being used by itithetical, he suggested that the antigens , detected were encoded by alleles, C and c. The reactions of the other two antibodies did not suggest an allelic relationship and he called these anti-D and -E. Three closely linked loci producing D or d, C or c, and E or e were postulated and these could be assembled into eight different gene complexes or haplotypes [12] (Table 5.2). Subsequent identification of anti-e [16] and of the rare haplotype dCE [17] supported Fisher's hypothesis, but anti-d has never been found. Although some of the rare haplotypes found later could not be accommodated easily, the Fisher–Race CDE language is the clearest for interpretation of the majority of serological reactions and for the communication of results. Where applicable, it is this notation that will be used in this book.

5.3.2 Wiener's theory

In an alternative theory, Wiener [18] suggested a series of multiple alleles (R^1, R^2, R^0, etc., Table 5.2) at a single locus. Each gene encodes an agglutinogen (antigen) composed of several blood factors (serological determinants). For example, the agglutinogen produced by R^1 expresses at least three blood factors, Rh_o, rh', and hr'' (D, C, and e in Fisher–Race terminology).

5.3.3 Numerical notation

Rosenfield *et al.* [19] considered that the descriptive notations based on different genetical theories had ob-

structed critical immunological interpretation. They introduced a numerical terminology, which recorded serological data 'free of bias and divorced from speculative implication', and which was ideal for computer storage and manipulation. This system avoided the assumptions often made in the older notations: for example, in CDE language the presumed genotype DCe/DCe is often used to describe D+C+c–E–red cells, even though they may not have been tested with anti-e.

Anti-D in CDE language, anti-Rh_o in Rh–Hr notation, became anti-Rh1. D+ cells were Rh:1 and D– were Rh:–1. The alleles producing these phenotypes were designated R^1 and R^{-1}, respectively. This numerical notation, slightly modified, is now the basis for the International Society of Blood Transfusion (ISBT) terminology for all blood groups (Chapter 1). The present 46 Rh antigens are listed in Table 5.1, showing their numerical, CDE, and Rh–Hr alternatives where appropriate.

5.3.4 Tippett's two-locus model

In 1986, Tippett [20] proposed a new model, based on a wealth of serological data, proposing only two structural Rh genes: one encoding D, the other encoding the CcEe antigens. Mutation and unequal crossing-over between the two loci were considered as possible explanations for some of the rare Rh complexes that involve aberrant expression of Rh antigens. According to this model, an individual with a common D+ phenotype would have two Rh proteins, one expressing D,

Table 5.2 Eight Rh haplotypes and their frequencies in English, Nigerian, and Hong Kong Chinese populations.

Haplotype			Frequencies		
CDE	Rh–Hr	Numerical	English	Nigerian	Chinese
DCe	R^1	RH 1,2,–3,–4,5	0.4205	0.0602	0.7298
dce	r	RH –1,–2,–3,4,5	0.3886	0.2028	0.0232
DcE	R^2	RH 1,–2,3,4,–5	0.1411	0.1151	0.1870
Dce	$R^°$	RH 1,–2,–3,4,5	0.0257	0.5908	0.0334
dcE	r''	RH –1,–2,3,4,–5	0.0119	0	0
dCe	r'	RH –1,2,–3,–4,5	0.0098	0.0311	0.0189
DCE	R^z	RH 1,2,3,–4,–5	0.0024	0	0.0041
dCE	r^y	RH –1,2,3,–4,–5	0	0	0.0036

Results of testing with anti-D, -C, -c, -E, and -e, red cells from 2000 English donors [13], 274 Yoruba of Nigeria [14], and 4648 Cantonese from Hong Kong [15].

the other expressing C or c and E or e, whereas an individual with a rare haplotype such as *D(C)(e)*, *(D)c(e)*, or *D^{IV}(C)–* may have a hybrid protein produced by a fusion gene comprising part of the *D* gene and part of the *CcEe* gene.

Within a few years molecular analysis of the Rh genes disclosed the accuracy of Tippett's two-locus and fusion gene theories, by demonstrating that there are at least two homologous Rh genes, one encoding D and the other encoding C or c and E or e (Section 5.5.2). As with the MNS system (Chapter 3), the multifarious Rh variants appear to arise from processes involving mutation, unequal crossing-over, gene conversion, post-translational modification of proteins, and interaction with other, unlinked, genes.

5.4 Haplotypes, genotypes, and phenotypes

5.4.1 Frequencies

From Fisher's analysis [12], eight different Rh haplotypes were predicted and these have all been identified. The frequencies of these haplotypes vary in different populations (for summaries of data from many populations see [14,21]). Haplotype frequencies tend to differ little among Europeans, with *dce* slightly lower and *DcE* slightly higher in southern Europe than in northern Europe. In sub-Saharan Africa *Dce* dominates; in east Asia, the Pacific area, and among the indigenous people of the Americas, haplotypes lacking *D* are either rare or absent [14]. Estimates for three selected populations are given in Table 5.2. Calculating frequencies of Rh haplotypes is complicated. Fisher [22,23] devised a maximum likelihood method, but other methods have also been used [14,24]. The haplotype *dCE* (*r^y*) is exceedingly rare in all populations tested.

5.4.2 Genotypes and phenotypes

The eight haplotypes shown in Table 5.2 can be paired into (8/2)(8 + 1) or 36 genotypes. However, by using anti-D, -C, -c, -E, and -e only 18 phenotypes can be distinguished (Table 5.3). Only eight of these phenotypes represent a single genotype, the other 10 represent two, three, or six possible genotypes. In the CDE notation, phenotypes are often expressed in the form of genotypes (e.g. DcE/dce). Unless demonstrated by

family analysis this is not a true genotype (and not italicized), but the genotype deemed most likely on the basis of gene frequencies for the appropriate population. For example, a white English donor whose red cells give the reactions D+C–c+E+e+ is 16 times more likely to be *DcE/dce* than *DcE/Dce*, and 180 times more likely than *Dce/dcE*. Consequently, the probable genotype would be DcE/dce. However, in Africans *Dce* is more frequent than *dce* and the probable genotype for D+C–c+E+e+ would be DcE/Dce. True genotypes can often be established by tests on red cells from relatives.

In parentage testing it is always important to remember that probable genotypes may differ from true genotypes. For example, a family with the probable genotypes, mother DCe/DcE, child DCe/DcE, and putative father dce/dce, may appear to exclude paternity, whereas the true genotypes may be mother *DCE/dce*, child *DCE/dce*, and putative father *dce/dce*, providing no exclusion.

The phenotype D+C+c+E+e+ covers six genotypes, but can be subdivided by the use of anti-ce, -Ce, -CE, or -cE (Table 5.3), although these antibodies are rare and in short supply.

Recent molecular techniques have made it possible to distinguish *D/D* from *D/d* (see Section 5.7.1). In *D/d* individuals who are also heterozygous for *RHCE*, it is still not possible to determine which *RHCE* allele is *in cis* with the active *RHD*.

5.4.3 Inheritance

At the basic level the genetics of Rh is simple. Families may be analysed for inheritance of separate antigens, for D and lack of D, for C and c, and for E and e. Race and Sanger [25] summarized many families analysed in this manner, which confirmed that the Rh antigens are inherited in a Mendelian manner.

Families may also be analysed in terms of the haplotypes shown in Table 5.2. This is laborious because more than 100 phenotype matings are possible from the phenotypes shown in Table 5.3, and most phenotypes represent more than one genotype. The phenotype mating DCe/dce × DCe/dce, for example, represents six genotypically different matings with the combined possibility of 10 genetically different offspring. Some references to analyses of unselected families are [24,26–30] and some others are provided in Section 32.3.1.2.

Table 5.3 Rh phenotypes with possible genotypes and their frequencies in an English population (calculated from data in [13]). Reactions with some antibodies to compound antigens and with anti-G are also provided.

D	C	c	E	e	Phenotype		Genotypes		Frequency (%)	ce	Ce	CE	cE	G
+	+	−	−	+	DCe/DCe	R_1R_1	DCe/DCe	R^1/R^1	17.68	−	+	−	−	+
							DCe/dCe	R^1r'	0.82					
+	−	+	+	−	DcE/DcE	R_2R_2	DcE/DcE	R^2R^2	1.99	−	−	−	+	+
							DcE/dcE	R^2r''	0.34					
+	−	+	−	+	Dce/dce	R_0r	Dce/dce	R^0r	2.00	+	−	−	−	+
							Dce/Dce	R^0R^0	0.07					
+	+	−	+	−	DCE/DCE	R_zR_z	DCE/DCE	R^zR^z	<0.01	−	−	+	−	+
							DCE/dCE	R^zr^y	<0.01*					
+	+	+	−	+	DCe/dce	R_1r	DCe/dce	R^1r	32.68	+	+	−	−	+
							DCe/Dce	R^1R^0	2.16					
							Dce/dCe	R^0r'	0.05					
+	−	+	+	+	DcE/dce	R_2r	DcE/dce	R^2r	10.97	+	−	−	+	+
							DcE/Dce	R^2R^0	0.73					
							Dce/dcE	R^0r''	0.06					
+	+	−	+	+	DCe/DCE	R_1R_z	DCe/DCE	R^1R^z	0.20	−	+	+	−	+
							DCE/dCe	R^zr'	<0.01					
							DCe/dCE	R^1r^y	<0.01*					
+	+	+	+	−	DcE/DCE	R_2R_z	DcE/DCE	R^2R^z	0.07	−	−	+	+	+
							DCE/dcE	R^zr''	<0.01					
							DcE/dCE	R^2r^y	<0.01*					
+	+	+	+	+	DCe/DcE	R_1R_2	DCe/DcE	R^1R^2	11.87	−	+	−	+	+
							DCe/dcE	R^1r''	1.00	−	+	−	+	+
							DcE/dCe	R^2r'	0.28	−	+	−	+	+
							DCE/dce	R^zr	0.19	+	−	+	−	+
							Dce/DCE	R^0R^z	0.01	+	−	+	−	+
							Dce/dCE	R^0r^y	<0.01*	+	−	+	−	+
−	+	−	−	+	dCe/dCe	$r'r'$	dCe/dCe	$r'r'$	0.01	−	+	−	−	+
−	−	+	+	−	dcE/dcE	$r''r''$	dcE/dcE	$r''r''$	0.01	−	−	−	+	−
−	−	+	−	+	dce/dce	rr	dce/dce	rr	15.10	+	−	−	−	−
−	+	−	+	−	dCE/dCE	r_yr_y	dCE/dCE	r^yr^y	<0.01*	−	−	+	−	+
−	+	+	−	+	dCe/dce	$r'r$	dCe/dce	$r'r$	0.76	+	+	−	−	+
−	−	+	+	+	dcE/dce	$r''r$	dcE/dce	$r''r$	0.92	+	−	−	+	−
−	+	−	+	+	dCe/dCE	$r'r_y$	dCe/dCE	$r'r^y$	<0.01*	−	+	+	−	+
−	+	+	+	−	dcE/dCE	$r''r_y$	dcE/dCE	$r''r^y$	<0.01*	−	−	+	+	+
−	+	+	+	+	dcE/dCe	$r''r'$	dcE/dCe	$r''r'$	0.02	−	+	−	+	+
							dCE/dce	r^yr	<0.01*	+	−	+	−	+

*Extremely rare.

5.5 Biochemistry and molecular genetics of the Rh polypeptides

5.5.1 Identification and isolation of the Rh polypeptides

In early investigations, Green et al. [31–36] found that D is associated with protein and dependent on phospholipid and intact sulphydryl groups. Removal of phospholipid by detergent resulted in loss of D antigen; replacement of phospholipid, whether derived from D+ or D– cells, resulted in re-expression of D. Although isolation of membrane proteins in deoxycholate led to loss of Rh antigen activity, Lorusso et al. [36] noted that immune complexes of D with anti-D remained intact in the presence of the detergent. In 1982, Moore et al. [37] in Edinburgh, and Gahmberg [38] in Helsinki exploited this protective property of anti-D on the integrity of D in the presence of detergent to isolate D antigen. They sensitized ^{125}I surface-labelled D+ red cells or membranes with IgG polyclonal anti-D, solubilized the membranes in the non-ionic detergent Triton X100, and precipitated immune complexes with protein A-Sepharose. SDS polyacrylamide gel electrophoresis (PAGE) and autoradiography revealed a major component of apparent M_r 30 000 [37–41]. A high level of SDS binding suggested a very hydrophobic protein [37,38,42].

Gahmberg [42] demonstrated that the M_r 30 000 D-active structure could not be labelled by carbohydrate-dependent labelling techniques, was not degraded by endoglycosidase treatment or by mild alkali, and did not bind carbohydrate-specific lectins. This protein therefore broke the rule that mammalian cell surface proteins are glycosylated. Furthermore, unlike most red cell membrane proteins, it is not phosphorylated [42]. The D polypeptide is fatty acylated; palmitic acid chains are attached through thioester linkages to cysteine residues located near to the cytoplasmic leaflet of the lipid bilayer [43,44].

Immunoprecipitation of radioiodinated membrane proteins by polyclonal or monoclonal anti-c or -E, or by a monoclonal antibody (R6A) to a non-polymorphic epitope associated with CcEe, demonstrated that the CcEe antigens are also associated with a membrane protein of apparent M_r about 30 000 [37,39,41,45]. This component resembles the D polypeptide; it is hydrophobic [37], palmitoylated [43,44], and not glycosylated [41]. Its electrophoretic mobility differs slightly from that of the D polypeptide, with an apparent M_r about 2000 higher [37,39,41].

Confirmation that D and CcEe antigens are expressed on similar, but distinctly different polypeptides, came from one- and two-dimensional peptide mapping. This involved the use of either iodolabelled peptides produced by protease degradation of M_r 30 000 polypeptides from D+ and D– red cells [46,47] or of Rh polypeptides immunopurified with monoclonal anti-D, -c, or -E [48,49]. Minor differences (13/14 iodopeptides identical) in two-dimensional peptide maps of the tryptic and chymotryptic peptides isolated from DcE/DcE red cells with anti-c or -E were interpreted as demonstrating that Cc and Ee antigens are present on highly homologous, but distinct, polypeptides [49]. This conclusion, now considered erroneous, may have derived from incomplete digestion of the isolates.

With small quantities of immunoprecipitated ^{125}I-labelled D polypeptide acting as a tracer, M_r 30 000 Rh polypeptides were purified non-immunologically from solubilized membrane skeletons or membrane vesicles by hydroxylapatite chromatography, gel filtration, and preparative PAGE [47,50]. Nineteen of the first 20 N-terminal amino acid residues were identified, identical sequences being obtained from polypeptides isolated from either D+ or D– red cells [47].

D polypeptide was also purified by large-scale immunoprecipitation with monoclonal anti-D [48,51]. The CcEe polypeptide was purified by the same technique, with monoclonal antibodies of the R6A type [51]. Amino acid sequences obtained for the N-terminal 41 residues of the D and CcEe polypeptides were identical [52].

Although isolation of the Rh proteins from the membrane usually results in loss of antigenic activity, soluble preparations of RhD protein in zwitterionic buffers maintained D activity [53]. RhD protein prepared in this way adhered to plastic surfaces and adsorbed monoclonal anti-D.

5.5.2 Cloning of the Rh genes

In 1990, research teams in Bristol and Paris utilized the N-terminal amino acid sequence of D polypeptide to isolate and clone an Rh gene. Avent et al. [52] used degenerate oligonucleotide primers, corresponding to amino acid residues 28–35 (sense) and 54–47 (antisense) of the D polypeptide, in a polymerase chain reaction (PCR) with human reticulocyte cDNA as template. Chérif-Zahar *et al.* [54] used mixtures of primers corresponding to amino acid residues 3–7 and 32–27 of the D polypeptide in a PCR with splenic erythroblast cDNA. Human bone marrow cDNA libraries were screened with radiolabelled PCR products and both teams isolated an identical gene with an open reading frame representing 417 amino acids, but differing from the D polypeptide sequence. This cDNA has subsequently been shown to represent *RHCE* [55,56]. The deduced amino acid sequence is shown in Fig. 5.1.

In 1992, cDNA representing *RHD* was cloned by Le Van Kim *et al.* [57] after further screening of a human bone marrow cDNA library with *RHCE* cDNA. The nucleotide sequence also predicted a 417 amino acid polypeptide, with 92% sequence identity with the CcEe polypeptide (Fig. 5.1). *RHD* cDNA was cloned independently by Kajii *et al.* [58] and by Arce *et al.* [59].

5.5.3 The Rh polypeptides

Although the *RHD* and *RHCE* cDNA open reading frames encode 417 amino acid polypeptides, the N-terminal methionine, which represents the mRNA translation-initiation signal, is cleaved from the mature proteins [52,54]. The RhD and RhCcEe polypeptides differ by between 31 and 35 amino acids, according to *RHCE* allele. The N- and C-terminal regions are well conserved (Fig. 5.1).

The calculated M_r of the Rh polypeptides is 45 500 [52,54,57]. The much lower M_r of 30 000 estimated from SDS PAGE is probably caused by the abnormally high level of SDS binding to these very hydrophobic

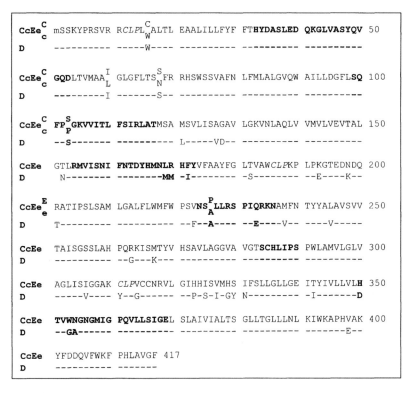

Fig. 5.1 Amino acid sequences of the CcEe and D polypeptides as deduced from cDNA nucleotide sequences [52,54,57–60]. Where the amino acid of both polypeptides is the same, that of the D polypeptide is shown by a dash (–). The N-terminal methionine (m at position 1) is cleaved from the mature proteins. The Cc and Ee polymorphisms are shown [56,60]. Proposed extracellular domains are shown in bold print, though the precise topology of the proteins in the membrane is not known [61–63]. Cys-Leu-Pro (CLP) motifs, probable sites for palmitoylation, are in italics.

proteins. Results of hydropathy analyses on the amino acid sequences suggested that the Rh polypeptides traverse the membrane lipid bilayer 12 times [52,58]. The sequence of the N-terminal domain, together with the lack of a cleaved N-terminal signal sequence, indicated that the N-terminus is located within the cytoplasm [52,54]. Avent *et al.* [64] demonstrated that the C-terminus is also cytoplasmic by raising an antibody in rabbits to a synthetic peptide representing the C-terminal domain of the Rh polypeptides. This antibody did not immunoprecipitate D and CcEe polypeptides from intact red cells, but did immunoprecipitate them from leaky red cell ghosts, which permit access of the antibody to the cytoplasmic side of the membrane. Furthermore, treatment of leaky ghosts with carboxypeptidase Y, an enzyme that cleaves the C-terminal region, resulted in loss of binding of the rabbit antibody, yet identical treatment of intact cells had no effect [64]. Similar experiments with antibodies raised to synthetic peptides have confirmed the intracellular location of the C-terminus [55,65] and led to general agreement that the D and CcEe polypeptides span the membrane 12 times and therefore have up to six extracellular domains (Fig. 5.2).

The D and CcEe polypeptides have five and six cysteine residues, respectively. Three of the cysteine residues in the CcEe polypeptide and two in the D polypeptide form Cys-Leu-Pro motifs at the point of entry of the polypeptide into the cytoplasmic leaflet of the lipid bilayer and probably represent the major sites for attachment of palmitic acid [43,44] (Fig. 5.2). Expression in erythroleukaemic (K562) cells of RhD polypeptide with the cysteine residues at positions 12, 186, 315, and 316 converted to alanine by site-directed mutagenesis demonstrated that intracellular cysteine residues are not essential for translocation and membrane assembly of RhD [67]. However, palmitoylation may play a part in maintaining the tertiary structure of the protein, as 11 of 20 monoclonal anti-D showed reduced reactivity with the mutated protein.

Both RhD and RhCcEe polypeptides have a cysteine residue at position 285 in the fifth extracellular loop. Cys285 has been considered essential for D, C, c, E, and e expression because red cell membranes lost antigen activity when treated with permeable and impermeable sulphydryl reagents [31,32,68,69], although these bulky cysteine-binding reagents might have created conformational changes in the Rh proteins that affected antigen expression or sterically blocked bind-

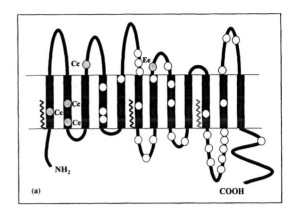

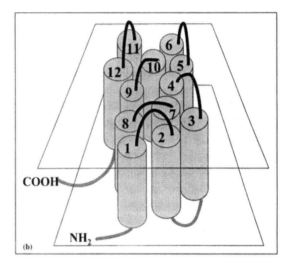

Fig. 5.2 Diagrammatic representations of the probable topology of the D and CcEe polypeptides within the red cell membrane showing 12 membrane spanning domains and cytoplasmic N- and C-termini. (a) The zig-zag lines represent probable sites of palmitoylation (Cys-Leu-Pro motifs); the third site at the tenth membrane spanning domain is only present on the CcEe polypeptide. The circles represent sites where the amino acid residues of the D and CcEe polypeptides may differ; those in grey marked Cc and Ee represent the Cc and Ee polymorphisms. (b) The diagram shows an attempt at a three-dimensional representation of the proteins in the membrane, with the numbered cylinders representing the 12 membrane-spanning domains (modified from [66]).

ing of antibodies. Subsequent work with intact red cells and sulphydryl reagents has suggested that Cys285 is not vital to expression of Rh antigens [70,71]. Furthermore, K562 cells transfected with

RHD cDNA with the Cys285 codon converted to alanine had normal expression of all D epitopes [72].

The D– phenotype results from absence of the RhD polypeptide from the membrane (Section 5.6.1). Most other Rh antigens are dependent on the conformation of the Rh protein in the membrane and may involve interactions between more than one extracellular domain. Their expression can be affected by relatively minor changes to the protein, such as a single amino acid substitution in a membrane-spanning domain of the protein, which could be remote from the sequence that is primarily responsible for expression of the antigen.

5.5.4 Organization of the Rh genes

The two Rh genes, *RHD* and *RHCE*, have almost identical genomic organization, each consisting of 10 exons, with exons 1–7 encoding 50–60 amino acids each and exons 8–10 encoding the last 58 residues [73,74] (Table 5.4). The regions of the Rh polypeptides encoded by the exons, according to the 12 membrane-spanning domain model, are shown in Fig. 5.3. *RHD* and *RHCE* share 93.8% homology over all introns and coding exons [75]. The most notable difference is in intron 4, where *RHD* has a deletion of about 600 bp, relative to *RHCE* [59,75–77]. Four other intronic insertions or deletions over 100 bp

were detected [75]. Various short tandem repeats are present [75], those in introns 2 and 8 being the most thoroughly analysed for polymorphism [78,79]. The 5′ flanking region of *RHCE* contains at least two erythroid-specific GATA-1 binding motifs, plus SP1 and Ets binding sites [73].

RHD and *RHCE* consist of 57 295 and 57 831 bp, respectively [75], and are separated by about 30 kb, which contains the gene *SMP1* (small membrane protein 1) [80] (Fig. 5.4). They are in tail-to-tail configuration (5′*RHD*3′–3′*RHCE*5′), with *RHD* centromeric of *RHCE* [80,81]. *RHD* is flanked by two 9 kb regions of 98.6% homology, named the *Rhesus boxes*

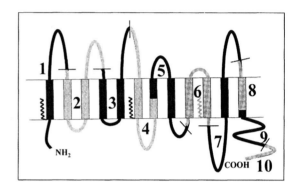

Fig. 5.3 Model of the RhD and RhCcEe polypeptides in the membrane showing the regions encoded by the 10 exons.

Table 5.4 Organization of *RHD*, *RHCE*, and *RHAG*.

	Codons		3′ intron size (bp)		
Exons	*RHD & RHCE*	*RHAG*	*RHD*	*RHCE*	*RHAG*
1	1–49	1–52	11 857	11 758	17 700
2	50–112	53–114	5 269	5 575 C 5 318 c	1 000
3	113–162	115–164	10 131	10 437	2 300
4	163–211	165–213	426	1 075	800
5	212–267	214–269	1 627	1 627	2 100
6	268–313	270–315	3 134	3 133	1 200
7	314–358	316–356	10 276	10 268	3 800
8	359–384	357–379	4 843	4 826	200
9	385–409	380–404	6 942	7 918	900
10	410–417	405–409			

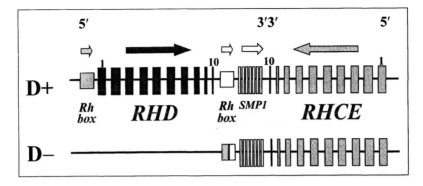

Fig. 5.4 Genomic organization of the Rh genes in typical D+ (above) and D− (below) haplotypes, showing *RHD*, the two homologous *Rh boxes*, and *SMP1* in 5′ to 3′ orientation, and *RHCE* in 3′ to 5′ orientation. In the D− haplotype, there is a deletion of part of each *Rh box* and of *RHD*.

(but called *Rh boxes* here). Deletion of *RHD*, the usual cause of the D− phenotype in white people, appears to have occurred between a 1463-bp region of identity in each of the *Rh boxes* [80] (Fig. 5.4).

In addition to the normal forms of *RHD* and *RHCE* mRNA containing sequence from all 10 exons, numerous alternative spliceoforms have been detected [82,83]. However, there is no evidence that they are represented by proteins in the membrane.

5.5.5 Genomic rearrangement of *RHD* and *RHCE*

Unequal crossing-over and gene conversion, as mechanisms for generating genomic recombination between closely linked homologous genes, are described in Section 3.10 for *GYPA* and *GYPB*, the genes for the MNS blood group antigens. Genomic rearrangements are associated with many examples of variant Rh phenotypes, with gene conversion appearing to be the predominant mechanism and resulting in the creation of *RHD–CE–D* and *RHCE–D–CE* hybrids. Macroconversion events give rise to an Rh gene in which a substantial segment is replaced by the equivalent segment from its homologue, whereas microconversion events can result in exchange of one or more small regions, often leading to single amino acid changes (see Fig. 5.6). In addition, the effects of gene conversion are often associated with untemplated mutations, which change nucleotides to those not derived from either gene. *D–CE* or *CE–D* breakpoints for *DVI*, *DFR*, $\bar{\bar{R}}^N$, and *Dc−* all occur within a recombination hotspot located in an *Alu*-S sequence and the 100 basepairs

immediately downstream of it, within intron 3 (see Figs 5.6 and 5.9) [85].

RHD and *RHCE* are in opposite orientation, so it is likely that the gene conversion events responsible for the generation of Rh hybrid genes occurred following the pairing of *RHD* and *RHCE*, *in cis* (Fig. 5.5). Consistent with this supposition, mutations in exons 5 and 7 of the *r′s* haplotype are present both in the *RHCE* gene and the *RHD–CE(exons 3–8)–D* gene (Section 5.13.2). Likewise, in the DVI type I haplotype, exons 5 of both *RHCE* and *RHD–CE(exons 4–5)–D* encode Pro226, characteristic of a E allele (Section 5.6.4.5).

5.5.6 *In vitro* expression of Rh genes

Following the cloning of the Rh genes, attempts at expressing Rh cDNA by transfection of eukaryotic cells with plasmid expression vectors met with very limited success [55,86]. In 1996 Smythe *et al.* [87] used a retroviral-mediated gene transfer method to express Rh gene products in K562 cells, erythroleukaemic cells that express the Rh-associated glycoprotein considered essential for expression of Rh antigens (Section 5.5.7). cDNA derived from *RHD* and from the *cE* allele of *RHCE* were cloned separately into pBabe puro retroviral vector and used to transfect K562 cells. Cells transfected with *RHD* cDNA expressed D and G; those transfected with *RHCE.cE* cDNA expressed c and E. Rh cDNA has subsequently been expressed by similar techniques in another myeloid leukaemic cell line, KU-812E [88].

205

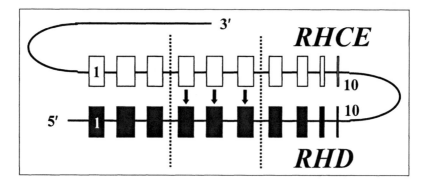

Fig. 5.5 Probable mechanism for Rh gene conversion, with pairing between *RHD* and *RHCE*, *in cis*. In this example exons 4–6 of *RHD* are being replaced by the equivalent exons from *RHCE* to produce the *RHD–CE–D* gene characteristic of DVI type II (see Fig. 5.6).

5.5.7 The Rh-associated glycoprotein (RhAG, CD241)

During the original isolation of the M_r 30000 Rh polypeptides, Moore *et al.* [37] noticed coprecipitating minor components of lower electrophoretic mobility. These components, with an apparent M_r varying between 35000 and 100000 were shown to be heterogeneously N-glycosylated glycoproteins with endo-β-galactosidase-degradable carbohydrate moieties that carry ABH determinants [41,51,89]. Treatment with endoglycosidase-F, which cleaves N-glycans, reduced their apparent M_r to about 30000 [89,90]. This glycoprotein has been referred to as Rh50 (after the molecular weight), but is now named the Rh-associated glycoprotein (RhAG).

A technique involving membrane solubilization in non-ionic detergent (Triton X100) and determination of the sedimentation velocity of membrane components through sucrose gradients indicated an M_r of 170 000 for the Rh polypeptides [44]. A similar estimation of molecular size was obtained by radiation inactivation [91]. These data were interpreted as implying that the Rh polypeptides exist in the membrane as a macromolecular complex, possibly a tetramer comprising two molecules of Rh polypeptides and two molecules of RhAG [44]. These four molecules might interact through their N-terminal domains [65,92]. Quantitative binding assays with monoclonal antibodies to the Rh polypeptides and with Duclos-like antibodies (Section 5.5.7.1) indicated that there are $1–2 \times 10^5$ copies of this complex per red cell [93].

Nucleotide sequences of cloned PCR products, amplified from genomic DNA with degenerate primers derived from the N-terminal amino acid sequence of RhAG, predicted a very hydrophobic 409 amino acid integral membrane protein with two potential extracellular N-glycosylation sites and no sites for palmitoylation. Hydropathy analysis suggested that RhAG closely resembles the Rh polypeptides with 12 membrane spanning domains [94]. Only Asn37, on the first extracellular loop, is N-glycosylated [65]. There is a high degree of sequence similarity between the Rh polypeptides and RhAG, but no indication of polymorphism in RhAG [94].

Organization of *RHAG*, the gene encoding RhAG, is very similar to that of *RHD* and *RHCE* (Table 5.4) [95–97]. Most of the sequence homology is confined to exons 2–9. The 5' promoter region contains several putative *cis*-acting elements including an inverted GATA sequence at position –58 to –53, which acted as an erythroid-specific promoter [95,98]. In addition, there is an erythroid-specific hypersensitive site 10 kb upstream from the translation-initiating codon, with powerful *RHAG*-transcription enhancing activity in K562 cells [99]. This site could be responsible for the erythroid-dominant expression of *RHAG*. Somatic cell hybridization studies showed that *RHAG* is located at 6p21–qter [94]; the genes controlling the Rh polymorphisms are on chromosome 1.

Presence of RhAG in the red cell membrane is a requirement for expression of Rh antigens. Homozygosity for inactivating mutations in *RHAG* is the most common cause of the rare Rh_{null} phenotype, in which none of the antigens of the Rh system is expressed (Section 5.16.2).

K562 erythroleukaemic cells express RhAG in their membranes, although this may be underglycosylated and has an M_r of 32 000 [100]. Transfection of these cells with *RHD* or *RHCE* cDNA results in the expression of Rh antigens [87,88] (Section 5.5.6). When K562 cells transfected with *RHD* cDNA were treated with a phorbol ester, TPA, endogenous *RHAG* expression was down-regulated, but *RHD* transfection was enhanced [101]. Despite this, D expression was reduced and only expression of recombinant RhAG could rescue membrane expression of D. Successful transfection of non-erythroid cells with *RHAG* and *RHD* cDNA did not result in D expression [88,102]. Transfection of non-erythroid cells with constructs designed to produce a fluorescently labelled RhD polypeptide resulted in fluorescent staining of the membrane, with or without RhAG being present [103]. It appears therefore that RhAG is not necessary for insertion of Rh proteins into the membrane, but is necessary for the conformation required for binding of Rh antibodies.

During erythropoiesis *ex vivo*, RhAG appears on the erythroid precursors well before the D or CcEe antigens [104–106]. RhAG on erythroid precursors is not fully glycosylated and has an apparent M_r of 32 000 [107]. The *N*-glycan of RhAG is smaller in Rh$_{null}$ cells, inferring that RhAG moves to the surface faster in the absence of the Rh polypeptides [90].

Human homologues of RhAG, named RhBG and RhCG (or RhGK), have been recognized in non-erythroid cells, and others are present in other species [97,108,109]. Thus, an Rh family in humans currently comprises five proteins encoded by the genes *RHD*, *RHCE*, *RHAG*, *RHBG*, and *RHCG* (*RHGK*).

5.5.7.1 Duclos antigen (901013)

Duclos is 901013 of the high frequency antigens. Apart from the cells of Mme Duclos, the sole maker of anti-Duclos, the Duclos antigen is lacking only from those red cells that are Rh$_{null}$ or Rh$_{mod}$ and also U–. Mme Duclos had an apparently normal DCe/dce phenotype, but a U antigen slightly weaker than normal [110]. A monoclonal antibody, MB-2D10, raised to human red cells, showed a Duclos-like specificity by reacting with all cells except those of Rh$_{null}$ U– and Rh$_{mod}$ U– phenotypes [111]; it differed from the Duclos antibody by reacting with the red cells of Mme Duclos [112]. Immunoblotting demonstrated that the MB-2D10 epitope is located on RhAG [113], so Duclos is likely to be on RhAG.

5.5.8 Rh accessory glycoproteins

Several other red cell membrane glycoproteins are associated with the Rh system by virtue of a partial or total absence of blood group antigens from Rh$_{null}$ red cells (Section 5.16.5). LW glycoprotein is totally absent from Rh$_{null}$ cells and LW antigens have a higher level of expression on D+ than D– cells (Chapter 16). In addition, monoclonal anti-LW coprecipitates LW glycoprotein and Rh polypeptide [114]. Fy5 antigen of the Duffy system (Section 8.4.3) is also totally absent from Rh$_{null}$ cells, though there is no evidence of reduced expression of the Duffy glycoprotein or other Duffy antigens.

Rh$_{null}$ cells have a 60–70% reduction in glycophorin B (GPB) [115], reflected as reduced levels of S, s, and U antigens (Section 3.22). Association between Rh and GPB was supported by an antibody that only reacted with red cells bearing both D and S antigens, found in a multiply transfused DCe/DcE S–s+ man [116]. The RhAG of GPB-deficient (S–s–U–) red cells is more heavily glycosylated than normal [90]. GPB might facilitate transport of RhAG to the cell surface membrane which, in the absence of GPB, remains in the intracellular membrane system longer, permitting more glycosylation [90].

CD47 or integrin-associated protein (IAP) is a widely distributed, heavily *N*-glycosylated, glycoprotein of apparent M_r 47 000–52 000 (reducing conditions) in red cell membranes [89]. It is present in reduced quantity (75% of normal) on Rh$_{null}$ red cells [89,117,118]. CD47 is a member of the immunoglobulin superfamily, with an extracellular N-terminal immunoglobulin domain and five hydrophobic membrane-spanning C-terminal domains [119]. It may function on red cells as a marker of self by binding signal regulatory protein α (SIRPα) on macrophages, generating a negative signal that prevents phagocytosis of the red cells [120]. Splenic macrophages in mice transfused with murine CD47-null (CD47$^{-/-}$) red cells rapidly eliminated the transfused cells from the peripheral blood [120]. The *CD47* gene is located on chromosome 3q13.1–q13.2 [117,118].

There is no evidence that antigens of the Diego system show altered expression in Rh$_{null}$ cells, but an association between band 3 (the Diego antigen) and Rh has been demonstrated by cotransfection experiments. K562 cells transfected with *RHD* or *RHCE.cE* cDNA express D or c and E antigens, respectively [87].

When these cells are subsequently transfected with cDNA encoding band 3, the levels of D or c and E, and of endogenously produced RhAG, are substantially increased [121,122]. This enhancing effect of band 3 expression appears to be greater on RhCcEe–RhAG complexes than on RhD–RhAG complexes [122]. The effect is reduced when K562 cells are transfected with band 3 cDNA containing the South-East Asian ovalocytosis (SAO) mutation, providing a possible explanation for reduced expression of Rh antigens on SAO red cells (see Section 10.8). Beckmann *et al.* [122] suggest that an interaction between band 3 and the Rh–RhAG complexes either enhances their translocation to the cell surface or affects their conformation in the plasma membrane.

The associations described in this section have led to proposals that the Rh polypeptides, their coprecipitating associated glycoproteins, and accessory glycoproteins exist in the red cell membrane as a protein cluster [115,123]. The nature of any association within the membrane between these structures is still a matter for conjecture. Only RhAG appears to be a requirement for expression of Rh antigens. Rh antigens are expressed normally on red cells with null phenotypes for LW, GPB (and GPA plus GPB), and Duffy. No human CD47-deficiency phenotype is known, but red cell membranes of CD47 knockout mice contained normal quantities of murine Rh and RhAG proteins [124]. There is no report of tests for Rh antigens in a band 3-deficient individual, or in band 3 knockout mice.

5.5.9 Association of the Rh complex with the membrane skeleton

Association of the Rh polypeptides, RhAG, and CD47 with the insoluble red cell membrane skeletal matrix during isolation in the non-ionic detergent Triton X100 has led to the conclusion that the Rh complex is linked to the membrane skeleton [125–128]. More direct evidence that the Rh complex is firmly linked to the membrane skeleton came from fluorescence-imaged microdeformation, which quantifies redistribution of fluorescently labelled proteins during membrane deformation induced by aspiration of the cell into a micropipette [129]. Red cells labelled with anti-D or -c Fab fragments gave results intermediate between those obtained for actin, a component of the membrane skeleton, and for band 3, a membrane glycoprotein that is firmly attached to the skeleton. The

mechanism for attachment and the components of the Rh protein complex involved are unknown.

5.6 D and variants of D

D is the most immunogenic of the Rh antigens and is the most important clinically. About 80% of D− recipients of large volumes of D+ blood make anti-D and, until the introduction of immunoglobulin prophylaxis, anti-D was a common cause of severe HDN.

D+ and D− phenotypes are often referred to as Rh+ and Rh−. Between 82% and 88% of Europeans and white North Americans are D+; around 95% of black Africans are D+ [14,21]. D is a high frequency antigen in the Far East, reaching 100% in some populations. By normal blood grouping techniques, 99.7% of Hong Kong Chinese [130] and a similar proportion of Japanese [14] appear D+, but a substantial proportion of those classified as D− have a very weak D antigen called DEL (Section 5.6.4.13).

D antigen expression varies quantitatively, with a continuum of antigen strength from the greatly enhanced expression associated with D−− to weak D, the most extreme of which is DEL. Even among the common phenotypes there is readily detectable quantitative variation of D. Less D is expressed in the presence of C [131–135]; in titrations with anti-D, DcE/DcE cells give higher scores than DCe/DCe cells. Fluorescence flow cytometry with monoclonal and polyclonal anti-D demonstrated the following decreasing order of strength of D antigen: DcE/DcE > DCe/DcE > DCe/DCe > DcE/dce > DCe/dce [136–138]. Further discussion on quantitative aspects of D is found in Section 5.6.8.

5.6.1 Molecular genetics of the D polymorphism

Outside of the ABO system, the most important blood group polymorphism from a clinical viewpoint is D. D− phenotype represents a total absence of D polypeptide from the red cell membrane and, consequently, absence of all epitopes of the D antigen. This explains why d, an antigen allelic to D, has never been found.

5.6.1.1 Europeans

By Southern analysis of genomic DNA with the entire CcEe cDNA probe and with several exon specific probes, Colin *et al.* [139] found that two highly homologous genes of identical genetic organization are present in the genome of D+ individuals, but that only one is present in D– people. Absence of the D gene from the genome of D– people was confirmed after cloning of *RHD* [57,59]. Numerous tests by a variety of techniques (see Section 5.7) have shown that homozygosity for a deletion of *RHD* is the most common cause of the D– phenotype in white people, other molecular backgrounds being rare. The deletion occurs between two 1463 bp regions of identity within the *Rh boxes* that flank *RHD* [80] (Fig. 5.4).

Tests with a technique that specifically detects intron 4 and exon 10 of *RHD* showed that all of 55 dce/dce British blood donors lacked both regions, but that discordant results were commonly associated with *dCe* and *dcE* haplotypes [76,140,141]. Of 33 dCe/dce donors, two had *RHD* intron 4 and exon 10, one had *RHD* intron 4 but not exon 10, and six had *RHD* exon 10 but not intron 4. Of three dcE/dce donors, two had *RHD* intron 4 and exon 10 and one had *RHD* intron 4 but not exon 10. Sequencing revealed that a dCe/dCe donor had a complete *RHD*, but with a nonsense mutation (Gln41stop) in exon 1 [76]. A white Australian with dCe/dce red cells had a 4-bp deletion at the 5′ end of *RHD* exon 4, which introduced a frameshift and a premature stop codon in exon 4 [142].

The frequency of the *RHD* deletion in a predominantly white English population can be estimated at about 0.39 (from data in Table 5.2).

5.6.1.2 Africans

In black Africans the most common molecular background for D– is homozygosity or hemizygosity (with an *RHD* deletion) for a complete, but inactive, *RHD* [141,143]. This inactive gene, called the *RHD* pseudogene or *RHDΨ*, contains a 37-bp sequence duplication consisting of the last 19 nucleotides of intron 3 and the first 18 nucleotides of exon 4 [143]. This duplication could generate a reading frameshift and introduce a premature translation stop codon. Alternatively, if a potential splice site at the 3′ end of the inserted intronic sequence in exon 4 were utilized, the sequence of exon 4 would remain unchanged. *RHDΨ* also has a nonsense mutation in exon 6 (Tyr269stop), which ensures that no RhD protein is present in the red cell membrane [143]. No transcript derived from *RHDΨ* was detected. *RHDΨ* is usually *in cis* with a *ce* allele of *RHCE*.

Another abnormal gene that is relatively common in D– Africans is *RHD–CE–Dˢ*, a hybrid gene comprising exons 1, 2, and the 3′ end of exon 3 of *RHD*, the 5′ end of exon 3 and exons 4–7 of *RHCE*, and exons 9 and 10 of *RHD* (exon 8 undetermined) [144–146]. This gene produces no D, but probably produces abnormal C. *RHD–CE–Dˢ* is associated with the VS+V– phenotype and the *d(C)ceˢ* (*rˢ*) haplotype (Section 5.13).

From tests on 100 black South African donors, the following frequencies of the D– alleles can be roughly estimated: *RHD* deletion, 0.10; *RHDΨ*, 0.07; *RHD–CE–Dˢ*, 0.04 [143,146]. Of 82 D– black Africans, 67% had *RHDΨ*, 15% had *RHD–CE–Dˢ*, and 18% had no *RHD*. For 54 D– African Americans the corresponding figures were 24%, 22%, and 54%, [143].

5.6.1.3 Asians

The existence of *RHD* in some D– Asians was originally indicated by the detection of *RHD* cDNA derived from erythroid progenitors from D– Japanese [58,147,148]. The molecular basis of the D– phenotype in Eastern Asia remains unclear. This is partly because of the presence of an extremely weak D antigen, called DEL, which can only be detected by very sensitive techniques, in particular adsorption and elution (Section 5.6.4.13).

In one study of 130 Japanese D– donors (DEL not found), 63% had no *RHD*, 28% (all C+) had an intact *RHD*, and two samples had probable *RHD–CE–D* hybrid genes [77]. All exons and the promoter region of the intact *RHD* genes were sequenced, but no explanation for the inactivity of these genes was found. In another study of 306 Japanese donors with an apparent D– phenotype, no *RHD* was detected in 67%; the remainder were DEL [149]. Of 87 apparent D– donors from the People's Republic of China, 60% lacked *RHD*, 25% (all C+) appeared to have an intact *RHD*, and 15% (all C+) had at least one exon of *RHD* [150]. In two studies of 230 and 204 Taiwanese, the following results were obtained: 63% and 74% with no *RHD*; 33% and 20% DEL; 4 and 6% apparent *RHD–CE–D* hybrid genes [151,152]. Where analysed, the hybrid gene comprises exons 1, 2, and 10 of *RHD* and exons 3–9 of *RHCE* [152].

209

5.6.2 Weak D (Dᵘ) and partial D

Stratton [153] first coined the term Dᵘ for a D antigen detected by only some anti-D. Dᵘ was subdivided into 'high grade', in which the cells were directly agglutinated by some anti-D, and 'low grade', in which the D antigen could only be detected in an antiglobulin test [154,155]. Dᵘ was shown to be inherited, the *Dᵘ* allele being dominant over *d*, but recessive to normal *D* [153,155,156] (but also see Section 5.6.6). The definition of Dᵘ evolved to become the D of those red cells that are not agglutinated by IgM anti-D, but which react with IgG anti-D in an antiglobulin test. With the introduction of modern, more potent, anti-D reagents, most red cells that would previously have been classified as Dᵘ would not now be considered as having an abnormal D by routine testing.

Dᵘ has been considered a purely quantitative variant of D, differing from normal D purely on the number of antigen sites per red cell [157–161]. Consequently, there can be no Dᵘ antigen and no anti-Dᵘ, so 'Dᵘ' was replaced with the term 'weak D' in the 1990s [162].

The definition of weak D has often depended on the anti-D reagents and techniques used, so it is difficult to provide frequencies for the weak D phenotype. One estimate gave frequencies for weak D as 0.3% and 1.7% in white and black North London donors, respectively [163]. Molecular definitions of weak D permit more accurate determination of the frequency of weak D (Section 5.6.4.12).

If weak D (Dᵘ) is considered a purely quantitative variant of D, then another type of D variant, now usually referred to as partial D [164,165], is a qualitative variant. Since the publication by Argall *et al.* [166] in 1953, it has been clear that rare D+ individuals can make a form of alloanti-D. Many different types of partial D antigen have been identified (Section 5.6.4). The D antigen can be regarded as a mosaic of epitopes. People whose red cells lack part of the D mosaic can, when exposed to a complete D antigen, make antibody to the missing epitopes. This antibody behaves as anti-D when tested against normal (complete) D.

Weak D red cells are considered to have all epitopes of D, expressed weakly. Partial D red cells have some epitopes missing, the remainder being expressed normally. Partial weak D cells have some epitopes missing, the remainder being expressed weakly. These divisions, however, are often not distinct and are difficult to differentiate, although the ability to make alloanti-D in

partial D phenotypes, but not in weak D phenotypes, is probably the most suitable definition if one is required. However, some individuals with red cell phenotypes initially regarded to be weak D have produced alloanti-D [167]. Weak D is often associated with *RHD* mutations encoding amino acid substitutions in the cytoplasmic or membrane-spanning domains of the D protein, whereas partial D is usually caused by changes in the extracellular loops [63]. However, this is not absolute and is dependent, to some extent, on the model for the conformation of the Rh proteins in the membrane used. The terms 'weak D' and 'partial D' are retained here to assist in providing some degree of order to the large number of aberrant D antigens, but there is a compelling argument in favour of scrapping the terms and replacing them with 'D variant'.

5.6.3 Partial D and the epitopes of D

The pioneering work on the subdivision of D, from which our current understanding of the immunologic profile of the D antigen is derived, was by Tippett and Sanger in the 1960s and 1970s [168,169]. They divided partial D antigens into six categories (I–VI) from the patterns of reactions between the red cells and antibodies of D+ people who made anti-D. Family studies showed all categories to be inherited. A seventh category was added later and category I is now obsolete [165,170]. Many cases of D+ people who made anti-D were also studied by Wiener and Unger [171–173]. They called the components of Rh₀ (D in Wiener's language), RhᴬΑ, Rhᴮ, Rhᶜ, and Rhᴰ. These subdivisions of Rh₀ could not be correlated with Tippett and Sanger's categories because there was no exchange of material between the two groups and they are now obsolete.

Tippett and Sanger excluded weak D antigens from their categories and only used potent anti-D made by category members for studying the categories. The partial D antigen of a person cannot be categorized on the basis of their anti-D alone, because the immune response within a category is not consistent. Associated low frequency antigens have subdivided categories IV, V, and VI, and assist in the definition of categories III and VII, and the partial D antigens DFR, DBT, and DHAR (Table 5.5).

In the 1980s, immunological analysis of antigens was revolutionized by the introduction of monoclonal antibody technology. A plethora of monoclonal anti-D has been produced. Testing these antibodies against

Table 5.5 Variant D antigens.

Name	Molecular basis*	Exons	EC† loops	LFA‡	RHCE	Anti-D	No. D sites/cell¶	Ethnic group	References
DII	RHD A354D	7	6		Ce	Yes	3 200	White	[170,174]
DIIIa	*RHD N152T§, T201R§, F223V§	3,4,5	0	DAK	ce	Yes	12 300	Black	[170,175,176]
DIIIb	*RHD–CE–D	2	2		ce	Yes	22 300	Black	[170,177]
DIIIc	*RHD–CE–D	3	0		Ce	Yes	33 255	White	[170,179]
DIII type IV	*RHD L62F, A137V, N152T§	2,3	0			Yes		White	[167]
DIVa	*RHD L62F, N152T§, D350H§	2,3,7	6	Go^a	ce	Yes	9 300	Black	[170,180]
DIVb	*RHD–CE–D	7–9	6	Evans	Ce, cE	Yes	4 000	White, Japanese	[170,180,181]
DIV type III	*RHD–CE–D	6–9	6		Ce		607	White	[63,167]
DIV type IV	*RHD D350H§, G353W§, A354N§	7	6		Ce			White	[182]
DVa	*RHD–CE–D	5	4	D^w	ce, Ce, CE	Yes	9 400	White, Black, Japanese	[170,180,183,200]
DVI type I	*RHD–CE–D	4,5	3,4		cE	Yes	300	White	[170,185]
DVI type II	*RHD–CE–D	4–6	3,4	BAR C	Ce	Yes	1 600	White, Japanese	[170,186]
DVI type III	*RHD–CE–D	3–6	3,4		Ce		14 502	White	[187]
DVII	RHD L110P	2	2	TAR	Ce	Yes	3 600	White	[170,188]
DAR	*RHD T201R§, F223V§, I342T	4,5,7	0		ce	Yes		Black	[189]
DBT type I	*RHD–CE–D	5–7	3,4	Rh32	Ce, ce	Yes	4 300	White, Black, Japanese	[190,191]
DBT type II	*RHD–CE–D	5–9	3,4,6	Rh32	Ce			Japanese	[190,192]
DCS	*RHD–CE–D	5	4		Ce			White	[193,194]
DFR	*RHD M169L§, M170R§, I172F§	4	3	FPTT	Ce, cE	Yes	5 300	White	[180,195,213]
DFW	RHD H166P	4	3		Ce			White	[182]
DHAR	*RHCE–D–CE	5	4	Rh33, FPTT	ce	Yes		White	[196–199]
DHK (DYO)	RHD E233K	5	4		ce			Japanese	[183,184,200]
DHMI	RHD T283I	6	5		cE	Yes	2 400	White	[201,202]
DHO	RHD K235T	5	4		Ce		1 300	White	[203]
DHR	RHD R229K	5	4		cE		3 800	White	[204]
DIM	RHD C285Y	6	5		cE		192	White	[167]
DMH	RHD L54P	1	1		ce			White	[205]
DNB	RHD G355S	7	6		ce	Yes		White	[182]

Continued p. 212

Table 5.5 *Continued.*

Name	Molecular basis*	Exons	ECt loops	LFA‡	RHCE	Anti-D	No. D sites/cell¶	Ethnic group	References
DNU	*RHD* G353R	7	6		Ce		10000	White	[174]
DOL	*RHD* M170T, F223V§	4,5	3		ce	Yes	4700	Black	[194,205]
Weak D type 1	*RHD* V270G	6	0		Ce		1285	White	[63,167]
Weak D type 2	*RHD* G385A	8	0		cE		489	White	[63,167]
Weak D type 3	*RHD* S3C	1	0		Ce		1932	White	[63,167]
Weak D type 4	*RHD* T201R§, F223V§	4,5	0		ce		2288	White	[63,167]
Weak D type 4.1	*RHD* W16C§, T201R§, F223V§	1,4,5	0				3811	White	[167]
Weak D type 5	*RHD* A149D	3	0		cE		296	White	[63,167]
Weak D type 6	*RHD* R10Q	1	0		Ce		1053	White	[63,167]
Weak D type 7	*RHD* G339E	7	0		Ce		2407	White	[63,167]
Weak D type 8	*RHD* G307R	6	0		Ce		972	White	[63,167]
Weak D type 9	*RHD* A294P	6	0		cE		248	White	[63,167]
Weak D type 10	*RHD* W393R	9	0		cE		1186	White	[63,167]
Weak D type 11	*RHD* M295I	6	0		ce		183	White	[63,167]
Weak D type 12	*RHD* G277E	6	0		Ce		96	White	[63,167]
Weak D type 13	*RHD* A276P	6	0		Ce		956	White	[63,167]
Weak D type 14	*RHD* S182T§, K198N§, T201R§	4	0		cE			White	[63]
Weak D type 15	*RHD* G282D	6	0		cE	Yes	297	White	[63,167]
Weak D type 16	*RHD* W220R	5	0		cE		235	White	[63,167]
Weak D type 17	*RHD* R114W	3	2**				66	White	[167]
Weak D type 18	*RHD* R7W	1	0					White	[206]
Weak D type 21	*RHD* P313L	6	0		Ce		5200	White	[203]
Weak D type 22	*RHD* W408C	9	0					White	[206]
DEL	**RHD* exon 9 del	9	0		Ce			Taiwanese	[151]
DEL	*RHD* splice site mutation	1?	0		Ce			Japanese	[207]
DEL	*RHD* splice site mutation	9?	0		Ce			Japanese	[207]

*See Fig. 5.5.

†Predicted extracellular loops involved.

‡Associated low frequency antigens.

¶Information obtained from [167,194,208].

§Encoded by *RHCE* sequence.

**Extracellular according to one model [61], in a membrane-spanning domain according to others [62,63].

red cells with partial D antigens led to different patterns of reactions, considered to represent different epitopes of the D antigen (epD). Lomas *et al.* [209] defined seven D reaction patterns (epD1–epD7) by testing 29 monoclonal anti-D against red cells representing most of the category D antigens, and two more epitopes were added later [210–212]. Although epD6 and epD7 had been shown to differ by inhibition studies with radiolabelled antibodies [178], they could not be distinguished by agglutination techniques and were referred to as epD6/7. Eighteen of the 29 antibodies were anti-epD6/7 [209].

In 1994, Lomas *et al.* [213] gave the name DFR to a new partial D antigen, identified with the assistance of monoclonal antibodies. They refrained from making DFR category VIII because it was no longer possible to carry out all the necessary cross-testing as some of the defining anti-D made by D category members were no longer available. Since then numerous other partial D antigens have been identified (Table 5.5), creating many subsplits of the original reaction patterns. A 30-epitope model [214] was upgraded to 37 at an international workshop for monoclonal antibodies [215]. The definition of some of these reaction patterns, however, depended on the use of enzyme modified red cells. As protease modification of the D protein might affect epitope conformation, Scott [215] proposed excluding patterns that were dependent on enzyme treatment of cells from the numbering. Using only those patterns confirmed in the 1996 workshop, 24 epitopes of D could be identified [215]. The latest pattern of reactions between partial D antigens and monoclonal antibodies, shown in Table 5.6, was produced in 2001 for the fourth international workshop on monoclonal antibodies to red cell surface antigens [216]. It includes 30 epitopes, with a terminology consisting of the original epD1–epD9 (excluding epD7) [209–212], followed by numbers representing subdivisions of the epitopes (e.g. epD6.4). It is important to remember that the D epitopes really only represent reaction patterns and are not absolute. Reaction patterns may be dependent on antibody concentrations, particularly with epitopes of low affinity, so different batches of the same antibody could produce different results. Other factors, such as reaction temperature or pH, might appear to alter specificity.

5.6.4 Characteristics of D variants

Listed below and in Table 5.5 are serological and molecular characteristics of D variants. Much of the serological information is taken from a variety of publications [30,165,168–170,209,210,212,213,217] and from unpublished observations. The molecular bases for D variants involving gene rearrangements are shown in Fig. 5.6.

5.6.4.1 DII, DNU, DNB

Category II originally contained three unrelated propositi with DII travelling with *Ce* in the two families tested. The rediscovery of the original category II propositus led to the subdivision of epD3 [212]. DII is associated with an Ala354Asp substitution in the sixth extracellular loop of RhD [174]. DNU and DNB are D variants with similar epitope profiles to DII: DNU is associated with Gly353Arg [174]; DNB with Gly355Ser [182].

5.6.4.2 DIII and the DAK antigen

This is the only D category that cannot be defined by monoclonal anti-D, because category III red cells react with all monoclonal anti-D (Table 5.6). There are four subcategories of DIII. Most DIIIa and DIIIb individuals are black and the partial D travels with *ce* in families. Some members have an abnormal VS and V phenotype: their red cells react with all anti-VS, but not with all anti-V.

DIIIa cells express the low frequency antigen DAK, which is also expressed by cells with the $\bar{R}^N$ phenotype [175] (Section 5.14.1.1). DIIIa is associated with *RHD* encoding three amino acid substitutions [176] (Fig. 5.6); changes that probably represent templated microconversion events, as Thr152, Arg201, and Val223 are encoded by *RHCE*. It is possible that none of these amino acids is in an extracellular domain, though positions 152 and 223 are close to the third and fourth extracellular loops, respectively. Tests on 93 African Americans and 63 African Brazilians, by a PCR RFLP procedure, revealed frequencies for the *RHDIIIa* allele of 0.11 and 0.19, respectively [218].

Unlike most D+ red cells, DIIIb cells are G– (see Section 5.11). Two DIIIb individuals have *RHD* in which exon 2 is replaced by exon 2 from a *c* allele of *RHCE* [177] (Fig. 5.6). This results in three amino acid

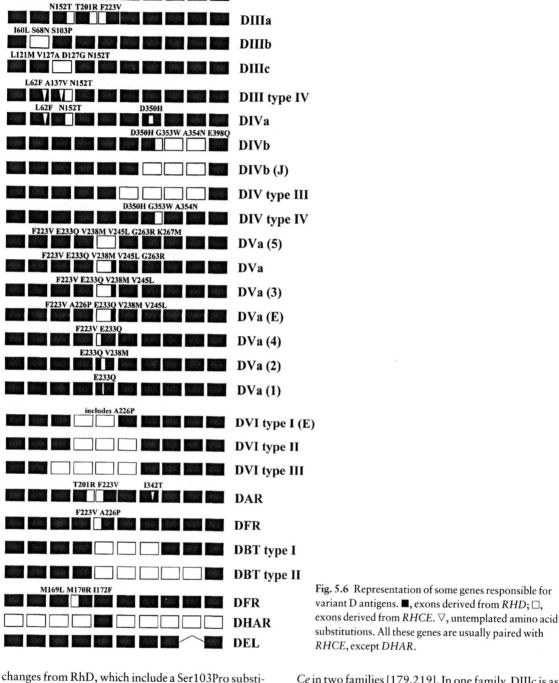

Fig. 5.6 Representation of some genes responsible for variant D antigens. ■, exons derived from *RHD*; □, exons derived from *RHCE*. ▽, untemplated amino acid substitutions. All these genes are usually paired with *RHCE*, except *DHAR*.

changes from RhD, which include a Ser103Pro substitution in the second extracellular loop. Ser103, encoded by *RHD* or the *C* allele of *RHCE*, is responsible for the G antigen. DIIIb has Pro103 and expresses no G.

DIIIc propositi are white and DIIIc is inherited with

Ce in two families [179,219]. In one family, DIIIc is associated with *RHD* in which exon 3 is replaced by exon 3 from *RHCE* [179] (Fig. 5.6). It is likely that none of the four changed amino acids is in an extracellular loop, although positions 121 and 152 are close to the second and third extracellular loops, respectively.

Table 5.6 Reactions of monoclonal antibodies defining 30 epitopes of D with partial D antigens (Fourth International Workshop on Monoclonal Antibodies against Human Red Cell Surface Antigens [216]).

Anti-EpD	Partial D antigen																			
	DII	DIII	DIVa	DIVb	DVa1	DVa2	DVa3	DVa4	DVa5	DVI	DVII	DFR	DBT	DHAR	DHMi	DNB	DAR	DNU	DOL	DHK
1.1	+	+	–	–	–	–	–	–	–	–	+	+	–	–	+	+	V	V	V	–
1.2	+	+	–	–	–	–	–	–	–	–	+	+	–	–	+	+	–	–	–	V
2.1	+	+	–	+	+	+	+	+	–	–	+	+	–	–	+	+	+	+	+	V
2.2	+	+	–	+	+	+	+	+	–	–	+	–	–	–	–	+	–	+	+	V
3.1	+	+	–	+	+	+	+	+	+	+	+	+	–	–	+	V	+	+	+	+
4.1	–	+	+	+	+	+	+	+	+	+	+	+	–	–	+	+	+	+	+	+
5.1	+	+	+	+	–	–	+	–	–	–	+	+	–	–	+	+	+	+	+	–
5.2	+	+	+	+	+	+	+	+	+	–	+	–	–	+	+	+	+	+	+	–
5.3	+	+	+	+	–	–	–	–	–	–	+	+	+	+	+	+	–	+	V	–
5.4	+	+	+	+	+	–	–	–	–	–	+	–	–	–	+	+	+	+	–	–
5.5	+	+	+	+	–	–	–	–	–	–	+	–	–	–	–	–	–	–	–	+
6.1	+	+	+	+	+	+	+	+	+	–	+	+	+	+	+	+	+	+	+	+
6.2	+	+	+	+	+	+	+	+	+	–	+	+	+	–	+	+	+	+	+	V
6.3	+	+	+	+	+	+	+	+	+	–	+	+	+	+	+	+	+	+	+	V
6.4	+	+	+	+	+	+	+	+	+	–	+	–	+	+	+	+	+	+	+	V
6.5	+	+	+	+	+	+	+	+	+	–	+	–	–	–	+	+	+	+	+	+
6.6	+	+	+	+	+	+	+	+	+	–	+	+	+	+	V	+	+	+	V	V
6.7	+	+	+	+	+	+	+	+	–	–	+	–	–	–	+	+	+	+	+	V
6.8	+	+	+	+	+	+	+	+	+	–	–	–	–	–	V	+	+	+	+	V
8.1	+	+	+	+	+	+	+	+	+	–	–	+	+	–	V	+	+	–	+	V
8.2	+	+	+	+	+	+	+	+	+	–	–	+	+	–	V	+	+	+	+	+
8.3	+	+	+	+	+	+	+	–	+	–	+	–	–	–	+	–	+	+	+	–
9.1	–	+	–	+	+	+	+	+	+	+	+	+	+	+	+	+	+	–	+	+
10.1	+	+	+	–	–	–	–	–	–	–	–	–	–	–	+	–	+	–	+	–
11.1	+	+	+	–	–	–	–	–	+	–	–	–	+	–	–	–	–	–	–	–
12.1	+	+	+	+	+	+	+	+	+	–	+	–	+	–	–	–	–	–	–	–
13.1	+	+	+	–	+	+	+	+	+	–	+	–	–	–	–	+	+	+	+	–
14.1	+	+	+	–	+	–	–	–	–	+	+	+	–	–	+	–	–	–	–	–
15.1	+	+	+	–	+	+	+	+	+	+	+	+	–	+	+	+	+	+	+	–
16.1	+	+	+	+	+	–	–	–	–	+	+	+	+	–	+	–	–	–	–	–

V, variable reactions with different antibodies.
For five types of DVa, see Fig. 5.6.

DIII type IV was added in 2000 [167]. The red cells reacted with all monoclonal anti-D and did not react with anti-D from a DIIIc individual; the anti-D from the DIII type IV patient did not react with DIIIc cells. Three amino acid substitutions encoded by *RHD* are associated with DIII type IV [167] (Fig. 5.6). Two result from untemplated mutations, whereas Asn152Thr is identical to one of the changes present in DIIIa. None is predicted to be in an extracellular loop.

5.6.4.3 DIV and the Go^a antigen (RH30)

The partial D antigen of the first DIV propositus was originally called D^{Cor} [221]. DIV appears to be elevated as judged by a few selected incomplete anti-D, which agglutinate saline suspensions of DIV red cells. DIV was initially subdivided by reactions with anti-Go^a, an antibody to a low frequency antigen [222–224]. DIVa and DIVb cells, which are Go(a+) and Go(a–), respectively, can be distinguished by monoclonal anti-D: DIVb, but not DIVa cells, lack epD4 (Table 5.6).

DIVa individuals are mostly black. DIVa travels with *ce* in most families tested, but is also present in the very rare complex DIV(C)– (Section 5.15.5). Three amino acid changes distinguish DIVa from D [180] (Fig. 5.6): two, encoded by exons 3 and 7, probably represent microconversion events; Leu62Phe (exon 2) represents an untemplated mutation. His350 (exon 7) is in the sixth extracellular loop.

Approximately 2% of African Americans are Go(a+) [225,226].

Sub-category IVb is heterogeneous; there is great variation in the strength of the partial D antigen. At least some DIVb cells have the low frequency antigen Evans (RH37) [227]. DIVb travelled with *Ce* in two families and with *cE* in three families [170]. DIVb is associated with an *RHD–CE–D* gene in which the 3′ end of exon 7, exon 9, and probably exon 8 are derived from a *RHCE* gene [180] (Fig. 5.6). All known DIVb propositi were white until four DIVb individuals were found among 5 million Japanese blood donors [228]. In Japanese, DIVb (J) results from an *RHD–CE–D* gene in which the whole of exons 7 and 9 are *RHCE*-derived [181] (Fig. 5.6).

DIV type III and type IV were defined primarily on a molecular basis. Both have an *RHD–CE–D* gene: in type III exons 6–9 have the *RHCE* sequence [63]; in type IV only part of exon 7 is exchanged [182] (Fig. 5.6).

Both types of DIVb and DIV types III and IV have Asp350His, Gly353Trp, and Ala354Asn changes in the sixth extracellular loop.

5.6.4.4 DV and the D^w antigen (RH23)

Category V has been subdivided by reactions with an antibody to a low frequency Rh antigen, anti-D^w [229]. DVa red cells are D^w+. DVa is usually produced by a *D^{Va}ce* haplotype in black families and by *D^{Va}Ce* in white and Japanese families; *D^{Va}cE* is rare [170,230]. The strength of DVa antigen is very variable. The molecular background to DVa is heterogeneous, but always involves replacement of all or part of exon 5 of *RHD* by the equivalent region of *RHCE* (Fig. 5.6) [180,183,184,200,203,230]. All forms involve Glu233Gln, predicted to be in the fourth extracellular loop, and one has only Glu233Gln. All give rise to a typical DVa phenotype, so the Glu233Gln substitution must be the key to D^w expression and loss of epD1, epD5.1, and epD5.3 (Table 5.6). Red cells with the DHK phenotype, in which there is a Glu233Lys substitution, lack epD1 and some epD5 epitopes, but are D^w– [184]. One of the DVa variants, DVa(E) (Fig. 5.6), has Pro226, suggesting that the *RHCE*-derived segment of exon 5 originated from a *E* allele [231]. The red cells expressed an abnormal E antigen, despite no *E* allele of *RHCE* being present, suggesting that the *RHD–CE–D* hybrid produced some E.

Sub-category Vb contained one propositus whose red cells did not react with any anti-D from category VI individuals and were D^w– [232]. The anti-D from this propositus reacted with some DVa red cells.

5.6.4.5 DVI and the BARC antigen (RH52)

DVI has very few D epitopes and most monoclonal anti-D do not react with category VI cells (Table 5.6). A minority of anti-D from D– people react with DVI cells, which may reflect a quantitative rather than a qualitative effect [170].

Most DVI propositi are white or Japanese. DVI travels with *Ce* in most families and less commonly with *cE*. Anti-BARC, an antibody to a low frequency antigen, is a marker for the *D^{VI}Ce* haplotype. Seventy-six of 78 *D^{VI}Ce* samples were BARC+; all of 21 *D^{VI}cE* samples were BARC– [170,233].

Molecular genetic analysis has revealed three types of *RHD–CE–D* encoding DVI (Fig. 5.6). The DVI type

I gene, which is always part of a $D^{VI}cE$ haplotype, has exons 4 and 5 derived from a E allele of RHCE (encoding Pro226) [185,220,234]. (The previously reported DVI gene with a deletion of exons 4–6 [186] does not exist.) DVI type II and III genes, which are part of $D^{VI}Ce$ haplotypes, have exons 4–6 and 3–6, respectively, from an e allele of RHCE (Ala226) [185–187]. DVI genes of types II and III, but not type I, produce BARC, suggesting that the presence of Ala226 in the hybrid Rh protein is important in BARC expression. Apart from the polymorphism at residue 226, all three types have the same amino acid changes from normal D in predicted extracellular loops: Met169Leu, Met170Arg, and Ile172Phe in loop 3; Glu233Gln in loop 4. Quantitative differences, in terms of numbers of D sites per cell, exist between these DVI types: type I is low with about 500 sites; type II has about 2400 sites; and type III is about normal for a DCe complex with 12 000–14 000 sites [167,187].

A unique monoclonal anti-D (LOR-15C9) binds denatured RhD on protein blots and detects the product of exon 7, binding most specifically to the region of amino acids 323–331 [235,236]. This antibody distinguishes cells with the product of a D^{VI} allele (types I–III). In addition to the M_r 33 000 RhD band, DVI cells give an M_r 21 000 band, possibly the product of an alternatively spliced transcript [235].

By screening with monoclonal antibodies, the incidence of DVI in Europe, the USA, and Australia has been estimated between 0.015% and 0.04% and represents between 5% and 16% of weak D samples [237–241]. Only one DVI was found in over 5 million Japanese donors [228].

5.6.4.6 DVII and the Tar antigen (RH40)

Characteristic of DVII is a positive reaction with anti-Tar [242–245]. Tar was associated with a DCe haplotype in several families [242]. Of eight DVII individuals with anti-D, two were untransfused males and in four a weak anti-D was accompanied by a strong anti-E [170,246]. Red cells of one of 1585 D+ British donors failed to react with anti-D from a DVII individual; this sample also had DVII antigen [242]. DVII results from a mutation in RHD exon 2 encoding Leu110Pro in the second extracellular loop of RhD [188]. Of over 60 000 German blood donors, 68 had DVII phenotype; of 33 DVII donors analysed, all had the Leu110Pro mutation [247]. An unusual RHD in

two unrelated individuals encoded Leu110Pro and Pro103Ser (characteristic of c in RHCE) substitutions, and probably produced Tar and partial c (Section 5.8.4) [248].

5.6.4.7 DFR and the FPTT antigen (RH50)

Red cells with the partial D phenotype DFR react with an antibody to the low frequency Rh antigen FPTT [195,213] and give a different pattern of reactions from that seen with any of the category D red cells with anti-D from D+ and D– individuals [213]. In 23 propositi DFR was associated with a DCe haplotype and in two propositi with DcE; in two families DFR travelled with Ce and in one family with cE. Two of the DFR propositi had produced anti-D. Two of 3967 Australians, but only one of 60 000 Germans, had DFR [213,241].

DFR is associated with an RHD–CE–D gene in which the 5′ end of exon 4 is RHCE-derived [180] (Fig. 5.6). The three amino acid substitutions are located in the third extracellular loop. The molecular basis of FPTT expression is described in Section 5.17.2.

5.6.4.8 DBT and the Rh32 antigen

Rh32 is a low frequency antigen associated with the partial D antigen DBT [190] and with the $\bar{R}^N$ complex, which has normal D, but weak C and e (Section 5.14.1.1). Of eight DBT propositi tested, five had normal C and c, two had weak C (one of whom had a weak e), and one was C–c+. Three had made anti-D. The propositi were mostly of white European origin, but one was Moroccan, one Thai, and one Japanese.

In the Moroccan family, DBT is associated with RHD–CE–D in which the whole of exons 5–7 (and possibly 8) are RHCE-derived [191] (type I, Fig. 5.6). This gives rise to Glu233Gln in loop 4 and Asp350His, Gly353Trp, and Ala354Asn in loop 6. In the Japanese DBT family the RHCE segment of the RHD–CE–D gene represents exons 5–9 [192] (type II, Fig. 5.6). The product differs from that of the Moroccan DBT gene by only one amino acid change, Glu398Val, located in the cytoplasmic tail. The molecular basis of Rh32 expression is described in Section 5.17.2.

5.6.4.9 DHAR, R_o^{Har}, and the Rh33 antigen

R_o^{Har} is a rare complex consisting of a weak partial D

(DHAR), c, a very weak e, no G, and two low frequency antigens, Rh33 and FPTT [196–198] (Section
5.14.2.1). Generally, weak D antigens are most efficiently detected by an antiglobulin technique, but
DHAR is different: only 7% of anti-D reacted with
DHAR cells by the antiglobulin technique, although
27% reacted with enzyme-treated DHAR cells [196].
All four IgM, but only five of 24 IgG human monoclonal anti-D reacted with DHAR cells [210]. There
are three reports of women with DHAR producing
anti-D [198,249,250], one of which caused mild HDN
[249].

The R_o^{Har} 'haplotype' differs from all others described in this section in that it comprises only one
gene: there is no *RHD* or *RHCE*, but an *RHCE–D–CE*
hybrid with only exon 5 representing *RHD* [199] (Fig.
5.6). Only six amino acid residues in the encoded protein are characteristic of RhD, and only one of these,
Glu233, is predicted to be extracellular (loop 4). Exon
5 of *RHD* encodes Ala226, the amino acid characteristic of e, explaining the weak e expression.

5.6.4.10 DAR

DAR is a partial D antigen associated with three amino
acid substitutions in RhD: two, Thr201Arg and
Phe223Val, are *RHCE*-derived; Ile342Thr is untemplated [189] (Fig. 5.6). None is predicted to be extracellular, although amino acid 223 is very close to loop
4. DAR is relatively common in Africans: of 326 black
South African donors, 16 (4.9%) had the *DAR* gene
and five (1.5%) of these had the DAR phenotype. One
DAR individual has made alloanti-D [189]. Of the 16
individuals with the *DAR* gene, all but two had an
RHCE variant, named *ceAR*, in which most of exon 5
and the 5′ end of exon 6 is *RHD*-derived (see Section
5.13.2).

5.6.4.11 Other partial D antigens

Several other partial D antigens have been described
and these are listed in Table 5.5. DCS, DHMI, DHO,
DHR, DFW, DMH, DOL, DHK, and DIM are all associated with one or two amino acid substitutions in
the RhD protein.

5.6.4.12 Weak D

As mentioned in Section 5.6.2, weak D is generally

considered a complete D antigen, with all epitopes present, but expressed weakly. However, this is often difficult to determine because monoclonal anti-D could
fail to react with weak D cells because of low avidity of
the antibody, rather than complete loss of the epitope.

Initially, studies on the molecular basis of weak D revealed no changes in the sequence of *RHD* transcripts
or in the *RHD* promoter region (–600 to +41)
[251,252]. In 1999 Wagner *et al.* [63,167] sequenced
the 10 *RHD* exons from 161 weak D samples from
Germany, all with between 70 and 4000 antigen sites
per cell, and found nucleotide changes encoding
amino acid substitutions in all of them. Based on sequence changes, at least 21 types of weak D have been
classified (Table 5.5). All the amino acid substitutions
associated with weak D were in the predicted
membrane-spanning or cytoplasmic domains of the
RhD protein; none was extracellular [63] (although
the Trp114 of type 17 would be extracellular according to a different model [61]). Weak D of types 1–3
were the most frequent, representing 70%, 18%, and
5%, respectively, of the weak D samples tested. Identification of an individual with alloanti-D and weak D
type 15 red cells [167] demonstrates that the distinction between weak D and partial D is not clear, at least
if production of alloanti-D remains as a definition of
partial D. In fact, weak D type 4.2 is functionally identical to DAR (Section 5.6.4.10), also associated with
anti-D production [189], as the *RHD* sequences differ
by only a single, silent nucleotide change. Of 50
DCe/dce Australian blood donors with weak D, 76%
had the type 1 mutation and 6% the type 3 mutation,
whereas of 48 DcE/dce donors with weak D, 96% had
the type 2 mutation [253].

The molecular background of weak remains unclear. Quantitative reverse-transcriptase PCR has
shown that *RHD* genes responsible for weak D types
1, 2, and 3 have normal levels of transcription [254].
Furthermore, transfection experiments with K562
cells suggested that neither translation nor the configuration of RhD is influenced by the type 1 weak D
mutation [254].

5.6.4.13 DEL (D_{el})

A very weak form of D found in the Far East is called
DEL (originally D_{el}) and can only be detected reliably
by adsorption–elution tests. Between 10% and 33% of
Japanese and Chinese red cell samples shown to be D–

by conventional serological techniques were found to be DEL [130,149,151,152,255] yet, in some studies on Japanese donors, DEL was not found [77,79]. The DEL gene is almost exclusively *in cis* with a *Ce* allele of *RHCE*. In Taiwan, DEL was associated with a 1013-bp deletion of *RHD* extending from intron 8 to intron 9 and encompassing the whole of exon 9 [256] (Fig. 5.6). *RHD* mutations with the potential to disrupt RNA splicing were found in three Japanese with DEL phenotype. In one of the donors, homozygosity or hemizygosity for G to A in the first nucleotide of intron 1 in one donor could result in loss of exon 1 in most mRNA molecules. In the other two donors, a G1227A transition in the last nucleotide of exon 9 is a silent mutation, but might lead to abnormal splicing of exon 9.

5.6.5 A molecular approach to the structure of D epitopes

Relating the patterns of D epitope expression to the regions of D protein changed in the various partial D phenotypes has led to speculations on the structures of the D epitopes [257,258]. If the 30-epitope model (Table 5.6) is used, this can become an extremely complex exercise, especially as some epitopes appear to be dependent on a single extracellular loop, whereas others might require interactions between two or even three loops [257]. It is also important to remember that Rh epitopes are highly conformational and their expression can be affected by changes in regions of the protein other than those exposed directly to the antibody.

Liu *et al.* [259,260] approached the problem by combining the technologies of site-directed mutagenesis and the expression of cDNA constructs in K562 cells. They expressed cDNA representing the *cE* allele of *RHCE* after having changed nucleotides encoding amino acids characteristic of the third, fourth, or sixth extracellular loops of RhCcEe to those characteristic of RhD. D epitope expression was then evaluated by flow cytometry. The overall conclusions were that there are six epitope clusters, some of which are overlapping, but are located predominantly on the third, fourth, and sixth *RHD*-specific loops (Fig. 5.7, Table 5.7). None of these epitope clusters is more than 25 Å in diameter. According to this model, some anti-D recognize a 'footprint' consisting of a single extracellular loop, with others the 'footprint' could comprise two, three, or four loops.

Chang and Siegel [261] provided an alternative view of the way that monoclonal antibodies define D epitopes. They used D+ red cells to isolate Fab/phage anti-D libraries from the B cells of a producer of anti-D [262]. Information from a genetic and serological analysis of 53 unique anti-D chosen from 83 random clones demonstrated extensive genetic homology between antibodies directed against different D epitopes. Chang and Siegel [261] suggest that these antibodies would not have such similar sequences if they recognized spatially discrete and structurally unrelated regions of the D protein. They propose that antibodies to the various D epitopes bind to an 'identical footprint', which represents most or all of the extracellular expression of the protein, rather than spatially distinct epitopes. The specificity differences with partial D antigens would result therefore from conformational changes within the 'footprint'. Liu *et al.* [260], however, claim that the extracellular 'footprint' of RhD is too large to represent the whole binding site of an antibody molecule. X-ray crystallography of antibody–antigen complexes will probably be required to clarify whether D antibodies recognize a single identical 'footprint' or spatially distinct epitopes.

5.6.6 Weak D caused by the *trans* effect of C

A weak D phenotype that is not inherited in a regular fashion often occurs when the haplotype encoding the D antigen is *in trans* (on the opposite chromosome) with *dCe* or, rarely, *dCE* or *d(C)ce^s* (*r's*) [263,264]. That is, there is a *trans* effect from a haplotype encoding C, but not D. When the haplotype producing the weakly expressed D is partnered by a haplotype that encodes neither C nor D (*dce* or *dcE*) in another family member, the D is expressed normally. Some examples of DEL could result from the effect of *dCe* on a haplotype containing a weak D gene [265].

5.6.7 Elevated D antigens

Extra strong D antigens are detected by direct agglutination of red cells by incomplete anti-D, IgG antibodies that do not agglutinate red cells with normal D expression. Elevation of D associated with *D––* and related haplotypes (*Dc–*, *DC^w–*, *D··*) results from an increased number of D sites (Section 5.15). Elevation of D is also associated with some *D(C)(e)* haplotypes (Section 5.14.1) and with DIVa partial D (Section

Table 5.7 Locations of D epitopes, according to the model of Liu *et al.* [260].

D epitope	Extracellular loop required
epD2 (some)	3+4+6
epD3 (most)	6+other RhD-specific residues*
epD3 (some)	6
epD4	6+other RhD-specific residues*
epD5 (some)	3+4
epD5 (some)	3+4+6
epD5 (one)	4+6
epD6/7 (some)	3+4
epD6/7 (some)	3+4+6
epD8	1+2+3+5
epD9 (some)	6
epD9 (some)	6+other RhD-specific residues*

*Some epitopes also appear to require the presence of RhD-specific cytoplasmic and/or transmembrane residues to stabilize the configuration.

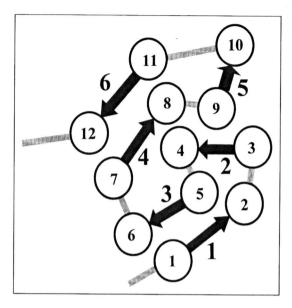

Fig. 5.7 Diagrammatic model of the RhD protein viewed from outside the membrane (i.e. from above), after [260]. Circles (numbered 1–12) represent the membrane-spanning domains, arrows (numbered 1–6) the extracellular loops, grey lines the cytoplasmic loops. See Table 5.7 for proposed location of the D epitopes.

5.6.4.3). Apparent elevation of D antigen, and of other Rh antigens, is observed in red cells with reduced sialic acid levels resulting from glycophorin A deficiency (Chapter 3).

5.6.8 Quantity of D antigen sites

The number of D sites on red cells, estimated by the use of radiolabelled anti-D and by fluorescence flow cytometry, has demonstrated that the site density differs within different phenotypes [157,167,208,266–268] (Table 5.8). As would be expected, less antigen sites were present on red cells with the weak D phenotype and the number detected was highly variable: the lowest numbers detected were about 100, the highest about 4000 [157,159,167,208]. Estimates for D site density on red cells with variant D phenotypes are shown in Table 5.5. Some partial D phenotypes, such as DIII and DIVa, have normal or greater than normal numbers of D sites per cell, whereas others, such as DVI types I and II, have very low D site density [161,167,208]. In any individual, there is a wide range in the number of D sites in each red cell [136,137].

Wagner *et al.* [167] have devised a 'Rhesus D similarity index', defined as the ratio of the 10 percentile and 90 percentile of the site densities for the various epitopes of D. Normal D antigens have an index approaching 1 as all epitopes are expressed strongly, whereas partial D antigens lacking most epitopes, such

as DVI, give an index of 0. Weak D red cells give an intermediate figure. Using this index, it may be possible to predict whether a new variant D phenotype is likely to be associated with anti-D alloimmunization.

5.6.9 D variants and transfusion practice

Traditionally, red cells from donors and patients were tested with IgM anti-D by an agglutination test and those not agglutinated retested by an antiglobulin test in order to detect weak D. It is now common practice to abandon the antiglobulin phase of D testing. If two potent agglutinating anti-D are used, almost all weak D samples will be classified as D+ and only the very weakest D samples will be inaccurately labelled D–. This is generally considered acceptable for the following reasons.

1 Although weak D donations may be mistaken for D– and transfused to D– patients, red cells with weak D phenotypes do not appear to be very immunogenic (but see below).

2 Weak D patients whose red cells are typed as D– will be given D– blood with no harmful effect.

3 Weak D perinatal patients typed as D– may be given

Table 5.8 Estimated number of D antigen sites per red cell for various Rh phenotypes [167,208,266,268].

Phenotype	D sites per cell (range)
DCe/dce	9 900–14 600
DcE/cde	12 000–19 700
Dce/dce	12 000–23 200
DCe/DCe	14 500–22 800
DCe/DcE	23 000–31 000
DcE/DcE	15 800–33 300
D--/D--	110 000–202 000

For numbers of C, c, and e sites, see Table 5.9.

Rh immunoglobulin unnecessarily, again harmless and advantageous should they have a partial D antigen.

4 A 'false' positive result in the antiglobulin test because of a positive direct antiglobulin reaction or the presence of a contaminating antibody could result in a D– patient being typed as weak D and either receiving D+ blood or failing to receive Rh immunoglobulin.

A unit of weak D type 2 red cells was responsible for primary anti-D immunization in a D– man with no previous history of transfusion [269]. Weak D type 2 cells have the lowest D antigen density of the more common types of weak D (Table 5.5), so Flegel et al. [269] recommend that weak D type 2 cells should represent the threshold of detection by anti-D typing reagents and should be used in the quality assurance of these reagents. Because weak D may also be responsible for secondary immunization, it has been recommended that D– donations should be checked for weak D by an antiglobulin test before transfusion to a patient with a history of anti-D [161]. A few cases of weak D involved in severe HDN and a fatal haemolytic transfusion reaction were all reported over 40 years ago, and it is likely that these examples of weak D would be considered normal D with modern reagents [270].

The most common partial D associated with anti-D is DVI. Most DVI cells have low density of D and behave like weak D. Although some polyclonal and monoclonal anti-D reagents agglutinate DVI and most weak D cells, many monoclonal anti-D agglutinate weak D, but not DVI cells. For D typing of patients, anti-D reagents that do not react with DVI cells should be selected, as it is preferable that DVI cells be typed as D–, so that DVI patients receive D– blood.

Anti-D in women with partial D has been responsible for severe HDN [190,179,228,271–275]. Anti-D immunoglobulin should be given to partial D women during and after pregnancy, because the anti-D constituent that does not bind to the mother's own partial D cells should suppress immunization by binding to the normal D of the fetus or baby [276]. This is particularly important in DVI mothers, whose red cells lack most D epitopes.

There is little information on the immunogenicity of partial D. No case of anti-D immunization by DVI red cells is reported. DVa stimulated production of anti-D in a D– woman during her first pregnancy and resulted in mild HDN of her second baby, who also appeared to have the partial D antigen [277]. The mother had received anti-D immunoglobulin after the first pregnancy.

5.7 Predicting D phenotype from DNA

A D+ fetus of a D– woman with anti-D is at risk from HDN (Section 5.18.1.3), so it is beneficial to be able to determine the D phenotype of the fetus at a fairly early stage of pregnancy. If the fetus is D+, the pregnancy can be managed appropriately; if D–, no further action is required. Now that the molecular basis for the D– phenotype is known, it is possible to predict, with a high level of accuracy, fetal D phenotype from fetal DNA derived from amniocytes, obtained by amniocentesis, chorionic villi, and even from maternal blood.

5.7.1 Methods for testing

Several PCR-based tests have been devised to predict D phenotype. The main difficulty in formulating these tests is the design of primers that distinguish between RHD and RHCE. Initially three tests were reported, all based on detecting the presence or absence of RHD. One exploited a sequence that is only present in the 3' untranslated region of RHD exon 10, to amplify a product from RHD, but not RHCE; a second pair of primers recognizing sequences common to exon 7 of both genes acted as a control for successful amplification [278]. Another test used sequence-specific primers to amplify products of different sizes from exons 7 of RHD and RHCE [279]. In a third method, a single pair of primers amplified across intron 4 of both genes, giving products of 600 and 1200 bp from

RHD and *RHCE*, respectively [59,280] (see Table 5.4). In each test, a D– phenotype was predicted by the absence of a band after electrophoresis of the PCR products.

Each of these methods detects a single region of *RHD*. Consequently, false results will be obtained in D variant phenotypes resulting from rearranged Rh genes. For example, DVI and DVa red cells are D+, yet the associated *RHD–CE–D* genes lack intron 4 from *RHD* and so will give a negative result in the intron 4 test (see Fig. 5.6). The *RHD–CE–D* gene responsible for DBT partial D lacks *RHD* exon 7 and so will give a negative result in the exon 7 test. The *RHD–CE–D* gene associated with d(C)ce^s produces no D, but has *RHD*-derived exon 10, and so gives a positive result in the exon 10 test (see Fig. 5.8). One way to avoid these errors is to test for more than one region of *RHD*, and multiplex tests enable both exon 10 and intron 4 of *RHD* to be detected in the same reaction [76,281]. Multiple (modular) or multiplex PCRs that distinguish all exons of *RHD* that differ from *RHCE* are useful for the identification of partial D antigens [282,283]. Many of the numerous publications on PCR-based D phenotype prediction are listed by Flegel *et al.* [284].

Recognition that an inactive *RHD* (*RHDΨ*), with all exons present, is a common cause of D– in people of African origin meant that this gene must be detected in any multiplex test for predicting D phenotype [143]. A PCR multiplex technique described by Singleton *et al.* [143] detects *RHD* exon 7 and intron 4, *RHDΨ*, and the C and c alleles of *RHCE*.

When the mother of a fetus is D–, knowledge of the *RHD* zygosity of the father will assist in predicting fetal D phenotype. If the father is homozygous for *RHD* then the fetus will be D+ and no test is required; if the father is hemizygous for *RHD*, there is an even chance that the fetus will be D+ or D–. Consequently, a test for determining *RHD* zygosity would be of value. All the methods described above (with the exception of that designed to detect *RHDΨ*) only predict a D– phenotype by detecting the absence of *RHD*, so they cannot distinguish homozygosity from hemizygosity for *RHD*. Identification of the DNA sequence across the breakpoint that occurs with the deletion of *RHD* in the D– haplotype has led to the design of PCR-based tests that detect the *RHD*-deletion haplotype directly, either by the use of sequence-specific primers or *Psf*I restriction endonuclease [80,285]. Other, more complex

methods, for determining *RHD* zygosity have involved Southern blotting methods with *Sph*I-digested DNA and exon-specific probes [286], real-time quantitative PCR [285], and *RHD* exon 10 amplification from single sperm [287].

5.7.2 Non-invasive methods for predicting fetal D phenotype

Amniocentesis and chorionic villus sampling are highly invasive techniques, which can lead to enhanced maternal sensitization, increasing the severity of HDN, or to fetal loss. In a population of European origin approximately 40% of D– pregnant women have a D– fetus yet, where the practice of antenatal anti-D immunoglobulin administration is employed, all receive the therapy. A reliable non-invasive technique for predicting fetal D phenotype will obviate the requirement for amniocentesis in patients with anti-D and could save wastage of immunoglobulin and spare patients from unnecessary treatment.

Lo *et al.* [288] showed that fetal DNA represents about 3% of total cell-free DNA in maternal plasma during the second trimester and increases throughout the pregnancy [289]. This fetal DNA is cleared rapidly from the maternal circulation after delivery, so there is no risk of carry-over to the next pregnancy [289]. Several studies have now demonstrated that fetal D type can be predicted reliably from fetal DNA in the plasma of D– pregnant women, from the beginning of the second trimester [289–292]. A flaw in this technology results from the large quantity of maternal DNA present in the DNA preparation, so that no internal control, to test for successful amplification of fetal DNA, can be included. PCR primers designed to amplify a sequence from a Y-borne gene (*SRY*) can be included in the test, but will only provide an internal control when the fetus is male [292].

Another approach to non-invasive fetal Rh testing has been to obtain DNA or mRNA (present in many more copies per cell than genomic DNA) from fetal erythroblasts, which represent about 50% of erythroblasts in maternal peripheral blood [293–299]. These cells survive in the presence of maternal anti-D [294], presumably because they are at too early a stage of erythroid development to express D. It is important that only erythroid cells are used, as fetal lymphoid (CD34$^+$ CD38$^+$) cells derived from a previous pregnancy may be present in the maternal blood [300]. In two studies, single fetal erythroblasts were isolated by micromanipulation and tested by a hemi-nested PCR specific for *RHD* exon 7 [296,299]. None of these approaches has proved sufficiently reliable for routine clinical application.

A method for testing single blastomeres obtained from cleavage-stage embryos has been developed for preimplantation diagnosis to prevent severe HDN [301].

5.8 C and c

5.8.1 C and c antigens

C and c are the products of alleles. C has a frequency of 68% and c a frequency of 81% in English blood donors, giving gene frequencies of 0.4327 and 0.5673 for C and c, respectively [13]. In black Africans the frequency of c is much higher and the frequency of C much lower, whereas in Eastern Asia the opposite is the case, C approaching 100% and c of low incidence [14,21].

Table 5.9 shows the estimated numbers of C, c, and e antigen sites on red cells of various Rh phenotypes [268,302]. The number of C sites is partially dependent on the nature of the anti-C used. The figures in Table 5.9 were obtained with anti-C serum that had been adsorbed with DcE/DcE cells to remove all traces of anti-G [302].

An antigen named C^u gave some, but not all, the reactions expected of weak C and was found in the complex DCe [303].

The *DCE* haplotype produces weak C. DCE/dce cells react weakly with most anti-C sera and DCE/DcE cells have a low number of C antigen sites [302] (Table 5.9). K562 cells transfected with cDNA representing the *Ce* allele of *RHCE* reacted strongly with three monoclonal anti-C, but when cDNA representing the *CE* allele was used, two of the anti-C did not react and the other reacted weakly [304]. It appears therefore that the Pro226Ala (E/e) polymorphism causes conformational changes to the protein that affect C expression.

5.8.2 The C/c polymorphism

The C/c polymorphism is usually associated with six nucleotide substitutions in *RHCE* resulting in four amino acid changes: Cys16Trp (C/c) encoded by exon

1; Ile60Leu, Ser68Asn, and Ser103Pro encoded by exon 2 [56,60] (Table 5.10). Only residue 103 is predicted to be outside the membrane, in the second extracellular loop (Fig. 5.2).

Ser103 is essential, but not sufficient, for C specificity. Exons 2 of *RHD* and the C allele of *RHCE* are identical and both encode Ser103. Any antibody specific for Ser103 would react with the products of *RHD* and the C allele of *RHCE*, so would be called anti-G, not anti-C (Section 5.11). C therefore is a very conformational antigen and anti-C are heterogeneous. For full expression of C, the protein must have Ser103, Cys16, and some other downstream amino acids characteristic of the RhCcEe protein. Cys16 is not a requirement for all epitopes of C. *RHD–CE–D^s*, part of the *d(C)ce^s* haplotype that is relatively common in Africans, has exons 1, 2, and the 5′ end of exon 3 derived from *RHD*, and so encodes Trp16 and Ser103 from *RHD*, but Thr152 and the amino acids of the third extracellular loop from *RHCE* [145]. *RHD–CE–D^s* produces weak C [144–146]. Likewise, the aberrant *RHCE* gene associated with *r^G*, which also produces weak partial C, encodes Ser103, but Trp16 [305]. Conversion of the codon for Cys16 to Trp by site-directed mutagenesis of cDNA representing the *Ce* allele of *RHCE*, and expression of the construct in K562 cells, resulted in about 50% reduction in binding of two anti-C, compared with wild type *Ce* cDNA [304]. The abnormal C associated with Ser103 and Trp16, could represent the antigen called C^G (RH21) [306,307].

The c antigen is determined, almost entirely, by the presence of Pro103, which is encoded by *RHCE* but not *RHD* (Table 5.10). The Cys16Trp polymorphism does not affect c expression—74% of C–c+ black Africans, with normal c, have Cys16 [308]—although Cys16 encoded by a *ce* allele does affect expression of some epitopes of e [309]. Cys16 was also present in 68% of white people with the Dce phenotype, but in none with dce/dce or DcE/DcE phenotypes [282]. Non-human primates with *RHCE* encoding Pro103, but no other amino acids characteristic of c, have c+ red cells [310,311]. Site-directed mutagenesis experiments have revealed that different anti-c have different amino acid requirements [260].

5.8.3 Predicting C/c phenotype from DNA

The defining difference between the *C* and *c* alleles of *RHCE* is a T307C change in exon 2. Exons 2 of *RHD*

Table 5.9 Estimated numbers of C, c, and e antigen sites per red cell [268,302].

Phenotype	Antigen sites per cell (range)		
	C	c	e
DCe/DCe	45 700–56 400		
dCe/dCe	42 200		
DCe/DcE	25 500–39 700	40 000–53 000	14 500
DCe/DCE			13 400
DCe/dce		37 000–42 000	24 400
DCe/dce C^w+	21 500–40 000		
dCe/dce	31 100		
DcE/DCE	8 500–9 800		
DcE/DcE		78 000–80 000	
dce/dce		70 000–85 000	18 200
d(C)ce^s/dce	7 200		

For numbers of D antigen sites, see Table 5.8.

and the C allele of *RHCE* have an identical sequence, so it is not possible to design allele-specific primers for identification of C (except in D– samples), although it is relatively straightforward to design them for *c* [143,282,312,313]. C48 in intron 1, encoding Cys16, does not correlate closely enough with C expression for use in predicting C phenotype (Section 5.8.2). Poulter *et al.* [314] identified a size polymorphism in intron 2 of *RHCE* that correlates closely with C/c expression. C/c genotyping has been achieved by performing two PCRs: one incorporating a primer complementary to a sequence within a C-specific 109 bp insert in *RHCE* intron 2; the other utilizing a primer specific for C307 (*c*) in exon 2 [143,315]. The *d(C)ce^s* haplotype gives a negative result in the intron 2 test despite producing C, because intron 2 from the *RHD–CE–D^s* gene that produces the abnormal C is *RHD*-derived (Section 5.17.2).

5.8.4 Partial c variants and Rh26

A variant c antigen was detected by its failure to react with one strong anti-c reagent. This antibody, which probably defines an epitope of c, was numbered anti-Rh26 [316]. Two further c+ Rh:–26 propositi, with the apparent phenotype DCe/dce, were found in tests with anti-Rh26 on 1900 C+ red cell samples. Enquiries revealed that two of the three propositi were related and all three were of Italian descent. Family studies showed that the unusual c was inherited in a haplotype that en-

Table 5.10 The C/c and E/e polymorphisms—amino acid substitutions in the RhCcEe polypeptide deduced from DNA sequences. The sequence of the D polypeptide is shown for comparison.

Polypeptide	Amino acid residue				
	16	60	68	103*	226*
ce	Trp	Leu	Asn	Pro	Ala
Ce	Cys	Ile	Ser	Ser	Ala
cE	Trp	Leu	Asn	Pro	Pro
CE	Cys	Ile	Ser	Ser	Pro
D	Trp	Ile	Ser	Ser	Ala

*Extracellular.

Amino acid residue 16 is encoded by exon 1 of *RHCE*; residues 60, 68, 103 by exon 2; residue 226 by exon 5.

coded e, but no D. Most anti-c sera appeared to contain mixtures of anti-c and -Rh26.

A DCe/dce Dutch woman made anti-Rh26 during her first pregnancy. Screening with the antibody revealed a second Dutch propositus with DCe/dce Rh:–26 red cells [317]. All c+ Rh:–26 family members had weak expression of c, but normal ce. They all had a *ce* allele of *RHCE* containing a G286A transition in exon 2, encoding a Gly96Ser substitution in the third membrane-spanning domain, close to the second extracellular loop [317]. Two of 10 monoclonal anti-c behaved as anti-Rh26 as they did not react with c+ Rh:–26 cells [317].

Analysis of the family of one c+ Rh:–26 patient showed that the haplotype encoding the variant c antigen did not produce any E, e, or ce, and was most likely *Dc*– [318].

D+C+c+E–e+ red cells of two unrelated white individuals had an abnormal weak c, as determined by polyclonal and monoclonal anti-c [248]. Their phenotype differed from c+ Rh:–26. The cells were also Tar+. Molecular analyses suggested that these two individuals were *DCe/DCe*, with normal *Ce* alleles of *RHCE* and one normal *RHD*, but with a variant *RHD* containing mutations encoding Pro103Ser, characteristic of c in *RHCE*, and Leu110Pro, characteristic of DVII and Tar (Section 5.6.4.6) [248].

5.8.5 Cc antibodies

The well-known heterogeneity of anti-C sera (lacking anti-D and -G) has been demonstrated by tests against a variety of C+ phenotypes [30]. This heterogeneity can only be partly interpreted in terms of varying quantities of anti-C, -Ce, and -CE [30,319]. Most immune 'anti-C' made by D+ people are predominantly anti-Ce (Section 5.10.2). Grouping reagents made from IgM anti-C found in sera of D– people, together with 'incomplete' anti-D, often contain anti-G [319].

5.9 E and e

5.9.1 E and e antigens

E and e, another pair of antithetical antigens within the Rh system, are encoded by *RHCE*, the same gene as that encoding C and c. In all populations e has a significantly higher frequency than E [14,21]. The following are antigen and gene frequencies in an English population: E 29%; e 98%; *E* 0.1554; *e* 0.8446 [13]. The figures for most other populations do not differ substantially from these.

Hughes-Jones *et al.* [268] found that E antigen site densities varied considerably, depending both on red cell phenotype and source of anti-E: estimates ranged between 450 and 25 600 sites per cell. Masouredis *et al.* [320] recorded 27 500 E sites on DcE/DcE cells and 17 900 on DcE/dce cells. Estimates of e antigen site densities are shown in Table 5.9.

A regularly inherited form of weak E has been called E^u [321–323].

5.9.2 The E/e polymorphism

The E/e polymorphism is associated with a C676G change in exon 5 of *RHCE*, predicting a Pro226Ala substitution in the fourth extracellular loop of the RhCcEe protein [56,60] (Table 5.10). Like C, the e antigen must be conformational because Ala226 is also encoded by *RHD*, though the *RHD* product does not express e. Many different changes to *RHCE* will affect e expression, as will become apparent in subsequent sections of this chapter. For example, the presence of VS antigen, which results from a Leu245Val substitution encoded by an *e* allele of *RHCE*, is associated with e weakness (Section 5.13) [145,146,324].

When C is *in cis* with E, as in the relatively rare *DCE* haplotype, the expression of C is often very weak (Section 5.8.1). Pro226 therefore appears to suppress C expression [304]. However, the C/c polymorphism has no obvious effect on the expression of E [304].

5.9.3 Predicting E/e phenotype from DNA

Occasionally anti-E and, rarely, anti-e cause HDN (Section 5.18.2), so a mechanism for predicting fetal E/e phenotype can be useful. The presence of an E allele can be detected by PCR with an allele-specific primer [312]. Detecting e is slightly more complex because G676, the nucleotide characteristic of the e allele of *RHCE*, is also present in *RHD*. This difficulty is easily resolved by using a primer specific for G676 paired with a primer to an *RHCE*-specific nucleotide in exon 5 (e.g. A787) [282,325]. Alternatively, E/e genotyping could be achieved by *Mnl*I digestion of an *RHCE*-specific PCR product. Steers *et al.* [324] amplified the whole of exon 5 of *RHCE* and *RHD* then used denaturing-gradient gel electrophoresis to distinguish *RHD* and the E, e, and e^s alleles of *RHCE*. Allele-specific PCR has been used to predict fetal E/e genotype from fetal erythroblasts isolated from maternal blood [326].

5.9.4 E variants

Red cells with the very rare antigen E^w (RH11) are reactive with some, but not all, anti-E sera. All known examples of anti-E^w are red cell immune and anti-E^w has been responsible for HDN [327,328]. Family studies of only five E^w+ propositi have been reported

[327–331]; three of these five propositi were German. E^w is always associated with *DcE*.

Several other qualitative variants of E have been reported. Red cells of 65% of E+ Aborigines from the Australian Western Desert did not react with a single anti-E, called anti-E^T, found in the serum of a DCe/DcE Australian aboriginal man [332]. The partial E antigen was inherited in a straightforward manner. Anti-E^T is no longer available for further studies.

E+ red cells of a white man of Dutch origin did not react with two of 12 polyclonal anti-E or with one of three monoclonal anti-E [333]. His mother and sister also had the abnormal E, inherited as part of a DcE complex. A similar, but distinctly different, unusual E+ phenotype was found in eight of 58 250 E+ Japanese blood donors by screening with a human IgM monoclonal anti-E [334]. These E+ red cells failed to react with two of eight monoclonal anti-E and with four of 22 polyclonal anti-E. A family study showed that the unusual E was inherited in a DcE complex expressing normal D and c.

Four categories of E variants (EI–EIV) were revealed by testing monoclonal anti-E against red cells with unusual E antigens. The variant E proteins all had Pro226. EI had a Met167Lys substitution in the third extracellular loop; EII had exons 1–3 derived from *RHD*; EIII had Gln233Glu and Met238Val substitutions in the fourth extracellular loop, encoded by a segment of exon 5 derived from *RHD*; and EIV had an Arg201Thr exchange in a membrane-spanning domain [335,336].

Seven patterns of reactions were recognized by testing monoclonal anti-E with E variants at a workshop in 2001 [216].

5.9.5 e Variants: hr^S, hr^B, and related antigens

Some e+ people, most of them of African origin, have made antibodies that resemble anti-e in tests with red cells of common Rh phenotypes. The categorization of e variants has been prevented by the scarcity of avid e reagents, the complexity of the antibody response by e+ people who make 'anti-e', and the large variety of these aberrant e antigens. Two of the possible categories, hr^S and hr^B, are well investigated. As will become clear from the text below, to consider these antigens strictly as e variants is a gross oversimplification.

5.9.5.1 hr^S (RH19) and Hr (RH18)

The antibody that defined the blood factor hr^S was the first alloanti-e-like found in the serum of a e+ person (Shabalala) [337]. The serum reacted with all cells of common Rh phenotype, but more strongly with E–e+ cells than with E+e– cells. After adsorption with E+e– cells, the serum no longer reacted with e– cells, but still reacted with e+ cells, with the exception of the red cells of about 1% of e+ black South Africans, which were considered hr^S–. Shapiro [337] estimated that about 6% of Bantu Rh haplotypes were *Dce* or *dce* encoding no hr^S. The antibody removed by adsorption of Shabalala serum with E+e– cells defines a high frequency antigen called Hr (also Hr^S and RH18). Hr is present on all red cells except those rare e+ cells that lack hr^S, cells with D–– and related phenotypes, and Rh$_{null}$ cells. Anti-Hr may also be a component of anti-Hr$_o$, the immune response of immunized D–– individuals (Section 5.15.6).

Moores [338] believes that the antibody referred to as anti-hr^S results purely from the partial adsorption of anti-Hr (the antibody to a high frequency antigen) to the point where it no longer reacts with E+e– cells, which have weak Hr. Others have confirmed the presence of two antibodies in Shabalala serum by adsorption experiments [339–341].

Other examples of anti-hr^S have been described [340,342], although many other antibodies labelled anti-hr^S will have been inaccurately identified. The immune response of hr^S– people is highly variable and antibodies behaving like anti-e in the serum of e+hr^S– individuals are often assumed to be anti-hr^S even when the critical cells for correct identification are not available. Anti-hr^S appears to be a component of many anti-e sera [337]. The ability of anti-e made by e– people to react with e+hr^S– cells is variable: some antibodies are negative with e+hr^S– cells, but are not anti-hr^S as demonstrated by reactions with other unusual e+ cells [217].

Anti-Hr has caused HDN [338].

As might be expected from the serological description, the molecular basis for the e+hr^S– phenotype is heterogeneous. Met238 encoded by exon 5 of a *ce* allele of *RHCE* appears to be an essential factor in hr^S expression, as a Met238Val substitution encoded by an allele named *ceMO* was associated with an e+hr^S– phenotype [343].

5.9.5.2 hr^B (RH31), Hr^B, and Rh34

Description of the blood factor hr^B is very similar to the hr^S story. Anti-hr^B was found in the serum of a black South African (Bastiaan), together with an antibody to a high frequency antigen, anti-Hr^B [344]. Anti-hr^B was made by adsorbing the serum with E+e– red cells. Sera that appear to contain anti-hr^B in the absence of any anti-Hr^B do exist [341]. However, Bastiaan serum probably contains a single antibody, the specificity called anti-hr^B resulting from the partial adsorption of anti-Hr^B to a level where it no longer reacts with e– cells, which have weak expression of Hr^B [345,346]. The number anti-Rh34 denotes the total immune response of Bastiaan and therefore represents anti-Hr^B plus anti-hr^B, if the latter exists.

A family study showed that Bastiaan had the unusual Rh genotype *d(C)ce^s/D^{III}ce* [344]. *Dce* haplotypes that produce neither hr^B nor Hr^B (i.e. no Rh34) have also been detected [344,346]. Of 65 e+hr^B– blood samples, 59 were VS+, greatly in excess of the number expected if there were no association. It is likely that the *d(C)ce^s* haplotype, which produces VS, but not V (Section 5.13), do not produces hr^B [347]. Twelve of 65 hr^B– blood samples were hr^S–, also substantially in excess of the expected figure [348].

A monoclonal antibody produced from lymphocytes of a white multiparous woman with anti-Ce behaved as anti-Ce by an antiglobulin test with untreated red cells, but when papain-treated cells were used the antibody reacted with all e+ red cells except e+hr^B– cells (and some other rare phenotypes such as D–– and Rh$_{null}$) [349]. When red cells of 982 Africans were tested by the papain method, 26 samples were non-reactive, 17 of which were E+e– and nine e+hr^B–.

Anti-hr^B was detected in the sera of two patients who had transient loss of hr^B [350]. The apparent alloantibodies were later found to be autoantibodies when hr^B reappeared.

5.9.5.3 Other variant e antigens

Many other examples of e-like antibodies have been detected in people with e+ red cells [217,340,341, 351]. To demonstrate the diversity of these phenotypes, Issitt [341] attempted to classify the e antigens of 16 e+ individuals with anti-e, but ended up with 12 categories. Two broad categories can be defined:

1 those with partial e who make an e-like antibody; and

2 those with partial e and partial Hr$_o$ (RH17) who make antibodies that react with all red cells save those of similar unusual phenotypes, Rh$_{null}$ cells, and cells with D–– and related phenotypes.

A separable e-like antibody may also be present in the sera of the second type. It is probable that cells of the first category come from individuals heterozygous for a rare *Dce* haplotype encoding a partial e antigen and for normal *DcE* (or *dcE*), which produces no e, but does produce the related high frequency antigen. Cells of the second category could then come from individuals homozygous for a rare haplotype, which produces partial e and no related high frequency antigen (or heterozygous for two similar haplotypes of this type). An excellent account on the complexities of the e mosaic is provided by Issitt [341].

5.9.5.4 STEM (RH49), a low frequency antigen associated with some hr^S– and hr^B– phenotypes

Further heterogeneity of hr^S– and hr^B– phenotypes was revealed by anti-STEM, an antibody to a determinant present on the red cells of 3–6% of black and mixed race people of Natal, but only very rarely present in white people [352]. Family studies suggested that STEM is associated with some *Dce* haplotypes that do not produce either hr^S or hr^B. Red cells of approximately 65% of hr^S–Hr– and 30% of hr^B–Hr^B–individuals are STEM+. People with hr^S+ STEM+ or hr^B+ STEM+ red cells may be heterozygous for an hr^S-deficient or hr^B-deficient *Dce* haplotype. Therefore, STEM may be marker for some partial e or 'partial Hr$_o$' antigens.

5.9.6 Ee antibodies

Anti-E occurs more commonly than anti-C in the sera of D+ people. Unlike other Rh antibodies, anti-E often appears to be 'naturally occurring' [270]. Many anti-E are only reactive with protease treated E+ red cells [353–356] (Section 5.18.3).

Anti-e is not a common antibody because only 3% of people are e–. Sera containing anti-e often contain anti-Ce or anti-ce (Section 5.10).

5.10 Compound CE antigens

Some Rh antigens, known as compound antigens, are only expressed when c and e, or C and e, or C and E, or c and E are produced by the same *RHCE* gene. Reactions of antibodies to these antigens are shown in Table 5.3. Antibodies to these compound antigens probably recognize conformational differences in the RhCcEe protein that result from the amino acid substitutions associated with both the C/c and E/e polymorphisms. This is consistent with a model of the Rh proteins in the membrane, in which extracellular loops 2 and 4 are close (within 20 Å) to each other [260] (Fig. 5.7).

5.10.1 ce or f (RH6)

Anti-ce (–f) reacts with the products of the *ce* allele of *RHCE*. It also reacts with d(C)ce^s cells (Section 5.13). Reactions of the products of some aberrant haplotypes with anti-ce are contrary to predictions based on their reactions with anti-c and -e. For example, some *Dc–* haplotypes express ce antigen, but no e [30] (Section 5.15.3).

The first two examples of anti-ce were detected in multitransfused DCe/DcE patients [357,358]. Anti-ce is a common component of anti-c and -e sera [357,359], but is only rarely found as a single specificity. Three cases of HDN caused by anti-ce have been reported [360–362] (although one of the sera also contained anti-c [360]). Anti-ce has also been implicated in a delayed haemolytic transfusion reaction [363]. One autoanti-ce in a DCe/dce patient could only be detected in an acidified antiglobulin test; its role in the patient's transfusion reaction was uncertain [364].

5.10.2 Ce (RH7) and Rh41

Recognition of the compound antigen Ce, or rh$_i$ as it was originally called [365], provided an explanation for the observation that certain anti-C sera distinguish C produced by *DCe* and *dCe* from that produced by *DCE* and *dCE* [366].

The original anti-Ce, together with a weak anti-e, was found in the serum of an immunized DcE/DcE woman; the anti-e was removed by adsorption with Dce or dce/dce cells [365]. Most immune anti-C made by D+ people are predominantly anti-Ce [345] and most anti-C and -CD sera contain at least some anti-Ce [319].

Anti-Ce has caused HDN, requiring treatment by exchange transfusion [367,368], and may have contributed to a haemolytic transfusion reaction [369]. Other examples of anti-Ce might have proved clinically significant, but were identified as anti-C. IgA anti-Ce in a DCe/DCe woman was responsible for autoimmune haemolytic anaemia [370].

Anti-Rh41, an antibody made by a DCC^{w}e/DcE woman, was similar to anti-Ce in reacting with cells from people carrying C and e produced by the same gene, but differed from anti-Ce by reacting with d(C)ce^s/dce, but not with DCC^{w}e/dce, DCC^{w}e/DcE, or dCC^{w}e/dce cells [371].

5.10.3 CE (RH22)

Anti-CE is a very rare antibody that reacts with the products of the rare haplotypes *DCE* and *dCE*. The first example was found together with anti-C in the serum of a dce/dce woman who had never been transfused and had a dce/dce husband and child [372]. A second example of anti-CE plus a weak anti-C also appeared to be 'naturally occurring' (P. Booth, personal communication).

5.10.4 cE (RH27)

Anti-cE (together with anti-E and -S) was first identified with confidence in the serum of a DCe/DCe woman [373]. Another example of anti-cE, detected in the serum of a DCC^{w}e/DCE man, appeared to be a 'naturally occurring' antibody and was unusual for an Rh antibody because it bound complement [374].

5.11 G (RH12)

With only rare exceptions, anti-G only reacts with red cells that express D, or C, or both. Ser103, encoded by *RHD* and by the C allele of *RHCE* is the key to G reactivity (see Table 5.10).

Existence of G was postulated to explain the unexpected reactions of the red cells of a white American blood donor, which were apparently C–D–, yet reacted with most anti-CD sera [375]. This very rare phenotype was represented as r^{G}r (r^G/dce). Positively reacting 'anti-CD' sera were assumed to contain an anti-G component and to be anti-D+G, anti-C+D+G, or anti-C+G. Anti-G could be isolated from these sera by adsorption and elution from the r^G/dce red cells.

Homozygosity for r^G was found in a man whose parents were first cousins [306]. The r^G gene produces G, very weak C detected by about one in three anti-C from D+ individuals (initially called anti-C^G [307]), and weak e [306,307,375]. It also produces the low frequency antigen JAHK (RH53) [376]. JAHK was detected on the red cells of three unrelated r^G/dce individuals, an r^G/r^G person, and three other propositi with the likely phenotype r^G/DcE. Anti-JAHK was found in several sera containing multiple antibodies to low frequency antigens.

The r^G gene represents $RHCE$ encoding Trp16 (characteristic of c and RHD) in exon 1 and Ile60, Ser68, and Ser103 (characteristic of C and RHD) in exon 2 [305] (see Table 5.10). This gene could represent a ce allele of $RHCE$ in which exon 2 is substituted by exon 2 from RHD or from a C allele of $RHCE$. This could have been formed as the result of gene conversion (see Section 5.5.5) or by crossing-over within intron 1, between c and Ce alleles of $RHCE$ (because exons 3–10 of c and C alleles are identical).

Confirmation that G was a distinct Rh antigen and basically represented Ser103 in either RhD or RhCcEe was provided by exceptions to the rule that all cells that have D and/or C are G+. DcE producing normal D, but no G, was found in three generations of a white family, studied because of HDN caused by anti-C+G [377]. In two unrelated individuals with DcE/dce G− red cells, also with apparently normal D, the RHD gene had a T307C change encoding a Ser103Pro substitution [378]. Red cells with the partial D antigen DIIIb express most epitopes of D, but are G− (Section 5.6.4.2) and their immune response sometimes includes a separable anti-G [165,169]. DIIIb is produced by RHD in which exon 2 is replaced by exon 2 from a c allele of $RHCE$ and therefore encodes Leu60, Asn68, and Pro103 (see Fig. 5.6) [177].

The haplotype labelled r''^G produces G, E and, possibly, very weak C, but no D, c, or JAHK [376,379]. The amount of G produced by r''^G in different families is variable [30,217]. The r''^G gene represents RHD–CE–D in which exons 4–8 derive from a E allele of $RHCE$ [378]. This gene encodes Trp16 and Ser103.

Only one example of C+ cells lacking G is reported: a D+C+c+E+e+G− woman who had made anti-G [380].

Skov [381] estimated the number of G antigen sites per red cell: DCe/DCe 9900–12 200; dCe/dCe 8200–9700; DCE/DCE 5400; DcE/DcE 3600–5800; Dce/Dce 4500–5300; DcE/dce 4200; and four unrelated dcE/dce G+ (r''^G/r) 600–3600. Anti-G blocks C and D sites [375] and, on occasion, e sites [382].

Anti-G was originally found in the sera of dce/dce people, together with anti-D and/or -C [375,383,384]. Issitt and Tessel [319] detected anti-G in 30% of single donor 'anti-CD' sera and in all commercial anti-CD and -CDE reagents. Anti-G can be isolated by adsorption–elution techniques with r^G/dce or r''^G/dce cells [375,381]. Because these phenotypes are rare, a double elution method has proved useful: 'anti-CD' is adsorbed onto and eluted from dCe/dce (D−C+G+) cells to isolate anti-C and -G, then this eluate, which contains no anti-D, is adsorbed onto and eluted from Dce/dce (D+C−G+) to isolate anti-G [385]. Anti-G has been found in the sera of D+G− people [169,377,386,387]. A thorough serological analysis of 27 sera from immunized women with apparent anti-D+C revealed three anti-D+C, 13 anti-D+C+G, seven anti-D+G, and four anti-C+G [388]. The clinical significance of anti-G is discussed in Section 5.18.2.

The concept of G has helped to sort out some previous serological puzzles. It explained why some dce/dce women immunized only by pregnancy appeared to have made anti-C+D, even though their husbands were C−; their antibody was anti-D+G. It provided an explanation for the apparent anti-C+D in the serum of two dce/dce mothers who had delivered dCe/dce children [383,384]; their antibodies were anti-C+G. Recognition of anti-G also explained the apparent ability of Dce/dce cells to adsorb anti-C activity from anti-C+D sera; such sera were anti-D+G. An apparent anti-C+D made by a D− woman transfused with eight units of D− blood was shown to be anti-C+G and one of the donors was identified as dCe/dce [389].

5.12 C^w, C^x, and MAR

C^w and C^x were initially thought to represent alleles of C and c, but were subsequently found to have an allelic relationship with the high incidence antigen MAR [390]. C^w and C^x result from single nucleotide changes in exon 1 of $RHCE$ (usually a Ce allele) encoding amino acid substitutions in the first extracellular loop: Gln41Arg in C^w; Ala36Thr in C^x [391]. These amino acid changes probably cause conformational alterations in the protein that are responsible for quantitative and qualitative abnormalities of C.

5.12.1 C^w (RH8)

Callender and Race [392] found the first example of anti-C^w in the serum of a DCe/DCe patient who had been transfused with DCe/DCe C^w+ red cells. In an English population C^w has an occurrence of 2.6% [13]; similar frequencies are found in most other northern European and white American populations [14]. The highest frequency of C^w (7–9%) has been found in Latvians, Lapps, and Finns [30]; in most other populations it is very much lower [14, 21].

C^w+ red cells are almost always C+, but the C antigen associated with C^w is weaker than normal C, though recognition of this weakness depends on the anti-C used. Although C^w is usually produced by a *DCe* haplotype, C^w associated with *dCe* [392], *dCE* [393], and *DCE* [394] have also been found. A person with apparently normal DCC^{w}e/dce red cells made anti-C that did not react with DCC^{w}e/dce or dCC^{w}e/dce cells [395]. Similar antibodies have been detected in the sera of DCC^{w}e/DCC^{w}e and DCC^{w}e/DcE individuals [396,397].

Studies with ^{125}I-labelled human monoclonal anti-C^w provided the following estimates of C^w sites per red cell: DCC^{w}e/DCC^{w}e 32 000; DCC^{w}e/DCe 15 200; DCC^{w}e/DcE 19 800; DCC^{w}e/dce 15 300; dCC^{w}e/dce 26 200 [398]. Similar studies with monoclonal anti-C did not reveal any obvious reduction in C antigen density in C^w+ cells compared with C^w– cells [398].

Very rarely, C^w is produced by *RHCE* that produces c and e [391,399,400]. In one individual with C^w+C–c+ red cells, the cells were also D– and G– (dcC^{w}e/dce) (G. Wittman, R. Zimmermann, M. Wallace, P. Tippett, personal communication). C^w is usually produced by a *Ce* allele of *RHCE* encoding Arg41; C^w associated with c is produced by a *ce* allele encoding Arg41 and Cys16 [391]. *CC^{w}e* and *cC^{w}e* alleles therefore have exons 1 of identical sequence (see Table 5.10) and *cC^{w}e* could have arisen by recombination between *CC^{w}e* (exon 1) and *ce* (exons 2–10) alleles of *RHCE*. The *DC^w–* haplotype, which produces C^w but no C, c, E, or e, is described in Section 5.15.4.

Anti-C^w is not an uncommon antibody and often results from no known red cell immunizing stimulus. One in 1100 pregnant Manitoban women had anti-C^w [401]. Anti-C^w has been responsible for several cases of HDN, but this has seldom been severe (reviewed in [401]). Bowman and Pollock [401] conclude that

neonatal deaths as a result of anti-C^w reported in 1947 [402] probably resulted from kernicterus caused by absence of exchange transfusion. PCR-based methods for predicting fetal C^w phenotype are useful in the management of potential HDN caused by anti-C^w [391,403].

5.12.2 C^x (RH9)

Like C^w, C^x is usually produced by a *DCe* haplotype that produces abnormal C. C^x+ red cells react with some, but not all, anti-C. Two very rare haplotypes also encode C^x: *dCC^{x}e* [30] and, in four of 513 unrelated Somalis, *dcC^{x}e^s*, which produces c, V, and VS, but no C or ce [404].

Seven C^x-positives were found among 5919 (0.12%) British donors [405,406] and 202 were found among 70 503 (0.29%) Americans [407]. C^x has a much higher incidence in Finland: 37 of 2060 (1.8%) Finns were C^x+ [390].

The first anti-C^x caused mild HDN, as have other examples since [405,406]. Some anti-C^x appear to be 'naturally occurring' [408]. Anti-C in the serum of a transfused DCC^{x}e/dce patient reacted with most C+ cells, including DCC^{w}e/dce cells, but not with DCC^{x}e/dce, DCC^{x}e/DcE, or DCC^{x}e/DCC^{x}e cells [409].

5.12.3 MAR (RH51)

Anti-MAR was found in a Finnish woman whose red cells were C^w+C^x+D+C+c–E–e+ and who was probably heterozygous DCC^{w}e/DCC^{x}e [390]. Testing of 10 045 Finnish donors revealed 21 MAR-negatives: nine were C^w+C^x– (probably *C^w/C^w*), three were C^w–C^x+ (*C^x/C^x*), and nine were C^w+C^x+ (*C^w/C^x*). In eight families, all 20 children of MAR– parents were either C^w+ or C^x+. Anti-MAR reacted weakly with many examples of C^w+C^x– and C^w–C^x+ cells. It did not react with Rh$_{null}$, D––, or DC^w– cells. As C^w and C^x usually result from Gln41Arg and Ala36Thr substitutions in the RhCe protein, respectively [391], it is probable that both Gln41 and Ala36 are required for MAR expression.

Two other antibodies to high frequency antigens, produced in probable C^x [407] and C^w [410] homozygous women, resembled anti-MAR in their serological reactions. However, the antibody from the C^w homozygote reacted weakly with DCC^{x}e/DCC^{x}e cells and the antibody from the C^x homozygote reacted strongly with DCC^{w}e/DCC^{w}e cells [410]. The antibody of the probable C^x homozygote caused HDN [407].

5.13 VS (RH20) and V (RH10)

5.13.1 Serology

Anti-V, first reported in 1955 [411], and anti-VS, described 5 years later [412], define antigens that are common on the red cells of Africans, but are very rare in other populations. V and VS are associated with a weak e called e^s, though e and e^s are often difficult to distinguish. As a general rule, VS is produced by the haplotypes Dce^s, dce^s, and $d(C)ce^s$, whereas V is produced by Dce^s and dce^s, but not $d(C)ce^s$.

The haplotype $d(C)ce^s$ produces normal c, e^s, ce (f), a weak partial C (sometimes called C^G), G, and VS; it does not produce D, Ce, or V. The symbol r^s was used for $d(C)ce^s$, but is inappropriate as the haplotype produces normal c. In addition, anti-Rh42, an antibody found in the serum of a DCe/Dce mother of Dce/d(C)ce^s and DCe/d(C)ce^s children, only reacts with the product of $d(C)ce^s$ [413]. Some individuals with d(C)ce^s phenotype have produced alloanti-C, confirming that the weak C is a partial C antigen [414]. VS is also associated with the hr^B– phenotype (Section 5.9.5.2): of 65 e+hr^B– samples, 59 were VS+ [348].

Many examples of anti-VS [30,217,340,415] and -V [411,415–417] have been found, often in sera containing other antibodies. The heterogeneity of anti-VS is widely reported and has been thoroughly investigated by Tregellas and Issitt [415]: some antibodies react preferentially with VS+V– cells, some prefer VS+V+ cells, and others react equally well with both types [30,217,340]. Heterogeneity of anti-VS probably provides an explanation for the specificity called anti-hr^H (RH28) [386]. Heterogeneity of V antibodies is also observed when they are tested against red cells of unusual phenotypes [217,386,415]. Clinically significant anti-VS or -V have not been reported. Anti-VS and -V are usually reactive by an antiglobulin technique, but a saline active anti-V is recorded [417].

A number of phenotypes that do not fit the serological rules described above have been reported. A D–C–V–VS+ donor [146] and a VS–V+ (ceAR) phenotype [146,189] are described in the section on molecular genetics (Section 5.13.2). Some DIIIa red cells are C– and react with all anti-VS, but only some anti-V sera [168,169,217]. Two propositi had the aberrant phenotype DCe/DCe VS+V+ [30,340; M. Reid and P. Tippett, personal communication].

Of 100 black South African blood donors, 34 were VS+V+, 9 were VS+V–, and four were VS–V+, with weak V (ceAR) [146]. The incidence of V in two surveys of African Americans was 27% [411] and 39% [418], respectively, and was 40% in West Africans [411]. V is not an exclusively African characteristic: there was no trace of African ancestry in two English families with V antigen [411].

Weakness of D in red cells of DcE/d(C)ce^s individuals demonstrated that $d(C)ce^s$ has a depressing effect on D in trans, similar to the effect of dCe (see Section 5.6.6) [30].

A haplotype named r^{Gs} appears remarkably similar to $d(C)ce^s$ [345]. No individual is reported with r^{Gs} in trans with a common haplotype encoding C, so it is not known whether r^{Gs} produces c.

5.13.2 Molecular genetics

VS is associated with single nucleotide change in exon 5 of a ce allele of RHCE, encoding a Leu245Val substitution. This has been demonstrated on genomic DNA from over 100 VS+ blood samples [145,146,324] and by sequencing of mRNA transcripts [145]. In dce^s and Dce^s haplotypes, no other mutation has been detected (Fig. 5.8). Val245 is present in the RhD protein, so a microconversion event may have been involved in the formation of the VS gene. Amino acid 245 is predicted to be in the eighth membrane-spanning domain, after the fourth extracellular domain, which contains Ala226, the residue primarily responsible for e expression (see Figs 5.1 and 5.2). It is likely that VS expression and the associated weakness of e (e^s) result from conformational changes to the protein caused by the Leu245Val substitution.

The $d(C)ce^s$ haplotype contains a hybrid gene, RHD–CE–D^s, consisting of exons 1, 2, part of 3 (including codons 121, 127, and 128), 9, and 10 from RHD and the remainder of exon 3 (including codon 152) and exons 4–7 from RHCE (e) [144,145] (Fig. 5.8). The origin of exon 8 is not known. RHD–CE–D^s encodes the following amino acid substitutions: Leu62Phe (exon 2), Ala137Val (exon 3), Leu245Val (exon 5), and Gly336Cys (exon 7) [145,146].

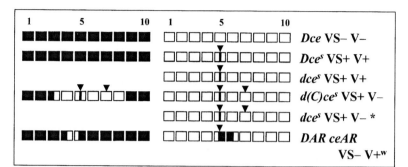

Fig. 5.8 Representation of the 10 exons of *RHD* ■ and *RHCE* □ in VS+ and/or V+ phenotypes. ▼ Codons for Val245 in exon 5 and Cys336 in exon 7. *Genotype not confirmed by transcript analysis.

RHD–CE–D^s is paired with a *ce* allele of *RHCE* which also encodes the Leu245Val (VS) and Gly336Cys substitutions (Fig. 5.8) [145,146]. The presence of Ser103 encoded by exon 2 of *RHD–CE–D^s* together with downstream sequences characteristic of *RHCE*, is probably responsible for C expression by d(C)ce^s, its weakness being caused by tryptophan, and not cysteine, at position 16 (Section 5.8.2). Both *RHD–CE–D^s* and its paired *RHCE* gene encode Val245 and Ala226 (e) and are likely to produce VS and e^s. Both genes also encode cysteine instead of glycine at position 336, a mutation not present in VS+V+ phenotypes [146]. It is possible that anti-VS and -V both recognize Val245 in an Rhce protein, but that anti-V is more conformationally dependent than anti-VS and does not react with the protein when Cys336 is also present. The presence of identical mutations in codons 245 and 336 in the *RHCE* segment of *RHD–CE–D^s* and *RHCE* on the same chromosome suggests that the hybrid gene originally arose from gene conversion between *RHD* and *RHCE in cis* (see Section 5.5.5 and Fig. 5.5).

A black English blood donor had the unusual phenotype D–C–c+E–e+G–V–VS+. Although no transcript analysis was possible, genomic studies suggested that this donor did not have *RHD–CE–D^s*, but did have the *RHCE* gene characteristic of d(C)ce^s, encoding Val245 and Cys336 [146] (Fig. 5.8). This strongly supports the suggestion that *RHD–CE–D^s* produces weak C and that the presence of Cys336, and not the hybrid Rh protein, is responsible for the absence of V in the d(C)ce^s phenotype.

Four individuals with an unusual phenotype, VS– and weak expression of V, were found in a survey of 100 black South African blood donors [146]. One also had a new partial D antigen. The VS–V+^{w} phenotype resulted from an *RHCE–D–CE* gene (called *ceAR*)

with codons for Val238, Val245 (VS), Gly263, and Lys267 derived from exon 5 of *RHD* and Val306 from exon 6 of *RHD* [146,189] (Fig. 5.8). In a survey of 326 black South Africans, 20 (6.1%) had *ceAR*, and 14 of these also had the *DAR* allele of *RHD* [189] (see Section 5.6.4.10).

5.14 Haplotypes producing depressed expression of CcEe antigens

Gathered together in this section are some haplotypes that result in weak expression of Rh antigens. It should be remembered that weak antigens (denoted by parentheses) can only be observed on red cells of people homozygous for the rare haplotype or on those of people with a suitable antithetical Rh haplotype: for example, weak C will not be detected if a normal C is produced by the opposite gene, but will be detected if the opposite gene produces c. Some depressed haplotypes also produce low frequency marker antigens. Some details of antibodies to low frequency Rh antigens are provided in Section 5.17 and Table 5.14. Those depressed complexes involving partial e antigens, described in Section 5.9.5, are omitted from this section. Homozygosity for some of the haplotypes described in this section has revealed that they do not encode certain high incidence Rh antigens, such as Hr$_0$ and Rh46, which are produced by all normal Rh haplotypes.

5.14.1 *DCe* haplotypes

5.14.1.1 R^N ($\bar{\bar{R}}^N$) or *D(C)(e)*: Rh32 and Rh46

$\bar{\bar{R}}^N$ was the name given by Rosenfield *et al.* [698] to a haplotype encoding weak C and weak e in an African American family. Because of word processing complications, the symbol R^N is now often used and will be

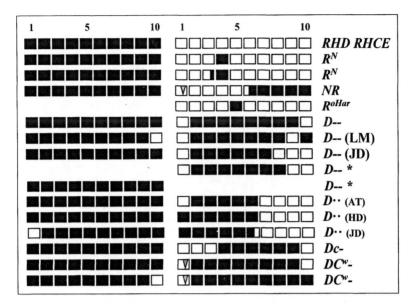

Fig. 5.9 Representation of the 10 exons of *RHD* ■ and *RHCE* □ in some haplotypes containing rearranged genes encoding either partial Hr$_o$ or no Hr$_o$. ▽, exon 1 encoding Arg41 and C^w. *Proposed haplotypes in one D–– propositus [84].

employed here. In addition to weak C and weak e, R^N encodes D and G, which have been shown to be elevated in some studies [251,425,699], and the low frequency antigen Rh32; R^N does not produce any c, E, ce, or, usually, Ce. However, in one family Ce was detected in two D(C)(e)/dce (or D(C)(e)/Dce) children, but not in their father who also had R^N [421]. The Hr$_o$-like high frequency antigen Rh46, produced by most Rh haplotypes, is not produced by R^N [430,699]. The low frequency antigen DAK, which is associated with DIIIa partial D, also appears to be produced by R^N [175].

R^N is most commonly found in people of African origin. It was estimated that Rh32 is present on red cells of about 1% of African Americans, but it has only been found as a rarity in white people [422,430]. Numerous R^N homozygotes are recorded; some found because of immune antibody in their serum (anti-Rh46), others because their weak C and e antigens were detected during routine Rh typing [40,430,699].

In two R^N homozygotes, R^N was associated with *RHD* paired with an *RHCE–D–CE* gene with exon 4 derived from *RHD*, the remainder of the gene having the *RHCE* (*Ce* allele) sequence (Fig. 5.9) [251]. One other individual, apparently heterozygous for R^N, had a similar hybrid gene, but with the 3′ end of exon 3, encoding Asn152, also derived from *RHD* (Fig. 5.9) [251]. These hybrid genes effect Leu169Met,

Arg170Met, and Phe172Ile changes in the third predicted extracellular loop of RhCcEe. The molecular basis for Rh32 expression is described in Section 5.17.2.

Rh32 did not show regular inheritance in a white Canadian Mennonite family: the DcE/D(C)(e) Rh:32 propositus was the child of DCe/DCe Rh:–32 and DCe/DcE Rh:–32 parents [422]. Chown *et al.* [422] proposed that the unusual phenotype of this propositus had arisen by mutation.

Homozygous R^N individuals can make, if immunized by pregnancy or transfusion, anti-Rh46, which reacts with red cells of almost all Rh phenotypes except R^N, Rh$_{null}$, D––, and related phenotypes [165,339,699]. Anti-Rh46 has been responsible for serious HDN [699]. Mouse and human monoclonal antibodies with Rh46 specificity have been produced [431,432].

5.14.1.2 Two more *D(C)(e)* haplotypes and Rh35

A depressed haplotype similar to R^N, but not producing Rh32, was found in six unrelated Swedes [433]. The families of four of the propositi showed the weak C to be inherited. Selected anti-C and -e sera distinguished the Swedish type D(C)(e) cells from R^N cells, even before anti-Rh32 had been identified [434]. Four

233

more propositi with the Swedish *D(C)(e)* haplotype were reported [435], but in one propositus and his mother, unlike the others, the depressed haplotype was associated with enhanced D expression. Existence of two Swedish *D(C)(e)* haplotypes was confirmed by the identification of an antibody, anti-Rh35, specific for Swedish D(C)(e) complex with normal D [425]. The weak C and enhanced D found on red cells of an English blood donor may represent a second example of the *D(C)(e)* haplotype producing enhanced D [436]. Families with similar haplotypes were also found in white Canadian families [29].

The original anti-Rh35 [425] is still the only example and very little of it remains.

5.14.1.3 *D(C)(e)* and JAL (RH48)

A multilaboratory investigation of the serum of a mother whose baby had DAT-positive red cells culminated in the recognition of a new low frequency antigen, JAL (RH48) [702]. Two of the nine propositi had a notably weak expression of C, which was inherited with JAL in their families. Analysis of the families of Swiss JAL+ donors demonstrated that the unusual haplotype produced weak C, weak e, and normal or slightly enhanced D and G; it did not produce any c, E, or ce [437]. These family studies also proved that JAL is encoded by *RH* (lod score of 6.69 at a recombination fraction of 0).

The *D(C)(e) JAL* haplotype has a frequency of 0.0003 in French-speaking Swiss; no JAL+ individual was found among more than 50 000 German-speaking Swiss [437].

JAL was associated with a haplotype producing weak c and weak e in black JAL+ individuals [702] (Section 5.14.2.2).

5.14.1.4 FPTT-associated haplotypes

Several new unusual Rh phenotypes were recognized during the investigation of a serum (Mol), which contained antibodies to several low incidence antigens [195]. Results of adsorption and elution tests suggested that a single antibody, anti-FPTT, was reacting with cells of three propositi, each with a 'new' phenotype. None of the families was large enough to define the new complexes completely. FPTT is also associated with R_o^{Har} (Sections 5.6.4.9 and 5.14.2.1) and DFR (Section 5.6.4.7).

One haplotype encoded weak C, detected by one of six anti-C, very weak e, and FPTT, but no ce. The haplotype was not paired with *dce* or *DCe*, so whether it produces D and/or G is not known and lack of c and E is not proven [195]. The reactions were similar to those of r^G cells, but r^G cells are not FPTT+.

The family of the second propositus showed that their FPTT-associated haplotype produced D, G, weak C, weak e, and atypical VS; it did not produce any E, ce, or V [195]. The groups of the family were uninformative about c production.

Red cells of the third propositus expressed weak e, but normal C. The family did not add any further information [195].

FPTT antigen is very variable in expression and is inherited in a normal way. FPTT has a frequency of about 0.01% in the south of France [195].

5.14.1.5 Other depressed *DCe* haplotypes

A single base change in a *Ce* allele of *RHCE*, encoding an Arg114Trp substitution in the second extracellular loop, was found in a white person whose D+ red cells had weak C and e, and were Rh:−32 [438].

Moores *et al.* [439] proposed that a German Rh:33 propositus was heterozygous for two Rh33-producing haplotypes: one, R^{oHar} (Section 5.14.2.1); the other, called R^{1Lisa}, producing Rh33, D, weak C, very weak or no e, and no Hr$_o$. The evidence for the *DCe*-like haplotype producing Rh33 was based solely on antigen strength.

Red cells of a white woman (NR) with anti-Hr$_o$ were D+C+c−E−e+C^W+, with weak expression of C and e, and were Rh:−32, but reacted with a serum containing inseparable anti-D^w/Rh32 [339,440,441]. She was considered to have the genotype D(C)C^w(e)/D−−; her daughter was *D−−/dce* and her husband *dce/dce* [339,440]. Molecular analysis revealed three transcripts:
1 *RHD*;
2 *RHCE−D*, with only exon 1 derived from *RHCE* (reported previously in *D··* and *DC^w−* [442,443]);
3 *RHCE−D*, with exons 1–5 and the 5′ end of exon 6 derived from a *CC^{w}e* allele of *RHCE* and the remainder of exon 6 and exons 7–10 derived from *RHD* [441] (Fig. 5.9).

The family of a Norwegian blood donor revealed a haplotype that was responsible for normal D, weak C, weak C^w, and weak e [444].

5.14.2 *Dce* haplotypes

5.14.2.1 R^{oHar} or *DHARc(e)* and Rh33

A new, low frequency Rh antigen associated with a *Dce*-like haplotype, named R^{oHar}, was found in two unrelated white people and numbered Rh33 [196]. In addition to Rh33, R^{oHar} produces a partial weak D, called DHAR (Section 5.6.4.9), normal c, very weak e, weak ce, and the low frequency antigen FPTT; it produces no C, E, G, or hr^S [195,196]. R^{oHar} consists solely of an *RHCE–D–CE* gene, in which only exon 5 is derived from *RHD* [199] (Fig. 5.9).

Two Rh:33 individuals, both Germans, appeared to be homozygous for R^{oHar} [196,445]. Their red cells did not react with about 50% of immune sera from D–– people (anti-Hr_o), suggesting they have a partial Hr_o antigen [339,440]. Red cells of another German propositus, believed to be heterozygous for R^{oHar} and for a unique *D(C)(e)* gene (R^{1Lisa}, Section 5.14.1.5), had abnormal Hr_o [439]. A black woman who had made anti-Hr_o appeared to be heterozygous for R^{oHar} and another abnormal *Dce* haplotype, R^{oJoh}, which produced normal D [446].

R^{oHar} is probably less rare in Germany than elsewhere. Seven of 14 000 apparently D– German donors gave discrepant results with anti-D; all seven turned out to be Rh:33 [30]. None of 1060 English blood donors screened with anti-Rh33 was Rh:33 [196]. One of 42 600 donors tested in southern France was Rh:33 and appeared to have the R^{oHar} haplotype [195].

5.14.2.2 *D(c)(e)* JAL

Red cells of four of nine JAL+ propositi, all of African ancestry, had very weak expression of c, in contrast to the weak C associated with JAL+ white people (Section 5.14.1.3) [702]. The unusual haplotype appeared to produce enhanced D, weak c, weak e, and JAL; it did not produce C, E, or ce. In families of three of the JAL+ propositi, JAL was inherited with weak c [702].

5.14.2.3 Other depressed *Dce* haplotypes

Several other depressed *Dce* haplotypes, often represented as *Dc(e)* or *Dc((e))*, are distinguished by the weak e antigens they produce. Cells with the very weak expression of e produced by *Dc((e))* could be mistyped as Dc– if strong anti-e reagents were not used by the

most effective methods [340]. Some *Dc(e)* haplotypes appear to produce Hr_o, others do not [340,447]. One apparent homozygous *Dc((e))* individual, was homozygous for *RHD* plus a *ce* allele of *RHCE* with a deletion of the codon for Arg229 in exon 5 [448]. Arg229 is very close to Ala226, characteristic of e, and therefore is probably important in the expression of e.

5.14.3 *dce* Haplotypes

Some abnormal *dce* haplotypes producing VS and weak e, and often containing an *RHCE–D–CE* gene producing weak C, are described in Section 5.13.

5.14.3.1 *d(c)(e)*: r^L and r^t

The family of a Swiss donor disclosed a new haplotype, r^L, which results in weak expression of c and e, but normal expression of ce [449]. Further examples of the phenotype in two Swedish families confirmed that r^L does not encode D [435,450].

The haplotype r^t, present in three generations of a British family, produces weak c, weak e, and weak ce [217]. Red cells of an Australian donor gave identical reactions with critical Rh antisera and revealed a second example of r^t [30]. The pattern of reactions with anti-c of cells representing r^L/*DCe* differed from those representing r^t/*DCe* [217].

5.14.3.2 *d(c)(e)* and Be^a (RH36)

The low frequency antigen Be^a (Berrens) was first described in 1953 [426]. Twenty years later, a case of HDN led to a family investigation that demonstrated that Be^a belongs to the Rh system [30]. In three generations of the family, four Be(a+) members had an unusual *dce* haplotype that produced slightly depressed c, e, and ce.

Anti-Be^a has been implicated in severe HDN [427–429].

5.14.3.3 *d(c)(e)*: Rh:–32, –46

Absence of the high frequency antigen Rh46 is usually associated with expression of Rh32, in the R^N phenotype (Section 5.14.1.1), or with absence of both E and e, in Rh_{null}, D––, and related phenotypes. Red cells of a man of Italian descent, who had made anti-Hr_o despite never having been transfused, were D–C–c+E–e+Hr_o–

Rh:–32, Rh:–46. There was weakened expression of c and e, though the weakness was only easily detected by flow cytometry [451].

5.14.3.4 $d(C)(c)(E)$ or r^{yn}

Like $d(C)ce^s$ (r^s, originally called r^n, Section 5.13), r^{yn} produces both C and c [452]. The haplotype encodes weak C, weak c, and weak E, though the weakness of c and E was only slight; there is no mention of G in the publication; r^{yn} does not make any D, Ce, ce, cE, or VS.

5.14.4 *DcE* or *dcE* haplotypes

Depression of c and E was observed in two generations of a Norwegian family [453]; $D(c)(E)$ or $d(c)(E)$ was traced in five other members of the family. Two other families carrying similar haplotypes have been reported; in one the haplotype was shown to encode D. A Japanese propositus with weak c, E, and Hr_o was considered to have the genotype $D(c)(E)/D$–– or $d(c)(E)/D$––, because of slightly elevated D on his red cells and those of his father (proposed genotype DCe/D––) [454]. The mother also had weak c and E antigens.

5.14.5 *dCE* haplotype

The unusual haplotype named r^M was found in three generations of a British family [455]. C, E, and G produced by r^M are weak and may also be qualitatively different from normal; r^M produces no c or ce.

5.15 Haplotypes producing neither E nor e; D–– and related phenotypes

This section includes haplotypes, often referred to as 'deleted' or 'partially deleted', that encode neither E nor e; some also produce neither C nor c. All encode D, which is usually exalted in expression. Most of these haplotypes were initially identified in individuals, homozygous for the haplotype, who had produced antibodies to high frequency antigens collectively known as anti-Hr_o. When the terms D––, Dc–, DC^w–, etc. are used to denote phenotypes, they usually represent homozygosity for the corresponding haplotype.

Most of these haplotypes consist of a complete, or almost complete, *RHD*, paired with a hybrid gene containing a substantial portion of *RHD* (Fig. 5.9). This may provide an explanation for the enhanced D expression.

Race and Sanger [456] remarked on the high incidence of consanguinity of parents of D––, DC^w–, and Dc– propositi, compared with other phenotypes resulting from homozygosity for rare genes. They also noted that there were more D–– (D––/D––) sibs of D–– propositi than would be expected if *D*–– were inherited in a straightforward manner. Information from later families supports Race and Sanger's unexpected findings [457]. No satisfactory explanation has been offered for these observations.

5.15.1 *D*––

The first propositus with the D–– phenotype, in which the red cells expressed D, but no C, c, E, or e, had consanguineous parents and was presumed by Race *et al.* [458,459] to be homozygous for a very rare haplotype, *D*––. Despite the rarity of this haplotype, many other examples of the D–– phenotype have been found [30,460–467]. The phenotype has been identified in many different populations: white Americans and Europeans, Native Americans, African Americans, Japanese, Chinese, Koreans, and Asian Indians. Almost all D–– propositi have been ascertained through the presence of anti-Hr_o in their serum (Section 5.15.6). Many propositi heterozygous for *D*–– and a common Rh haplotype have been found, often being disclosed by apparent parentage exclusions [468–471], including four South African families of mixed race [471]. Analysis of a large Canadian family revealed that two sisters with the D–– phenotype, and whose parents were not consanguineous, had the genotype *D*––/–– (heterozygous for *D*–– and the Rh amorph gene, Section 5.16.1) [465].

The frequency of the *D*–– haplotype was roughly estimated as 0.0005 in Sweden [472], but about 10 times that (0.0047) in Iceland [466]. Seven of 692 000 (0.001%) Japanese donors had the D–– phenotype, a frequency of 0.0032 for the *D*–– gene [473].

D–– produces only three Rh antigens: D, G, and Rh29. Red cells of individuals homozygous or heterozygous for *D*–– express more D antigen than normal D+ cells and are directly agglutinated by some incomplete (usually non-agglutinating) anti-D. Most incomplete polyclonal anti-D will directly agglutinate cells of D–– homozygotes, but only carefully selected antibodies will distinguish cells of D–– heterozygotes from DcE/DcE cells. This elevated expression of D is attributed to an increased number of D sites per red cell (Table 5.8).

The molecular genetic background of the D−− phenotype is heterogeneous. A French D−− donor [474] and two D−members of a Native American family [475] appeared to have intact *RHD* and *RHCE* genes, though inactivating or splice site mutations within *RHCE* might not have been detected. Homozygosity for *RHCE–D–CE* hybrid genes appears to account for several other examples of D−− (Fig. 5.9). In D−− individuals from Iceland, Britain, and Italy, only exons 1 and 10 were *RHCE*-derived [475,476]. Studies on two D−− members of an Italian family (LM) suggested that two hybrid genes were present:

1 *RHCE–D–CE–D*, with only exons 1 and 9 *RHCE*-derived; and

2 *RHD–CE*, with only exon 10 *RHCE*-derived [475,477,478].

Transcript analyses on a family (JD) whose propositus was heterozygous for D−− and D·· (Section 5.15.2) revealed *RHD* paired with *RHCE–D–CE*, with exons 2–6 (or 3–6) *RHD*-derived [442].

A thorough molecular analysis on a Japanese family (* in Fig. 5.9) with a D−− propositus, whose parents were not consanguineous, suggested that she was heterozygous for two abnormal Rh haplotypes [84]. In one, inherited from the father, there is an *RHCE–D–CE* gene with exons 2 (or 3) to 7 derived from *RHD*, but no normal *RHD* (Fig. 5.9). The other comprises *RHD*, but no *RHCE*. *D1S80* is a gene marker on chromosome 1, telomeric to the *RH* loci. As the propositus has received no *D1S80* allele from her mother, Okuda *et al.* [84] propose that a region of chromosome 1, containing *RHCE* and *D1S80*, was deleted during maternal gametogenesis.

A *cE* allele of *RHCE* (named *cEMI*) in a D+C+c+E−e+ black individual contained a nine-nucleotide deletion in exon 3 and appeared to produce no Rh polypeptide at the red cell surface [343]. There is no evidence that it was linked to *RHD*.

Like Rh$_{null}$ cells, D−− cells have a substantial reduction in content of CD47 (Section 5.5.8 and see Table 5.13), but only slight reduction on RhAG [479].

An unusual form of D−− produced Tar (RH40) [243], a low frequency antigen usually associated with DVII (Section 5.6.4.6). The D antigen produced by this D−− haplotype was stronger than that usually associated with Tar, but weaker than normal D.

5.15.2 *D··* and Evans (RH37)

Similarity between *D−−* and the Rh haplotype producing the low frequency antigen Evans, recognized during studies on the first two Evans+ propositi, led to the Evans haplotype being denoted *D··* [701]. Inheritance of the haplotype was straightforward. Testing of apparent D−− red cell samples with anti-Evans led to discovery of the first person homozygous for *D··* (HD) [480]. Positive reactions of apparent D−− red cells with immune sera from D−− individuals disclosed a second *D··* homozygote [481]. Families with *D··* have all been white, mostly British.

The antigens produced by *D··* are D, G, Evans, and the high frequency antigens Rh29 and Dav (RH47) [440]. The D antigen is elevated, but less so than that produced by D−− [480]. The number of D antigen sites per red cell were estimated to be 56 000 for *D··/D··*, compared with 110 000–202 000 for *D−−/D−−* and 21 000 for *DcE/DcE* [480].

Molecular analyses on a Scottish family (AT) with five Evans+ members in three generations demonstrated that *D··* comprised *RHCE–D–CE*, with exons 2 (or 3) to 6 derived from *RHCE*, paired with *RHD* [482] (Fig. 5.9). A very similar haplotype, but with exon 1 and the 5′ untranslated region of the hybrid gene also derived from *RHD*, was present in a *D··* homozygote (HD) [478] (although a different result was obtained on the same individual in another study [475]). In another family study, in which the propositus (JD) was heterozygous for *D··* and D−−, the haplotype producing Evans comprised *RHCE–D*, with only exon 1 derived from *RHCE*, plus *RHD–CE*, with the 3′ end of exon 6 (encoding Cys311) and exons 7–10 derived from *RHCE* [442]. The amino acid sequence encoded by the junction of the 5′ end of *RHD* exon 6 and the 3′ end of *RHCE* exon 7 creates a unique amino acid sequence in the fifth cyt oplasmic domain of the protein (Table 5.11). Conformational changes resulting from this sequence are probably responsible for Evans expression. The gene encoding the partial D antigen DIVb also has this exon 6–7 junction and also encodes Evans (Section 5.6.4.3 and Fig. 5.6) [227].

5.15.3 *Dc−*

The first homozygous *Dc−* propositus was found in an inbred white American family of French extraction [483]. His parents were double first cousins and two of

Table 5.11 Amino acid sequences Leu303 to Cys316 encoded by the 3' end of exon 6 and the 5' end of exon 7 of *RHD*, *RHCE*, and two hybrid genes encoding Evans. The important residues in Evans expression appear to be Val/Ile306 and Gly/Val314, but not Tyr/Cys310.

Gene	Exon 6													Exon 7		
				306				310						314		
RHD	...	L	I	S	V	G	G	A	K	Y	L	P		G	C	C ...
RHCE	...	–	–	–	I	–	–	–	–	C	–	–		V	–	– ...
RHD-CE Evans (AT & HD)	...	–	–	–	I	–	–	–	–	–	–	–		V	–	– ...
RHD-CE Evans (JD)	...	–	–	–	–	–	–	–	–	C	–	–		V	–	– ...

–, Identical residue to that encoded by RHD.

his four sibs were also *Dc–/Dc–*. Three other propositi with the Dc– phenotype have been reported: Japanese [484], French [485], and Argentinian [486]. The four Dc– propositi were ascertained through the presence anti-Hr$_0$ in their serum.

Dc– produces D, G, c, Rh29, and, sometimes, ce. The strength of the D antigen is elevated and that of c is depressed; the c antigen may also differ qualitatively from normal c [340,483]. Dc– is serologically heterogeneous: red cells of the Japanese propositus expressed no ce; those of the French and American propositi reacted with anti-ce made in DCe/DcE individuals [30].

Transcript analysis on the French Dc– homozygote revealed *RHD* plus *RHCE–D–CE*, with exons 4–9 derived from *RHD* [474] (Fig. 5.9). Exon 2 encoded Pro103, explaining the c expression. It is possible that the weak expression of ce is caused by Ala226, encoded by the *RHD*-derived exon, explaining the absence of e.

Some haplotypes dubbed *Dc–* should, more accurately, be called Dc(e) or Dc((e)), as e can be detected by adsorption–elution tests or even by direct testing [30,340,487,488] (Section 5.14.2.3). These haplotypes, mostly found in black people, have normal c and either normal or only slightly enhanced D.

5.15.4 DC^w–

A propositus identified as homozygous for *DC^w–* was a member of a large Canadian family [489]. Her parents were second cousins and four of her eight sibs were also *DC^w–/DC^w–*. *DC^w–* produces D, G, C^w, and Rh29; the D antigen is elevated in strength [489] and the C^w is depressed [490]. Unlike other haplotypes

producing C^w, *DC^w–* makes neither C nor c. One other apparent *DC^w–* homozygote has been reported [443].

The original *DC^w–/DC^w–* propositus had transcripts representing *RHD* and *RHCE–D–CE*, with exons 2 (or 3) to 9 derived from *RHD* [474] (Fig. 5.9). The second propositus had *RHCE–D*, with only exon 1 derived from *RHCE*, paired (or possibly *in trans*) with *RHD–CE* with only exon 10 derived from *RHCE* [443] (Fig. 5.9). In both individuals, the *RHCE*-derived exon 1 encoded Arg41, characteristic of C^w (Section 5.12).

5.15.5 DIV(C)– and Riv (RH45)

Homozygosity for a haplotype denoted *DIV(C)–* was proposed to explain the reactions of red cells of a woman from the Ivory Coast (Mme Nou), whose third child had fatal HDN [491]. Her two children had the same weak expression of C as their mother. The following antigens are produced by *DIV(C)–*: partial D giving the reactions of a strong DIV antigen; apparently normal G; very depressed C; Go^a (a low frequency antigen always associated with DIVa, Section 5.6.4.3); three other low frequency antigens, Rh33, Riv, and FPTT [195,700]; and three high frequency antigens, Rh29, Nou (RH43), and Dav (RH47) [440,492,493]. Three of 10 anti-e sera reacted with DIV(C)– cells, but were not proven to lack anti-Ce [447].

No other *DIV(C)–* homozygote has been found, but the association with low frequency antigens has led to the identification of three propositi heterozygous for *DIV(C)–*, all of African ancestry [700]. The unusual haplotype and the low frequency antigens were inherited together.

5.15.6 Anti-Hr$_o$ (-RH17) and related antibodies

People with D–– and related phenotypes, who have been exposed to red cells of common phenotype by transfusion or pregnancy, usually have antibodies to high frequency Rh antigens.

Red cells and immune sera of D––, Dc–, and DC^w– people are mutually compatible, showing that there is no anti-C^w or -c component. All such sera are non-reactive with Rh$_{null}$ cells. In tests with red cells of common Rh phenotypes, these sera appear to contain an antibody to a single high frequency determinant, named Hr$_o$ and numbered RH17. In some of the sera, separable anti-e has also been identified [339,440, 459,494].

Heterogeneity within anti-Hr$_o$ specificity is demonstrated by the variable reactions of different anti-Hr$_o$ with red cells of phenotypes representing homozygosity for certain rare Rh haplotypes, DIV(C)–, D··, r^G, R^{oHar}, and also with Rh$_{mod}$ cells [339,340,434,440]. Adsorption and elution tests showed that those D–– sera reactive with DIV(C)– cells contained at least two antibodies to high frequency antigens, one that reacted with the DIV(C)– cells, named anti-Nou (anti-RH44), and one that did not [492,493]. Similar tests with D·· cells revealed an antibody, named anti-Dav (anti-RH47), in some D–– sera [440]. Anti-Dav reacted with cells of common Rh phenotype and with D·· cells. Other antibodies to high frequency antigens, non-reactive with Rh$_{null}$ and D–– cells, have been identified in individuals with unusual Rh phenotypes, such as those homozygous for R^N (anti-Rh46), or for genes producing partial e antigens (anti-Hr, -Hr^B) [340,341,430,699]. As polyclonal anti-D represents a mixture of antibodies directed at numerous epitopes on different regions of the D protein (Section 5.6.3), so anti-Hr$_o$ represents antibodies to epitopes on different regions of the CcEe protein. D–– cells lack the whole Hr$_o$ mosaic and, when immunized, D–– people can make a variety of antibodies to different parts of the mosaic, collectively referred to as anti-Hr$_o$ and including anti-Nou, -Dav, -Hr, and -Hr^B.

Anti-Hr$_o$ in the sera of D––, Dc–, DC^w–, and DIV(C)– mothers has been responsible for severe, and often fatal, HDN [459,462–464,467,483,489, 491,495]. In one case of fatal HDN the mother admitted no previous history of pregnancy or blood transfusion [463].

Monoclonal antibodies that behave as anti-Hr$_o$ were produced in a mouse immunized with human red cells [431] and in a crab-eating macaque immunized with gorilla and human red cells [496]. These antibodies detect non-polymorphic epitopes on the RhCcEe protein, but not on RhD.

5.16 Rh-deficiency phenotypes: Rh$_{null}$ and Rh$_{mod}$

The Rh$_{null}$ phenotype, in which no Rh antigens can be detected on the red cells, was first described by Vos et al. [497] in 1961. Rh$_{null}$ is very rare, as reflected by the high consanguinity rate among parents of Rh$_{null}$ propositi. Two types of Rh$_{null}$, with an identical Rh phenotype, are distinguished on the basis of their inheritance and molecular genetics.

1 The amorph type represents apparent homozygosity for silent genes at RHD and RHCE loci, resulting from inactivating mutations in RHCE and a deletion of RHD.

2 In the regulator type the Rh genes are normal, but there is homozygosity (or double heterozygosity) for inactivating mutations in RHAG, the gene encoding the Rh-associated glycoprotein (RhAG), without which Rh antigens are not expressed (Section 5.5.7). Some mutations in RHAG give rise to low level expression of Rh antigens, a phenotype called Rh$_{mod}$.

5.16.1 Rh$_{null}$ of the amorph type

The amorph type of Rh$_{null}$ is extremely rare, with only four propositi reported: Japanese [498–500], German [501,502,703], Norwegian Lapp [30], and Spanish [503,703]. Family analyses suggested that their unusual phenotype was caused by homozygosity for a silent or amorph gene at the RH locus and the symbol –––/––– was used for the genotype. The parents and children of amorph Rh$_{null}$ individuals are obligate heterozygotes for the amorph gene and consequently always appear, from serological results, to be homozygous at the RH locus. The presence of a silent haplotype may be demonstrated if, for example, an apparent DCe/DCe parent (DCe/–––) has an apparent DcE/DcE child (DcE/–––).

Titration of anti-c and -e with red cells of 1803 German donors revealed four apparent ––– heterozygotes, verified by family studies [501]. A frequency of 0.0001–0.0002 was estimated for ––– in Sweden [472].

Table 5.12 Mutations associated with Rh-deficiency phenotypes.

Name	Population	Mutation		References
Rh$_{null}$ amorph				
DR	German	*RHCE.Ce*	TCA→C, frameshift after Ile322	[501,502,703]
	Japanese	*RHCE.ce*	Deletion TCTTC, frameshift after Leu26	[498,500]
DAA	Spanish	*RHCE.ce*	Intron 4 5′ splice site	[503,703]
Rh$_{null}$ regulator				
SF, JL	White South African	*RHAG*	CCTC→GA, frameshift after Tyr51	[479,504]
TB	Swiss	*RHAG*	Heterozygous A deletion, frameshift after Ala362 + no detectable transcript	[479]
HT	Japanese	*RHAG*	Val270 Ile, Gly280Arg	[505]
WO	Japanese	*RHAG*	Gly380Val (partial exon 9 skipping)	[505]
YT	Australian	*RHAG*	Heterozygous Gly279Glu + intron 1 5′ splice site	[506–508]
TT	Japanese	*RHAG*	Intron 7 5′ splice site, frameshift after Thr315	[96]
AL	White American	*RHAG*	Intron 1 5′ splice site	[479,704]
AC	Spanish, Japanese	*RHAG*	Intron 6 3′ splice site, frameshift after Thr315	[509,704]
Rh$_{mod}$				
SM	Russian Jewish	*RHAG*	Met1Ile	[510]
VL	White American	*RHAG*	Ser79Asn	[479,511]
CB	French	*RHAG*	Heterozygous Asp399Tyr + ?	[512]

The pertinent mutations have been resolved for three of the amorph Rh$_{null}$ individuals (Table 5.12). In each there is no *RHD*, but homozygosity for a grossly intact *RHCE* gene containing an inactivating mutation. In the German [502,703] and Japanese [500] propositi, respectively, dinucleotide (exon 7) and pentanucleotide (exon 1) deletions predict reading frameshifts and premature termination of translation. If translated, the gene with the exon 1 mutation would produce a protein of only 31 amino acids. The gene with the exon 7 mutation would give rise to a 398-residue protein (compared with 417 residues in the normal protein), with a completely changed C-terminal 76 amino acid sequence. If the 398-residue protein were produced, it would be abnormally folded and unlikely to be inserted in the membrane. Alternatively, the protein might be inserted in the membrane, but not accessible to antibodies.

The Spanish propositus had a mutation in the intron 4 donor spice site of *RHCE*, giving rise to aberrant transcripts [703]. Both parents, three brothers, and three children of the propositus were heterozygous for the mutation.

5.16.2 Rh$_{null}$ of the regulator type

The first Rh$_{null}$ propositus, an Australian aboriginal woman, was found during an anthropological survey [497,513]. No close relative was available for testing. The second Rh$_{null}$ propositus was a member of a large family [514]. The Rh groups showed that her rare phenotype resulted from inhibition of her *RH* genes: her husband was dce/dce, yet their daughter was DCe/dce and must have received D and C from her Rh$_{null}$ mother. Race and Sanger [30] coined the term 'regulator' for this type of Rh$_{null}$. The regulator type of Rh$_{null}$ can be recognized when a parent or child of the Rh$_{null}$ propositus is heterozygous at the *RH* locus; that is, when they have both C and c, and/or both E and e antigens.

Although Rh$_{null}$ remains very rare, many examples of the families displaying the regulator type have been reported. These have been people of white European origin [504,506,507,514–521,704] or Japanese [96, 505,522,523]. No Rh$_{null}$ of black African origin has been found.

The regulator gene was called X°*r* by Levine *et al.*

[514], an unfortunate terminology as the X-chromosome is not involved. Family studies showed that the regulator locus is not part of the *RH* complex locus [30]. In 1996, Chérif-Zahar *et al.* [479] showed that Rh_{null} of the regulator type was associated with inactivating mutations in *RHAG*, making *RHAG* a prime candidate for the regulator locus. Several other *RHAG* inactivating mutations, in other Rh_{null} individuals, have confirmed the association (Table 5.12). Some Rh_{null} individuals are homozygous, others doubly heterozygous, for *RHCE*-inactivating mutations. In all cases except one, normal *RHD* and *RHCE* were present, the exception having no *RHD* [512]. The *RHAG* mutations include frameshift mutations, which predict truncated proteins [479], and splice site mutations, which give rise to abnormally spliced transcripts [96,479,506–509,704] (Table 5.12). As with the Rh proteins, it is possible that the predicted proteins, if translated, are not transported to the membrane or cannot be inserted into the membrane.

Some cases of Rh_{null} result from single or double missense mutations in *RHAG* [505–508] (Table 5.12). The encoded amino acid substitutions are predicted to be in the fourth cytoplasmic domain (Val270 Ile) and the ninth (Gly279Glu and Gly380Val) and twelfth (Gly380Val) membrane-spanning domains. Why these apparently minor changes to the protein prevent expression of the Rh antigens is unclear. The missense mutation encoding Gly380Val is in the first nucleotide of exon 9 and also causes partial splicing of exon 9 [505].

Evidence exists that RhAG is not required for insertion of the Rh proteins in the membrane, but that in the absence of RhAG the Rh proteins are conformationally changed and cannot be detected with antibodies (Section 5.5.7).

In some families, heterozygosity for the regulator allele resulted in weakened expression of some Rh antigens [504,513–517,521].

5.16.3 Rh_mod

A phenotype associated with modified expression of antigens produced by both *RH* haplotypes was called Rh_{mod} by Chown *et al.* [511]. Red cells with this phenotype could easily be mistaken for Rh_{null} if only limited testing were carried out. Initially, the original propositus appeared to be r^G, but extensive tests revealed weak D, C, c, E, and e on her cells. Her parents

were consanguineous and her rare phenotype was attributed to homozygosity for a modifier gene (called X^Q), at a locus separate from the Rh complex locus [511]. Reports on several other Rh_{mod} propositi have been published [510,524–528]. About half of the known propositi are Japanese and the parents of most Rh_{mod} propositi are consanguineous.

Rh_{mod} is a heterogeneous phenotype. Apart from G, the Rh antigens of the first propositus were only detected by adsorption–elution tests with selected sera [511]. The Rh antigens of the second propositus were much stronger and the C, c, and G antigens could be detected by direct testing [434,524]. In contrast, the third propositus was originally called Rh_{null}, although D was revealed by adsorption and elution, the only Rh antigen to be detected [525]. Rh_{mod} cells are most easily distinguished from Rh_{null} by immune sera from some people with D–– and related phenotypes (anti-Hr$_o$) and by some anti-Rh29 [434]. Relatives of Rh_{mod} individuals, heterozygous for the modifier gene, may have reduced expression of Rh antigens [524,527].

Molecular analyses on three Rh_{mod} propositi have suggested that the modifying gene is *RHAG*, the same gene as that responsible for the regulator type of Rh_{null} (Table 5.12) [479,510,512]. All three propositi have missense mutations in *RHAG*; two of them are homozygous, the other heterozygous with any mutation in the *trans* gene still to be elucidated. In the Jewish family of Russian origin the mutation converts the translation-initiating methionine codon to an isoleucine codon. It is probable that the small quantity of RhAG produced is translated from the ATG triplet that normally encodes Met8 [510]. The amino acid substitutions in the other two Rh_{mod} individuals are in the first cytoplasmic loop of RhAG (position 79) [479] and in the C-terminal cytoplasmic tail (position 399) [512]. All three propositi had low quantities of RhAG in their red cell membranes [479,510,512].

5.16.4 Antibodies in the sera of Rh_null people

Anti-Rh29 (anti 'total Rh'), an antibody found in the serum of some immunized Rh_{null} individuals, reacts with red cells of all Rh phenotypes apart from Rh_{null} [501,504,518–521,523]. Anti-Rh29 has been made by people with Rh_{null} of both types. Not all Rh_{null} individuals make anti-Rh29 when immunized; two Rh_{null} sisters had no Rh antibody although they had a total of nine children [30]. Other immunized Rh_{null} individuals are reported to have made anti-e [514] or -Hr$_o$ [503]. Antibodies in the sera of two Rh$_{null}$ donors who had received no known immunizing stimulus behaved as anti-Hr$_o$, reacting with all red cell samples save those of Rh$_{null}$ and D−− phenotypes [522,529].

Anti-Rh29 has been responsible for mild HDN [504,519] and for severe HDN, which was successfully managed by repeated exchange transfusions with D− blood of common Rh phenotypes [520]. Anti-Hr$_o$ in an Rh$_{null}$ woman was also responsible for HDN [503]. A haemolytic transfusion reaction caused by anti-Rh29 may have contributed to the death of an elderly Rh$_{null}$ patient transfused with D− blood of common phenotype [530].

A variety of mouse monoclonal antibodies behave like anti-Rh29 and probably define epitopes common to both Rh polypeptides (Section 5.18.6).

5.16.5 Other antigens affected in Rh deficiency phenotypes

Affects of the Rh deficiency phenotypes extend beyond the Rh blood group system. Several red cell antigens are lacking, or at least show reduced expression, on Rh$_{null}$ and Rh$_{mod}$ red cells (Sections 5.5.7 and 5.5.8).

RhAG is not detected on Rh$_{null}$ red cells of the regulator type and is expressed in reduced quantity on Rh$_{mod}$ cells (Table 5.13). Indeed, as described above, it is the absence or altered conformation of RhAG that is primarily responsible for these phenotypes. RhAG is present on Rh$_{null}$ cells of the amorph type, but in reduced quantity [479]. Duclos antigen, which is probably located on RhAG (Section 5.5.7.1), is also absent from most Rh$_{null}$ cells.

The high frequency antigens of the LW system, LW^a and LW^{ab}, are absent from all Rh$_{null}$ cells and weakly expressed on Rh$_{mod}$ cells (Chapter 16). Anti-Fy5 of the Duffy system behaves like anti-Fy3, except that it does not react with Rh-deficiency cells, none of which are Fy:−3 (Chapter 8). Rh-deficiency cells have reduced expression of glycophorin B and are often U− (Sections 5.5.9 and 3.22). CD47, a glycoprotein on red cells with no blood group activity, is also present in reduced quantity on Rh-deficiency cells (Table 5.13).

Glycophorin A antigens, M, N, and En^a, are reported to be slightly enhanced in the regulator type of Rh$_{null}$ (amorph type not mentioned) [30,531]; some increase in strength of Jk^a, Jk^b, and Do^a has also been found [30]. Elevation of i antigen on Rh-deficiency

Table 5.13 Estimated numbers of RhAG and CD47 molecules on Rh-deficiency and D−− cells [479,703,704].

Phenotype	Number of molecules per cell (range)	
	RhAG	CD47
Rh$_{null}$ regulator	0	2 900–3 900
Rh$_{null}$ amorph	44 000–58 000	2 000–3 000
Rh$_{mod}$	43 000	6 600
D−−	180 000–206 000	8 000–12 000
D+	220 000–280 000	35 000–50 000

phenotype cells probably results from bone marrow stress caused by the associated anaemia [532]. Antibodies that reacted with Rh$_{null}$ cells and with cells of other 'null' phenotypes, but not with cells of 'normal' phenotypes unless they had been papain treated, were found in three patients with anaemia [533,534].

Many human autoantibodies are considered Rh-related because they do not react with Rh$_{null}$ cells. Weiner and Vos [631] called these antibodies anti-pdl (anti-partially deleted), to distinguish them from anti-dL (anti-deleted), which react with all red cells, and anti-nl (antinormal), which react with all red cells except for Rh$_{null}$ and D−− cells.

5.16.6 Rh-deficiency syndrome

Schmidt et al. [532,535] were first to recognize that Rh$_{null}$ red cells are morphologically and functionally abnormal. Most Rh$_{null}$ and Rh$_{mod}$ individuals have some degree of haemolytic anaemia, the severity of which varies from severe enough to merit splenectomy to a fully compensated state requiring sophisticated tests to demonstrate shortened red cell survival. Typical symptoms of Rh-deficiency syndrome are the presence of stomatocytes (cup-shaped red cells) and some spherocytes, reduced survival of autologous red cells, increased red cell osmotic fragility, increased reticulocyte counts, increased fetal haemoglobin, enhanced i antigen strength, and reduced haemoglobin and haptoglobin levels (reviews in [512,536]).

Investigation of Rh$_{null}$ red cell membranes did not reveal any obvious aberration of their structural components compared with normal cells [518,537]. Rh$_{null}$ red cells have an abnormal organization of their membrane phospholipids [538], increased cation permeability, partially compensated by an increase in the number of K^+Na^+ pumps [539], reduced cation and water contents [518], and reduced membrane cholesterol content [518]. It is not known whether any of these defects accounts directly for the autohaemolyis in Rh-deficiency syndrome. Issitt [540] points out that the haemolytic anaemia is alleviated by splenectomy, so whatever the ultimate cause of stomatocytosis in Rh-deficiency syndrome, it is the early sequestration of these abnormally shaped cells that is responsible for the anaemia. Binding of CD47 on red cells to SIRPα on macrophages generates a negative signal that protects against phagocytosis of the red cells (Section 5.5.8), so reduced CD47 levels on Rh_{null} cells could be involved in their elimination [120].

5.17 Low frequency Rh antigens and the antibodies that define them

5.17.1 Low frequency antigens

Twenty antigens of low incidence belong to the Rh system (Table 5.14). Without exception, the presence of these antigens is associated with abnormal (usually partial or depressed) expression of one or more of the DCcEe antigens. Consequently, the low frequency antigens make useful markers for rare haplotypes. Although an oversimplification, as reference to the appropriate sections of this chapter reveals, the low frequency antigens can be loosely classified as follows:

D^w, Go^a, Rh32, Rh33, Evans, Tar, FPTT, BARC, DAK: associated with partial D (Section 5.6.4)

C^w, C^x: associated with abnormal C (Section 5.12)

E^w: associated with abnormal E (Section 5.9.4)

V, VS, Rh42, STEM: associated with abnormal e (Sections 5.9.5, 5.13)

Rh32, Rh35, JAL, FPTT, DAK: associated with abnormal *DCe* (Section 5.14.1)

Rh33, JAL: associated with abnormal *Dce* (Section 5.14.2)

Be^a: associated with abnormal *dce* (Section 5.14.3.2)

JAHK: associated with abnormal *dCe* (Section 5.11)

Evans: associated with abnormal *D−−* (Section 5.15.2)

Go^a, Rh33, Riv, FPTT: associated with *DIV(C)−* (Section 5.15.5).

Family studies have shown that expression of these low frequency antigens is controlled by the *RH* com-

plex locus. It is not safe to assume that an antigen belongs to the Rh system simply because it is associated with abnormal expression of Rh antigens. The Ol(a+) members of a large family had weak expression of some Rh antigens while the Rh antigens of the Ol(a−) members were normal, yet the family showed that Ol^a is not inherited at the *RH* complex locus [541]. It is feasible, but purely speculative, that Ol^a arises from a mutation in *RHAG*. Two other low incidence antigens, HOFM (700050) and LOCR (700053), are associated with abnormal expression of Rh antigens in families, but insufficient evidence has prevented their elevation to the Rh system. HOFM is associated with depressed C antigen in the only family in which it has been detected [542]. All six members of the family were HOFM+ and had depressed C: in the C+c+ members this weakness was easily detected; in the C+c− members the scores with anti-C were comparable to C/c heterozygotes. LOCR is transmitted with *dce* in all three families tested; in two families it is associated with weakened c and in the other family with weakened e [543]. Lod scores at θ = 0.0 for *RH* and the gene controlling LOCR are only 2.107, still short of statistical significance. DAK appears to be associated with DIIIa, respectively, but this remains to be confirmed [175]. Regrettably, the antigen Crawford [544] received the number RH43, although there is no evidence that it is an Rh antigen.

Most of the antigens listed in Table 5.14 are of low incidence in all populations tested, but the frequencies of some vary in different populations. C^w and VS would not be considered private antigens in white and black populations, respectively.

5.17.2 Speculation on the molecular basis of Rh32 and FPTT

The molecular backgrounds to some of the Rh low frequency antigens can be speculated on from the changes to the *RHD* and *RHCE* genes associated with their expression. These are described in other sections of this chapter. Two antigens, Rh32 and FPTT, are each associated with two serologically very different phenotypes and these will be described in more detail here.

Rh32 is associated with the partial D antigen DBT, usually together with C and e (Section 5.6.4.8). R^N produces Rh32 together with slightly elevated D, weak C, and weak e (Section 5.14.1.1). DBT arises from

Table 5.14 Antibodies to low frequency Rh antigens.

Antigen		Red cell immune	'Naturally occurring'	Other antibodies present	HDN	No. of examples	References
C^w	RH8	Yes	Yes	Yes	Yes	Many	[392,395,401]
C^x	RH9	Yes	Yes	Yes	Mild	Many	[405,406,408]
V	RH10	Yes	No	Yes	No	Many	[411,415–417]
E^w	RH11	Yes	No	No	Yes	Several	[327,328]
VS	RH20		Yes	Yes	No	Many	[412,415]
D^w	RH23		Yes	Yes*	No	Several	[229,419]
Go^a	RH30	Yes	Yes	Yes*	Yes	Several	[225,420]
Rh32	RH32	Yes	Yes	Yes*	Yes	Several	[421–423]
Rh33	RH33		Yes	Yes	No	3	[196,424]
Rh35	RH35		Yes	Yes	No	1	[425]
Be^a	RH36	Yes	No	No	Yes	Several	[426–429]
Evans	RH37	Yes	Yes	Yes*	Yes	Several	[701]
Tar	RH40	Yes	Yes	Yes	Yes	3	[243–245]
Rh42	RH42	Yes	No	No	Mild	2	[413]
Riv	RH45	Yes	No	Yes	Mild	1	[700]
JAL	RH48	Yes	Yes	Yes	Mild	3	[702]
STEM	RH49	Yes	No	Yes	Mild	Several	[352]
FPTT	RH50		Yes	Yes	No	1	[195]
BARC	RH52		Yes	Yes	No	1	[233]
JAHK	RH53		Yes	Yes	No	Several	[376]
DAK			Yes	Yes	No	Several	[175]

*Not always separable from other Rh specificities, see text.

an *RHD–CE–D* gene in which exons 5–7 (or 5–9) are *RHCE*-derived (Fig. 5.10). R^N consists of *RHD* and *RHCE–D–CE* in which exon 4 is *RHD*-derived. From comparison of the abnormal hybrid genes in the *DBT* and in the R^N haplotypes it appears that Rh32 could result from the conformation of an Rh polypeptide with the product of *RHD* exon 4 fused to the product of *RHCE* exon 5. However, Rh32 does not simply arise from a unique linear amino acid sequence resulting from the gene rearrangements. A sequence of 21 amino acids spanning the junction of the products of exons 4 of *RHD* and exon 5 of *RHCE* is identical in the polypeptides encoded by the two genes. Rh32 must be a discontinuous antigen involving two extracellular loops of the Rh protein. The abnormal genes in both *DBT* and R^N produce a polypeptide in which the three amino acid residues characteristic of a D polypeptide within the third extracellular loop (Met169, Met170, Ile172) could interact with the one amino acid characteristic of a CcEe polypeptide in the fourth extracellular loop (Gln233), to create Rh32 (Fig. 5.10).

FPTT is associated with the rare R^{oHar} gene, which also produces a partial D antigen (DHAR), c, very weak e, and another low frequency antigen, Rh33 (Sections 5.6.4.9 and 5.14.2.1). FPTT is also associated with DFR, another partial D antigen (Section 5.6.4.7). R^{oHar} is an *RHCE–D–CE* gene in which only exon 5 is *RHD*-derived. DFR is produced by *RHD–CE–D* in which part of exon 4 is *RHCE*-derived. FPTT appears to be the opposite to Rh32, resulting from the interaction of a third extracellular loop encoded by *RHCE*-derived exon 4 and a fourth extracellular loop encoded by *RHD*-derived exon 5 (Fig. 5.10).

5.17.3 Antibodies to low frequency antigens

Table 5.14 summarizes published and unpublished information available to the author; other examples of these antibodies may well exist. Some antibodies have caused severe HDN, but where antibodies are shown to have caused mild HDN, in a few cases this may only represent a positive DAT on the baby's red cells. Anti-Go^a is implicated in a delayed haemolytic transfusion reaction [545].

Although some specificities, for example anti-Go^a

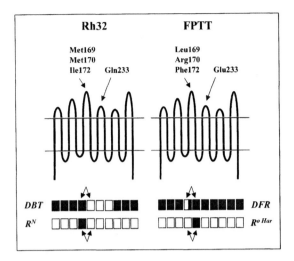

Fig. 5.10 Molecular bases of the low frequency Rh antigens Rh32 and FPTT. Rh32 probably results from the interaction between a third extracellular (EC) loop encoded by an *RHD*-derived exon 4 and a fourth EC loop encoded by an *RHCE*-derived exon 5 in the hybrid genes associated with DBT and R^N. FPTT probably results from the interaction between a third EC loop encoded by an *RHCE*-derived exon 4 and a fourth EC loop encoded by an *RHD*-derived exon 5 in the hybrid genes associated with DFR and R$_o$^{Har}.

and anti-Rh32, are each found as the sole antibody in some sera and may have caused HDN, in other sera they occur together and are 'naturally occurring'. When these two specificities are found together they are generally not separable by adsorption. To take a specific example, the Tillett serum contained antibodies to many low incidence antigens, although Mrs Tillett had not been exposed to these antigens. Anti-Go^a, -Evans, and, sometimes, anti-Rh32 were present in Tillett serum, but these specificities could not be isolated from each other by adsorption and elution: adsorption with Rh:32 Go(a–) Evans– cells removed activity against Go(a+) and Evans+ cells, as well as against Rh:32 cells. Adsorption with Rh:32 cells of a later batch of Tillett serum, which no longer contained anti-Rh32, did not affect the strength of the anti-Go^a and -Evans, but adsorption with either Evans+ or Go(a+) cells removed all activity for those cells [165]. Presumably conformational similarities exist between Rh32, Evans, and Go^a determinants and some antibodies detect a common feature of these determinants whereas others can distinguish between them.

Some anti-D^w are specific for the product of a *DVa* gene, in which the presence of Gln233 in an RhD pro-

tein appears to be the key factor (Section 5.6.4.4). However, most anti-D^w also react with Rh:32 cells, some reacting only weakly with the Rh:32 cells and some reacting as strongly with Rh:32 cells as with D^w+ cells [546]. Comparison of *DVa* genes, which produce D^w, with *DBT* and *R^N* genes, which produce Rh32 (Figs 5.6 and 5.9), reveals that all involve exon 5 encoding Gln233 (*RHCE*) adjacent to exon 4 derived from *RHD*.

5.18 Rh antibodies

Most details on the specificities of Rh antibodies are to be found in the preceding sections, where the antigens they define are described. Provided here are more general comments on Rh antibodies, polyclonal and monoclonal, and on their clinical significance.

Rh antibodies are usually produced in response to red cell immunization resulting from blood transfusion or pregnancy, although 'naturally occurring' Rh antibodies are not unknown. Rh antibodies generally react optimally at 37°C, their reactivity being enhanced by protease treatment of the cells. Most Rh antibodies, in the absence of an enhancing medium, do not directly agglutinate untreated antigen-positive red cells.

Most Rh antibodies should be considered potential agents of HDN and of haemolytic transfusion reactions. Transfusion reactions may be immediate or delayed.

5.18.1 Anti-D

5.18.1.1 Alloanti-D

Anti-D are mostly IgG, but some sera may contain an IgM component. Sera containing IgM anti-D usually agglutinate saline suspended D+ cells, as do some sera containing relatively high concentrations of IgG anti-D alone [270]. Most anti-D sera from hyperimmunized subjects also contain an IgA component [270]. IgG1 and IgG3 are the predominant anti-D subclasses; IgG1 is nearly always present and, in individuals who have received multiple immunizations, both subclasses are generally detected [270,547,548]. IgG2 and IgG4 anti-D are also found occasionally [548–550].

The failure of almost all anti-D to activate complement is attributed to the distance between antigen sites, which prevents the collaboration between IgG molecules required for C1q binding [270]. D+ red cells that had been very heavily coated with anti-D bound up to 1600 molecules of C1q, yet the classical complement pathway was not activated [551]; however, there are exceptions. For example, one well-investigated anti-C+D (Ripley) would haemolyse D+ cells through the activation of complement [552,553] and a complement binding anti-D was found in the serum of a woman with a weak partial D [554].

Examples of IgG anti-D in the sera of untransfused men have been described [555,556], but these are rare. 'Naturally occurring' IgG anti-D that were only detectable in an AutoAnalyser, were reported to be relatively common [557].

Human anti-D was produced in mice with severe combined immunodeficiency (SCID), which had been reconstituted with peripheral blood mononuclear cells obtained from D– people who had recently been sensitized with D+ red cells [558]. When mononuclear cells were used from donors many years after sensitization, no anti-D was produced in the mice even though anti-D was still present in the donor's plasma. It appears that long-lived or memory cells are not present in the peripheral blood of individuals who have not been recently boosted.

5.18.1.2 Monoclonal anti-D

The development of the mouse hybridoma technique in the late 1970s and 1980s led to the production of murine monoclonal antibodies to a host of blood group antigens, yet mouse monoclonal anti-D has never been made. Failure to make anti-D in mice stimulated attempts to produce human monoclonal antibodies, primarily to replace polyclonal antibodies as grouping reagents and for prophylactic use. The hybridoma technique of Köhler and Milstein [559] was not very successful when applied to humans, but an alternative approach, that of immortalizing human B lymphocytes by *in vitro* transformation with Epstein–Barr virus (EBV) [560], did bring success.

Crawford *et al.* [561] were the first to clone EBV-transformed lymphoblastoid cells to produce a stable cell line secreting anti-D. Although some cell lines producing anti-D made in this way have survived for several years [237,561–565], these cell lines are often unstable [566] and difficult to grow in large-scale culture. To overcome these problems, EBV-transformed lymphoblastoid cells are usually fused with myeloma

cells to produce a hybridoma [567]. Fusion partners used for the production of monoclonal anti-D have been mouse myelomas [564,568–571], mouse–human heterohybridomas [572,573], and human lymphoblastoid cell lines [564,570]. CD40 activation of lymphocytes can be used to replace EBV transformation [574]. One monoclonal anti-D produced by a human × human hybridoma, with no EBV or CD40 activation, is reported [575]. Greatest success in producing monoclonal anti-D has been achieved when lymphocytes from recently rebooted antibody makers were used (for reviews see [576–579]).

Of the 52 cell lines secreting anti-D summarized by McCann *et al.* [578], 17 were IgM and 35 IgG; of the 33 IgG subclassed, 24 were IgG1, eight IgG3, and one IgG2. The predominance of IgG1 and IgG3 molecules reflects the antibody profile of the lymphocyte donors. EBV-transformation followed by fusion appeared to increase the probability of making IgM anti-D [578]. IgA monoclonal anti-D has been reported [568].

Reactions of monoclonal anti-D with red cells expressing partial D antigens has identified numerous epitopes on the RhD protein (Table 5.6 and Section 5.6.3). Most monoclonal anti-D do not react with category VI cells. Leader *et al.* [237] succeeded in making three monoclonal anti-D for detecting DVI antigen by using DVI red cells for rosetting in the production and maintenance of their transformed cell lines.

Idiotype-specific antibodies produced in rabbits immunized with a purified monoclonal anti-D completely inhibited that anti-D, but no other monoclonal or polyclonal anti-D [580]. The idiotype antibodies brought about agglutination of D+ red cells coated with only four of 118 examples of incomplete polyclonal anti-D. Three monoclonal antibodies made by immunizing mice with BRAD-5 monoclonal anti-D detected three different idiotopes on the anti-D [581]. The antibodies bound to BRAD-5 and other antibodies from clones derived from the same donor, but to no other anti-D, including three with the same D epitope specificity.

The IgM heavy chain variable region gene segment V4-34 is present in cold agglutinins with I and i specificity (Section 25.7.1.1). About 85% of IgM monoclonal anti-D are encoded by V4-34 and these antibodies agglutinate papain-treated D– red cells; some will agglutinate untreated D– cells at 4°C [582,583]. This cold agglutination is usually i-specific, but can be I-specific. V4-34 IgM monoclonal anti-D also exhibit tissue multireactivity, mostly directed against intracellular components, in particular cytoplasmic intermediate filament proteins [583,584]. Clearly, the cold agglutinin characteristics of IgM anti-D must be a consideration in the development of reagents. Although multireactivity is pertinent to the development of monoclonal anti-D as HDN prophylactic agents, antibodies required for this purpose are IgG, where multireactivity is much less prevalent.

Anti-D monoclonals and blends of monoclonals are now generally used as Rh grouping reagents. IgM monoclonal anti-D reagents agglutinate all but the weakest of weak D samples, although most do not agglutinate DVI cells (Section 5.6.9 and reviewed in [214,585]). The potential use of monoclonal anti-D in HDN prophylaxis is discussed in the section below.

Human immunoglobulin V-gene cDNA derived from peripheral blood lymphocytes can been amplified and cloned, and the V_H and V_L gene repertoires linked together at random to encode of single chain Fv (scFv) antibody fragments. These synthetic scFv cDNAs are inserted into phage vectors so that they can be incorporated into filamentous phages. By linking the scFv cDNA to a gene for a phage coat protein the encoded scFv molecules are represented at the surface of the phage, which then behaves like an antibody. Phages containing genetic information for variable regions that bind to a specific antigen can then be isolated, by selecting with an appropriate solid phase antigen. Red cells can be used for this purpose. *Escherichia coli* can then be transduced with these genes, cloned, and the single chain variable region fragments are secreted [586]. By this technique, antibody fragments specific for D and E were produced from non-immunized donors, but these antibodies were of low affinity [587,588]. Subsequently, similar phage repertoire cloning techniques have led to the production of Fab fragments with D antigen binding characteristics identical to those of the parental antibodies [589,590].

Genetically engineered IgG anti-D molecules, secreted by insect or mammalian cell lines, have a functional Fc domain and behave normally in immunological functional assays [590,591]. Such engineered antibodies could be candidates for use in HDN prophylaxis.

Sequencing of the genes encoding the variable regions of the light and heavy chains (V_L and V_H) of monoclonal IgG anti-D, revealed an extremely restricted use of germline genes [261,592–595]. The germline V_H segments used in IgG anti-D are among the most cationic available in the human V_H repertoire [593]. This would explain the relatively high isoelectric point of anti-D, compared with that of serum IgG, which may be an important factor in binding to the D antigen, which is located close to the membrane lipids.

5.18.1.3 Clinical significance of anti-D

Clinically, D is the most important red cell antigen after A and B. Anti-D has the potential to cause severe haemolytic transfusion reactions. D+ red cells must never be transfused to patients with anti-D and red cells of donors and recipients should always be typed for D, except in populations where the D– phenotype is very rare. About 85% of D– individuals make anti-D following infusion of 200 mL or more of D+ red cells [270], so D+ cells should not be transfused to D– patients, except in an emergency, and must never be transfused to D– girls and women of child-bearing age. The same criteria should be applied to blood products that may be contaminated with red cells.

Before the 1970s, HDN caused by anti-D was a significant cause of fetal and neonatal morbidity and mortality. In 1970, the incidence of infant deaths and stillbirths from HDN caused by anti-D in England and Wales was 1.2 per 1000 births; by 1989 the figure had fallen to 0.02 per 1000 births [596]. This remarkable fall in prevalence is predominantly the result of immunoprophylaxis with anti-D immunoglobulin, which prevents the production of maternal anti-D following D-incompatible pregnancies. The mechanism for this antibody-mediated immune suppression is not known, but is probably dependent on interactions with an IgG Fcγ receptors (reviewed in [597]). All D– women must receive anti-D immunoglobulin within 72 h of delivery of a D+ baby, the dose of anti-D being related to the size of the transplacental haemorrhage. In addition, it has been recommended that anti-D immunoglobulin be given to all pregnant D– women at 28 and 34 weeks' gestation, to protect against antenatal immunization [598–600].

The severity of anti-D HDN is highly variable. The most severely affected fetuses die *in utero* from about the 17th week of gestation onwards. In less severe cases, hydrops fetalis may occur. In severely affected infants who are born alive, jaundice may develop rapidly and lead to kernicterus. About 70% of infants who develop kernicterus die within a few days; of those who survive, many have permanent cerebral damage [270]. For reviews on Rh HDN, its treatment, and prevention see [270,579,596,598,601,602].

IgG1 and IgG3 anti-D both appear capable of causing HDN, although which of these subclasses is responsible for the more severe disease is controversial [598,602]. A variety of assays has been developed in an attempt to predict the severity of HDN during the course of a pregnancy, to assist in management of the disease. In addition to IgG subclassing and anti-D quantification in an AutoAnalyser, cellular functional assays model the *in vivo* destruction of antibody-coated red cells following interaction with Fcγ-receptors of the mononuclear phagocyte system. Functional cellular assays include:

1 monocyte monolayer assays, which measure adhesion and phagocytosis;

2 chemiluminescence assays, which measure the metabolic response of monocytes during phagocytosis; and

3 monocyte and lymphocyte (K cell) antibody-dependent cell-mediated cytotoxicity (ADCC) assays, which measure haemolysis (reviews in [270,602]).

Despite the sophistication of these tests, none has proved entirely satisfactory [602–604].

The success of the Rh immunoglobulin prophylaxis programme has created a problem: very few D– women become immunized to make anti-D, creating a shortage of the immunoglobulin necessary to prevent their immunization. This shortage has been exacerbated by the introduction of antenatal prophylaxis programmes. The solution, in the short term at least, must lie with monoclonal anti-D, in which an almost infinite volume of immunoglobulin can be produced *in vitro* from one immunization (reviewed in [579]). These potential therapeutic reagents are currently undergoing clinical trials. Radiolabelled D+ red cells were coated, *in vitro*, with varying quantities of two human monoclonal anti-D, one IgG1 (FOG-1) and one IgG3 (BRAD-3), and returned to their donor. Both antibodies mediated immune clearance of the coated cells, but substantially fewer IgG3 molecules were required than IgG1, and there was no synergistic effect when both antibodies were used [605]. When D– volunteers were given intramuscular injections of monoclonal anti-D followed by infusions of radiolabelled D+ red cells, IgG3 anti-D (BRAD-3) induced clearance at a rate slower than polyclonal anti-D, but IgG1 anti-D (BRAD-5) gave a similar clearance rate to

the polyclonal antibody [606]. In another trial, 95 D–male volunteers were injected with 5 mL of D+ red cells and then, 24 h later, received an intramuscular injection of a cocktail of BRAD-3 and -5. The monoclonal antibody appeared generally successful in preventing D immunization, though there was one failure and one possible failure [607].

Peptide immunotherapy, the use of peptides derived from the RhD protein to render D-specific helper T cells tolerant, is another potential approach to preventing anti-D HDN. This technology is currently at an early stage of investigation [608].

Occasional unexpectedly mild cases of HDN occur in the D+ fetuses of women with anti-D and a history of severe HDN in previous pregnancies. This can occur as the result of maternal HLA antibodies blocking Fc receptors on fetal macrophages, protecting sensitized fetal red cells from destruction [609,610]. FcγRI-blocking antibodies could have a potential for the treatment of HDN.

5.18.2 Anti-C, -c, -E, -e, and -G

The numerous complexities of the specificities of antibodies described as anti-C, -c, -E, and -e are described in Sections 5.8 and 5.9. These antibodies share many of the characteristics of anti-D. They are generally immune antibodies, mostly IgG, and predominantly IgG1, although IgG2, IgG3, and IgG4 have all been detected [548]. Antibodies of all these specificities have been involved in haemolytic transfusion reactions, particularly of the delayed type [270]. Anti-c is clinically the most important Rh antigen after anti-D and may cause severe HDN. In three series of studies, between 14% and 21% of c+ babies born to women with anti-c required exchange transfusion [611–613]. Anti-C, -E, -e, and -G have all caused HDN, but the occurrence is rare and the outcome seldom severe [270]. The clinical significance of antibodies with compound CcEe specificities is described in Section 5.10. Anti-G may be mistaken for anti-C+D (Section 5.11). It is important that pregnant women with anti-G or anti-C+G receive anti-D immunoglobulin, to prevent them making anti-D. Unlike other Rh specificities, apparently 'naturally occurring' anti-E are not uncommon [355,356].

Intravascular haemolytic transfusion reactions have been associated with specific Rh antigens in the absence of any detectable Rh antibody [614]. Rh association was inferred because transfusion of red cells positive for a particular Rh antigen resulted in haemolysis, whereas transfusion of antigen-negative cells resulted in normal red cell survival. C, c, and e have been implicated in this type of reaction [614].

Human monoclonal antibodies to C, c, E, e, and G have been produced by cloning of EBV-transformed lymphoblastoid cell lines or by cloning of heterohybridomas produced from a fusion of EBV-transformed cells with mouse myeloma cells (see Section 5.18.1.2) [564,615,616]. One monoclonal anti-C was derived from a heterohybridoma involving untransformed lymphocytes [617]. Mouse monoclonal antibodies with anti-e-like specificity are described below (Section 5.18.6).

5.18.3 'Enzyme-only' antibodies

Some Rh antibodies, often referred to as 'enzyme only' antibodies, agglutinate red cells treated with protease enzymes, but are not detected by conventional antiglobulin tests with untreated cells. Although these antibodies are most often 'naturally occurring' anti-E [353–356], 'enzyme-only' anti-D, -C, -c, -e, and -ce and have also been identified [618–622]. 'Enzyme-only' antibodies are generally clinically insignificant [618,620,621] and are not detected when tests employing protease-treated red cells for antibody screening are avoided; however, there are rare exceptions. Single examples of 'enzyme only' anti-c, -e+ce, and -C (which bound C3) caused haemolytic transfusion reactions [618,619,622]. One 'enzyme-only' anti-E became active by an indirect antiglobulin test during pregnancy and caused HDN requiring exchange transfusion [623].

5.18.4 Rh autoantibodies

Rh antigens are the most common targets for warm autoantibodies [624,625]. The involvement of Rh antibodies in autoimmune haemolytic anaemia (AIHA) was first appreciated when autoantibodies with anti-e specificity were recognized [626]. Of the 'simple' Rh-specific autoantibodies, anti-e is the most common, but anti-c, -E, -D, and -C also occur, roughly in that order of prevalence [624,627,628]. These specificities occasionally occur alone, but more often adsorption tests with Rh-phenotyped red cells are necessary to determine the specificities present on the red cells and in the serum of AIHA patients. Some Rh antibodies with apparently simple specificities, dubbed 'mimicking antibodies' by Issitt et al. [629], can be totally adsorbed by 'antigen-negative' red cells, demonstrating a broader specificity. Cold type AIHA resulting from complement activating IgM autoanti-D has been described [630].

Use of red cells with the rare Rh phenotypes Rh_{null} and D–– showed that antibodies to high incidence Rh antigens often occur as autoantibodies [631]. Rh-related antibodies may also be involved in some cases of drug-induced AIHA [270,624,625]. Loss or weakness of some Rh antigens has been reported in a few patients with AIHA [350,632,633].

Some D+ patients developed anti-D and a positive DAT after transfusion of D+ blood [634–636]. The anti-D was transient, although an injection of D+ blood in one patient restimulated the antibody [635]. Autoanti-D may occur concurrently with alloanti-D in immunized individuals with partial D antigens [637,638] and, rarely, before the alloanti-D can be detected [639].

5.18.5 Transplant donor-derived Rh antibodies

Anti-D derived from donor lymphocytes in D+ recipients of solid organ transplants (kidney, liver, heart–lung) has been responsible for haemolysis, sometimes severe [640–646]. The donor origin of such anti-D has been demonstrated by Gm grouping [641,646]. Chimerism was demonstrated by the presence of leucocytes of donor origin, identified by HLA Class II genotyping, in the peripheral blood of a heart–lung recipient 2 months after transplantation [646]. Anti-c, -E, and -e have also been detected in similar circumstances [642–644,647]. Acute haemolysis caused by anti-D plus -E occurred in a D+ recipient of the liver from a D– donor. Anti-D, -E, and -K were detected in the recipient of a kidney and the pancreas from the same donor, but a third D+ patient, who received the donor's other kidney, did not develop anti-D [643].

Anti-D has been observed in D+ recipients of D– bone marrow [648–651], in one case not appearing until immunosuppression for graft-vs.-host disease had been discontinued, 2 years after transplantation [650]. Anti-D, -E, and -G were detected in the serum of a DcE/dce patient 4 months after he received bone marrow from his sister, presumably the result of immunization of the donor-derived lymphocytes by the patient's D+E+ red cells [651].

5.18.6 Rh-related murine monoclonal antibodies

No mouse monoclonal anti-D, -C, -c, -E, or -e has been produced. Many murine antibodies to high frequency red cell antigens are Rh-related, because they do not react, or react only weakly, with Rh_{null} cells. Some of these antibodies react with D– and D–– cells, suggesting they define epitopes common to the RhCcEe and RhD polypeptides (anti-Rh29-like), others do not react with D–– cells, suggesting that they define RhCcEe-specific epitopes (anti-Rh17-like) [89, 210,431,652]. Some mouse monoclonal antibodies that react with all red cells except those of Rh_{null} and D–– phenotypes show a preference for e+ red cells over e– cells and, under certain conditions, behave as anti-e [210,653–655]. Despite reacting only weakly with DcE/DcE cells, one of these antibodies (BS58) reacted as strongly with DCE/DCE cells as with dce/dce cells [655].

5.19 Rh mosaics and acquired phenotype changes

5.19.1 Malignancy

Abnormal expression of some Rh antigens has occasionally been observed in patients with myeloid leukaemias, polycythaemia, and other myeloproliferative disorders. In most cases these patients appear to be mosaics with two populations of red cells of different Rh phenotype [137,656–661], although a few have complete loss of certain Rh antigens [662–665]. One patient with myeloid metaplasia, previously known to be D+ , was found to be D– and had made anti-D plus -C [663]. Most of these patients are afflicted with conditions that are clonal in origin and their unusual Rh types are attributed to clones of monosomic cells. The strength of antigen expression and proportions of the two cell populations can vary over a period of time [656,661,664]. A myelofibrosis patient with a mixture of DCe/dce and dce/dce cells (father dce/dce, mother DCe/DCe) had an aberrant karyotype, a cytogenetic mixture with an abnormal population containing a balanced translocation involving

chromosomes 1, 4, and 7 [662]. However, in most cases no abnormality of chromosome 1, which contains the Rh genes, was observed.

A D+ woman became D– over a 3-year period, during which she was treated with irradiation for breast cancer and diagnosed with chronic myeloid leukaemia [665]. Reticulocyte transcript analysis revealed *RHD* with a deletion of G600 in exon 4, introducing a reading frameshift and premature stop codon, plus *Ce* and *ce* alleles of *RHCE*. The *RHD* mutation, which was present in neutrophils and cultured erythroblasts, but not lymphoid cells, probably resulted from a somatic mutation in a myeloid stem cell.

5.19.2 Healthy people

Although rare, there are many examples known of apparently healthy people whose blood appears to contain two red cell populations, as judged by tests with Rh antisera, but have no sign of mosaicism in tests for other genetic markers [30,660,666–668]. The Rh mosaicism is not a transient condition. Families of four propositi eliminated chimerism as a possible explanation [30]. Screening with anti-D+C of blood from 552 individuals over 60 years old disclosed one Rh mosaic [668]. These unusual phenotypes could result from somatic mutation or from proliferation of clones monosomic for *RH*. Karyotypes of two propositi were examined and appeared normal [30,660].

Two individuals with Rh mosaicism were also mosaics for another chromosome 1 marker, the Duffy blood group [669,670]. Jenkins and Marsh [669] found 30% DCe/dce Fy(a+) and 70% dce/dce Fy(a–) red cell populations in a male blood donor. The results of testing his family showed that he could not be dce/dce: his father was DCe/DCe Fy(a+b–), his mother DCe/dce Fy(a–b+), and his sister DCe/dce Fy(a+b+). Extensive serological investigation led to the conclusion that the father had a homozygous dose of C and e antigens. Eight years later the phenotype showed the same mosaicism and the donor's karyotype appeared normal [671]. In another case, 30% of red cells were D+C+Fy(b+) and 70% D–C–Fy(b–), but no other sign of mosaicism was observed in the many markers studied (including red cell groups, HLA, plasma proteins, and isozymes) [670]. The karyotype determined on lymphocyte and fibroblast cultures was normal. A simple deletion of part of chromosome 1 could not provide the explanation for these two cases as *RH* and *FY* are not within measurable distance of each other and loss of both loci would involve a visible change to the chromosome (see Chapter 32).

5.20 Development and distribution of Rh antigens

5.20.1 Fetal red cells

Rh antigens are readily detected on cord red cells; no surprise considering the part they play in HDN. D, C, c, E, and e antigens have been detected on fetal red cells at the eighth week of gestation [672] and no variation in D antigen density was apparent between weeks 10 and 40 [673]. No D antigen or *RHD* mRNA transcript was detected in trophoblasts between 8 and 40 weeks' gestation [674].

5.20.2 Erythroid precursors

RhAG appears at an early stage of erythropoiesis on erythroid blast-forming units (BFU-E). During the course of *in vitro* erythroid culture from isolated CD34+ cells, RhAG appears after glycophorin C and Kell glycoprotein, but before glycophorin A and band 3. The Rh antigens appear substantially later, after glycophorin A and band 3 [104–106]. The products of *RHD* and *RHCE* appear at the same time, although some D epitopes appear later than others [106,675], which could reflect conformational changes to the Rh protein complex that might occur during the erythropoietic process. Pronormoblasts from D+ bone marrows have about 25% of the quantity of D antigen present on mature D+ red cells, the quantity increasing during red cell maturation [676].

5.20.3 Other cells and tissues

Rh antigens appear to be erythroid specific. No D, C, c, E, or e antigen could be detected on granulocytes, lymphocytes, monocytes, or platelets by radioimmunoassay and fluorescent flow cytometry [677,678]. There is no evidence of Rh antigens on cells of other tissues.

RhAG may also be erythroid-specific, but homologueues of RhAG (RhBG and RhCG or RhGK) are present in kidney, liver, skin, and testis [97,108,109].

5.21 Functional aspects of the Rh membrane complex

Functions of the Rh proteins, or of the Rh membrane complex, are unknown. The predicted topology of the Rh proteins in the cell membrane—polytopic, with cytoplasmic N- and C-termini—is characteristic of membrane transporters. RhAG bears even closer resemblance to red cell membrane transporters, as it has a single *N*-glycan on one of its extracellular loops. There is now some evidence to suggest that RhAG, and other members of the Rh protein family, could function as ammonium transporters.

Ammonium may be friend or foe. It is utilized by prokaryotes and lower eukaryotes as a source of nitrogen, whereas in mammals it is toxic and must be metabolized and excreted. A family of ammonium transporters, the Mep/Amt proteins, is ubiquitous in lower organisms, including bacteria, yeast, and plants [679,680]. These proteins are polytopic and generally have 11 membrane-spanning domains and an extracellular N-terminus [681]. RhAG shares between 20% and 27% sequence identity with proteins of the Mep/Amt family [682].

Yeast (*Saccharomyces cerevisae*) cells have three membrane ammonium transporters: Mep1, Mep2, Mep3. Yeast cells lacking all three Mep proteins (triple-*mepΔ*) fail to grow in low levels (5 mM) of ammonium, though any one of the Mep proteins can restore growth. Marini *et al.* [109] demonstrated that the growth defect in triple-*mepΔ* yeast cells could be repaired by transfection of the cells with *RHAG* cDNA or with cDNA encoding a kidney homologue, RhGK (also called RhCG). These transformed cells grew in 1 mM ammonium. Furthermore, transfection of yeast cells with *RHAG* or *RHGK* cDNA conferred resistance to a toxic concentration of methylammonium, suggesting that the human proteins are involved in the export of the ammonium analogue.

No evidence exists that the Rh complex functions to facilitate transfer of ammonium in or out of the red cells. Ammonium concentration is three times higher in red cells than in plasma. It is tempting to speculate that RhAG promotes retention of ammonium in red cells for transport to the liver or kidney and subsequent removal from the body, thus protecting against ammonium toxicity in the brain [109,683]. RhAG homologues in the kidney are likely to be involved in ammonium secretion by the renal proximal tubule [97,108,109]. Mep2 has the highest level of homology with RhAG of the three yeast Mep proteins [512]. In addition to being an ammonium transporter, Mep2 also acts as an ammonium sensor [683], fuelling speculation that Rh-family proteins may function as human ammonium sensors.

Red cells with Rh-deficiency phenotypes are usually morphologically and functionally abnormal (Section 5.16.6), and a number of anomalies have been associated with Rh deficiency including abnormal organization of membrane phospholipids [538]. The lipid bilayer of normal cells is asymmetrical: phosphatidylcholine and sphingomyelin are found predominantly in the outer leaflet, while almost all phosphatidylethanolamine and phosphatidylserine molecules are in the inner leaflet. This asymmetry is maintained, in part, by an aminophospholipid translocator, a cysteine-containing, non-glycosylated, integral membrane polypeptide of apparent M_r 32 000 (reviewed in [684,685]). Although there have been suggestions that Rh polypeptides are involved in trans-bilayer movement of phosphatidylserine [684], Rh_{null} red cells have normal aminophospholipid translocator activity and the aminophospholipid translocator and Rh polypeptides have now been shown to be different molecules [686,687].

5.22 Evolutionary aspects

Ancestors of the genes of the Rh family appear to be primitive, non-erythroid homologues of *RHAG*, present in slime mould and throughout the animal kingdom [62,97]. The degree of homology between *RHAG* and homologous human and some non-human genes is shown Table 5.15. *RHAG* has a higher level of homology with its slime mould homologue, than with the Rh genes, *RHCE* and *RHD*. Gene duplications and subsequent chromosomal translocations have produced at least five human, four murine, and two nematode (*Caenorhabditis elegans*) genes of the Rh family. Single Rh-family genes have been found in the marine sponge, *Geodia cydonium*, and the slime mould, *Dictyostelium discoideum* [62]. Genes of the Rh family are also homologous to genes encoding ammonium transporters of the Mep/Amt family in plants and lower animals (see Section 5.21), but these show substantially lower levels of identity [682].

The ancestral *RH* (*RHCE* and *RHD*, or *RH30*)

genes were formed, almost certainly, by duplication of an ancestral *RHAG*-like (or *RH50*) gene. Analyses of the numbers of synonymous and non-synonymous substitutions in the *RH* and *RHAG* genes in human, macaque, mouse, and rat suggested that Darwinian selection had acted on both genes, but that *RHAG* is more conserved than the *RH* genes, having evolved 2–3 times more slowly [688,689]. This suggests that *RHAG* has greater functional significance than *RH*. Duplication of an *RHAG*-like gene to form an ancestral *RH* gene is estimated to have occurred between 240 and 346 million years ago, about the time of the divergence of mammals and birds [688,689]. However, a more recent study suggests that the duplication occurred earlier, 510 million years ago, before divergence of jawless fish and jawed vertebrates [690]. *RH* gene homologues have been detected in all mammals studied and, at low stringency, Southern analysis with an *RH* gene-specific PCR product revealed an *RH*-

Table 5.15 Percentage of identity between human *RHAG* and other genes of the human Rh family and *RHAG* homologues in other species [97].

Species	Gene	Percentage identity to *RHAG*
Homo sapiens (human)	*RHAG*	100.0
	RHCG (RHGK)	50.9
	RHBG	49.9
	RHCE	33.0
	RHD	32.8
Mus musculus (mouse)	*Rhag*	76.5
Danio rerio (zebrafish)	*Rhg*	43.0
Drosophila melanogaster (fruit fly)	*Rhp*	41.4
Caenorhabditis elegans (nematode)	*Rhp-1*	35.9
	Rhp-2	43.0
Geodia cydonium (marine sponge)	*Rhg*	41.8
Dictyostelium discoideum (slime mould)	*RhgA*	34.5

related fragment in the DNA of chickens [691]. M_r 32 000 non-glycosylated polypeptides shown to be 30–60% identical to human Rh polypeptides by two-dimensional peptide mapping, have been purified by non-immunological techniques from membrane vesicles prepared from rhesus monkey, cow, cat, and rat red cells [692].

Rh-related mRNA transcripts were isolated from the bone marrow of chimpanzee, gorilla, gibbon, crab-eating macaque (*Macaca fascicularis*), and rhesus monkey (*M. mulatta*), by reverse-transcriptase PCR using primers designed from the sequence of human Rh genes [310,693]. The cDNA sequences demonstrated a high degree of homology to the human sequence and predicted proteins of 417 amino acids. Like most humans, chimpanzees and gorillas have at least two *RH* genes; other primates, including orang-utans and gibbons, Old World and New World monkeys, and prosimians, have only one *RH* gene per haploid genome [694]. Consequently, the duplication of the ancestral *RH* gene that led to the evolution of *RHCE* and *RHD* in man must have occurred in the common ancestor of humans, chimpanzees, and gorillas, between 8 and 11 million years ago [695,696]. Perception of the mechanism involved in the duplication event is complicated by the observation that *RHCE* and *RHD* are in opposite orientation on the chromosome (Fig. 5.4) [80].

Antigens similar to Rh antigens are found on the red cells of some non-human primates. Anti-c reacts with red cells of chimpanzees, gorillas, and gibbons, whereas anti-D detects polymorphisms on the red cells of chimpanzees (R^c of the R–C–E–F system), gorillas (D^{gor}), and orang-utans (Rh$_o$^{Or}). There are no reports of C, E, or e on red cells of non-human primates (reviewed in [694,696]).

A series of events are predicted to have generated the present Rh haplotypes [75,695]. Duplication of an ancestral *RH* gene, followed by divergence resulting from mutations and complex recombination events, generated genes resembling *RHD* and the *ce* allele of *RHCE*. *Dce* therefore is the root of the human Rh system (Fig. 5.11). Deletion or inactivation of *RHD* then created *dce*, non-reciprocal recombination of *RHD* sequences in the exon 2 region into the *ce* allele of *RHCE* could have produced *DCe*, and a point mutation in the *ce* allele would have produced *DcE*. In harmony with the thesis of Fisher and Race [697] from 1946, Carritt *et al.* [695] proposed that *dCe* arose from recombina-

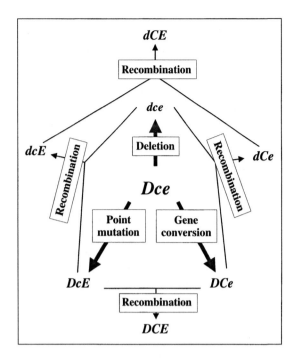

Fig. 5.11 Scheme to show the proposed derivation of the eight Rh haplotypes from the ancestral haplotype, *Dce* (after [695]). The haplotype *dce* resulted from deletion of *RHD*, *DcE* from a point mutation within *RHCE*, and *DCe* from a gene conversion event between *RHD* and *RHCE*. The less common haplotypes *dcE*, *dCe*, and *DCE*, then arose from recombination events involving *dce*, *DcE*, and *DCe*. The very rare haplotype *dCE* resulted from recombination between *dcE* and *dCe*.

tion between *DCe* and *dce*, *dcE* from recombination between *DcE* and *dce*, and *DCE* from recombination between *DCe* and *DcE*. The very rare haplotype *dCE* must have arisen from recombination between the uncommon haplotypes, *dCE* and *dcE*.

The Rh blood groups are highly polymorphic, particularly in Africans where there are three relatively common genetic backgrounds to D– (Section 5.6.1.2). If the Rh complex were to function as an ammonium transporter, trivial changes to the Rh complex caused by mutations in the *RH* genes could result in altered ammonium concentration within the cells, which might affect the suitability of the cells as a host for malarial parasites. In this way a delicate evolutionary balance between the parasite and its host could be responsible for the high level of Rh polymorphism.

References

1 Levine P, Stetson RE. An unusual case of intra-group agglutination. *J Am Med Assoc* 1939;**113**:126–7.

2 Landsteiner K, Wiener AS. An agglutinable factor in human blood recognized by immune sera for Rhesus blood. *Proc Soc Exp Biol NY* 1940;**43**:223.

3 Landsteiner K, Wiener AS. Studies on an agglutinogen (Rh) in human blood reacting with anti-rhesus sera and with human isoantibodies. *J Exp Med* 1941;**74**:309–20.

4 Wiener AS, Peters HR. Hemolytic reactions following transfusions of blood of the homologous group, with three cases in which the same agglutinogen was responsible. *Ann Int Med* 1940;**13**:2306–22.

5 Levine P, Burnham L, Katzin EM, Vogel P. The role of iso-immunization in the pathogenesis of erythroblastosis fetalis. *Am J Obst Gynecol* 1941;**42**:925–37.

6 Fisk RT, Foord AG. Observations on the Rh agglutinogen of human blood. *Am J Clin Pathol* 1942;**12**:545.

7 Levine P, Celano MJ, Wallace J, Sanger R. A human 'D-like' antibody. *Nature* 1963;**198**:596–7.

8 Race RR, Taylor GL, Cappell DF, McFarlane MN. Recognition of a further common Rh genotype in man. *Nature* 1944;**153**:52–3.

9 Wiener AS. Genetic theory of the Rh blood types. *Proc Soc Exp Biol Med* 1943;**54**:316–19.

10 Levine P, Katzin EM, Burnham L. Isoimmunization in pregnancy: its possible bearing on the etiology of erythroblastosis foetalis. *J Am Med Assoc* 1941;**116**:825–7.

11 Levine P, Vogel P, Katzin EM, Burnham L. Pathogenesis of erythroblastosis fetalis: statistical evidence. *Science* 1941;**94**:371–2.

12 Race RR. An 'incomplete' antibody in human serum. *Nature* 1944;**153**:771–2.

13 Race RR, Mourant AE, Lawler SD, Sanger R. The Rh chromosome frequencies in England. *Blood* 1948;**3**:689–95.

14 Mourant AE, Kopec AC, Domaniewska-Sobczak K. *The Distribution of the Human Blood Groups and Other Polymorphisms*, 2nd edn. London: Oxford University Press, 1976.

15 Mackay JF, Wang JC, Wong KS. The incidence of blood groups in 4648 southern Chinese from Toishan district and its vicinity. *J Hong Kong Med Tech Assoc* 1969;**1**:11–14.

16 Mourant AE. A new Rhesus antibody. *Nature* 1945;**155**:542.

17 Van den Bosch C. The very rare Rh genotype *Ryr* (*CdE/cde*) in a case of erythroblastosis foetalis. *Nature* 1948;**162**:781.

18 Wiener AS, Wexler IB. *An Rh–Hr Syllabus*, 2nd edn. New York: Grune & Stratton, 1963.

19 Rosenfield RE, Allen FH, Swisher SN, Kochwa S. A review of Rh serology and presentation of a new terminology. *Transfusion* 1962;**2**:287–312.

20 Tippett P. A speculative model for the Rh blood groups. *Ann Hum Genet* 1986;**50**:241–7.

21 Tills D, Kopec AC, Tills RE. *The Distribution of the Human Blood Groups and Other Polymorphisms* (Suppl. 1). Oxford: Oxford University Press, 1983.

22 Fisher RA. The fitting of gene frequencies to data on Rhesus reactions. *Ann Eugen* 1946;**13**:150–5.

23 Fisher RA. Note on the calculation of the frequencies of Rhesus allelomorphs. *Ann Eugen* 1947;**13**:223–4.

24 Lewis M, Kaita H, Chown B. The inheritance of the Rh blood groups. I. Frequencies in 1000 unrelated Caucasian families consisting of 2000 parents and 2806 children. *Vox Sang* 1971;**20**:500–8.

25 Race RR, Sanger R. *Blood Groups in Man*, 4th edn. Oxford: Blackwell Scientific Publications, 1962.

26 Sanger R, Race RR, Walsh RJ, Montgomery C. An antibody which subdivides the human MN blood groups. *Heredity* 1948;**2**:131–9.

27 Lawler SD, Bertinshaw D, Sanger R, Race RR. Inheritance of the Rh blood groups: 150 families tested with anti-*C–c–C^w–D–E* and anti-*e*. *Ann Eugen* 1950;**15**:258–70.

28 Mohr J. Genetics of fourteen marker systems: associations and linkage relations. *Acta Genet* 1966;**16**:1–58.

29 Chown B, Lewis M, Kaita H. The inheritance of the Rh blood groups. II. Expression of the Rh antigens in random unrelated Caucasian families. *Vox Sang* 1971;**21**:126–34.

30 Race RR, Sanger R. *Blood Groups in Man*, 6th edn. Oxford: Blackwell Scientific Publications, 1975.

31 Green FA. Studies of the Rh(D) antigen. *Vox Sang* 1965;**10**:32–53.

32 Green FA. Erythrocyte membrane sulfhydryl groups and Rh antigen activity. *Immunochemistry* 1967;**4**:247–57.

33 Green FA. Phospholipid requirement for Rh antigenic activity. *J Biol Chem* 1968;**243**:5519–24.

34 Green FA. Erythrocyte membrane lipids and Rh antigen activity. *J Biol Chem* 1972;**247**:881–7.

35 Lorusso DJ, Green FA. Reconstitution of Rh(D) antigen activity from human erythrocyte membranes solubilized by deoxycholate. *Science* 1975;**188**:66–7.

36 Lorusso DJ, Binette JP, Green FA. The Rh antigen system and disaggregated human erythrocyte membranes. *Immunochemistry* 1977;**14**:503–8.

37 Moore S, Woodrow CF, McClelland DBL. Isolation of membrane components associated with human red cell antigens Rh(D), (c), (E) and Fy^a. *Nature* 1982;**295**:529–31.

38 Gahmberg CG. Molecular identification of the human Rh$_o$ (D) antigen. *FEBS Lett* 1982;**140**:93–7.

39 Ridgwell K, Roberts J, Tanner MJA, Anstee DJ. Absence of two membrane proteins containing extracellular thiol groups in Rh$_{null}$ human erythrocytes. *Biochem J* 1983;**213**:267–9.

40 Bloy C, Blanchard D, Lambin P *et al.* Human mono-

clonal antibody against Rh(D) antigen: partial characterization of the Rh(D) polypeptide from human erythrocytes. *Blood* 1987;69:1491–7.

41 Moore S, Green C. The identification of specific Rhesus-polypeptide–blood-group-ABH-active-glycoprotein complexes in the human red-cell membrane. *Biochem J* 1987;244:735–41.

42 Gahmberg CG. Molecular characterization of the human red cell Rh_o (D) antigen. *EMBO J* 1983;2:223–7.

43 de Vetten MP, Agre P. The Rh polypeptide is a major fatty acid-acylated erythrocyte membrane protein. *J Biol Chem* 1988;263:18193–6.

44 Hartel-Schenk S, Agre P. Mammalian red cell membrane Rh polypeptides are selectively palmitoylated subunits of a macromolecular complex. *J Biol Chem* 1992;267:5569–74.

45 Bloy C, Blanchard D, Lambin P *et al.* Characterization of the D, c, E and G antigens of the Rh blood group system with human monoclonal antibodies. *Mol Immunol* 1988;25:925–30.

46 Krahmer M, Prohaska R. Characterization of human red cell Rh (Rhesus-)specific polypeptides by limited proteolysis. *FEBS Lett* 1987;226:105–8.

47 Saboori AM, Smith BL, Agre P. Polymorphism in the M_r 32 000 Rh protein purified from Rh(D)-positive and -negative erythrocytes. *Proc Natl Acad Sci USA* 1988;85:4042–5.

48 Bloy C, Blanchard D, Dahr W *et al.* Determination of the N-terminal sequence of human red cell Rh(D) polypeptide and demonstration the Rh(D), (c), and (E) antigens are carried by distinct polypeptide chains. *Blood* 1988;72:661–6.

49 Blanchard D, Bloy C, Hermand P *et al.* Two-dimensional iodopeptide mapping demonstrates that erythrocyte Rh D, c, and E polypeptides are structurally homologous but nonidentical. *Blood* 1988;72:1424–7.

50 Agre P, Saboori AM, Asimos A, Smith BL. Purification and partial characterization of the M_r 30 000 integral membrane protein associated with the erythrocyte Rh(D) antigen. *J Biol Chem* 1987;262:17497–503.

51 Avent ND, Ridgwell K, Mawby WJ *et al.* Protein-sequence studies on Rh-related polypeptides suggest the presence of at least two groups of proteins which associate in the human red-cell membrane. *Biochem J* 1988;256:1043–6.

52 Avent ND, Ridgwell K, Tanner MJA, Anstee DJ. cDNA cloning of a 30 kDa erythrocyte membrane protein associated with Rh (Rhesus)-blood-group-antigen expression. *Biochem J* 1990;271:821–5.

53 Yared MA, Moise KJ, Rodkey LS. Stable solid-phase Rh antigen. *Transfus Med* 1997;7:311–17.

54 Chérif-Zahar B, Bloy C, Le Van Kim C *et al.* Molecular cloning and protein structure of a human blood group Rh polypeptide. *Proc Natl Acad Sci USA* 1990; 87:6243–7.

55 Hermand P, Mouro I, Huet M *et al.* Immunochemical characterization of Rhesus proteins with antibodies raised against synthetic peptides. *Blood* 1993; 82:669–76.

56 Mouro I, Colin Y, Chérif-Zahar B, Cartron J-P, Le Van Kim C. Molecular genetic basis of the human Rhesus blood group system. *Nature Genet* 1993;5:62–5.

57 Le Van Kim C, Mouro I, Chérif-Zahar B *et al.* Molecular cloning and primary structure of the human blood group RhD polypeptide. *Proc Natl Acad Sci USA* 1992;89:10925–9.

58 Kajii E, Umenishi F, Iwamoto S, Ikemoto S. Isolation of a new cDNA clone encoding an Rh polypeptide associated with the Rh blood group system. *Hum Genet* 1993;91:157–62.

59 Arce MA, Thompson ES, Wagner S *et al.* Molecular cloning of RhD cDNA derived from a gene present in RhD-positive, but not RhD-negative individuals. *Blood* 1993;82:651–5.

60 Simsek S, de Jong CAM, Cuijpers HTM *et al.* Sequence analysis of cDNA derived from reticulocyte mRNAs coding for Rh polypeptides and demonstration of E/e and C/c polymorphisms. *Vox Sang* 1994;67:203–9.

61 Anstee DJ, Tanner MJA. Biochemical aspects of the blood group Rh (Rhesus) antigens. *Baillière's Clin Haematol* 1993;6:401–22.

62 Huang C-H, Liu PZ, Cheng JG. Molecular biology and genetics of the Rh blood group system. *Semin Hemat* 2000;37:150–65.

63 Wagner FF, Gassner C, Müller TH *et al.* Molecular basis of weak D phenotypes. *Blood* 1999;93:385–93.

64 Avent ND, Butcher SK, Liu W *et al.* Localization of the C termini of the Rh (Rhesus) polypeptides to the cytoplasmic face of the human erythrocyte membrane. *J Biol Chem* 1992;267:15134–9.

65 Eyers SAC, Ridgwell K, Mawby WJ, Tanner MJA. Topology and organization of human Rh (Rhesus) blood group-related polypeptides. *J Biol Chem* 1994;269:6417–23.

66 Avent ND. Molecular biology of the Rh blood group polymorphisms. In: M-J King, ed. *Human Blood Cells: Consequences of Genetic Polymorphisms and Variations.* London: Imperial College Press, 2000, 105–47.

67 Smythe JS, Anstee DJ. The role of palmitoylation in RhD expression [Abstract]. *Transfus Med* 2000;10(Suppl. 1):30.

68 Abbott RE, Schachter D. Impermeant maleimides: oriented probes of erythrocyte membrane proteins. *J Biol Chem* 1976;251:7176–83.

69 Schmitz G, Sonneborn HH, Ernst M *et al.* The effect of cysteine modification and proteinases on the major antigens (D, C, c, E and e) of the Rh blood group system. *Vox Sang* 1996;70:34–9.

70 Suyama K, Lunn R, Goldstein J. Red cell surface cysteine residue (285) of D polypeptide is not essential for D antigenicity. *Transfusion* 1995;35:653–9.

71 Dahr W, Schmitz G, Ernst M, Gielen W, Sonneborn

H-H. Rh antigens and cysteine modification. *Biotest Bull* 1997;**5**:451–7.

72 Smythe JS, Anstee DJ. K562 cells expressing Rh D polypeptide with a Cys 285 to Ala mutation have normal D antigen [Abstract]. *Transfus Med* 1997;**7**(Suppl. 1):29.

73 Chérif-Zahar B, Le Van Kim C, Rouillac C *et al*. Organization of the gene (*RHCE*) encoding the human blood group RhCcEe antigens and characterization of the promoter region. *Genomics* 1994;**19**:68–74.

74 Chérif-Zahar B, Raynal V, Cartron J-P. RH gene structure: reassignment of two exon–exon junctions. *Blood* 1997;**89**:4661–2.

75 Okuda H, Suganuma H, Kamesaki T *et al*. The analysis of nucleotide substitutions, gaps, and recombination events between *RHD* and *RHCE* through complete sequencing. *Biochem Biophys Res Commun* 2000;**274**:670–83.

76 Avent ND, Martin PG, Armstrong-Fisher S *et al*. Evidence of genetic diversity underlying Rh D⁻, weak D (Dᵘ), and partial D phenotypes as determined by multiplex polymerase chain reaction analysis of the *RHD* gene. *Blood* 1997;**89**:2568–77.

77 Okuda H, Kawano M, Iwamoto S *et al*. The *RHD* gene is highly detectable in RhD-negative Japanese donors. *J Clin Invest* 1997;**100**:373–9.

78 Kemp TJ, Poulter M, Carritt B. Microsatellite variation within the human RHCE gene. *Vox Sang* 1999;**77**:159–63.

79 Fujiwara H, Okuda H, Omi T *et al*. The STR polymorphisms in intron 8 may provide information about the molecular evolution on *RH* haplotypes. *Hum Genet* 1999;**104**:301–6.

80 Wagner FF, Flegel WA. *RHD* gene deletion occurred in the *Rhesus box*. *Blood* 2000;**95**:3662–8.

81 Suto Y, Ishikawa Y, Hyodo H, Uchikawa M, Juji T. Gene organization and rearrangements at the human Rhesus blood group locus revealed by fiber-FISH analysis. *Hum Genet* 2000;**106**:164–71.

82 Le Van Kim C, Chérif-Zahar B, Raynal V *et al*. Multiple Rh messenger RNA isoforms are produced by alternative splicing. *Blood* 1992;**80**:1074–8.

83 Kajii E, Umenishi F, Omi T, Ikemoto S. Intricate combinatorial patterns of exon splicing generate multiple Rh-related isoforms in human erythroid cells. *Hum Genet* 1995;**95**:657–65.

84 Okuda H, Fujiwara H, Omi T *et al*. A Japanese propositus with D–– phenotype characterized by the deletion of both the *RHCE* gene and D1S80 locus situated in chromosome 1p and the existence of a new *CE–D–CE* hybrid gene. *J Hum Genet* 2000;**45**:142–53.

85 Matassi G, Chérif-Zahar B, Mouro I, Cartron J-P. Characterization of the recombination hot spot involved in the genomic rearrangement leading to the hybrid *D–CE–D* gene in the Dᵛᴵ phneotype. *Am J Hum Genet* 1997;**60**:808–17.

86 Suyama K, Roy S, Lunn R, Goldstein J. Expression of the 32-Kd polypeptide of the Rh antigen. *Blood* 1993;**82**:1006–9.

87 Smythe JS, Avent ND, Judson PA *et al*. Expression of *RHD* and *RHCE* gene products using retroviral transduction of K562 cells establishes the molecular basis of Rh blood group antigens. *Blood* 1996;**87**:2968–73.

88 Iwamoto S, Yamasaki M, Kawano M *et al*. Expression analysis of human rhesus blood group antigens by gene transduction into erythroid and non-erythroid cells. *Int J Hematol* 1998;**68**:257–68.

89 Avent N, Judson PA, Parsons SF *et al*. Monoclonal antibodies that recognize different membrane proteins that are deficient in Rh$_{null}$ human erythrocytes. *Biochem J* 1988;**251**:499–505.

90 Ridgwell K, Eyers SAC, Mawby WJ, Anstee DJ, Tanner MJA. Studies on the glycoprotein associated with Rh (Rhesus) blood group antigen expression in the human red blood cell membrane. *J Biol Chem* 1994;**269**:6410–16.

91 Folkerd EJ, Ellory JC, Hughes-Jones NC. A molecular size determination of Rh(D) antigen by radiation inactivation. *Immunochemistry* 1977;**14**:529–31.

92 Avent ND, Liu W, Warner K *et al*. Immunochemical analysis of the human erythrocyte Rh polypeptides. *J Biol Chem* 1996;**271**:14233–9.

93 Gardner B, Anstee DJ, Mawby WJ, von Tanner MJA, dem Borne AEGK. The abundance and organization of polypeptides associated with antigens of the Rh blood group system. *Transfus Med* 1991;**1**:77–85.

94 Ridgwell K, Spurr NK, Laguda B *et al*. Isolation of cDNA clones for a 50 kDa glycoprotein of the human erythrocyte membrane associated with Rh (Rhesus) blood-group antigen expression. *Biochem J* 1992;**287**:223–8.

95 Matassi G, Chérif-Zahar B, Raynal V, Rouger P, Cartron JP. Organization of the human *RH50A* gene (RHAG) and evolution of base composition of the RH gene family. *Genomics* 1998;**47**:286–93.

96 Huang C-H. The human Rh50 glycoprotein gene. *J Biol Chem* 1998;**273**:2207–13.

97 Liu Z, Chen Y, Mo R *et al*. Characterization of human RhCG and mouse Rhcg as novel nonerythroid Rh glycoprotein homologues predominantly expressed in kidney and testis. *J Biol Chem* 2000;**275**:25641–51.

98 Iwamoto S, Omi T, Yamasaki M *et al*. Identification of 5′ flanking sequence of *RH50* gene and the core region for erythroid-specific expression. *Biochem Biophys Res Commun* 1998;**243**:233–40.

99 Iwamoto S, Suganuma H, Kamesaki T, Omi T, Okuda H, Kajii E. Cloning and characterization of erythroid-specific DNase I-hypersensitive site in human Rhesus-associated glycoprotein gene. *J Biol Chem* 2000;**275**:27324–31.

100 Suyama K, Lunn R, Smith BL, Haller S. Expression of

the Rh-related glycoprotein (Rh50). *Acta Haematol* 1998;100:181–6.

101 Mouro-Chanteloup J, D'Ambrosio AM, Gane P, Raynal V. Post transcriptional regulation of recombinant RhD membrane expression by the RhAG glycoprotein in K562 cells [Abstract]. *Vox Sang* 2000;78(Suppl. 1):O016.

102 Suyama K, Zhu A. Surface expression of Rh-associated glycoprotein (RhAG) in nonerythroid COS-1 cells. *Blood* 2000;95:336–41.

103 Liu Z, Chen Y, Huang C-H. Insertion of Rh30 polypeptides in the plasma membrane does not require coexpression of Rh50 glycoprotein [Abstract]. *Blood* 1999;94(Suppl. 1):188a.

104 Southcott MJG, Tanner MJA, Anstee DJ. The expression of human blood group antigens during erythropoiesis in a cell culture system. *Blood* 1999;93:4425–35.

105 Bony V, Gane P, Bailly P, Cartron J-P. Time-course expression of polypeptides carrying blood group antigens during human erythroid differentiation. *Br J Haematol* 1999;107:263–74.

106 Daniels G, Green C. Expression of red cell surface antigens during erythropoiesis. *Vox Sang* 2000;78(Suppl. 2):149–53.

107 Suyama K, Li H, Zhu A. Expression of Rh30 and Rh-related glycoproteins during erythroid differentiation in a two-phase liquid culture system. *Transfusion* 2000;40:214–21.

108 Liu Z, Peng J, Mo R, Hui C, Huang C-H. Rh type B glycoprotein is a new member of the Rh superfamily and a putative ammonia transporter in mammals. *J Biol Chem* 2001;276:1424–33.

109 Marini a-M, Matassi G, Raynal V *et al.* The human Rhesus-associated RhAG protein and a kidney homologue promote ammonium transport in yeast. *Nature Genet* 2000;26:341–4.

110 Habibi B, Fouillade MT, Duedari N *et al.* The antigen Duclos: a new high frequency red cell antigen related to Rh and U. *Vox Sang* 1978;34:302–9.

111 von dem Borne AEGK, Bos MJE, Lomas C *et al.* Murine monoclonal antibodies against a unique determinant of erythrocytes, related to Rh and U antigens: expression on normal and malignant erythrocyte precursors and Rh_null red cells. *Br J Haematol* 1990;75:254–61.

112 Le Pennec PY, Klein MT, Le Besnerais M *et al.* Immunological characterization of 18 monoclonal antibodies directed against Rh, G and LW molecules. *Rev Franc Transfus Immuno-Hémat* 1988;31:123–31.

113 Mallinson G, Anstee DJ, Avent ND *et al.* Murine monoclonal antibody MB-2D10 recognizes Rh-related glycoproteins in the human red cell membrane. *Transfusion* 1990;30:222–5.

114 Bloy C, Blanchard D, Hermand P *et al.* Properties of the blood group LW glycoprotein and preliminary comparison with Rh proteins. *Mol Immunol* 1989;26:1013–19.

115 Dahr W, Kordowicz M, Moulds J *et al.* Characterization of the Ss sialoglycoprotein and its antigens in Rh_null erythrocytes. *Blut* 1987;54:13–24.

116 Le Pennec PY, Rouger Ph, Klein MT, Le Besnerais M, Salmon C. An antibody supporting the evidence of an association between the Rh polypeptides and glycophorin B on the red cell membrane [Abstract]. *Joint Congr Int Soc Blood Transfus and Am Ass Blood Banks* 1990, 29.

117 Lindberg FP, Lublin DM, Telen MJ *et al.* Rh-related antigen CD47 is the signal-transducer integrin-associated protein. *J Biol Chem* 1994;269:1567–70.

118 Miller YE, Daniels GL, Jones C, Palmer DK. Identification of a cell-surface antigen produced by a gene on human chromosome 3 (cen-q22) and not expressed by Rh_null cells. *Am J Hum Genet* 1987;41:1061–70.

119 Lindberg FP, Gresham HD, Schwarz E, Brown EJ. Molecular cloning of integrin-associated protein: an immunoglobulin family member with multiple membrane-spanning domains implicated in $\alpha_v\beta_3$-dependent ligand binding. *J Cell Biol* 1993;123:485–96.

120 Oldenborg P-A, Zheleznyak A, Fang Y-F *et al.* Role of CD47 as a marker of self on red blood cells. *Science* 2000;288:2051–4.

121 Beckman R, Smythe JS, Anstee DJ, Tanner MJA. Functional cell surface expression of band 3, the human red blood cell anion exchange protein (AE1), in K562 erythroleukemia cells: band 3 enhances the cell surface reactivity of Rh antigens. *Blood* 1998;92:4428–38.

122 Beckmann R, Smythe JS, Anstee DJ, Tanner MJA. Coexpression of band 3 mutants and Rh polypeptides: differential effects of band 3 on the expression of the Rh complex containing D polypeptide and the Rh complex containing CcEe polypeptide. *Blood* 2001;97:2496–505.

123 Cartron JP, Bailly P, Le Van Kim C *et al.* Insights into the structure and function of membrane polypeptides carrying blood group antigens. *Vox Sang* 1998;74(Suppl. 2):29–64.

124 Mouro-Chanteloup J, Johansen M, Brown EJ, Cartron JP, Colin Y. Normal red cell membrane expression of Rh and RhAG polypeptides in CD47-deficient mice [Abstract]. *Vox Sang* 2000;78(Suppl. 1):P030.

125 Gamhberg CG, Karhi KK. Association of Rh_o (D) polypeptides with the membrane skeleton in Rh_o (D)-positive human red cells. *J Immunol* 1984;133:334–7.

126 Ridgwell K, Tanner MJA, Anstee DJ. The Rhesus (D) polypeptide is linked to the human erythrocyte cytoskeleton. *FEBS Lett* 1984;174:7–10.

127 Paradis G, Bazin R, Lemieux R. Protective effect of the membrane skeleton on the immunologic reactivity of the human red cell Rh_o (D) antigen. *J Immunol* 1986;137:240–4.

128 Gane P, Le Van Kim C, Bony V *et al.* Flow cytometric analysis of the association between blood group-related proteins and the detergent-insoluble material of K562

cells and erythroid precursors. *Br J Haematol* 2001; 113:680–8.

129 Gimm A, Mouro I, Lambin P, Mohandas N, Cartron JP. Direct evidence for *in situ* interaction between Rh complex and membrane skeleton in intact cells [Abstract]. *Vox Sang* 2000;78(Suppl. 1):O014.

130 Mak KH, Yan KF, Cheng SS, Yuen MY. Rh phenotypes of Chinese blood donors in Hong Kong, with special reference to weak D antigens. *Transfusion* 1993; 33:348–51.

131 Levine P, Celano M, Lange S, Stroup M. The influence of gene interaction on dosage effects with complete anti-D sera. *Vox Sang* 1959;4:33–9.

132 Masouredis SP, Chi CA, Ferguson E. Relationship between Rh_o (D) genotype and quantity of I^{131} anti-Rh_o (D) bound to red cells. *J Clin Invest* 1960;39:1450–62.

133 Silber R, Gibbs MB, Jahn EF, Akeroyd JH. Quantitative hemagglutination studies in the Rh blood group system. II. A study of the D (Rh_o) agglutinogen. *Blood* 1961; 17:291–301.

134 Gibbs MB, Rosenfield RE. Immunochemical studies of the Rh system. IV. Hemagglutination assay of antigenic expression regulated by interaction between paired Rh genes. *Transfusion* 1966;6:462–74.

135 Araszkiewicz P, Szymanski IO. Quantitative studies on the Rh-antigen D: effect of the C gene. *Transfusion* 1987;27:257–61.

136 Hughes-Jones NC, Bloy C, Gorick B *et al.* Evidence that the c, D and E epitopes of the human Rh blood group system are on separate polypeptide molecules. *Mol Immunol* 1988;25:931–6.

137 van Bockstaele DR, Berneman ZN, Muylle L, Cole-Dergent J, Peetermans ME. Flow cytometric analysis of erythrocytic D antigen density profile. *Vox Sang* 1986;51:40–6.

138 Nicholson G, Lawrence A, Ala FA, Bird GWG. Semi-quantitative assay of D antigen site density by flow cytometric analysis. *Transfus Med* 1991;1:87–90.

139 Colin Y, Chérif-Zahar B, Le Van Kim C *et al.* Genetic basis of the RhD-positive and RhD-negative blood group polymorphism as determined by Southern analysis. *Blood* 1991;78:2747–52.

140 Hyland CA, Wolter LC, Saul A. Three unrelated Rh D gene polymorphisms identified among blood donors with Rhesus CCee (r'r') phenotypes. *Blood* 1994; 84:321–4.

141 Aubin J-T, Le Van Kim C, Mouro I *et al.* Specificity and sensitivity of RHD genotyping methods by PCR-based DNA amplification. *Br J Haematol* 1997;98:356–64.

142 Andrews KT, Wolter LC, Saul A, Hyland CA. The RhD⁻ trait in a white patient with the RhCCee phenotype attributed to a four-nucleotide deletion in the *RHD* gene. *Blood* 1998;92:1839–40.

143 Singleton BK, Green CA, Avent ND *et al.* The presence of an *RHD* pseudogene containing a 37 base pair duplication and a nonsense mutation in most Africans with the Rh D-negative blood group phenotype. *Blood* 2000;95:12–18.

144 Blunt T, Daniels G, Carritt B. Serotype switching in a partially deleted RHD gene. *Vox Sang* 1994;67: 397–401.

145 Faas BHW, Beckers EAM, Wildoer P *et al.* Molecular background of VS and weak C expression in blacks. *Transfusion* 1997;37:38–44.

146 Daniels GL, Faas BHW, Green CA *et al.* The Rh VS and V blood group polymorphisms in Africans: a serological and molecular analysis. *Transfusion* 1998;38:951–8.

147 Kajii E, Umenishi F, Ikemoto S. A cDNA clone encoding an Rh polypeptide detected in RhD-negative erythroid cells. *Vox Sang* 1993;64:196.

148 Umenishi F, Kajii E, Ikemoto S. Molecular analysis of Rh polypeptides in a family with RhD-positive and RhD-negative phenotypes. *Biochem J* 1994;299: 207–11.

149 Fukumori Y, Hori Y, Ohnoki S *et al.* Further analysis of D_{el} (D-elute) using polymerase chain reaction (PCR) with *RHD* gene-specific primers. *Transfus Med* 1997;7: 227–31.

150 Lan JC, Chen Q, Wu DL *et al.* Genetic polymorphism of RhD-negative associated haplotype in the Chinese. *J Hum Genet* 2000;45:224–7.

151 Sun C-F, Chou C-S, Lai N-C, Wang W-T. RHD gene polymorphisms among RhD-negative Chinese in Taiwan. *Vox Sang* 1998;75:52–7.

152 Chang J-G, Shih MC, Wang J-C. *et al.* Molecular basis for the RHD negative phenotype in Taiwanese [Abstracts]. *10th Regional Congr Int Soc Blood Transfus Western Pacific Region*: 1999: 254.

153 Stratton F. A new Rh allelomorph. *Nature* 1946; 158:25–6.

154 Stratton F, Renton PH. Rh genes allelomorphic to D. *Nature* 1948;162:293–4.

155 Race RR, Sanger R, Lawler SD. The *Rh* antigen D^u. *Ann Eugen* 1948;14:171–84.

156 Renton PH, Stratton F. Rhesus type D^u. *Ann Eugen* 1950;15:189–209.

157 Bush M, Sabo B, Stroup M, Masouredis SP. Red cell D antigen sites and titration scores in a family with weak and normal D^u phenotypes inherited from a homozygous D^u mother. *Transfusion* 1974;14:433–9.

158 Cunningham NA, Zola AP, Hui HL, Taylor LM, Green FA. Binding characteristics of anti Rh_o (D) antibodies to Rh_o (D) -positive and D^u red cells. *Blood* 1985;66:765–8.

159 Szymanski IO, Araszkiewicz P. Quantitative studies on the D antigen of red cells with the D^u phenotype. *Transfusion* 1989;29:103–5.

160 Merry AH, Hodson C, Moore S. Variation in the level of Rh(D) antigen expression. *Transfusion* 1988;28:397–8.

161 Gorick B, McDougall DCJ, Ouwehand WH *et al.* Quan-

titation of D sites on selected 'weak D' and 'partial D' red cells. *Vox Sang* 1993;65:136–40.

162 Agre PC, Davies DM, Issitt PD *et al*. A proposal to standardize terminology for weak D antigen. *Transfusion* 1992;32:86–7.

163 Contreras M, Knight RC. Controversies in transfusion medicine: testing for D^u: Con. *Transfusion* 1991;31:270–2.

164 Salmon C, Cartron J-P, Rouger P. *The Human Blood Groups*. New York: Masson, 1984.

165 Tippett P. Rh blood group system: the D antigen and high- and low-frequency Rh antigens. In: V Vengelen-Tyler, S Pierce, eds. *Blood Group Systems: Rh*. Arlington: American Association of Blood Banks, 1987, 25–53.

166 Argall CI, Ball JM, Trentelman E. Presence of anti-D antibody in the serum of a D^u patient. *J Lab Clin Med* 1953;41:895–8.

167 Wagner FF, Frohmajer A, Ladewig B *et al*. Weak D alleles express distinct phenotypes. *Blood* 2000;95:2699–708.

168 Tippett P, Sanger R. Observations on subdivisions of the Rh antigen D. *Vox Sang* 1962;7:9–13.

169 Tippett P, Sanger R. Further observations on subdivisions of the Rh antigen D. *Ärztl Lab* 1977;23:476–80.

170 Tippett P, Lomas-Francis C, Wallace M, The Rh antigen D: partial D antigens and associated low incidence antigens. *Vox Sang* 1996;70:123–31.

171 Wiener AS, Unger LJ. Rh factors related to the Rh$_0$ factor as a source of clinical problems. *J Am Med Assoc* 1959;169:696–9.

172 Unger LJ, Wiener AS. Some observations on blood factors Rh^A, Rh^B, and Rh^C of the Rh–Hr blood group system. *Blood* 1959;14:522–34.

173 Wiener AS, Unger LJ. Further observations on the blood factors Rh^A, Rh^B, Rh^C and Rh^D. *Transfusion* 1962;2:230–3.

174 Avent ND, Jones JW, Liu W *et al*. Molecular basis of the D variant phenotypes DNU and D^{II} allows localization of critical amino acids required for expression of Rh D epitopes epD3, 4 and 9 to the sixth external domain of the Rh D protein. *Br J Haematol* 1997;97:366–71.

175 Sausais L, Oyen R, Rios M *et al*. DAK, a low incidence antigen shared by D^{IIIa} and R$^{=N}$ RBCs [Abstract]. *Transfusion* 1999;39(Suppl.):79S.

176 Huang C-H, Chen Y, Reid M. Human D^{IIIa} erythrocytes: RhD protein is associated with multiple dispersed amino acid variations. *Am J Hematol* 1997;55:139–45.

177 Rouillac C, Le Van Kim C, Blancher A *et al*. Lack of G blood group antigen in D^{IIIb} erythrocytes is associated with segmental DNA exchange between *RH* genes. *Br J Haematol* 1995;89:424–6.

178 Gorick BD, Thompson KM, Melamed MD, Hughes-Jones NC. Three epitopes on the human Rh antigen D recognized by ^{125}I-labelled human monoclonal IgG antibodies. *Vox Sang* 1988;55:165–70.

179 Beckers EAM, Faas BHW, Ligthart P *et al*. Characterization of the hybrid *RHD* gene leading to the partial D category IIIc phenotype. *Transfusion* 1996;36:567–74.

180 Rouillac C, Colin Y, Hughes-Jones NC *et al*. Transcript analysis of D category phenotypes predicts hybrid Rh D-CE-D proteins associated with alteration of D epitopes. *Blood* 1995;85:2937–44.

181 Hyodo H, Ishikawa Y, Tsuneyama H *et al*. New RhD^{IVb} identified in Japanese. *Vox Sang* 2000;79:116–17.

182 Wagner FF, Gassner C, Eicher N, Lonicer C, Flegel WA, Characterization of D category IV type IV, DFW, and DNB [Abstract]. *Transfusion* 1998;38(Suppl.):63S.

183 Omi T, Takahashi J, Tsudo N *et al*. The genomic organization of the partial D category D^{Va}: the presence of a new partial D associated with the D^{Va} phenotype. *Biochem Biophys Res Commun* 1999;254:786–94.

184 Omi T, Okuda H, Iwamoto S *et al*. Detection of Rh23 in the partial D phenotype associated with the D^{Va} category. *Transfusion* 2000;40:256–8.

185 Avent ND, Liu W, Jones JW *et al*. Molecular analysis of Rh transcripts and polypeptides from individuals expressing the D^{VI} variant phenotype: and *RHD* gene deletion event does not generate all D^{VI}ccEe phenotypes. *Blood* 1997;89:1779–86.

186 Mouro I, Le Van Kim C, Rouillac C *et al*. Rearrangements of the blood group RhD gene associated with the D^{VI} category phenotype. *Blood* 1994;83:1129–35.

187 Wagner FF, Gassner C, Müller TH *et al*. Three molecular structures cause Rhesus D category VI phenotypes with distinct immunohematologic features. *Blood* 1998;91:2157–68.

188 Rouillac C, Le Van Kim C, Beolet M, Cartron J-P, Colin Y. Leu110Pro substitution in the RhD polypeptide is responsible for the D^{VII} category blood group phenotype. *Am J Hematol* 1995;49:87–8.

189 Hemker MB, Ligthart PC, Berger L *et al*. DAR, a new RhD variant involving exons 4, 5, and 7, often in linkage with ceAR, a new Rhce variant frequently found in African blacks. *Blood* 1990;94:4337–42.

190 Wallace M, Lomas-Francis C, Beckers E *et al*. DBT: a partial D phenotype associated with the low-incidence antigen Rh32. *Transfus Med* 1997;7:233–8.

191 Beckers EAM, Faas BHW, Simsek S *et al*. The genetic basis of a new partial D antigen: D^{DBT}. *Br J Haematol* 1996;93:720–7.

192 Huang CH, Chen Y, Reid ME, Okubo Y. Evidence for a separate genetic origin of the partial D phenotype DBT in a Japanese family. *Transfusion* 1999;39:1259–65.

193 Pisacka M, Vytisková J, Hejná J, Gassner Ch. A new variant of Rh(D) antigen: revealed by reactions of anti-ep12 monoclonal antibodies and lacking exon 5 D-specific reaction of exon-scanning RHD/CE PCR-SSP. *Vox Sang* 1998;74(Suppl. 1):Abstract 1332.

194 Avent ND. The Rhesus blood group system: insights

from recent advances in molecular biology. *Transfus Med Rev* 1999;13:245–66.

195 Bizot M, Lomas C, Rubio F, Tippett P. An antiserum identifying a red cell determinant expressed by Rh:33 and by some 'new' depressed Rh phenotypes. *Transfusion* 1988;28:342–5.

196 Giles CM, Crossland JD, Haggas WK, Longster G. An Rh gene complex which results in a 'new' antigen detectable by a specific antibody, anti-Rh33. *Vox Sang* 1971;21:289–301.

197 Wallace M, Lomas-Francis C, Tippett P. The D antigen characteristic of R_0^{Har} is a partial D antigen. *Vox Sang* 1996;70:169–72.

198 Beckers EAM, Porcelijn L, Ligthart P et al. The R_0^{Har} antigen complex is associated with a limited number of D epitopes and alloanti-D production: a study of three unrelated persons and their families. *Transfusion* 1996;36:104–8.

199 Beckers EAM, Faas BHW, von dem Borne AEGK et al. The R_0^{Har} Rh:33 phenotype results from substitution of exon 5 of the *RHCE* gene by the corresponding exon of the *RHD* gene. *Br J Haematol* 1996;92:751–7.

200 Hyodo H, Ishikawa Y, Kashiwase K et al. Polymorphisms of RhD^{Va} and a new RhD^{Va}-like variant found in Japanese individuals. *Vox Sang* 2000;78:122–5.

201 Jones J. Identification of two new D variants, D^{HMi} and D^{HMii} using monoclonal anti-D. *Vox Sang* 1995;69:236–41.

202 Liu W, Jones JW, Scott ML, Voak D, Avent ND. Molecular analysis of two D-variants, D^{HMi} and D^{HMii} [Abstract]. *Transfus Med* 1996;6(Suppl. 2):21.

203 Müller TH, Wagner FF, Trockenbacher A et al. PCR screening for common weak D types shows different distributions in three Central European populations. *Transfusion* 2001;41:45–52.

204 Jones JW, Finning K, Mattock R et al. The serological profile and molecular basis of a new partial D phenotype, DHR. *Vox Sang* 1997;73:252–6.

205 Avent ND, Poole J, Singleton B et al. Studies of two partial Ds: DMH and DOL [Abstract]. *Transfus Med* 1999;9(Suppl. 1):33.

206 The Rhesus site. http://www.uni-ulm.de/~wflegel/RH/.

207 Singleton BK, Green CA, Kimura K et al. Two new *RHD* mutations associated with DEL phenotype [Abstract]. *Transfus Clin Biol* 2001;8(Suppl. 1):9S.

208 Jones JW, Lloyd-Evans P, Kumpel BM. Quantitation of Rh D antigen sites on weak D and D variant red cells by flow cytometry. *Vox Sang* 1996;71:176–83.

209 Lomas C, Tippett P, Thompson KM, Melamed MD, Hughes-Jones NC. Demonstration of seven epitopes on the Rh antigen D using human monoclonal anti-D antibodies and red cells from D categories. *Vox Sang* 1989;57:261–4.

210 Tippett P, Moore S. Monoclonal antibodies against Rh and Rh related antigens. *J Immunogenet* 1990;17:309–19.

211 Tippett P. Serologically defined Rh determinants. *J Immunogenet* 1990;17:247–57.

212 Lomas C, McColl K, Tippett P. Further complexities of the Rh antigen D disclosed by testing category D^{II} cells with monoclonal anti-D. *Transfus Med* 1993;3:67–9.

213 Lomas C, Grässmann W, Ford D et al. FPTT is a low-incidence Rh antigen associated with a 'new' partial Rh D phenotype, DFR. *Transfusion* 1994;34:612–16.

214 Jones J, Scott ML, Voak D. Monoclonal anti-D specificity and Rh D structure: criteria for selection of monoclonal anti-D reagents for routine typing of patients and donors. *Transfus Med* 1995;5:171–84.

215 Scott M. Rh serology: coordinator's report. *Transfus Clin Biol* 1996;6:333–7.

216 Scott ML. Rh serology: co-ordinator's report. 4th International Workshop Monoclonal Antibodies against Human Red Cell Surface Antigens, Paris. *Transfus Clin Biol* 2002;9:23–9.

217 Tippett P. *Serological study of the inheritance of unusual Rh and other blood group phenotypes.* PhD thesis, University of London, 1963.

218 Rios M, Storry JR, Hue-Roye K et al. Incidence of partial D, DIIIa, in black donors as determined by PCR-RFLP analysis [Abstract]. *Transfusion* 1998;38(suppl):63S.

219 Rossi U, Lomas C, Tippett P et al. Inheritance of a D^{IIIc} antigen: study of an Italian family. *Trasfusione Sangue* 1991;36:566–70.

220 Huang C–H. Human D^{VI} category: erythrocytes: correlation of the phenotype with a novel hybrid RhD–CE–D gene but not an internally deleted RhD gene. *Blood*, 1997: 89: 1834–5.

221 Rosenfield RE, Haber G, Gibbel N. A new Rh variant. *Proc 6th Congr Int Soc Blood Transfus* 1956: 90–5.

222 Lewis M, Chown B, Kaita H et al. Blood group antigen Go^a and the Rh system. *Transfusion* 1967;7:440–1.

223 Chown B, Lewis M, Kaita H et al. On the antigen Go^a and the Rh system. *Vox Sang* 1968;15:264–71.

224 Lassiter GR, Issitt PD, Garris ML, Welborn R. Further studies on the D^{Cor} (Go^a) antigen of the Rh system [Abstract]. *Transfusion* 1969;9:282.

225 Alter AA, Gelb AG, Chown B, Rosenfeld RE, Cleghorn TE. Gonzales (Go^a), a new blood group character. *Transfusion* 1967;7:88–91.

226 Lovett DA, Crawford MN. Js^b and Go^a screening of Negro donors. *Transfusion* 1967;7:442.

227 Lomas-Francis C, Reid ME. The Rh blood group system: the first 60 years of discovery. *Immunohematology* 2000;16:7–17.

228 Okubo Y, Seno T, Yamano H, Yamaguchi H, Lomas C, Tippett P. Partial D antigens disclosed by a monoclonal anti-D in Japanese blood donors. *Transfusion* 1991; 31:782.

229 Chown B, Lewis M, Kaita H. A new Rh antigen and antibody. *Transfusion* 1962;2:150–4.

230 Legler TJ, Wiemann V, Ohto H et al. D^{Va} category phe-

notype and genotype in Japanese families. *Vox Sang* 2000;78:194–7.

231 Avent ND, Finning KM, Liu W, Scott ML. Molecular biology of partial D phenotypes. *Transfus Clin Biol* 1996;6:511–16.

232 Sacchi R, Tippett P, Reali G, Sermasi G. Su un nuovo caso di D anti-D (D^{Vb}). *Trasfusione Sangue* 1974; 19:699–702.

233 Green CA, Lomas-Francis C, Wallace M, Gooch A, Simonsen AC. Family evidence confirms that the low frequency antigen BARC is an Rh antigen [Abstract]. *Transfus Med* 1996;6(Suppl. 2):26.

234 Maaskant-van Wijk PA, Beckers EAM, van Rhenen DJ *et al*. Evidence that the *RHD^{VI}* deletion genotype does not exist. *Blood* 1997;90:1709–20.

235 Apoil PA, Reid ME, Halverson G *et al*. A human monoclonal anti-D antibody which detects a nonconformation-dependent epitope on the RhD protein by immunoblot. *Br J Haematol* 1997;98:365–74.

236 Zhu A, Haller S, Li H *et al*. Use of RhD fusion protein expressed on K562 cell surface in the study of molecular basis for D antigenic epitopes. *J Biol Chem* 1999; 274:5731–7.

237 Leader KA, Kumpel BM, Poole GD *et al*. Human monoclonal anti-D with reactivity against category D^{VI} cells used in blood grouping and determination of the incidence of the category D^{VI} phenotype in the D^U population. *Vox Sang* 1990;58:106–11.

238 van Rhenen DJ, Thijssen PMHJ, Overbeeke MAM. Serological characteristics of partial D antigen category VI in 8 unrelated blood donors. *Vox Sang* 1994; 66:133–6.

239 Beck ML, Hardman JT. Incidence of D category VI among D^U donors in the USA [Abstract]. *Transfusion* 1991;31(Suppl.):25S.

240 Watt J. The incidence of category VI amongst weak Rh (D) positive Sydney blood donors [Abstract]. *Transfus Med* 1993;3:72.

241 Flegel WA, Wagner FF. The frequency of RHD protein variants in Caucasians [Abstract]. *Transfus Clin Biol* 1996;3(spécial):10s.

242 Lewis M, Kaita H, Allerdice PW *et al*. Assignment of the red cell antigen, Targett (Rh40), to the Rh blood group system. *Am J Hum Genet* 1979;31:630–3.

243 Humphreys J, Stout TD, Kaita H, Lewis M. A family in which the Targett (Rh: 40) antigen is carried with R° (–D–). *Vox Sang* 1980;39:277–81.

244 Levene C, Sela R, Grunberg L *et al*. The Rh antigen Tar (Rh40) causing haemolytic disease of the newborn. *Clin Lab Haematol* 1983;5:303–5.

245 Lylloff K, Lundsgaard A, Lomas C, Green C. Third example of anti-Tar and segregation of the Tar (Targett, Rh40) antigen in a Danish family. *Hum Hered* 1984;34:194–6.

246 Lomas C, Bruce M, Watt A *et al*. Tar+ individuals with anti-D, a new category D^{VII} [Abstract]. *Transfusion* 1986;26:560.

247 Flegel WA, Hillesheim B, Kerowgan M, Kasulke D, Wagner FF. Lack of heterogeneity in the molecular structure of RHD category VII [Abstract]. *Transfusion* 1996;36(Suppl.):50S.

248 Faas BHW, Beuling EA, von Ligthart PC *et al*. Expression of RHc from the RHD polypeptide. *Transfusion* 2001;41:1136–42.

249 Hazenberg CAM, Beckers EAM, Overbeeke MAM. Hemolytic disease of the newborn caused by alloanti-D from an R$_o$^{Har}r Rh: 33 mother. *Transfusion* 1996;36: 478–9.

250 Petershofen EK, Teixidor D, Rabold U *et al*. Alloanti-D antibody production in a RH33 R$_o$^{Har} patient, a case report [Abstract]. *Vox Sang* 2000;78(Suppl. 1):P033.

251 Rouillac C, Gane P, Cartron J *et al*. Molecular basis of the altered antigenic expression of RhD in weak D (D^u) and RhC/c in R^N phenotypes. *Blood* 1996;87:4853–61.

252 Beckers EAM, Faas BHW, Lightart P *et al*. Lower antigen site density and weak D immunogenicity cannot be explained by structural genomic abnormalities or regulatory defects of the *RHD* gene. *Transfusion* 1997; 37:616–23.

253 Cowley NM, Saul A, Hyland CA. *RHD* gene mutations and the weak D phneotype: an Australian blood donor study. *Vox Sang* 2000;79:251–2.

254 Hemker MB, Berger L, van der Schoot CE, van Rhenen DJ, Maaskant-van Wijk PA. A transfection model for weak rhesus D expression [Abstract]. *Transfus Med* 2000;10:332.

255 Okubo Y, Yamaguchi H, Tomita T, Nagao N. A D variant, D$_{el}$? *Transfusion* 1984;24:542.

256 Chang J-G, Wang J-C, Yang T-Y *et al*. Human RhD^{el} is caused by a deletion of 1013 bp between introns 8 and 9 including exon 9 of RHD gene. *Blood* 1998;92:2602–4.

257 Scott ML, Voak D, Jones JW *et al*. A structural model for 30 Rh D epitopes based on serological and DNA sequence data from partial D phenotypes. *Transfus Clin Biol* 1996;6:391–6.

258 Cartron J-P, Rouillac C, Le Van Kim C, Mouro I, Colin Y. Tentative model for the mapping of D epitopes on the RhD polypeptide. *Transfus Clin Biol* 1996;6:497–503.

259 Liu W, Smythe JS, Scott ML *et al*. Site-directed mutagenesis of the human D antigen. definition of D epitopes on the sixth external domain of the D protein expressed on K562 cells. *Transfusion* 1999;39:17–25.

260 Liu W, Avent ND, Jones JW, Scott ML, Voak D. Molecular configuration of Rh D epitopes as defined by site-directed mutagenesis and expression of mutant Rh constructs in K562 erythroleukemia cells. *Blood* 1999;94:3986–96. Also see *Blood* 2000;96:1197–9.

261 Chang TY, Siegel DL. Genetic and immunological properties of phage-displayed human anti-Rh(D) antibodies: implications for Rh(D) epitope topology. *Blood* 1998; 91:3066–78. Also see *Blood* 2000;96:1196–7.

262 Siegel DL, Chang TY, Russell SL, Bunya VY. Isolation of cell surface-specific human monoclonal antibodies

using phage display and magnetically-activated cell sorting: applications in immunohematology. *J Immunol Methods* 1997;**206**:73–85.

263 Ceppellini R, Dunn LC, Turri M. An interaction between alleles at the Rh locus in man which weakens the reactivity of the Rh$_0$ factor (D^u). *Proc Natl Acad Sci USA* 1955;**41**:283–8.

264 McGee R, Levine P, Celano M. First example of genotype r^{y}r^y: a family study. *Science* 1957;**125**:1043.

265 Hasekura H, Ota M, Ito S *et al.* Flow cytometric studies of the D antigen of various Rh phenotypes with particular reference to D^u and D$_{el}$. *Transfusion* 1990;**30**:236–8.

266 Rochna E, Hughes-Jones NC. The use of purified ^{125}I-labelled anti-γglobulin in the determination of the number of D antigen sites on red cells of different phenotypes. *Vox Sang* 1965;**10**:675–86.

267 Masouredis SP, Dupuy ME, Elliot M. Relationship between Rh$_0$ (D) zygosity and red cell Rh$_0$ (D) antigen content in family members. *J Clin Invest* 1967;**46**:681–94.

268 Hughes-Jones NC, Gardner B, Lincoln PJ. Observations of the number of available c, D, and E antigen sites on red cells. *Vox Sang* 1971;**21**:210–16.

269 Flegel WA, Khull SR, Wagner FF. Primary anti-D immunization by weak D type 2 RBCs. *Transfusion* 2000;**40**:428–34.

270 Mollison PL, Engelfriet CP, Contreras M. *Blood Transfusion in Clinical Medicine*, 10th edn. Oxford: Blackwell Science, 1997.

271 Lowes BCR. Hemolytic disease of the newborn due to anti-Rh14 (Rh^B). *Vox Sang* 1969;**16**:231–2.

272 Hill Z, Vacl J, Kalasová E, Calábková M, Pintera J. Haemolytic disease of new-born due to anti-D antibodies in a D^u-positive mother. *Vox Sang* 1974;**27**:92–4.

273 Lacey PA, Caskey CR, Werner DJ, Moulds JJ. Fatal hemolytic disease of a newborn due to anti-D in an Rh-positive D^u variant mother. *Transfusion* 1983;**23**:91–4.

274 White CA, Stedman CM, Frank S. Anti-D antibodies in D– and D^u-positive women: a cause of hemolytic disease of the newborn. *Am J Obstet Gynecol* 1983;**145**:1069–75.

275 Østgård P, Fevang F, Kornstad L. Anti-D in a 'D positive' mother giving rise to severe haemolytic disease of the newborn. *Acta Paediat Scand* 1986;**75**:175–8.

276 Lubenko A, Contreras M, Habash J. Should anti-Rh immunoglobulin be given to D variant women? *Br J Haematol* 1989;**72**:429–33.

277 Mayne K, Bowell P, Woodward T *et al.* Rh immunization by the partial D antigen of category D^{Va}. *Br J Haematol* 1990;**76**:537–9.

278 Bennett PR, Le Van Kim C, Colin Y *et al.* Prenatal determination of fetal RhD type by DNA amplification. *N Engl J Med* 1993;**329**:607–10.

279 Wolter LC, Hyland CA, Saul A. Rhesus D genotyping using polymerase chain reaction. *Blood* 1993;**82**:1682–3.

280 Simsek S, Faas BHW, Bleeker MAM *et al.* Rapid Rh D

genotyping by polymerase chain reaction-based amplification of DNA. *Blood* 1995;**85**:2975–80.

281 Pope J, Navarrete C, Warwick R, Contreras M. Multiplex PCR, analysis of RhD gene. *Lancet* 1995;**346**:375–6.

282 Gassner C, Schmarda A, Kilga-Nogler S *et al.* RHD/CE typing by polymerase chain reaction using sequence-specific primers. *Transfusion* 1997;**37**:1020–6.

283 Maaskant-van Wijk PA, Faas BHW, de Ruijter JAM *et al.* Genotyping of *RHD* by multiplex polymerase chain reaction analysis of six *RHD*-specific exons. *Transfusion* 1998;**38**:1015–21.

284 Flegel WA, Wagner FF, Müller TH, Gassner C. Rh phenotype prediction by DNA typing and its application to practice. *Transfus Med* 1998;**8**:281–302.

285 Chiu RW, Murphy MF, Fidler C *et al.* Determination of RhD zygosity: comparison of a double amplification refractory mutation system approach and a multiplex real-time quantitative PCR approach. *Clin Chem* 2001;**47**:667–72.

286 Huang C-H, Reid ME, Chen Y, Coghlan G, Okubo Y. Molecular definition of red cell Rh haplotypes by tightly linked *Sph*I RFLPs. *Am J Hum Genet* 1996;**58**:133–42.

287 Reubinoff BE, Avner R, Rojansky N *et al.* RhD genotype determination by single sperm cell analysis. *Am J Obstet Gynecol* 1996;**174**:1300–5.

288 Lo YMD, Corbetta N, Chamberlain PF *et al.* Presence of fetal DNA in maternal plasma and serum. *Lancet* 1997;**350**:485–7.

289 Lo YMD. Fetal RhD genotyping from maternal plasma. *Ann Med* 1999;**31**:308–12.

290 Faas BHW, Beuling EA, von Christiaans GCML, dem Borne AEGK, van der Schoot CE. Detection of fetal *RHD*-specific sequences in maternal plasma. *Lancet* 1998;**352**:1196.

291 Lo YMD, Hjelm NM, Fidler C *et al.* Prenatal diagnosis of fetal RhD status by molecular analysis of maternal plasma. *N Engl J Med* 1998;**339**:1734–8.

292 Zhong XY, Holzgreve W, Hahn S. Detection of fetal Rhesus D and sex using fetal DNA from maternal plasma by multiplex polymerase chain reaction. *Br J Obstet Gynaecol* 2000;**107**:766–9.

293 Lo Y-MD, Bowell PJ, Selinger M *et al.* Prenatal determination of fetal RhD status by analysis of peripheral blood of rhesus negative mothers. *Lancet* 1993;**341**:1147–8.

294 Lo Y-MD, Noakes P, Bowell PJ, Fleming KA, Wainscoat JS. Detection of fetal RhD sequence from peripheral blood of sensitized RhD-negative pregnant women. *Br J Haematol* 1994;**87**:658–60.

295 Geifman-Holtzman O, Bernstein IM, Berry SM *et al.* Fetal RhD genotyping in fetal cells flow sorted from maternal blood. *Am J Obstet Gynecol* 1996;**174**:818–22.

296 Sekizawa A, Watanabe A, Kimura T *et al.* Prenatal diagnosis of the fetal RhD blood type using a single fetal nucleated erythrocyte from maternal blood. *Obstet Gynecol* 1996;**87**:501–5.

297 Al-Mufti R, Howard C, Overton T *et al.* Detection of fetal messenger ribonucleic acid in maternal blood to determine fetal RhD status as a strategy for noninvasive prenatal diagnosis. *Am J Obstet Gynecol* 1998;**179**: 210–14.

298 Cunningham J, Yates Z, Hamlington J *et al.* Noninvasive RNA-based determination of fetal Rhesus D type: a prospective study based on 96 pregnancies. *Br J Obstet Gynaecol* 1999;**106**:1023–8.

299 Troeger C, Zhong XY, Burgemeister R *et al.* Approximately half of the erythroblasts in maternal blood are of fetal origin. *Mol Hum Reprod* 1999;**5**:1162–5.

300 Bianchi DW, Zickwolf GK, Weil GJ, Sylvester S, DeMaria MA. Male fetal progenitor cells persist in maternal blood for as long as 27 years postpartum. *Proc Natl Acad Sci USA* 1996;**93**:705–8.

301 Van den Veyver IB, Chong SS, Cota J *et al.* Single-cell analysis of the RhD blood type for use in preimplantation diagnosis in the prevention of severe hemolytic disease of the newborn. *Am J Obstet Gynecol* 1995; **172**:533–40.

302 Skov F, Hughes-Jones NC. Observations of the number of available C antigen sites on red cells. *Vox Sang* 1977;**33**:170–4.

303 Race RR, Sanger R, Lawler SD. Rh genes allelomorphic to C. *Nature* 1948;**161**:316.

304 Smythe JS, Anstee DJ. Expression of C antigen in transduced K562 cells. *Transfusion* 2001;**41**:24–30.

305 Mouro I, Colin Y, Gane P *et al.* Molecular analysis of blood group Rh transcripts from a r^{G}r variant. *Br J Haematol* 1996;**93**:472–4.

306 Levine P, Rosenfield RE, White J. The first example of the Rh phenotype r^{G}r^G. *Am J Hum Genet* 1961; **13**:299–305.

307 Rosenfield RE, Levine P, Heller C. Quantitative Rh typing of r^{G}r^G with observations on the nature of G (Rh12) and anti-G. *Vox Sang* 1975;**28**:293–304.

308 Avent ND, Daniels GL, Martin PG *et al.* Molecular investigation of the Rh C/c polymorphism [Abstract]. *Transfus Med* 1997;**7**(Suppl. 1):18.

309 Westhoff CM, Silberstein LE, Wylie DE, Skavdahl M, Reif ME. 16Cys encoded by the *RHce* gene is associated with altered expression of the e antigen and is frequent in the R$_0$ haplotype. *Br J Haematol* 2001;**113**:666–71.

310 Salvignol I, Calvas P, Socha WW *et al.* Structural analysis of the RH-like blood group gene products in nonhuman primates. *Immunogenet* 1995;**41**:271–81.

311 Westhoff CM, Silberstein LE. Wylie DE. Evidence supporting the requirement for two proline residues for expression of c. *Transfusion* 2000;**40**:321–4.

312 Le Van Kim C, Mouro I, Brossard Y *et al.* PCR-based determination of Rhc and RhE status of fetuses at risk of Rhc and RhE haemolytic disease. *Br J Haematol* 1994;**88**:193–5.

313 Geifman-Holtzman O, Kaufman L, Gonchoroff N, Bernstein I, Holtzman EJ. Prenatal diagnosis of the fetal

Rhc genotype from peripheral maternal blood. *Obstet Gynecol* 1998;**91**:506–10.

314 Poulter M, Kemp TJ, Carritt B. DNA-based Rhesus typing: simultaneous determination of RHC and RHD status using the polymerase chain reaction. *Vox Sang* 1996;**70**:164–8.

315 Rozman P, Dovc T, Gassner C. Differentiation of autologous *ABO, RHD, RHCE, KEL, JK,* and *FY* blood group genotypes by analysis of peripheral blood samples of patients who have recently received multiple transfusions. *Transfusion* 2000;**40**:936–42.

316 Huestis DW, Catino ML, Busch S. A 'new' Rh antibody (anti-Rh 26) which detects a factor usually accompanying hr'. *Transfusion* 1964;**4**:414–18.

317 Faas BHW, Ligthart PC, Lomas-Francis C *et al.* Involvement of Gly96 in the formation of the Rh26 epitope. *Transfusion* 1997;**37**:1123–30.

318 Moulds JJ, Case J, Anderson TD, Cooper ES. The first example of allo-anti-c produced by a c-positive individual [Abstracts]. *17th Congr International Soc Blood Transfus* 1982:289.

319 Issitt PD, Tessel JA. On the incidence of antibodies to the Rh antigens G, rh$_i$ (Ce), C, and C^G in sera containing anti-CD or anti-C. *Transfusion* 1981;**21**:412–18.

320 Masouredis SP, Sudora EJ, Mahan L, Victoria EJ. Antigen site densities and ultrastructural distribution patterns of red cell Rh antigens. *Transfusion* 1976;**16**:94–106.

321 Ceppellini R. L'antigène Rh E^u. *Rev Hemat* 1950; **5**:285–93.

322 O'Riordan JP, Wilkinson JL, Huth MC, Wilson TE, Mourant AE, Giles CM. The Rh gene complex cdE^u. *Vox Sang* 1962;**7**:14–21.

323 Sussman LN. The rare blood factor rh(") or E^u. *Blood* 1955;**10**:1241–5.

324 Steers F, Wallace M, Johnson P, Carritt B, Daniels G. Denaturing gradient gel electrophoresis: a novel method for determining Rh phenotype from genomic DNA. *Br J Haematol* 1996;**94**:417–21.

325 Faas BHW, Simsek S, Bleeker PMM *et al.* Rh E/e genotyping by allele-specific primer amplification. *Blood* 1995;**85**:829–32.

326 Geifman-Holtzman O, Makhlouf F, Kaufman L, Gonchoroff NJ, Holtzman EJ. The clinical utility of fetal cell sorting to determine prenatally fetal E/e or e/e Rh genotype from peripheral maternal blood. *Am J Obstet Gynecol* 2000;**183**:462–8.

327 Greenwalt TJ, Sanger R. The Rh antigen E^w. *Br J Haematol* 1955;**1**:52–4.

328 Grobel RK, Cardy JD. Hemolytic disease of the newborn due to anti-E^w: a fourth example of the Rh antigen, E^w. *Transfusion* 1971;**11**:77–8.

329 Kaita H, Lewis M, Chown B. The Rh antigen E^w. *Transfusion* 1964;**4**:118–19.

330 Winter N, Milkovich L, Konugres AA. A third example of the Rh antigen, E^w. *Transfusion* 1966;**6**:271–2.

331 Henke J, Kasulke D. The first example of the Rh antigen E^w in Western Europe. *Vox Sang* 1976;30: 305–7.

332 Vos GH, Kirk RL. A 'naturally-occurring' anti-E which distinguishes a variant of the E antigen in Australian Aborigines. *Vox Sang* 1962;7:22–32.

333 Lubenko A, Burslem SJ, Fairclough LM *et al.* A new qualitative variant of the RhE antigen revealed by heterogeneity among anti-E sera. *Vox Sang* 1991;60: 235–40.

334 Okubo Y, Yamano H, Nagao N *et al.* A partial E in the Rh system? *Transfusion* 1994;34:183.

335 Noizat-Pirenne F, Mouro I, Gane P *et al.* Heterogeneity of blood group RhE variants revealed by serological analysis and molecular alteration of the *RHCE* gene and transcript. *Br J Haematol* 1998;103:429–36.

336 Noizat-Pirenne F, Mouro I, Le Pennec P *et al.* Molecular basis of category EIV variant phenotype [Abstract]. *Transfusion* 1999;39(Suppl.):103S.

337 Shapiro M. Serology and genetics of a new blood factor: hr^S. *J Forens Med* 1960;7:96–105.

338 Moores P. Rh18 and hr^S blood group and antibodies. *Vox Sang* 1994;66:225–30.

339 Daniels GL. *Blood group antigens of high frequency: a serological and genetical study.* PhD thesis, University of London, 1980.

340 Issitt PD, Anstee DJ. *Applied Blood Group Serology,* 4th edn. Durham: Montgomery Scientific Publications, 1998.

341 Issitt PD. An invited review: the Rh antigen e, its variants, and some closely related serological observations. *Immunohematology* 1991;7:29–36.

342 Grobbelaar BG, Moores PP. The third example of anti-hr^S. *Transfusion* 1963;3:103–4.

343 Noizat-Pirenne F, Mouro I, Le Pennec P-Y *et al.* Two new alleles of the *RHCE* gene in black individuals: the *RHce* allele ceMO and the *RHcE* allele cEMI. *Br J Haematol* 2001;113:672–9.

344 Shapiro M, le Roux M, Brink S. Serology and genetics of a new blood factor: hr^B. *Haematologia* 1972;6: 121–8.

345 Case J. Compound and complex Rh antigens. In: V Vengelen-Tyler, SR Pierce, eds. *Blood Group Systems: Rh.* Arlington: American Association of Blood Banks, 1987: 55–75.

346 Moores P, Smart E. Serology and genetics of the red blood cell factor Rh34. *Vox Sang* 1991;61:122–9.

347 Beal CL, Oliver CK, Mallory DM, Issitt PD. The r′ gene is overrepresented in hr^B-negative individuals. *Immunohematology* 1995;11:74–7.

348 Reid ME, Storry JR, Issitt PD *et al.* Rh haplotypes that make e but not hr^B usually make VS. *Vox Sang* 1997;72:41–4.

349 Blancher AP, Reid ME, Alié-Daram SJ, Dugoujon J-MH, Roubinet EL. Chatacterization of human anti-

350 Vengelen-Tyler V, Mogck N. Two cases of 'hrB-like' autoantibodies appearing as alloantibodies. *Transfusion* 1991;31:254–6.

hr^B-like monoclonal antibody. *Immunohematology* 1996;12:119–22.

351 Lewis M, Kaita H, Chown B *et al.* Inheritance of the Rh complex 'Santi', R$^{ou\,(GV)\,1}$. *Vox Sang* 1976;30:282–90.

352 Marais I, Moores P, Smart E, Martell R. STEM, a new low-frequency Rh antigen associated with the e-variant phenotypes hr^S– (Rh: –18,–19) and hrB– (Rh: –31,–34). *Transfus Med* 1993;3:35–41.

353 Heistö H. An anti-E antibody reacting strongly with enzyme-treated cells, but showing no signs of agglutination or absorption with untreated cells. *Acta Path Microbiol Scand* 1955;26:381–4.

354 Vogt E, Krystad E, Heistö H, Myhre K. A second example of a strong anti-E reacting *in vitro* almost exclusively with enzyme treated E positive cells. *Vox Sang* 1958;3:118–23.

355 Dybkjaer E. Anti-E antibodies disclosed in the period 1960–66. *Vox Sang* 1967;13:446–8.

356 Harrison J. The 'naturally occurring' anti-E. *Vox Sang* 1970;19:123–31.

357 Sanger R, Race RR, Rosenfield RE, Vogel P, Gibbel N. Anti-f and the 'new' Rh antigen it defines. *Proc Natl Acad Sci USA* 1953;39:824–34.

358 Grundorfer J, Kopchik W, Tippett P, Sanger R. Anti-f in the serum of a *CDe/cDE* person: the second example. *Vox Sang* 1961;6:618–19.

359 Jones AR, Steinberg AG, Allen FH, Diamond LK, Kriete B. Observations on the new Rh agglutinin anti-f. *Blood* 1954;9:117–22.

360 Levine P, White J, Stroup M, Zmijewski CM, Mohn JF. Hæmolytic disease of the newborn probably due to anti-f. *Nature* 1960;185:188–9.

361 Freda VJ, D'Esopo DA, Rosenfield RE, Haber GV. Erythroblastosis due to anti-Rh6. *Transfusion* 1963; 3:281–2.

362 Spielmann W, Seidl S, von Pawel J. Anti-ce (anti-f) in a *CDe/cD*– mother, as a cause of haemolytic disease of the newborn. *Vox Sang* 1974;27:473–7.

363 O'Reilly RA, Lombard CM, Azzi RL. Delayed hemolytic transfusion reaction associated with Rh antibody anti-f: first reported case. *Vox Sang* 1985;49:336–9.

364 Lucia SP, Wild GM, Hunt ML. Anti-f sensitization detected by an acidified indirect Coombs test. *Vox Sang* 1960;5:377–82.

365 Rosenfield RE, Haber GV. An Rh blood factor, rh$_i$ (Ce), and its relationship to hr (ce). *Am J Hum Genet* 1958;10:474–80.

366 Race RR, Sanger R, Levine P *et al.* A position effect of the *Rh* blood group genes. *Nature* 1954;174:460–1.

367 Wagner T, Resch B, Legler TJ *et al.* Severe HDN due to anti-Ce that required exchange transfusion. *Transfusion* 2000;40:571–4.

368 Malde R, Stanworth S, Patel S, Knight R. Haemolytic disease of the newborn due to anti-Ce. *Transfus Med* 2000;**10**:305–6.

369 Molthan L, Matulewicz TJ, Bansal-Carver B, Benz EJ. An immediate hemolytic transfusion reaction due to anti-C and a delayed hemolytic transfusion reaction due to anti-Ce+e: hemoglobinemia, hemoglobinuria and transient impaired renal function. *Vox Sang* 1984;**47**:348–53.

370 Lee E, Knight RC. A case of autoimmune haemolytic anaemia with an IgA anti-Ce autoantibody [Abstract]. *Vox Sang* 2000;**78**(Suppl. 1):P130.

371 Svoboda RK, Van West B, Grumet FC. Anti-Rh41, a new Rh antibody found in association with an abnormal expression of chromosome 1 genetic markers. *Transfusion* 1981;**21**:150–6.

372 Dunsford I. A new Rh antibody: anti CE. *Proc 8th Congr Europ Soc Haemat* 1961: 491.

373 Keith P, Corcoran PA, Caspersen K, Allen FH. A new antibody; anti-Rh[27] (cE) in the Rh blood group system. *Vox Sang* 1965;**10**:528–35.

374 Kline WE, Sullivan CM, Pope M, Bowman RJ. An example of a naturally occurring anti-cE (Rh27) that binds complement. *Vox Sang* 1982;**43**:335–9.

375 Allen FH, Tippett PA. A new Rh blood type which reveals the Rh antigen G. *Vox Sang* 1958;**3**:321–30.

376 Green C, Coghlan G, Bizot M, *et al.* JAHK: a low frequency antigen associated with the r^G complex of the Rh blood group system. *Transfus Med* 2002: **12**:55–61.

377 Stout TD, Moore BPL, Allen FH, Corcoran P. A new phenotype: D+G– (Rh:1,–12). *Vox Sang* 1963;**8**:262–8.

378 Faas BHW, Beckers EAM, Simsek S *et al.* Involvement of Ser103 of the Rh polypeptides in G epitope formation. *Transfusion* 1996;**36**:506–11.

379 Case J. Quantitative variation in the G antigen of the Rh blood group system. *Vox Sang* 1973;**25**:529–39.

380 Kusnierz-Alejska G. Anti-G alloantibody produced by C-positive D-positive G-negative patient [Abstract]. *Vox Sang* 1994;**67**(Suppl.2):53.

381 Skov F. Observations of the number of available G (rh^G, Rh12) antigen sites on red cells. *Vox Sang* 1976;**31**:124–30.

382 Allen FH, Tippett PA. Blocking tests with the Rh antibody anti-G. *Vox Sang* 1961;**6**:429–34.

383 Jakobowicz R, Simmons RT. Iso-immunization in a mother which demonstrates the 'new' Rh blood antigen G (rh^G) and anti-G (rh^G). *Med J Aust* 1959;**ii**:357–8.

384 Jakobowicz R, Whittingham S, Barrie JU, Simmons RT. A further investigation of polyvalent anti-C (rh′) and anti-G (rh^G) antibodies produced by iso-immunization in pregnancy. *Med J Aust* 1962;**i**:895–6.

385 Vos GH. The evaluation of specific anti-G (CD) eluate obtained by a double absorption and elution procedure. *Vox Sang* 1960;**5**:472–8.

386 Shapiro M. Serology and genetics of a 'new' blood factor: hr^H. *J Forensic Med* 1964;**11**:52–66.

387 Zaino EC. A new Rh phenotype Rh$_o$rh, G-negative. *Transfusion* 1965;**5**:320–1.

388 Palfi M, Gunnarsson C. The frequency of anti-C+ anti-G in the absence of anti-D in alloimmunized pregnancies. *Transfus Med* 2001;**11**:207–10.

389 Smith TR, Sherman SP, Nelson CA, Taswell HF. Formation of anti-G by the transfusion of D-negative blood [Abstract]. *Transfusion* 1978;**18**:388.

390 Sistonen P, Sareneva H, Pirkola A, Eklund J. MAR, a novel high-incidence Rh antigen revealing the existence of an allelic sub-system including C^W (Rh8) and C^x (Rh9) with exceptional distribution in the Finnish population. *Vox Sang* 1994;**66**:287–92.

391 Mouro I, Colin Y, Sistonen P *et al.* Molecular basis of the RhC^W (Rh8) and RhC^x (Rh9) blood group specificities. *Blood* 1995;**86**:1196–201.

392 Callender ST, Race RR. A serological and genetical study of multiple antibodies formed in response to blood transfusion by a patient with lupus erythematosus diffusus. *Ann Eugen* 1946;**13**:102–17.

393 Dunsford I, Aspinall P. Th Rh chromosome C^{w}dE (Ry^w) occurring in three generations. *Nature* 1951;**168**:954–5.

394 Prokop O, Rackwitz A. Eine weitere Beobachtung von R$_z$^{w} in der seltenen Kombination R$_z$^{w}R$_1$^{w} mit einer Bemerkung über den Dosiseffekt von C^w. *Blut* 1959;**5**:279–81.

395 Leonard GL, Ellisor SS, Reid ME, Sanchez PD, Tippett P. An unusual Rh immunization. *Vox Sang* 1976;**31**:275–6.

396 Watt J, Pepper R. Anti-C in an Rl^{w}Rl^w patient [Abstract]. *Joint Congr Int Soc Blood Transfus and Am Ass Blood Banks* 1990: 80.

397 Govoni M, Battistini I, Menini C. A rare case of Rh immunization. *Vox Sang* 1990;**58**:137.

398 Thorpe SJ, Boult CE, Thompson KM. Immunochemical characterization of the Rh C^w antigen using human monoclonal antibodies. *Vox Sang* 1997;**73**: 174–81.

399 Sachs HW, Reuter W, Tippett P, Gavin J. An Rh gene complex producing both C^w and c antigen. *Vox Sang* 1978;**35**:272–4.

400 Giannetti M, Stadler E, Rittner C, Lomas C, Tippett P. A rare Rh haplotype producing C^w and c, and D and e in a German family. *Vox Sang* 1983;**44**:319–21.

401 Bowman JM, Pollock J. Maternal C^w alloimmunization. *Vox Sang* 1993;**64**:226–30.

402 Lawler SD, van Loghem JJ. The Rhesus antigen C^w causing hæmolytic disease of the newborn. *Lancet* 1947;**ii**:545–6.

403 Reiner AP, Teramura G, Aramaki KM. Use of PCR-based assay for fetal C^w antigen genotyping in a patient with a history of moderately severe hemolytic disease of the newborn due to anti-C^w. *Am J Perinatol* 1999;**16**:277–81.

404 Sistonen P, Aden Abdulle O, Sahid M. Evidence for a

'new' Rh gene complex producing the rare C^x (Rh9) antigen in the Somali population of East Africa. *Transfusion* 1987;27:66–8.

405 Stratton F, Renton PH. Haemolytic disease of the newborn caused by a new Rh antibody, anti-C^x. *Br Med J* 1954;i:962–5.

406 Finney RD, Blue AM, Willoughby MLN. Haemolytic disease of the newborn caused by the rare Rhesus antibody anti-C^x. *Vox Sang* 1973;25:39–42.

407 Mougey R, Martin J, Hackbart C. A new high frequency Rh red cell antigen associated with the Rh antigen C^x [Abstract]. *Transfusion* 1983;23:410.

408 Plaut G, Booth PB, Giles CM, Mourant AE. A new example of the Rh antibody, anti-C^x. *Br Med J* 1958;i:1215–7.

409 Bradford MF, Porter M, Lacey PA, Moulds JJ. Further complexities of anti-C: an antibody produced by an R$_1$^{x}r individual [Abstract]. *Transfusion* 1985;25: 471.

410 O'Shea KP, Øyen R, Sausais L *et al*. A MAR-like antibody in a DC^{w}e/DC^{w}e person. *Transfusion* 2001;41: 53–5.

411 DeNatale A, Cahan A, Jack JA, Race RR, Sanger R. V, a 'new' Rh antigen, common in Negroes, rare in white people. *J Am Med Assoc* 1955;159:247–50.

412 Sanger R, Noades J, Tippett P, Race RR, Jack JA, Cunningham CA. An Rh antibody specific for V and R$'$s. *Nature* 1960;186:171.

413 Moulds JJ, Case J, Thornton S, Pulver VB, Moulds MK. Anti-Ce^s: a previously undescribed Rh antibody [Abstract]. *Transfusion* 1980;20:631–2.

414 Lomas C, Storry JR, Spruell P, Moulds M. Apparent alloanti-C produced by r$'$S people: five examples [Abstract]. *Transfusion* 1994;34(Suppl.):25S.

415 Tregellas WM, Issitt PD. An investigation of the relationship between the V (hr^V), VS, and hr^H antigens. *Transfusion* 1978;18:15–20.

416 Giblett ER, Chase J, Motulsky AG. Studies on anti-V. A recently discovered Rh antibody. *J Lab Clin Med* 1957;49:433–9.

417 Cheng MS. Saline-reactive anti-V. *Transfusion* 1982; 22:401.

418 Byrne PC, Howard JH. The incidence of V (Rh10) and Js^a (K6) in the contemporary African American blood donor. *Immunohematology* 1994;10:136–8.

419 Spruell P, Lacey P, Bradford MF *et al*. Incidence of hemolytic disease of the newborn due to anti-D^w [Abstract]. *Transfusion* 1997;37(Suppl.):43S.

420 Leschek E, Pearlman SA, Boudreaux I, Meek R. Severe hemolytic disease of the newborn caused by anti-Gonzales antibody. *Am J Perinat* 1993;10:362–4.

421 Issitt PD, Gutgsell NS, Martin PA, Ferguson JR. Hemolytic disease of the newborn caused by anti-Rh32 and demonstration that $\bar{\bar{R}}^N$ encodes rh$_i$ (Ce,Rh7). *Transfusion* 1991;31:63–6.

422 Chown B, Lewis M, Kaita H. The Rh system: an anomaly of inheritance, probably due to mutation. *Vox Sang* 1971;21:385–96.

423 Orlina AR, Unger PJ, Lacey PA. Anti-Rh32 causing severe hemolytic disease of the newborn. *Rev Franc Transfus Immuno-Hémat* 1984;27:613–18.

424 Issitt PD, Wren MR, McDowell MA, Strohm PL, Roberts TM. Anti-Rh33, the second separable example, also made by a person who made anti-D and has C+ red cells. *Transfusion* 1986;26:506–10.

425 Giles CM, Skov F. The *CDe* Rhesus gene complex; some considerations revealed by a study of a Danish family with an antigen of the Rhesus gene complex *(C)D(e)* defined by a 'new' antibody. *Vox Sang* 1971;20:328–34.

426 Davidsohn I, Stern K, Strauser ER, Spurrier W. Be, a new 'private' blood factor. *Blood* 1953;8:747–54.

427 Stern K, Davidsohn I, Jensen FG, Muratore R. Immunologic studies on the Be^a factor. *Vox Sang* 1958;3:425–34.

428 Clark J, Yorek H, Schuler S, Milam JD. Hemolytic disease of the newborn due to anti-Berrens antibody: the third reported case [Abstract]. *Joint Congr Int Soc Blood Transfus and Am Ass Blood Banks* 1990:81.

429 Amil M, Casais C, Vicente I *et al*. Severe hemolytic disease of the new born caused by anti-Rh36 [Abstract]. *Vox Sang* 2000;78(Suppl.):P122.

430 Issitt PD, Gutgsell NS, McDowell MA, Tregellas WM. Studies on anti-Rh46 [Abstract]. *Blood* 1987;70(Suppl.1):110a.

431 Rouger P, Edelman L. Murine monoclonal antibodies associated with Rh17, Rh29, and Rh46 antigens. *Transfusion* 1988;28:52–5.

432 Le Pennec PY, Buffière F, Gane P *et al*. Study of a human monoclonal anti-RH46 [Abstract]. *Transfusion* 1996;36(Suppl.):54S.

433 Broman B, Heiken A, Tippett PA, Giles CM. The *D(C)(e)* gene complex revealed in the Swedish population. *Vox Sang* 1963;8:588–93.

434 Tippett P. Depressed Rh phenotypes. *Rev Franc Transfus Immuno-Hémat* 1978;21:135–50.

435 Heiken A, Giles CM. On the Rh gene complexes D––, D(C)(e) and d(c)(e). *Hereditas* 1965;53:171–86.

436 Renton PH, Hancock JA. An individual of unusual Rh type. *Vox Sang* 1955;5:135–42.

437 Poole J, Hustinx H, Gerber H *et al*. The red cell antigen JAL in the Swiss population: family studies showing that JAL is an Rh antigen (RH48). *Vox Sang* 1990;59: 44–7.

438 Noizat-Pirenne F, Le Pennec P-Y, Mouro I *et al*. The molecular basis of a D(C)(e) complex probably associated with the RH35 low frequency antigen [Abstract]. *Transfusion* 1999;39(Suppl.):103S.

439 Moores P, Smart E, Sternberger J, Schneider W. Rh33 in two of three German siblings with D+C+c+E+e– red cells. *Transfusion* 1991;31:759–61.

440 Daniels GL. An investigation of the immune response of homozygotes for the Rh haplotype: –D– and related

haplotypes. *Rev Franc Transfus Immuno-Hémat* 1982;**25**:185–97.

441 Westhoff CM, Skavdahl M, Walker PS, Storry JR, Reid ME. A new hybrid *RHCE* gene that is responsible for expression of a novel antigen [Abstract]. *Transfusion* 2000;**40**(Suppl.):7S.

442 Cheng G-J, Chen Y, Reid ME, Huang C-H. Evans antigen: a new hybrid structure occurring on background of D·· and D–– Rh complexes. *Vox Sang* 2000;**78**:44–51.

443 Huang C-H. Alteration of *RH* gene structure and expression in human dCCee and DC^w– red blood cells: phenotypic homozygosity versus genotypic heterozygosity. *Blood* 1996;**88**:2326–33.

444 Kornstad L, Heier Larsen AM. A possible *D(C^w)(e)* gene complex of the Rh system. *Vox Sang* 1973;**25**: 385–9.

445 Schneider W, Tippett P. Rh33, another possible homozygote [Abstract]. *Transfusion* 1978;**18**:392.

446 Issitt PD, Gutgsell NS. A new gene, *R^o Job*, that makes Rh33 and normal D [Abstract]. *Blood* 1987; **70**(Suppl.1):110a.

447 Issitt PD, Smith DL, McCollister LS, Wren MR, Ballas SK. Studies on the blood of a *Dc(e)* homozygote and her family. *Transfusion* 1988;**28**:439–43.

448 Huang C-H, Reid ME, Chen Y, Novaretti M. Deletion of Arg229 in RhCE polypeptide alters expression of RhE and CE-associated Rh6 antigens [Abstract]. *Blood* 1997;**90**(Suppl.1):272a.

449 Metaxas MN, Metaxas-Bühler M. An Rh gene complex which produces weak c and e antigens in a mother and her son. *Vox Sang* 1961;**6**:136–41.

450 Broman B, Heiken A, Giles CM. An unusual Rh gene complex producing a weak c antigen. *Vox Sang* 1964;**9**:741–5.

451 Storry JR, Gorman M, Maddox NI *et al*. First example of Rh:–32,–46 red cell phenotype. *Immunohematology* 1994;**10**:130–3.

452 Morton NE, Rosenfield RE. A new Rh allele, *r^yn* (*R^-1,2,w3,w4*). *Transfusion* 1967;**7**:117–19.

453 Kornstad L, Øyen R. An Rh gene complex producing weak c and E antigens. *Vox Sang* 1967;**13**:417–22.

454 Enomoto T, Ohmura K, Hando K. *et al*. Studies on the blood of a *(c)D(E)/-D-* propositus and her family [Abstract]. *24th Congr International Soc Blood Transfus* 1996: 144.

455 Tippett PA, Sanger R, Dunsford I, Barber M. An Rh gene complex, *r^M*, in some ways like *r^G*. *Vox Sang* 1961;**6**:21–33.

456 Race RR, Sanger R. Consanguinity and certain rare blood groups. *Vox Sang* 1960;**5**:383–4.

457 Daniels G. *Human Blood Groups*. Oxford: Blackwell Science, 1995.

458 Race RR, Sanger R, Selwyn JG. A probable deletion in a human Rh chromosome. *Nature* 1950;**166**:520.

459 Race RR, Sanger R, Selwyn JG. A possible deletion in a human Rh chromosome: a serological and genetical study. *Br J Exp Pathol* 1951;**32**:124–35.

460 Waller RK, Sanger R, Bobbitt OB. Two examples of the –D–/–D– genotype in an American family. *Br Med J* 1953;i:198–9.

461 Buchanan DI, McIntyre J. Consanguinity and two rare matings. –D–/–D–×CDe/–D– and CDe/–D–× cDe/–D–. *Br J Haematol* 1955;**1**:304–7.

462 Yokoyama M, Solomon JM, Kuniyuki M, Stroup M. R^=o (D––) in two Japanese families with a note on its genetic interpretation. *Transfusion* 1961;**1**:273–9.

463 De Torregrosa MV, Rullán MM, Cecile C, Sabater A, Alberto C. Severe erythroblastosis in a primigravida associated with absence of Rh chromosomes. *Am J Obstet Gynecol* 1961;**82**:1375–8.

464 Badakere SS, Bhatia HM. Haemolytic disease of the newborn in a –D–/–D– Indian woman. *Vox Sang* 1973;**24**:280–2.

465 Kendrick L, Dunstan-Adams C, Humphreys J *et al*. The rare Rh haplotypes –D– and. ––– in a family with a –D–/––– propositus. *J Immunogenet* 1981;**8**:243–7.

466 Ólafsdóttir S, Jensson O, Thordarson G, Sigurdardóttir S. An unusual Rhesus haplotype, –D–, in Iceland. *Forensic Sci Int* 1983;**22**:183–7.

467 Whang DH, Kim HC, Hur M *et al*. A successful delivery of a baby from a D––/D–– mother with strong anti-Hr₀. *Immunohematology* 2000;**16**:112–14.

468 Henningsen K. Significance of –D– chromosome in a legal paternity case. *Vox Sang* 1957;**2**:399–405.

469 Lawler SD, Marshall R. A serological study of –D– heterozygotes in the same family. *Vox Sang* 1962;**7**:305–14.

470 Heiken A, Giles CM. A study of a family possessing the Rh gene complex D–– in the heterozygous state. *Acta Genet* 1966;**16**:155–61.

471 Mulvihal M, Moores P. The Rh haplotype D–– identified in five Cape Colored families. *Transfusion* 1991;**31**:188–9.

472 Rasmuson M, Heiken A. Frequency of occurrence of the human Rh complexes D(C)(e), d(c)(e), D–– and –––. *Nature* 1966;**212**:1377–9.

473 Okubo Y, Tomita T, Nagao N, Yamaguchi H, Tanaka M. Mass screening donors for –D– and Jk(a–b–) using the Groupamatic-360. *Transfusion* 1983;**23**:362–3.

474 Chérif-Zahar B, Raynal V, D'Ambrosio A-M, Cartron JP, Colin Y. Molecular analysis of the structure and expression of the RH locus in individuals with D––, Dc–, and DC^w– gene complexes. *Blood* 1994;**84**:4354–60.

475 Kemp TJ, Poulter M, Carritt B. A recombination hot spot in the Rh genes revealed by analysis of unrelated donors with the rare D–– phenotype. *Am J Hum Genet* 1996;**59**:1066–73.

476 Blunt T, Steers F, Daniels G, Carritt B. Lack of RH C/E expression in the Rhesus D–– phenotype is the result of a gene deletion. *Ann Hum Genet* 1994;**58**:19–24.

267

477 Huang C-H, Reid ME, Chen Y. Identification of a partial internal deletion in the *RH* locus causing the human erythrocyte D–– phenotype. *Blood* 1995;**86**:784–90.

478 Cherif-Zahar B, Raynal V, Cartron J-P. Lack of RHCE-encoded proteins in the D–– phenotype may result from homologous recombination between the two *RH* genes. *Blood* 1996;**88**:1518–20.

479 Cherif-Zahar B, Raynal V, Gane P *et al.* Candidate gene acting as a suppressor of the *RH* locus in most cases of Rh-deficiency. *Nature Genet* 1996;**12**:168–73.

480 Contreras M, Armitage S, Daniels GL, Tippett P. Homozygous ·D·. *Vox Sang* 1979;**36**:81–4.

481 Skradski K, Sabo B, Daniels G. A second homozygous ·D·. *Transfusion* 1981;**21**:472.

482 Huang C-H, Chen Y, Reid ME, Ghosh S. Genetic recombination at the human *RH* locus: a family study of the red-cell Evans phenotype reveals a transfer of exons 2–6 from the *RHD* to the *RHCE* gene. *Am J Hum Genet* 1996;**59**:825–33.

483 Tate H, Cunningham C, McDade MG, Tippett PA, Sanger R. An Rh gene complex *Dc*–. *Vox Sang* 1960;**5**: 398–402.

484 Yamaguchi H, Okubo Y, Tomita T, Yamano H, Tanaka M. A case of Rh gene complex cD–/cD– found in a Japanese. *Proc Jpn Acad* 1969;**45**:618–20.

485 Delmas-Marsalet Y, Goudemand M, Tippett P. Un nouvel exemple de génotype rhésus cD–/cD–. *Rev Franc Transfus* 1969;**12**:233–8.

486 Cotorruelo C, Biondi C, Garcia Rosasco M, Foresto P, Racca A, Valverde J. Deletion of E and e antigens in a pregnant woman. *Transfusion* 1996;**36**:191.

487 Leyshon WC. The Rh gene complex *cD*– segregating in a Negro family. *Vox Sang* 1967;**13**:354–6.

488 Moores P, Vaaja U, Smart E. D–– and Dc– gene complexes in the Coloureds and Blacks of Natal and the Eastern Cape and blood group phenotype and gene frequency studies in the Natal Coloured population. *Hum Hered* 1991;**41**:295–304.

489 Gunson HH, Donohue WL. Multiple examples of the blood genotype C^wD–/C^wD– in a Canadian family. *Vox Sang* 1957;**2**:320–31.

490 Tippett P, Gavin J, Sanger R. The antigen C^W produced by the gene complex C^WD–. *Vox Sang* 1962;**7**:249–50.

491 Salmon C, Gerbal A, Liberge G *et al.* Le complexe génique D^{IV} (C)–. *Rev Franc Transfus* 1969;**12**:239–47.

492 Perrier P, Habibi B, Salmon C. Allo antibodies in partially silent Rh phenotypes: evidence for a possibly new high frequency Rh antigen. *Rev Franc Transfus Immuno-Hémat* 1980;**23**:327–39.

493 Habibi B, Perrier P, Salmon C. Antigen Nou: a new high frequency Rh antigen. *Rev Franc Transfus Immuno-Hémat* 1981;**24**:117–20.

494 Hackel E. Rh antibodies in the serum of two –D–/–D– people. *Vox Sang* 1957;**2**:331–41.

495 Buchanan DI. Blood genotypes –D–/–D– and CDe/–D–:

496 Blancher A, Roubinet F, Reid ME *et al.* Characterization of a macaque anti-Rh17-like monoclonal antibody. *Vox Sang* 1998;**75**:58–62.

497 Vos GH, Vos D, Kirk RL, Sanger R. A sample of blood with no detectable Rh antigens. *Lancet* 1961;**i**: 14–15.

498 Ishimori T, Hasekura H. A Japanese with no detectable Rh blood group antigens due to silent Rh alleles or deleted chromosomes. *Transfusion* 1967;**7**:84–7.

499 Hasekura H, Ishimori T, Furusawa S *et al.* Haematological observations on the r̄h(––– / –––) propositus, the homozygote of amorphic Rh blood group genes. *Proc Jpn Acad* 1971;**47**:579–83.

500 Kato-Yamazaki M, Okuda H, Kawano M *et al.* Molecular genetic analysis of the Japanese amorph Rh_{null} phenotype. *Transfusion* 2000;**40**:617–18.

501 Seidl S, Spielmann W, Martin H. Two siblings with Rh_{null} disease. *Vox Sang* 1972;**23**:182–9.

502 Huang C-H, Chen Y, Reid ME, Seidl C. Rh_{null} disease: the amorph type results from a novel double mutation in RhCe gene on D-negative background. *Blood* 1998;**92**:664–71.

503 Pérez-Pérez C, Taliano V, Mouro I *et al.* Spanish Rh_{null} family caused by a silent Rh gene: hematological, serological, and biochemical studies. *Am J Hematol* 1992;**40**:306–12.

504 Gibbs BJ, Moores P. Rh_{null} red cells and pregnancy. *Vox Sang* 1983;**45**:83–6.

505 Huang C-H, Cheng G, Liu Z *et al.* Molecular basis for Rh_{null} syndrome: identification of three new missense mutations in the Rh50 glycoprotein gene. *Am J Hematol* 1999;**62**:25–32.

506 Huang C-H, Liu Z, Cheng G, Chen Y. Rh50 glycoprotein gene and Rh_{null} disease: a silent splice donor is *trans* to a Gly_{279}→Glu missense mutation in the conserved transmembrane segment. *Blood* 1998;**92**:1776–84.

507 Hyland CA, Chérif-Zahar B, Cowley N *et al.* A novel single missense mutation identified along the RH50 gene in a composite heterozygous Rh_{null} blood donor of the regulator type. *Blood* 1998;**91**:1458–63.

508 Cowley NM, Saul A, Cartron J-P, Hyland CA. A single point mutation at a splice site generates a silent *RH50* gene in a composite heterozygous Rh_{null} blood donor. *Vox Sang* 1999;**76**:247–8.

509 Kawano M, Iwamoto S, Okuda H, Fukuda S, Hasegawa N, Kajii E. A splicing mutation of the *RHAG* gene associated with the Rh_{null} phenotype. *Ann Hum Genet* 1998;**62**:107–13.

510 Huang C-H, Cheng G-J, Reid ME, Chen Y. Rh_{mod} syndrome: a family study of the translation-initiator mutation in the Rh50 glycoprotein gene. *Am J Hum Genet* 1999;**64**:108–17.

511 Chown B, Lewis M, Kaita H, Lowen B. An unlinked modifier of Rh blood groups: effects when heterozygous

transfusion therapy and some effects of multiple pregnancy. *Am J Clin Pathol* 1956;**26**:21–8.

and when homozygous. *Am J Hum Genet* 1972; 24:623–37.

512 Cartron J-P. *RH* blood group system and molecular basis of Rh-deficiency. *Baillière's Clin Haematol* 1999;12:655–89.

513 Boettcher B, Hasekura H. Rh blood groups of Australian Aborigines in the tribe containing the original Rh$_{null}$ propositus. *Vox Sang* 1971;21: 200–9.

514 Levine P, Celano MJ, Falkowski F, White Chambers J, Hunter OB, English CT. A second example of --- / --- or Rh$_{null}$ blood. *Transfusion* 1965;5:492–500.

515 Senhauser DA, Mitchell MW, Gault DB, Owens JH. Another example of phenotype Rh$_{null}$. *Transfusion* 1970;10:89–92.

516 Gomez Casal G, Poderos Baeta C, Romero Colas MS *et al*. Déficit de antigenos eritrocitarios como causa de patologia. II. Enfermedad del Rh-null. *Rev Clin Espanola* 1983;171:19–21.

517 Sistonen P, Palosuo T, Snellman A. Identical twins with the Rh$_{null}$ phenotype of the regulator type in a Finnish Lapp family. *Vox Sang* 1985;48:174–7.

518 Ballas SK, Clark MR, Mohandas N *et al*. Red cell membrane and cation deficiency in Rh null syndrome. *Blood* 1984;63:1046–55.

519 Gabra GS, Bruce M, Watt A, Mitchell R. Anti-Rh29 in a primigravida with Rhesus null syndrome resulting in haemolytic disease of the newborn. *Vox Sang* 1987;53:143–6.

520 Lubenko A, Contreras M, Portugal CL *et al*. Severe haemolytic disease in an infant born to an Rh$_{null}$ proposita. *Vox Sang* 1992;63:43–7.

521 Snowden JA, Poole J, Bates AJ *et al*. The Rh$_{null}$ phenotype in an English individual: haematological, serological and immunochemical studies. *Clin Lab Haematol* 1997;19:143–8.

522 Naoki K, Uda M, Uchiyama B *et al*. Rh$_{null}$ with naturally occurring antibody. *Transfusion* 1984;24:182–3.

523 Kishi K, Yasuda T, Uchida M. A Japanese patient with the rare Rh$_{null}$ phenotype of the 'regulator type'. *J Immunogenet* 1987;14:261–4.

524 McGuire Mallory D, Rosenfield RE, Wong KY *et al*. Rh$_{mod}$, a second kindred (Craig). *Vox Sang* 1976;30: 430–40.

525 Stevenson MM, Anido V, Tanner AM, Swoyer J. Rh 'null' is not always null. *Br Med J* 1973;i:417.

526 Yamaguchi H, Okubo Y, Tanaka M, Tokunaga E, Amari S. Rare blood type Rh$_{mod}$ occurring in two Japanese families. *Proc Jpn Acad* 1975;51:763–6.

527 Saji H, Hosoi T. A Japanese Rh$_{mod}$ family: serological and haematological observations. *Vox Sang* 1979;37:296–304.

528 Steers FJ, Wallace M, Mora L *et al*. Rh$_{mod}$ phenotype. a parentage problem solved by denaturing gradient gel electrophoresis of Genomic DNA. *Immunohematology* 1996;12:154–8.

529 Nagel V, Kneiphoff H, Pekker S *et al*. Unexplained appearance of antibody in an Rh$_{null}$ donor. *Vox Sang* 1972;22:519–23.

530 Badon SJ, DeLong EN, Cable RG, Jagathambal K. Rh$_{null}$ disease: a case report [Abstract]. *Transfusion* 1998;38(Suppl.):35S.

531 Sturgeon P. Haematological observations on the anemia associated with blood type Rh$_{null}$. *Blood* 1970;36:310–20.

532 Schmidt PJ, Lostumbo MM, English CT, Hunter OB. Aberrant U blood group accompanying Rh$_{null}$. *Transfusion* 1967;7:33–4.

533 McGinniss MH, Kaplan HS, Bowen AB, Schmidt PJ. Agglutinins for 'null' red blood cells. *Transfusion* 1969;9:40–2.

534 McGinniss MH, Schmidt PJ, Perry MC. An autoagglutinin for 'null' red blood cells [Abstract]. *26th Ann Mtg Am Ass Blood Banks* 1973: 114–15.

535 Schmidt PJ, Vos GH. Multiple phenotypic abnormalities associated with Rh$_{null}$ (---/---). *Vox Sang* 1967;13:18–20.

536 Nash R, Shojania AM. Hematological aspect of Rh deficiency syndrome: a case report and a review of the literature. *Am J Hematol* 1987;24:267–75.

537 Smith JA, Lucas FV, Martin AP, Senhauser DA, Vorbeck ML. Lipid–protein interactions of erythrocyte membranes. comparison of normal, O,Rh(D) positive with the rare O,Rh$_{null}$. *Biochem Biophys Res Commun* 1973;54:1015–23.

538 Kuypers F, van Linde-Sibenius-Trip M, Roelofsen B *et al*. Rh$_{null}$ human erythrocytes have an abnormal membrane phospholipid organization. *Biochem J* 1984;221:931–4.

539 Lauf PK, Joiner CH. Increased potassium transport and ouabain binding in human Rh$_{null}$ red blood cells. *Blood* 1976;48:457–68.

540 Issitt PD. Null red blood cell phenotypes: associated biological changes. *Transfus Med Rev* 1993;7:139–55.

541 Kornstad L. A rare blood group antigen, Ol^a (Oldeide), associated with weak Rh antigens. *Vox Sang* 1986;50:235–9.

542 Hoffman JJML, Overbeeke MAM, Kaita H, Loomans AAH. A new, low incidence red cell antigen (HOFM), associated with depressed C antigen. *Vox Sang* 1990;59:240–3.

543 Coghlan G, McCreary J, Underwood V, Zelinski T. A 'new' low-incidence red cell antigen, LOCR, associated with altered expression of Rh antigens. *Transfusion* 1994;34:492–5.

544 Cobb ML. Crawford: investigation of a new low frequency red cell antigen [Abstract]. *Transfusion* 1980;20:631.

545 Larson PJ, Lukas MB, Friedman DF, Manno CS. Delayed hemolytic transfusion reaction due to anti-Go^a, an antibody against the low-prevalence Gonzalez antigen. *Am J Hematol* 1996;53:248–50.

546 Reid ME, Sausais L, Zaroulis CG *et al*. Two examples of an inseparable antibody that reacts equally well with D^w+ and Rh32+ red blood cells. *Vox Sang* 1998;**75**:230–3.

547 Devey ME, Voak D. A critical study of the IgG subclasses of Rh anti-D antibodies formed in pregnancy and in immunized volunteers. *Immunology* 1974;**27**:1073–9.

548 Hardman JT, Beck ML. Hemagglutination in capillaries: correlation with blood group specificity and IgG subclass. *Transfusion* 1981;**21**:343–6.

549 Frame M, Mollison PL, Terry WD. Anti-Rh activity of human γG4 proteins. *Nature* 1970;**225**:641–3.

550 Abramson N, Schur PH. The IgG subclasses of red cell antibodies and relationship to monocyte binding. *Blood* 1972;**40**:500–8.

551 Hughes-Jones N, Ghosh S. Anti-D-coated Rh-positive red cells will bind the first component of the complement pathway, C1q. *FEBS Lett* 1981;**128**:318–20.

552 Waller M, Lawler SD. A study of the properties of the Rhesus antibody (Ri) diagnostic for the rheumatoid factor and its application to Gm grouping. *Vox Sang*, 1962; **7**:591–606.

553 Harboe M, Müller-Eberhard HJ, Fudenberg H, Polley MJ, Mollison PL. Identification of the components of complement participating in the antiglobulin reaction. *Immunology* 1963;**6**:412–20.

554 Ayland J, Horton MA, Tippett P, Waters AH. Complement binding anti-D made in a D^u variant woman. *Vox Sang* 1978;**34**:40–2.

555 Contreras M, de Silva M, Teesdale P, Mollison PL. The effect of naturally occurring Rh antibodies on the survival of serologically incompatible red cells. *Br J Haematol* 1987;**65**:475–8.

556 Algora M, Barbolla L, Contreras M. Naturally occurring anti-D, anti-K, anti-Fy^a, and anti-Le^ab. *Vox Sang* 1991;**61**:141.

557 Perrault RA, Högman CF. Low concentration red cell antibodies. III. 'Cold' IgG anti-D in pregnancy: incidence and significance. *Acta Universitatis Uppsaliensis*, 1972:120.

558 Leader KA, Macht LM, Steers F, Kumpel BM, Elson CJ. Antibody responses to the blood group antigen D in SCID mice reconstituted with human blood mononuclear cells. *Immunology* 1992;**76**:229–34.

559 Köhler G, Milstein C. Continuous cultures of fused cells secreting antibody of predefined specificity. *Nature* 1975;**256**:495–7.

560 Steinitz M, Klein G, Koskimies S, Makel O. EB virus-induced B lymphocyte cell lines producing specific antibody. *Nature* 1977;**269**:420–2.

561 Crawford DH, Barlow MJ, Harrison JF, Winger L, Huehns ER. Production of human monoclonal antibody to Rhesus D antigen. *Lancet* 1983;**i**:386–8.

562 Doyle A, Jones TJ, Bidwell JL, Bradley BA. *In vitro* development of human monoclonal antibody-secreting plasmacytomas. *Hum Immunol* 1985;**13**:199–209.

563 Paire J, Monestier M, Rigal D, Martel F, Desgranges C. Establishment of human cell lines producing anti-D monoclonal antibodies: identification of rhesus D antigen. *Immunol Lett* 1986;**13**:137–41.

564 Goossens D, Champomier F, Rouger P, Salmon C. Human monoclonal antibodies against blood group antigens. Preparation of a series of stable EBV immortalized B clones producing high levels of antibody of different isotypes and specificities. *J Immunol Methods* 1987;**101**:193–200.

565 Kumpel BM, Poole GD, Bradley BA. Human monoclonal anti-D antibodies. I. Their production, serology, quantitation and potential use as blood grouping reagents. *Br J Haematol* 1989;**71**:125–9.

566 Melamed MD, Gordon J, Ley SJ, Edgar D, Hughes-Jones NC. Senescence of a human lymphoblastoid clone producing anti-Rhesus (D). *Eur J Immunol* 1985;**15**:742–6.

567 Kozbor D, Roder JC, Chang TH, Steplewski Z, Koprowski H. Human anti-tetanus toxoid monoclonal antibody secreted by EBV-transformed human B cells fused with murine myeloma. *Hybridoma* 1982;**1**:323–8.

568 Thompson KM, Hough DW, Maddison PJ, Melamed MD, Hughes-Jones N. The efficient production of stable, human monoclonal antibody-secreting hybridomas from EBV-transformed lymphocytes using the mouse myeloma X63-Ag8.653 as a fusion partner. *J Immunol Methods* 1986;**94**:7–12.

569 Thompson KM, Melamed MD, Eagle K *et al*. Production of human monoclonal IgG and IgM antibodies with anti-D (rhesus) specificity using heterohybridomas. *Immunology* 1986;**58**:157–60.

570 MacDonald G, Primrose S, Biggins K *et al*. Production and characterization of human–human and human–mouse hybridomas secreting Rh(D)-specific monoclonal antibodies. *Scand J Immunol* 1987;**25**:477–83.

571 Melamed MD, Thompson KM, Gibson T, Hughes-Jones NC. Requirements for the establishment of heterohybridomas secreting monoclonal human antibody to rhesus (D) blood group antigen. *J Immunol Methods* 1987;**104**:245–51.

572 Bron D, Feinberg MB, Teng NNH, Kaplan HS. Production of human monoclonal IgG antibodies against Rhesus (D) antigen. *Proc Natl Acad Sci USA* 1984;**81**: 3214–17.

573 Foung SKH, Blunt JA, Wu PS *et al*. Human monoclonal antibodies to Rho (D). *Vox Sang* 1987;**53**:44–7.

574 Thompson JM, Lowe J, McDonald DF. Human monoclonal anti-D secreting heterohybridomas from peripheral B lymphocytes expanded in the CD40 system. *J Immunol Methods* 1994;**175**:137–40.

575 Lowe AD, Green SM, Voak D, Gibson T, Lennox ES. A human-human monoclonal anti-D by direct fusion with a lymphoblastoid line. *Vox Sang* 1986;**51**:212–6.

576 James K, Bell GT. Human monoclonal antibody pro-

duction: current status and future prospects. *J Immunol Methods* 1987;**100**:5–40.

577 Crawford DH, Azim T, Daniels GL, Huehns ER. Monoclonal antibodies to the Rh D antigen. In: Cash, JD, ed. *Progress in Transfusion Medicine*, Vol. 3. Edinburgh: Churchill Livingstone, 1988: 175–97.

578 McCann MC, James K, Kumpel BM. Production and use of human monoclonal anti-D antibodies. *J Immunol Methods* 1988;**115**:3–15.

579 Scott ML. Monoclonal anti-D for immunoprophylaxis. *Vox Sang* 2001;**81**:213–8.

580 Lambin P, Rouger P, Goossens D *et al*. Idiotypic specificity of a human monoclonal anti-Rhesus(D) antibody. *Ann Inst Pasteur/Immunol* 1986;**137D**:383–90.

581 Walker RY, Andrew S, Kumpel BM, Austin EB. Murine monoclonal antibodies reactive with a human monoclonal anti-RhD antibody (BRAD-5). *Transfus Med* 2000;**10**:225–31.

582 Thorpe SJ, Boult CE, Stevenson FK *et al*. Cold agglutinin activity is common among human monoclonal IgM Rh system antibodies using the V_{4-34} heavy chain variable segment. *Transfusion* 1997;**37**:1111–16.

583 Thorpe SJ, Turner CE, Stevenson FK *et al*. Human monoclonal antibodies encoded by the V4–34 gene segment show cold agglutinin activity and variable multireactivity which correlates with the predicted charge of the heavy-chain variable region. *Immunology* 1998;**93**:129–36.

584 Thorpe SJ, Boult CE, Bailey SW, Thompson KM. The basis of unexpected cross-reactions shown by human monoclonal antibodies against blood group antigens as revealed by immunohistochemistry. *Appl Immunohistochem* 1996;**4**:190–200.

585 Williams M. Monoclonal reagents for Rhesus-D typing of Irish patients and donors: a review. *Br J Biomed Sci* 2000;**57**:142–9.

586 Hoogenboom HR, Marks JD, Griffiths AD, Winter G. Building antibodies from genes. *Immunol Rev* 1992;**130**:41–68.

587 Marks JD, Ouwehand WH, Bye JM *et al*. Human antibody fragments specific for human blood group antigens from a phage display library. *Bio/Technology* 1993;**11**:1145–9.

588 Hughes-Jones NC, Gorick BD, Bye JM *et al*. Characterization of human blood group scFv antibodies derived from a V gene phage-display library. *Br J Haematol* 1994;**88**:180–6.

589 Dziegiel M, Nielsen LK, Andersen PS *et al*. Phage display used for gene cloning of human recombinant antibody against the erythrocyte surface antigen, rhesus D. *J Immunol Methods* 1995;**182**:7–19.

590 Edelman L, Margaritte C, Chaabihi H *et al*. Obtaining a functional recombinant anti-rhesus (D) antibody using the baculovirus-insect cells expression system. *Immunology* 1997;**91**:13–19.

591 Miescher S, Zahn-Zabal M, De Jesus M *et al*. CHO expression of a novel human recombinant IgG1 anti-RhD antibody isolated by phage display. *Br J Haematol* 2000;**111**:157–66.

592 Bye JM, Carter C, Cui Y *et al*. Germline variable region gene segment derivation of human monoclonal anti-Rh (D) antibodies. Evidence for affinity maturation by somatic hupermutation and repertoire shift. *J Clin Invest* 1992;**90**:2481–90.

593 Boucher G, Broly H, Lemieux R. Restricted use of cationic germline V_H gene segments in human Rh(D) red cell antibodies. *Blood* 1997;**89**:3277–86.

594 Hughes-Jones NC, Bye JM, Gorick BD, Marks JD. Synthesis of Rh Fv phage-antibodies using VH and VL germline genes. *Br J Haematol* 1999;**105**:811–16.

595 Perera WS, Moss MT, Urbaniak SJ. V(D)J germline gene repertoire analysis of monoclonal D antibodies and the implication for D epitope specificity. *Transfusion* 2000;**40**:846–55.

596 Tovey LAD. Towards the conquest of Rh haemolytic disease: Britain's contribution and the role of serendipity. *Transfus Med* 1992;**2**:99–109.

597 Kumpel BM, Elson CJ. Mechanism of anti-D-mediated immune suppression: a paradox awaiting resolution? *Trend Immunol* 2001;**22**:26–31.

598 Urbaniak SJ, Greiss MA. RhD haemolytic disease of the fetus and the newborn. *Blood Rev* 2000;**14**:44–61.

599 Royal College of Physicians of Edinburgh and Royal College of Obstetricians and Gynaecologists. Statement from the Consensus Conference on Anti-D Prophylaxis. *Vox Sang* 1998;**74**:127–8 and *Transfusion* 1998;**38**:97–9.

600 Lee D, Contreras M, Robson SC, Rodeck CH, Whittle MJ. Recommendations for the use of anti-D immunoglobulin for Rh prophylaxis. *Transfus Med* 1999;**9**:93–7.

601 Bowman JM. The prevention of Rh immunization. *Transfus Med Rev* 1988;**2**:129–50.

602 Hadley AG. In vitro assays to predict the severity of hemolytic disease of the newborn. *Transfus Med Rev* 1995;**9**:302–13.

603 Report from nine collaborating laboratories. Results of tests with different cellular bioassays in relation to severity of RhD haemolytic disease. *Vox Sang* 1991;**60**:225–9.

604 Garner SF, Gorick BD, Lai WYY *et al*. Prediction of the severity of haemolytic disease of the newborn: quantitative IgG anti-D subclass determinations explain the correlation with functional assay results. *Vox Sang* 1995;**68**:169–76.

605 Thomson A, Contreras M, Gorick B *et al*. Clearance of Rh D-positive red cells with monoclonal anti-D. *Lancet* 1990;**336**:1147–9.

606 Kumpel B, Goodrick J, Pamphilon DH *et al*. Human Rh D monoclonal antibodies (BRAD-3 and BRAD) cause accelerated clearance of Rh D⁺ red blood cells and sup-

pression of Rh D immunization in Rh D⁻ volunteers. *Blood* 1995;**86**:1701–9.

607 Smith NA, Ala FA, Lee D *et al.* A multi-centre trial of monoclonal anti-D in the prevention of Rh-immunisation of RhD– male volunteers by RhD+ red cells [Abstract]. *Transfus Med* 2000;**10**(Suppl.1):8.

608 Stott L-M, Barker RN, Urbaniak SJ. Identification of alloreactive T-cell epiotpes on the Rhesus D protein. *Blood* 2000;**96**:4011–19.

609 Dooren MC, Kuijpers RWAM, Joekes EC *et al.* Protection against immune haemolytic disease of newborn infants by maternal monocyte-reactive IgG alloantibodies (anti-HLA-DR). *Lancet* 1992;**339**:1067–70.

610 Shepard SL, Noble AL, Filbey D, Hadley AG. Inhibition of the monocyte chemiluminescent response to anti-D-sensitized red cells by FcγRI-blocking antibodies which ameliorate the severity of haemolytic disease of the newborn. *Vox Sang* 1996;**70**:157–63.

611 Astrup J, Kornstad L. Presence of anti-c in the serum of 42 women giving birth to c positive babies: serological and clinical findings. *Acta Obstet Gynecol Scand* 1977;**56**:185–8.

612 Hardy J, Napier JAF. Red cell antibodies detected in antenatal tests on Rhesus positive women in south and mid Wales, 1948–78. *Br J Obstet Gynaecol* 1981;**88**:91–100.

613 Kozlowski CL, Lee D, Shwe KH, Love EM. Quantitation of anti-c in haemolytic disease of the newborn. *Transfus Med* 1995;**5**:37–42.

614 Harrison CR, Hayes TC, Trow LL, Benedetto AR. Intravascular hemolytic transfusion reaction without detectable antibodies: a case report and review of the literature. *Vox Sang* 1986;**51**:96–101.

615 Foung SKH, Blunt J, Perkins S, Winn L, Grumet FC. A human monoclonal antibody to rh^G. *Vox Sang* 1986;**50**:160–3.

616 Thompson K, Barden G, Sutherland J, Beldon I, Melamed M. Human monoclonal antibodies to C, c, E, e and G antigens of the Rh system. *Immunology* 1990;**71**:323–7.

617 Mannessier L, Horbez C, Broly H. Caractérisation et validation d'un anticorps monoclonal humain anti-C. *Rev Franc Transfus Hémobiol* 1991;**34**:403–8.

618 Issitt PD, Combs MR, Bredehoeft SJ *et al.* Lack of clinical significance of 'enzyme-only' red cell alloantibodies. *Transfusion* 1993;**33**:284–93.

619 Devenish A, Kay LA. Hemolytic transfusion reactions due to anti-e+f detectable only by nonstandard serologic techniques. *Immunohematology* 1994;**10**:120–3.

620 Jemmolo G, Malferrari F, Tazzari PL, Conte R. Critical review of protease-treated red cell tests for the detection of irregular blood group antibodies during pregnancy. *Vox Sang* 1995;**69**:144.

621 Hundric-Haspl Z, Jurakovic-Loncar N, Grgicevic D. Enzyme-only blood group alloantibodies in pregnancy. *Transfusion* 1998;**38**:318.

622 Judd WJ, Davenport RD, Suchi M. An'enzyme-only' IgG C3-binding alloanti-C causing an acute hemolytic trnasfusion reaction [Abstract]. *Transfusion* 2000; **40**(Suppl.):119S.

623 Garner SF, Devenish A, Barber H, Contreras M. The importance of monitoring 'enzyme-only' red cell antibodies during pregnancy. *Vox Sang* 1991;**61**:219–20.

624 Garratty G. Target antigens for red-cell-bound autoantibodies. In: SJ Nance, ed. *Clinical and Basic Science Aspects of Immunohematology.* Arlington: American Association of Blood Banks, 1991: 33–72.

625 Garratty G. Specificity of autoantibodies reacting optimally at 37°C. *Immunohematology* 1999;**15**:24–40.

626 Weiner W, Battey DA, Cleghorn TE, Marson FGW, Meynell MJ. Serological findings in a case of haemolytic anaemia with some general observations on the pathogenesis of this syndrome. *Br Med J* 1953;**ii**:125–8.

627 Bell CA, Zwicker H, Sacks HJ. Autoimmune hemolytic anemia: routine serologic evaluation in a general hospital population. *Am J Clin Pathol* 1973;**60**:903–11.

628 Issitt PD, Pavone BG, Goldfinger D *et al.* Anti-Wr^b, and other autoantibodies responsible for positive direct antiglobulin tests in 150 individuals. *Br J Haematol* 1976;**34**:5–18.

629 Issitt PD, Zellner DC, Rolih SD, Duckett JB. Autoantibodies mimicking alloantibodies. *Transfusion* 1977;**17**:531–8.

630 Longster GH, Johnson E. IgM anti-D as auto-antibody in a case of 'cold' auto-immune haemolytic anaemia. *Vox Sang* 1988;**54**:174–6.

631 Weiner W, Vos GH. Serology of acquired hemolytic anemias. *Blood* 1963;**22**:606–13.

632 van't Veer MB, van Wieringen PMV, van Leeuwen I *et al.* A negative direct antiglobulin test with strong IgG red cell autoantibodies present in the serum of a patient with autoimmune haemolytic anaemia. *Br J Haematol* 1981;**49**:383–6.

633 Issitt PD, Gruppo RA, Wilkinson SL, Issitt CH. A typical presentation of acute pahse, antibody-induced haemolytic anaemia in an infant. *Br J Haematol* 1982;**52**:537–43.

634 Anderson LD, Race GJ, Owen M. Presence of anti-D antibody in an Rh(D) -positive person. *Am J Clin Pathol* 1958;**30**:228–9.

635 Chown B, Kaita H, Lewis M, Roy RB, Wyatt L. A 'D-positive' man who produced anti-D. *Vox Sang* 1963;**8**:420–9.

636 Krikler SH, Ferguson DJ, Akabutu JJ, Lomas CG. Transient anti-D in an Rh-positive patient with congenital dyserythropoietic anemia type II. *Transfusion* 1984;**24**:169–70.

637 Lalezari P, Talleyrand NP, Wenz B, Schoenfeld ME, Tippett P. Development of direct antiglobulin reaction accompanying alloimmunization in a patient with Rh^d (D, Category III) phenotype. *Vox Sang* 1975;**28**:19–24.

638 Macpherson CR, Stevenson TD, Gayton J. Anti-D in a D-positive man, with positive direct Coombs test and normal red cell survival. *Am J Clin Pathol* 1966;45:748–50.

639 Church A, Storry J, Jefferies LC. Uncommon presentation of auto anti-D in a D mosaic individual [Abstract]. *Transfusion* 1991;31(Suppl.):28S.

640 Ramsey G, Israel L, Lindsay GD, Mayer TK, Nusbacher J. Anti-Rho (D) in two Rh-positive patients receiving kidney grafts from an Rh-immunized donor. *Transplantation* 1986;41:67–9.

641 Swanson J, Sebring E, Sastamoinen R, Chopek M. Gm allotyping to determine the origin of the anti-D causing hemolytic anemia in a kidney transplant recipient. *Vox Sang* 1987;52:228–30.

642 Ramsey G. Red cell antibodies arising from solid organ transplants. *Transfusion* 1991;31:76–86.

643 Ramsey G, Kiss JE, Sacher RA, Fernandez C, Starzl TE. Rh antibodies in two patients receiving liver and kidney-pancreas grafts from the same Rh-sensitized donor [Abstract]. *Joint Congr Int Soc Blood Transfus and Am Assoc Blood Banks* 1990: 198.

644 Kim BK, Whitsett CF, Hillyer CD. Donor origin Rh antibodies as a cause of significant hemolysis following ABO-identical orthotopic liver transplantation. *Immunohematology* 1992;8:100–1.

645 Lee J-H, Mintz PD. Graft versus host anti-Rho (D) following minor Rh-incompatible orthotopic liver transplantation. *Am J Hematol* 1993;44:168–71.

646 Knoop C, Andrien M, Antoine M et al. Severe hemolysis due to a donor anti-D antibody after heart–lung transplantation: association with lung and blood chimerism. *Am Rev Respir Dis* 1993;148:504–6.

647 Larrea L, de la Rubia J, Arriaga F, Sanchez J, Marty ML. Severe hemolytic anemia due to anti-E after renal transplantation. *Transplantation* 1997;64:550–1.

648 Lasky LC, Warkentin PI, Kersey JH et al. Hemotherapy in patients undergoing blood group incompatible bone marrow transplantation. *Transfusion* 1983;23:277–85.

649 Hows J, Beddow K, Gordon-Smith E et al. Donor-derived red blood cell antibodies and immune hemolysis after allogeneic bone marrow transplantation. *Blood* 1986;67:177–81.

650 Gandini G, Franchini M, de Gironcoli M et al. Detection of an anti-RhD antibody 2 years after sensitization in a patient who had undergone an allogeneic BMT. *Bone Marrow Transplant* 2000;25:457–9.

651 Heim MU, Schleuning M, Eckstein R et al. Rh antibodies against the pretransplant red cells following Rh-incompatible bone marrow transplantation. *Transfusion* 1988;28:272–5.

652 Anstee DJ, Edwards PAW. Monoclonal antibodies to human erythrocytes. *Eur J Immunol* 1982;12:228–32.

653 Bourel D, Lecointre M, Genetet N, Gueguen-Duchesne M, Genetet B. Murine monoclonal antibody suitable for use as an Rh reagent, anti-e. *Vox Sang* 1987;52:85–8.

654 Fraser RH, Inglis G, Allan JC et al. Murine monoclonal antibody with e-like specificity: suitability for screening for e-negative cells. *Transfusion* 1990;30:226–9.

655 Sonneborn H-H, Ernst M, Tills D et al. Comparison of the reactions of the Rh-related murine monoclonal antibodies BS58 and R6A. *Vox Sang* 1990;58:219–23.

656 Tovey GH, Lockyer JW, Tierney RBH. Changes in Rh grouping reactions in a case of leukaemia. *Vox Sang* 1961;6:628–31.

657 Levan A, Nichols WW, Hall B et al. Mixture of Rh positive and Rh negative erythrocytes and chromosomal abnormalities in a case of polycythemia. *Hereditas* 1964;52:89–105.

658 Mannoni P, Bracq C, Yvart J, Salmon C. Anomalie de fonctionnement du locus Rh au cours d'une myélofibrose. *Nouv Rev Franc Hémat* 1970;10:381–8.

659 Callender ST, Kay HEM, Lawler SD et al. Two populations of Rh groups together with chromosmally abnormal cell lines in the bone marrow. *Br Med J* 1971;i:131–3.

660 Habibi B, Lopez M, Salmon C. Two new cases of Rh mosaicism: selective study of red cell populations. *Vox Sang* 1974;27:232–42.

661 Bracey AW, McGinniss MH, Levine RM, Whang-Peng J. Rh mosaicism and aberrant MNSs antigen expression in a patient with chronic myelogenous leukemia. *Am J Clin Pathol* 1983;79:397–401.

662 Marsh WL, Chaganti RSK, Gardner FH et al. Mapping human autosomes. evidence supporting assignment of Rhesus to the short arm of chromosome 1. *Science* 1974;183:966–8.

663 Cooper B, Tishler PV, Atkins L, Breg WR. Loss of Rh antigen associated with acquired Rh antibodies and a chromosome translocation in a patient with myeloid metaplasia. *Blood* 1979;54:642–7.

664 Mohandas K, Najfield V, Gilbert H, Azar P, Skerrett D. Loss and reappearance of Rh_o (D) antigen in an individual with acute myelogenous leukemia. *Immunohematology* 1994;10:134–5.

665 Chérif-Zahar B, Bony V, Steffensen R et al. Shift from Rh-positive to Rh-negative phenotype caused by a somatic mutation within the *RHD* gene in a patient with chronic myelocytic leukaemia. *Br J Haematol* 1998;102:1263–70.

666 Vogt E. Norsk forening for medisinsk blodtypeserologi. *Nordisk Med* 1964;71:510.

667 Muller A, Seger J, Garretta M et al. Mosaïcisme Rh par mutation dans une gémellité monozygote. *Rev Franc Transfus Immuno-Hémat* 1978;21:151–63.

668 Salaru NNR, Lay WH. Rh blood group mosaicism in a healthy elderly woman. *Vox Sang* 1985;48:362–5.

669 Jenkins WJ, Marsh WL. Somatic mutation affecting the Rhesus and Duffy blood group systems. *Transfusion* 1965;5:6–10.

670 Northoff H, Goldmann SF, Lattke H, Steinbach P. A patient, mosaic for Rh and Fy antigens lacking other signs

of chimerism or chromosomal disorder. *Vox Sang* 1984;**47**:164–9.

671 Marsh WL, Chaganti RSK. Blood group mosaicism involving the Rhesus and Duffy blood groups. *Transfusion* 1973;**13**:314–5.

672 Gemke RJBJ, Kanhai HHH, Overbeeke MAM *et al.* ABO and Rhesus phenotyping of fetal erythrocytes in the first trimester of pregnancy. *Br J Haematol* 1986;**64**:689–97.

673 Garritsen HSP, Benachi A, Surbek D *et al.* Rhesus D antigen expression during fetal development [Abstract]. *Infusionsther Transfusionmed* 1997:**24**:190–3.

674 Benachi A, Garritsen HSP, Howard CM, Bennett P, Fisk NM. Absence of expression of RhD by human trophoblast cells. *Am J Obstet Gynecol* 1998;**178**:294–9.

675 Green CA, Daniels GL. The development of Rh antigens on erythroid precursor cells [Abstract]. *Transfusion* 1998;**38**(Suppl.):62S.

676 Rearden A, Masouredis SP. Blood group D antigen content of nucleated red cell precursors. *Blood* 1977;**50**:981–6.

677 Dunstan RA, Simpson MB, Rosse WF. Erythrocyte antigens on human platelets. Absence of Rh, Duffy, Kell, Kidd, and Lutheran antigens. *Transfusion* 1984:**24**:243–6.

678 Dunstan RA. Status of major red cell blood group antigens on neutrophils, lymphocytes and monocytes. *Br J Haematol* 1986;**62**:301–9.

679 Marini A-M, Vissers S, Urrestarazu A, André B. Cloning and expression of the *MEP1* gene encoding an ammonium transporter in *Saccharomyces cerevisae*. *EMBO J* 1994;**13**:3456–63.

680 Ninnemann O, Jauniaux J-C, Frommer WB. Identification of a high affinity NH_4^+ transporter from plants. *EMBO J* 1994;**13**:3864–471.

681 Thomas GH, Mullins JG, Merrick M. Membrane topology of the Mep/Amt family of ammonium transporters. *Mol Microbiol* 2000;**37**:331–44.

682 Marini A-M, Urrestarazu A, Beauwens R, André B. The Rh (Rhesus) blood group polypeptides are related to NH_4^+ transporters. *Trends Biochem Sci* 1997;**22**:460–1.

683 Heitman J, Agre P. A new face of the Rhesus antigen. *Nature Genet* 2000;**26**:258–9.

684 Schroit AJ, Bloy C, Connor J, Cartron J-P. Involvement of Rh blood group polypeptides in the maintenance of aminophospholipid asymmetry. *Biochemistry* 1990;**29**:10303–6.

685 Zachowski A. Phospholipids in animal eukaryotic membranes. transverse asymmetry and movement. *Biochem J* 1993;**294**:1–14.

686 Smith RE, Daleke DL. Phosphatidylserine transport in Rh_{null} erythrocytes. *Blood* 1990;**76**:1021–7.

687 Geldwerth D, Chérif-Zahar B, Helley D *et al.* Phosphatidylserine exposure and aminophospholipid

688 Kitano T, Sumiyama K, Shiroishi T, Saitou N. Conserved evolution of the Rh50 gene compared to its homologous Rh blood group gene. *Biochem Biophys Res Commun* 1998; **249**:78–85.

689 Matassi G, Chérif-Zahar B, Pesole G, Raynal V, Cartron JP. The members of the *RH* gene family (*RH50* and *RH30*) followed different evolutionary pathways. *J Mol Evol* 1999;**48**:151–9.

690 Kitano Y, Saitou N. Evolutionary history of the *Rh* blood group-related genes in vertebrates. *Immunogenetics* 2000;**51**:856–62.

691 Westhoff CM, Wylie DE. Investigation of the human Rh blood group system in nonhuman primates and other species with serologic and Southern blot analysis. *J Mol Evol* 1994;**39**:87–92.

692 Saboori AM, Denker BM, Agre P. Isolation of proteins related to the Rh polypeptides from nonhuman erythrocytes. *J Clin Invest* 1989;**83**:187–91.

693 Mouro I, Le Van Kim C, Cherif-Zahar B *et al.* Molecular characterization of the Rh-like locus and gene transcripts from the Rhesus monkey (*Macaca mulatta*). *J Mol Evol* 1994;**38**:169–76.

694 Blancher A, Reid ME, Socha WW. Cross-reactivity of antibodies to human and primate red cell antigens. *Transfus Med Rev* 2000;**14**:161–79.

695 Carritt B, Kemp TJ, Poulter M. Evolution of the human *RH* (rhesus) blood group genes: a 50 year old prediction (partially) fulfilled. *Hum Molec Genet* 1997;**6**:843–50.

696 Blancher A, Socher WW. The Rhesus system. In: A Blancher, J Klein, WW Socha, eds. *Molecular Biology and Evolution of Blood Group and MHC Antigens in Primates*. Berlin: Springer, 1997: 147–218.

697 Fisher RA, Race RR. Rh gene frequencies in Britain. *Nature* 1946;**157**:48–9.

698 Rosenfield RE, Haber GV, Schroeder R, Ballard R. Problems in Rh typing as revealed by a single Negro family. *Am J Hum Genet* 1960;**12**:147–59.

699 Le Pennec PY, Rouger P, Klein MT *et al.* A serologic study of red cells and sera from 18 Rh: 32, –46 ($\bar{R}^N/\bar{R}^N$) persons. *Transfusion* 1989;**29**:798–802.

700 Delehanty CL, Wilkinson SL, Issitt PD *et al.* Riv: a new low incidence Rh antigen [Abstract]. *Transfusion* 1983;**23**:410.

701 Contreras M, Stebbing B, Blessing M, Gavin J. The Rh antigen Evans. *Vox Sang* 1978;**34**:208–11.

702 Lomas C, Poole J, Salaru N *et al.* A low-incidence red cell antigen JAL associated with two unusual Rh gene complexes. *Vox Sang* 1990;**59**:39–43.

703 Chérif-Zahar B, Matassi G, Raynal V *et al.* Molecular defects of the *RHCE* gene in the Rh-deficient individuals of the amorph type. *Blood* 1998;**92**:639–46.

704 Chérif-Zahar B, Matassi G, Raynal V, *et al.* Rh-deficiency of the regulator type caused by splicing mutations in the human *RH50* gene. *Blood* 1998;**92**:2535–40.

6 Lutheran blood group system

6.1 Introduction

The Lutheran system consists of 18 antigens: LU1–LU20 in the numerical notation, with two declared obsolete (Table 6.1). Four pairs of these antigens have allelic relationships: Lu^a (LU1) and Lu^b (LU2); Lu6 and Lu9; Lu8 and Lu14; and Au^a (LU18) and Au^b (LU19). Red cells of a null phenotype, Lu_null or Lu(a–b–), lack all Lutheran system antigens, as determined by agglutination techniques. Lu_null may arise from any of three genetic backgrounds: homozygosity for an autosomal-recessive amorph gene; heterozygosity for a dominant suppressor gene; or hemizygosity for a recessive X-linked suppressor gene. Only the autosomal-recessive type of Lu_null is a true null phenotype, as weak Lutheran antigens may be detected by adsorption and elution techniques on Lu_null red cells of the other two types, but all three types are referred to as Lu_null here. The high frequency antigen Lu3 is present on all red cells save those of the Lu_null phenotype. Nine other antigens, all of very high frequency, are absent (or expressed very weakly) on Lu_null cells, but have not been shown to be controlled by the *LU* locus.

Lutheran antigens are located on two red cell membrane glycoproteins (CD239) of apparent M_r 78 000 and 85 000, which belong to the immunoglobulin superfamily of receptors and adhesion molecules. The Lutheran glycoproteins are ligands for the extracellular matrix glycoprotein, laminin.

The Lutheran locus is situated on chromosome 19 and is part of a linkage group that includes the loci for Secretor, Lewis, H, and LW (Chapter 32).

6.2 The Lutheran glycoproteins and the gene that encodes them

6.2.1 The Lutheran glycoproteins (Lu-glycoproteins)

Components of apparent M_r 85 000 and 78 000 were revealed by immunoblotting of red cell membranes with monoclonal anti-Lu^b or with alloanti-Lu^a, -Lu^b, -Lu3, -Lu4, -Lu6, -Lu8, -Lu12, -Au^a, or -Au^b [1–3]. There was a small reduction in the apparent M_r of these structures following sialidase treatment of the red cells [2]. The two components were not apparent when Lu_null red cells were used and were not present in cytoskeleton preparations. No bands were seen when membranes were prepared under reducing conditions, suggesting the importance of intact disulphide bonds in antigen integrity. Immunoblots from membranes of red cells treated with endoglycosidase-F did not show the 85 000 and 78 000 components, but two new faint bands of M_r 73 000 and 66 000 became apparent, interpreted as representing the loss of one or more N-linked oligosaccharide chains [1].

Parsons *et al.* [4] purified the Lu-glycoproteins by immunoaffinity chromatography with a monoclonal antibody, BRIC 221. From the amino acid sequence obtained, they designed redundant oligonucleotide primers and used the product of a PCR to isolate a cDNA clone of 2417 bp from a human placental cDNA library. The predicted mature protein consists of 597 amino acids: 518 comprising an extracellular domain, 19 a single transmembrane domain, and 59 a cytoplasmic domain. This structure represents the M_r 85 000 isoform. The cytoplasmic tail may be directly attached to the membrane skeleton [5]. Immunoprecipitation experiments with a rabbit antiserum prepared to an amino acid sequence of the cytoplasmic domain

Table 6.1 Lutheran system antigens.

No.	Name	Frequency	Allelic antigen	Lu-glycoprotein IgSF domain	Molecular basis*
LU1	Lu^a	Polymorphic	Lu^b	1	His77 (Arg)
LU2	Lu^b	High	Lu^a	1	Arg77 (His)
LU3	Lu3	High			
LU4	Lu4	High		2	
LU5	Lu5	High		1	Arg109 (His)
LU6	Lu6	High	Lu9	3	Ser275 (Pho)
LU7	Lu7	High		4	
LU8	Lu8	High	Lu14	2	Met204 (Lys)
LU9	Lu9	Low	Lu6	3	Phe275 (Ser)
LU11	Lu11	High			
LU12	Lu12	High		1 or 2	
LU13	Lu13	High		5	Ser447 (Leu)
LU14	Lu14	Low	Lu8	2	Lys204 (Met)
LU16	Lu16	High			
LU17	Lu17	High			
LU18	Au^a	Polymorphic	Au^b	5	Thr539 (Ala)
LU19	Au^b	Polymorphic	Au^a	5	Ala539 (Thr)
LU20	Lu20	High		3	Thr302 (Met)

*[10,11,V. Crew and G. Daniels, unpublished observations]. Shown in parentheses are the amino acids associated with an antigen-negative phenotype.
Obsolete: LU10, previously Singleton; LU15, AnWj (now 901009).

showed that the M_r 78 000 structure lacks part of the cytoplasmic domain [4] (Fig. 6.1). A cDNA clone encoding an epithelial cancer antigen (B-CAM) [6] was subsequently shown to represent the M_r 78 000 isoform, with a 19 amino acid cytoplasmic tail [7].

6.2.2 The Lu-glycoproteins belong to the immunoglobulin superfamily (IgSF)

The immunoglobulin superfamily (IgSF) is a large collection of glycoproteins, abundant on leucocytes, but also present on other cells, which contain repeating extracellular domains with sequence homology to immunoglobulin variable (V) or constant (C1 or C2) domains. Each IgSF domain consists of approximately 100 amino acids and is structured into two β-sheets stabilized by a conserved disulphide bond. IgSF glycoproteins mostly function as receptors and adhesion molecules, and may be involved in signal transduction [8,9].

The extracellular domain of the Lu-glycoproteins is organized into two V and three C2 IgSF domains [4,6] (Fig. 6.1). There are five potential N-glycosylation sites, one in the third domain and the other four in the

fourth domain. At least four other IgSF glycoproteins are present in the red cell surface membrane: LW glycoprotein (Chapter 16), CD147 (Ok-glycoprotein; Chapter 22), CD47 (Chapter 5), and CD58 (LFA-3). For discussion on functional aspects of the Lu-glycoproteins see Section 6.7.

Parsons *et al.* [10] constructed a series of *LU* cDNA deletion mutants, each encoding Lu-glycoprotein lacking one, two, three, or four of the IgSF domains. K562 erythroleukaemia cell cultures expressing one of the deletion mutant constructs or the whole *LU* cDNA were analysed by flow cytometry with a variety of antibodies to Lutheran-system antigens, in order to determine the location of those antigens on the Lu-glycoproteins. The deduced locations are shown in Fig. 6.1.

6.2.3 Organization of the *LU* gene

The *LU* gene is 12.5 kb organized into 15 exons (Fig. 6.1, Table 6.2). Exon 1 encodes the signal peptide; exons 2–12 the five IgSF domains (two exons per domain except domain 2, which is encoded by exons 4–6); exon 13 the transmembrane domain and the

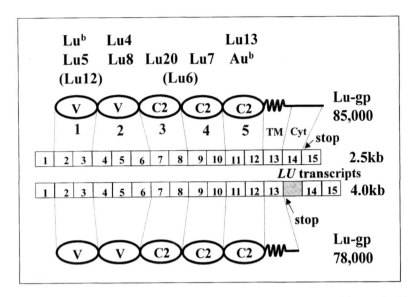

Fig. 6.1 Diagrammatic representation of the 15 exons of the 2.5 and 4.0 kb *LU* transcripts and the unspliced intron 13 (shaded box) in the 4.0 kb transcript [10,11]. The two isoforms of the Lu-glycoprotein (Lu-gp), the products of the two transcripts, are shown. Translation stop codons are present near the 5′ end of exon 15 of the 2.5 kb transcript and at the 5′ end of the unspliced intron 13 of the 4.0 kb transcript, explaining the longer cytoplasmic domain in the product of the 2.5 kb transcript [11]. Location of the Lutheran-system antigens on the IgSF domains (V and C2) of the Lu-glycoproteins is also shown. The precise location of Lu12 and Lu6 was not conclusive [10]. TM, transmembrane domain.

Table 6.2 Exon/intron organization of *LU* [10,11].

Exon	Domain encoded	Exon size (bp)	Intron size (kb)
1	5′ UT + leader	105	2.0
2	1 IgSF (V)	122	0.7
3	1 IgSF (V)	229	0.09
4	2 IgSF (V)	71	0.5
5	2 IgSF (V)	95	0.09
6	2 IgSF (V)	185	0.53
7	3 IgSF (C2)	137	0.31
8	3 IgSF (C2)	157	3.5
9	4 IgSF (C2)	116	0.1
10	4 IgSF (C2)	142	0.17
11	5 IgSF (C2)	137	0.15
12	5 IgSF (C2)	145	0.09
13	TM + 19 residues cyt	145	0.97
14	cyt (85 000 isoform)	118	0.09
15	1 residue cyt (85 000 isoform)	498	

TM, transmembrane; cyt, cytoplasmic.

cytoplasmic domain common to both isoforms; exons 14 and 15 the C-terminal 40 amino acids of the larger isoform [10,11]. Two *LU* transcripts have been isolated, one of 2.5 kb encoding the larger Lu-glycoprotein isoform (85 000) and one of 4.0 kb encoding the smaller (B-CAM, 78 000) isoform [7]. The two transcripts differ as a result of alternative splicing of intron 13. In the 2.5 kb transcript intron 13 has been removed by splicing and exons 14 and 15 encode the C-terminal 40 amino acids of the larger isoform. In the 4.0 kb transcript intron 13 remains, explaining the larger size of the transcript. The 5′ end of the intron contains a UGA translation-stop codon, so the unspliced intron 13 and exons 14 and 15 are not translated and the protein product has a cytoplasmic domain consisting only of the 19 amino acids encoded by exon 13 [11] (Fig. 6.1).

The 5′ flanking region of *LU* does not contain TATA or CAAT boxes, but showed an organization typical of ubiquitous genes with several potential binding sites for the SP1 transcription factor. The region between –673 and –764 upstream of the coding region contains binding sequences for GATA and CACCC or SP1 transcription factors [11].

6.3 Lu^a and Lu^b (LU1 and LU2)

The first Lutheran antibody, anti-Lu^a, was described in 1945 by Callender et al. [12] and in more detail the following year by Callender and Race [13]. Ten years later the antithetical antibody, anti-Lu^b, was described by Cutbush and Chanarin [14].

6.3.1 Frequencies of Lu^a and Lu^b

The early estimates of Lu^a frequency were based on studies performed before the discovery of anti-Lu^b. Estimates of the gene, genotype, and phenotype frequencies derived from the first three reports of tests on unrelated English people [13,15,16] are shown in Table 6.3; of 1373 samples, 7.65% were Lu(a+).

Other studies from around the world are listed by Mourant et al. [17]. Lu^a is widely distributed amongst Europeans, Africans, and North Americans with a frequency of around 8%, but is very rare or absent from all other indigenous populations studied [17].

Of 1456 Manitoban white people tested with anti-Lu^a and -Lu^b, 93.06% were Lu(a–b+), 6.80% Lu(a+b+), and 0.14% Lu(a+b–) [18,19]. These data fit well with those predicted from the gene frequencies in Table 6.3. Similar results were obtained from tests on 1201 white Bostonians [20]. Of 922 Chinese in Taiwan tested with anti-Lu^a and -Lu^b, all were Lu(a–b+) [21].

In two large surveys, in which donor red cells were screened with anti-Lu^b and all negatives tested with anti-Lu^a, the following results were obtained: South of England, approximately 250 000 tested, 230 Lu(a+b–), 72 Lu(a–b–) [22]; South Wales, 75 614 tested, 39 Lu(a+b–), 15 Lu(a–b–) [23]. Therefore, in a predominantly European population, roughly one in 1000 is Lu(b–); approximately two-thirds of these being Lu(a+b–) and one-third Lu(a–b–) (see Section 6.4).

6.3.2 Inheritance of Lu^a and Lu^b

Numerous family studies have demonstrated that Lu^a and Lu^b are inherited as codominant allelic characters [18,24,25]. In a substantial series of Canadian families tested with anti-Lu^a and -Lu^b [18], the observed numbers of different mating types and their offspring fit perfectly with the expected figures calculated from the frequency data on Manitobans [18,19], supporting straightforward inheritance of Lu^a and Lu^b.

6.3.3 Molecular basis for Lu^a and Lu^b

The Lu^a/Lu^b polymorphism results from a single base change in exon 3 of LU, encoding an amino acid substitution in the first IgSF domain of the Lu-glycoproteins: Lu^a A252, His77; Lu^b G252, Arg77 [10,11]. The importance of this amino acid substitution in Lu^a/Lu^b expression was confirmed by in vitro site-directed mutation experiments [11]. The nucleotide change is associated with an AciI restriction-site polymorphism [11].

6.3.4 Variation in antigenic strength

The Lutheran antigens are very variable in strength. Lu(a+) cells from different families may vary quantitatively in the amount of antigen they carry, but the antigenic strength remains roughly constant within the family [24]. The strength of the Lutheran antigens often shows zygosity dosage [14,26–29]. Occasionally adsorption and elution tests are required to detect weak Lu^b on Lu(a+b+) cells.

Heterogeneity of Lutheran antigen strength between individual red cells within a person can also be detected. This accounts for the mixed field agglutination patterns (characteristic clumps of agglutinated cells in the presence of many free cells) usually seen with Lutheran antisera, especially anti-Lu^a [13,14], and the wide range of survival times of Lu(b+) cells introduced into an Lu(a+b–) person with anti-Lu^b [57].

The abundance of Lu^b antigens on red cells, as determined by Scatchard analysis with purified monoclonal

Table 6.3 Gene, genotype, and phenotype frequencies calculated from results of tests with anti-Lu^a on red cells of 1373 English people [13,15,16].

Gene frequency	Genotype frequency	Phenotype frequency
Lu^a 0.0390	Lu^a/Lu^a 0.0015 ⎫	
	Lu^a/Lu^b 0.0765 ⎬	Lu(a+) 0.0750
Lu^b 0.9610		
	Lu^b/Lu^b 0.9235	Lu(a–) 0.9235

anti-Lu^b (BRIC 108), is relatively low and shows wide variation, confirming many previous serological studies [30]. The number of Lu^b sites was estimated at 1640–4070 on Lu(a–b+) cells and 850–1820 on Lu(a+b+) cells [30].

6.3.5 Development of Lutheran antigens

Red cells from cord samples and from infants in the first year of life have markedly weakened expression of Lu^a and Lu^b compared with those from adults [28,29,31]. Ten of 155 cord blood samples had the phenotype Lu(a–b–), which is very rare in adults [31]. Adult levels of Lu^a and Lu^b antigenic expression are reached by the age of 15 years [29].

The only extensive study of fetal blood also indicates gradual development of Lutheran antigens [32]. Red cells from four of 82 fetuses reacted with anti-Lu^a compared with those of 18 of 87 of their parents. Lu^a has been detected in a 12-week fetus [24]; Lu^b has been found in two fetuses of 10 weeks, but not in fetuses of 6–9 weeks [32].

6.3.6 Anti-Lu^a and -Lu^b

6.3.6.1 Anti-Lu^a

The first example of anti-Lu^a was found in a multiply transfused patient with lupus erythematosus diffusus, together with anti-c, -C^w, -Kp^c, and -N [13]. The antibody had been stimulated by transfusion of blood from a donor named Lutheran. The titre rapidly declined after transfusion and attempts to regenerate the antibody with small injections of blood failed.

Anti-Lu^a has been reported after pregnancy and/or transfusion [13,26,29,33–35], and often appears together with other antibodies [13], especially red cell reactive HLA antibodies (anti-Bg) [36]. Anti-Lu^a may also be 'naturally occurring' [26,37], and in some cases a 'naturally occurring' antibody may be augmented by transfusion [38,39]. Anti-Lu^a suitable for grouping reagents is uncommon.

Lu^a antibodies are usually IgM, but, like other Lutheran-system antibodies, often have IgG and IgA components [40,41]. Anti-Lu^a often agglutinate Lu(a+) red cells directly, with a thermal optimum well below 37°C. Some also react in an antiglobulin test, and a few, predominantly IgG examples, are reactive only by an antiglobulin test [33,40].

6.3.6.2 Anti-Lu^b

Despite being a relatively rare antibody, many examples of anti-Lu^b have been described [26–29,42–48] since the first report in 1956 [14]. Anti-Lu^b is often found as a single antibody. Anti-Lu^b has been stimulated by transfusion and by pregnancy; 'naturally occurring' examples have not been found.

Anti-Lu^b are often optimally active in the antiglobulin test [26,29,43,44,46,48–50], but directly agglutinating anti-Lu^b have been described [14,27–29], many with a temperature optimum of about 20°C. Most anti-Lu^b are mixtures of IgG and IgM, although IgA may also be present [40,41,45,46]. IgG anti-Lu^b may be predominantly IgG1 [46,50], although IgG2 and IgG4 may be present [48,50,51].

Two monoclonal anti-Lu^b (BRIC 108 and LM342/767.31) have been produced from mice immunized with Lu(b+) red cells [1,52]. The antibodies agglutinated Lu(a–b+) and Lu(a+b+) cells, but not Lu(a+b–) cells or Lu$_{null}$ cells, although adsorption and elution tests demonstrated some binding of BRIC 108 to Lu(a+b–) cells and to Lu$_{null}$ cells of dominant and recessive types [53–55].

6.3.6.3 Clinical significance of anti-Lu^a and -Lu^b

Lutheran antibodies are not clinically important. No case of haemolytic disease of the newborn (HDN) caused by anti-Lu^a or -Lu^b and requiring any treatment other than phototherapy is reported, although raised bilirubin or a positive direct antiglobulin test (DAT) may be detected [28,33,35,43,44,46,47]. Poor development of Lutheran antigens on neonatal red cells (Section 6.3.5) may be the reason for Lutheran antibodies not being implicated in HDN, but there is another possible explanation. Babies of mothers with high-titre IgG1 anti-Lu^b and -Lu6 (Section 6.5.1) had no sign of HDN, their red cells gave negative DATs, and Lutheran antibody could not be detected in their sera [50]. Maternal IgG1 antibodies usually become concentrated in the fetal circulation by active placental transfer. As Lu-glycoprotein is present on placental tissue [4], it is possible that Lutheran antibodies are adsorbed by placental cells, preventing their transfer to the fetus.

Lutheran antibodies have not been implicated in immediate haemolytic transfusion reactions, although they may have been responsible for mild delayed reactions and post-transfusion jaundice [26,40,43,56]. Radiolabelled Lu(a+) red cells injected into a patient with anti-Lu^a survived normally [34]. Similar survival tests in patients with anti-Lu^b showed that at least a proportion of injected Lu(b+) cells could be removed fairly rapidly [45,57,58].

6.4 Lutheran-null phenotypes (Lu$_{null}$)

Like most blood group systems, Lutheran has a null phenotype. This null phenotype, first described by Crawford *et al.* [59] in 1961, is often called Lu(a–b–), but will be referred to as Lu$_{null}$ here. Lu$_{null}$ has at least three genetic backgrounds:

1 homozygosity for a recessive allele at the *LU* locus;
2 heterozygosity for a dominant suppressor gene unlinked to *LU*; and
3 hemizygosity for an X-linked suppressor gene (Table 6.4).

The very rare recessive type is the only true null phenotype as weak expression of Lutheran antigens may be detected on red cells of the other two types.

6.4.1 Frequency of Lu$_{null}$

Several large surveys in England and Wales have shown that the incidence of Lu$_{null}$ varies between 0.005% and 0.032% [22,23,60,61] (Table 6.5). A frequency of 0.027% was found in African Americans from Detroit [62].

The dominant type of Lu$_{null}$ is by far the least rare type. Analysis of the families of 50 Lu$_{null}$ propositi demonstrated that 41 were of the dominant type; the genetical background of the other nine could not be determined, but serological tests suggested that most of these were also of the dominant type [22,23]. Screening red cells from Houston blood donors with monoclonal anti-CD44 gave an incidence for Lu$_{null}$ of 0.02% [63], but screening with anti-AnWj in Portland, Oregon gave a much higher incidence of 0.12% [64]. Both antibodies would reveal Lu$_{null}$ only of the dominant type (Table 6.5).

6.4.2 Lu$_{null}$ of the recessive type and anti-Lu3

Lu$_{null}$ with a recessive mode of inheritance was first

Table 6.4 Three types of Lu$_{null}$.

Mode of inheritance	Gene responsible	Lu system antigens	AnWj	P1, i, CD44, etc.
Recessive	*Lu*	None	+	Normal
Dominant	*In(Lu)*	Extremely weak*	–*	Reduced
X-linked	*XS2*	Extremely weak*	+	Normal†

*Antigens may be detected by adsorption/elution tests.
†i Antigen may be enhanced.

Table 6.5 Frequency of Lu$_{null}$ in several populations.

Population	No. tested	No. of Lu$_{null}$	Incidence of Lu$_{null}$	Antibodies used for screening	References
South London, UK	~250 000	79	~0.0003	Anti-Lu^b (-Lu^a)	[22]
Sheffield, UK	18 069	1	0.0001	Anti-Lu3	[60]
Cambridge, UK	3 197	1	0.0003	Not stated	[61]
South Wales	75 614	15	0.0002	Anti-Lu^b (-Lu^a)	[23]
Houston, USA	42 000	8	0.0002	Anti-CD44*	[63]
Portland, USA	2 400	3	0.0012	Anti-AnWj*	[64]
Detroit, USA; African Americans	7 314	2	0.0003	Not stated	[62]
Taiwan Chinese	1 922	1	0.0005	Anti-Lu^b, -Lu^a	[21,149]

*Only dominant [In(Lu)] type of Lu$_{null}$ detected.

found by Darnborough *et al.* [60] in an English woman (Mrs L.B.) with an antibody to a high frequency antigen in her serum. The antibody did not react with Lu_{null} cells from members of the original Lu_{null} family [59]. No other example of Lu_{null} was found in Mrs L.B.'s family and titrations with anti-Lu^b suggested that her Lu(a–b+) children had only a single dose of Lu^b. Her Lu_{null} phenotype appeared to result from homozygosity for a recessive amorph gene (*Lu*) at the *LU* locus.

This example was followed by three Lu_{null} members of a Canadian family (Mo.) [65], two in a Japanese family (Fuj.) [66], and one in each of two other Japanese families [67]. The sera of five of these additional seven Lu_{null} individuals contained an antibody, anti-Lu3, reactive with all red cells save those of the Lu_{null} phenotype. There were consanguineous matings in three of the families and the Lutheran groups proved recessive inheritance. One of the Lu(a–b–) members of the Mo. family, married to an Lu(a+b+) husband and with Lu(a+b–) and Lu(a–b+) children, was ascertained independently of the propositus of this family because of her anti-Lu3 [65]. The five Lu_{null} individuals ascertained through production of anti-Lu3 have a total of six Lu(a–b+) and one Lu(a–b–) sibs. None of the 10 offspring from Lu_{null} ×not-Lu_{null} matings had the Lu_{null} phenotype.

The presence of anti-Lu3 in the serum of an African American woman with the Lu_{null} phenotype suggested that she may also have the recessive type, but no family study was possible [68]. Further evidence for a silent allele at the Lutheran locus is provided by a family in which the Lu(a+b+) (Lu^a/Lu^b) and Lu(a–b+) (presumed Lu^b/Lu) parents had two Lu(a+b–) (presumed Lu^a/Lu) children [65].

Lu_{null} cells of the recessive type lack all Lutheran system antigens. Lutheran antigens cannot be detected on the cells by adsorption and elution tests.

In one Japanese family, the Lu(a–b–) propositus with anti-Lu3 was homozygous for a C733A missense mutation in exon 6 of *LU*, converting the codon for Cys237 to a translation stop codon [67]. His parents were heterozygous for the mutation.

6.4.2.1 Anti-Lu3

All recessive Lu_{null} propositi have been found following the detection of an antibody to a high frequency antigen originally called anti-Lu^aLu^b and later re-

named anti-Lu3 [69]. Anti-Lu3 has a single specificity and reacts equally strongly with Lu(a+b–), Lu(a+b+), and Lu(a–b+) cells. Adsorption with Lu(a+b–) cells will remove the activity for Lu(a–b+) cells and *vice versa* [60,66]. Lu3 is present on all red cells that express any Lutheran antigen. Anti-Lu3 does not react with Lu_{null} cells by agglutination tests, direct or indirect, but can be adsorbed and eluted from Lu_{null} cells of dominant and X-linked types (Sections 6.4.3 and 6.4.5).

Two murine monoclonal antibodies (BRIC 221 and BRIC 224) behave serologically like anti-Lu3. They react with all red cells except Lu_{null} cells [4].

6.4.3 Lu_{null} of the dominant type and the *In(Lu)* gene

Examination of the pedigree of the first Lu_{null} propositus (MNC) showed that the rare phenotype was dominantly inherited through three generations [59]. Since this first family, numerous other examples have been found [22,23,61,70–73]. Unlike recessive Lu_{null} individuals, these propositi have usually been found in searches of random donors.

Fifty-two propositi of families with dominant Lu_{null} had 63 Lu_{null} and 61 not-Lu_{null} sibs [22–24,61]. An analysis of Lu_{null}×not-Lu_{null} matings revealed 64 Lu_{null} and 61 not-Lu_{null} children. Both counts are very close to the 1:1 ratio expected for dominant inheritance.

In(Lu) was the name given by Taliano *et al.* [72] for the rare unlinked suppressor of the Lutheran antigens, dominant in effect over the common allele *in(Lu)*. The discovery that *In(Lu)* also inhibited expression of P1 and i antigens led Race and Sanger [24] to say, 'This new finding has, of course, made the notation *In(Lu)* less appropriate, and no doubt in time someone will think of a better.' Marsh *et al.* [74] proposed that the *In(Lu)* locus be renamed *SYN-1* (for synthesis), with *SYN-1 B* the rare dominant allele that prevents normal biosynthesis of a number of red cell determinants and *SYN-1 A* the common allele that, in the absence of *SYN-1 B*, permits normal biosynthesis. A new name implying that *In(Lu)* modifies antigen synthesis is premature while the mechanism of the effect of this gene remains undetermined [75]. For this reason, the term *In(Lu)* will continue to be used here and In(Lu) is also used to denote the phenotype resulting from the presence of an *In(Lu)* gene.

Red cells of individuals with an *In(Lu)* gene are not true Lu$_{null}$ cells as they will bind selected Lutheran antibodies, as determined by adsorption and elution tests [70,76–78]. Failure to adsorb and elute Lutheran antibodies from Lu$_{null}$ cells, however, cannot be taken as proof of recessive inheritance because in some studies Lutheran antibodies were not eluted from In(Lu) cells [59,71].

Adsorption and elution tests with anti-Lu^a and -Lu^b have permitted the determination of the true Lutheran genotype in some In(Lu) members of families. Figure 6.2 shows how elucidation of Lutheran phenotypes by this method demonstrated that *In(Lu)* is a suppressor gene, which is not inherited at the *LU* locus [72]. Other families have demonstrated recombination between *In(Lu)* and *LU*, and between *In(Lu)* and the loci governing ABO, MNS, P1, Rh, Kell, Kidd, Yt, Colton, Secretor, and HLA [22,23]. Statistical analysis of family data has not suggested close linkage with any blood group locus [22,23].

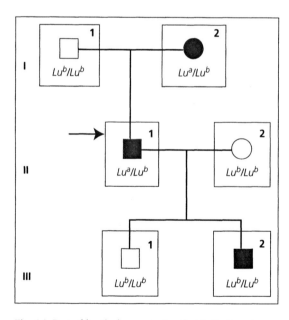

Fig. 6.2 Part of family demonstrating that *In(Lu)* is not part of the *LU* locus [72]. Phenotypes were determined by agglutination tests: ■● Lu(a–b–) (Lu$_{null}$); ○ Lu(a–b+). Genotypes were determined by adsorption and elution tests with anti-Lu^a and -Lu^b. II-1 inherited *Lu^a* together with *In(Lu)* from his mother (I-2); II-1 passed his *Lu^b* gene to both of his children (III-1 and III-2), but only passed *In(Lu)* to one of them. Recombination must have occurred between *LU* and *In(Lu)*.

No Lutheran-system antibody has been detected in the serum of any person with an *In(Lu)* gene, presumably because of the weak expression of Lutheran system antigens on their red cells. Sera of at least 12 In(Lu) women with not-Lu$_{null}$ children have been tested [22,71].

6.4.4 Other effects of *In(Lu)*

In(Lu) suppresses expression of all high incidence Lutheran antigens. *In(Lu)* also suppresses a number of other red cell antigens, which do not belong to the Lutheran system and appear to be expressed normally on recessive Lu$_{null}$ cells (Table 6.6).

6.4.4.1 P1 antigen

The effect of *In(Lu)* on expression of P1 antigen is less obvious than that on Lutheran antigens. Amongst 236 members of 41 In(Lu) families the distribution of P$_1$ and P$_2$ among the Lu$_{null}$ members was significantly different from that observed in the not-Lu$_{null}$ members and in the general population [22,61,79] (Table 6.7). The 36 Lu$_{null}$ P$_1$ people may have possessed a strong *P1$^+$* allele, or been homozygous for *P1$^+$*, or both. There is no evidence that P1 antigen is suppressed in recessive Lu$_{null}$ individuals [79]. Three families in which P$_2$ Lu$_{null}$ and P$_2$ Lu(a–b+) parents have a P$_1$ Lu(a–b+) child confirm the effect of *In(Lu)* on P1 [22,23,73] (Fig. 6.3).

Table 6.6 Red cell antigens modified by *In(Lu)*.

Very depressed (antigens usually only detectable by adsorption/elution techniques)
Lutheran system antigens
AnWj

Moderately depressed (titration and family studies often required to detect weakness)
P1
i
CD44, In^b
Knops system antigens and Cs^a (disputed)
MER2

Elevated
CDw75

Table 6.7 Suppression of P1 by *In(Lu)*. Propositi and relatives from 41 families [22,61,79]. Numbers in parentheses represent expected values calculated from frequencies given by Race and Sanger [24].

	P_1	P_2
Lu_{null}	36 (95)	84 (25)
Not-Lu_{null}	86 (91)	30 (25)

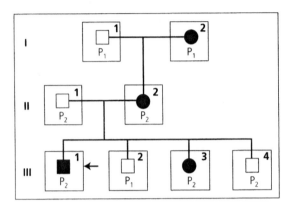

Fig. 6.3 Sardinian In(Lu) family showing P1 groups [73]. ■● Lu(a–b–) (Lu$_{null}$); □ Lu(a–b+). III-2 is P_1 despite having P_2 parents. II-2 is presumed to have a *P1+* gene, which is suppressed by *In(Lu)*. I-2 is probably homozygous for *P1+* and expresses P1 in the presence of *In(Lu)*.

6.4.4.2 i Antigen

The monomorphic i antigen is also suppressed by *In(Lu)*, as judged by selected anti-i [22,73,79]. Red cells of neonates have a strong i antigen and this is not dramatically suppressed in red cells of babies with an *In(Lu)* gene [80]. The i antigen was of normal strength in two recessive Lu$_{null}$ people [79]. I antigen is unaffected by *In(Lu)* [79].

6.4.4.3 CD44 and In^b antigens

CD44 represents a cluster of monoclonal antibodies that define epitopes on a glycoprotein present on a variety of tissues, including red cells. CD44 glycoprotein carries the In^a and In^b antigens (Chapter 21). The expression of CD44, and consequently of the high incidence In^b antigen, is suppressed by *In(Lu)*, although these determinants are still easily detected on In(Lu)

cells [77,81]. CD44 and In^b are expressed normally on Lu$_{null}$ cells of the recessive type [81,82].

6.4.4.4 AnWj antigen

AnWj is an antigen of very high incidence, which may be associated with the CD44 glycoprotein (Chapter 21). It is not expressed, or at least is expressed only very weakly, on red cells of individuals with an *In(Lu)* gene. AnWj was initially given the number LU15, but this became obsolete when AnWj was found to be expressed normally on recessive Lu$_{null}$ cells [83]. The one family showing inheritance of AnWj, also demonstrated recombination between the genes for AnWj and Lu^a [84].

6.4.4.5 Other antigens suppressed by *In(Lu)*

Analysis of a series of families suggested that In(Lu) red cells are more often weak for the Knops system antigens, Kn^a, McC^a, Sl^a, and Yk^a, and for Cs^a antigen, than are red cells from the general population [85], but this was not confirmed [78]. Antigens of the Knops system reside on the C3/C4 receptor, CR1 (Chapter 20), but CR1 expression does not appear to be regulated by *In(Lu)* [78].

MER2 is a red cell polymorphism defined by monoclonal antibodies and human alloantibodies (Chapter 23). Strength of expression of MER2 is variable. When MER2 antibodies were titrated with red cells from members of a large three generation Sardinian family with the *In(Lu)* gene, the following scores were obtained: nine Lu$_{null}$ members varied from 0 to 15 with a mean of 6; 12 Lu(a–b+) members varied from 12 to 21 with a mean of 16 [86].

Equine anti-lymphocyte globulin is used in the prevention of immunological rejection of organ grafts following transplantation. It reacts with red cells, but reacts less strongly with In(Lu) cells than cells of common Lutheran type or Lu$_{null}$ cells of the recessive type [87,88].

Agglutination with concanavalin A lectin of red cells of all five In(Lu) individuals from two families was reduced, compared with cells of the other family members [63]. The anion exchange protein, band 3, is the major concanavalin A binding protein, so this reduction in binding was interpreted as suggesting an abnormality in glycosylation of band 3 in In(Lu) cells [63].

6.4.4.6 CDw75

CDw75 is a determinant on lymphocytes and red cells defined by several monoclonal antibodies [89]. Although its biochemistry and function are not known, N-glycans containing α2,6-sialic acid residues are essential components of the CDw75 determinant [90]. CDw75 is unique as a red cell antigen in being enhanced by presence of the *In(Lu)* gene. Guy and Green [91] showed by haemagglutination tests and radiobinding assays that there was a substantial increase in expression of CDw75 on In(Lu) red cells compared with cells of common Lutheran type. Lu$_{null}$ red cells of the recessive type have normal CDw75 expression, but Lu$_{null}$ cells of the X-linked type (Section 6.4.5) are negative for CDw75 [92]. Cord red cells, including In(Lu) cord cells, do not react with CDw75 monoclonal antibodies [92]. Protease treatment of red cells did not abolish the CDw75 determinant; one CDw75 monoclonal antibody reacted with sialidase-treated red cells, but two others did not [92].

6.4.4.7 Abnormal red cell morphology and electrolyte metabolism associated with *In(Lu)*

Individuals with an *In(Lu)* gene are generally healthy with no obvious anaemia or reticulocytosis, although a degree of acanthocytosis has been associated with *In(Lu)* in three families [63,93]. Autologous *in vivo* survival of In(Lu) red cells is normal [93].

Osmotic fragility of In(Lu) cells is normal, although incubation of these cells in plasma for 24 h at 37°C resulted in significant resistance to osmotic lysis compared with cells of common Lutheran type, in which osmotic fragility increases [63]. Before incubation, In(Lu) and control cells had similar concentrations of Na$^+$ and K$^+$ ions; during incubation, In(Lu) cells, but not control cells, lost K$^+$ and, to a lesser extent, gained Na$^+$ ions. This reduction in total cation content in In(Lu) red cells could explain their relative resistance to osmotic lysis [63]. Significant haemolysis of In(Lu) cells was observed within a few days of storage at 4°C in modified Alsever's solution [93]. This haemolysis could be reduced by the addition of glucose or ATP.

6.4.4.8 How does *In(Lu)* suppress expression of so many red cell surface antigens?

Dominant genes suppressing expression of genes at

another locus are unusual in human genetics; such an inhibitor gene affecting blood group genes at several different loci is unique. Consequently, there are no existing models on which to base an explanation for the mechanism of *In(Lu)*, which remains a matter for speculation.

Marcus *et al.* [94] proposed that the dominant type of Lu$_{null}$ might result from the presence of a glycosyltransferase, which adds an extraneous sugar to a backbone structure shared by determinants suppressed by *In(Lu)*. Udden *et al.* [63] added that decreased expression of concanavalin A receptor suggests abnormality of glycosylation of band 3, further evidence for *In(Lu)* being responsible for aberrant glycosylation of a common carbohydrate sequence present in many glycoproteins and some glycolipids. However, it should be pointed out that there is no evidence that any membrane structure affected by *In(Lu)* has abnormal glycosylation. An alternative effect of *In(Lu)*, suggested by Shaw and Tippett [75], could be to alter membrane conformation indirectly thus reducing the quantity of antigen presented to the antibody or impeding antigen binding.

Another explanation could be that *In(Lu)* encodes a DNA binding protein or transcription factor that down-regulates genes encoding those membrane structures depressed in In(Lu) phenotype or up-regulates genes that modify those structures.

6.4.4.9 Variable effects of *In(Lu)*

The typical phenotype of individuals with an *In(Lu)* gene is Lu(a−b−) with Lutheran system and AnWj antigens only detectable by extremely sensitive methods and P1, i, In^b and some other antigens depressed to a lesser extent. In some families a dominantly inherited depression of Lutheran antigens is less extreme, and weakly expressed Lutheran system antigens and AnWj can be detected by direct testing [95,96]. It is tempting to speculate that this Lu$_{weak}$ phenotype results from a less effective allele of *In(Lu)*.

6.4.5 Lu$_{null}$ of the X-linked type

In 1986, Norman *et al.* [97] described a large Australian family (Fig. 6.4) in which five members had an Lu$_{null}$ phenotype with serological features characteristic of both dominant and recessive types of Lu$_{null}$. The red cells were Lu(a−b−) and lacked the other

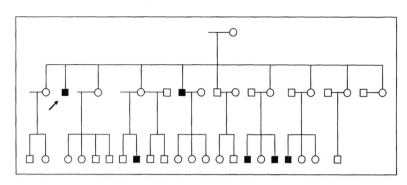

Fig. 6.4 Part of the family demonstrating recessive X-linked inheritance of Lu_{null} [97]. ■ Lu(a–b–) (Lu_{null}); ○ Lu(a–b+). All Lu_{null} members are male and, presumably, hemizygous *XS2/Y*, having received their *XS2* gene from their heterozygous *XS1/XS2* mothers.

Lutheran antigens, yet anti-Lu^b could be adsorbed and eluted from the cells. The cells were AnWj+ and appeared to have slightly enhanced i antigen. They also had weak P1 antigens, although this may have been caused by the presence of a weak *P1$^+$* gene in the family.

The feature that clearly distinguishes this new Lu$_{null}$ phenotype from the other types of Lu$_{null}$ is its mode of inheritance. Lu$_{null}$ in this family could not be caused by a dominant inhibitor (*In(Lu)*) because three of the Lu$_{null}$ members had Lu(a–b+) parents; it could not be caused by homozygosity for a recessive amorph gene because five unrelated people would have to be carriers of the extremely rare amorph gene. The mode of inheritance of Lu$_{null}$ in this family showed the features of resulting from a recessive X-borne inhibitor gene. All the Lu$_{null}$ members are males and, although the Lu$_{null}$ phenotype occurs in successive generations, there is no example of transmission of the phenotype from parent to child (Fig. 6.4). The regulator locus is called *XS*; *XS1* is the common allele and *XS2* is the rare inhibitor allele. Lu$_{null}$ members of this family are hemizygous for *XS2* (because they are male, there being no *XS* locus on the Y-chromosome) and their Lu(a–b+) mothers are heterozygous *XS1/XS2*. See Chapter 32 for linkage relations of *XS*.

6.4.6 Acquired Lu$_{null}$

A bizarre case is reported of an autoimmune thrombocytopenic purpura (AITP) patient with an antibody resembling anti-Ku, whose red cells had temporarily lost their Kell system antigens [98]. These red cells had normal expression of Lu^a, Lu^b, and LW^a. One year later the Kell antigens had returned to normal and the anti-Ku-like had disappeared, but now the cells lacked Lutheran antigens and the patient had produced an antibody resembling anti-Lu3. Expression of LW^a was also extremely depressed. Lu(a–b+) red cells of another patient with AITP became Lu(a–b–), but retained normal AnWj and LW expression [99]. This patient also had an Lu-related antibody.

6.5 Other Lutheran antigens

In addition to Lu^a, Lu^b, and Lu3, the Lutheran system contains 15 other antigens: 11 of high frequency, two of low frequency, and two polymorphic (Table 6.1). Three pairs of allelic antigens—Lu6 and Lu9, Lu8 and Lu14, and Au^a and Au^b—have been shown to be inherited at the *LU* locus. Recombination as a result of crossing-over has never been observed within the Lutheran system. Lu4, Lu5, Lu7, Lu12, Lu13, and Lu20 are antigens of very high incidence. They are absent from Lu$_{null}$ cells of the recessive, dominant, and X-linked type (except Lu20, which has not been tested for on Lu$_{null}$ cells of the X-linked type), but they have not been shown to be inherited at the *LU* locus. All except Lu20 have been shown to be inherited. Like Lu^a, Lu^b, and Lu3, Lu4, Lu5, Lu6, Lu7, Lu8, Lu12, Lu13, Lu14, Au^a, Au^b, and Lu20 have been shown, by immunoblotting and/or by flow cytometry with K562 cells transfected with *LU* cDNA, to be located on the Lu-glycoproteins [2,3,10,100,101]. All of these Lutheran antigens are expressed less strongly on cord red cells than red cells of adults.

Lu11, Lu16, and Lu17 are antigens of high frequency absent from Lu$_{null}$ cells of recessive and In(Lu) types. Only Lu17 has been tested with Lu$_{null}$ cells of the X-linked type, which are Lu:–17. Lu11, Lu16, and Lu17 have not been shown to be inherited and have not been shown to be located on the Lu-glycoproteins. Consequently, the evidence that they belong to the Lutheran system is limited and they are referred to here as para-Lutheran antigens.

285

Antibodies to none of the antigens described in this section have been incriminated in a serious haemolytic transfusions reaction or in HDN. All of the antibodies have been produced in Lu(a–b+) individuals, with the exception of anti-Lu16.

6.5.1 Lu4

Bove et al. [69] described the only known example of anti-Lu4. Two sibs of the Lu:–4 propositus, a white woman, were also Lu:–4. All of about 2700 predominantly white donors were Lu:4. Lu4 is located on the second IgSF domain of the Lu-glycoproteins [10] (Fig. 6.1).

6.5.2 Lu5

Anti-Lu5, -Lu6, and -Lu7, were initially found at an AABB 'wet' workshop and reported by Marsh [95]. At least 10 examples of anti-Lu5 have been identified and have been found in black and in white people [36,95,102,103]. Two of the Lu:–5 propositi each had an Lu:–5 sib [102,103]. None of 423 mostly white donors was Lu:–5 [95]. Like Lu^a and Lu^b, Lu5 is located on the N-terminal IgSF domain of the Lu-glycoproteins [10] (Fig. 6.1).

Results of a chemiluminescent functional assay suggested that one anti-Lu5 might cause increased clearance of transfused Lu:5 red cells [103].

6.5.3 Lu6 and Lu9

Lu6 and Lu9, Lutheran antigens of high and low frequency, respectively, have an allelic relationship. Anti-Lu6 was first described by Marsh et al. [95] and other examples have since been reported [50,104–108]. Lu6 is absent from Lu_{null} cells of all three types [95,97]. Two sibs of the original Lu:–6 propositus were also Lu:–6.

In vivo red cell survival studies, macrophage binding assays, and transfusion of Lu:6 cells to patients with anti-Lu6 have all suggested that anti-Lu6 is not clinically significant [106,108]. Similar assays in an elderly white woman, however, suggested that her IgG1 anti-Lu6 was clinically significant; she was transfused with Lu_{null} cells, which had normal or near normal survival [107]. Red cells of the baby of a woman with high-titre IgG1 anti-Lu6 gave a negative DAT and no anti-Lu6 could be detected in the baby's serum, sug-

gesting that the antibody was unable to cross the placenta [50] (see Section 6.3.6.3).

The original anti-Lu9 was found, together with anti-Lu^a, in the serum of a white woman (Mrs Mull) [109]. The anti-Lu9 was responsible for a weak direct antiglobulin reaction with the red cells of her three babies. Red cells of Mrs Mull's husband were Lu(a+b+) and Lu:9. Study of his family showed that Lu9 expression was controlled by the LU locus, although it did not represent an allele of Lu^a and Lu^b. The only other example of anti-Lu9 was found in a multitransfused woman [110]. Of 521 random donors tested with the Mull serum, nine (1.7%) were considered Lu:9 [109]. This figure may be inaccurate, however, as the serum has since been shown to contain anti-HLA-B7 (-Bg^a) [36]. Tests on 200 random red cell samples with the second anti-Lu9 unearthed only one Lu:9 sample (0.5%) [110].

Cells of the original Lu:–6 propositus, those of her two Lu:–6 sibs, and those of the second Lu:–6 propositus, were all strongly reactive with anti-Lu9, suggesting homozygosity for Lu9. With the exception of Lu_{null}, all Lu:–6 individuals have been Lu:9. Red cells of one Lu:–6 propositus reacted only weakly with anti-Lu9 [105]. Her Lu^b antigen was of normal strength. Cells of an Lu:–6 sib reacted strongly with anti-Lu9 and those of her mother reacted more weakly than would be expected for an $Lu6/Lu9$ heterozygote. The variation in strength of Lu9 in this family is unexplained.

Lu6 appears to be on either the third or fourth IgSF domain of the Lu-glycoprotein, but the results were inconclusive [10] (Fig. 6.1).

6.5.4 Lu7

The original anti-Lu7 was found in an Lu:–7 woman with an Lu:–7 brother [95]. An IgG3 antibody in an Lu(a–b+) Lu:–7 Latino woman was assumed to be another example of anti-Lu7, but Lu:–7 cells were not available for confirmation [101]. Her baby's red cells did not give a positive DAT. None of 285 mostly white donors was Lu:–7 [95].

Lu7 is located on the fourth IgSF domain of the Lu-glycoproteins [10] (Fig. 6.1).

6.5.5 Lu8 and Lu14

Anti-Lu8, an antibody to a high frequency antigen absent from Lu$_{null}$ cells, was first described by MacIlroy *et al.* [111] in 1972. Several other examples have since been reported [112–114]. One gave positive results in monocyte monolayer assays and was responsible for a mild transfusion reaction [113].

Lu8 was located on the second IgSF domain of the Lu-glycoproteins [10] (Fig. 6.1).

In 1977, Judd *et al.* [115] described an antibody in the serum of a multiply transfused dialysis patient (Mrs Hof), which reacted with red cells of 14 of 580 (2.4%) random white donors. The antibody, numbered anti-Lu14, reacted strongly with Lu:–8 red cells of three unrelated individuals. Thus Lu14 and Lu8 appeared antithetical, and this was supported by family studies [115]. Lu14 also appeared to have a higher frequency in Lu(a–b+) than in Lu(a+b+) samples, suggestive of allelic association [115]. Monoclonal anti-Lu^b (BRIC 108) gave consistently higher titration scores with Lu:14 cells than with Lu:–14 cells [116].

The frequency of Lu14 in 610 Danish donors and 600 English donors was 1.5% and 1.8%, respectively (F. Skov, J. Jørgensen, L. Torreggiani, J. Poole, C. Green, P. Tippett, unpublished observations, 1982).

Two other examples of anti-Lu14 are reported [117,118], and at least eight more are known [36]. One IgG anti-Lu14 was apparently 'naturally occurring'.

6.5.6 Lu12

The first example of anti-Lu12 was produced by Mrs Much, a woman of Polish and Ukrainian extraction [119]. The red cells of Mrs Much were Lu(a–), but had only weak expression of Lu^b. Red cells of her father, which had a weak Lu12 antigen, and of her Lu:–12 sister, were also Lu(a–b+^{w}) and, like the cells of Mrs Much, had only weak expression of other high frequency Lutheran antigens. Red cells from all except one of 1050 Canadian donors reacted strongly with anti-Lu12; those from the exceptional donor reacted weakly and were Lu(a–b+^{w}). The Much pedigree revealed recombination between the genes controlling Lu12 and ABH secretion, providing odds of at least 9:1 against Lu12 being governed by the *LU* locus [119].

The second example of anti-Lu12 was found in an Lu:–12 white woman with two Lu:–12 sibs [120]. An *in vivo* red cell survival test suggested that this anti-

body had the potential to cause accelerated destruction of transfused Lu:12 cells.

Analysis of expressed *LU* cDNA deletion mutants was inconclusive about the precise location of the Lu12 epitope on the Lu-glycoproteins, but a monoclonal antibody-specific immobilization of erythrocyte antigens (MAIEA) assay suggested that Lu12 is located close to Lu^b on the first IgSF domain [10] (Fig. 6.1).

6.5.7 Lu13

The original anti-Lu13 (Hughes) was unpublished. A second anti-Lu13 was found in a Finnish woman, but anti-Lu13 was not available for testing her red cells [121]. A family in which three of five sibs were Lu:–13 has been mentioned briefly [122]. Lu13 is located on the fifth IgSF domain of the Lu-glycoproteins [10] (Fig. 6.1).

6.5.8 The Auberger antigens, Au^a (LU18) and Au^b (LU19)

Au^a and Au^b represent a fourth pair of alleles at the *LU* locus, and are numbered LU18 and LU19. For many years the Auberger antigens were considered to represent a system independent of Lutheran, mainly because of results on one family, which showed recombination between *Au^a* and *Lu^a* [123]. When the family was retested for Au^a and tested for Au^b, errors in the original testing were discovered and the family now supported linkage between Auberger and Lutheran [124]. Family studies confirmed that Auberger and Lutheran antigens are controlled by a single gene (combined lod scores of 10.83 at a recombination fraction of zero) [125]. Lu$_{null}$ cells of all three types are Au(a–b–) [79,97,126].

The first anti-Au^a was identified in 1961 by Salmon *et al.* [127] in the serum of a multitransfused woman, which also contained anti-E, -K, -Fy^a, and -Bg (-HLA). Only two other examples of anti-Au^a are reported, also in sera containing multiple antibodies to red cell antigens [24,128]. The antithetical antibody was not found until 1989, when Frandson *et al.* [126] identified anti-Au^b in a serum containing anti-Lu^a. Three further examples of anti-Au^b, all in sera containing anti-Lu^a, were soon found [129].

Au^a has an incidence of between 80% and 90% in European populations [127,128]. Au^b has an inci-

Table 6.8 Phenotype and deduced genotype frequencies as determined by tests with anti-Au^a and -Au^b.

Population	Phenotypes (numbers tested)				Gene frequencies		
	Au(a+)	Au(a−)	Au(b+)	Au(b−)	Au^a	Au^b	References
Paris	315	74			0.5638	0.4362	[127]
London	131	24			0.6065	0.3935	[127]
Copenhagen	362	38			0.6918	0.3082	[128]
London			112	108	0.7006	0.2994	[126]
African American			59	28	0.5673	0.4327	[126]

dence of about 50% in a European population and 68% in an African American population [126] (Table 6.8).

Au^a and Au^b were shown, by immunoblotting and immunoprecipitation techniques, to be expressed on the Lu-glycoproteins [3] and Au^b was found to be on the IgSF domain closest to the membrane [10] (Fig. 6.1). Sequence analysis of exons 11 and 12 of *LU* cDNA demonstrated an A1637G single base substitution in exon 12, encoding Thr539 in Au^a and Ala539 in Au^b[10].

6.5.9 Lu20

Anti-Lu20 was identified in the serum of an Israeli thalassaemic patient [100]. The serum also contained anti-C, -K, and -Fy^b. Lu20 has not been shown to be inherited. It is located on the third IgSF domain of the Lu-glycoproteins [10] (Fig. 6.1).

6.5.10 Para-Lutheran antigens

6.5.10.1 Lu11

The first example of anti-Lu11, an IgM antibody, was present in the serum of a white woman [130]. At least two other examples have been identified since [36]. There is no evidence that Lu11 is inherited. All of 500 predominantly white donors were Lu:11 [130].

6.5.10.2 Lu16

Anti-Lu16 was found, together with anti-Lu^b, in the sera of three Lu(a+b−) black women [131]. Only one family study was conducted and this was uninformative regarding the inheritance of Lu16.

6.5.10.3 Lu17

The only example of anti-Lu17 was found in an Italian woman [132]. There is no evidence that Lu17 is inherited. *In vivo* studies suggested that anti-Lu17 might be capable of causing a modest reduction in survival of transfused Lu:17 red cells [133].

6.5.10.4 Other antigens

Several other examples of antibodies to high frequency antigens, which could qualify for para-Lutheran status, have been studied in many laboratories, but as these have not been published or numbered they will not be described here. An antibody to a low frequency antigen called Singleton was, at one time, thought to have an antithetical relationship with anti-Lu5 and was numbered Lu10. As this relationship could not be substantiated, LU10 has become obsolete.

6.6 Effects of enzymes and reducing agents on Lutheran antigens

Lutheran antigens are destroyed by treatment of red cells with trypsin or α-chymotrypsin; papain has little effect [86]. Monoclonal anti-Lu^b did not agglutinate red cells treated with endoglycosidase F, which catalyses the cleavage of *N*-glycosidically linked oligosaccharides from glycoproteins, although the antibody could be adsorbed and eluted from the modified cells [1].

Sulphydryl reducing agents, such as 2-aminoethylisothiouronium bromide (AET) and dithiothreitol (DTT), break inter- and intra-polypeptide chain disulphide bonds resulting in the unfolding of the protein. Red cells treated with 6% AET or

200 mM DTT at pH 8.0 did not react with most Lutheran antibodies tested, including many examples of anti-Lu^a and -Lu^b [1,86,134]. This is to be expected, considering that the Lutheran antigens are located in the disulphide-bonded IgSF domains of the Lu-glycoproteins.

6.7 Distribution and functions of the Lutheran glycoproteins

Lu^b was not detected on lymphocytes, granulocytes, monocytes, platelets, or the erythroleukaemic cell lines K562 and HEL [1,135,136]. The Lu-glycoproteins are widely distributed. They are under developmental control in the liver, with a high level of expression on fetal hepatic epithelial cells during the first trimester. They are also present in placenta, in arterial walls of a variety of adult tissues, including tongue, trachea, oesophagus, skin, cervix, ileum, colon, stomach, and gall bladder, and in the basement membrane region of superficial epithelia and around mucous glands [4]. Both LU transcripts were detected in all tissues analysed, with the 2.5 kb transcript, encoding the larger (M_r 85 000) isoform, predominant except in a colon carcinoma cell line [7].

The Lu-glycoproteins are members of the immunoglobulin superfamily of adhesion molecules, receptors, and signal transducers [8,9]. The V-V-C2-C2-C2 organization of the IgSF domains of the Lu-glycoproteins (Fig. 6.1) is the same as that of MUC18 (CD146), a marker for melanoma progression, ALCAM (CD166), a human antigen of activated leucocytes that binds CD6, and chicken and rat neural adhesion molecules (reviewed in [137]). The cytoplasmic domain of the M_r 85 000 isoform, but not the M_r 78 000 isoform, contains an SH3 binding motif and five potential phosphorylation sites, suggesting possible receptor and signal-transduction functions [4]. Interaction between the cytoplasmic domain and the cytoskeleton could be critical to signal transduction [138]. The cytoplasmic domain of the M_r 85 000 isoform also contains a Leu-Leu motif that may be important for targeting expression of the glycoprotein to the basolateral membrane of polarized epithelial cells [139].

Laminins are a family of extracellular matrix glycoproteins present in all basement membranes. They are heterotrimers composed of three genetically distinct chains, α, β, and γ [140]. Twelve laminin isoforms may exist, derived from combinations of five different α chains, three β chains, and three γ chains. The Lu-glycoproteins bound laminin on immunoblots and in a monoclonal antibody-specific immobilization of erythrocyte antigens (MAIEA) assay [141]. Lu$_{null}$ red cells of the recessive type, which have no Lu-glycoproteins, but normal expression of the other putative laminin binding protein CD44, bound no laminin [141]. Both isoforms of the Lutheran glycoprotein had the same laminin binding capacity [142,143]. Transfection of human and murine erythroleukaemia cell lines with LU cDNA induced binding of solubilized and immobilized laminin [138,141,142]. The Lu-glycoproteins bind specifically and with high affinity to LN-10/11, isoforms of laminin that contain α5 chains [138]. Laminin-binding experiments with Lu-glycoprotein constructs lacking different IgSF domains have produced conflicting evidence: two suggested that the N-terminal three domains were critical for laminin binding [138,144]; another that it is the fifth domain that binds laminin [143] (see Fig. 6.1). Perhaps there are two laminin-binding sites on the Lu-glycoproteins.

Red cells of patients with sickle cell disease, which express about 67% more Lu-glycoprotein than normal cells, bind increased quantities of laminin [141–143]. The Lu-glycoproteins could be involved in the adherence of red cells to vascular endothelial cells and, consequently, in the vascular occlusion that is an important factor in the pathology of sickle cell disease.

During *in vitro* erythropoiesis, the Lu-glycoproteins appear on the erythroid cells after band 3 and the Rh proteins, at about the orthochromatic erythroblast stage [145–147]. This late appearance of the Lu-glycoproteins correlates with laminin binding [142]. The presence of LN-10/11 on the bone marrow sinusoidal endothelium has led to speculation that the Lutheran glycoproteins are involved in facilitating movement of maturing erythroid cells from the bone marrow, across the sinusoidal endothelium to the peripheral blood [137,138,145]. The Lutheran glycoproteins may also have a role in the migration of erythroid progenitors from the fetal liver to the bone marrow [4,137].

A mouse gene encoding a protein with 72% identity to human Lu glycoprotein binds LN-10/11 [138,148]. Genetic knockout experiments in mice could prove valuable in determining the functions of the Lu-glycoproteins.

References

1 Parsons SF, Mallinson G, Judson PA *et al.* Evidence that the Lu^b blood group antigen is located on red cell membrane glycoproteins of 85 and 78 kd. *Transfusion* 1987;27:61–3.

2 Daniels G, Khalid G. Identification, by immunoblotting, of the structures carrying Lutheran and para-Lutheran blood group antigens. *Vox Sang* 1989;57: 137–41.

3 Daniels G. Evidence that the Auberger blood group antigens are located on the Lutheran glycoproteins. *Vox Sang* 1990;58:56–60 and unpublished observations.

4 Parsons SF, Mallinson G, Holmes CH *et al.* The Lutheran blood group glycoprotein, another member of the immunoglobulin superfamily, is widely expressed in human tissues and is developmentally regulated in human liver. *Proc Natl Acad Sci USA* 1995;92: 5496–500.

5 Gane P, Le Van Kim C, Bony V *et al.* Flow cytometric analysis of the association between blood group-related proteins and the detergent-insoluble material of K562 cells and erythroid precursors. *Br J Haematol* 2001; 113:680–8.

6 Campbell IG, Foulkes WD, Senger G *et al.* Molecular cloning of the B-CAM cell surface glycoprotein of epithelial cancers: a novel member of the immunoglobulin superfamily. *Cancer Res* 1994;54:5761–5.

7 Rahuel C, Le Van Kim C, Mattei MG, Cartron JP, Colin Y. A unique gene encodes spliceoforms of the B-cell adhesion molecule cell surface glycoprotein of epithelial cancer and of the Lutheran blood group glycoprotein. *Blood* 1996;88:1865–72.

8 Williams AF, Barclay AN. The immunoglobulin superfamily: domains for cell surface recognition. *Ann Rev Immunol* 1988;6:381–405.

9 Barclay AN, Brown MH, Law SKA *et al. The Leucocyte Antigen Facts Book*, 2nd edn. London: Academic Press, 1997.

10 Parsons SF, Mallinson G, Daniels GL *et al.* Use of domain-deletion mutants to locate Lutheran blood group antigens to each of the five immunoglobulin superfamily domains of the Lutheran glycoprotein: elucidation of the molecular basis of the Lu^a/Lu^b and the Au^a/Au^b polymorphisms. *Blood* 1997;88:4219–25.

11 El Nemer W, Rahuel C, Colin Y *et al.* Organization of the human *LU* gene and molecular basis of the Lu^a/Lu^b blood group polymorphism. *Blood* 1997;89:4608–16.

12 Callender S, Race RR, Paykoc ZV. Hypersensitivity to transfused blood. *Br Med J* 1945;ii:83.

13 Callender ST, Race RR. A serological and genetical study of multiple antibodies formed in response to blood transfusion by a patient with lupus erythematosus diffusus. *Ann Eugen* 1946;13:102–17.

14 Cutbush M, Chanarin I. The expected blood-group antibody, anti-Lu^b. *Nature* 1956;178:855–6.

15 Mainwaring UR, Pickles MM. A further case of anti-Lutheran immunization with some studies on its capacity for human sensitization. *J Clin Pathol* 1948;1: 292–4.

16 Bertinshaw D, Lawler SD, Holt HA, Kirman BH, Race RR. The combination of blood groups in a sample of 475 people in a London hospital. *Ann Eugen* 1950; 15:234–42.

17 Mourant AE, Kopec AC, Domaniewska-Sobczak K. *The Distribution of Human Blood Groups and Other Polymorphisms*, 2nd edn. London: Oxford University Press, 1976.

18 Chown B, Lewis M, Kaita H. The Lutheran blood groups in two Caucasian population samples. *Vox Sang* 1966;11:108–10.

19 Chown B, Lewis M, Kaita H, Philipps S. Some blood group frequencies in a Caucasian population. *Vox Sang* 1963;8:378–81.

20 Dublin TD, Bernanke AD, Pitt EL *et al.* Red blood cell groups and ABH secretor system as genetic indicators of susceptibility to rheumatic fever and rheumatic heart disease. *Br Med J* 1964;2:775–9.

21 Yung CH, Chow MP, Hu HY *et al.* Blood group phenotypes in Taiwan. *Transfusion* 1989;29:233–5.

22 Shaw MA, Leak MR, Daniels GL, Tippett P. The rare Lutheran blood group phenotype Lu(a–b–): a genetic study. *Ann Hum Genet* 1984;48:229–37 and unpublished observations.

23 Rowe GP, Gale SA, Daniels GL, Green CA, Tippett P. A study on Lu-null families in South Wales. *Ann Hum Genet* 1992;56:267–72.

24 Race RR, Sanger R. *Blood Groups in Man*, 6th edn. Oxford: Blackwell Scientific Publications, 1975.

25 Lawler SD. The inheritance of the Lutheran blood groups in forty-seven English families. *Ann Eugen* 1950;15:255–7.

26 Greenwalt TJ, Sasaki T. The Lutheran blood groups: a second example of anti-Lu^b and three further examples of anti-Lu^a. *Blood* 1957;12:998–1003.

27 Metaxas MN, Metaxas-Bühler M, Dunsford I, Holländer L. A further example of anti-Lu^b together with data in support of the Lutheran-Secretor linkage in man. *Vox Sang* 1959;4:298–307.

28 Kissmeyer-Nielsen F. A further example of anti-Lu^b as a cause of a mild haemolytic disease of the newborn. *Vox Sang* 1960;5:532–7.

29 Greenwalt TJ, Sasaki TT, Steane EA. The Lutheran blood groups: a progress report with observations on the development of the antigens and characteristics of the antibodies. *Transfusion* 1967;7:189–200.

30 Merry AH, Gardner B, Parsons SF, Anstee DJ. Estimation of the number of binding sites for a murine mono-

clonal anti-Lu[b] on human erythrocytes. *Vox Sang* 1987;53:57–60.

31 Henke J, Basler M, Baur MP. Further data on the development of red blood cell antigens Lu[a], Lu[b], and Co[b]. *Forensic Sci Int* 1982;20:233–6.

32 Toivanen P, Hirvonen T. Antigens Duffy, Kell, Kidd, Lutheran and Xg[a] on fetal red cells. *Vox Sang* 1973;24:372–6.

33 Francis BJ, Hatcher DE. Hemolytic disease of the newborn apparently caused by anti-Lu[a]. *Transfusion* 1961; 1:248–50.

34 Greendyke RM, Chorpenning FW. Normal survival of incompatible red cells in the presence of anti-Lu[a]. *Transfusion* 1962;2:52–7.

35 Inderbitzen PE, Windle B. An example of HDN probably due to anti-Lu[a]. *Transfusion* 1982;22:542.

36 Crawford MN. The Lutheran Blood Group System: serology and genetics. In: SR Pierce, CR Macpherson, eds. *Blood Group Systems: Duffy, Kidd and Lutheran.* Arlington: American Association of Blood Banks, 1988: 93–117.

37 Hartmann O, Heier AM, Kornstad L, Weisert O, Örjasæter H. The frequency of the Lutheran blood group antigens, as defined by anti-Lu[a], in the Oslo population. *Vox Sang* 1965;10:234–8.

38 Gonzenbach R, Hässig A, Rosin S. Über posttransfusionelle Bildung von Anti-Lutheran-Antikörpen. Die Häufigkeit des Lutheran-Antigens Lu[a] in der Bevölkerung Nord-, West- und Mitteleuropas. *Blut* 1955;1:272–4.

39 Shaw S, Mourant AE, Ikin EW. Hypersplenism with anti-Lutheran antibody following transfusion. *Lancet* 1954;ii:170–1.

40 Mollison PL, Engelfriet CP, Contreras M. *Blood Transfusion in Clinical Medicine*, 10th edn. Oxford: Blackwell Scientific Publications, 1997.

41 Adkins D. Immunoglobulin composition of Lutheran system antibodies [Abstract]. *Transfusion* 1989; 29(Suppl.):16S.

42 Croucher BEE, Scott JG, Crookston JH. A further example of anti-Lu[b]. *Vox Sang* 1962;7:492–5.

43 Molthan L, Crawford MN. Three examples of anti-Lu[b] and related data. *Transfusion* 1966;6:584–9.

44 Scheffer H, Tamaki HT. Anti-Lu[b] and mild hemolytic disease of the newborn: a case report. *Transfusion* 1966;6:497–8.

45 Peters B, Reid ME, Ellisor SS, Avoy DR. Red cell survival studies of Lu[b] incompatible blood in a patient with anti-Lu[b][Abstract]. *Transfusion* 1978;18:623.

46 Dube VE, Zoes CS. Subclinical hemolytic disease of the newborn associated with IgG anti-Lu[b]. *Transfusion* 1982;22:251–3.

47 Boulton FE. No clinical effect of Lutheran antibodies on a susceptible neonate. *Vox Sang* 1990;59:61.

48 Novotny VMJ, Kanhai HHH, Overbeeke MAM *et al.* Misleading results in the determination of haemolytic

disease of the newborn using antibody titration and ADCC in a woman with anti-Lu[b]. *Vox Sang* 1992;62: 49–52.

49 Chattoraj A, Gilbert R, Josephson AM. On the detection of anti-Lu[b]. *Transfusion* 1967;7:355–6.

50 Herron B, Reynolds W, Northcott M, Herborn A, Boulton FE. Data from two patients providing evidence that the placenta may act as a barrier to the maternofetal transfer of anti-Lutheran antibodies [Abstract]. *Transfus Med* 1996;6(Suppl.2):24.

51 Hardman JT, Beck ML. Hemagglutination in capillaries: correlation with blood group specificity and IgG subclass. *Transfusion* 1981;21:343–6.

52 Inglis G, Fraser RH, Mitchell R. The production and characterization of a mouse monoclonal anti-Lu[b] (LU2) [Abstract]. *Transfus Med* 1993;3(Suppl.1):94.

53 Daniels G. Lutheran related antibodies. *Rev Franc Transfus Immuno-Hémat* 1988;31:447–52.

54 Telen M. Serological and biochemical characterization of monoclonal antibodies against red cell markers related to expression of Lutheran blood group antigens. *Rev Franc Transfus Immuno-Hémat* 1988;31:421–8.

55 Judson PA, Spring FA, Parsons SF, Anstee DJ, Mallinson G. Report on group 8 (Lutheran) antibodies. *Rev Franc Transfus Immuno-Hémat* 1988;31:433–40.

56 Castillo L, Leveque C. Delayed hemolytic transfusion reaction due to anti-Lu[a] [Abstract] *Joint Congr Int Soc Blood Transfus and Am Assoc Blood Banks*, 1990:162.

57 Cutbush M, Mollison PL. Relation between characteristics of blood-group antibodies *in vitro* and associated patterns of red-cell destruction *in vivo. Br J Haematol* 1958;4:115–37.

58 Tilley CA, Crookston MC, Haddad SA, Shumak KH. Red blood cell survival studies in patients with anti-Ch[a], anti-Yk[a], anti-Ge, and anti-Vel. *Transfusion* 1977;17: 169–72.

59 Crawford MN, Greenwalt TJ, Sasaki T *et al.* The phenotype Lu(a–b–) together with unconventional Kidd groups in one family. *Transfusion* 1961;1:228–32.

60 Darnborough J, Firth R, Giles CM, Goldsmith KLG, Crawford MN. A 'new' antibody anti-Lu[a]Lu[b] and two further examples of the genotype Lu(a–b–). *Nature* 1963;198:796.

61 Gibson T. Two kindred with the rare dominant inhibitor of the Lutheran and P$_1$ red cell antigens. *Hum Hered* 1976;26:171–4.

62 Winkler MM, Hamilton JR. Previously tested donors eliminated to determine rare phenotype frequencies [Abstract] *Joint Congr Int Soc Blood Transfus and Am Assoc Blood Banks*, 1990:158.

63 Udden MM, Umeda M, Hirano Y, Marcus DM. New abnormalities in the morphology, cell surface receptors, and electrolyte metabolism of In(Lu) erythrocytes. *Blood* 1987;69:52–7.

64 Lukasavage T. Donor screening with anti-AnWj. *Immunohematology* 1993;9:112.

65 Brown F, Simpson S, Cornwall S *et al.* The recessive Lu(a–b–) phenotype: a family study. *Vox Sang* 1974;26: 259–64.

66 Myhre B, Thompson M, Anson C, Fishkin B, Carter PK. A further example of the recessive Lu(a–b–) phenotype. *Vox Sang* 1975;29:66–8.

67 Mallinson G, Green CA, Okubo Y, Daniels GL. The molecular background of recessive Lu(a–b–) phenotype in a Japanese family [Abstract]. *Transfus Med* 1997; 7(Suppl.1):18.

68 Melonas K, Noto TA. Anti-Lu^{a}Lu^b imitating a panagglutinin [Abstract]. *Transfusion* 1965;5:370 and unpublished observations.

69 Bove JR, Allen FH, Chiewsilp P, Marsh WL, Cleghorn TE. Anti-Lu4: a new antibody related to the Lutheran blood group system. *Vox Sang* 1971;21:302–10.

70 Stanbury A, Francis B. The Lu(a–b–) phenotype: an additional example. *Vox Sang* 1967;13:441–3.

71 Wright J, Moore BPL. A family with 17 Lu(a–b–) members. *Vox Sang* 1968;14:133–6.

72 Taliano V, Guévin R-M, Tippett P. The genetics of a dominant inhibitor of the Lutheran antigens. *Vox Sang* 1973;24:42–7.

73 Contreras M, Tippett P. The Lu(a–b–) syndrome and an apparent upset of P$_1$ inheritance. *Vox Sang* 1974;27: 369–71.

74 Marsh WL, Johnson CL, Mueller KA. Proposed new notation for the *In(Lu)* modifying gene. *Transfusion* 1984;24:371–2.

75 Shaw MA, Tippett P. Proposed new notation for *In(Lu)* modifying gene: another view. *Transfusion* 1985;25: 170–1.

76 Tippett P. A case of suppressed Lu^a and Lu^b antigens. *Vox Sang* 1971;20:378–80.

77 Telen MJ, Eisenbarth GS, Haynes BF. Human erythrocyte antigens: regulation of expression of a novel erythrocyte surface antigen by the inhibitor Lutheran *In(Lu)* gene. *J Clin Invest* 1983;71:1878–86.

78 Moulds JM, Shah C. Complement receptor 1 red cell expression is not controlled by the *In(Lu)* gene. *Transfusion* 1999;39:751–5.

79 Crawford MN, Tippett P, Sanger R. Antigens Au^a, i and P$_1$ of cells of the dominant type of Lu(a–b–). *Vox Sang* 1974;26:283–7.

80 Crawford MN, Wilfert K, Tippett P. Cord samples from *In(Lu)* type Lu-null babies: expression of i antigen [Abstract]. *Transfusion* 1992;32(Suppl.):20S.

81 Spring FA, Dalchau R, Daniels GL *et al.* The In^a and In^b blood group antigens are located on a glycoprotein of 80,000 MW (the CDw44 glycoprotein) whose expression is influenced by the *In(Lu)* gene. *Immunology* 1988;64:37–43.

82 Telen MJ, Green AM. Human red cell antigens. V. Expression of *In(Lu)* -related p80 antigens by recessive-type Lu(a–b–) red cells. *Transfusion* 1988;28: 430–4.

83 Poole J, Giles CM. Observations on the Anton antigen and antibody. *Vox Sang* 1982;43:220–2.

84 Poole J, Levene C, Bennett M *et al.* A family showing inheritance of the Anton blood group antigen AnWj and independence of AnWj from Lutheran. *Transfus Med* 1991;1:245–51.

85 Daniels GL, Shaw MA, Lomas CG, Leak MR, Tippett P. The effect of *In(Lu)* on some high-frequency antigens. *Transfusion* 1986;26:171–2.

86 Daniels G. The Lutheran blood group system: monoclonal antibodies, biochemistry and the effect of *In (Lu)*. In: SR Pierce, CR Macpherson, eds. *Blood Group Systems: Duffy, Kidd and Lutheran.* Arlington: American Association of Blood Banks, 1988:119–47.

87 Anderson HJ, Aubuchon JP, Draper EK, Ballas SK. Transfusion problems in renal allograft recipients: anti-lymphocyte globulin showing Lutheran system specificity. *Transfusion* 1985;25:47–50.

88 Postoway N, Garratty G. Mechanisms causing positive antiglobulin tests subsequent to anti-lymphocyte globulin (ALG) administration [Abstract]. *Transfusion* 1984; 24:427.

89 Guy K, Andrew JM. Expression of the CDw75 (β-galactoside α2,6-sialyltransferase) antigen on normal blood cells and in B-cell chronic lymphocytic leukaemia. *Immunology* 1991;74:206–14.

90 Bast BJEG, Zhou L-J, Freeman GJ *et al.* The HB-6, CDw75, and CD76 differentiation antigens are unique cell-surface carbohydrate determinants generated by the β-galactoside α2,6-sialyltransferase. *J Cell Biol* 1992;116:423–35.

91 Guy K, Green C. The influence of the *In(Lu)* gene on expression of CDw75 antigens on human red blood cells. *Immunology* 1992;75: 713–6.

92 Tippett P, Guy K. Apparent lack of CDw75 antigen from red cells of cord bloods and of rare *XS2* Lu-null phenotype [Abstract]. *Transfusion* 1993;33(Suppl.): 48S.

93 Ballas SK, Marcolina MJ, Crawford MN. *In vitro* storage and *in vivo* survival studies of red cells from persons with the *In(Lu)* gene. *Transfusion* 1992;32: 607–11.

94 Marcus DM, Kundu SK, Suzuki A. The P blood group system: recent progress in immunochemistry and genetics. *Semin Hematol* 1981;18:63–71.

95 Marsh WL. Anti-Lu5, anti-Lu6 and anti-Lu7: three antibodies defining high frequency antigens related to the Lutheran blood group system. *Transfusion* 1972;12: 27–34.

96 Tippett P. Regulator genes affecting red cell antigens. *Transfus Med Rev* 1990;4:56–68.

97 Norman PC, Tippett P, Beal RW. An Lu(a–b–) phenotype caused by an X-linked recessive gene. *Vox Sang* 1986;51:49–52.

98 Williamson LM, Poole J, Redman C *et al.* Transient loss of proteins carrying Kell and Lutheran red cell antigens

during consecutive relapses of autoimmune thrombocytopenia. *Br J Haematol* 1994;87:805–12.

99 Poole J, Skidmore I, Carter L, Win N, Gillett DS. Transient loss of Lutheran antigens in an AITP patient [Abstract]. *Vox Sang* 2000;78(Suppl. 1):P124.

100 Levene C, Gekker K, Poole J *et al*. Lu20, a new high incidence 'para'-Lu antigen in the Lutheran blood group system [Abstract]. *Rev Paulista Medical* 1992:110: IH–13.

101 Reid ME, Hoffer J, Øyen R *et al*. The second example of Lu:–7 phenotype: serology and immunochemical studies. *Immunohematology* 1996;12:66–8.

102 Bowen AB, Haist AL, Talley LL, Reid ME, Marsh WL. Further examples of the Lutheran Lu(–5) blood type. *Vox Sang* 1972;23:201–4.

103 Smart E, Poole J, Banks J, Fogg P, Reddy V. Anti-Lu5 and the rare Lu:–5 phenotype encountered in two patients in South Africa [Abstract]. *VI Regional Eur Congr Int Soc Blood Transfus*, 1999:82.

104 Wrobel DM, Moore BPL, Cornwall S *et al*. A second example of Lu(–6) in the Lutheran system. *Vox Sang* 1972;23:205–7.

105 Dybkjaer E, Lylloff K, Tippett P. Weak Lu9 antigen in one Lu:–6 member of a family. *Vox Sang* 1974;26:94–6.

106 Gibson M, Devenish A, Daniels GL, Contreras M. A transfusion problem in a thalassaemic infant with anti-Lu6 [Abstract]. *Ann Mtg Br Blood Transfus Soc* 1983: no. 27.

107 Issitt PD, Valinsky JE, Marsh WL, DiNapoli J, Gutgsell NS. *In vivo* red cell destruction by anti-Lu6. *Transfusion* 1990;30:258–60.

108 Ellis M, Yahalom V, Yashar Z *et al*. Anti-Lu:6: a clinically significant antibody? [Abstract]. *VI Reg Eur Congr Int Soc Blood Transfus*, 1999:82.

109 Moltan L, Crawford MN, Marsh WL, Allen FH. Lu9, another new antigen of the Lutheran blood-group system. *Vox Sang* 1973;24:468–71.

110 Champagne K, Moulds M, Schmidt J. Anti-Lu9: the finding of the second example after 25 years. *Immunohematology* 1999;15:113–16.

111 MacIlroy M, McCreary J, Stroup M. Anti-Lu8, an antibody recognizing another Lutheran-related antigen. *Vox Sang* 1972;23:455–7.

112 Shirey RS, Buck S, Niebyl J *et al*. Anti-Lu8 detected during pregnancy [Abstract]. *18th Congr Int Soc Blood Transfus*, 1984: 168.

113 Kobuszewski M, Wallace M, Moulds M *et al*. Clinical significance of anti-Lu8 in a patient who received Lu:8 red cells [Abstract]. *Transfusion* 1988;28(Suppl.): 37S.

114 Watt J, Jones ML, Rose P, Pepper R. Significance of anti-LU8 in pregnancy. *Vox Sang* 1995;68:130–1.

115 Judd WJ, Marsh WL, Øyen R *et al*. Anti-Lu14: a Lutheran antibody defining the product of an allele at the Lu8 blood group locus. *Vox Sang* 1977;32:214–19.

116 Zelinski T, Kaita H, Lewis M. Preliminary serological studies of 4 monoclonal antibody samples with 'Lutheran' specificities. *Rev Franc Transfus Immuno-Hémat* 1988;31:429–32.

117 Marsh WL, Øyen R, Rosso M, Gruber D, Cooper J. A second example of anti-Lu14. *Transfusion* 1976;16: 633–5.

118 Cantrell H, Escobar R, Indrikovs AJ. Naturally occurring anti-Lu14 in a pregnant woman [Abstract]. *Proc 50th Ann Mtg Am Assoc Blood Banks*, 1997: 154S.

119 Sinclair M, Buchanan DI, Tippett P, Sanger R. Another antibody related to the Lutheran blood group system (Much.). *Vox Sang* 1973;25:156–61.

120 Shirey RS, Oyen R, Heeb KN, Kickler TS, Ness PM. ^{51}Cr radiolabeled survival studies in a patient with anti-Lu12 [Abstract]. *Transfusion* 1988;28(Suppl.):37S.

121 Sistonen P, Sareneva H, Siitonen S, Pirkola A. Second example of anti-Lu13 antibody [Abstract]. *Vox Sang* 2000;78(Suppl.1):P019.

122 Marsh WL, Johnson CL, Mueller KA, Mannessier L, Rouger P. First example of the Wj-negative phenotype [Abstract]. *Transfusion* 1983;23:423.

123 Salmon C, Rouger P, Liberge G, Streiff F. A family demonstrating the independence between Lutheran and Auberger loci. *Rev Franc Transfus Immuno-Hémat* 1981;24:339–43.

124 Daniels GL, Le Pennec PY, Rouger P, Salmon C, Tippett P. The red cell antigens Au^a and Au^b belong to the Lutheran system. *Vox Sang* 1991;60:191–2.

125 Zelinski T, Kaita H, Coghlan G, Philipps S. Assignment of the Auberger red cell antigen polymorphism to the Lutheran blood group system: genetic justification. *Vox Sang* 1991;61:275–6.

126 Frandson S, Atkins CJ, Moulds M *et al*. Anti-Au^b: the antithetical antibody to anti-Au^a. *Vox Sang* 1989;56: 54–6.

127 Salmon C, Salmon D, Liberge G *et al*. Un nouvel antigène de groupe sanguin érythrocytaire présent chez 80% des sujets de race blanche. *Nouv Rev Franc Hémat* 1961;1:649–61.

128 Drachmann O, Thyme S, Tippett P. Serological characteristics of the third anti-Au^a. *Vox Sang* 1982;43: 259–62.

129 Moulds M, Moulds J, Frandson S *et al*. Anti-Au^b, the antithetical antibody to anti-Au^a, detected in four individuals [Abstract]. *Transfusion* 1988;28(Suppl.): 20S.

130 Gralnick MA, Goldfinger D, Hatfield PA, Reid ME, Marsh WL. Anti-Lu 11: another antibody defining a high-frequency antigen related to the Lutheran blood group system. *Vox Sang* 1974;27:52–6.

131 Sabo B, Pancoska C, Myers M *et al*. Antibodies against two high frequency antigens of the Lutheran system. Lu:2 and Lu:16, made by Lu(a+b–) Black females [Abstract]. *Transfusion* 1980;20:630.

132 Turner C. Anti-Lu17 (anti-Pataracchia): a new antibody

to a high frequency antigen in the Lutheran system. *Can J Med Tech* 1979;41:43–7.

133 Heddle N, Murphy W. Anti-Lu17. *Transfusion* 1986; **26**:306.

134 Levene C, Karniel Y, Sela R. 2-Aminoethylisothiouronium bromide-treated red cells and the Lutheran antigens Lu^a and Lu^b. *Transfusion* 1987;**27**:505–6.

135 Dunstan RA, Simpson MB, Rosse WF. Erythrocyte antigens on human platelets: absence of Rh, Duffy, Kell, Kidd, and Lutheran antigens. *Transfusion* 1984;24:243–6.

136 Dunstan RA. Status of major red cell blood group antigens on neutrophils, lymphocytes and monocytes. *Br J Haematol* 1986;62:301–9.

137 Parsons SF, Spring FA, Chasis JA, Anstee DJ. Erythroid cell adhesion molecules Lutheran and LW in health and disease. *Baillière's Best Prac Res Clin Haematol* 1999;12:729–45.

138 Parsons SF, Lee G, Spring FA *et al.* Lutheran blood group glycoprotein and its newly characterized mouse homologue specifically bind α5 chain-containing human laminin with high affinity. *Blood* 2001;97:312–20.

139 El Nemer W, Colin Y, Bauvy C *et al.* Isoforms of the Lutheran/basal cell adhesion molecule glycoprotein are differentially delivered in polarized epithelial cells. *J Biol Chem* 1999;274:31903–8.

140 Ayad S, Boot-Handford RP, Humphries MJ, Kadler KE, Shuttleworth CA. *The Extracellular Matrix Facts Book*, 2nd edn. London: Academic Press, 1998.

141 Udani M, Zen Q, Cottman M *et al.* Basal cell adhesion molecule/Lutheran protein: the receptor critical for sickle cell adhesion to laminin. *J Clin Invest* 1998;**101**:2550–8.

142 El Nemer WE, Gane P, Colin Y *et al.* The Lutheran blood group glycoproteins, the erythroid receptors for laminin, are adhesion molecules. *J Biol Chem* 1998;**273**:16686–93.

143 Zen Q, Cottman M, Truskey G, Fraser R, Telen MJ. Critical factors in basal cell adhesion molecule/Lutheran-mediated adhesion to laminin. *J Biol Chem* 1999;274:728–34.

144 El Nemer W, Gane P, Colin Y *et al.* Characterization of the laminin binding domains of the Lutheran blood group glycoprotein. *J Biol Chem* 2001;**276**:23757–62.

145 Southcott MJG, Tanner MJA, Anstee DJ. The expression of human blood group antigens during erythropoiesis in a cell culture system. *Blood* 1999;93:4425–35.

146 Bony V, Gane P, Bailly P, Cartron J-P. Time-course expression of polypeptides carrying blood group antigens during human erythroid differentiation. *Br J Haematol* 1999;107:263–74.

147 Daniels G, Green C. Expression of red cell surface antigens during erythropoiesis. *Vox Sang* 2000; 78(Suppl.1):149–53.

148 Rahuel C, Colin Y, Goosens D *et al.* Characterization of a mouse laminin receptor gene homologous to the human blood group Lutheran gene. *Immunogenetics* 1999;50:271–7.

149 Broadberry RE, Lin-Chu M, Chang FC. The first example of the Lu(a–b–) phenotype in Chinese [Abstract]. *20th Congr Int Soc Blood Transfus*, 1988:301.

7.1 Introduction

Kell was the first of many blood group systems disclosed by the antiglobulin test [1]. When Allen *et al.* [2] described the fourth Kell system antigen, Kpᵇ, they concluded prophetically, 'There is, probably, much still to be learned about the Kell blood group system.' There are now 24 antigens in the Kell system (Table 7.1), and at least two independent systems, Kx and Gerbich, are related through epistatic interactions.

There are five sets of antigens in the Kell system with allelic relationships: K and k; Kpᵃ, Kpᵇ, and Kpᶜ; Jsᵃ and Jsᵇ; K11 and K17 (Wkᵃ); and K14 and K24. There are an additional seven high frequency antigens, K12, K13, K18, K19, K22, TOU, and RAZ, and three low frequency antigens, Ulᵃ, K23, and VLAN. All have been shown to be governed by the *KEL* locus and/or to be expressed on the Kell glycoprotein. No *KEL* haplotype has been found that produces more than one of the lower frequency antigens. Recombination as a result of crossing-over has never been observed within the *KEL* complex.

None of the Kell antigens is expressed on cells of the Kell-null phenotype, K₀, which arises from homozygosity for a silent gene at the *KEL* locus. Ku antigen is present on all cells save those of the K₀ phenotype (Section 7.7).

Several rare phenotypes occur in which all or most of the high frequency Kell antigens are expressed only weakly. Some are caused by epistasis, such as the McLeod phenotype and depressed Kell associated with some Gerbich-negative phenotypes, and some are caused by interactions within the *KEL* gene. In some depressed Kell phenotypes the exact mode of inheritance is unclear (K₍ₘₒd₎). In patients with Kell-related autoantibodies, the depressed Kell phenotype may be acquired and transient (Section 7.10).

The Kell antigens are located on CD238, a red cell transmembrane glycoprotein of apparent M_r 93 000, a metalloendopeptidase (Section 7.2). The molecular bases for most of the Kell antigens are known and all the Kell system polymorphisms result from single amino acid substitutions (Table 7.1). *KEL* is situated on chromosome 7q32–q36 (Chapter 32).

McLeod syndrome is a form of neuroancanthocytosis, which includes an abnormal Kell red cell phenotype. McLeod phenotype red cells have depressed Kell antigens and lack the high frequency antigen Kx. The inheritance of Kx is controlled by an X-borne gene, *XK*, and represents a blood group system (the Kx system) independent of Kell. The Kx protein and Kell glycoprotein are linked by a disulphide bond. Because of its phenotypic and biochemical associations with Kell, the Kx system is described in this chapter (Section 7.14).

7.1.1 Notation

A numerical notation for the Kell system, first proposed by Allen and Rosenfield [3], is now used in many publications and is shown in a modified form in Table

Table 7.1 Antigens of the Kell and Kx blood group systems.

No.	Name	Relative frequency	Allelic antigens	Molecular basis*
KEL1	K	Low	k	Met193 (Thr)
KEL2	k	High	K	Thr193 (Met)
KEL3	Kpª	Low	Kpᵇ, Kpᶜ	Trp281 (Arg or Gln)
KEL4	Kpᵇ	High	Kpª, Kpᶜ	Arg281 (Trp or Gln)
KEL5	Ku	High		Complex
KEL6	Jsª	Low	Jsᵇ	Pro597 (Leu)
KEL7	Jsᵇ	High	Jsª	Leu597 (Pro)
KEL10	Ulª	Low		Val494 (Glu)
KEL11	K11 (Côté)	High	K17	Val302 (Ala)
KEL12	K12 (Boc)	High		His548 (Arg)
KEL13	K13	High		
KEL14	K14 (San)	High	K24	Arg180 (Pro, His, or Cys)
KEL16	'k-like'	High		
KEL17	K17 (Wkª)	Low		Ala302 (Val)
KEL18	K18	High		Arg130 (Trp or Gln)
KEL19	K19 (Sub)	High		Arg492 (Gln)
KEL20	Km	High		
KEL21	Kpᶜ	Low	Kpª, Kpᵇ	Gln281 (Arg or Trp)
KEL22	K22	High		Ala322 (Val)
KEL23	K23	Low		Arg382 (Gln)
KEL24	K24 (Cls)	Low	K14	Pro180 (Arg)
KEL25	VLAN	Low		Arg248 (Gln)
KEL26	TOU	High		Arg406 (Gln)
KEL27	RAZ	High		Glu299 (Lys)
XK1	Kx	High		Complex

*Shown in parentheses are the amino acids associated with an antigen-negative phenotype.
Obsolete: KEL8, previously Kw; KEL9, previously KL; KEL15, Kx (now XK1).

7.1. Although the arguments in favour of using this notation are cogent, the more traditional notation is generally employed in this chapter, as it is the most widely used notation and will make the chapter more accessible for most readers. Furthermore, allelic relationships are more clearly demonstrated by the original notations: for example, the symbols Kpª, Kpᵇ, and Kpᶜ indicate allelic antigens; not so KEL3, KEL4, and KEL21.

7.2 The Kell glycoprotein and the gene that encodes it

7.2.1 The Kell glycoprotein

Two groups independently isolated a red cell membrane glycoprotein of M_r 93 000 by immunoprecipitation with antibodies to Kell system antibodies [4–6]. Redman *et al.* [5] sensitized intact red cells with anti-K,

-k, -Jsᵇ, or -K22 and subsequently solubilized the membranes with Triton X-100 and deoxycholate, whereas Wallas *et al.* [6] added anti-K to Triton-solublized K+ red cell membranes. Treatment of the Kell glycoprotein with an *N*-glycanase reduced the apparent M_r by about 15 000, whereas *O*-glycanase had little effect. Consequently, the Kell antigens appeared to be located on a glycoprotein with several *N*-glycans, but an insubstantial number of *O*-glycans [7]. The Kell glycoprotein is phosphorylated, but not palmitoylated [8,9]. All of the Kell system antigens (except K24) have been shown to reside on the Kell glycoprotein [10–15]. Kell antibodies do not generally react with isolated Kell glycoprotein by immunoblotting, although mouse monoclonal and rabbit antibodies, produced by immunizing animals with purified Kell glycoprotein, detect the M_r 93 000 Kell glycoprotein on immunoblots [4,16]. No Kell glycoprotein was detected on blots of K_o cells or isolated from K_o cells by immunoprecipitation with a variety of polyclonal and monoclonal Kell antibodies [4,16].

Amino acid sequencing of purified Kell polypeptide was hampered by a blocked N-terminus. Lee *et al.* [17] isolated three tryptic peptides. Based on the amino acid sequence of one of the peptides, primers were synthesized and a specific oligonucleotide probe prepared by the polymerase chain reaction (PCR). This probe was used to screen a human bone-marrow cDNA library and a clone was isolated with an open reading frame encoding a 732 amino acid polypeptide containing all the known Kell amino acid sequences. Rabbit antibody prepared to a synthetic 30 amino acid peptide derived from the cDNA sequence bound to Kell glycoprotein on an immunoblot.

Hydropathy analysis indicated a type II membrane protein with a single hydrophobic membrane-spanning region, a highly hydrophilic N-terminal cytoplasmic domain of 47 amino acids (or 28 amino acids if the codon for Met20 is used for translation initiation), and a large, 665-amino acid, C-terminal extracellular domain (Fig. 7.1). The N-terminal methionine residue is probably cleaved from the mature protein. The extracellular domain has six Asn-Xxx-Ser/Thr putative N-glycosylation sites (positions 94, 115, 191, 345, 627, and 724), although Asn724 is unlikely to be glycosylated as residue 725 is proline, which usually inhibits glycosylation. There are 15 extracellular cysteine residues, suggesting the presence of seven intramolecular disulphide bonds, resulting in extensive folding of the molecule. The Kell protein has structural and sequence homology with a family of zinc-binding endopeptidases (for functional aspects see Section 7.13).

Kell glycoprotein is closely associated in the membrane with the Kx protein and an M_r 120 000 heterodimer may be isolated by immunoprecipitation under non-reducing conditions [18]. The two proteins are linked by disulphide bonding between Cys72 of Kell and Cys347 of Kx [19] (Section 7.14.2).

7.2.2 Organization of the *KEL* gene

KEL spans about 21.5 kb organized into 19 exons of coding sequence [20] (Table 7.2). Exon 1 encodes a possible translation initiating methionine residue and SP1 and GATA-1 binding sites. The exon 1 region is involved in negative regulation of the promoter in non-erythroid tissue [21]. Exon 2 encodes the cytoplasmic

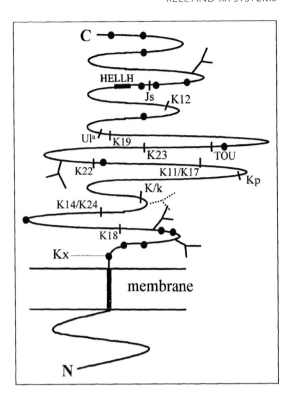

Fig. 7.1 Diagrammatic representation of the Kell glycoprotein showing the relative positions of the N-glycans (Y), cysteine residues (●), the HELLH sequence characteristic of zinc neutral endopeptidases, and the amino acid substitutions responsible for the Kell polymorphisms, absence of high frequency antigens, or presence of low frequency antigens. It must be emphasized that the conformation of the extracellular domain is not known.

domain and a second possible translation initiation site at Met20, exon 3 the membrane-spanning domain, and exons 4–19 the large extracellular domain. The 5′ flanking region to nucleotide –176 contains two GATA-1 binding sites and a CACCC box [20].

7.3 K and k (KEL1 and KEL2)

In 1946, in the first report on the applications of the direct antiglobulin test (DAT), Coombs *et al.* [1] described an antibody of new specificity. This antibody, originally called anti-Kell and subsequently anti-K or anti-KEL1, reacted with the red cells of the husband and two children of the antibody producer and with about 7% of random blood samples [22].

Three years later, Levine *et al.* [23] described anti-Cellano, an antibody antithetical to anti-K. As *k* had

Table 7.2 Exon/intron organization of *KEL*.

Exon	Codons	3' intron size (kb)	Comments
1	5'UT Met1	0.34	
2	2–27	0.29	Cytoplasmic
3	28–74	0.26	Transmembrane
4	75–133	~2.6	K18
5	134–175	0.33	
6	176–224	~3.2	K14/K24 K/k
7	225–245	0.093	
8	246–308	0.23	Kpa/Kpb/ Kpc K11/K17 VLAN RAZ
9	309–358	~1.3	K22
10	359–401	~6	K23
11	402–438	~1.6	TOU
12	439–471	0.24	
13	472–497	0.44	K19 Ula
14	498–531	0.19	
15	532–568	0.15	K12
16	569–590	0.23	HELLH
17	591–647	0.35	Jsa/Jsb
18	648–679	~1.3	
19	680–732 3'UT		

HELLH, consensus sequence for zinc neutral endopeptidases; UT, untranslated.

already been used [24] to represent the common allele of *K*, the symbol k was subsequently adopted for the product of that gene [23]. K and k are the products of codominant alleles, confirmed by numerous family studies [24–27].

Kell antigens are well developed at birth. K was found in fetuses of 10–11 weeks' and k at 6–7 weeks' gestation [28].

7.3.1 Frequency of K and k

In tests on nearly 10 000 English blood donors (mostly white), 9.02% were K+ [25]. From this figure the following gene and genotype frequencies have been calculated: *K* 0.0462; *k* 0.9538; *K/K* 0.0021; *K/k* 0.0881; *k/k* 0.9097 (assuming *k* is the only allele of *K*). K is much less common in Africans and extremely rare in Eastern Asia and in Native Americans [29] (Table 7.3). K achieves its highest level among people of the Arabian and Sinai peninsulas, where up to 25% may be K+.

The k antigen has a high incidence in all populations. From the gene frequencies given above it can be estimated that the incidence of K+k– would be one in 476. The incidence of k– was found to be one in 549 South London donors [43], but only one in 1340 South Wales donors [44].

Table 7.3 Frequency of Kell system antigens and genes of relative low frequency.

Antigen	Population	No. tested	Positive (%)	Gene frequency	References
K	English	9875	9.02	0.0462	[25]
	Parisians	81 962	8.55	0.0437	[30]
	Finns	5 000	4.10	0.0207	[31]
	African Americans	4079	1.50	0.0075	[32]
	Japanese	14 541	0.02	0.0001	[33]
Kpa	White people	18 934	2.28	0.0114	[25,34,35,36]
Kpc	Japanese (Osaka)	4442	0.32	0.0016	[*]
	Japanese (Miyagi)	5974	0.18	0.0009	[37]
Jsa	African Americans	1298	15.87	0.0828	[32,38,39]
	Black Africans	593	15.68	0.0818	[40]
Ula	Finns	2620	2.6	0.0131	[31]
	English	5 000	0	0.0000	[31]
	Swedes	501	0.2	0.0011	[31]
	Chinese	12	1 pos.		[31]
	Japanese	8 000	0.46	0.0023	[41]
K17	English	11 044	0.29	0.0058	[42]

*H. Yamaguchi, Y. Okuba, T. Seno, unpublished observations.

7.3.2 The molecular basis of the K/k polymorphism and K/k genotyping

The K/k polymorphism results from a T698C transition within exon 6 of the *KEL* gene, which gives rise to an amino acid substitution in the Kell glycoprotein: Met193 in K and Thr193 in k [45,46]. This affects glycosylation of the molecule. In the *k* product, Asn-Arg-Thr193 is a consensus sequence for N-glycosylation of Asn191, whereas Asn-Arg-Met in the product of *K* is not. Immunoblotting revealed that K-active glycoprotein migrated faster than the k-active molecule, strongly suggesting that the former is less heavily glycosylated than the latter. This glycosylation difference may explain the strong immunogenicity of K compared with other Kell system antigens. Responsibility of the single base change for K or k expression has been confirmed by site-directed mutagenesis experiments [47].

Anti-K is a relatively common cause of severe haemolytic disease of the newborn (HDN) (Section 7.3.5.2). In pregnant women with anti-K, it is advantageous to be able to make a prediction of fetal K phenotype from fetal cells, such as amniocytes. Several PCR-based techniques have been devised for this purpose and for determining K/k genotype. Some exploit the *Bsm*I (*Bsa*MI) restriction site in the *K*, but not the *k* allele [45,48,49], others involve the use of allele-specific primers [49–51] or hybridization of allele-specific oligonucleotides [270]. All these tests may give a false prediction if a *K°* allele is present.

7.3.3 Kell antigen site density

By use of radioiodinated polyclonal and monoclonal anti-K, the number of K antigen sites per red cell has been estimated as 4000–6200 on K+k– cells and 2500–3500 on K+k+ cells [12,52]. With Fab fragments of three monoclonal antibodies directed at epitopes on the Kell glycoprotein, figures of 4000–8000 sites per cell were obtained, but Fab fragments from a fourth antibody gave a figure of 18000 sites per cell [53].

7.3.4 Unusual K and k expression

Two examples of inherited qualitative K variants have been reported. A K+ woman had an antibody resembling anti-K in the serum. Her red cells and those of her daughter expressed a weak K antigen, which did not react with her K-like antibody, whereas the cells of her son, like those of his father, appeared to have normal K antigen and did react with the mother's antibody [54]. Red cells of a white man reacted with eight of 72 anti-K reagents, the strength of reaction being slightly less than that of control K+k+ cells [55]. Adsorption and elution tests confirmed that the reactivity was a result of anti-K. Red cells of his three sisters had the same unusual K antigen, but no other example was found from screening 55000 donors.

Weakened K expression in four generations of a family was associated normal expression of k, Kp^b, and Js^b [56]. The term K_mod was used for four individuals with K that could only be detected by adsorption and elution, no k, and weak expression of high frequency Kell system antigens [57]. All four were homozygous for a *KEL* mutation encoding Thr193Arg. Like the Thr193Met substitution usually associated with K, this Thr193Arg would not support N-glycosylation of Asn191. Weakness of other Kell antigens was a result of reduced quantity of Kell glycoprotein. Weak expression of K has also occurred in the McLeod [58] and Gerbich-negative [59] phenotypes (Section 7.10).

During a terminal episode of sepsis, red cells of a patient previously known to be K–k+ became K+, as did K– transfused cells [60]. Post-mortem blood samples contained a Gram-positive organism, *Streptococcus faecium*. K– red cells incubated with a culture containing disrupted *S. faecium* were converted to K+.

Weakness of k is detected in a variety of phenotypes in which all the high frequency Kell antigens are depressed (Section 7.10) and in the K+k+ Kp(a+b+) phenotype, where *k* is *in cis* with *Kp^a* (Section 7.10.3). A C1388T mutation in exon 11 of *KEL*, encoding an Ala423Val substitution is purported to be responsible for weak k expression, but no serological details are provided [46].

7.3.5 Anti-K

7.3.5.1 Alloanti-K

Anti-K is the most common immune red cell antibody outside of the ABO and Rh systems; about two-thirds of non-Rh red cell immune antibodies are anti-K [61]. Giblett [62] estimated the relative potency of antigens in stimulating the formation of antibodies and, excluding ABO and D, K attained the highest score with a relative potency of twice that for c, about 20 times that for Fy^a, and over 100 times that for S. Anti-K is often found in sera containing antibodies to high incidence Kell system antigens. Seventy-five per cent of people with IgG autoantibodies related to the Kell system also have alloanti-K in their serum [63].

Anti-K, like other Kell system antibodies, are generally IgG, and predominantly IgG1 [64]. Although IgG anti-K may occasionally agglutinate K+ red cells directly, the antiglobulin test is usually the method of choice. Anti-K often react poorly in low ionic strength solutions (LISS) [65,66] and fewer molecules of anti-K bind to red cells in LISS than in normal strength saline [67]. Problems in detecting anti-K have also been encountered in automated systems [68].

7.3.5.2 Clinical significance of anti-K

All Kell system antibodies must be considered clinically significant. Anti-K can be responsible for severe haemolytic transfusion reactions [61,69,70], including reactions caused by incompatibility between donations given to the same patient [71,72].

K antibodies can cause severe HDN [1,22,61, 69,73–76]. In one series of tests [73], maternal anti-K was detected in 127 of 127 076 pregnancies (0.1%). Thirteen of the pregnancies with maternal anti-K produced a K+ baby, five (38%) of whom were severely affected with HDN. Most anti-K appear to be induced by blood transfusion and it is becoming common practice for girls and women of child-bearing age to be transfused only with K– red cells. It has been suggested that anti-K stimulated by transfusion causes less severe disease than anti-K stimulated by previous pregnancy [73], although this has been disputed [76].

The pathogenesis of anti-K HDN differs from that resulting from anti-D. Severity of the anti-K disease is harder to predict than the anti-D disease. There is very little correlation between anti-K titre and severity of disease [61], although severe HDN caused by anti-K of titre less than 32 is extremely rare [75]. Anti-K HDN is associated with lower concentrations of amniotic fluid bilirubin than in anti-D HDN of equivalent severity, and postnatal hyperbilirubinaemia is not prominent in babies with anaemia caused by anti-K [73,77,78]. There is also reduced reticulocytosis and erythroblastosis in the anti-K disease, compared with anti-D HDN [77,78]. These symptoms suggest that anti-K HDN is

associated with a lower degree of haemolysis. Fetal anaemia in anti-K HDN therefore appears to result predominantly from a suppression of erythropoiesis [77,78]. Kell glycoprotein appears on erythroid progenitors very early in erythropoiesis, whereas the Rh proteins are late to appear [79–81]. Vaughan et al. [82] found that in vitro growth of K+ erythroid blast-forming units (BFU-E) and colony-forming units (CFU-E) was specifically inhibited by monoclonal and polyclonal anti-K. As the Kell glycoprotein is an endopeptidase (Section 7.13), they speculated that it might be involved in regulating the growth and differentiation of erythroid progenitors, possibly by modulating peptide growth factors on the cell surface. Consequently, binding of anti-K to the Kell glycoprotein might impede its enzymatic activity and suppress erythropoiesis. Unfortunately, this theory does not take into account the K_o phenotype, in which no Kell glycoprotein is present on the surface of erythroid cells, yet erythropoiesis is apparently normal. It is more likely therefore that anti-K suppresses erythropoiesis through the immune destruction of early erythroid progenitors. Daniels et al. [83] have used a functional assay to demonstrate that early erythroid progenitors cultured from CD34+ cells derived from K+ neonates expressed K and elicited a strong response from monocytes in the presence of anti-K; no response was obtained with anti-D because Rh antigens do not appear on erythroid cells until much later, when they have become haemoglobinized erythroblasts [81].

In addition to inhibiting erythropoiesis [82,84], Kell antibodies also inhibit in vitro proliferation of granulocyte-monocyte and megakaryocyte progenitors (CFU-GM and CFU-MK) [84,85]. Substantial thrombocytopenia was detected in three cases of HDN caused by anti-K [85].

7.3.5.3 Anti-K and microbial infection

Most examples of anti-K are stimulated by pregnancy or transfusion, but a few cases of apparently non-red cell immune anti-K have been described. In some cases the antibodies were found in untransfused, healthy, male blood donors and no mechanism to explain the presence of anti-K could be found [86,87]; in others microbial infection was implicated.

A 20-day-old child with *Escherichia coli* enterocolitis had an IgM anti-K, yet the infant had not been transfused and no anti-K could be detected in her mother's serum [88]. When the baby recovered, the bacteria disappeared as did the anti-K. An uncommon variant of *E. coli* was found in stool cultures. Cell-free preparations from these cultures inhibited IgM anti-K and K antigens were detected on the bacterial cells. Savalonis *et al.* [89] detected K on one *E. coli* subtype, but not on 23 other species of Gram-negative bacteria. No pathogenic coliforms could be isolated from stools of another baby with IgM anti-K and clinical symptoms of septicaemia [90]. Mycobacterium, responsible for pulmonary tuberculosis, *Enterococcus faecalis*, and *Morganella morganii*, have all been implicated in K immunization [91–94]. The anti-K in a patient with *M. morganii* infection was entirely IgA, prompting a suggestion that previously described 'naturally occurring' anti-K classified as IgM on the basis of their denaturation by reducing agents, may really have been IgA [94].

7.3.5.4 'Mimicking' autoanti-K

Autoantibodies that appear to have K specificity, but which can be adsorbed and eluted from K– cells, have been detected in the serum and red cell eluates of three K– patients [95–97]. These antibodies caused strong direct antiglobulin reactions and were not associated with any weakening of high frequency Kell system antigens.

7.3.5.5 Monoclonal anti-K

Murine monoclonal anti-K have been produced by immunizing mice with plasmids encoding K, followed by a boost injection of plasmid-transfected cells [98]. IgG and IgM human monoclonal anti-K are reported [99–101].

7.3.6 Anti-k

Less than two in 1000 people are k– and therefore capable of making anti-k, yet many examples of this rare antibody have been described [102]. Most anti-k are IgG (often IgG1 [64]) and work best by the antiglobulin test, but cold agglutinating IgM anti-k are known [103,104]. Anti-k has been responsible for haemolytic transfusion reactions [69,102], including severe intravascular haemolysis [105], and for HDN [69,102,106].

IgG1 and IgG2a monoclonal anti-k, which could not be adsorbed and eluted from k– red cells, have been raised in mice [107–109]. Some murine monoclonal antibodies react with red cells of all Kell phenotypes except K_o, but react more strongly with K–k+ and K+k+ cells than with K+k– cells and may behave as anti-k at an appropriate dilution [98,101, 109,110].

7.4 Kp^a, Kp^b, and Kp^c (KEL3, KEL4, and KEL21)

In 1957, Allen and Lewis [34] described anti-Kp^a and its probable antithetical antibody anti-Kp^b. Kell became a complex blood group system in the following year when Kp^a and Kp^b alleles were shown to be linked to K and k [2]. Family evidence confirmed this very close linkage; K+ Kp(a+) people never receive both K and Kp^a from the same parent and never pass them on to the same child [2,35,111,112]. Despite numerous studies of families with K+ Kp(a+) propositi, the KKp^a gene complex has never been found: K is always *in cis* with Kp^b, and Kp^a is always *in cis* with k; the common gene complex is kKp^b.

Tests with anti-Kp^a on just under 19 000 white people from Europe and North America [25,34–36], showed 2.28% to be Kp(a+), a gene frequency of 0.0114 for Kp^a [25] (Table 7.3). Only 1.21% of K+ people are Kp(a+) [25]. Although about 9% of white people are K+, only 2.7% of Kp(a+) Bostonians (mostly white) were K+ [34]. Very little is known about the frequency of Kp^a in other ethnic groups [29]; Kp^a has not been found in black people or in Japanese. Kp^b is a public antigen in all populations studied.

The suppressive effect of Kp^a on other Kell antigens expressed on the same molecule is described in Section 7.10.3.

In 1979, Yamaguchi *et al.* [113] found that the red cells of a Japanese blood donor were Kp(a–b–) with otherwise unremarkable Kell antigens. Her red cells reacted with the serum containing anti-Levay [114], an antibody to the first inherited private red cell antigen, originally reported in 1945 [115,116]. Study of the informative family of the Japanese propositus proved that Levay is the product of Kp^c, a third allele at the Kp sublocus.

Several more Kp^c homozygotes have been found in Japan following identification of anti-Kp^b in their serum [117, H. Yamaguchi, Y. Okubo and T. Seno, unpublished observations]. In one Japanese family, two Kp(a–b–c+) members appeared to be heterozygous for Kp^c and the Kell-null gene K^o [37]. The incidence of Kp^c in Japan is shown in Table 7.3. Other than the original Levay-positive propositus and her family, only one Kp(c+) individual has been found outside Japan, a Kp(a+b–c+) Spanish American with anti-Kp^b (J. Lawson, J. Gavin, unpublished observations).

Kp^a and Kp^c differ from the common allele, Kp^b, by single nucleotide changes at adjacent sites within the same codon in exon 8 [118]. Kp^b has CGG at codon 281 encoding arginine, Kp^a has TGG encoding tryptophan, and Kp^c has CAG encoding glutamine. The Kp^a and Kp^c mutations introduce NlaIII and PvuII restriction sites, respectively, that can be utilized in PCR-based genotyping methods [118,119]. Site-directed mutagenesis experiments have been used to confirm that the single base change is responsible for the Kp^a/Kp^b polymorphism [47].

7.4.1 Anti-Kp^a

Many examples of anti-Kp^a are known. The first (Penney) appeared to be 'naturally occurring' but, as with most anti-Kp^a, reacted best by the antiglobulin test [25,34]. Anti-Kp^a very rarely causes HDN severe enough to require transfusion [120], but one case of hydrops fetalis attributed to anti-Kp^a has been reported [121].

Murine monoclonal anti-Kp^a have been produced by immunizing mice with plasmid DNA followed by a boost injection of plasmid-transfected cells [98].

7.4.2 Anti-Kp^b

The first anti-Kp^b (Rautenberg) was found during routine crossmatching [2]; the serum also contained anti-K, as do some other examples [25]. Although anti-Kp^b is usually IgG (IgG1+IgG4 [64]), Race and Sanger [25] mention two examples which appear to be 'naturally occurring' and did not react by the antiglobulin test.

Serious HDN caused by anti-Kp^b is very rare, but two cases are reported where obstetric intervention and, in one case, transfusion, were required [122,123]. Both mothers had been transfused during childhood. In vivo red cell survival studies and monocyte mono-

layer assays predict that anti-Kp^b has the potential to cause reduced survival of transfused Kp(b+) cells [124,125]. Anti-Kp^b has been responsible for a delayed haemolytic transfusion reaction [124]. Kp(b+) units of blood have been administered to patients with anti-Kp^b, with no indications of transfusion reaction or reduced red cell survival [126–128], although one of these antibodies subsequently became clinically significant, as determined by an in vitro functional assay and an in vivo red cell survival test [128].

Autoanti-Kp^b has been responsible for autoimmune haemolytic anaemia [129,130], in one case in a 12-week-old infant [130]. Autoantibodies to Kell system antigens are often associated with weakened expression of Kell (Section 7.10.5).

A murine monoclonal antibody (BRIC 203) defined an epitope shared by Kp^b and Kp^c, but not Kp^a [53]. A human single-chain Fv (scFv) antibody fragment specific for Kp^b has been isolated from a V gene phage-display library derived from non-immunized donors [131] (see Section 5.18.1.2).

7.4.3 Anti-Kp^c

The first anti-Kp^c, called anti-Levay for 34 years, was made by a patient with lupus erythematosus diffusus in response to transfusion [115,116]. This patient had already made the first examples of incomplete anti-c, -Lu^a, -C^w, and human anti-N. Several more anti-Kp^c, all immune and all in Japanese, have since been found [117].

7.5 Js^a and Js^b (KEL6 and KEL7)

Giblett in 1958 [132] and Giblett and Chase [38] the following year, described a new antigen, Js^a, present on the red cells of about 20% of African Americans in the Seattle area. None of 500 white people was Js(a+). Js^a segregated from most of the blood group systems but, because of the low incidence of K and Kp^a in black people, it was clear that it would be difficult to show independence from the Kell system.

In 1963, Walker et al. [133,134] found an antibody to a high frequency antigen in the serum of a Js(a+) black woman with four Js(a+) children. This antibody failed to react with the red cells of 13 of 1269 black donors. Twelve of the 13 were tested with anti-Js^a and all were positive. The antibody did not react with the Js(a+) red cells of two sisters, believed to be homozygous for *Js^a* because all of their 10 children were Js(a+). The antibody was therefore called anti-Js^b.

The first hint that Js^a and Js^b might belong to the Kell system came from the observation that cells of the Kell-null phenotype (K_o) were Js(a–b–) [32]. A search of 4000 black donors revealed six K+ Js(a+) propositi and the subsequent family studies suggested control of Js^a and Js^b at the *KEL* locus. This was confirmed by four large Brazilian families with K+ Js(a+) propositi [135].

Js^a is almost completely confined to people of African origin [29]. The incidence of Js^a among African Americans is about 16%, giving a frequency of 8% for the *Js^a* gene (Table 7.3). Js^a is very rare, although not unknown [25], in white people. It has not been found in Japanese [136]. Of 11 000 African Americans tested with anti-Js^b, 34 were Js(b–) [137]. The phenotype Js(a+b–) has not been reported in a person of non-African origin.

The Js^a/Js^b polymorphism is associated with two nucleotide changes in exon 17 of *KEL*, one encoding an amino acid substitution: *Js^a*, C1910 Pro597, G2019 Leu633; *Js^b*, T1910 Leu597, A2019 Leu633 [138]. Responsibility of the C1910T change for the Js^a/Js^b polymorphism has been confirmed by site-directed mutagenesis experiments [47]. The T1910C and A2019G mutations eliminated *Mnl*I and *Dde*I restriction sites, respectively, in the *Js^a* allele. The Leu597Pro substitution is between two cysteine residues and could affect disulphide bonding and, consequently, folding of the molecule.

7.5.1 Anti-Js^a

Anti-Js^a generally react best by the antiglobulin test and are red cell immune in origin [25]. An apparently 'naturally occurring' IgM anti-Js^a in a Japanese woman directly agglutinated Js(a+) cells [136].

Anti-Js^a has been responsible for HDN [139,140]. Two anti-Js^a, barely detectable by routine serological tests, caused delayed haemolytic transfusion reactions [141,142].

7.5.2 Anti-Js^b

All examples of anti-Js^b have been found in black people. They generally work best by the antiglobulin test. Anti-Js^b has caused severe HDN [143–146], resulting in fatal hydrops fetalis [145,146]. The mother

of a hydropic baby received a transfusion of 275 mL Js(b+) red cells and suffered no symptoms of transfusion reaction, although the survival of the Js(b+) cells was substantially reduced [145]. Alloanti-Js^b in a Js(a+b+) patient was responsible for a delayed haemolytic transfusion reaction [147].

Autoanti-Js^b, enhanced by polyethylene glycol, was detected in the serum of a Js(a–b+) renal patient whose red cells gave a weakly positive DAT [148].

A potent murine monoclonal anti-Js^b was raised by immunizing a mouse with a murine erythroleukaemia (MEL) cell line expressing recombinant human Kell glycoprotein [149].

7.6 Ul^a (KEL10)

Anti-Ul^a was found, by Furuhjelm *et al.* [31] in 1968, through an incompatible crossmatch and shown to react with the red cells of 2.6% of Helsinki blood donors. Despite the relatively low frequency of K in Helsinki (4.1%), by the following year three families with K+ Ul(a+) members had virtually proven that Ul^a is another antigen belonging to the Kell system [150]. There was no recombinant and 13 non-recombinants between *Ul^a* and *k*, giving a lod score of 3.3 at a recombination fraction of zero. An antibody antithetical to anti-Ul^a has not been found. Ul^a is often considered a predominantly Finnish characteristic, but 0.46% of Japanese [41] and one of 12 Chinese [31] were Ul(a+) (Table 7.3).

Ul^a results from an A1601T transversion in exon 13 of *KEL*, encoding a Glu494Val substitution and acquiring an *Acc*I restriction site [118].

7.6.1 Anti-Ul^a

Anti-Ul^a is very rare. No anti-Ul^a was detected in the serum of 19 Ul(a–) mothers of Ul(a+) children [31]. One case of HDN caused by anti-Ul^a is reported [151].

7.7 The Kell-null phenotype, K_o, and anti-Ku (-KEL5)

7.7.1 K_o phenotype

In the same year as the discovery of Kp^a and Kp^b [34], Chown *et al.* [152] found a new Kell phenotype, K–k–Kp(a–b–), in two sisters. The consanguineous parents and two other sisters were of the common Kell phenotype K–k+ Kp(a–b+). The propositus had made an antibody that reacted with all but K–k– Kp(a–b–) cells. This antibody was used to search for another example of the new phenotype [153,154]: the 3122nd blood tested did not react and was also K–k– Kp(a–b–). The parents of this donor were first cousins and because of this parental consanguinity it was assumed that homozygosity for a rare gene, named $K°$ by Allen *et al.* [2], was responsible for the K–k– Kp(a–b–) or K_o phenotype.

Family studies showed that K_o results from apparent homozygosity for an amorph gene at the *KEL* locus [25]. In several families heterozygosity for a silent gene producing no K or k explains abnormal inheritance. The molecular basis for K_o has been determined for nine unrelated propositi, who are either homozygous for inactivating mutations in the *KEL* gene or heterozygous for two such mutations [155,156] (Table 7.4). The splice site mutations result in skipping of exon 3 and introduction of a reading frameshift and premature termination of translation. The Ser363Asn and Ser676Asn mutants, expressed in human embryonic kidney cells, were retained in a pre-Golgi compartment and not transported to the cell surface [156]. The Arg128Stop mutations, homozygous in two African Americans, were present in *Js^a* alleles of the *KEL* gene.

K_o cells lack expression of all Kell antigens, including, by definition, Ku and Km. The strength of Kx anti-

Table 7.4 *KEL* mutations responsible for K_o phenotype.

Mutation	Origin	Reference
Cys83Stop (exon 4)	Yugoslavia	[156]
Arg128Stop (exon 4)	African Americans	[156]
Arg192Stop (exon 6)*	USA	[156]
Gln348Stop (exon 9)	Portugal	[156]
Ser363Asn (exon 10)†	USA	[156]
Ser676Asn (exon 18)	Israel, America	[156]
g to a, intron 3 5′ splice site	Réunion Island, USA	[156]
g to c, intron 3 5′ splice site	Taiwan	[155]

*In heterozygote with Ser363Asn.
†In heterozygote with Arg192Stop or 5′ intron 3 mutation.

gen detected on the surface of intact K_o red cells is reported to be enhanced [157], yet the quantity of Kx protein is reduced [158] (Section 7.14.2). K_o red cells demonstrate no morphological abnormality [159] or unusual expression of antigens belonging to other blood group systems, except Kx. No Kell glycoprotein, either in a complete or truncated form, could be detected in K_o red cell membranes by immunoblotting with antibodies to determinants on the Kell glycoprotein [4,16,156].

Only one K_o was found from testing 16 518 white donors with the serum of the original K_o propositus [36]. Several studies provided only one example of K_o from 24 953 white people [25]. These results suggest a frequency of about 0.007 for the $K°$ gene in white people. One K_o was found among 14 541 Japanese, suggesting a similar gene frequency [33].

7.7.2 Anti-Ku (-KEL5)

Anti-Ku is the typical antibody of immunized K_o individuals and detects an antigen present on all red cells apart from those of the K_o phenotype. It appears to be a single specificity and cannot be separated, by adsorption and elution, into components of other Kell specificity [160]. Race and Sanger [25] list 10 examples of anti-Ku and many more have since been found. Exceptional K_o individuals with anti-Kp^b or -k have been reported [10,25].

The original anti-Ku caused both HDN and a haemolytic transfusion reaction [152]. Anti-Ku was also responsible for a severe transfusion reaction resulting in jaundice, renal failure, and anuria [161].

A number of murine monoclonal antibodies to epitopes on the Kell glycoprotein resemble anti-Ku by reacting with all red cells save those of the K_o phenotype [53,101,109,110,162]. Two similar murine monoclonal antibodies, produced by immunizing a mouse with MEL cell line expressing *KEL* cDNA, reacted only very weakly with K+k– and with Kp(a+b–) cells [149].

7.8 Other Kell system antigens

In addition to the Kell polymorphisms—K/k, Kp^a/Kp^b/Kp^c, Js^a/Js^b, and Ul^a—a number of other Kell system antigens are known, all of either high frequency or low frequency (Table 7.1). They are absent from K_o cells and expressed either weakly or not at all on McLeod phenotype cells. All except K24 have been shown by immunochemical means to be located on the Kell glycoprotein [10–15] and the molecular background is known for all except K13 and K25.

7.8.1 K11 and K17 (Wk^a)

The original anti-K11 was found, by Guévin et al. [163], in the serum of a French-Canadian woman (Mrs Côté). It reacted with all red cells tested except for her own, those of two sibs, and K_o phenotype cells. McLeod phenotype cells, which show reduced expression of Kell antigens, did not react with Côté serum by the antiglobulin test, but did adsorb the antibody. Thus Côté serum appeared to contain an antibody recognizing a new high frequency antigen related to the Kell system.

Strange et al. [42] noticed that an antibody to a low frequency antigen, anti-Wk^a, reacted with red cells of 0.3% of English blood donors (Table 7.3), but with those of only 0.1% of K+ donors. None of 1000 Kp(a+) donors was Wk(a+). Six months of testing all K+ samples in two transfusion centres with anti-Wk^a revealed seven K+ Wk(a+) donors. Studies of the families of five of these donors showed that Wk^a was always inherited with k; there was no recombinant and 13 non-recombinants. Thus Wk^a appeared to be a new low frequency Kell antigen and was numbered K17.

K:–11 red cells were found to be Wk(a+) and the allelic status of *K11* and *Wk^a* was confirmed by family studies [42,164]. As K11 has never been called Wk^b, the numerical notation of K17 will now be used here for Wk^a.

K11 and *K17* differ by a single nucleotide in exon 8 of *KEL*. C1025 encodes Val302 in *K11*; C1025 encodes Arg302 in *K17* [118]. This mutation creates an additional *Msc*I restriction site in the *K17* allele.

7.8.1.1 Anti-K11 and -K17 (-Wk^a)

Anti-K11 is a rare antibody. A patient with anti-K11 was transfused with 11 units of K:11 red cells with no adverse clinical outcome [165]. ^{51}Cr-labelled K:11 cells survived normally and there was no increase in reactive monocytes in a monocyte monolayer assay. The second child of a woman with anti-K11 was stillborn, autopsy revealing some symptoms of HDN, and the red cells of her third child gave a direct antiglobulin reaction, although no treatment was required [164].

The original anti-K17 is the only published example [42], although others are known.

7.8.2 K12

Five examples of anti-K12 and four K:–12 propositi are reported [166–169]. All are white (although one was originally described as black [170]). Two of the propositi each had a K:–12 sib [168,169]. One of the K:–12 propositi and her K:–12 sister suffered from gastrointestinal ulcers; both had been transfused and both had anti-K12 [168]. Two of the propositi were transfused with K:12 blood with no evidence of *in vivo* destruction [168,169].

Two unrelated K:–12 individuals had an A1763G transition in exon 15, encoding Arg548 in place of histidine and abolishing an *Nla*III restriction site [46].

7.8.3 K13

Marsh et al. [171] described the first example of anti-K13 and the only reported K:–13 propositus, a much transfused man of Italian parentage. The antibody in his serum did not react with the red cells of one of his five sibs, who had not made anti-K13 despite having seven children. The red cells of the K:–13 propositus and his sister displayed weakened expression of k, Kp^b, Js^b, Ku, and K12 and gave an enhanced score with anti-Kx (typical of cells from a K^o heterozygote). It was proposed that the K:–13 siblings are heterozygous for *K–13* and *K^o*, and that the absence of K13 for the Kell glycoprotein has the effect of suppressing expression of other Kell system antigens on the same molecule [171]. This would be a similar effect to that already known to occur in individuals with *Kp^a* on one chromosome and *K^o* on the other (Section 7.10.3). The parents of the K:–13 sibs were not known to be consanguineous.

The molecular basis for K:–13 is not known, but K13 has been shown, by immunoprecipitation, to be located on the Kell glycoprotein [10].

The second example of anti-K13 was an IgG autoantibody eluted from the red cells of a K:13 woman with autoimmune haemolytic anaemia [172].

7.8.4 K14 and K24

After an earlier brief mention [166], the original

anti-K14, found in the serum of a white woman, was described by Wallace *et al.* [173] in 1976. K14 was shown to be an inherited character retrospectively when Dp, a previously described public antigen [174], was found to be K14 [175]. The K:–14 propositus, a white woman with consanguineous parents, had four K:14 and two K:–14 sibs [174].

At least three IgG murine monoclonal anti-K14 have been produced [101,107].

An antibody in the serum of a white woman, which reacted with the red cells of her baby and the baby's sister, father, two paternal uncles, and paternal grandfather, appeared to be antithetical to anti-K14 and was numbered anti-K24 [176]. Anti-K24 reacted with all three K:–14 samples tested, but with none of 700 other red cell samples, and gave a higher titre with K:–14,24 cells than with K:14,24 cells.

Two unrelated K:–14,24 individuals had a G659C transversion in exon 6 of *KEL* introducing a *Hae*III restriction site [177]: K14 represents Arg180; K24 represents Pro180. DNA analysis on two unrelated K:–14 Japanese revealed two other mutations: G659A encoding Arg180His; and C658T encoding Arg180Cys [178].

7.8.5 K18

K18 is the only Kell antigen not shown to be inherited. The only two known K:–18 individuals (who do not have the K_o phenotype) were both white and made the only two examples of anti-K18 [11,179]. Despite being serologically identical, the two unrelated propositi had different single base mutations in the same codon in exon 4, encoding different amino acid substitutions: C508T, Arg130Trp; and G509A, Arg130Gln [46]. The two mutations created *Eco*57I and *Taq*II restriction sites, respectively. No example of K:–18 was revealed by tests on 54 450 blood donors [180].

In vivo survival studies and mononuclear phagocyte assays predicted that the original anti-K18 would not cause an acute haemolytic transfusion reaction, but that transfusion therapy with K:18 red cells would be ineffective in all but an emergency [180].

7.8.6 K19

The first anti-K19 was found in a K:–19 woman with a K:–19 brother and two K:19 sisters [181]. The second

anti-K19, identified in the serum of a black man, caused a delayed haemolytic transfusion reaction, eliminating four units of incompatible blood [182]. None of 10 757 donors tested with anti-K19 was K:–19 [182]. Two unrelated K:–19 individuals had G1595A transitions in exon 13 encoding Arg492Gln [46].

7.8.7 K22

Anti-K22 was found in the serum of an Israeli woman of Iranian Jewish origin [183]. One of her three sisters was also K:–22. The family of the second K:–22 propositus, also an Iranian Jew living in Israel, provided some evidence of genetic linkage between *K22* and *k* [184]. Three unrelated K:–22 individuals had a C1085T transition encoding Ala322Val [46].

Anti-K22 in the second K:–22 propositus was responsible for mild HDN in her fourth and fifth children and severe HDN in her sixth child, requiring exchange transfusion with the mother's washed red cells [184,185]. The IgG isotype was IgG1 during the fourth and fifth pregnancies and IgG1 plus IgG3 during the sixth.

7.8.8 K23

An antibody in the serum of a white woman of Italian ancestry reacted with red cells of her two children, her husband, and his mother, but with none of 2100 reference samples [186]. The antibody precipitated Kell glycoprotein from the husband's red cells and the antigen was designated K23. Red cells lacking high frequency Kell antigens were all K:–23. Two K:23 family members were heterozygous for an A1265G transition, encoding Gln382Arg and creating a *Bcn*I restriction site [46].

Anti-K23 caused a strongly positive DAT on the red cells of the third baby of the propositus, but did not cause HDN [186].

7.8.9 VLAN (KEL25)

VLAN is a low frequency antigen detected on the red cells of a Dutch blood donor when they were cross-matched with the serum of a patient of unknown transfusion history [15]. Two sisters and a niece of the donor were also VLAN+. VLAN was shown to be located on the Kell glycoprotein by a monoclonal antibody-specific immobilization of erythrocyte antigens (MAIEA) analysis. A G863A mutation encoding Arg 248Gln is responsible for VLAN [272]. Anti-VLAN consisted of IgG1 and IgG2 isotypes and directly agglutinated VLAN+ red cells. None of 1068 donors was VLAN+.

7.8.10 TOU (KEL26)

TOU is an antigen of high frequency absent from K_o cells and shown to be located on the Kell glycoprotein by a MAIEA analysis [14]. Two examples of anti-TOU have been identified, one in a Native American man and the other in a Latino woman [14]. Neither had been transfused, but the woman had been pregnant twice. In three TOU– samples from two families, a G1337A transition in exon 11 was detected, encoding Arg406Gln [46]. A monocyte monolayer assay suggested that the original anti-TOU was not clinically significant [14].

7.8.11 RAZ (KEL27)

RAZ is a high frequency antigen, not present on K_o cells and located on the Kell glycoprotein as determined by a MAIEA assay [187]. Anti-RAZ was found in a Kenyan-Indian woman, the only RAZ– person known. She is homozygous for G865A, which encodes a Glu249Lys substitution [272].

7.9 Spatial arrangement of Kell antigens on the Kell glycoprotein

The Kell glycoprotein is highly folded and the shape of its large extracellular domain is unknown. Kell system antigens are destroyed by disulphide-bond reducing agents (Section 7.11) and so must be dependent on the native conformation of the molecule. Some may also be discontinuous; that is, dependent on two linearly discrete regions of the polypeptide chain that come to proximity because of folding of the protein.

In competitive binding assays, Parsons et al. [53] showed that the monoclonal antibodies BRIC 18, BRIC 68, and BRIC 203 (anti-Kp^{bc}) define an overlapping set of epitopes whereas BRIC 107 (anti-k-like) defines a separate, discrete epitope. The MAIEA assay, in which antibodies are incubated with intact cells before solubilization, has proved ideal for the study of Kell system antigens. Antigens of the Kell system have been studied by MAIEA with many monoclonal antibodies to epitopes on the Kell glycoprotein. Figure 7.2 represents information obtained from several studies with MAIEA performed with these and other monoclonal antibodies, together with human alloantibodies to Kell system antibodies [13–15,169,187,188]. The diagram indicates positions of the Kell system antigens relative to each other, based on the assumption that an unexpected negative result represents mutual blocking between the antibodies. Although these data suggest a spatial relationship between many of the Kell system antigens on the Kell glycoprotein, two antigens in close proximity on the native protein may be far apart on the linear sequence of the protein. Like $Kp^a/Kp^b/Kp^c$ and VLAN, K23 and TOU belong to the same cluster and are linearly close, but no other correlation between spatial positioning as determined by MAIEA and linear positioning is obvious.

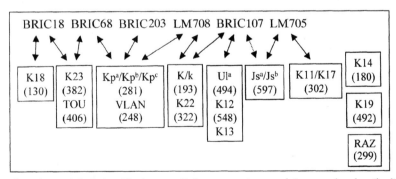

Fig. 7.2 Diagram to show the spatial relationships between Kell system antigens and six monoclonal antibodies to the Kell glycoprotein as suggested by MAIEA. The double-headed arrows show where blocking has occurred between antibodies to the antigens in the boxes and the monoclonal antibodies above. The amino acid positions for the substitutions involved in expression of the antigens are indicated in parentheses and show that the spatial relationships are not linear.

Despite numerous family studies, no *KEL* gene encoding more than one of the lower frequency antigens has been found. Expression in human embryonic kidney of a cDNA construct encoding both K and Js^a shows that there is no conformational restraint to K and Js^a being expressed on the same molecule [47].

7.10 Depressed Kell phenotypes

There are a number of rare phenotypes in which most or all of the high frequency Kell antigens are expressed weakly. The degree of depression varies. These depressed Kell phenotypes arise from different genetic backgrounds and some appear to be acquired and possibly transient. The inherited depressed phenotypes will be considered first.

7.10.1 McLeod phenotype

The McLeod phenotype results from hemizygosity for rare alleles or deletions at an X-borne locus, *XK*. The high incidence antigen Kx, product of *XK*, is not a Kell system antigen, but is the sole antigen of Kx system. The Kx system, including the McLeod phenotype and the Kx antigen, is discussed in Section 7.14.

7.10.2 Gerbich-negatives

Another depressed Kell phenotype resulting from inheritance of a rare gene at an independent locus is that accompanying some Gerbich-negative phenotypes. This phenomenon was first recognized in a K+ woman and her brother with the rare Ge:−2,−3 phenotype [59]. Both showed weakened expression of K, k, and

Kp^b. Nine of 11 red cell samples from Ge:−2,−3 people showed at least some degree of weakening of Kell antigens [271]. In some cases only K11 appeared to be affected whereas in others all Kell antigens were depressed, although to a lesser extent than that found in the McLeod phenotype. All six Ge:−2,3 samples had normal expression of Kell antigens. Cells of the Ge:−2,−3,−4 Leach phenotype also demonstrated depression of at least some of the Kell system antigens [189,190]. Red cells with the K$_o$, K$_{mod}$, and McLeod phenotypes have normal expression of Gerbich antigens. Jaber *et al.* [12] used monoclonal anti-K to estimate that K+k+ Ge:−2,−3 red cells had about half the number of K antigen sites of K+k+ Ge:2,3 cells. The biochemical nature of the phenotypic association between Gerbich and Kell is not understood, but probably involves the absence of exon 3 of *GYPC* in the Ge:−2,−3,4 and Ge:−2,−3,−4 phenotypes (Chapter 18).

7.10.3 The Kp^a effect

In the original description of Kp^a, Allen and Lewis [34] noted some difficulty in k typing some K+ Kp(a+) family members. This was probably a result of weakening of k because of a depressing effect of Kp^a on k and the other Kell system antigens on the same molecule [25]. This effect can only be recognized under certain conditions:

1 when an alternative allele, such as *K*, is present on the opposite chromosome;
2 when there is a *K°* gene *in trans*; or
3 with difficulty, when there is homozygosity for *Kp^a*.
Families, such as the one represented in Fig. 7.3, have shown that the Kp^a effect is most obvious in those

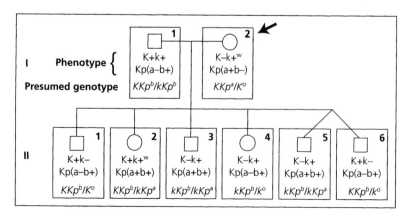

Fig. 7.3 Family demonstrating depressing effect of Kp^a on k expressed on the same molecule [191]. Weakness of k was apparent in I-2, who has a *K°* gene, and in II-2, who has a *K* allele, *in trans* with k. All high frequency Kell antigens were depressed in I-2 who has the *Kp^a/K°* genotype.

Kp(a+b–c–) individuals who are heterozygous for $K°$; that is, $Kp^a/K°$ [191,192].

Tippett [193] reported the results of titrations of selected anti-k and -Js^a with five examples of Kp(a+b–) red cells. One cell sample gave markedly reduced scores and was assumed to be $Kp^a/K°$; the other four, presumably Kp^a/Kp^a, showed a slight reduction in the strength of their k and Js^b antigens. Kp^c, a low incidence allele of Kp^a, does not appear to produce a similar effect when *in trans* with $K°$ [37].

The Kp^a effect results from a reduced quantity in the red cell membrane of Kell glycoprotein produced by the Kp^a allele, rather than conformational changes preventing optimum binding of antibodies to Kell system antigens. This was demonstrated by immunoblotting with antibodies to denatured Kell glycoprotein [47,119]. Expression of cDNA constructs in human embryonic kidney cells showed that the Kp^a mutation causes retention of most of the Kell glycoprotein in a pre-Golgi compartment because of differential processing, suggesting aberrant transport of the Kell glycoprotein to the cell surface [47]. Arg281 (Kp^b) or Glu281 (Kp^c) therefore appears to be a requirement for effective trafficking of Kell glycoprotein to the cell surface.

In an unusual case, a man whose red cells initially appeared to lack all Kell antigens was shown not to have K$_o$ phenotype for three reasons:

1 anti-k could be adsorbed onto and eluted from his red cells;

2 his red cells were Kx-negative; and

3 he had three Kp(a+b+) children and therefore could not have passed a $K°$ gene to any of them [119]. Analysis of *KEL* exon 8 with *Nla*III demonstrated that he was homozygous for Kp^a. He also had a splice site mutation in his *XK* gene and so had the McLeod phenotype (Section 7.14.4). Presumably the Kell weakening effects arising both from Kp^a homozygosity and from Kx deficiency led to his K$_o$-like phenotype.

7.10.4 K$_{mod}$ phenotype

Marsh and Redman [7] introduced K$_{mod}$ as an umbrella term to describe phenotypes in which Kell antigens are expressed very weakly, often requiring adsorption–elution tests for detection, and in which Kx antigen expression is elevated [194–198]. K$_{mod}$ cells have reduced quantity of the Kell glycoprotein [198]. Some K$_{mod}$ individuals make an antibody, which resembles

anti-Ku, but differs from anti-Ku by being non-reactive with K$_{mod}$ cells [7,194,195,197,198].

K$_{mod}$ is probably inherited as a recessive character, but the precise mode of inheritance has not been confirmed. In one family the aberrant phenotype was detected in the propositus and in two of his four brothers, but in none of his seven children and 13 grandchildren [195]. A K$_{mod}$ woman had a brother with a similar weak Kell phenotype [197].

Four individuals with weak Kell antigens, including very weak K, were homozygous for a *KEL* mutation encoding Thr193Arg [57] (see Section 7.3.4).

Weak Kp^b and k antigens could only be detected by adsorption and elution tests in two K–k+ Kp(a+b+^{w}) sibs and a third K+k+^{w} Kp(a–b+) sib in a Swiss family. Poole *et al.* [199] suggested that they were heterozygous for K^{mod} and either kKp^a or KKp^b. A similar explanation probably accounts for the Kp(a+b+^{w}), Allen phenotype [200]. In 13 of 70 apparent Kp(a+b–) samples weak Kp^b could be detected by adsorption and elution of anti-Kp^b [199]. These 13 individuals are probably heterozygous for K^{mod}, indicating that the K^{mod} gene is not uncommon.

7.10.5 Acquired and transient depressed Kell phenotypes

In 1972, Seyfried *et al.* [129] described the case of a boy with severe autoimmune haemolytic anaemia whose red cells gave a weakly positive DAT and had weak expression of k, Kp^b, Js^b, and Ku. His serum contained a potent anti-Kp^b, responsible for a haemolytic transfusion reaction. Within 16 weeks of the start of the investigation, his positive DAT had virtually disappeared, there was no sign of the anti-Kp^b, and his Kell antigens were back to normal strength. Similar examples of Kell-related autoantibodies associated with weak Kell antigens have since been described [201–205]. Degradation of Kell system antigens by enzymes of microbial origin has been proposed to explain this phenomenon [201,202].

Anti-Kp^b was responsible for a positive DAT on the cells of a patient who was genetically Kp(a+b–) [203]. Her k and Js^b antigens were weakly expressed, but she had strong Kp^a. Nine months later the DAT was negative, the anti-Kp^b undetectable, and her k and Js^b back to the strength expected for Kp(a+b–) cells. Her own anti-Kp^b, stored frozen from the initial study, no longer reacted with her cells. Manny *et al.* [203] suggested that Kp^b-like antigen was of microbial origin and may have become adsorbed onto the red cells and stimulated antibody production.

A patient with idiopathic thrombocytopenic purpura (ITP) had a potent antibody to a high frequency Kell antigen. His red cells gave a negative DAT and displayed profound depression of Kell system antigens. Transfused cells also lost their Kell antigens. Five months later the antibody had disappeared and the patient's Kell antigens had returned to normal. Again an environmental agent, possibly of microbial origin, appeared to be responsible [206]. Another similar case in an ITP patient is reported [207]; in remission his Kell antibody disappeared and his Kell antigens returned to normal, but his red cells lost their Lutheran antigens during a subsequent relapse (see Chapter 6). The possibility that Kell glycoprotein is expressed on megakaryocytes [85] might provide an explanation for the ITP in these patients.

7.11 Effects of enzymes and reducing agents on Kell antigens

Treatment of red cells with the proteases papain, ficin, or trypsin does not reduce expression of Kell antigens; the effects of α-chymotrypsin and pronase are variable [208]. Treatment of red cells with a mixture of trypsin and chymotrypsin, with trypsin followed by chymotrypsin, or vice versa, abolishes activity of Kell antigens [208,209], but some Kell-related monoclonal antibodies continue to agglutinate red cells treated in this way [53].

The Kell glycoprotein has 15 cysteine residues in its extracellular domain (see Fig. 7.1) and thiol-reducing agents, which dissociate disulphide bonds between cysteine residues, destroy Kell antigens on intact red cells. All Kell antigens are destroyed by 100–200 mM dithiothreitol (DTT) and by 6% 2-aminoethylisothiouronium bromide (AET) at pH 8 [210,211]. Js^a and Js^b are inactivated by substantially lower concentrations of DTT (<2 mM) [210]. Two cysteine residues flank the position of the amino acid substitution associated with the Js^a/Js^b polymorphism (residue 597) and probably form part of the Js^a and Js^b epitopes [138] (see Fig. 7.1). Like natural K$_o$ cells, artificial K$_o$ cells produced by AET treatment of red cells have enhanced expression of Kx antigen [211]. AET treatment of red cells is not a reliable way of identifying Kell system antibodies as AET destroys many other red cell antigens,

including the Lutheran, Yt, Dombrock, LW, Knops, and JMH antigens.

Glycine-HCl-EDTA treatment of red cells for dissociation of IgG also denatures Kell system antigens [212].

7.12 Kell antigens on other cells and in other species

7.12.1 Other cells and other tissues

For some time Kell was considered erythroid-specific. No Kell system antigen or Kell glycoprotein was detected on human lymphocytes, granulocytes, monocytes, or platelets, by flow cytometry with several Kell-related monoclonal antibodies [213] or by immunoblotting with a monoclonal antibody to purified Kell glycoprotein [16]. Cells of the human erythroleukaemic line, K562, did not express Kell antigens [213,214], unless induced to synthesize haemoglobin by hemin, after which k, Kp^b, Js^b, and Ku were detected [214]. Kell mRNA transcripts were detected in haemopoietic tissue, bone marrow and fetal liver, and in peripheral blood leucocytes [215]. There is also indirect evidence that Kell glycoprotein could be present on progenitors of granulocytes, monocytes, and megakaryocytes [84,85] (Section 7.3.5.2).

KEL mRNA transcripts were found to be about equally abundant in erythroid tissues and testis, and were detected in lesser amounts in lymph node, brain, colon, spleen, skeletal muscle, and several other tissues [21,215]. Immunoblotting and immunohistochemistry revealed Kell glycoprotein in testis, lymphoid tissues, and skeletal muscle [21,215]. Kell glycoprotein was co-isolated with Kx protein in skeletal muscle [215].

7.12.2 Evolutionary aspects

Chimpanzees (*Pan troglodyte*) have the Kell phenotype K–k+ Kp(a–b+) Ku+ Js(a+b–) Ul(a–) K:11,12,13,14,18,19,22 Kx+ [216]. Antigens k, Kp^b, and Js^a are also present on the red cells of gorilla and gibbon, K and Js^a on those of Old World monkeys, and k on those of New World monkeys [217].

The mouse *KEL* homologue, *Kel*, has been cloned [218]. Mouse and human Kell glycoprotein share 74% amino acid sequence identity and the mouse Kell glycoprotein is disulphide-linked to Kx protein.

7.13 Functional aspects

Kell protein shares a pentameric zinc-binding motif, His-Glu-Xxx-Xxx-His (HEXXH, HELLH in Kell, Fig. 7.1), with zinc-dependent endopeptidases [17]. Closest homology is with the neprilysin family consisting of at least six other enzymes, including neutral endopeptidase 24.11 (NEP or CD10), two endothelium-converting enzymes (ECE-1 and ECE-2), and PEX, an enzyme associated with X-linked hypophosphataemia [219]. These enzymes process a variety of biologically active peptides. ECE-1 and ECE-2 cleave big endothelin (ET)-1, big ET-2, and big ET-3, inactive peptides of about 40 amino acids, to create 21-amino-acid peptides with vasoconstrictor activity, ET-1, ET-2, and ET-3. A *KEL* cDNA construct lacking the regions encoding the cytoplasmic and membrane-spanning domains was expressed in insect (sf9) cells and a truncated Kell glycoprotein was secreted. This secreted glycoprotein cleaved big ET-3 at Trp21-Ile22 to produce ET-3. It could also process ET-1 and ET-2 from big ET-1 and big ET-2, but to a much lesser extent [220]. Secreted Kell glycoprotein was inactivated by mutating the HELLH motif, essential for catalytic activity, to HGLLH. Red cells of normal Kell phenotype, but not those of the K_o phenotype, were also capable of processing ET-3. ET-3 is a biologically active peptide with multiple roles, so the function of the Kell glycoprotein remains unclear. It is not known whether the Kell glycoprotein processes any other biopeptides.

Kell glycoprotein appears on erythroid progenitor cells at an early stage of erythropoiesis, before glycophorin A or band 3 [79–81]. When K562 erythroleukaemia cell line is stimulated with hemin to develop as an erythroid line it expresses Kell but no NEP, but when stimulated into megakaryocyte development with phorbol ester it expresses NEP but no Kell [221]. Kell may therefore play a part in erythropoiesis (but see Section 7.3.5.2).

7.14 The Kx system

The Kx system consists of one antigen, Kx (XK1 or 019001), encoded by an X-linked gene, *XK*. Absence of Kx from red cells results in severe reduction in expression of Kell antigens, the McLeod phenotype.

7.14.1 The Kx protein and the gene that encodes it

Kx, a red cell membrane protein of apparent M_r 37 000, was isolated from red cells by immunoprecipitation with human alloanti-Kx [222]. Kx protein is not glycosylated [18,223]; it is phosphorylated and palmitoylated [8,9].

Patients with McLeod syndrome (MLS) lack Kx and occasionally have interstitial deletions of chromosome Xp21. Ho *et al.* [223] assembled a cosmid contig of 360 kb covering the region between *DXS709* and *CYBB*, genes that flank *XK*. They then hybridized the cosmids with genomic DNA from patients with MLS and identified the breakpoints of a deletion of about 50 kb. Genomic fragments that spanned deletion endpoints were used to screen human cDNA libraries and a consensus full-length transcript for a candidate *XK* gene was derived from seven cDNA clones. The open reading frame predicted a 444 amino acid polypeptide with no N-glycosylation site and a calculated M_r of 50 913 [223]. Rabbit antibodies raised to synthetic peptides with sequences corresponding to the *XK* cDNA clone bound to the M_r 37 000 Kx protein on immunoblots of membrane proteins derived from red cells of common phenotype, but not to blots of proteins from McLeod phenotype red cells [158]. The N-terminal 22 amino acids of the M_r 37 000 Kx protein were in accordance with the corresponding nucleotide sequence of the cDNA clone [18].

Hydropathy analysis of the amino acid sequence of the Kx protein revealed 10 hydrophobic regions of 21 amino acids [223]. The protein probably spans the membrane 10 times, with internal N- and C-termini (Fig. 7.4) and has the structural appearance of a membrane transporter. The predicted topographical arrangement is identical to that of members of a family of proteins that cotransport a neurotransmitter together with Na^+ and Cl^- ions [224], the amino acid sequence bearing closest resemblance to an Na^+-dependent glutamate transporter [223]. Kx protein also shares similarity with CED-8, a protein of the nematode *Caenorhabditidis elegans*, which is involved in the regulation of apoptosis [225].

XK is organized into three exons, encoding amino acids 1–82, 83–168, and 169–444, respectively [223]. *XK* mRNA showed widespread distribution, with high levels of expression detected in fetal liver and in adult skeletal muscle, brain, and heart [223].

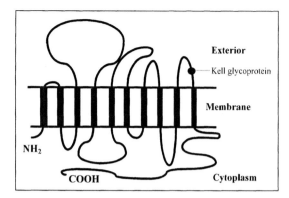

Fig. 7.4 Diagrammatic representation of the topology of the Kx protein in the red cell membrane, showing cytoplasmic termini, 10 membrane-spanning domains, and (●) Cys347, which is linked by a disulphide bond with Cys72 of the Kell glycoprotein (Fig. 7.1).

A mouse homologue of *XK* encodes a protein with 82% identity to human Kx protein with 10 predicted membrane-spanning domains [226].

7.14.2 Association of Kx protein and Kell glycoprotein

When immunoprecipitation experiments were performed under non-reducing conditions with monoclonal anti-K and K+ red cells, a disulphide-bonded heterodimer comprising the M_r 93 000 Kell glycoprotein and the M_r 37 000 Kx protein was detected [18]. Rabbit antibody raised to the purified complex reacted with both components on immunoblots and precipitated the Kx protein from K_o red cells, but not from McLeod phenotype cells.

Precipitation with a rabbit antibody raised to a peptide representing the second extracellular loop of Kx protein (Fig. 7.4) isolated the Kell–Kx complex from COS-1 mammalian cells cotransfected with *KEL* and *XK* cDNA. Conversion of cysteine residues to serine by site-directed mutagenesis demonstrated that Cys347 on the fifth extracellular loop of the Kx protein is linked by a single disulphide bond to Cys72 of the Kell glycoprotein [19]. Time–course studies on the *KEL* and *XK* transfected COS-1 cells demonstrated that the Kell–Kx complex is assembled in the endoplasmic reticulum and transported to the cell surface [227].

The relative amount of Kx protein in K_o is lower than in cells of common Kell type [156,158]. In con-

trast, Kx antigen, as determined by serological techniques with alloanti-Kx, is expressed more strongly on K_o cells than on cells of common Kell type [157], suggesting that the presence of the Kell glycoprotein may impair access of anti-Kx to the Kx protein in intact cells. Unlike Kell system antigens, Kx is not denatured by the disulphide-bond reducing agents DTT and AET. On the contrary, red cells treated with the appropriate concentrations of these chemicals resemble K_o cells and have enhanced serological expression of Kx [211,228].

If Kx is a transporter, it is possible that it can only function as the light chain of a complex with the Kell glycoprotein, as seen in the permease family of amino acid transporters [229].

7.14.3 McLeod phenotype and McLeod syndrome (MLS)

Routine tests on medical students led Allen *et al.* [230] to recognize that one of the students, Mr McLeod, had an unusual Kell phenotype. In the McLeod red cell phenotype all high frequency Kell antigens are expressed weakly, the degree of depression of these antigens varying in different individuals. K is also weakly expressed when present [58]. McLeod phenotype red cells lack the Kx and Km (KEL20) antigens (Section 7.14.5).

McLeod phenotype is very rare and no frequency estimate has been published. Two unrelated men with the McLeod phenotype were found as a result of testing, with anti-k, red cells from many thousands of donors from south-east England [231]. All reported McLeod phenotype individuals have been white [7] or Japanese [232–234], except one African American [235].

McLeod phenotype is only one of a number of characteristics that collectively make up a wider phenomenon known as McLeod syndrome (MLS). McLeod cells are acanthocytic [231,236,237] with decreased whole cell deformability [238] and reduced *in vivo* survival [239]. A variety of muscular and neurological defects, including muscle wasting, diminished deep tendon reflex, choreiform movements, and cardiomyopathy, have been associated with MLS; elevated serum creatine phosphokinase is a constant feature. A thorough review of 22 affected males is provided by Danek *et al.* [240]. In some cases the symptoms may be severe, leading to premature death. In one family, five of seven affected males presented with psychiatric disorders [241]. The reason for the association between Kx deficiency and neuroacanthocytosis and muscular defects is unknown, but the relationship of Kx protein to mammalian neurotransmitter transporters could provide a clue. Acanthocytosis associated with neuropathy, in the absence of the McLeod red cell phenotype, is well known [237].

MLS red cells appear biochemically and physiologically relatively normal, despite their grossly abnormal morphology and the virtual absence of Kell system antigens. The protein profile, as determined by SDS PAGE is normal, suggesting no defect of the membrane skeleton [222,242,243]. Phospholipid content is essentially normal [244,245], but there is evidence for abnormalities in the composition of the membrane lipid bilayers [246] and enhanced transbilayer mobility of phosphatidylcholine [245]. Electrolyte transport in McLeod cells is normal, but osmotic water permeability is reduced [244].

7.14.4 Inheritance and molecular genetics of Kx and the McLeod phenotype

Expression of Kx antigen, present on all red cells save those of the McLeod phenotype, is controlled by an X-borne gene. MLS is therefore inherited as an X-linked recessive disease. With only one exception [237], McLeod has always been found in males and the rare gene is inherited from the mother, not the father.

Hemizygosity for a variety of inactivating mutations has been associated with MLS (Table 7.5). A deletion of exon 2 of *XK* was detected in a man with MLS and in his grandson, predicting that the boy will be afflicted with the disease in the future [247]. A mutation in the fifth nucleotide of the 5' donor splice site of intron 2, a nucleotide that is 82% conserved in the splice consensus sequence, was found in a man with almost no Kell antigens on his red cells and in his two daughters [119]. This mutation would also be expected to cause some degree of abnormal splicing. This man did not have neuroacanthocytosis or muscle defects, possibly because of some degree of normal *XK* RNA splicing. The extreme reduction in Kell antigen was attributed to the combined effects of homozygosity for a *Kpᵃ* allele and the Kx deficiency [119] (Section 7.10.3). A nonsense mutation in *XK* exon 3 of a man with MLS was probably a new mutation as it was not present in his mother or sister [251].

Table 7.5 *XK* mutations associated with McLeod syndrome.

Mutation	References
Deletion of whole gene*	[223,254–259]
Deletion of promoter and exon 1	[223]
Deletion of exon 1	[240]
Deletion of exon 2	[247]
Deletion of intron 2 and exon 3	[240,248]
Trp36Stop (exon 1)	[240]
Single nt (T) deletion, codon 90 (exon 2)	[249]
Arg133Stop (exon 2)	[240,250]
Gln145Stop (exon 2)	[240]
Single nt (C) insertion, codon 151 (exon 2)	[234]
Trp236Stop (exon 3)	[240]
Double nt (TT) deletion, codon 229	[240]
Single nt (G) deletion, codon 257 (exon 3)	[240]
5 nt (CTCTA) deletion, codon 285 (exon 3)	[240]
Cys294Arg (exon 3)	[240]
Gln299Stop (exon 3)	[241]
14 nt deletion, codon 313 (exon 3)	[240]
Trp314Stop (exon 3)	[251]
Single nt (T) deletion, codon 338 (exon 3)	[233]
g to c, intron 1 5' splice site	[252]
g to a, intron 2 5' splice site	[223]
g to a, at nt 5, intron 2 5' splice site	[119]
g to a, intron 2 3' splice site	[223]

*Deletion often encompasses other X-linked genes.
nt, nucleotide.

Chronic granulomatous disease (CGD), an inherited disorder that may be either autosomal or X-linked, impairs the functioning of phagocytes resulting in severe susceptibility to infection. A small minority of CGD patients, all of the X-linked type, have MLS. X-linked CGD results from deletion of the gene (*CYBB*) for the gp91^{phox} subunit of flavocytochrome b_{558}, or from mutations within that gene [253]. The locus for X-linked CGD and the *XK* locus are discrete and the association of MLS with CGD results from a deletion of part of the X-chromosome that encompasses both genes [253–259] (see Section 32.3.15.2). Three of 46 patients with X-linked CGD had MLS. All three had large interstitial deletions of Xp21.1, whereas the other 40 had simple mutations within *CYBB* [258].

Adsorption studies demonstrating the presence of Kx antigen on leucocytes from most people, but not on those from patients with X-linked CGD, suggested that Kx on leucocytes may be an important factor in the phagocytic process [157,159]. However, more recent studies with more sophisticated techniques have failed to demonstrate Kx on human granulocytes [260].

7.14.4.1 X-chromosome inactivation

XK is subject to the phenomenon of X-chromosome inactivation (Lyonization), in which all somatic cells in female mammals have one active X-chromosome and one inactive X-chromosome (described in Section 12.7.1). Mixed populations of Kx+ and Kx− red cells, or of red cells with strong and weak Kell antigen expression, have been recognized in many female carriers of genes responsible for the McLeod phenotype or of *XK* gene deletions [117,236,239,261]. The proportion of McLeod phenotype red cells in female McLeod carriers usually varies from 5% to 85% [7]. This dual population of red cells is often difficult to detect serologically, especially if Kell antibodies and not anti-Kx are used, but flow cytometry permits an accurate estimation of the two red cell populations [7,262].

The only female with MLS [237] was found to be heterozygous for a single basepair deletion in exon 2 of *XK* [249] (Table 7.5). Her severe neurological and muscular defects and weakening of her Kell antigens were attributed to extreme skewing of inactivation of her X-chromosome carrying the normal *XK* gene.

7.14.5 Anti-Kx and -Km (-KEL20)

A 5-year-old boy afflicted with recurrent infections (later presumed to be CGD), the second example of the McLeod phenotype, suffered a haemolytic transfusion reaction caused by anti-KL. The antibody reacted with all cells tested, except for his own and those of Mr McLeod [263]. The term anti-KL was shown to represent two separable antibodies, anti-Kx and -Km [157,263,264]. Anti-Kx reacts strongly with K_o cells, weakly with red cells of common Kell phenotype, and not at all with McLeod phenotype cells [157] (Table 7.6). Adsorption of 'anti-KL' serum with K_o cells removes anti-Kx and isolates anti-Km. The anti-Kx can be recovered by elution. Unfortunately, the separation of anti-Kx from anti-Km is often difficult to achieve

Table 7.6 Expression of Kx, Km, and Ku on red cells of common, K_o, McLeod, and K_{mod} phenotypes.

Phenotype	Kx	Km	Ku*
Common	Weak	Strong	Strong
K_o	Strong	Negative	Negative
McLeod	Negative	Negative	Weak
K_{mod}	Strong	Not tested	Weak

*Ku represents all high frequency Kell antigens.

and sera containing these antibodies are in very short supply. Anti-Km reacts with red cells of common Kell phenotype, but not with K_o or McLeod phenotype red cells [157] (Table 7.6). Km is probably a discontinuous antigen, the product of interaction between Kell glycoprotein and Kx protein for expression. Although Km has been numbered KEL20, it could belong to the Kx system.

Anti-Kx+-Km is the typical immune response of McLeod phenotype CGD patients following transfusion [157,263,265], and has been responsible for a haemolytic transfusion reaction [239,263]. An untransfused McLeod phenotype CGD patient made anti-Km during septic shock [266]. Two transfused McLeod individuals without CGD made anti-Km, but no anti-Kx [267,268]. When one of these patients required further transfusion, a monocyte monolayer assay was strongly positive and no radiolabelled red cells of common Kell phenotype survived, *in vivo*, 24 h after injection. Consequently, the patient received four units of K_o and one unit of K_{mod} blood. The transfusion was successful and, despite receiving strongly Kx-positive red cells, the patient did not make anti-Kx [268]. A man with severe MLS made anti-Kx following transfusion of four units for gastrointestinal haemorrhage [252]. Whether the molecular background to MLS affects the immune response is not clear.

An IgG autoanti-Kx in a man with common Kell phenotype did not cause haemolysis of his own or transfused Kx+ cells [269].

References

1   Coombs RRA, Mourant AE, Race RR. *In-vivo* isosensitisation of red cells in babies with haemolytic disease. *Lancet* 1946;i:264–6.
2   Allen FH, Lewis SJ, Fudenberg H. Studies of anti-Kp^b, a new antibody in the Kell blood group system. *Vox Sang* 1958;3:1–13.

3 Allen FH, Rosenfield RE. Notation for the Kell blood-group system. *Transfusion* 1961;1:305–7.

4 Redman CM, Avellino G, Pfeffer SR *et al*. Kell blood group antigens are part of a 93 000-Dalton red cell membrane protein. *J Biol Chem* 1986;261:9521–5.

5 Redman CM, Marsh WL, Mueller KA, Avellino GP, Johnson CL. Isolation of Kell-active protein from the red cell membrane. *Transfusion* 1984;24:176–7.

6 Wallas C, Simon R, Sharpe MA, Byler C. Isolation of a Kell-reactive protein from red cell membranes. *Transfusion* 1986;26:173–6.

7 Marsh WL, Redman CM. Recent developments in the Kell blood group system. *Transfus Med Rev* 1987;1:4–20.

8 Carbonnet F, Hattab C, Cartron J-P, Bertrand O. Kell and Kx, two disulphide-linked proteins of the human erythrocyte membrane are phosphorylated *in vivo*. *Biochem Biophys Res Commun* 1998;247:569–75.

9 Carbonnet F, Hattab C, Callebaut I *et al*. Kx, a quantitatively minor protein from human erythrocytes, is palmitoylated *in vivo*. *Biochem Biophys Res Commun* 1998;250:569–74.

10 Marsh WL, Redman CM. The Kell blood group system: a review. *Transfusion* 1990;30:158–67.

11 Pehta JC, Valinsky J, Redman C, Marsh WL. Biochemical and flow cytometric analysis of the second example of anti-K18 [Abstract]. *Joint Congr Int Soc Blood Transfus and Am Assoc Blood Banks* 1990:57.

12 Jaber A, Blanchard D, Goossens D *et al*. Characterization of the blood group Kell (K1) antigen with a human monoclonal antibody. *Blood* 1989;73:1597–602.

13 Petty AC, Daniels GL, Tippett P. Application of the MAIEA assay to the Kell blood group system. *Vox Sang* 1994;66:216–24.

14 Jones J, Reid ME, Oyen R *et al*. A novel common Kell antigen, TOU, and its spatial relationship to other Kell antigens. *Vox Sang* 1995;69:53–60.

15 Jongerius JM, Daniels GL, Overbeeke MAM *et al*. A new low-incidence antigen in the Kell blood group system: VLAN (KEL25). *Vox Sang* 1996;71:43–7.

16 Jaber A, Loirat M-J, Willem C *et al*. Characterization of murine monoclonal antibodies directed against the Kell blood group glycoprotein. *Br J Haematol* 1991;79:311–15.

17 Lee S, Zambas ED, Marsh WL, Redman CM. Molecular cloning and primary structure of Kell blood group protein. *Proc Natl Acad Sci USA* 1991;88:6353–7.

18 Khamlichi S, Bailly P, Blanchard D *et al*. Purification and partial characterization of the erythrocyte Kx protein deficient in McLeod patients. *Eur J Biochem* 1995;228:931–4.

19 Russo D, Redman C, Lee S. Association of XK and Kell blood group proteins. *J Biol Chem* 1998;273:13950–6.

20 Lee S, Zambas E, Green ED, Redman C. Organization of the gene encoding the human Kell blood group protein. *Blood* 1995;85:1364–70.

21 Camara-Clayette V, Rahuel C, Lopez C *et al*. Transcriptional regulation of the *KEL* gene and Kell protein expression in erythroid and non-erythroid cells. *Biochem J* 2001;356:171–80.

22 Race RR. A summary of present knowledge of human blood-groups, with special reference to serological incompatibility as a cause of congenital disease. *Br Med Bull* 1946;4:188–93.

23 Levine P, Backer M, Wigod M, Ponder R. A new human hereditary blood property (Cellano) present in 99.8% of all bloods. *Science* 1949;109:464–6.

24 Sanger R, Bertinshaw D, Lawler SD, Race RR. Les groupes sanguins humains Kell: fréquences géniques et recherches génétiques. *Rev Hémat* 1949;4:32–5.

25 Race RR, Sanger R. *Blood Groups in Man*, 6th edn. Oxford: Blackwell Scientific Publications, 1975.

26 Lewis M, Chown B, Kaita H. Inheritance of blood group antigens in a largely Eskimo population sample. *Am J Hum Genet* 1963;15:203–8.

27 Lewis M, Kaita H, Chown B. The inheritance of the Kell blood groups in a Caucasian population sample. *Vox Sang* 1969;17:221–3.

28 Toivanen P, Hirvonen T. Antigens Duffy, Kell, Kidd, Lutheran and Xg^a on fetal red cells. *Vox Sang* 1973;24:372–6.

29 Mourant AE, Kopec AC, Domaniewska-Sobczak K. *The Distribution of the Human Blood Groups and Other Polymorphisms*, 2nd edn. London: Oxford University Press, 1976.

30 Garretta M, Gener J, Muller A. Analyse de 280 000 déterminations du facteur Kell sur les équipements Groupamatic. *Rev Franc Transfus Immuno-Hémat* 1978;21:379–86.

31 Furuhjelm U, Nevanlinna HR, Nurkka R *et al*. The blood group antigen Ul^a (Karhula). *Vox Sang* 1968;15:118–24.

32 Stroup M, MacIlroy M, Walker R, Aydelotte JV. Evidence that Sutter belongs to the Kell blood group system. *Transfusion* 1965;5:309–14.

33 Hamilton HB, Nakahara Y. The rare Kell blood group phenotype K^o in a Japanese family. *Vox Sang* 1971;20:24–8.

34 Allen FH, Lewis SJ. Kp^a (Penney), a new antigen in the Kell blood group system. *Vox Sang* 1957;2:81–7.

35 Dichupa PJ, Anderson C, Chown B. A further search for hypothetic K^p of the Kell-system. *Vox Sang* 1969;17:1–4.

36 Chown B, Lewis M, Kaita H, Philipps S. Some blood group frequencies in a Caucasian population. *Vox Sang* 1963;8:378–81.

37 Kikuchi M, Endo N, Seno T, Okubo Y, Yamaguchi H. A Japanese family with two Kp(a–b–c+) members, presumed genotype Kp^c/K^o. *Transfusion* 1983;23:254–5.

38 Giblett ER, Chase J. Js^a, a 'new' red-cell antigen found in Negroes; evidence for an eleventh blood group system. *Br J Haematol* 1959;5:319–26.

39 Jarkowski TL, Hinshaw CP, Beattie KM, Silberberg B. Another example of anti-Js^a. *Transfusion* 1962;2:423–4.

40 Spielmann W, Teixidor D, Renninger W, Matznetter T. Blutgruppen und Lepra bei moçambiquanischen Völkerschaften. *Humangenetik* 1970;10:304–17.

41 Okubo Y, Yamaguchi H, Seno T *et al*. The first example of anti-Ul^a and Ul (a+) red cells found in Japan. *Transfusion* 1986;26:215.

42 Strange JJ, Kenworthy RJ, Webb AJ, Giles CM. Wk^a (Weeks), a new antigen in the Kell blood group system. *Vox Sang* 1974;27:81–6.

43 Ball M, Cant B, Garwood P *et al*. Evaluation of a murine monoclonal anti-k (BS45). *Biotest Bull* 1989;4:15–18.

44 Gale SA, Rowe GP, Northfield FE. Application of a microtitre plate antiglobulin technique to determine the incidence of donors lacking high frequency antigens. *Vox Sang* 1988;54:172–3.

45 Lee S, Wu X, Reid M, Zelinski T, Redman C. Molecular basis of the Kell (K1) phenotype. *Blood* 1995; 85:912–16.

46 Lee S. Molecular basis of Kell blood group phenotypes. *Vox Sang* 1997;73:1–11 and *Vox Sang* 1998; 74:58.

47 Yazdanbakhsh K, Lee S, Lu Q, Reid ME. Identification in a defect in the intracellular trafficking of a Kell blood group variant. *Blood* 1999;94:310–18.

48 Murphy MY, Fraser RH, Goddard JP. Development of a PCR-based diagnostic assay for the determination of *KEL* genotype in donor blood samples. *Transfus Med* 1996;6:133–7.

49 Lee SH, Bennett PR, Overton T *et al*. Prenatal diagnosis of Kell blood group genotypes: *KEL1* and *KEL2*. *Am J Obstet Gynecol* 1996;175:455–9.

50 Hessner MJ, McFarland JG, Endean DJ. Genotyping of *KEL1* and *KEL2* of the human Kell gene blood group system by the polymerase chain reaction with sequence-specific primers. *Transfusion* 1996;36: 495–9.

51 Avent ND, Martin PG. Kell typing by allele-specific PCR (ASP). *Br J Haematol* 1996;93:728–30.

52 Hughes-Jones NC, Gardner B. The Kell system studied with radioactively-labelled anti-K. *Vox Sang* 1971; 21:154–8.

53 Parsons SF, Gardner B, Anstee DJ. Monoclonal antibodies against Kell glycoprotein: serology, immunochemistry and quantitation of antigen sites. *Transfus Med* 1993;3:137–42.

54 McDowell MA, Mann JM, Milakovic K. Kell-like antibody in a Kell positive patient [Abstract]. *Transfusion* 1978;18:389.

55 Skradski K, Reid ME, Mount M *et al*. A novel variant of the human blood group K1 antigen. *Vox Sang* 1994;66:68–71.

56 Kline WE, Sullivan CM, Bowman RJ. A rare example of weakened expression of the Kell (K1) antigen. *Vox Sang* 1984;47:170–3.

57 Uchikawa M, Onodera T, Tsuneyama H *et al*. Molecular basis of unusual K$_{mod}$ phenotype with K+^{w}k– [Abstract]. *Vox Sang* 2000;78(Suppl.1):O011.

58 Marsh WL, Schnipper EF, Johnson CL, Mueller KA, Schwartz SA. An individual with McLeod syndrome and the Kell blood group antigen K (K1). *Transfusion* 1983;23:336–8.

59 Muller A, André-Liardet J, Garretta M, Brocteur J, Moullec J. Observations sur un anticorps rare. l'anti-Gerbich. *Rev Franc Transfus* 1973;16:251–7.

60 McGinniss MH, MacLowry JD, Holland PV. Acquisition of K:1-like antigen during terminal sepsis. *Transfusion* 1984;24:28–30.

61 Mollison PL, Engelfriet CP, Contreras M. *Blood Transfusion in Clinical Medicine*, 10th edn. Oxford: Blackwell Science, 1997.

62 Giblett ER. A critique of the thoretical hazard of inter vs. intra-racial transfusion. *Transfusion* 1961;1: 233–8.

63 Marsh WL, Mueller KA, Johnson CL. Use of AET-treated cells in the investigation of Kell related autoimmunity [Abstract]. *Transfusion* 1982;22:419.

64 Hardman JT, Beck ML. Hemagglutination in capillaries: correlation with blood group specificity and IgG subclass. *Transfusion* 1981;21:343–6.

65 Molthan L, Strohm PL. Hemolytic transfusion reaction due to anti-Kell undetectable in low-ionic-strength solutions. *Am J Clin Pathol* 1981;75:629–31.

66 Voak D, Downie M, Haigh T, Cook N. Improved antiglobulin tests to detect difficult antibodies: detection of anti-Kell by LISS. *Med Lab Sci* 1982;39: 363–70.

67 Merry AH, Thomson EE, Lagar J *et al*. Quantitation of antibody binding to erythrocytes in LISS. *Vox Sang* 1984;47:125–32.

68 West NC, Jenkins JA, Johnston BR, Modi N. Interdonor incompatibility due to anti-Kell antibody undetectable by automated antibody screening. *Vox Sang* 1986;50:174–6.

69 Schultz MH. Serology and clinical significance of Kell blood group system antibodies. In: B Laird-Fryer, G Daniels, J Levitt, eds. *Blood Group Systems: Kell*. Arlington: American Association of Blood Banks, 1990: 37–68.

70 Ottensooser F, Mellone O, Biancalana A. Fatal transfusion reaction due to the Kell factor. *Blood* 1953;8: 1029–33.

71 Zettner A, Bove JR. Hemolytic transfusion reaction due to interdonor incompatibility. *Transfusion* 1963; 3:48–51.

72 Reiner AP, Sayers MH. Hemolytic transfusion reaction due to interdonor Kell incompatibility. *Arch Pathol Lab Med* 1990;114:862–4.

73 Caine ME, Mueller-Heubach E. Kell sensitization in pregnancy. *Am J Obstet Gynecol* 1986;154:85–90.

74 Leggat HM, Gibson JM, Barron SL, Reid MM. Anti-Kell in pregnancy. *Br J Obstet Gynecol* 1991; 98:162–5.

75 McKenna DS, Nagaraja HN, O'Shaughnessy R. Management of pregnancies complicated by anti-Kell isoimmunization. *Obstet Gynecol* 1999;93: 667–73.

76 Grant SR, Kilby MD, Meer *et al*. The outcome of pregnancy in Kell alloimmunisation. *Br J Obstet Gynecol* 2000;107:481–5.

77 Vaughan JI, Warwick R, Letsky E *et al*. Erythropoietic suppression in fetal anemia because of Kell alloimmunization. *Am J Obstet Gynecol* 1994;171:247–52.

78 Weiner CP, Widness JA. Decreased fetal erythropoiesis and hemolysis in Kell hemolytic anemia. *Am J Obstet Gynecol* 1996;174:547–51.

79 Southcott MJG, Tanner MJA, Anstee DJ. The expression of human blood group antigens during erythropoiesis in a cell culture system. *Blood* 1999;93: 4425–35.

80 Bony V, Gane P, Bailly P, Cartron J-P. Time-course expression of polypeptides carrying blood group antigens during human erythroid differentiation. *Br J Haematol* 1999;107:263–74.

81 Daniels G, Green C. Expression of red cell surface antigens during erythropoiesis. *Vox Sang* 2000; 78(Suppl.1):149–53.

82 Vaughan JI, Manning M, Warwick RM *et al*. Inhibition of erythroid progenitor cells by anti-Kell antibodies in fetal alloimmune anemia. *N Engl J Med* 1998;338:798–803.

83 Daniels GL, Hadley AG, Green CA. Fetal anaemia due to anti-K may result from immune destruction of early erythroid progenitors [Abstract]. *Transfus Med* 1999;9(Suppl.):16.

84 Wagner T, Berer A, Lanzer G, Geissler K. Kell is not restricted to erythropoietic lineage but is also expressed on myeloid progenitor cells. *Br J Haematol* 2000; 110:409–11.

85 Wagner T, Bernaschek G, Geissler K. Inhibition of megakaryopoiesis by Kell-related antibodies. *N Engl J Med* 2000;343:72.

86 Morgan P, Bossom EL. 'Naturally occurring' anti-Kell (K1): two examples. *Transfusion* 1963;3:397–8.

87 Clark A, Monaghan WP, Martin CA. Two additional examples of non-transfusion-stimulated anti-Kell. *Am J Med Tech* 1981;47:983–4.

88 Marsh WL, Nichols ME, Øyen R *et al*. Naturally occurring anti-Kell stimulated by *E. Coli* enterocolitis in a 20-day-old child. *Transfusion* 1978;18:149–54.

89 Savalonis JM, Kalish RI, Cummings EA, Ryan RW, Aloisi R. Kell blood group activity of gram-negative bacteria. *Transfusion* 1988;28:229–32.

90 Judd WJ, Walter WJ, Steiner EA. Clinical and laboratory findings on two patients with naturally occurring anti-Kell agglutinins. *Transfusion* 1981;21:184–8.

91 Tegoli J, Sausais L, Issitt PD. Another example of a 'naturally-occurring' anti-K1. *Vox Sang* 1967;12: 305–7.

92 Kanel GC, Davis I, Bowman JE. 'Naturally-occurring' anti–K1: possible association with mycobacterium infection. *Transfusion* 1978;18:472–3.

93 Doelman CJA, Westermann WF, van Voorst tot Voorst E, Miedema K. An anti-K apparently induced by *Enterococcus faecalis* in a 30-year-old man. *Transfusion* 1992;32:790.

94 Pereira A, Monteagudo J, Rovira M *et al*. Anti-K1 of the IgA class associated with *Morganella morganii* infection. *Transfusion* 1989;29:549–51.

95 Garratty G, Sattler MS, Petz LD, Flannery EP. Immune hemolytic anemia associated with anti-Kell and a carrier state for chronic granulomatous disease. *Rev Franc Transfus Immuno-Hémat* 1979;22:529–49.

96 Hare V, Wilson MJ, Wilkinson S, Issitt PD. A Kell system antibody with highly unusual characteristics [Abstract]. *Transfusion* 1981;21:613.

97 Viggiano E, Clary NL, Ballas SK. Autoanti-K antibody mimicking an alloantibody. *Transfusion* 1982;22: 329–32.

98 Tearina Chu T-H, Halverson GR, Yazdanbakhsh K, Øyen R, Reid ME. A DNA-based immunization protocol to produce monoclonal antibodies to blood group antigens. *Br J Haematol* 2001;113:32–6.

99 Goossens D, Champomier F, Rouger P, Salmon C. Human monoclonal antibodies against blood group antigens: preparation of a series of stable EBV immortalized B clones producing high levels of antibody of different isotypes and specificities. *J Immunol Methods* 1987;101:193–200.

100 Paire-Dante J, Martel F, Montcharmont P, Vignal M, Rigal D. Generation of a human lymphoblastoid cell line producing anti-Kell monoclonal antibodies. In: P Rouger, C Salmon, eds. *Monoclonal Antibodies Against Human Red Blood Cells and Related Antigens*. Paris: Arnette, 1989:293–5.

101 Daniels G, ed. Third International Workshop on Monoclonal Antibodies Against Human Red Blood Cell and Related Antigens. *Transfus Clin Biol* 1997;4:99–114 (4 papers).

102 Kluge A, Jungfer H. Anti-K2 (Cellano) blood group antibodies: typing as IgG and IgA with a review of their clinical significance. *Blut* 1970;21:357–65.

103 Thomas MJ, Konugres AA. An anti-K2 (Cellano) serum with unusual properties. *Vox Sang* 1966;11: 227–9.

104 Dinning G, Doughty RW, Collins AK. A further exam-

ple of IgM anti-K2 (Cellano). *Vox Sang* 1985;48: 317–18.

105 Mullis NC, Harris DF, Roberts C *et al*. Intravascular hemolysis caused by anti-K2 [Abstract]. *Transfusion* 1999;39(Suppl.):47S.

106 Bowman JM, Harman FA, Manning CR, Pollock JM. Erythroblastosis fetalis produced by anti-k. *Vox Sang* 1989;56:187–189 and *Vox Sang* 1990;58:139.

107 Nichols ME, Rosenfield RE, Rubenstein P. Monoclonal anti-K14 and anti-K2. *Vox Sang* 1987;52:231–5.

108 Chester MA, Johnson U, Lundblad A *et al*. *Proceedings of the 2nd International Workshop on Monoclonal Antibodies Against Human Red Blood Cell and Related Antigens* 1990:126–138.

109 Rouger P, Anstee D, Salmon C, eds. First International Workshop on Monoclonal Antibodies Against Human Red Blood Cell and Related Antigens. *Rev Franc Transfus Immuno-Hémat* 1988;31:381–418.

110 Inglis G, Fraser RH, McTaggart S *et al*. Monoclonal antibodies to high incidence Kell epitopes: characterization and application in automated screening of donor samples. *Transfus Med* 1994;4:209–12.

111 Lewis M, Kaita H, Duncan D, Chown B. Failure to find hypothetic K^a (KKp^a) of the Kell blood group system. *Vox Sang* 1960;5:565–7.

112 Wright J, Cornwall SM, Matsina E. A second example of hemolytic disease of the newborn due to anti-Kp^b. *Vox Sang* 1965;10:218–21.

113 Yamaguchi H, Okubo Y, Seno T, Matsushita K, Daniels GL. A 'new' allele, *Kp^c*, at the *Kell* complex locus. *Vox Sang* 1979;36:29–30.

114 Gavin J, Daniels GL, Yamaguchi H, Okubo Y, Seno T. The red cell antigen once called Levay is the antigen Kp^c of the Kell system. *Vox Sang* 1979;36:31–3.

115 Callender S, Race RR, Paykoc ZV. Hypersensitivity to transfused blood. *Br Med J* 1945;ii:83.

116 Callender ST, Race RR. A serological and genetical study of multiple antibodies formed in response to blood transfusion by a patient with lupus erythematosus diffusus. *Ann Eugen* 1946;13:102–17.

117 Daniels GL. *Blood group antigens of high frequency: a serological and genetical study*. PhD thesis, University of London, 1980.

118 Lee S, Wu X, Son S *et al*. Point mutations characterize *KEL10*, the *KEL3*, *KEL4*, and *KEL21* alleles, and the *KEL17* and *KEL11* alleles. *Transfusion* 1996;36:490–4.

119 Daniels GL, Weinauer F, Stone C *et al*. A combination of effects of rare genotypes at the *XK* and *KEL* blood group loci results in absence of Kell system antigens from the red blood cells. *Blood* 1996;88:4045–50.

120 Costamagna L, Barbarini M, Viarengo GL *et al*. A case of hemolytic disease of the newborn due to anti-Kp^a. *Immunohematology* 1997;13:61–2.

121 Smoleniek J, Anderson N, Poole GD. Hydrops fetalis caused by anti-Kp^a, an antibody not usually detected in routine screening [Abstract]. *Transfus Med* 1994;4(Suppl.1):48.

122 Dacus JV, Spinnato JA. Severe erythroblastosis fetalis secondary to anti-Kp^b sensitization. *Am J Obstet Gynecol* 1984;150:888–9.

123 Gorlin JB, Kelly L. Alloimmunisation via previous transfusion places female Kp^b-negative recipients at risk for having children with clinically significant hemolytic disease of the newborn. *Vox Sang* 1994;66:46–8.

124 Wren MR, Issitt PD. The monocyte monolayer assay and *in vivo* antibody activity [Abstract]. *Transfusion* 1986;26:548.

125 Eby CS, Cowan JL, Ramos RR, Chaplin H. *In-vivo* and *in-vitro* studies of anti-Kp^b allo-antibody [Abstract]. *Joint Congr Int Soc Blood Transfus and Am Assoc Blood Banks* 1990:156.

126 Kohan AI, Reybaud JF, Salamone HJ *et al*. Management of a severe transfusional problem in a patient with alloantibody to Kp^b (K4). *Vox Sang* 1990; 59:216–17.

127 Watt JM, Chatfield SY, Moffitt P. Transfusion against anti-Kp^b [Abstract]. *Transfus Med* 1992;2:171.

128 Mazzara R, Lozano M, Salmerón JM *et al*. Transfusion of incompatible RBCs to a patient with alloanti-Kp^b. *Transfusion* 2001;41:611–4.

129 Seyfried H, Górska B, Maj S *et al*. Apparent depression of antigens of the Kell blood group system associated with autoimmune acquired haemolytic anaemia. *Vox Sang* 1972;23:528–36.

130 Win N, Kaye T, Mir N, Damain-Willems C, Chatfield C. Autoimmune haemolytic anaemia in infancy with anti-Kp^b specificity. *Vox Sang* 1996;71:187–8.

131 Hughes-Jones NC, Gorick BD, Bye JM *et al*. Characterization of human blood group scFv antibodies derived from a V gene phage-display library. *Br J Haematol* 1994;88:180–6.

132 Giblett ER. Js, a 'new' blood group antigen found in Negroes. *Nature* 1958;181:1221–2.

133 Walker RH, Argall CI, Steane EA, Sasaki TT, Greenwalt TJ. Anti-Js^b, the expected antithetical antibody of the Sutter blood group system. *Nature* 1963;197:295–6.

134 Walker RH, Argall CI, Steane EA, Sasaki TT, Greenwalt TJ. Js^b of the Sutter blood group system. *Transfusion* 1963;3:94–9.

135 Morton NE, Krieger H, Steinberg AG, Rosenfield RE. Genetic evidence confirming the localization of Sutter in the Kell blood-group system. *Vox Sang* 1965; 10:608–13.

136 Ito K, Mukumoto Y, Konishi H. An example of 'naturally occurring' anti-Js^a (K6) in a Japanese female. *Vox Sang* 1979;37:350–1.

137 Beattie KM, Shafer AW, Sigmund K, Cisco S. Mass screening of American Black donors to identify high

incidence antigen-negative bloods [Abstract]. *19th Congr Int Soc Blood Transfus* 1986:312.

138 Lee S, Wu X, Reid M, Redman C. Molecular basis of the K:6,−7 [Js(a+b−)] phenotype in the Kell blood groups system. *Transfusion* 1995;35:822−5.

139 Donovan LM, Tripp KL, Zuckerman JE, Konugres AA. Hemolytic disease of the newborn due to anti-Js^a. *Transfusion* 1973;13:153.

140 Levene C, Rudolphson Y, Shechter Y. A second case of hemolytic disease of the newborn due to anti-Js^a. *Transfusion* 1980;20:714−15.

141 Taddie SJ, Barrasso C, Ness PM. A delayed transfusion reaction caused by anti-K6. *Transfusion* 1982;22:68−9.

142 Anderson RR, Sosler SD, Kovach J, DeChristopher PJ. Delayed hemolytic transfusion reaction due to anti-Js^a in an alloimmunized patient with a sickle cell syndrome. *Am J Clin Pathol* 1997;108:658−61.

143 Lowe RF, Musengezi AT, Moores P. Severe hemolytic disease of the newborn associated with anti-Js^b. *Transfusion* 1978;18:466−8.

144 Purohit DM, Taylor HL, Spivey MA. Hemolytic disease of the newborn due to anti-Js^b. *Am J Obstet Gynecol* 1978;131:755−6.

145 Ratcliff D, Fiorenza S, Culotta E, Arndt P, Garratty G. Hydrops fetalis (HF) and a material hemolytic transfusion reaction associated with anti-Js^b. [Abstract]. *Transfusion* 1987;27:534.

146 Gordon MC, Kennedy MS, O'Shaughnessy RW, Waheed A. Severe hemolytic disease of the newborn due to anti-Js^b. *Vox Sang* 1995;69:140−1.

147 Waheed A, Kennedy MS. Delayed hemolytic transfusion reaction caused by anti-Js^b in a Js(a+b+) patient. *Transfusion* 1982;22:161−2.

148 Eveland D. Autoanti-Js^b enhanced by polyethylene glycol [Abstract]. *Joint Congr Int Soc Blood Transfus and Am Assoc Blood Banks* 1990: 156.

149 Chu T-HT, Yazdanbakhsh K, Øyen R, Smart E, Reid ME. Production and characterization of anti-Kell monoclonal antibodies using transfected cells as the immunogen. *Br J Haematol* 1999;106:817−23.

150 Furuhjelm U, Nevanlinna HR, Nurkka R, Gavin J, Sanger R. Evidence that the antigen Ul^a is controlled from the Kell complex locus. *Vox Sang* 1969;16:496−9.

151 Sakuma K, Suzuki H, Ohto H, Tsuneyama H, Uchikawa M. First case of hemolytic disease of the newborn due to anti-Ul^a antibodies. *Vox Sang* 1994;66:293−4.

152 Chown B, Lewis M, Kaita K. A 'new' Kell blood-group phenotype. *Nature* 1957;180:711.

153 Kaita H, Lewis M, Chown B, Gard E. A further example of the Kell blood group phenotype K−,k−,Kp(a−b−). *Nature* 1959;183:1586.

154 Chown B, Lewis M, Kaita H, Nevanlinna HR, Soltan HC. The pedigrees of two people already reported as of

phenotype K−, k−, Kp(a−b−). *Vox Sang* 1961;6:620−3.

155 Yu L-C, Twu Y-C, Chang C-Y, Lin M. Molecular basis of the Kell-null phenotype: a mutation at the splice site of human *KEL* gene abolishes the expression of Kell blood group antigens. *J Biol Chem* 2001;276:10247−52.

156 Lee S, Russo DCW, Reiner AP *et al.* Molecular defects underlying the Kell null phenotype. *J Biol Chem* 2001;276:27281−9.

157 Marsh WL, Øyen R, Nichols ME, Allen FH. Chronic granulomatous disease and the Kell blood groups. *Br J Haematol* 1975;29:247−62.

158 Carbonnet F, Hattab C, Collec E *et al.* Immunochemical analysis of the Kx protein from human red cells of different Kell phenotypes using antibodies raised against synthetic peptides. *Br J Haematol* 1997;96:857−63.

159 Marsh WL, Øyen R, Nichols ME. Kx antigen, the McLeod phenotype, and chronic granulomatous disease: further studies. *Vox Sang* 1976;31:356−62.

160 Corcoran PA, Allen FH, Lewis M, Chown B. A new antibody, anti-Ku (anti-Peltz), in the Kell blood group system. *Transfusion* 1961;1:181−3.

161 Nunn HD, Giles CM, Dormandy KM. A second example of anti-Ku in a patient who has the rare Kell phenotype, K^o. *Vox Sang* 1966;11:611−19.

162 Parsons SF, Judson PA, Anstee DJ. BRIC 18: a monoclonal antibody with a specificity related to the Kell blood group system. *J Immunogenet* 1982;9:377−80.

163 Guévin RM, Taliano V, Waldmann O. The Côté serum (anti-K11), an antibody defining a new variant in the Kell system. *Vox Sang* 1976;31(Suppl.1):96−100.

164 Sabo B, McCreary J, Gellerman M *et al.* Confirmation of K^{11} and K^{17} as alleles in the Kell blood group system. *Vox Sang* 1975;29:450−5.

165 Kelley CM, Karwal MW, Schlueter AJ, Olson JD. Outcome of transfusion of K:11 erythrocytes in a patient with anti-K11 antibody. *Vox Sang* 1998;74:205−8.

166 Heistø H, Guévin R-M, Taliano V *et al.* Three further antigen-antibody specificities associated with the Kell blood group system. *Vox Sang* 1973;24:179−80.

167 Marsh WL, Stroup M, Macilroy M *et al.* A new antibody, anti-K12, associated with the Kell blood group system. *Vox Sang* 1973;24:200−5.

168 Beattie KM, Heinz B, Korol S, Oyen R, Marsh WL. Anti-K12 in the serum of two brothers: inheritance of the K:−12 phenotype. *Rev Franc Transfus Immuno-Hémat* 1982;25:611−8.

169 Reid ME, Øyen R, Redman CM *et al.* K12 is located on the Kell blood group protein in proximity to K/k and Js^a/Jsb. *Vox Sang* 1995;68:40−5.

170 Taylor HL. Anti-K12 in a Black? *Transfusion* 1979;19:787−8.

171 Marsh WL, Jensen L, Øyen R *et al.* Anti-K13 and the K:−13 phenotype. *Vox Sang* 1974;26:34−40.

172 Marsh WL, DiNapoli J, Øyen R. Auto-immune hemolytic anemia caused by anti-K13. *Vox Sang* 1979;**36**:174–8.

173 Wallace ME, Bouysou C, de Jongh DS *et al*. Anti-K14: an antibody specificity associated with the Kell blood group system. *Vox Sang* 1976;**30**:300–4.

174 Frank S, Schmidt RP, Baugh M. Three new antibodies to high-incidence antigenic determinants (anti-E1, anti-Dp, and anti-So). *Transfusion* 1970;**10**:254–7.

175 Sabo B, McCreary J, Harris P. Anti-Dp is anti-K14. *Vox Sang* 1982;**43**:56.

176 Eicher C, Kirkley K, Porter M, Kao Y. A new low frequency antigen in the Kell system: K24 (Cls) [Abstract]. *Transfusion* 1985;**25**:448.

177 Lee S, Naime Reid M, Redman C. The *KEL24* and *KEL14* alleles of the Kell blood group system. *Transfusion* 1997;**37**:1035–8.

178 Uchikawa M, Onodera T, Tsuneyama H *et al*. Different point mutations in the same codon of KEL:–14 phenotype [Abstract]. *Transfusion* 1999;**39**(Suppl.): 50S.

179 Barrasso C, Eska P, Grindon AJ, Øyen R, Marsh WL. Anti-K18: an antibody defining another high-frequency antigen related to the Kell blood group system. *Vox Sang* 1975;**29**:124–7.

180 Barrasso C, Baldwin ML, Drew H, Ness PM. *In vivo* survival of K:18 red cells in a recipient with anti-K18. *Transfusion* 1983;**23**:258–9.

181 Sabo B, McCreary J, Stroup M, Smith DE, Weidner JG. Another Kell-related antibody, anti-K19. *Vox Sang* 1979;**36**:97–102.

182 Marsh WL, DiNapoli J, Øyen R *et al*. Delayed hemolytic transfusion reaction caused by the second example of anti-K19. *Transfusion* 1979;**19**:604–8.

183 Bar Shany S, Ben Porath D, Levene C, Sela R, Daniels GL. K22, a 'new' para-Kell antigen of high frequency. *Vox Sang* 1982;**42**:87–90.

184 Manny N, Levene C, Harel N *et al*. The second example of anti-K22 and a family genetically informative for *K* and *K22*. *Vox Sang* 1985;**49**:135–7.

185 Levene C, Sela R, DaCosta Y, Manny N. Clinical significant of anti-K22 [Abstract]. *20th Congr Int Soc Blood Transfus* 1988:295.

186 Marsh WL, Redman CM, Kessler LA *et al*. A low-incidence antigen in the Kell blood group system identified by biochemical characterization. *Transfusion* 1987;**27**:36–40.

187 Daniels GL, Petty A, Reid M *et al*. Demonstration by the MAIEA assay that a new red cell antigen belongs to the Kell blood group system. *Transfusion* 1994;**34**:818–20.

188 Petty AC, Green CA, Daniels GL. The monoclonal antibody-specific immobilisation of erythrocyte antigens assay (MAIEA) in the investigation of human red cell antigens and their associated membrane proteins. *Transfus Med* 1997;**7**:179–88.

189 Anstee DJ, Ridgwell K, Tanner MJA, Daniels GL, Parsons SF. Individuals lacking the Gerbich blood-group antigen have alterations in the human erythrocyte membrane sialoglycoproteins β and γ. *Biochem J* 1984;**221**:97–104.

190 Daniels GL, Shaw M-A, Judson PA *et al*. A family demonstrating inheritance of the Leach phenotype: a Gerbich-negative phenotype associated with elliptocytosis. *Vox Sang* 1986;**50**:117–21.

191 Walsh TJ, Daniels GL, Tippett P. A family with unusual Kell genotypes. *Forensic Sci Int* 1981;**18**:161–3.

192 Ford DS, Knight AE, Smith F. A further example of Kpª/Kº exhibiting depression of some Kell group antigens. *Vox Sang* 1977;**32**:220–3.

193 Tippett P. Some recent developments in the Kell and Lutheran systems. In: *Human Blood Groups, 5th Int Convoc Immunol, Buffalo NY*. Basel: Karger, 1977: 401–9.

194 Brown A, Berger R, Lasko D *et al*. The Day phenotype: a 'new' variant in the Kell blood group system. *Rev Franc Transfus Immuno-Hémat* 1982;**25**:619–27.

195 Peloquin P, Yochum G, Hagy L, Øyen R, Johnson C. The Mullins phenotype: another RBC phenotype characterized by weak Kell antigens [Abstract]. *Transfusion* 1988;**28**(Suppl.):19S.

196 Winkler MM, Beattie KM, Cisco SL *et al*. The K_{mod} blood group phenotype in a healthy individual. *Transfusion* 1989;**29**:642–5.

197 Pehta JC, Johnson CL, Giller RL, Gay A, Marsh WL. Evidence that K_{mod} is an inherited condition [Abstract]. *Transfusion* 1989;**29**(Suppl.):15S.

198 Byrne PC, Deck M, Oyen R *et al*. Serological and biochemical studies on a previously undescribed K_{mod} individual [Abstract]. *Transfusion* 1993;**33**(Suppl.):55S.

199 Poole J, Hustinx H, Rodriguez M. Kmod: incidence and inheritance [Abstract]. *Transfus Med* 1995; **5**(Suppl.1):28.

200 Norman PC, Daniels GL. Unusual suppression of Kell system antigens in a healthy blood donor. *Transfusion* 1988;**28**:460–2.

201 Beck ML, Marsh WL, Pierce SR *et al*. Auto-anti-Kpᵇ associated with weakened antigenicity in the Kell blood group system: a second example. *Transfusion* 1979;**19**:197–202.

202 Marsh WL, Øyen R, Alicea E, Linter M, Horton S. Autoimmune hemolytic anemia and the Kell blood groups. *Am J Hematol* 1979;**7**:155–62.

203 Manny N, Levene C, Sela R *et al*. Autoimmunity and the Kell blood groups: auto-anti-Kpᵇ in a Kp(a+b–) patient. *Vox Sang* 1983;**45**:252–6.

204 Puig N, Carbonell F, Marty ML. Another example of mimicking anti-Kpᵇ in a Kp(a+b–) patient. *Vox Sang* 1986;**51**:57–9.

205 Rowe GP, Tozzo GG, Poole J, Liew YW. The elucidation of a Kell-related autoantibody using ZZAP-treated red cells. *Immunohematology* 1989;**5**:79–82.

206 Vengelen-Tyler V, Gonzalez B, Garratty G *et al.* Acquired loss of red cell Kell antigens. *Br J Haematol* 1987;**65**:231–4.

207 Williamson LM, Poole J, Redman C *et al.* Transient loss of proteins carrying Kell and Lutheran red cell antigens during consecutive relapses of autoimmune thrombocytopenia. *Br J Haematol* 1994;**87**: 805–12.

208 Daniels G. Kell related antibodies. *Rev Franc Transfus Immuno-Hémat* 1988;**31**:395–405.

209 Judson PA, Anstee DJ. Comparative effect of trypsin and chymotrypsin on blood group antigens. *Med Lab Sci* 1977;**34**:1–6.

210 Branch DR, Muensch HA, Sy Siok Hian AL, Petz LD. Disulfide bonds are a requirement for Kell and Cartwright (Yt^a) bood group antigen integrity. *Br J Haematol* 1983;**54**:573–8.

211 Advani H, Zamor J, Judd WJ, Johnson CL, Marsh WL. Inactivation of Kell blood group antigens by 2-aminoethylisothiouronium bromide. *Br J Haematol* 1982;**51**:107–15.

212 Judd WJ. *Methods in Immunohematology.* Miami: Montgomery Scientific Publications, 1988.

213 Parsons SF, Judson PA, Spring FA, Mallinson G, Anstee DJ. Antibodies with specificities related to the Kell blood group system. *Rev Franc Transfus Immuno-Hémat* 1988;**31**:401–5.

214 McGinniss MH, Dean A. Expression of red cell antigens by K562 human leukemia cells before and after induction of hemoglobin synthesis by hemin. *Transfusion* 1985;**25**:105–9.

215 Russo D, Wu X, Redman CM, Lee S. Expression of Kell blood group protein in non-erythroid tissues. *Blood* 2000;**96**:340–6.

216 Redman CM, Lee S, Ten Bokkel Huinink D *et al.* Comparison of human and chimpanzee Kell blood group systems. *Transfusion* 1989;**29**:486–90.

217 Blancher A, Reid ME, Socha WW. Cross-reactivity of antibodies to human and primate red cell antigens. *Transfus Med Rev* 2000;**14**:161–79.

218 Lee S, Russo DCW, Pu J, Ho M, Redman CM. The mouse Kell blood group gene (*Kel*): cDNA sequence, genomic organization, expression, and enzymatic function. *Immunogenetics* 2000;**52**:53–62.

219 Turner AJ, Isaac RE, Coates D. The neprilysin (NEP) family of zinc metallopeptidases: genomics and function. *Bioessays* 2001;**23**:261–9.

220 Lee S, Lin M, Mele A *et al.* Proteolytic processing of big endothelin-3 by the Kell blood group protein. *Blood* 1999;**94**:1440–50.

221 Belhacène N, Maulon L, Guérin S *et al.* Differential expression of the Kell blood group and CD10 antigens: two related membrane metallopeptidases during differentiation of K562 cells by phorbol ester and hemin. *FASEB J* 1998;**12**:531–9.

222 Redman CM, Marsh WL, Scarborough A *et al.* Biochemical studies on McLeod phenotype red cells and isolation of Kx antigen. *Br J Haematol* 1988;**68**:131–6.

223 Ho M, Chelly J, Carter N *et al.* Isolation of the gene for McLeod syndrome that encodes a novel membrane transport protein. *Cell* 1994;**77**:869–80.

224 Amara SG, Kuhar MJ. Neurotransmitter transporters: recent progress. *Ann Rev Neurosci* 1993;**16**:73–93.

225 Stanfield GM, Horvitz HR. The *ced-8* gene controls the timing of programmed cell deaths in *C. elegans*. *Mol Cell* 2000;**5**:423–33.

226 Collec E, Colin Y, Carbonnet F *et al.* Structure and expression of the mouse homologue of the *XK* gene. *Immunogenetics* 1999;**50**:16–21.

227 Russo D, Lee S, Redman C. Intracellular assembly of Kell and XK blood group proteins. *Biochim Biophys Acta* 1999;**1461**:10–18.

228 Branch DR, Sy Siok Hian AL, Petz LD. Unmasking of Kx antigen by reduction of disulphide bonds on normal and McLeod red cells. *Br J Haematol* 1985;**59**:505–12.

229 Mastroberardino L, Spindler B, Pfeiffer R *et al.* Amino-acid transport by heterodimers of 4F2hc/CD98 and members of the permease family. *Nature* 1998;**395**:288–91.

230 Allen FH, Krabbe SMR, Corcoran PA. A new phenotype (McLeod) in the Kell blood-group system. *Vox Sang* 1961;**6**:555–60.

231 Swash M, Schwartz MS, Carter ND *et al.* Benign X-linked myopathy with acanthocytes (McLeod syndrome): its relationship to X-linked muscular dystrophy. *Brain* 1983;**106**:717–33.

232 Uchida K, Nakajima K, Shima H *et al.* The first example of the McLeod phenotype in a Japanese baby with chronic granulomatous disease. *Transfusion* 1992;**32**:691.

233 Hanaoka N, Yoshida K, Nakamura A *et al.* A novel frameshift mutation in the McLeod syndrome gene in a Japanese family. *J Neurol Sci* 1999;**165**:6–9.

234 Ueyama H, Kumamoto T, Nagao S *et al.* A novel mutation in the McLeod syndrome gene in a Japanese family. *J Neurol Sci* 2000;**176**:151–4.

235 Fikrig SM, Phillipp JCD, Smithwick EM, Øyen R, Marsh WL. Chronic granulomatous disease and McLeod syndrome in a Black child. *Pediatrics* 1980;**66**:403–4.

236 Wimer BM, Marsh WL, Taswell HF, Galey WR. Haematological changes associated with the McLeod phenotype of the Kell blood group system. *Br J Haematol* 1977;**36**:219–24.

237 Hardie RJ, Pullon HWH, Harding AE *et al.* Neuroacanthocytosis: a clinical, haematological and pathological study of 19 cases. *Brain* 1991;**114**: 13–49.

238 Ballas SK, Bator SM, Aubuchon JP *et al.* Abnormal

membrane physical properties of red cells in McLeod syndrome. *Transfusion* 1990;30:722–7.

239 Brzica SM, Rhodes KH, Pineda AA, Taswell HF. Chronic granulomatous disease and the McLeod phenotype: successful treatment of infection with granulocyte transfusions resulting in subsequent hemolytic transfusion reaction. *Mayo Clin Proc* 1977;52:153–6.

240 Danek A, Rubio JP, Rampoldi L *et al*. McLeod neuroacanthocytosis: genotype and phenotype. *Ann Neurol* 2001;50:755–64.

241 Jung HH, Hergersberg M, Kneifel S *et al*. McLeod syndrome: a novel mutation, predominant psychiatric manifestations, and distinct striatal imaging findings. *Ann Neurol* 2001;49:384–92.

242 Tang LL, Redman CM, Williams D, Marsh WL. Biochemical studies on McLeod phenotype erythrocytes. *Vox Sang* 1981;40:17–26.

243 Glaubensklee CS, Evan AP, Galey WR. Structural and biochemical analysis of the McLeod erythrocyte membrane. I. Freeze fracture and discontinuous polyacrylamide gel electrophoresis analysis. *Vox Sang* 1982;42:262–71.

244 Galey WR, Evan AP, Van Nice PS *et al*. Morphology and physiology of the McLeod erythrocyte. I. Scanning electron microscopy and electrolyte and water transport properties. *Vox Sang* 1978;34:152–61.

245 Kuypers FA, van Linde-Sibenius Trip M, Roelofsen B *et al*. The phospholipid organisation in the membranes of McLeod and Leach phenotype erythrocytes. *FEBS Lett* 1985;184:20–4.

246 Redman CM, Huima T, Robbins E, Lee S, Marsh WL. Effect of phosphatidylserine on the shape of McLeod red cell acanthocytes. *Blood* 1989;74:1826–35.

247 Singleton BK, Green CA, Renaud S *et al*. McLeod syndrome: a Swiss family with a novel exon deletion in the *XK* gene [Abstract]. *Transfus Med* 2000;10(Suppl.1):30.

248 Kawakami T, Takiyami Y, Sakoe K *et al*. A case of McLeod syndrome with unusually severe myopathy. *J Neurol Sci* 1999;166:36–9.

249 Ho MF, Chalmers RM, Davis MB, Harding AE, Monaco AP. A novel point mutation in the McLeod syndrome gene in neuroacanthocytosis. *Ann Neurol* 1996;39:672–5.

250 Dotti MT, Battisti C, Malandrini A *et al*. McLeod syndrome and neuroacanthocytosis with a novel mutation in the XK gene. *Mov Disord* 2000;15:1282–5.

251 Supple SG, Iland HJ, Barnett MH, Pollard JD. A spontaneous novel *XK* gene mutation in a patient with McLeod syndrome. *Br J Haemat* 2001;115:369–72.

252 Russo DC, Øyen R, Powell VI *et al*. First example of anti-Kx in a person with the McLeod phenotype and without chronic granulomatous disease. *Transfusion* 2000;40:1371–5.

253 Heyworth PG, Curnutte JT, Rae J *et al*. Hematologi-

254 Francke U, Ochs HD, de Martinville B *et al*. Minor Xp21 chromosome deletion in a male associated with expression of Duchenne muscular dystrophy, chronic granulomatous disease, retinitis pigmentosa, and McLeod syndrome. *Am J Hum Genet* 1985; 37:250–67.

255 Frey D, Mächler M, Seger R, Schmid W, Orkin SH. Gene deletion in a patient with chronic granulomatous disease and McLeod syndrome: fine mapping of the Xk gene locus. *Blood* 1988;71:252–5.

256 de Saint-Basile G, Bohler MC, Fischer A *et al*. Xp21 DNA microdeletion in a patient with chronic granulomatous disease, retinitis pigmentosa, and McLeod phenotype. *Hum Genet* 1988;80:85–9.

257 Bertelson CJ, Pogo AO, Chaudhuri A *et al*. Localization of the McLeod locus (XK) within XP21 by deletion analysis. *Am J Hum Genet* 1988;42:703–11.

258 Curnutte J, Bemiller L. Chronic granulomatous disease with McLeod phenotype: an uncommon occurrence [Abstract]. *Transfusion* 1995;35(Suppl.):60S.

259 El Nemer W, Colin Y, Collec E *et al*. Analysis of deletions in three McLeod patients: exclusion of the *XS* locus from the Xp21.1–Xp21.2 region. *Eur J Immunogenet* 2000;27:29–33.

260 Branch DR, Gaidulis L, Lazar GS. Human granulocytes lack red cell Kx antigen. *Br J Haematol* 1986;62:747–55.

261 Symmans WA, Shepherd CS, Marsh WL *et al*. Hereditary acanthocytosis associated with the McLeod phenotype of the Kell blood group system. *Br J Haematol* 1979;42:575–83.

262 Øyen R, Reid ME, Rubenstein P, Ralph H. A method to detect McLeod phenotype red blood cells. *Immunohematology* 1996;12:160–3.

263 van der Hart M, Szaloky A, van Loghem JJ. A 'new' antibody associated with the Kell blood group system. *Vox Sang* 1968;15:456–8.

264 Marsh WL. Letter. *Vox Sang* 1979;36:375–6.

265 Giblett ER, Klebanoff SJ, Pincus SH *et al*. Kell phenotypes in chronic granulomatous disease: a potential transfusion hazard. *Lancet* 1971;i:1235–6.

266 Carstairs K, Ruthledge Harding S, Lue K, Johnson CL, Marsh WL. Anti-K9 in an untransfused McLeod individual [Abstract]. *Transfusion* 1988;28(Suppl.):20S.

267 White W, Washington ED, Sabo BH *et al*. Anti-Km in a transfused man with McLeod syndrome. *Rev Franc Transfus Immuno-Hémat* 1980;23:305–17.

268 Sharp D, Rogers S, Dickstein B, Johnson C, Toy E. Successful transfusion of K$_o$ blood to a Km–Kx– patient with anti-Km [Abstract]. *Transfusion* 1988; 28(Suppl.):37S.

269 Sullivan CM, Kline WE, Rabin BI, Johnson CL, Marsh

WL. The first example of autoanti-Kx. *Transfusion* 1987;27:322–4.

270 Mifsud NA, Haddad AP, Sparrow RL, Condon JA. Use of the polymerase chain reaction-sequence specific oligonucleotide technique for the detection of the K1/K2 polymorphism of the Kell blood groups system. *Blood* 1997;89:4662–3.

271 Daniels GL. Studies on Gerbich negative phenotypes and Gerbich antibodies [Abstract]. *Transfusion* 1982;22:405.

272 Lee S, Reid ME, Redman CM. Point mutations in KEL exon 8 determine a high-incidence (RAZ) and a low-incidence (KEL25, VLAN) antigen of the Kell blood group system. *Vox Sang* 2001;81:259–63.

8 Duffy blood group system

8.1 Introduction

Fy^a and Fy^b are the products of alleles, which give rise to three phenotypes in white people: Fy(a+b–), Fy(a+b+), and Fy(a–b+). Another allele, Fy^x, produces a weak Fy^b antigen. In people of African origin the most common Duffy phenotype is Fy(a–b–), the result of homozygosity for an apparently silent gene, Fy. Fy(a–b–) is extremely rare in white people and other races.

Fy3, Fy5, and Fy6 are high frequency antigens in white and Mongoloid people, polymorphic in African Americans, and private antigens in parts of West Africa. Fy3 and Fy6 are expressed on red cells of all Duffy phenotypes apart from Fy(a–b–). Fy3 is defined by alloantibodies occasionally made by Fy(a–b–) individuals; Fy6 is defined by murine monoclonal antibodies. Fy5 resembles Fy3, but is not present on Fy:3 Rh$_{null}$ cells. The single example of anti-Fy4 behaved as if it detected a product of the Fy allele. The antigens of the Duffy system are listed in Table 8.1.

Duffy antigens are located on a glycoprotein of apparent M_r between 35 000 and 50 000, a chemokine receptor of the G protein-coupled family (Sections 8.2 and 8.7). Fy^a and Fy^b result from a Gly42Asp substitution within the Duffy glycoprotein (Section 8.3.2). Duffy glycoprotein is present on endothelial cells of postcapillary venules and on other cells throughout the body (Section 8.6).

The Fy(a–b–) phenotype in black people is caused by homozygosity for a mutation within an erythroid-specific, GATA-1, transcription-factor binding site upstream of the coding region of the Duffy gene (Section 8.4.1.1). This mutation prevents expression of the Duffy glycoprotein on red cells, but not on other cells.

Individuals with the Fy(a–b–) phenotype are resistant to infection by the malarial parasite *Plasmodium vivax*, and Fy(a–b–) red cells are refractory to invasion by *P. vivax in vitro*. Interaction between the Duffy glycoprotein and receptors on *P. vivax* merozoites are essential, but not sufficient, for red cell invasion (Section 8.8).

The Duffy (*FY*) locus is on chromosome 1q21–q25 (Chapter 32).

8.2 The Duffy glycoprotein and the gene that encodes it

Storage of red cells in saline for 2 weeks at 12°C results in a small loss of Fy^a, Fy^b, and Fy3 activity and substances with specific inhibitory activity for the appropriate Duffy antibodies can be detected in the saline [1]. By radioimmunoprecipitation, Moore *et al.* [2] found that Fy^a was associated with components of apparent M_r 39 500, 64 000, and 88 000. Immunoblotting with anti-Fy^a revealed a broad band with an intense region of apparent M_r 35 000–43 000 [3] or 40 000–50 000 [4]. Molecules electroeluted from the 35 000–43 000 region of the gel inhibited anti-Fy^a [3]. Immunoblotting with monoclonal anti-Fy6 produced a similar broad band [5,6].

Treatment of red cells with endo F, an *N*-glycanase that cleaves *N*-linked oligosaccharides, prior to solubilization and immunoblotting with anti-Fy^a, resulted in a dramatic reduction in apparent M_r and sharpening of the band on the blot [4]. Sialidase treatment of the red cells reduced the apparent M_r by about 4000 [3,4], and sialidase treatment of endo F-treated cells resulted in no alteration of electrophoretic mobility. Similar results were obtained by treatment of purified Duffy

Table 8.1 Antigens of the Duffy system.

No.	Name	Relative frequency		Comments
		White people	Black people	
FY1	Fy^a	Polymorphic	Polymorphic	Allelic to Fy^b (FY2), Gly42
FY2	Fy^b	Polymorphic	Polymorphic	Allelic to Fy^a (FY1), Asp42
FY3	Fy3	High	Polymorphic	Absent from Fy(a–b–) cells
FY4	Fy4	Low	Polymorphic	Possibly antithetical to Fy3
FY5	Fy5	High	Polymorphic	Absent from Fy(a–b–) and Rh$_{null}$ cells
FY6	Fy6	High	Polymorphic	Very similar to Fy3. Defined by monoclonal antibodies

glycoprotein or of tryptic peptide derived from it [6,7]. The Duffy glycoprotein therefore is N-glycosylated, but has no, or very little, O-glycosylation. Variation in the degree of N-glycosylation probably accounts for the range of molecular weight. The Duffy glycoprotein aggregates readily *in vitro* [3,8], and may exist in the membrane in a multimeric form [8].

Chaudhuri *et al.* [8] purified the Duffy glycoprotein following immunoprecipitation with monoclonal anti-Fy6. They isolated a protein of apparent M_r 36 000–46 000, together with its higher molecular weight oligomers, which reacted with anti-Fy6 on immunoblots. Several other proteins, which co-purified with the M_r 36 000–46 000 component, were not immunostained by anti-Fy6. Minor differences were detected on two-dimensional peptide maps between Duffy protein from Fy(a+b–) and Fy(a–b+) red cells.

From an internal peptide sequence obtained from purified Duffy glycoprotein, Chaudhuri *et al.* [9] constructed degenerate oligonucleotide primers and amplified, by polymerase chain reaction (PCR), a segment of cDNA derived from Fy(a–b+) individuals. This amplified product was then used to isolate cDNA clones from a human bone marrow library. An open reading frame of 1267 bp, predicting a 338 amino acid polypeptide of M_r 35 733, was identified. Hydropathy analysis suggested that the mature protein has seven membrane-spanning α-helices, an extracellular N-terminus, and a cytoplasmic C-terminus [10] (Fig. 8.1). This arrangement is characteristic of the G protein-coupled superfamily of receptors, which includes chemokine receptors [12,13]. The 65-amino acid extracellular domain contains three potential N-glycosylation sites, at residues 16, 27, and 33. Anti-

Fy6 reacted with a synthetic peptide representing part of the N-terminal domain of the Duffy glycoprotein.

The first *FY* cDNA to be cloned was encoded by a single exon [14–16]. Subsequently, Iwamoto *et al.* [17] showed that the predominant transcript in all tissues tested represented two exons separated by a 479-bp intron, the first exon encoding the seven N-terminal amino acids of Duffy glycoprotein, including the translation-initiating methionine codon. Furthermore, the sequence of the minor transcript that encodes the nine N-terminal amino acid residues is part of the intron of the predominant, spliced transcript. The N-terminal sequence of the majority of Duffy glycoprotein molecules is therefore MGNCLHRAEL [17] and not MASSGYVLQAEL [14], and the former protein is two amino acids shorter than the latter. The major erythroid transcription start point is 34 bp upstream of the first methionine codon in erythroid cells, but 82 bp upstream in lung and kidney [17]. In this chapter, nucleotides and amino acids will be numbered from the translation-initiating methionine residue of the major form of the glycoprotein.

The 5′ upstream region of *FY* contains no TATA or CAAT boxes, but it does contain several transcription-factor binding site motifs, including those for SP1 and GATA [15,16].

8.3 Fy^a and Fy^b (FY1 and FY2)

Anti-Fy^a was discovered in the serum of a transfused haemophiliac, Mr Duffy, by Cutbush *et al.* in 1950 [18,19]. Only 1 year elapsed before Ikin *et al.* [20] identified the antithetical antibody, anti-Fy^b. Fy^x is the name given by Chown *et al.* [21] for a quantitative variant of Fy^b.

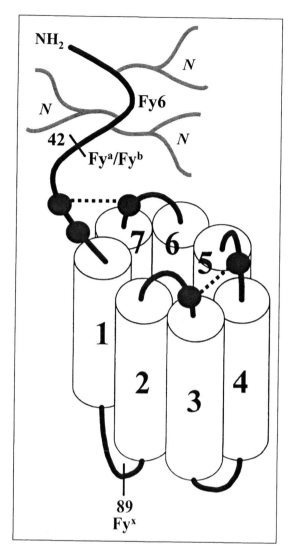

Fig. 8.1 Three-dimensional representation of the Duffy glycoprotein in the red cell membrane as proposed by Mallinson *et al.* [11]. An extracellular N-terminal domain of 61 amino acids, containing three N-glycosylation sites (*N*) and the site of the Fy^a/Fy^b polymorphism at position 42, is followed by seven membrane-spanning domains, represented as cylinders, and a cytoplasmic C-terminal domain. The first cytoplasmic loop contains the site of the amino acid substitution responsible for the Fy^x phenotype. There are five extracellular cysteine residues (●). Dotted lines represent the likely positions of disulphide bridges between cysteine residues in the N-terminal domain and the third loop and between the first and second loops.

8.3.1 Frequency of Fy^a and Fy^b

Fy^a and Fy^b are useful anthropological markers (Table 8.2). Results of numerous population studies carried out with anti-Fy^a have been tabulated by Mourant *et al.* [22]. Studies employing anti-Fy^a and -Fy^b are far fewer because of the scarcity of good anti-Fy^b reagents. An extensive study of 2182 white Canadians, in which anti-Fy^b capable of detecting Fy^x was included (see Section 8.3.4), provided the following phenotype and gene frequencies: Fy(a+b–) 0.1823; Fy(a+b+) 0.4735; Fy(a+b+^{w}) 0.0136; Fy(a–b+) 0.3302; Fy(a–b+^{w}) 0.0004; Fy(a–b–) 0; *Fy^a* 0.425; *Fy^b* 0.557; *Fy^x* 0.016; *Fy* 0.002 [21,23].

The frequencies of *Fy^a* and *Fy^b* in African Americans and in Africans are variable, but low compared with Europeans because of the high frequency of the silent allele *Fy* (Table 8.2). As in Northern Europeans, *Fy^b* is more common than *Fy^a*. In the Far East, *Fy^b* has a far lower frequency than *Fy^a* [22,24,25] (Table 8.2). Weak *Fy^a* was detected in Indonesia [25].

Table 8.3 shows genotype and allele frequencies in black South Africans and white Swedes, determined by a PCR-based method on genomic DNA [26] (Section 8.5).

8.3.2 Inheritance of Fy^a and Fy^b and the molecular basis of the Duffy polymorphism

Fy^a and Fy^b are inherited in a straightforward Mendelian fashion as products of codominant alleles. In a series of 1091 Manitoban families tested with anti-Fy^a and anti-Fy^b, a good fit was obtained between observed results and those predicted from the gene frequencies [21,23]. The few black families studied will be mentioned in Section 8.4.1.1.

Sequencing of PCR products derived from reticulocyte cDNA and representing the entire coding sequence for the Duffy glycoprotein revealed a single base change at position 159 encoding an amino acid substitution representing the Fy^a/Fy^b polymorphism: Fy^a is associated with Gly42, Fy^b with Asp42 [11,14,15,27] (Table 8.4, Fig. 8.1). This was confirmed by expressing the appropriate cDNA clones in simian COS-7 cells and detecting Fy^a or Fy^b by flow cytometry [27]. The *Fy^a* sequence creates a *Ban*I restriction site.

An Ala100Thr (G298A) polymorphism in the second membrane-spanning domain does not appear

Table 8.2 Typical Duffy phenotype frequencies and associated genotypes (compiled from [22]).

Phenotype	Genotype	Frequencies (%)		
		Europeans	Africans	Japanese
Fy(a+b−)	Fy^a/Fy^a or Fy^a/Fy	20	10	81
Fy(a+b+)	Fy^a/Fy^b	48	3	15
Fy(a−b+)	Fy^b/Fy^b or Fy^b/Fy	32	20	4
Fy(a−b−)	Fy/Fy	0	67	0

Table 8.3 Genotype and allele frequencies in black South African and white Swedish populations, determined by molecular analysis of the Duffy genes of 100 individuals from each population [26].

Phenotype	Genotype (%)			Allele (%)		
		Black	White		Black	White
Fy(a+b−)	Fy^a/Fy^a	0	21	Fy^a	3	41
	Fy^a/Fy	4	0	Fy^b	17.5	59
Fy(a+b+)	Fy^a/Fy^b	2	40	Fy	79.5	0
Fy(a−b+)	Fy^b/Fy^b	2	39			
	Fy^b/Fy	29	0			
Fy(a−b−)	Fy/Fy	63	0			

Fy^x cannot be distinguished from Fy^b by this method.

Table 8.4 The four FY alleles affecting red cell surface antigen expression.

Allele	nt −67	nt 125 aa 42	nt 265 aa 89	nt 298 aa 100
Fy^a	T	G Gly	C Arg	G Ala
Fy^b	T	A Asp	C Arg	G or A Ala or Thr
Fy^x	T	A Asp	T Cys	A Thr
Fy	C	A Asp	C Arg	G Ala

aa, amino acid; nt, nucleotide.
Numbering from the major translation-initiating methionine residue [17].

to affect antigenic expression [9–11]. In Swedish donors, the allele encoding Thr100 was detected in 22% of Fy(a−b+), 9% of Fy(a+b+), but in 0% of Fy(a+b−) [28]. None of 100 black South Africans had Thr100 [28].

Duffy glycoprotein homologues are present in non-human primates, with amino acid sequence homology of 99% between human and chimpanzee and 93–94% between human and squirrel, rhesus, and dourocouli monkeys [14]. All non-human primates have Duffy genes encoding Asp42, suggesting that Fy^b is the ancestral allele [14,29].

8.3.3 Effects of enzymes on Fy^a and Fy^b

Fy^a and Fy^b are very sensitive to most proteolytic enzymes; they are completely destroyed by papain, ficin, bromelin, pronase, and chymotrypsin treatment of the red cells, but trypsin does not abolish Fy^a and Fy^b activity [30–32]. Use of impure preparations of

327

trypsin containing chymotrypsin probably accounts for some early reports that Duffy antigens are trypsin-sensitive. Sialidase treatment of red cells does not affect the activity of Duffy antigens [33,34].

8.3.4 Fy^x

Fy^x behaves as a weak Fy^b antigen; there is no anti-Fy^x. Fy^x is inherited as an allele of Fy^a and Fy^b; codominant with Fy^a and recessive to Fy^b [21,23]. Some anti-Fy^b sera react weakly with red cells of Fy^a/Fy^x individuals, whereas others, particularly directly agglutinating anti-Fy^b, do not agglutinate those cells. The presence of Fy^x may be confirmed by adsorption and elution of anti-Fy^b [21,35]. It is not generally possible to distinguish Fy^b/Fy^x from Fy^b/Fy^b except by pedigree or DNA analysis.

Fy^x has mostly been described in white populations, where it is not especially rare. Eleven Fy(a+b+^{w}) and one Fy(a–b+^{w}) were found among 1108 white people and the estimated gene frequencies were Fy^x 0.015 and Fy 0.001 [23]. Fy^x has also been detected in a Canadian Cree kindred [36]. Several probable Fy^x homozygotes have been reported [23,35,37–39]; two of the Fy^x/Fy^x individuals were originally thought to be Fy(a–b–) [35,39].

In addition to Fy^b, there is a very marked depression of Fy3, Fy5, and Fy6 in Fy^x homozygotes [11,28,33,36,37,40–42]. Flow cytometric analysis produced the following estimations of Fy6 site numbers per red cell: Fy(a–b+) (Fy^b/Fy^b) 2200–2400; Fy(a–b+^{w}) (Fy^x/Fy) 150; and Fy(a–b+^{w}) (Fy^x/Fy^x) 250 [41]. Reduced levels of Fy6 binding associated with Fy^x were also detected by immunoblotting of Duffy glycoprotein isolated from the red cell membrane [41,42]. This suggests that Fy^x represents reduced levels of Duffy glycoprotein in the membrane rather than an altered Fy^b determinant or conformational changes affecting several determinants.

Fy^x and Fy^b have the same coding sequence apart from a single nucleotide change (C265T) encoding an Arg89Cys substitution [28,29,41,43] (Table 8.4). This amino acid substitution is located in the first cytoplasmic loop of the Duffy glycoprotein (Fig. 8.1). The replacement of a positively charged arginine residue by a neutral cysteine residue results in protein instability and might compromise the insertion of the molecule in the red cell membrane. Mammalian cells transfected with FY cDNA constructs in which the Cys89 codon

had been introduced by site-directed mutagenesis had substantially reduced expression of Fy^b, Fy3, and Fy6, compared with cells transfected with normal Fy^b cDNA [41,42] or with with Fy^b cDNA in which Arg89 had been replaced with positively charged lysine [44]. The Fy^x mutation abolishes an AciI restriction site. Fy^x encodes threonine at the site of the Ala100Thr polymorphism (Table 8.4 and Section 8.3.2) [28,39] and also has a C to T change at nucleotide 190 of the FY intron [43]. Site-directed mutation experiments confirmed that the Ala100Thr polymorphism does not affect expression of Duffy antigens [42]. Fy^x, as determined by the presence of the Arg89Cys mutation, has an allele frequency of 0.025 in 100 white Swedish donors and of 0.015 in 300 white Austrians, but was not found in 100 black South Africans [28,43]. However, Fy^x appears to be associated with some degree of genetic heterogeneity. In some Fy^x individuals no change from the Fy^b allele was detected in the coding region of the gene [11] and Fy^x has also been associated with a single base deletion in an SP1 transcription factor binding site upstream of the transcription start position [45].

8.3.5 Anti-Fy^a

The original anti-Fy^a of Mr Duffy was reported in 1950 [18,19] and three other examples were reported the same year [46–48]. Anti-Fy^a is estimated to be three times less frequent than anti-K [49], and Fy^a 40 times less immunogenic than K [33]. There is substantial evidence, from several different centres in the USA, that Fy^a is less immunogenic in black than in white people [49–52], although one survey disputes this [53] (for a full discussion on this issue see [54]). Anti-Fy^a often accompanies or precedes anti-Fy3 in Fy(a–b–) black people [55–58] (Section 8.4.2.2).

Some anti-Fy^a may have been stimulated by pregnancy, but most arise from blood transfusion. 'Naturally occurring' anti-Fy^a are very rare [48,59]. Although anti-Fy^a may occur alone, it is often found in mixtures of antibodies. Anti-Fy^a are usually IgG antibodies [49], mostly IgG1 [60,61]. They generally react best by an antiglobulin test, but rarely anti-Fy^a may be directly agglutinating [62,63]. About 50% of anti-Fy^a activate complement up to the C3 stage [49].

Anti-Fy^a has been incriminated in immediate [48] and delayed [53,64] haemolytic transfusion reactions.

Although generally mild, a few immediate reactions have proved fatal [65,66]. The majority of radiolabelled Fy(a+) red cells injected into a patient with anti-Fy^a were eliminated within 10 min [67]. Anti-Fy^a in a donor blood was responsible for a transfusion reaction in a Fy(a+b+) patient [68]. Haemolytic disease of the newborn (HDN) caused by anti-Fy^a is usually mild, but is occasionally severe [69–72]. In a survey of 68 pregnancies in which the mother has anti-Fy^a, three resulted in a severely anaemic fetus, two requiring intrauterine transfusion [72].

Murine monoclonal anti-Fy^a has been produced from lymphocytes derived from transgenic mice expressing Fy^b and immunized with a transfected human embryonic kidney cell line expressing Fy^a [73].

8.3.6 Anti-Fy^b

Anti-Fy^b, a relatively rare antibody, is estimated to be 20 times less common than anti-Fy^a [33]. It is usually found only in mixtures of red cell antibodies. Anti-Fy^b has been stimulated by pregnancy [20,74], transfusion [75,76] and, in a mother, by intrauterine transfusion [77]; two apparently 'naturally occurring' anti-Fy^b have been found [54,78]. Often consisting entirely of IgG1 [60,61], Fy^b antibodies generally react best by an antiglobulin test, but directly agglutinating examples are known [21]. Some anti-Fy^b bind complement [33].

Anti-Fy^b has been responsible for a fatal haemolytic transfusion reaction [79] and for a delayed transfusion reaction [80]. The single reported case of HDN caused by anti-Fy^b was treated by phototherapy and two transfusions [81].

Four cases of Fy(a+b–) patients with autoantibodies mimicking anti-Fy^b have been described [82–84]; one responsible for autoimmune haemolytic anaemia [82]. The antibodies reacted more strongly with Fy(a–b+) and Fy(a+b+) cells than with Fy(a+b–) cells, and not at all with Fy(a–b–) cells. In one case, pure anti-Fy^b specificity was subsequently found [82].

Murine monoclonal anti-Fy^b was produced by immunizing mice with synthetic peptides (12 amino acids) representing the Fy^b epitope [85].

8.4 Fy(a–b–) phenotype; Fy3, Fy5, Fy6, and Fy4 antigens

8.4.1 Fy(a–b–) phenotype

8.4.1.1 Fy(a–b–) in people of African origin

The Fy(a–b–) phenotype came to light when Sanger et al. [86], testing the red cells of African American blood donors with anti-Fy^a and -Fy^b, found that cells of nearly 70% failed to react with both antibodies. Fy, a new allele recessive to Fy^a and Fy^b, was postulated in order to account for this null phenotype. Fy(a–b–) has a frequency of about 63% in black New Yorkers, West Indians [87], and South Africans [26], but the frequency is higher in some African populations [22] (Tables 8.2 and 8.3). All of 1168 donors from rural Gambia were Fy(a–b–) [88].

Data from black families analysed with anti-Fy^a and -Fy^b, involving a total of 53 matings, are consistent with Fy being an allele of Fy^a and Fy^b [87]. Anti-Fy^a capable of demonstrating gene dosage show that Fy(a+b–) cells from white people generally give a 'double dose' reaction compared with a 'single dose' for most red cells of that phenotype from black people [86].

Although Fy(a–b–) red cells lack Duffy glycoprotein [5,8], Duffy glycoprotein was expressed in endothelial cells lining postcapillary venules of soft tissues and splenic sinusoids from black Fy(a–b–) individuals [89]. Duffy mRNA was not detected in the bone marrow of Fy(a–b–) individuals, but was present in their lung, spleen, and colon [14]. The coding sequence of Fy is identical to that of an Fy^b allele [9,11,14,15,27,89], but a T to C change is present in the promoter region of the gene, 33 bp upstream of the erythroid transcription start point and 67 bp upstream of the major translation start codon (position –67), introducing a StyI restriction site [16,90]. This mutation is within a GATA consensus sequence (CTTATCT to CTTACCT), disrupting binding of the erythroid-specific GATA-1 transcription factor and preventing expression of the gene in erythroid cells, but not in other cells. A human erythroid cell line (HEL) and human microvascular endothelial cells transfected with a construct consisting of the promoter region of the Fy^b allele and the reporter gene chloramphenicol acetyltransferase (CAT) had high levels of CAT activity. Transfection with a construct containing the Fy

329

allele T–33C GATA mutation abolished CAT activity in the HEL cells [16,90], but not in the endothelial cells [90].

Twenty-three of 1062 individuals from the East Sepik of Papua New Guinea were heterozygous for an *FY* allele with the *Fy^a* sequence (encoding Gly42), but with the GATA mutation characteristic of *Fy*, an allele frequency of 0.022 [91]. This allele is probably silent in erythroid cells and red cells of these individuals had lower levels of Fy6 than those homozygous for the normal *Fy^a* allele.

Resistance of people with the Fy(a–b–) red cell phenotype to the malarial parasite *Plasmodium vivax* is described in Section 8.8.

8.4.1.2 Fy(a–b–) in other racial groups

Fy(a–b–) is very rare in racial groups not originating from Africa [22]. None of 6000 white Australian donors was Fy(a–b–), as determined by testing red cells with the original anti-Fy3 [34]. Chown *et al.* [21,23] estimated the frequency of the *Fy* allele in white people as being in the order of 0.001, giving an incidence of one in a million for Fy(a–b–). Anomalous inheritance of Fy^a and Fy^b in some white families has been explained by invoking a silent allele, but is probably due to undetected presence of *Fy^x* [21].

Most examples of non-African Fy(a–b–) have been found through the presence of strong anti-Fy3. The molecular background to the Fy(a–b–) phenotype has been determined in four non-Africans with anti-Fy3, all of whom had been transfused and/or pregnant. The *FY* gene of a white Australian woman [34] contains a 14-bp deletion resulting in a reading frameshift and introduction of a translation stop codon [11]. Homozygosity for nonsense mutations that introduced translation stop codon was found in three examples: a white British woman with G408A (Trp136Stop) in *Fy^a* [92]; a Lebanese Jewish woman with G407A (Trp136Stop) in *Fy^b* [92]; and a native Canadian (Cree) with G287A (Trp96Stop) in *Fy^a* [36,92].

An Fy(a–b–) Japanese woman without anti-Fy3, but who had never been transfused or pregnant, was homozygous for an *Fy^a* allele with a deletion of C327, which introduces a stop signal 12 codons downstream at codon 120 [93]. Each of these mutations would be expected to result in no expression of Duffy antigen in

red cells or, unlike the GATA mutation responsible for the African Fy(a–b–) phenotype, in any other parts of the body.

Fy(a–b–) phenotype without anti-Fy3 in Czech gypsies [94,95] and in a white woman of Scottish and Swiss ancestry [92] resulted from homozygosity for the GATA mutation characteristic of African Fy(a–b–).

8.4.2 Fy3 and anti-Fy3

8.4.2.1 Fy3 antigen

Fy3 is present on all red cells apart from those of the Fy(a–b–) phenotype. Fy3 is a public antigen in people of European and Asian origin, polymorphic in many black populations, and a private antigen in some parts of Africa. In contrast to Fy^a and Fy^b, Fy3 is resistant to the treatment of red cells with proteases [34,36,55,96]. Red cells of some primates have Fy3, but not Fy^a or Fy^b (see Table 8.6).

8.4.2.2 Anti-Fy3

The original anti-Fy3 was found by Albrey *et al.* [34] in the serum of an Fy(a–b–) white Australian woman during her third pregnancy. She had been transfused following her second delivery. The antibody reacted equally strongly with Fy(a+b–), Fy(a+b+), and Fy(a–b+) cells, and could not be separated into anti-Fy^a and -Fy^b components. It did not react with Fy(a–b–) cells (Table 8.5). Four other examples of anti-Fy3 have been produced by people who are not black [36,92,96], one of which appeared to show a preference for Fy(a+) cells [96].

Anti-Fy3 is rare in Fy(a–b–) black people, though several examples have been reported [53,55–57, 105,106]. Most anti-Fy3 in black people are found in mixtures of antibodies to red cell antigens, which often include anti-Fy^a. In some black patients with anti-Fy3, anti-Fy^a had preceded development of anti-Fy3 but was no longer detected when the anti-Fy3 was present [58]. Anti-Fy^a is a far more common antibody in the serum of multiply transfused black patients than anti-Fy3. Antibody screening tests on sera from 566 transfused Fy(a–b–) black patients in France revealed no Duffy antibodies [107].

Fy(a–b–) black people are homozygous for an *Fy* allele containing a mutation in the GATA-1 erythroid

Table 8.5 Reactions of anti-Fy3 (from different ethnic groups), anti-Fy5, and monoclonal anti-Fy6 with red cells of various phenotypes.

Race and phenotype	Anti-Fy3		Anti-Fy5	Anti-Fy6
	Black	Other		
All races				
Fy(a+b−)	+	+	+	+
Fy(a+b+)	+	+	+	+
Fy(a−b+)	+	+	+	+
Cord cells*	− or +	+	+	+
Papain-treated cells*	+	+	+	−
Black				
Fy(a−b−)	−	−	−	−
White				
Fy(a−b−)	−	−	+†	nt
Fy(a−b+^{w}) (Fy^x/Fy^x)	w	w	w	w
Rh$_{null}$*	+	+	−	+
D−−*	+	+	w	+

*Not Fy(a−b−) cells.
†White Australian [34,110].
nt, not tested; w, weakly positive.

transcription factor binding motif (Section 8.4.1.1). Their red cells are Fy:−3, but they have Duffy glycoprotein in other parts of the body [89]. Apart from the GATA mutation, *Fy* is identical to an *Fy^b* allele, so it is likely that *Fy* homozygotes express Fy3 and Fy^b in non-erythroid tissues, explaining the rarity of anti-Fy3, the absence of anti-Fy^b, and the relatively common occurrence of anti-Fy^a in transfused Fy(a−b−) black people. Unless the Fy(a−b−) phenotype of black people who make anti-Fy3 has a different genetic background from that of the common *Fy/Fy* genotype, anti-Fy3 made in black people must be able to recognize a subtle difference between the Duffy glycoprotein expressed in different tissues, possibly a glycosylation or conformational difference. Anti-Fy3 made by black people react either very weakly or not at all with cord cell samples [56,57,105], whereas anti-Fy3 from three non-black women all reacted equally strongly with red cells of adults and newborn infants [36,96]. Perhaps Duffy antigen on fetal red cells resembles that on adult endothelial cells.

Anti-Fy3 is potentially haemolytic and has been responsible for immediate and delayed transfusion reactions [58,96,106]. The third child of the white Australian and the eighth child of the Cree woman with anti-Fy3 showed signs of HDN, but in neither case was any treatment beyond phototherapy required [34,36].

Mouse monoclonal antibodies have been produced that resemble anti-Fy3 in reactivity and detect protease-resistant epitopes on the Duffy glycoprotein [108]. Studies on insect cells transfected with cDNA constructs encoding chimeric molecules containing different regions of both Duffy glycoprotein and an interleukin-8 receptor demonstrated that monoclonal anti-Fy3-like detects an epitope on the third extracellular loop [109] (see Fig. 8.1). However, it is likely that polyclonal human alloanti-Fy3 detects epitopes on more than one region of the molecule.

8.4.3 Fy5 and anti-Fy5

Fy5 closely resembles Fy3 (Table 8.5); it differs by its absence from Fy:3 Rh$_{null}$ cells (amorph and regulator type), weak expression on red cells of *D−−* homozygotes, and presence on Fy(a−b−) cells from people of non-African origin. Like Fy3, Fy5 is a protease-resistant antigen [110,111]. Fy5 is expressed equally strongly on red cells of adults and newborns [110, 111]. The reactions of anti-Fy5 suggest that the Duffy glycoprotein may be associated in the membrane with the Rh proteins or Rh-associated glycoprotein (see Chapter 5).

At least six examples of anti-Fy5 have been reported, all in multiply transfused black Fy(a−b−) patients, mostly with sickle cell disease [58,110–113]. All were present with a mixture of other red cell antibodies; in two anti-Fy^a was present [111,113] and in another two anti-Fy^a had preceded anti-Fy5 but was no longer detectable [58]. Anti-Fy5 could not be separated into other antibody components by adsorption and elution. Some Rh e-variant red cells also have weak Fy5 antigen [114]. Red cells from *Fy^x* homozygotes have depressed Fy5 [33].

Anti-Fy5 has been incriminated in delayed haemolytic transfusion reactions [58,112,113]. One patient had two separate reactions, one as a result of anti-Fy^a, the other anti-Fy5 [113].

8.4.4 Monoclonal anti-Fy6

At least two monoclonal antibodies produced by immunizing mice with red cells have a specificity very similar to that of anti-Fy3 [5,6]. They were named anti-Fy6 because, unlike anti-Fy3, the determinant they detect is destroyed by papain (Table 8.5), ficin, and chymotrypsin; Fy6 is resistant to trypsin. Both anti-Fy6 were shown, by peptide scanning and by site-directed mutagenesis, to recognize a linear epitope comprising amino acid residues 19–25 (QLDFEDV) on the N-terminal extracellular domain of the Duffy glycoprotein (see Fig. 8.1) [115]. In its distribution on red cells of non-human primates, Fy6 differs from Fy^a, Fy^b, and Fy3, but shows close accord with susceptibility to *Plasmodium vivax* invasion (see Section 8.8 and Table 8.6). Monoclonal anti-Fy6 has proved invaluable in the isolation of Duffy glycoprotein [6,8].

8.4.5 Fy4 and anti-Fy4

When Sanger *et al.* [86] postulated a silent allele, *Fy*, to account for the high frequency of Fy(a–b–) amongst black people, an unsuccessful attempt was made to find 'anti-Fy' or 'anti-Fy^c' in white people who had been transfused with blood from black donors. In 1973, Behzad *et al.* [116] described an antibody, produced by an Fy(a+b+) black girl with sickle cell anaemia, which gave most of the reactions expected of anti-Fy^c, although weak reactions confused some of the results. The antibody was numbered anti-Fy4. No second example of anti-Fy4 has been found. The reaction of anti-Fy4 with Fy:4 cells is enhanced by papain treatment of the cells [116].

Compiled data from three laboratories of tests with anti-Fy4 on red cells of 150 black donors, including 114 with the Fy(a–b–) phenotype, and 107 white donors, fitted reasonably well with anti-Fy4 representing 'anti-Fy', although there were some anomalous reactions [116]. Unfortunately, no families were tested. Fy(a–b–) red cells from the white Australian and Cree propositi reacted with anti-Fy4, those of the former reacting only weakly [36,116]. Duffy glycoprotein is not present on Fy(a–b–) cells, but Fy4 could represent a conformation of an associated membrane component that occurs in the absence of Duffy glycoprotein.

8.5 Duffy genotype determination

Knowledge of the nucleotide changes that define the

Fy^a, Fy^b, and *Fy* alleles has made it possible to devise PCR-based techniques for determining Duffy genotype and therefore for predicting Duffy phenotype. Such methods are valuable for the determination of Duffy phenotype of fetuses of mothers with anti-Fy^a, in order to assist in assessing the risk of HDN [72]. The G159A substitution associated with the Fy^a/Fy^b polymorphism creates a *Ban*I restriction site in the Fy^a allele [11,14,15,27,117] and the T–67C substitution associated with the Fy/Fy^{ab} polymorphism creates a *Sty*I restriction site in the *Fy* allele [16,90]. Genotypes can be obtained by digestion of PCR-amplified gene segments incorporating the two polymorphic sites.

Genotyping methods have been developed utilizing allele-specific primers: two alternative sense primers, specific for C–67 (*Fy*) or T–67 (Fy^a or Fy^b); and two alternative antisense primers, specific for G159 (Fy^a) or A159 (Fy^b or *Fy*) (Fig. 8.2) [26,118,119]. By using the four possible combinations of primer pairs, the presence of any of the three alleles is revealed by an amplification product of about 700 bp with the appropriate primer pair. Allele frequencies in black and white populations, obtained by this method, are provided in Table 8.3.

Sickle cell disease patients are regularly transfused and often make multiple red cell antibodies, which make subsequent transfusion difficult. Phenotype-matched blood is therefore often requested for these patients and Duffy genotyping might assist in providing matched blood. Fy(a+b–) patients who are Fy^a/Fy^a would be capable of making anti-Fy^b, but those who are Fy^a/Fy would not, as the *Fy* allele probably produces Fy^b in non-erythroid tissues.

8.6 Site density, development, and distribution of Duffy antigens

Fy(a+b–) and Fy(a–b+) red cells were estimated, by quantitative immunoferritin microscopy, to have 13 000–14 000 Fy^a or Fy^b sites; Fy(a+b+) cells have about half that number of Fy^a sites [120]. More than 85% of the sites were lost after papain treatment. With two radioiodinated monoclonal anti-Fy6, estimates of 12 200 and 6000 sites per red cell were obtained [5,6].

Fy^a and Fy^b are fully developed at birth and have been detected on red cells from embryos as early as 6–7 weeks' gestation [121,122]. The expression of Fy^a and Fy^b is as strong on red cells of very young fetuses as on those of adults, and remains unmodified throughout fetal life.

There is some dispute regarding the appearance of Duffy glycoprotein (Fy6) during erythropoiesis, *in vitro*. In one-stage serum-free methods of cell culture Fy6 appeared quite late, about the same time as the Lutheran glycoprotein [123,124], whereas in a two-stage method, Fy6 appeared early, at about the same time as glycophorin C [125]. There is almost 50% higher level of expression of Fy6 on reticulocytes than on mature erythrocytes [126].

In addition to its presence on red cells, Duffy glycoprotein, detected with anti-Fy6, is abundant on endothelial cells lining postcapillary venules throughout the body, except for liver [127,128], and on Purkinje neurones of the cerebellum [129]. Sequence analyses of cDNA indicate that the renal and erythroid isoforms of the Duffy polypeptide are identical and any small differences in M_r of the glycoproteins are probably accounted for by altered glycosylation [10,127,128]. Duffy glycoprotein was also detected, with a rabbit polyclonal antibody specific for the glycosylation of Duffy glycoprotein, on some other vascular endothelial cells and on epithelial cells of renal collecting ducts and pulmonary alveoli [128]. The effect of the GATA mutation in the *Fy* allele is erythroid-specific, so Duffy glycoprotein is present on non-erythroid tissues in black people with the Fy(a–b–) red cell phenotype [89] (Section 8.4.1.1).

An mRNA transcript was detected by hybridization with Duffy cDNA, in bone marrow from individuals with Fy(a+b–), Fy(a–b+), and Fy(a+b+) red cells, but not from those with Fy(a–b–) cells [9,14]. Duffy mRNA has been detected in lung, muscle, spleen, colon, heart, pancreas, kidney and brain [10,14,127]. This transcript is present in tissues from Fy(a–b–) black individuals [14]. Although the major transcript is about 1.35 kb, Le Van Kim *et al.* [130] found that a 7.5-kb transcript was predominant in cerebellum. The two transcripts differ in the length of their 5′ untranslated regions, but encode the same polypeptide. However, Neote *et al.* [10] report that an 8.5-kb transcript in fetal brain changes into a 1.35-kb transcript in adult brain.

Fy^a and Fy^b are not present on lymphocytes, monocytes, granulocytes, or platelets [131,132].

8.7 The Duffy glycoprotein is a chemokine receptor

The Duffy glycoprotein binds a variety of proinflammatory chemokines and is known as the Duffy antigen receptor for chemokines (DARC). Chemokines are chemotactic cytokines that are involved in many cellular processes, especially the recruitment and activation of leucocytes [133]. There are three main classes of chemokines, called C-X-C, C-C, and C on the basis of the position of highly conserved cysteine residues at their N-termini. Most chemokine receptors belong to a very large family of integral cell membrane glycoproteins, G protein-coupled receptors, which traverse the membrane seven times and have an extracellular N-terminal domain

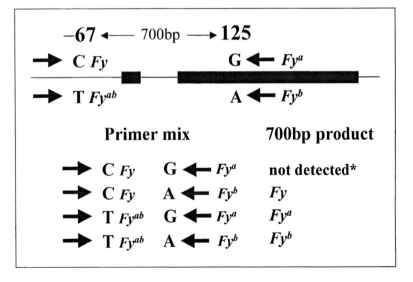

Fig. 8.2 PCR-based method with allele-specific primers for determination of Duffy genotype [26,118]. Two allele-specific sense primers (→C *Fy* and →T *Fy^{ab}*) are paired in four different combinations with two antisense primers (G ←*Fy^a* and A ←*Fy^b*). An internal positive-control primer pair is included in each primer mix. Amplification of a product of about 700 bp in the appropriate reactions reveals the alleles present and is visualized by agarose gel electrophoresis. *A 700-bp product would be expected in this reaction with DNA from the Melanesians with the C–67, G125 allele [91].

(Fig. 8.1) [12,13]. G protein-coupled receptors mediate the actions of extracellular signals as diverse as light, odourants, neurotransmitters, and peptide hormones such as chemokines. Most chemokine receptors are specific for one or more chemokines of a single class, but the Duffy glycoprotein, a promiscuous receptor, binds chemokines of the C-X-C and C-C classes [134–136]. Examples of C-X-C chemokines are interleukin-8 (IL-8) and melanoma growth stimulatory activity (MGSA), and of C-C chemokines are regulated on activation, normal T expressed and secreted (RANTES) and monocyte chemotactic protein-1 (MCP-1). Duffy glycoprotein does not bind the C chemokine, lymphotactin [137]. Unlike almost all other G protein-coupled receptors, the Duffy glycoprotein lacks the Asp-Arg-Tyr (DRY) motif in the second cytoplasmic loop and does not appear to be coupled to a guanosine triphosphate-binding protein (G-protein) [138].

Fy(a–b–) red cells do not bind chemokines [41,139]. Fy(a–b+^{w}) (Fy^x/Fy^x) bind chemokines in substantially reduced quantities compared with Fy(a–b+) cells [41,42].

The chemokine-binding pocket of the Duffy glycoprotein appears to include sequences in the first and fourth extracellular domains, which are brought into close vicinity by a disulphide bridge between Cys51 and Cys276 [140] (Fig. 8.1). IL-8 binding was diminished by 60% by treatment of the cells with the disulphide bond reducing agent DTT [140]. Anti-Fy^a, -Fy^b, and -Fy6, which bind to the first extracellular domain of the Duffy glycoprotein, and monoclonal anti-Fy3-like, which binds the fourth extracellular domain, all compete with chemokines for binding [109,137,139–142] (although in one study anti-Fy3-like did not inhibit chemokine binding [109]). IL-8 bound to red cells treated with trypsin, sialidase, or N-glycanase, but not to cells treated with papain or α-chymotrypsin [143], which cleave the N-terminal extracellular domain of the Duffy glycoprotein (see Section 8.3.3). Glycosylation of the protein therefore is not required for chemokine binding.

The function of the Duffy glycoprotein is not known. It has been suggested that it may act as a clearance receptor for inflammatory mediators and that Duffy-positive red cells function as a 'sink' or as scavengers for the removal of unwanted chemokines [134]. If so, this function must be of limited importance as Duffy is not present on the red cells of most Africans.

IL-8 released into the plasma after acute myocardial infarction binds to red cells, resulting in only transient elevation of plasma IL-8 [144].

Duffy glycoprotein is present on many cells throughout the body, in both Duffy-positive people and Fy(a–b–) Africans (Section 8.6). The kidney isoform binds chemokines with the same affinity as the red cell isoform [127]. Hadley and Peiper [138] point to the conservation of the gene encoding Duffy glycoprotein across species as evidence for the importance of the protein. They speculate that endothelial Duffy glycoprotein may interact with other membrane components, to elicit tissue specific responses to ligand binding. K562 erythroid cells transfected with Duffy cDNA bind chemokines [10,141] and are able to endocytose the ligand [89]. Duffy glycoprotein has been detected as a transmembrane protein in caveolae of endothelial cells [128] and may participate in receptor-mediated endocytosis, possibly generating the chemotactic gradient essential for leucocyte attraction [138]. Significant up-regulation of Duffy glycoprotein was detected in renal tissues of children with HIV nephropathy and haemolytic uraemic syndrome, suggesting that the Duffy glycoprotein plays a part in the pathogenesis of renal inflammation [145].

Genes homologous to FY have been cloned from non-human primates, cow, pig, rabbit, and mouse [14,138,146]. Mouse red cells bind murine and human chemokines [137], as do K562 cells transfected with cDNA derived from Dfy, the mouse homologue of FY [146]. Dfy$^{-/-}$ (knockout) mice, deficient in the Duffy homologue, were healthy and apparently identical to wild-type mice [147,148]. Analyses of their response to inflammatory agents, particularly with respect to leucocyte migration, brought conflicting results [147,148].

Five people have the Fy(a–b–) red cell phenotype because of homozygosity for inactivating mutations within the coding region of their Duffy genes (Section 8.4.1.2). None of these individuals would be expected to have Duffy glycoprotein in any of their tissues, yet all were apparently healthy. Consequently, if Duffy glycoprotein has an important function, some other structure must be able to perform the same role.

8.8 Duffy antigens and malaria

Plasmodium vivax is the pathogen responsible for

tertian malaria, a widely distributed form of malaria, but less severe than that resulting from infection by *P. falciparum* (see Section 3.23.1). For several decades it had been known that most black people are resistant to *P. vivax* infection. When Miller *et al.* [31] showed that Fy(a–b–) red cells are refractory to invasion by the simian parasite *P. knowlesi*, which can invade human red cells *in vitro*, it was not long before the association between the Fy(a–b–) phenotype and resistance to *P. vivax* infection became apparent [97]. For many years, before *P. vivax* could be cultured [98], *P. knowlesi* was used as a model for *P. vivax* experiments *in vitro* (reviews in [138,149]).

Amongst 11 black and six white volunteers exposed to *P. vivax*, all became infected except for the five Fy(a–b–) black subjects [97]. In a study of 420 Hondurans, 247 of whom were Fy(a–b–), none of the 14 (seven black, seven white) with *P. vivax* infection was Fy(a–b–) [150]. Antibodies to *P. vivax* were found almost exclusively in Duffy-positive people, whereas antibodies to *P. falciparum* were almost equally distributed between Duffy-positive and -negative individuals [150].

It is probable that the high incidence of the *Fy* allele in Africa results from the selective advantage it confers in the homozygous state by providing resistance to *P. vivax* malaria. In parts of West Africa the frequency of *Fy* is almost 100%, yet *P. vivax* is not present in these areas [88]. The parasite might have been eliminated because of disruption of its life cycle resulting from a shortage of susceptible hosts.

In vitro, Fy(a–b–) human red cells are refractory to invasion by *P. knowlesi* and *P. vivax* merozoites, whereas Fy(a+b+) cells are invaded [31,98,99]. This is not a purely racial characteristic as Fy(a–b–) red cells from two Cree Indians and a white Australian (Section 8.4.1.2) were not invaded by *P. knowlesi* [151]. *P. knowlesi* merozoites are able to attach to Fy(a–b–) cells, but they cannot enter the cells and eventually become detached [31,100,151]. Invasion of Duffy-positive red cells by *P. knowlesi* and *P. vivax* can be blocked by the presence of monoclonal anti-Fy6; invasion of Fy(a+) cells can be partially blocked by anti-Fy[a] [31,98]. The chemokines IL-8 and MGSA, for which the Duffy glycoprotein is a receptor (Section 8.7), blocked invasion of Duffy-positive cells by *P. knowlesi* [139]. Treatment of Duffy-positive red cells with chymotrypsin renders them resistant to invasion by *P. knowlesi* and *P. vivax*, whereas trypsin treatment

has no effect [31,98]. This parallels the effects of these proteases on Fy[a], Fy[b], and Fy6 antigens, but not on Fy3 and Fy5, which are resistant to chymotrypsin cleavage. Surprisingly, trypsin or sialidase-treated Fy(a–b–) cells were invaded by *P. knowlesi* merozoites [151]. *P. vivax* prefers to invade reticulocytes, which have about 50% more Fy6 sites than mature erythrocytes [126].

Table 8.6 shows the Duffy phenotypes of some non-human primates and the susceptibility of their red cells to invasion by *P. knowlesi* and *P. vivax*. Despite being Fy(b+) and Fy:3, red cells of the Old World rhesus monkey are Fy:–6 and are not invaded by *P. vivax*, but are invaded by *P. knowlesi*. New World capuchin monkey cells are Fy(a–b–) Fy:3,6 and are not invaded by *P. knowlesi* or *P. vivax* merozoites. These data suggest that the Fy6 epitope is important for the invasion of *P. vivax*.

Proteins that bind Duffy-positive human red cells, but not Fy(a–b–) cells, have been isolated from the supernatants of cultured *P. knowlesi* and *P. vivax* at the time of merozoite release and reinvasion [101,102] (Table 8.6). The protein isolated from *P. knowlesi* and *P. vivax* cultures are of M_r 135 000 and 140 000, respectively. Binding could be inhibited by anti-Fy6 and by the chemokines IL-8 and MGSA [101–103]. Chymotrypsin treatment of Duffy-positive red cells abrogates binding of the Duffy-associating proteins, whereas trypsin treatment has little effect (Table 8.6). Trypsin-treated Fy(a–b–) cells, which are invaded by *P. knowlesi* [151], did not bind the protein isolated from *P. knowlesi* [101]. The purified parasite proteins bound specifically to purified Duffy glycoprotein. Genes encoding both proteins were cloned and the extracellular domains of each protein have been classified into six regions of amino acid homology [104]. COS-7 cells expressing the cysteine-rich region II formed rosettes with Duffy-positive, but not Fy(a–b–), red cells [152]. This rosetting could be blocked by a synthetic peptide representing amino acid residues 8–42 of the N-terminal domain of the Duffy glycoprotein [153]. Red cells of individuals heterozygous for the silent allele, *Fy*, bind substantially less *P. vivax* Duffy-binding protein than those of individuals with two active *FY* alleles, suggesting that heterozygosity for *Fy* may have a selective advantage in areas where *P. vivax* is endemic [154]. Region II of the *P. vivax* and *P. knowlesi* Duffy-binding proteins also shares extensive sequence homology with the *P. falciparum* gly-

Table 8.6 Invasion of red cells of various Duffy phenotypes by *Plasmodium knowlesi* and *P. vivax* merozoites, and binding of the Duffy-binding protein derived from these parasites. Data compiled from [5,31,33,98,101–103,149,151,157,158].

Red cells	Duffy phenotype				Invasion by		Binds Duffy-binding protein from	
	Fyª	Fyᵇ	Fy3	Fy6	*P. knowlesi*	*P. vivax*	*P. knowlesi*	*P. vivax*
Human (*Homo sapiens*)	+	+	+	+	+	+	+	+
	+	−	+	+	+	+	+	+
	−	+	+	+	+	+	+	+
	−	−	−	−	−	−	−	−
Trypsin-treated*	+	+	+	+	+	+	+	+
Chymotrypsin treated*	−	−	+	−	−	−	−	−
Old World monkey								
Rhesus (*Macaca mulatta*)	−	+	+	−	+	−	+	−
New World monkeys								
Squirrel (*Saimiri sciureus*)	−	−	+	+	+	+	+	−
Capuchin (*Cebus apella*)	−	−	+	−	−	−	+	−
Dourocouli (*Aotus triviratus*)	−	+	+	+	+	+	+	+
Subprimate	−	−	−	−	−	−	−	−

*Fy(a+b+) Fy:3,6 before treatment.

cophorin A-binding protein, EBA-175 [104] (Section 3.23.1). Analysis of the Duffy-binding ligands has led to the identification of the *var* genes that encode the variant endothelial cytoadherence proteins of *P. falciparum* (for review see [138]).

Singh *et al.* [155] have devised a method for expressing the functional region of *P. vivax* Duffy-binding protein (PvRII) in *Escherichia coli*, and refolding it to make it functionally active. Refolded PvRII is a candidate vaccine for *P. vivax* malaria as it elicits high titre antibodies that can inhibit binding of *P. vivax* binding protein to red cells. Any advantage of vaccinating against *P. vivax* malaria, however, must be weighed against evidence that *P. vivax* infection in infants might act as a natural vaccine against *P. falciparum* malaria [156].

References

1 Williams D, Johnson CL, Marsh WL. Duffy antigen changes on red blood cells stored at low temperature. *Transfusion* 1981;21:357–9.

2 Moore S, Woodrow CF, McClelland DBL. Isolation of membrane components associated with human red cell antigens Rh(D), (c), (E) and Fyª. *Nature* 1982; 295:529–31.

3 Hadley TJ, David PH, McGinniss MH, Miller LH.

Identification of an erythrocyte component carrying the Duffy blood group Fyª antigen. *Science* 1984;223:597–9.

4 Tanner MJA, Anstee DJ, Mallinson G *et al.* Effect of endoglycosidase F-Peptidyl *N*-glycosidase F preparations on the surface components of the human erythrocyte. *Carbohydr Res* 1988;173:203–12.

5 Nichols ME, Rubinstein P, Barnwell J *et al.* A new human Duffy blood group specificity defined by a murine monoclonal antibody. Imunogenetics and association with susceptability to *Plasmodium vivax*. *J Exp Med* 1987;166:776–85.

6 Riwom S, Janvier D, Navenot JM *et al.* Production of a new murine monoclonal antibody with anti-Fy6 specificity and characterization of the immunopurified *N*-glycosylated Duffy-active molecule. *Vox Sang* 1994;66:61–7.

7 Wasniowska K, Eichenberger P, Kugele F, Hadley TJ. Purification of a 28 kD non-aggregating tryptic peptide of the Duffy blood group protein. *Biochem Biophys Res Commun* 1993;192:366–72.

8 Chaudhuri A, Zbrzezna V, Johnson C *et al.* Purification and characterization of an erythrocyte membrane protein complex carrying Duffy blood group antigenicity: possible receptor for *Plasmodium vivax* and *Plasmodium knowlesi* malaria parasite. *J Biol Chem* 1989;264:13770–4.

9 Chaudhuri A, Polyakova J, Zbrzezna V *et al.* Cloning of glycoprotein D cDNA, which encodes the major subunit

of the Duffy blood group system and the receptor for the *Plasmodium vivax* malaria parasite. *Proc Natl Acad Sci USA* 1993;**90**:10793–7.

10 Neote K, Mak JY, Kolakowski LF, Schall TJ. Functional and biochemical analysis of the cloned Duffy antigen: identity with the red blood cell chemokine receptor. *Blood* 1994;**84**:44–52.

11 Mallinson G, Soo KS, Schall TJ, Pisacka M, Anstee DJ. Mutations in the erythrocyte chemokine receptor (Duffy) gene: the molecular basis of the Fy^a/Fy^b antigens and identification of a deletion in the Duffy gene of an apparently healthy individual with the Fy (a–b–) phenotype. *Br J Haematol* 1995;**90**:823–9.

12 Ji TH, Grossman M, Ji I. G protein-coupled receptors. I. Diversity of receptor–ligand interactions. *J Biol Chem* 1998;**273**:17299–302.

13 Murdoch C, Finn A. Chemokine receptors and their role in inflammation and infectious diseases. *Blood* 2000;**95**:3032–43.

14 Chaudhuri A, Polyakova J, Zbrzezna V, Pogo AO. The coding sequence of Duffy blood group gene in humans and simians: restriction fragment length polymorphism, antibody and malarial parasite specificities, and expression in nonerythroid tissues in Duffy-negative individuals. *Blood* 1995;**85**:615–21.

15 Iwamoto S, Omi T, Kajii E, Ikemoto S. Genomic organization of the glycoprotein D gene: Duffy blood group Fy^a/Fy^b alloantigen system is associated with a polymorphism at the 44-amino acid residue. *Blood* 1995;**85**:622–6.

16 Tournamille C, Colin Y, Cartron JP, Le Van Kim C. Disruption of a GATA motif in the *Duffy* gene promoter abolishes erythroid gene expression in Duffy-negative individuals. *Nature Genet* 1995;**10**:224–8.

17 Iwamoto S, Li J, Omi T, Ikemoto S, Kajii E. Identification of a novel exon and spliced form of Duffy mRNA that is the predominant transcript in both erythroid and postcapillary venule endothelium. *Blood* 1996;**87**:378–85.

18 Cutbush M, Mollison PL, Parkin DM. A new human blood group. *Nature* 1950;**165**:188–9.

19 Cutbush M, Mollison PL. The Duffy blood group system. *Heredity* 1950;**4**:383–9.

20 Ikin EW, Mourant AE, Pettenkofer HJ, Blumenthal G. Discovery of the expected hæmagglutinin, anti-Fy^b. *Nature* 1951;**168**:1077.

21 Chown B, Lewis M, Kaita H. The Duffy blood group system in Caucasians: evidence for a new allele. *Am J Hum Genet* 1965;**17**:384–9.

22 Mourant AE, Kopec AC, Domaniewska-Sobczak K. *Distribution of Human Blood Groups and Other Polymorphisms*, 2nd edn. London: Oxford University Press, 1976.

23 Lewis M, Kaita H, Chown B. The Duffy blood group system in Caucasians: a further population sample. *Vox Sang* 1972;**23**:523–7.

24 Lewis M, Kaita H, Chown B. The blood groups of a Japanese population. *Am J Hum Genet* 1957;**9**:274–83.

25 Shimizu Y, Hiroko A, Soemantri A *et al.* Sero- and molecular typing of Duffy blood group in Southeast Asians and Oceanians. *Hum Biol* 2000;**72**:511–18.

26 Olsson ML, Hansson C, Avent ND *et al.* A clinically applicable method for determining the three major alleles at the Duffy (*FY*) blood group locus using polymerase chain reaction with allele-specific primers. *Transfusion* 1998;**38**:168–73.

27 Tournamille C, Le Van Kim C, Gane P, Cartron J-P, Colin Y. Molecular basis and PCR-DNA typing of the Fy^a/fy^b blood group polymorphism. *Hum Genet* 1995;**95**:407–10.

28 Olsson ML, Smythe JS, Hansson C *et al.* The Fy^x phenotype is associated with a missense mutation in the Fy^b allele predicting Arg89Cys in the Duffy glycoprotein. *Br J Haematol* 1998;**103**:1184–91.

29 Li J, Iwamoto S, Sugimoto N, Okuda H, Kajii E. Dinucleotide repeat in the 3′ flanking region provides a clue to the molecular evolution of the Duffy gene. *Hum Genet* 1997;**99**:573–7.

30 Morton JA. Some observations on the action of blood-group antibodies on red cells treated with proteolytic enzymes. *Br J Haematol* 1962;**8**:134–48.

31 Miller LH, Mason SJ, Dvorak JA, McGinniss MH, Rothman IK. Erythrocyte receptors for (*Plasmodium knowlesi*) malaria: Duffy blood group determinants. *Science* 1975;**189**:561–3.

32 Judson PA, Anstee DJ. Comparative effect of trypsin and chymotrypsin on blood group antigens. *Med Lab Sci* 1977;**34**:1–6.

33 Marsh WL. Present status of the Duffy blood group system. *CRC Clin Rev Clin Lab Sci* 1975;**5**:387–412.

34 Albrey JA, Vincent EER, Hutchinson J *et al.* A new antibody, anti-Fy3, in the Duffy blood group system. *Vox Sang* 1971;**20**:29–35.

35 Cedergren B, Giles CM. An Fy^{x}Fy^x individual found in Northern Sweden. *Vox Sang* 1973;**24**:264–6.

36 Buchanan DI, Sinclair M, Sanger R, Gavin J, Teesdale P. An Alberta Cree Indian with a rare Duffy antibody, anti-Fy3. *Vox Sang* 1976;**30**:114–21.

37 Habibi B, Fouillade MT, Levanra I *et al.* Antigène Fy^x: etude quantitative chez les sujets Fy^{b}Fy^x, Fy^{a}Fy^x et Fy^{x}Fy^x provenant de deux nouvelles familles. *Rev Franc Transfus Immuno-Hémat* 1977;**20**:427–38.

38 Cook PJL, Page BM, Johnston AW, Stanford WK, Gavin J. Four further families informative for 1q and the Duffy blood group. *Cytogenet Cell Genet* 1978;**22**:378–80.

39 Parasol N, Reid M, Rios M *et al.* A novel mutation in the coding sequence of the FY*B allele of the Duffy chemokine receptor gene is associated with an altered erythrocyte phenotype. *Blood* 1998;**92**:2237–43.

40 Habibi B, Perrier P, Salmon C. HD50 assay evaluation of the antigen Fy3 depression in Fy^x individuals. *J Immunogenet* 1980;**7**:191–3.

41 Tournamille C, Le Van Kim C, Gane P *et al.* Arg89Cys substitution results in very low membrane expression of the Duffy antigen/receptor for chemokines in Fy^x individuals. *Blood* 1998;**92**:2147–2156. Erratum in *Blood* 2000;**95**:2753.

42 Yazdanbakhsh K, Rios M, Storry JR *et al.* Molecular mechanisms that lead to reduced expression of Duffy antigens. *Transfusion* 2000;**40**:310–20.

43 Gassner C, Kraus RL, Dovc T *et al.* Fy^x is associated with two missense point mutations in its gene and can be detected by PCR-SSP. *Immunohematology* 2000;**16**:61–7.

44 Tamasauskas D, Powell V, Saksela K, Yazdanbakhsh K. A homologous naturally occurring mutation in Duffy and CCR5 leading to reduced receptor expression. *Blood* 2001;**97**:3651–4.

45 Moulds JM, Hayes S, Wells TD. DNA analysis of Duffy genes in American Blacks. *Transfusion* 1998; **74**:248–52.

46 Ikin EW, Mourant AE, Plaut G. A second example of the Duffy antibody. *Br Med J* 1950;i:584–5.

47 van Loghem JJ, van der Hart M. Een nieuwe bloedgroep. *Ned Tijdschr Geneeskd* 1950;**94**:748–9.

48 Rosenfield RE, Vogel P, Race RR. Un nouveau cas d'anti-Fy^a dans un sérum humain. *Rev Hémat* 1950;**5**: 315–7.

49 Mollison PL, Engelfriet CP, Contreras M. *Blood Transfusion in Clinical Medicine*, 10th edn. Oxford: Blackwell Science, 1997.

50 Issitt PD. Production of anti-Fy^a in Black Fy (a–b–) individuals. *Immunohematology* 1984;**1**:11–13.

51 Beattie KM. Letter. *Immunohematology* 1984;**1**:14.

52 Baldwin M, Shirey RS, Coyle K, Kickler TS, Ness PM. The incidence of anti-Fy^a and anti-Fy^b antibodies in Black and White patients [Abstract]. *Transfusion* 1986; **26**:546.

53 Sosler SD, Perkins JT, Fong K, Saporito C. The prevalence of immunization to Duffy antigens in a population of known racial distribution. *Transfusion* 1989; **29**:505–7.

54 Issitt PD, Anstee DJ. *Applied Blood Group Serology*, 4th edn. Durham: Montgomery Scientific Publications, 1997.

55 Oberdorfer CE, Kahn B, Moore V *et al.* A second example of anti-Fy3 in the Duffy blood group system. *Transfusion* 1974;**14**:608–11.

56 Molthan L, Crawford MN. Anti-Fy3: second example in a Black [Abstract]. *Transfusion* 1978;**18**:386.

57 Kosinski KS, Molthan L, White L. Three examples of anti-Fy3 produced in Negroes. *Rev Franc Transfus Immuno-Hémat* 1984;**27**:619–24.

58 Vengelen-Tyler V. Anti-Fy^a preceding anti-Fy3 or -Fy5: a study of five cases [Abstract]. *Transfusion* 1985;**25**:482.

59 Algora M, Barbolla L, Contreras M. Naturally occurring anti-D, anti-K, anti-Fy^a, and anti-Le^{ab}. *Vox Sang* 1991;**61**:141.

60 Hardman JT, Beck ML. Hemagglutination in capillaries: correlation with blood group specificity and IgG subclass. *Transfusion* 1981;**21**:343–6.

61 Szymanski IO, Huff SR, Delsignore R. An autoanalyzer test to determine immunoglobulin class and IgG subclass of blood group antibodies. *Transfusion* 1982; **22**:90–5.

62 Chown B, Lewis M, Kaita H. Atypical Duffy inheritance in three Caucasian families: a possible relationship to Mongolism. *Am J Hum Genet* 1962;**14**:301–308 and *Am J Hum Genet* 1965;**17**:188.

63 Race RR, Sanger R, Lehane D. Quantitative aspects of the blood-group antigen Fy^a. *Ann Eugen* 1953; **17**:255–66.

64 Pineda AA, Taswell HF, Brzica SM. Delayed hemolytic transfusion reaction: an immunologic hazard of blood transfusion. *Transfusion* 1978;**18**:1–7.

65 Freiesleben E. Fatal hemolytic transfusion reaction due to anti-Fy^a ('Duffy'). *Acta Path Microbiol Scand* 1951;**29**:283–6.

66 Badakere SS, Bhatia HM. A fatal transfusion reaction due to anti-Duffy (Fy^a): case report. *Indian J Med Sci* 1970;**24**:562–4.

67 Mollison PL, Cutbush M. Use of isotope-labelled red cells to demonstrate incompatibility *in vivo*. *Lancet* 1955;i:1290–5.

68 Gover PA, Morton JR. Transfusion reaction due to anti-Fy^a in donor blood. *Clin Lab Haematol* 1990;**12**:233–6.

69 Baker JB, Grewar D, Lewis M, Ayukawa H, Chown B. Haemolytic disease of the newborn due to anti-Duffy (Fy^a). *Arch Dis Child* 1956;**31**:298–9.

70 Greenwalt TJ, Sasaki T, Gajewski M. Further examples of haemolytic disease of the newborn due to anti-Duffy (anti-Fy^a). *Vox Sang* 1959;**4**:138–43.

71 Weinstein L, Taylor ES. Hemolytic disease of the neonate secondary to anti-Fy^a. *Am J Obstet Gynecol* 1975;**121**:643–5.

72 Goodrick MJ, Hadley AG, Poole G. Haemolytic disease of the fetus and newborn due to anti-Fy^a and the potential clinical value of Duffy genotyping in pregnancies at risk. *Transfusion Med* 1997;**7**:301–4.

73 Halverson GR, Reid ME, Yazdanbakhsh K, Pogo O, Chaudhuri A. The first murine monoclonal anti-Fy^a produced by a transgenic mouse expressing the human Fy^b antigen [Abstract]. *Transfusion* 1999;**39**(Suppl.): 92S.

74 Vetter O, Wegner H. A further case of anti-Fy^b and the frequency of Duffy-antigens in the population of the city of Leipzig. *Acta Genet* 1967;**17**:338–40.

75 Levine P, Sneath JS, Robinson EA, Huntington PW. A second example of anti-Fy^b. *Blood* 1955;**10**:941–4.

76 Giblett ER, Hillman RS, Brooks LE. Transfusion reaction during marrow suppression in a thalassemic patient with a blood group anomaly and an unusual cold agglutinin. *Vox Sang* 1965;**10**:448–59.

77 Contreras M, Gordon H, Tidmarsh E. A proven case of

maternal alloimmunization due to Duffy antigens in donor blood used for intrauterine transfusion. *Br J Haematol* 1983;**53**:355–6.

78 Michalewski B. Naturally occurring anti-Fy^b + C^w. *Vox Sang* 2001;**80**:235.

79 Badakere SS, Bhatia HM, Sharma RS, Bharucha Z. Anti-Fy^b (Duffy) as a cause of transfusion reaction: case report. *Indian J Med Sci* 1970;**24**:565–7.

80 Boyland IP, Mufti GJ, Hamblin TJ. Delayed hemolytic transfusion reaction caused by anti-Fy^b in a splenectomized patient. *Transfusion* 1982;**22**:402.

81 Carreras Vescio LA, Fariña D, Rogido M, Sóla A. Hemolytic disease of the newborn caused by anti-Fy^b. *Transfusion* 1987;**27**:366.

82 van't Veer MB, van Leeuwen I, Haas FJLM *et al.* Red-cell auto-antibodies mimicking anti-Fy^b specificity. *Vox Sang* 1984;**47**:88–91.

83 Harris T. Two cases of autoantibodies that demonstrate mimicking specificity in the Duffy blood group system. *Immunohematology* 1990;**6**:87–91.

84 Dickstein B, Kosanke J, Morris D *et al.* Report of an autoantibody with mimicking all anti-Fy^b specificity [Abstract]. *Transfusion* 1998;**38**(Suppl.):37S.

85 Colligan DA, Mackie A, Fraser RH. Production of murine monoclonal anti-Fy^b [Abstract]. *Transfus Med* 2000;**10**(Suppl.1):6.

86 Sanger R, Race RR, Jack J. The Duffy blood groups of New York Negroes: the phenotype Fy (a–b–). *Br J Haematol* 1955;**1**:370–4.

87 Race RR, Sanger R. *Blood Groups in Man*, 6th edn. Oxford: Blackwell Scientific Publications, 1975.

88 Welch SG, McGregor IA, Williams K. The Duffy blood group and malaria prevalence in Gambian West Africans. *Trans R Soc Trop Med Hyg* 1977;**71**:295–6.

89 Peiper SC, Wang Z, Neote K *et al.* The Duffy antigen/receptor for chemokines (DARC) is expressed in endothelial cells of Duffy-negative individuals who lack the erythrocyte receptor. *J Exp Med* 1995;**181**:1311–17.

90 Iwamoto S, Li J, Sugimoto N, Okuda H, Kajii E. Characterization of the Duffy gene promoter: evidence for tissue-specific abolishment of expression in Fy (a–b–) of black individuals. *Biochem Biophys Res Commun* 1996;**222**:852–9.

91 Zimmerman PA, Woolley I, Masinde GL *et al.* Emergence of *FY* * A^{null} in a *Plasmodium vivax*-endemic region of Papua New Guinea. *Proc Natl Acad Sci USA* 1999;**96**:13973–7.

92 Rios M, Chaudhuri A, Mallinson G *et al.* New genotypes in Fy(a–b–) individuals: nonsense mutations (Trp to stop) in the coding sequence of either *FY A* or *FY B*. *Br J Haematol* 2000;**108**:448–54.

93 Tsuneyama H, Uchikawa M, Shinozaki K *et al.* A deletion in the Duffy gene of an apparently healthy individual with the Fy(a–b–) phenotype [Abstract]. *Transfusion* 2000;**40**(Suppl.):116S.

94 Libich M, Kout M, Giles CM. Fy (a–b–) phenotype in Czechoslovakia. *Vox Sang* 1978;**35**:423–5.

95 Pisacka M, Vytiskova J, Latinakova A, *et al.* Molecular background of the Fy(a–b–) phenotype in gypsy population living in the Czech and Slovak Republics [Abstract]. *Transfusion* 2001;**41**:15S.

96 Mannessier L, Habibi B, Salmon C. Un nouvel example anti-Fy3 comportant une réactivité pseudo-anti-Fy^a. *Rev Franc Transfus Immuno-Hémat* 1979;**22**:195–8.

97 Miller LH, Mason SJ, Clyde DF, McGinniss MH. The resistance factor to *Plasmodium vivax* in Blacks: the Duffy blood group genotype, FyFy. *N Engl J Med* 1976;**295**:302–4.

98 Barnwell JW, Nichols ME, Rubinstein P. *In vitro* evaluation of the role of the Duffy blood group in erythrocyte invasion by *Plasmodium vivax*. *J Exp Med* 1989;**169**:1795–802.

99 Miller LH, Haynes JD, McAuliffe FM, Shiroishi T, Durocher JR, McGinniss MH. Evidence for differences in erythrocyte surface receptors for the malarial parasites, *Plasmodium falciparum* and *Plasmodium knowlesi*. *J Exp Med* 1977;**146**:277–81.

100 Miller LH, Aikawa M, Johnson JG, Shiroishi T. Interaction between cytochalasin B-treated malarial parasites and erythrocytes: attachment and junction formation. *J Exp Med* 1979;**149**:172–84.

101 Haynes JD, Dalton JP, Klotz FW *et al.* Receptor-like specificity of a *Plasmodium knowlesi* malarial protein that binds to Duffy antigen ligands on erythrocytes. *J Exp Med* 1988;**167**:1873–81.

102 Wertheimer SP, Barnwell JW. *Plasmodium vivax* interation with the human Duffy blood group glycoprotein: identification of a parasite receptor-like protein. *Exp Parasitol* 1989;**69**:340–50.

103 Miller LH, McAuliffe FM, Mason SJ. Erythrocyte receptors for malaria merozoites. *Am J Trop Med Hyg* 1977;**26**(6):204–8.

104 Adams JH, Kim Lee Sim B, Dolan SA *et al.* A family of erythrocyte binding proteins of malaria parasites. *Proc Natl Acad Sci USA* 1992;**89**:7085–9.

105 Oakes J, Taylor D, Johnson C, Marsh WL. Fy3 antigenicity of blood of newborns. *Transfusion* 1978;**18**:127–8.

106 Jensen N, Crosson J, Grotte D, Anderson D. Severe hemolytic reaction due to anti-Fy3 following partial red cell exchange for sickle cell disease (SCD) [Abstract]. *Transfusion* 1988;**28**(Suppl.):8S.

107 Le Pennec PY, Rouger P, Klein MT, Robert N, Salmon C. Study of anti-Fy^a in five black Fy(a–b–) patients. *Vox Sang* 1987;**52**:246–9.

108 Daniels G, ed. Third International Workshop on Monoclonal Antibodies Against Human Red Blood Cell and Related Antigens. *Transfus Clin Biol* 1997;**4**:99–114 (4 papers).

109 Lu Z, Wang Z, Horuk R *et al.* The promiscuous chemokine binding profile of the Duffy antigen/receptor

for chemokines is primarily localized to sequences in the amino-terminal domain. *J Biol Chem* 1995;270: 26239–45.

110 Colledge KI, Pezzulich M, Marsh WL. Anti-Fy5, an antibody disclosing a probable association between the Rhesus and Duffy blood group genes. *Vox Sang* 1973;24:193–9.

111 DiNapoli J, Garcia A, Marsh WL, Dreizin D. A second example of anti-Fy5. *Vox Sang* 1976;30:308–11.

112 Chan-Shu SA. The second example of anti-Duffy[5]. *Transfusion* 1980;20:358–60.

113 Bowen DT, Devenish A, Dalton J, Hewitt PE. Delayed haemolytic transfusion reaction due to simultaneous appearance of anti-Fy[a] and anti-Fy5. *Vox Sang* 1988; 55:35–6.

114 Meredith LC. Anti-Fy5 does not react with e variants [Abstract]. *Transfusion* 1985;25:482.

115 Wasniowska K, Blanchard D, Janvier D *et al.* Identification of the Fy6 epitope recognized by two monoclonal antibodies in the N-terminal extracellular portion of the Duffy antigen receptor for chemokines. *Mol Imuunol* 1996;33:917–23.

116 Behzad O, Lee CL, Gavin J, Marsh WL. A new antierythrocyte antibody in the Duffy system: anti-Fy4. *Vox Sang* 1973;24:337–42.

117 Murphy MT, Templeton LJ, Fleming J *et al.* Comparison of Fy[b] status as determined serologically and genetically. *Transfus Med* 1997;7:135–41.

118 Mullighan CG, Marshall SE, Fanning GC, Briggs DC, Welsh KI. Rapid haplotyping of mutations in the Duffy gene using the polymerase chain reaction and sequence-specific primers. *Tissue Antigens* 1998;51: 195–9.

119 Hessner MJ, Pircon RA, Johnson ST, Luhm RA. Prenatal genotyping of the Duffy blood group system by allele-specific polymerase chain reaction. *Prenat Diagn* 1999;19:41–5.

120 Masouredis SP, Sudora E, Mahan L, Victoria EJ. Quantitative immunoferritin microscopy of Fy[a], Fy[b], Jk[a], U, and Di[b] antigen site numbers on human red cells. *Blood* 1980;56:969–77.

121 Toivanen P, Hirvonen T. Fetal development of red cell antigens K, k, Lu[a], Lu[b], Fy[a], Fy[b], Vel and Xg[a]. *Scand J Haematol* 1969;6:49–55.

122 Toivanen P, Hirvonen T. Antigens Duffy, Kell, Kidd, Lutheran and Xg[a] on fetal red cells. *Vox Sang* 1973;24:372–6.

123 Southcott MJG, Tanner MJA, Anstee DJ. The expression of human blood group antigens during erythropoiesis in a cell culture system. *Blood* 1999;93: 4425–35.

124 Daniels G, Green C. Expression of red cell surface antigens during erythropoiesis. *Vox Sang* 2000; 78(Suppl.1):149–53.

125 Bony V, Gane P, Bailly P, Cartron J-P. Time-course expression of polypeptides carrying blood group antigens during human erythroid differentiation. *Br J Haematol* 1999;107:263–74.

126 Woolley IJ, Hotmire KA, Sramkoski RM, Zimmerman PA, Kazura JW. Differential expression of the Duffy antigen receptor for chemokines according to RBC age and *FY* genotype. *Transfusion* 2000;40:949–53.

127 Hadley TJ, Lu Z, Wasniowska K *et al.* Postcapillary venule endothelial cells in kidney express a multispecific chemokine receptor that is structurally and functionally identical to the erythroid isoform, which is the Duffy blood group antigen. *J Clin Invest* 1994;94:985–91.

128 Chaudhuri A, Nielsen S, Elkjaer M-L *et al.* Detection of Duffy antigen in the plasma membranes and caveolae of vascular endothelial and epithelial cells of nonerythroid organs. *Blood* 1997;89:701–12.

129 Horuk R, Martin AW, Wang Z *et al.* Expression of chemokine receptors by subsets of neurons in the central nervous system. *J Immunol* 1997;158:2882–90.

130 Le Van Kim C, Tournamille C, Kroviarski Y, Cartron JP, Colin Y. The 1.35-kb and 7.5-kb Duffy mRNA isoforms are differentially regulated in various regions of the brain, differ by the length of their 5′ untranslated sequence, but encode the same polypeptide. *Blood* 1997;70:2851–3.

131 Dunstan RA, Simpson MB, Rosse WF. Erythrocyte antigens on human platelets: absence of Rh, Duffy, Kell, Kidd, and Lutheran antigens. *Transfusion* 1984;24: 243–6.

132 Dunstan RA. Status of major red cell blood group antigens on neutrophils, lymphocytes and monocytes. *Br J Haematol* 1986;62:301–9.

133 Rollins BJ. Chemokines. *Blood* 1997;90:909–28.

134 Darbonne WC, Rice GC, Mohler MA *et al.* Red blood cells are a sink for interleukin 8, a leukocyte chemotaxin. *J Clin Invest* 1991;88:1362–9.

135 Neote K, Darbonne W, Ogez J, Horuk R, Schall TJ. Identification of a promiscuous inflammatory peptide receptor on the surface of red blood cells. *J Biol Chem* 1993;268:12247–9.

136 Horuk R, Colby TJ, Darbonne WC, Schall TJ, Neote K. The human erythrocyte inflammatory peptide (chemokine) receptor, biochemical characterization, solubilization, and development of a binding assay for the soluble receptor. *Biochemistry* 1993;32:5733–8.

137 Szabo MC, Soo KS, Zlotnik A, Schall TJ. Chemokine class differences in binding to the Duffy antigen-erythrocyte chemokine receptor. *J Biol Chem* 1995; 270:25348–51.

138 Hadley TJ, Peiper SC. From malaria to chemokine receptor: the emerging physiologic role of the Duffy blood group antigen. *Blood* 1997;89:3077–91.

139 Horuk R, Chitnis CE, Darbonne WC *et al.* A receptor for the malarial parasite *Plasmodium vivax*: the erythrocyte chemokine receptor. *Science* 1993;261: 1182–4.

140 Tournamille C, Le Van Kim C, Gane P *et al.* Close association of the first and fourth extracellular domains of the Duffy antigen/receptor for chemokines by a disulphide bond is required for ligand binding. *J Biol Chem* 1997;272:16274–80.

141 Chaudhuri A, Zbrzezna V, Polyakova J *et al.* Expression of the Duffy antigen in K562 cells. Evidence that it is the human erythrocyte chemokine receptor. *J Biol Chem* 1994;269:7835–8.

142 Hausman E, Dzik W, Blanchard D. The red cell chemokine receptor is distinct from the Fy6 epitope. *Transfusion* 1996;36:421–425.

143 Wasniowska K, Czerwinski M, Jachymek W, Lisowska E. Expression and binding properties of a soluble chimeric protein containing the N-terminal domain of the Duffy antigen. *Biochem Biophys Res Commun* 2000;273:705–11.

144 de Winter RJ, Manten A, de Jong YP *et al.* Interleukin 8 released after acute myocardial infarction is mainly bound to red cells. *Heart* 1997;78:598–602.

145 Liu X-H, Hadley TJ, Xu L, Peiper SC, Ray PE. Up-regulation of Duffy antigen receptor expression in children with renal disease. *Kidney Int* 1999;55:1491–500.

146 Luo H, Chaudhuri A, Johnson KR *et al.* Cloning, characterization, and mapping of a murine promiscuous chemokine receptor gene: homolog of the human Duffy gene. *Genome Res* 1997;7:932–41.

147 Luo H, Chaudhuri A, Zbrzezna Yu H, Pogo AO. Deletion of the murine Duffy gene (*Dfy*) reveals that the Duffy receptor is functionally redundant. *Mol Cell Biol* 2000;20:3097–101.

148 Dawson TC, Lentsch AB, Wang Z *et al.* Exaggerated response to endotoxin in mice lacking the Duffy antigen/receptor for chemokines (DARC). *Blood* 2000;96:1681–4.

149 Hadley TJ, Miller LH, Haynes JD. Recognition of red cells by malaria parasites: the role of erythrocyte-binding proteins. *Transfus Med Rev* 1991;5:108–22.

150 Spencer HC, Miller LH, Collins WE *et al.* The Duffy blood group and resistance to *Plasmodium vivax* in Honduras. *Am J Trop Med Hyg* 1978;27:664–70.

151 Mason SJ, Miller LH, Shiroishi T, Dvorak JA, McGinniss MH. The Duffy blood group determinants: their role in the susceptibility of human and animal erythrocytes to *Plasmodium knowlesi* malaria. *Br J Haematol* 1977;36:327–35.

152 Chitnis CE, Miller LH. Identification of the erythrocyte binding domains of *Plasmodium vivax* and *Plasmodium knowlesi* proteins involved in erythrocyte invasion. *J Exp Med* 1994;180:497–506.

153 Chitnis CE, Chaudhuri A, Horuk R, Pogo AO, Miller LH. The domain of the Duffy blood group antigen for binding *Plasmodium vivax and P. knowlesi* malarial parasites to erythrocytes. *J Exp Med* 1996;184:1531–6.

154 Michon P, Woolley I, Wood EM *et al.* Duffy-null promoter heterozygosity reduces DARC expression and abrogates adhesion of the *P. vivax* ligand required for blood-stage infection. *FEBS Lett* 2001;495:111–14.

155 Singh S, Pandey K, Chattopadhayay R *et al.* Biochemical, biophysical and functional characterization of bacterially expressed and refolded receptor binding domain of *Plasmodium vivax* Duffy-binding protein. *J Biol Chem* 2001;276:17111–6.

156 Williams TN, Maitland K, Bennett S *et al.* High incidence of malaria in α-thalassaemic children. *Nature* 1996;383:522–5.

157 Tippett P, Gavin J. Duffy groups and malaria in monkeys [Abstract]. *Transfusion* 1979;19:662.

158 Palatnik M, Rowe AW. Duffy and Duffy-related human antigens in primates. *J Hum Evol* 1984;13:173–9.

Kidd blood group system

9.1 Introduction

Jk^a and Jk^b of the Kidd system are the products of alleles and are polymorphic in all populations tested. The Jk^a/Jk^b polymorphism is associated with an Asp280Asn substitution in the Kidd antigen. Kidd antibodies are often difficult to work with. They are potentially dangerous, as they are a common cause of delayed haemolytic transfusion reactions.

A rare null phenotype, Jk(a–b–), is generally inherited recessively and is most commonly found in Polynesians. Jk(a–b–) cells lack the high incidence antigen Jk3. Five inactivating mutations, responsible for Jk(a–b–), have been found.

The Kidd glycoprotein functions as a urea transporter.

The *JK* (*SLC14A1*) locus is on chromosome 18 at 18q11–q12 (Chapter 32).

9.2 The Kidd glycoprotein and the gene that encodes it

Before the Kidd glycoprotein had been purified or the *JK* gene cloned, failure of Jk(a–b–) red cells to lyse in 2 M urea led to the supposition that the Kidd glycoprotein might be a red cell urea transporter (Section 9.4.2). A red cell membrane structure of apparent M_r 45 000 was isolated by affinity purified IgG anti-Jk^a, -Jk^b, and -Jk3 bound to nylon membranes [1]. Immunoprecipitation with anti-Jk3 isolated a glycoprotein of apparent M_r 46 000–60 000 from red cells of all phenotypes except Jk(a–b–) [2]. The M_r was reduced to 36 000 by removal of N-glycosylation with N-glycanase [2]. Jk(a+b–) red cells were estimated to have around 14 000 Jk^a antigen sites by immunoelectron microscopy with anti-Jk^a and ferritin labelled

anti-human IgG [3]. This is compatible with an estimate of less than 32 000 sites per cell obtained by determining the quantity of a mercurial required to inhibit facilitated urea transport [4].

Olivès *et al.* [5] produced a cDNA probe from human erythroblast mRNA by reverse transcriptase polymerase chain reaction (PCR) with primers derived from the amino acid sequence of a rabbit urea transporter. They used this probe to isolate a cDNA clone (*HUT11*) by screening a human bone marrow library. An M_r 36 000 polypeptide produced by coupled *in vitro* transcription-translation of the cDNA was immunoprecipitated by anti-Jk3. Immunoblotting with a rabbit antibody raised to peptides predicted from the cDNA sequence revealed M_r 46 000–60 000 components from human red cell membranes, except those of the Jk(a–b–) phenotype [2]. *HUT11* has subsequently been shown to be an aberrant transcript or a cloning artefact [6]. Another transcript (*HUT11A*) encoding glutamic acid in place of lysine at position 44 and two Val-Gly dipeptides instead of three after position 227, produces the Kidd glycoprotein and red cell urea transporter [6,7]. The predicted gene product is an M_r 43 000, 389 amino acid polypeptide with about 63% identity with the rabbit urea transporter. The protein contains 10 potential membrane-spanning domains (Fig. 9.1). Only one of two N-glycosylation consensus sequences (Asn211) is extracellular and is on the third extracellular loop.

The *JK* (*SLC14A1*) gene is 30 kb long and contains 11 exons [8,9]. Exons 1–3 and part of 4 represent the 3' untranslated region; exons 4–11 encode the mature protein (Table 9.1). The transcription initiation site is 335 bp upstream of the translation start codon in exon 4. The region between nucleotides –837 and –336 contains erythroid-specific GATA-1 and SP1 transcription

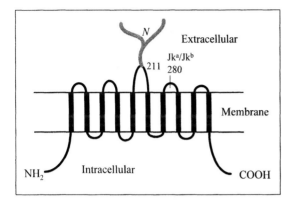

Fig. 9.1 Diagrammatic representation of the Kidd glycoprotein in the red cell membrane, showing 10 membrane-spanning domains, cytoplasmic N- and C-termini, a single *N*-glycan on the third extracellular loop, and the position of the Jk^a/Jk^b polymorphism on the fourth extracellular loop.

Table 9.1 Organization of the *JK* gene.

Exon	Size (bp)	Amino acids	Intron size (kb) [8]	Intron size (kb) [9]
1	93		0.7	
2	64		2.4	
3	157		3.1	
4	172	1–50	0.6	0.543
5	190	51–113	3.55	3.0
6	129	114–156	1.9	2.0
7	193	157–221	2.5	2.5
8	148	222–270	0.27	0.217
9	135	271–315	8.6	9.0
10	50	316–332	1.4	1.4
11	551	333–389		

factor binding sites, plus TATA and inverted CAAT boxes [8]. Two equally abundant erythroid transcripts, of 4.4 and 2.0 kb, have been identified, the smaller arising from skipping of exon 3 [8].

9.3 Jk^a and Jk^b (JK1 and JK2)

An antibody in the serum of an American woman, Mrs Kidd, was named anti-Jk^a in 1951 by Allen *et al.* [10], from the initials of Mrs Kidd's sixth child, who showed signs of haemolytic disease of the newborn (HDN).

The antibody reacted with the red cells of 77% of Bostonians. The anticipated antithetical antibody, anti-Jk^b, was found in England 2 years later by Plaut *et al.* [11].

9.3.1 Frequency of Jk^a and Jk^b

The following phenotype frequencies were obtained from six series of tests with anti-Jk^a on a total of 4275 Europeans [12]: Jk(a+), 76.4%; and Jk(a–), 23.6%. The following gene and genotype frequencies are derived from these figures: *Jk^a* 0.5142, *Jk^b* 0.4858; *Jk^a/Jk^a* 0.2644, *Jk^a/Jk^b* 0.4996, and *Jk^b/Jk^b* 0.2360. These gene frequencies are very similar to those obtained from tests with anti-Jk^a and -Jk^b on red cells from 2102 parents of 1051 Canadian families [12,13]: *Jk^a* 0.5162 and *Jk^b* 0.4838. Molecular analysis on DNA from 106 Swedes gave the allele frequencies *Jk^a* 0.53 and *Jk^b* 0.47 [7]. Numerous other population studies, many conducted with anti-Jk^a only, have been summarized [14,15]. The gene frequency of *Jk^a*, usually about 50% in Europeans, rises to 75% in some parts of Africa, but this frequency is by no means representative of all African populations. The frequency of *Jk^a* is around 30% in Chinese and falls to as low as 20% in some Japanese studies, but this low frequency does not occur throughout Asia.

9.3.2 Inheritance of Jk^a and Jk^b and the molecular basis of the Kidd polymorphism

Jk^a and *Jk^b* are inherited as codominant alleles. Analysis of over 2000 white families provided phenotype frequencies that fitted well with those calculated on the basis of two alleles [12,13]. The frequency of a silent allele, *Jk*, is too low to upset these calculations.

The *Jk^a/Jk^b* polymorphism results from a G838A transition, encoding an Asp280Asn substitution on the fourth extracellular loop of the Kidd glycoprotein [16] (Fig. 9.1). *Jk^a/Jk^b* is also associated with a silent G588A transition in exon 7 and another single nucleotide polymorphism at position –46 from the 3′ end of intron 9 [9]. G838 of the *Jk^a* allele introduces an *Mnl*I restriction site, which can be used for genotyping and Kidd phenotype prediction [6]. Other genotyping methods involve PCR with allele-specific primers [7,17]. In one of the methods, *Jk^a* and *Jk^b* are detected in a single multiplex PCR with a *Jk^a*-specific forward primer and a *Jk^b*-specific reverse primer, their corresponding reverse and forward primers being positioned to give amplification products of different sizes [7].

9.3.3 Effect of enzymes and reducing agents

Jk^a, Jk^b, and Jk3 are papain-, ficin-, trypsin-, chymotrypsin-, and pronase-resistant; treatment of red cells with these enzymes generally enhances reactivity with Kidd antibodies. Kidd antigens are not affected by sialidase or by 2-aminoethylisothiouronium bromide (AET).

9.3.4 Anti-Jk^a and -Jk^b

9.3.4.1 Alloantibodies

After the description of Mrs Kidd's antibody in 1951 [10], many reports of anti-Jk^a [18–23] and -Jk^b [11,24–27] soon followed. Numerous other examples have since been found, but neither antibody is common, anti-Jk^b being rarer than anti-Jk^a. They are often found in antibody mixtures, reflecting the relatively low immunogenicity of the Kidd antigens. Anti-Jk^a, in two Jk(a–b+) 9-month-old non-identical twins, detectable only by solid-phase method, are the only reported examples of 'naturally occurring' Kidd antibodies [28]. Anti-Jk^a has been found during the first pregnancy of an untransfused woman [20] and a case of anti-Jk^a sensitization following amniocentesis and intrauterine transfusion is reported [29].

Kidd antibodies are often difficult to detect. Some directly agglutinate antigen-positive cells, but the reactions are usually weak by this method [10,19,20,27,30–32]. Generally an antiglobulin test is required to detect Kidd antibodies. Use of enzyme-treated cells may be necessary to detect weaker antibodies. Anti-Jk^a detectable only by the manual Polybrene test was responsible for a haemolytic transfusion reaction, emphasizing the importance of detecting weak Kidd antibodies [33]. Many anti-Jk^a react more strongly with Jk(a+b–) than with Jk(a+b+) cells [12,34], and some anti-Jk^a can only be detected with Jk(a+b–) cells [22]. Panels for screening patient sera for antibodies should therefore contain Jk(a+b–) cells. Some anti-Jk^b also demonstrate a hint of dosage [11,31].

Kidd antibodies are usually IgG or a mixture of IgG and IgM; they are rarely pure IgM [35,36]. Most IgG anti-Jk^a are IgG3 or a mixture of IgG3 and IgG1, and occasionally IgG1 alone [36,37]. IgG2 may also be present [36]. Four anti-Jk^b contained IgG1; one also contained IgG3 and one IgG4 [37]. Around 40–50% of sera containing Kidd antibodies bind complement; some Kidd antibodies can only be detected in the antiglobulin test when polyspecific antiglobulin or anti-complement is used [38,39]. Some Kidd antibodies may not be detectable by techniques incorporating a diluent that binds calcium [40]. Only those Kidd sera with an IgM component are capable of complement binding as IgG Kidd antibodies are unable to fix complement [39].

9.3.4.2 Clinical significance

Kidd antibodies, which are often difficult to detect, are a hazard in blood transfusion. Anti-Jk^a has been responsible for severe and fatal immediate haemolytic transfusion reactions [19,32,33,41,42] and is regularly associated with delayed haemolytic transfusion reactions (DHTR) [38,43,44]. These DHTR may be severe, leading to oliguria, renal failure, and even death [43,44]. Anti-Jk^b has also been incriminated in severe DHTR [31,45]. Probably a major reason why Kidd antibodies are such a common cause of DHTR is their tendency to fall rapidly to low or undetectable levels in the plasma [18,19,31,46]. Pineda *et al.* [43,47] estimated that over one-third of DHTRs were caused by anti-Jk^a.

Clearance of incompatible red cells transfused to individuals with Kidd antibodies is generally rapid [33,48,49]. The reactivity of anti-Jk^a and -Jk^b in a monocyte monolayer assay is enhanced by the presence of complement [50,51].

Anti-Jk^a was responsible for haemolysis and drop in haemoglobin in a Jk(a+) recipient of a peripheral blood progenitor cell transplant from her Jk(a–) sister [52]. The antibody was probably produced by passenger lymphocytes derived from the donor. The patient was being treated with cyclosporin and methotrexate.

In contrast to the haemolytic activity of Kidd antibodies in incompatible blood transfusion, anti-Jk^a and -Jk^b are only very rarely responsible for severe HDN [53]. Only one such case is reported, this caused by anti-Jk^a and resulting in kernicterus [46]. The reason why Kidd antibodies so rarely cause HDN, even when present in relatively high titre, is unclear.

9.3.4.3 Autoantibodies

Several cases of autoanti-Jk^a associated with autoimmune haemolytic anaemia (AIHA) have been described [54–59]. Red cells of one patient, who also developed idiopathic thrombocytopenic purpura, were initially typed as Jk(a–b+), but later became Jk(a+b+), their true phenotype as demonstrated by family study [59]. AIHA in a Jk(a+) patient taking Aldomet (methyldopa), with anti-Jk^a in her serum and in an eluate from her red cells, declined on cessation of the drug and the autoantibody gradually disappeared [55]. A Jk(a+b+) patient taking chlorpropamide, a hypoglycaemic agent, had an apparent anti-Jk^a in her serum and acute haemolytic anaemia [57]. In a post-transfusion specimen the anti-Jk^a only reacted with Jk(a+b+) cells in the presence of chlorpropamide or related structures. The antibody could not be neutralized with chlorpropamide and drug–antibody complexes attaching preferentially to Jk(a+) red cells were proposed to explain the phenomenon [57]. The AIHA declined when chlorpropamide administration was stopped. The Kidd antigen is a urea transporter (Section 9.6), which may be pertinent as chlorpropamide contains a urea structure.

Autoanti-Jk^a has also been found in healthy individuals [60,61]. Four examples of benign autoanti-Jk^a reacted preferentially with red cells in the presence of parabens (butyl, ethyl, methyl, and propyl esters of *p*-hydroxybenzoate) or certain other neutral aromatic compounds [62,63]. The antibodies were detected because of the presence of parabens as preservatives in commercial low ionic-strength solutions. Judd *et al.* [62] suggested that either parabens cause a reversible structural alteration to the Jk^a antigen, which is recognized by the autoantibodies, or that the benzene rings of the parabens interact with aromatic amino acid residues involved in both the Jk^a antigen and the binding sites of the antibodies.

A Jk(a–b+) nephrectomy patient who had suffered from chronic proteus infections showed signs of a haemolytic transfusion reaction, although no transfusion had taken place [64]. The patient's serum contained autoanti-Jk^b. Jk(b–) red cells incubated with *Proteus mirabilis* reacted with anti-Jk^b reagents.

9.3.4.4 Monoclonal antibodies

IgM human monoclonal anti-Jk^a and -Jk^b have been produced by Epstein–Barr virus transformation of lymphocytes from immunized donors and fusion with mouse myeloma cells to form heterohybridomas [65,66]. Some of these antibodies make excellent agglutinating blood grouping reagents [66]. Kidd alloantibodies are notorious for being unstable, unreliable, and present in mixtures of antibodies to red cell antigens. As reagents, monoclonal antibodies are a welcome replacement.

9.4 Jk(a–b–) phenotype and Jk3 antigen

The Kidd null phenotype, Jk(a–b–), was first described by Pinkerton *et al.* in 1959 [67]. A Filipino woman of Chinese and Spanish ancestry, with two children, became jaundiced after blood transfusion. Her serum reacted with all cells save her own, which had the novel phenotype Jk(a–b–). Adsorption of her serum with Jk(a+b–) cells left some activity for Jk(a–b+) cells, but adsorption with Jk(a–b+) cells removed all antibody. Eluates from the adsorbing cells reacted with Jk(a+b–) and Jk(a–b+) cells. Thus, her serum contained a mixture of the first example of anti-Jk3, plus anti-Jk^b.

9.4.1 Jk(a–b–) of the recessive type

In this section a number of Jk(a–b–) individuals from a variety of ethnic groups are mentioned. Serological studies on some families have suggested that the phenotype results from homozygosity for a rare recessive gene [68–72]. In one family, for example, three Jk(a–b–) sibs had other sibs with the phenotypes Jk(a+b–), Jk(a–b+), and Jk(a+b+), suggesting that their parents had the genotypes *Jk^a/Jk* and *Jk^b/Jk* [69]. Examples of the Jk(a–b–) phenotype have been reported in Polynesians [9,68,71,73–76], Filipinos and Indonesians [15,77,78], Chinese [8,79], Japanese [80], Asian Indians [15,81], Native Brazilians [15,82], an African American [83], a Tunisian [84], and in Europeans, including Finns [9,76,85], French [70], Swiss [72], and English [72] families. Many were ascertained through the production of anti-Jk3 [68–70,72,73,78,79,85].

Jk(a–b–) is most abundant amongst Polynesians. Of 17 300 random Polynesian blood donors screened by the urea lysis method (Section 9.4.2) and confirmed serologically, 47 (0.27%) were Jk(a–b–) Jk:–3 [75]. The highest frequency was found in Niueans and Tongans, with 1.4 and 1.2% Jk(a–b–), respectively

[75]. The urea lysis method has been used to search for Jk(a–b–) in other ethnic groups. Of 638 460 Japanese donors in Osaka, 14 were Jk(a–b–), of whom 12 (0.002%) appeared to be of the recessive type [80]. Screening of 13 817 South African (Natal) blood donors disclosed a Jk(a–b–) donor of Indian origin [81]. Screening of 52 908 English and 120 000 predominantly European New Zealand blood donors by a urea lysis test revealed no European Jk(a–b–) [74,86], but 24 (0.03%) of 79 349 Finns were Jk:–3 [85]. Aberrant inheritance of *Jk^a* and *Jk^b*, supported by dosage studies, demonstrated the presence of a *Jk* allele in the original Lu_{null} family, a white American family [34], and in an African American family [87].

Homozygosity for five different mutations has been shown to be responsible for the Jk(a–b–) phenotype.

1 The Polynesian mutation is a G to A transition in the invariant 3′ acceptor splice site of intron 5 of a *Jk^b* allele, causing loss of exon 6 from mRNA transcripts [8,9]. The predicted, truncated Kidd glycoprotein could not be detected in *Xenopus* oocytes transfected with the abnormal transcript [8]. Of 46 Polynesians, eight were heterozygous for the intron 5 mutation, a gene frequency of 8.7%, which predicts an incidence of 0.76% for Jk(a–b–) [9]. This mutation was also found in Chinese, Australian, American, and European Jk(a–b–) individuals [76].

2 The Finnish mutation is a T871C transition in a *Jk^b* allele, encoding Ser291Pro [9,76]. Although this substitution disrupts a potential *N*-glycosylation site (Asn289-Ser-Ser to Asn-Ser-Pro), Asn289 is situated in the eighth predicted membrane-spanning domain and is not glycosylated [76]. When expressed in *Xenopus* oocytes, the mutated protein functions as a urea transporter, but does not appear to reach the membrane of erythroid cells [76].

3 In one Jk(a–b–) white French person, a G to T transversion in the donor splice site of intron 7 of a *Jk^b* allele led to skipping of exon 7 from the mRNA transcript [8].

4 A deletion of about 1.6 kb encompassing exons 4 and 5 of a *Jk^a* allele in two Jk(a–b–) English sisters and a Tunisian [72,84]. In the English sisters, no transcript contained exon 3 and the most abundant transcript lacked exons 3–5 (exon 4 contains the translation start codon) [72]. In the Tunisian, exons 4 and 5 were missing from the transcript, but were replaced by 136 bp of intron 3 sequence flanked by cryptic splice sites [84].

5 A nonsense mutation in exon 7 of a *Jk^a* allele converting the codon for Tyr194 to a stop codon in three Jk(a–b–) Swiss sisters. This mutation predicts a truncated polypeptide of 193 amino acids [72].

These five mutations can be detected by a multiplex PCR-based technique [72].

9.4.2 The urea lysis test for Jk(a–b–) phenotype

The urea lysis test for detecting Jk(a–b–) phenotype was discovered serendipitously by Heaton and McLoughlin [74] in 1982. A Samoan man with aplastic anaemia appeared to have excessively high platelet counts in an automated system, which was dependent on lysing red cells with 2 *M* urea. These false platelet counts were shown to result from a failure of his Jk(a–b–) red cells to lyse. Red cells of common Kidd phenotypes lysed within 1 min in 2 *M* urea; Jk(a–b–) red cells required at least 30 min for lysis. The urea lysis test has proved useful in screening for Jk(a–b–) [71,75,80,81,85,86]. Red cells of individuals heterozygous for the *Jk* allele demonstrated intermediate lysis time in a modified urea lysis test [88].

9.4.3 Anti-Jk3

Anti-Jk3, an antibody produced by the original Jk(a–b–) propositus, behaved as inseparable anti-Jk^aJk^b, with no preference for Jk(a+b–) or Jk(a–b+) cells [67]. Anti-Jk3 is a rare antibody, yet many examples of this antibody have been described [68,69,71,73,77–79,81,83].

Anti-Jk3 is not usually found in antibody mixtures, but may be accompanied by separable anti-Jk^a [79] or anti-Jk^b [67,78]. Only a minority of immunized Jk(a–b–) people produce anti-Jk3 [71,80]. An apparently 'naturally occurring' IgM anti-Jk3 was found in an untransfused male, the only reported example; his Jk(a–b–) sister had been pregnant seven times without making anti-Jk3 [69].

Jk3 antibodies react optimally by an antiglobulin test, the reaction being enhanced by enzyme treatment of the cells. Enzyme-treated cells may be haemolysed by anti-Jk3 in the presence of fresh serum [68]. Anti-Jk3 are usually IgG [71,73,74]. Like other Kidd antibodies, anti-Jk3 may decline rapidly *in vivo* [79].

Anti-Jk3 has been responsible for severe immediate [89] and delayed [71,77,79] haemolytic transfusion reactions. Most babies of mothers with anti-Jk3 are clinically unaffected, although the baby's red cells may give a positive direct antiglobulin test, and in a few cases phototherapy was administered [71,73,78,81].

Two examples of autoanti-Jk3, or mimicking autoanti-Jk3, have occurred during pregnancy [90,91]. In one, which was associated with autoimmune haemolytic anaemia, mimicking autoanti-Jk^b was also present [90]. Anti-Jk3 in a patient with transient Jk(a–b–) phenotype is described in Section 9.4.5.

9.4.4 Jk(a–b–) of the dominant type

Red cells from two of 14 Jk(a–b–) Japanese blood donors found by the urea lysis test (Section 9.4.2) proved to be different from those of the other 12 and from Jk(a–b–) cells previously reported [80]. A family study suggested a dominant mode of inheritance: the presence of a Jk(a+b+) mother of two Jk(a–b–) daughters, both with Jk(a–b–) children, excludes homozygosity of a silent gene. The dominant inhibitor gene proposed to account for these observations was named *In(Jk)*, as it was considered analogous to *In(Lu)* of the Lutheran system (Chapter 6). Although two further examples have been found in Japan, the recessive type of Jk(a–b–) is estimated to be six times more frequent than the dominant type in Japan [80].

Jk(a–b–) red cells of the dominant type can bind anti-Jk3 and anti-Jk^a and/or anti-Jk^b, as detected in adsorption and elution tests. Kidd genotypes deduced in this way demonstrated that *In(Jk)* is not inherited at the *JK* locus. In(Jk) cells are less readily lysed in the urea lysis test than cells of common Kidd type and less resistant to lysis than Jk(a–b–) cells of the recessive type [80].

9.4.5 Transient Jk(a–b–)

An 85-year-old Russian woman with myelofibrosis and bleeding secondary to colon carcinoma was found to be Jk(a–b–) and to have anti-Jk3, which was responsible for a severe haemolytic transfusion reaction [89]. Neither anti-Jk^a nor -Jk^b could be adsorbed and eluted from her red cells. Five weeks later her red cells had weak Jk^a, which became progressively stronger; her serum now contained anti-Jk^b and weak anti-Jk3. The following year her cells were again Jk(a–b–) (although this could be because of transfusions of Jk(a–b–) cells) but no anti-Jk3 could be detected. After another year her cells appeared to have a normal

Jk(a+b–) phenotype and no anti-Jk3 or -Jk^b was present.

9.5 Development and distribution of Kidd antigens

Jk^a and Jk^b are well developed on the red cells of neonates. Fetal cells have the same distribution of Kidd phenotypes as that found in the adult population [12,92]. Jk^a and Jk^b antigens have been detected on red cells of 11- and 7-week-old fetuses, respectively [92].

The Kidd glycoprotein was detected on endothelial cells of the vasa recta, the vascular supply of the renal medulla, but it is not present in renal tubules [93]. Rabbit antibodies raised to peptides at the N- and C-termini of the Kidd protein were used to detect the structure. A similar pattern of distribution of *JK* mRNA was demonstrated by *in situ* hybridization on human kidney sections [93]. A splice variant of *JK* mRNA is present on osteoblasts of bone explant cultures, but is down-regulated as the cells undergo adipogenesis [94].

Kidd antigens were not detected on lymphocytes, monocytes, granulocytes, or platelets [95–98]. Jk3 first appears on erythroblasts at a late stage of erythropoiesis [99].

9.6 The Kidd glycoprotein is the red cell urea transporter

Failure of Jk(a–b–) red cells to lyse in aqueous solutions of urea provided the first clue that the Kidd glycoprotein might function as a urea transporter (Section 9.4.2). Red cell lysis in the presence of urea is caused by osmotic imbalance. In cells of common Kidd phenotype urea is transported very rapidly across red cell membranes, so in 2 M urea these cells rapidly take up urea, become hypertonic, and lyse because of the rapid diffusion of water into the cell [100]. Jk(a–b–) red cells lack the Kidd glycoprotein. They take up urea slowly and therefore lyse very slowly in 2 M urea. Treatment of normal red cells with *p*-chloromercuribenzenesulphonic acid (*p*CMBS), an inhibitor of urea and water transport, resulted in a substantial retardation of lysis in 2 M urea (aqueous solution) [101]. Measurements of unidirectional urea and thiourea fluxes revealed that urea crosses the membrane of Jk(a–b–) red cells about 1000 times slower than normal cells [102].

The Kidd glycoprotein has substantial sequence homology with another human urea transporter (HUT2), present only on renal cells [103], and with a rabbit urea transporter [5].

Physiological levels of expression of Kidd (*HUT11A*) cDNA in *Xenopus* oocytes strongly facilitated urea transport, but not water permeability [6]. This activity is blocked by the urea transport inhibitors *p*CMBS and phloretin [5]. At higher levels of expression, an increased level of urea transport was observed, together with high water permeability and a selective uptake of small solutes [6].

Urea transporters in the kidney play an important part in concentrating urea in the renal medulla, while conserving water, in order to produce a concentrated urine [104]. A urea transporter in red cells has two main functions:

1 transporting urea rapidly in and out the cells to prevent shrinkage as they pass through the high urea concentration of the renal medulla, and to prevent swelling as they leave; and

2 to prevent the red cells from carrying urea away from the renal medulla, which would decrease the urea concentrating efficacy of the kidney [105].

The Kidd null phenotype is not associated with any clinical defect, although two unrelated Jk(a–b–) individuals had a urine concentrating defect [106]. This may be because other urea transporters compensate for the absence of the Kidd urea transporter in the kidney, and because maximal urea concentrating ability is rarely required under normal conditions.

References

1 Sinor LT, Eastwood KL, Plapp FV. Dot-blot purification of the Kidd blood group antigen. *Med Lab Sci* 1987;**44**:294–6.

2 Olivès B, Mattei M-G, Huet M *et al*. Kidd blood group and urea transport function of human erythrocytes are carried by the same protein. *J Biol Chem* 1995; **270**:15607–10.

3 Masouredis SP, Sudora E, Mahan L, Victoria EJ. Quantitative immunoferritin microscopy of Fy^a, Fy^b, Jk^a, U, and Di^b antigen site numbers on human red cells. *Blood* 1980;**56**:969–77.

4 Mannuzzu LM, Moronne MM, Macey RI. Estimate of the number of urea transport sites in erythrocyte ghosts using a hydrophobic mercurial. *J Membr Biol* 1993; **133**:85–97.

5 Olives B, Neau P, Bailly P *et al*. Cloning and functional expression of a urea transporter from human bone marrow cells. *J Biol Chem* 1994;**269**:31649–52.

6 Sidoux-Walter F, Lucien N, Olivès B *et al*. At physiological expression levels the Kidd blood group/urea transporter protein is not a water channel. *J Biol Chem* 1999;**274**:30228–35.

7 Irshaid NM, Thuresson B, Olsson ML. Genomic typing of the Kidd blood group locus by a single-tube allele-specific primer PCR technique. *Br J Haematol* 1998; **102**:1010–14.

8 Lucien N, Sidoux-Walter F, Olivès B *et al*. Characterization of the gene encoding the human Kidd blood group/urea transporter protein: evidence for splice site mutations in Jk$_{null}$ individuals. *J Biol Chem* 1998; **273**:12973–80.

9 Irshaid NM, Henry SM, Olsson ML. Genomic characterization of the Kidd blood group gene: different molecular basis of the Jk(a–b–) phenotype in Polynesians and Finns. *Transfusion* 2000;**40**:69–74.

10 Allen FH, Diamond LK, Niedziela B. A new blood-group antigen. *Nature* 1951;**167**:482.

11 Plaut G, Ikin EW, Mourant AE, Sanger R, Race RR. A new blood-group antibody, anti-Jk^b. *Nature* 1953;**171**:431.

12 Race RR, Sanger R. *Blood Groups in Man*, 6th edn. Oxford: Blackwell Scientific Publications, 1975.

13 Chown B, Lewis M, Kaita H. The Kidd blood group system in Caucasians. *Transfusion* 1965;**5**:506–7.

14 Mourant AE, Kopec AC, Domaniewska-Sobczak K. *The Distribution of the Human Blood Groups and Other Biochemical Polymorphisms*, 2nd edn. London: Oxford University Press, 1976.

15 Tills D, Kopec AC, Tills RE. *The Distribution of the Human Blood Groups and Other Polymorphisms* (Suppl. 1). Oxford: Oxford University Press, 1983.

16 Olivès B, Merriman M, Bailly P *et al*. The molecular basis of the Kidd blood group polymorphism and its lack of association with type 1 diabetes susceptibility. *Hum Mol Genet* 1997;**6**:1017–20.

17 Hessner MJ, Pircon RA, Johnson ST, Luhm RA. Prenatal genotyping of Jk^a and Jk^b of the human Kidd blood group system by allele-specific polymerase chain reaction. *Prenat Diagn* 1998;**18**:1225–31.

18 Rosenfield RE, Vogel P, Gibbel N, Ohno G, Haber G. Anti-Jk^a: three new examples of the isoantibody — frequency of the factor in Caucasians, Negroes and Chinese of New York City. *Am J Clin Pathol* 1953;**23**:1222–5.

19 Lundevall J. The Kidd blood group system: investigated with anti-Jk^a. *Acta Path Microbiol Scand* 1956;**38**:39–42.

20 Hunter L, Lewis M, Chown B. A further example of Kidd (Jk^a) hæmagglutinin. *Nature* 1951;**168**:790–1.

21 Milne GR, Wallace J, Ikin EW, Mourant AE. The Kidd (anti-Jk^a) hæmagglutinin: a third example. *Lancet* 1953;**i**:627.

22 van der Hart M, van Loghem JJ. A further example of anti-Jk^a. *Vox Sang* 1953;3:72–3.

23 Greenwalt TJ, Sasaki T, Sneath J. Haemolytic disease of the newborn caused by anti-Jk^a. *Vox Sang* 1956;1:157–60.

24 Rosenfield RE, Ley AB, Haber G, Harris JP. A further example of anti-Jk^b. *Am J Clin Pathol* 1954;24: 1282–4.

25 Sanger R, Race RR, Rosenfield RE, Vogel P. A serum containing anti-s and anti-Jk^b. *Vox Sang* (old series) 1953;4:71.

26 van Loghem JJ, Heier A-M, van der Hart M, Sanches VR. A serum containing anti-Jk^b, anti-C and anti-M. *Vox Sang* (old series) 1953;3:115–17.

27 Geczy A, Leslie M. Second example of hemolytic disease of the newborn caused by anti-Jk^b *Transfusion* 1961;1:125–7.

28 Rumsey DH, Nance SJ, Rubino M, Sandler SG. Naturally-occurring anti-Jk^a in infant twins. *Immunohematology* 1999;15:159–62.

29 Harrison KL, Popper EI. Maternal Jk^a sensitization following amniocentesis and intrauterine transfusion. *Transfusion* 1981;21:90–1.

30 Simmons RT, Graydon JJ, Jakobowicz R, Santamaria J, Garson M. Immunization by the blood antigen Kidd (Jk^a) in pregnancy and in blood transfusion. *Med J Aust* 1957;ii:933–5.

31 Morgan P, Wheeler CB, Bossom EL. Delayed transfusion reaction attributed to anti-Jk^b. *Transfusion* 1967;7:307–8.

32 Kronenberg H, Kooptzoff O, Walsh RJ. Hæmolytic transfusion reaction due to anti Kidd. *Aust Ann Med* 1958;7:34–5.

33 Maynard BA, Smith DS, Farrar RP, Kraetsch RE, Chaplin H. Anti-Jk^a, -C, and -E in a single patient, initially demonstrable only by the manual hexadimethrine bromide (Polybrene) test, with incompatibilities confirmed by ^{51}Cr-labeled red cell studies. *Transfusion* 1988;28:302–6.

34 Crawford MN, Greenwalt TJ, Sasaki T *et al.* The phenotype Lu(a–b–) together with unconventional Kidd groups in one family. *Transfusion* 1961;1:228–32.

35 Polley MJ, Mollison PL, Soothill JF. The role of 19S gamma-globulin blood-group antibodies in the antiglobulin reaction. *Br J Haematol* 1962;8:149–62.

36 Szymanski IO, Huff SR, Delsignore R. An autoanalyzer test to determine immunoglobulin class and IgG subclass of blood group antibodies. *Transfusion* 1982; 22:90–5.

37 Hardman JT, Beck ML. Hemagglutination in capillaries: correlation with blood group specificity and IgG subclass. *Transfusion* 1981;21:343–6.

38 Mollison PL, Engelfriet CP, Contreras M. *Blood Transfusion in Clinical Medicine*, 10th edn. Oxford: Blackwell Scientific Publications, 1997.

39 Yates J, Howell P, Overfield J *et al.* IgG anti-Jk^a/Jk^b antibodies are unlikely to fix complement. *Transfus Med* 1998;8:133–40.

40 O'Brien P, Hopkins L, McCarthy D, Murphy S. Complement-binding anti-Jk^a not detectable by DiaMed gels. *Vox Sang* 1998;74:53–5.

41 Degnan TJ, Rosenfield RE. Hemolytic transfusion reaction associated with poorly detectable anti-Jk^a. *Transfusion* 1965;5:245–7.

42 Polesky HF, Bove JR. A fatal hemolytic transfusion reaction with acute autohemolysis. *Transfusion* 1964; 4:285–92.

43 Pineda AA, Taswell HF, Brzica SM. Delayed hemolytic transfusion reaction: an immunologic hazard of blood transfusion. *Transfusion* 1978;18:1–7.

44 Ness PM, Shirey RS, Thoman SK, Buck SA. The differentiation of delayed serologic and delayed hemolytic transfusion reactions: incidence, long-term serologic findings, and clinical significance. *Transfusion* 1990;30: 688–93.

45 Holland PV, Wallerstein RO. Delayed hemolytic transfusion reaction with acute renal failure. *J Am Med Assoc* 1968;204:1007–8.

46 Matson GA, Swanson J, Tobin JD. Severe hemolytic disease of the newborn caused by anti-Jk^a. *Vox Sang* 1959;4:144–7.

47 Pineda AA, Vamvakas EC, Gorden LD, Winters JL, Moore SB. Trends in the incidence of delayed hemolytic and delayed serologic transfusion reactions. *Transfusion* 1999;39:1097–1103 and corrections in *Transfusion* 2000;40:891.

48 Cutbush M, Mollison PL. Relation between characteristics of blood-group antibodies *in vitro* and associated patterns of red-cell destruction *in vivo*. *Br J Haematol* 1958;4:115–37.

49 Howard JE, Winn LC, Gottlieb CE *et al.* Clinical significance of the anti-complement component of antiglobulin antisera. *Transfusion* 1982;22:269–72.

50 Nance SJ, Arndt PA, Garratty G. The effect of fresh normal serum on monocyte monolayer assay reactivity. *Transfusion* 1988;28:398–9.

51 Zupanska B, Brojer E, McIntosh J, Seyfried H, Howell P. Correlation of monocyte-monolayer assay results, number of erythrocyte-bound IgG molecules, and IgG subclass composition in the study of red cell alloantibodies other than D. *Vox Sang* 1990;58:276–80.

52 Leo A, Mytilineos J, Voso MT *et al.* Passenger lymphocyte syndrome with severe hemolytic anemia due to an anti-Jk^a after allogeneic PBPC transplantation. *Transfusion* 2000;40:632–6.

53 Dorner I, Moore JA, Chaplin H. Combined maternal erythrocyte autosensitization and materno-fetal Jk^a incompatibility. *Transfusion* 1974;14:212–19.

54 van Loghem JJ, van der Hart M. Varieties of specific auto-antibodies in acquired haemolytic anaemia. *Vox Sang* (old series) 1954;4:2–11.

55 Patten E, Beck CE, Scholl C, Stroope RA, Wukasch C.

Autoimmune hemolytic anemia with anti-Jk[a] specificity in a patient taking aldomet. *Transfusion* 1977; **17**:517–20.

56 Strikas R, Seifer MR, Lentino JR. Autoimmune hemolytic anemia and *Legionella pneumophila* pneumonia. *Ann Intern Med* 1983;**99**:345.

57 Sosler SD, Behzad O, Garratty G *et al.* Acute hemolytic anemia associated with a chlorpropamide-induced apparent auto-anti-*Jk[a]*. *Transfusion* 1984;**24**:206–9.

58 Sander RP, Hardy NM, Van Meter SA. Anti-Jk[a] autoimmune hemolytic anemia in an infant. *Transfusion* 1987;**27**:58–60.

59 Ganly PS, Laffan MA, Owen I, Hows JM. Auto-anti-Jk[a] in Evans' syndrome with negative direct antiglobulin test. *Br J Haematol* 1988;**69**:537–9.

60 Holmes LD, Pierce SR, Beck M. Autoanti-Jk[a] in a healthy blood donor [Abstract]. *Transfusion* 1976; **16**:521.

61 Issitt PD, Pavone BG, Frohlich JA, McGuire Mallory D. Absence of autoanti-Jk3 as a component of anti-dl. *Transfusion* 1980;**20**:733–6.

62 Judd WJ, Steiner EA, Cochran RK. Paraben-associated autoanti-Jk[a] antibodies: three examples detected using commercially prepared low-ionic-strength saline containing parabens. *Transfusion* 1982;**22**:31–5.

63 Halima D, Garratty G, Bueno R. An apparent anti-Jk[a] reacting only in the presence of methyl esters of hydroxybenzoic acid. *Transfusion* 1982;**22**:521–4.

64 McGinniss MH, Leiberman R, Holland PV. The JK[b] red cell antigen and gram-negative organisms [Abstract]. *Transfusion* 1979;**19**:663.

65 Lecointre-Coatmelec M, Bourel D, Ferrette J, Genetet B. A human anti-Jk[b] monoclonal antibody. *Vox Sang* 1991;**61**:255–7.

66 Thompson K, Barden G, Sutherland J, Beldon I, Melamed M. Human monoclonal antibodies to human blood group antigens Kidd Jk[a] and Jk[b]. *Transfus Med* 1991;**1**:91–6.

67 Pinkerton FJ, Mermod LE, Liles BA, Jack JA, Noades J. The phenotype Jk(a–b–) in the Kidd blood group system. *Vox Sang* 1959;**4**:155–60.

68 Yokoyama M, Mermod LE, Stegmaier A. Further examples of Jk(a–b–) blood in Hawaii. *Vox Sang* 1967; **12**:154–6.

69 Arcara PC, O'Connor MA, Dimmette RM. A family with three Jk(a–b–) members [Abstract]. *Transfusion* 1969;**9**:282.

70 Habibi B, Avril J, Fouillade MT *et al.* Jk(a–b–) phenotype in a French family: quantitative evidence for the inheritence of a silent allele (Jk). *Haematologia* 1976;**10**:403–10.

71 Woodfield DG, Douglas R, Smith J *et al.* The Jk(a–b–) phenotype in New Zealand Polynesians. *Transfusion* 1982;**22**:276–8.

72 Irshaid NM, Eicher NI, Hustinx H, Poole J, Olsson ML. Novel alleles at the JK blood group locus explain the ab-

73 Kuczmarski CA, Bergren MO, Perkins HA. Mild hemolytic disease of the newborn due to anti-Jk3: a serologic study of the family's Kidd antigens. *Vox Sang* 1982;**43**:340–4.

74 Heaton DC, McLoughlin K. Jk(a–b–) red blood cells resist urea lysis. *Transfusion* 1982;**22**:70–1.

75 Henry S, Woodfield G. Frequencies of the Jk(a–b–) phenotype in Polynesian ethnic groups. *Transfusion* 1995;**35**:277.

76 Sidoux-Walter F, Lucien N, Nissinen R *et al.* Molecular heterogeneity of the Jk[null] phenotype: expression analysis of the Jk(S291P) mutation found in Finns. *Blood* 2000;**96**:1566–73.

77 Marshall CS, Dwyre D, Eckert R, Russell L. Severe hemolytic reaction due to anti-JK3. *Arch Pathol Lab Med* 1999;**123**:949–51.

78 Pierce SR, Hardman JT, Steele S, Beck ML. Hemolytic disease of the newborn associated with anti-Jk3. *Transfusion* 1980;**20**:189–91.

79 Day D, Perkins HA, Sams B. The minus-minus phenotype in the Kidd system. *Transfusion* 1965;**5**:315–19.

80 Okubo Y, Yamaguchi H, Nagao N *et al.* Heterogeneity of the phenotype Jk(a–b–) found in Japanese. *Transfusion* 1986;**26**:237–9.

81 Smart EA, Moores PP, Reddy R, Calvert M. Anti-Jk3 and the Jk:–3 phenotype in Natal, South Africa [Abstract]. *Transfus Med* 1993;**3**(Suppl.1):84.

82 Silver RT, Haber JM, Kellner A. Evidence for a new allele in the Kidd blood group system in Indians of Northern Mato Grosso, Brazil. *Nature* 1960;**186**:481.

83 Oliver CK, Sexton T, Joyner J. Case study: a Jk:–3 phenotype in an African-American family [Abstract]. *Transfusion* 1993;**33**(Suppl.):23S.

84 Lucien N, Chiaroni J, Cartron J-P, Bailly P. Partial deletion of the JK locus causing a JK[null] phenotype. *Blood* 2002;**99**:1079–81.

85 Sareneva H, Pirkola A, Siitonen S, Sistonen P. Exceptionally high frequency of a gene for recessive Jk blood group null phenotype among the Finns [Abstract]. *6th Reg Eur Cong Int Soc Blood Transfus* 1999:96.

86 McDougall DCJ, McGregor M. Jk:–3 red cells have a defect in urea transport: a new urea-dependent lysis test. *Transfusion* 1988;**28**:197–8.

87 Behzad O, Wong C, Gaucys G, Lee CL. A possible Kidd antigen variant. *Transfusion* 1980;**20**:119–20.

88 Edwards-Moulds J, Kasschau MR. Methods for the detection of *Jk* heterozygotes: interpretations and applications. *Transfusion* 1988;**28**:545–8.

89 Issitt PD, Obarski G, Hartnett PL, Wren MR, Prewitt PL. Temporary suppression of Kidd system antigen expression accompanied by transient production of anti-Jk3. *Transfusion* 1990;**30**:46–50.

90 Ellisor SS, Reid ME, O'Day TO *et al.* Autoantibodies mimicking anti-Jk[b] plus anti-Jk3 associated with

sence of the erythrocyte urea transporter in European families. *Br J Haematol* 2002;**116**:445–54.

autoimmune hemolytic anemia in a primipara who delivered an unaffected infant. *Vox Sang* 1983;45: 53–9.

91 O'Day T. A second example of autoanti-Jk3. *Transfusion* 1987;27:442.

92 Toivanen P, Hirvonen T. Antigens Duffy, Kell, Kidd, Lutheran and Xgᵃ on fetal red cells. *Vox Sang* 1973;24:372–6.

93 Xu Y, Olivès B, Bailly P *et al.* Endothelial cells of the kidney vasa recta express the urea transporter HUT11. *Kidney Int* 1997;51:138–46.

94 Prichett WP, Patton AJ, Field JA *et al.* Identification and cloning of a human urea transporter HUT11, which is downregulated during adipogenesis of explant cultures of human bone. *J Cell Biochem* 2000;76:639–50.

95 Marsh WL, Øyen R, Nichols ME. Kidd blood-group antigens of leukocytes and platelets. *Transfusion* 1974;14:378–81.

96 Dunstan RA, Simpson MB, Rosse WF. Erythrocyte antigens on human platelets: absence of Rh, Duffy, Kell, Kidd, and Lutheran antigens. *Transfusion* 1984;24:243–6.

97 Dunstan RA. Status of major red cell blood group antigens on neutrophils, lymphocytes and monocytes. *Br J Haematol* 1986;62:301–9.

98 Gaidulis L, Branch DR, Lazar GS, Petz LD. The red cell antigens A, B, D, U, Ge, Jk3 and Ytᵃ are not detected on human granulocytes. *Br J Haematol* 1985;60:659–68.

99 Bony V, Gane P, Bailly P, Cartron J-P. Time-course expression of polypeptides carrying blood group antigens during human erythroid differentiation. *Br J Haematol* 1999;107:263–74.

100 Moulds JM. The Kidd blood group and urea transport. In: J-P Cartron, P Rouger, eds. *Blood Cell Biochemistry*, Vol. 6. New York: Plenum Press, 1995:267–79.

101 Edwards-Moulds J, Kasschau MR. The effect of 2 Molar urea on Jk(a–b–) red cells. *Vox Sang* 1988;55: 181–5.

102 Fröhlich O, Macey RI, Edwards-Moulds J, Gargus JJ, Gunn RB. Urea transport deficiency in Jk(a–b–) erythrocytes. *Am J Physiol* 1991;260:C778–83.

103 Olivès B, Martial S, Mattie M-G *et al.* Molecular characterization of a new kidney urea transporter in the human kidney. *FEBS Lett* 1996;386:156–60.

104 Sands JM, Timmer RT, Gunn RB. Urea transporters in kidney and erythrocytes. *Am J Physiol* 1997;273: F321–39.

105 Macey RI, Yousef LW. Osmotic stability of red cells in renal circulation required rapid urea transport. *Am J Physiol* 1988;254:C669–74.

106 Sands JM, Gargus JJ, Fröhlich O, Gunn RB, Kokko JB. Urinary concentrating ability in patients with Jk(a–b–) blood type who lack carrier-mediated urea transport. *J Am Soc Nephrol* 1992;2:1689–96.

351

10

Diego blood group system

10.1 Introduction

The Diego system consists of 21 antigens: two pairs of antithetical antigens, Diᵃ and Diᵇ, Wrᵃ and Wrᵇ, plus 17 antigens of very low frequency (Table 10.1). Diᵃ is a useful anthropological marker because it is polymorphic in most Mongoloid populations, but virtually absent from other ethnic groups. Diᵃ represents Leu854 and Diᵇ Pro854 in the red cell anion exchanger, band 3 or AE1 (CD233). The low frequency Wrᵃ (DI3) and high frequency Wrᵇ (DI4) antigens represent Lys658 and Glu658 in band 3, respectively. Glycophorin A (GPA)-deficient red cells are Wr(a–b–), as Wrᵇ requires the presence of both band 3 and GPA for expression. The other low frequency Diego system antigens are all associated with amino acid substitutions in band 3. No healthy person with a Diego null phenotype has been reported, reflecting the functional importance of band 3.

SLC4A1, the gene encoding band 3, is located on chromosome 17q12–q21 (Chapter 32).

10.2 Band 3, the red cell anion exchanger (AE1), and the gene that encodes it

Band 3, or anion exchanger 1 (AE1), or CD233, is a major intrinsic red cell membrane glycoprotein, with approximately 1.2 million copies per red cell. After sodium dodecyl sulphate polyacrylamide gel electrophoresis (SDS PAGE) of red cell membranes, band 3 is easily detected by Coomassie blue staining. It migrates as a diffuse band of about M_r 100 000 (reviews on band 3 in [1–3]).

The band 3 gene (*SLC4A1*) covers 18 kb of DNA and contains 20 exons [4] (Table 10.2). Cloning and sequencing of band 3 cDNA confirmed that the protein consists of three domains: a cytoplasmic N-terminal domain of 403 amino acids; a hydrophobic transmembrane domain of 479 amino acids; and a C-terminal cytoplasmic tail of 29 amino acids [5,6] (Fig. 10.1). The N-terminal domain interacts with ankyrin of the cytoskeleton. In the original model the transmembrane domain has 14 α-helical membrane spanning domains and cytoplasmic N- and C-termini [1,6], but this model has recently been challenged [7,8] (Fig. 10.1). The single N-linked oligosaccharide on Asn642, on the fourth extracellular loop, carries H, A, B, I, and i activity (Chapters 2 and 25). Variation in the number of repeating N-acetyllactosamine units accounts for the broadness of the band on SDS PAGE. Band 3 exists in the red cell membrane as dimers and higher oligomers, with tetramers being preferred for binding to ankyrin [9]. Associations between band 3 and glycophorin A are discussed in Section 10.4.2 and in Chapter 3.

10.3 Diᵃ and Diᵇ (DI1 and DI2)

Diᵃ was first described in a Venezuelan family by Layrisse *et al.* [10] in 1955. It soon became apparent that Diᵃ is relatively common in South American Indians, but rare in people of European origin [10,11]. Two examples of antibodies detecting an antithetical antigen, Diᵇ, were described by Thompson *et al.* [12] in 1967.

10.3.1 Frequencies

Frequency studies on Diᵃ are prodigious because of its usefulness as an anthropological marker. Diᵃ occurs

Table 10.1 Antigens of the Diego blood group system.

No.	Name	Relative frequency	Antithetical antigen	Molecular basis*
DI1	Di^a	Low†	Di^b (DI2)	Leu854 (Pro)
DI2	Di^b	High	Di^a (DI1)	Pro854
DI3	Wr^a	Low	Wr^b (DI4)	Lys658 (Glu)
DI4	Wr^b	High	Wr^a (DI3)	Glu658
DI5	Wd^a	Low		Met557 (Val)
DI6	Rb^a	Low		Leu548 (Pro)
DI7	WARR	Low		Ile552 (Thr)
DI8	ELO	Low		Trp432 (Arg)
DI9	Wu	Low		Ala565 (Gly)
DI10	Bp^a	Low		Lys569 (Asn)
DI11	Mo^a	Low		His656 (Arg)
DI12	Hg^a	Low		Cys656 (Arg)
DI13	Vg^a	Low		His555 (Tyr)
DI14	Sw^a	Low		Gln or Trp646 (Arg)
DI15	BOW	Low		Ser561 (Pro)
DI16	NFLD	Low		Asp429 (Glu); Ala561 (Pro)
DI17	Jn^a	Low		Ser566 (Pro)
DI18	KREP	Low		Ala566 (Pro)
DI19‡	Tr^a	Low		Asn551 (Lys)
DI20	Fr^a	Low		Lys480 (Glu)
DI21	SW1	Low		Trp646 (Arg)

*Common amino acid residue shown in parentheses.
†Polymorphic in people of Mongoloid origin.
‡Provisional assignment.

Table 10.2 Organization of the band 3 gene, *SLC4A1* [4].

Exon	Size (bp)	Amino acids	Intron size (kb)
1	582		>3
2	83	1–5	0.125
3	91	6–36	0.998
4	62	36–56	0.757
5	181	57–117	0.095
6	136	117–162	0.472
7	124	162–203	0.227
8	85	204–232	0.152
9	182	232–292	0.539
10	211	293–363	0.232
11	195	363–428	0.178
12	149	428–477	0.114
13	195	478–542	1.503
14	174	543–600	0.377
15	90	601–630	0.543
16	167	631–686	1.126
17	254	686–771	1.527
18	170	771–827	0.086
19	174	828–885	0.620
20	2146	886–911	

almost exclusively among Mongoloid people and it is often difficult to eliminate Mongoloid ancestry in the rare exceptions. Extensive reviews of the frequency data are provided elsewhere [13–15]; studies on selected populations are shown in Table 10.3.

In the papers describing the first anti-Di^a, Layrisse *et al.* [10,11] reported a high incidence of Di^a antigen among Venezuelan Indians. Since 1955, numerous studies of South American Indians have demonstrated that Di^a occurs in most of these populations. The frequency of Di(a+) is variable, reaching 60–70% in some populations. Di^a is also found in most Central and North American native populations, although the incidence in the northern continent is generally not as high as in the southern continent. Surprisingly, Di^a is rare among the Inuit of Alaska and Canada, but relatively common in Siberian Inuits. Di^a also occurs in South-East Asian populations where the frequency varies between about 2 and 12%, the incidence in Japan being generally higher than that in China [17,28].

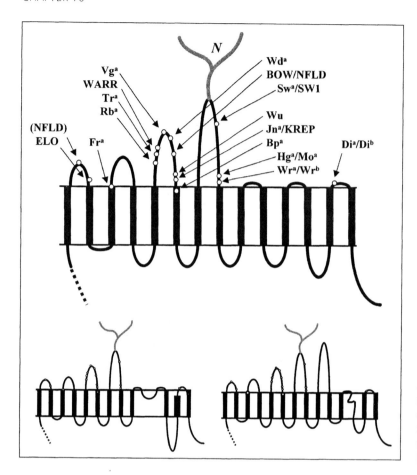

Fig. 10.1 Three models for the topography of the membrane domain of band 3 glycoprotein. In the conventional model (above) the protein spans the membrane 14 times and has cytoplasmic N- and C-terminal domains [1,6,7]. Positions of the amino acid substitutions associated with the Diego system antigens are shown. N represents the single N-glycan at Asn642. The large cytoplasmic N-terminal domain is not shown. Below are two alternative models (left [7], right [8]).

Very few Di(a+) white people with no apparent Mongoloid admixture are reported [10,29,30]. Invasion of parts of Poland by Tartars in the thirteenth to seventeenth centuries was used to explain Di^a in 0.46% of Poles [25]. Di^a appears to be absent from Australian Aborigines and many Pacific Oceanic populations, and absent, or extremely rare, among Africans (Table 10.3).

A few large surveys have been carried out with anti-Di^b [13,14,19,31]. All Di(b–) individuals were Di(a+); Di(a–b–) phenotype has not been described.

10.3.2 Inheritance and molecular basis of the Diego polymorphism

Family analyses have demonstrated that Di^a is inherited as a straightforward Mendelian dominant character [16,30,32–35].

When red cells are treated with pronase or chymotrypsin prior to SDS PAGE, a band 3 polymorphism can be detected [36]. In most cases an M_r 60 000 band is stained representing the N-terminal region of band 3, but in a minority of subjects a second band of reduced mobility (M_r 63 000) is also apparent. The variant band, called band 3 Memphis, results from a single-base mutation within exon 4, which encodes a Lys56Glu substitution within the cytoplasmic N-terminal domain of band 3 [37,38]. In rare individuals homozygous for the band 3 Memphis allele, only the M_r 63 000 band is present [39,40]. Band 3 Memphis was initially detected in 6–7% of random blood samples [37]; a higher incidence has been found in African Americans (16%), Native Americans (17–25%), Chinese (13%), Filipinos (17%), and Japanese (29%) [39,40]. The red cell anion exchange inhibitors diisothiocyanatostilbene (DIDS) and its dihydro derivative H$_2$DIDS bind covalently to Lys539 of band 3 [5]. In some individuals with band 3 Memphis, the variant band 3 has markedly increased binding of H$_2$DIDS [41]. This is called band 3 Memphis variant II

Table 10.3 Results of some selected studies on the frequency of Di^a.

Population	No. tested	No. Di(a+)	Di^a frequency	References
Carib Indians (Venezuela)	121	43	0.3554	[11]
Arawaco Indians (Venezuela)	152	8	0.0526	[11]
Kainganges Indians (Brazil)	48	26	0.5416	[11]
Mayan Indians (Guatemala)	255	57	0.2235	[16]
Chippewa Indians (USA)	148	16	0.1081	[17]
Penobscot Indians (USA)	249	20	0.0803	[18]
Inuits (Alaska, Cananda)	1477	2	0.0014	[13]
Inuits (Siberia)	86	18	0.2093	[13,14]
Mexicans (USA)	1685	172	0.1021	[19]
Japanese	2427	244	0.1005	[20]
Chinese	617	32	0.0519	[13]
Chinese (Taiwan)	1000	32	0.0320	[21]
Koreans	277	17	0.0614	[22]
Indian (North India)	377	15	0.0400	[13]
Europeans	4462	1	0.0002	[11,19,23,24]
Poles	9661	45	0.0047	[25]
White Americans	1000	0	0	[11]
African Americans	827	1	0.0012	[13]
Ghanaians	107	0	0	[26]
Australian Aborigines	1374	0	0	[27]
Papua New Guineans	1741	0	0	[27]

in order to distinguish it from band 3 Memphis variant I, which has normal H$_2$DIDS binding.

Spring et al. [42] recognized an association between band 3 and the Diego system when they found by SDS PAGE and H$_2$DIDS binding that Di(a+) red cells always have band 3 Memphis variant II. Band 3 Memphis from Di(a+) red cells bound about three times the normal quantity of radiolabelled H$_2$DIDS, whereas the band 3 Memphis from Di(a–) red cells bound normal quantities of H$_2$DIDS. Di^a is associated with band 3 Memphis variant II; Di^b is associated with both normal band 3 and with band 3 Memphis variant I.

Following PCR amplification of the entire coding region of band 3 cDNA, Bruce et al. [43] showed that Di^a expression and Memphis variant II are associated with a C2561T transition in exon 19: Di^a encodes Leu854; Di^b encodes Pro854. The Di^a allele is associated with loss of MspI and NaeI restriction sites. According to the 14 transmembrane-domain model, this amino acid substitution occurs in the seventh extracellular loop (Fig. 10.1). Amino acid 854 is also exposed at the cell surface in the two alternative models presented in Fig. 10.1. The enhanced H$_2$DIDS binding

occurring with Leu854 (Di^a) could be because of a localized conformational change that affects the rate of covalent cross-linking between Lys851 in the seventh extracellular loop and Lys539 in the fifth transmembrane domain [44].

MspI cleavage of PCR products to determine Di^a/Di^b genotype of 72 Parakana (Amazonian) Indians revealed 27 Di^a/Di^a, 26 Di^a/Di^b, and 19 Di^b/Di^b, giving gene frequencies of Di^a 0.56 and Di^b 0.44 [45]. Results of MnlI cleavage tests to analyse the Lys56Glu, Memphis polymorphism, was consistent with Di^a and Di^b being associated with Glu56 and Lys56 codons, respectively, apart from four Di^a/Di^a individuals being heterozygous for Glu56 and Lys56 codons.

Two Di(a+b–) individuals of European origin appeared, from molecular analyses, to be heterozygous Di^a/Di^b. The apparently silent Di^b allele contained a frameshift mutation in one and a nonsense mutation in the other [46].

10.3.3 Effect of enzymes and reducing agents

Di^a and Di^b are resistant to treatment of red cells with papain, trypsin, α-chymotrypsin, pronase, sialidase, and 2-aminoethylisothiouronium bromide (AET) [47].

10.3.4 Weak Di^b

A healthy Mexican woman with many weak red cell antigens initially appeared to have Di(a–b–) red cells but, on further testing, was shown to have weak Di^b [48]. Weaker than expected Di^b reactions were detected with red cells from several Di(a+) Mexican-Americans [19]. Issitt *et al.* [31] found that all of 784 Hispanic Americans were Di(b+); 11 had weaker than average Di^b antigens and were tested with anti-Di^a, but only one was Di(a+). Di^b is depressed in South-East Asian ovalocytosis [49] (Section 10.8).

10.3.5 Anti-Di^a and -Di^b

Di^a and Di^b are fully developed at birth [12,19,23,32,50–52]. The first three examples of anti-Di^a were responsible for severe and, in the original case, fatal HDN [11,34,50]. Many other examples of anti-Di^a have been identified since; most have been stimulated by pregnancy, often causing HDN [24,25,30,53,54]. One example of anti-Di^a, in a white Australian, was apparently 'naturally occurring' [29]. Anti-Di^a may have caused an immediate haemolytic transfusion reaction (HTR), but the presence of anti-c and incomplete information confused the picture [55], and is implicated in a delayed HTR [56]. Red cell panels used for antibody screening often do not contain Di(a+) cells and examples of anti-Di^a remain undetected, especially in America where the incidence of Di(a+) is quite high among the indigenous population [53]. In Brazil, four of 112 (3.6%) multitransfused patients had anti-Di^a [57].

One of the original two anti-Di^b may have been responsible for a delayed HTR [12]. Many other examples have been found, but there has been no other report of a transfusion reaction. There are three reports of HDN caused by anti-Di^b requiring exchange transfusion [58–60]. One anti-Di^b did not cause HDN, despite being IgG3 and responsible for neonatal red cells giving a strongly positive direct antiglobulin test (DAT) [61]. In monocyte monolayer assays with anti-Di^b, significantly higher scores of adherence and phagocytosis were obtained with Di(a–b+) red cells than with Di(a+b+) cells [62]. No example of 'naturally occurring' anti-Di^b is reported. Two of 74 sera

containing red cell autoantibodies contained autoanti-Di^b together with other autoantibodies [63]. One of the autoanti-Di^b may have been responsible for haemolytic anaemia.

Although anti-Di^a has been detected in sera containing multiple antibodies to low incidence antigens, anti-Di^a and -Di^b are most often found alone. They usually require antiglobulin to agglutinate cells, but directly agglutinating anti-Di^a [29] and -Di^b [64] have been described. Anti-Di^a and -Di^b are often IgG1 and IgG3 [24,25,53,54,61] and occasionally anti-Di^a binds complement and may haemolyse untreated cells [25,65].

Two monoclonal anti-Di^a were produced by human–mouse heterohybridomas incorporating lymphocytes derived from individuals with anti-Di^a [20]. One (IgM) directly agglutinated Di(a+) cells, the other (IgG1) required anti-human globulin.

10.4 Wright antigens

10.4.1 Wr^a and Wr^b (DI3 and DI4)

Wr^a, first described by Holman in 1953 [66], has an incidence of around 1 in 1000 in white populations (Table 10.4). Very few large surveys have been carried out on other ethnic groups. No Wr(a+) was found among 2000 Australian Aborigines or 2000 Papua New Guineans [27].

Many families have shown that Wr^a is inherited as an autosomal Mendelian character [66,68,70,71,77,78]. One family gave a suggestion of close linkage between the genes controlling Wr^a and Sd(a++) [77]. Wr^a shows individual variation in strength of expression and is fully developed at birth.

The name anti-Wr^b was provisionally used by Adams *et al.* [79] in 1971 for an antibody, in the serum of a Wr(a+) woman (Fr), which detected a high frequency antigen. Her red cells appeared to have a double dose of Wr^a antigen and the antibody reacted more strongly with Wr(a–) cells than with Wr(a+) cells. Red cells of a second Wr(a+b–) person with anti-Wr^b differed slightly from those of Fr as they reacted weakly with several monoclonal anti-Wr^b [80]. Wr^a and Wr^b dosage on Wr(a+b+), Wr(a–b+), and Wr(a+b–) cells was confirmed by an enzyme-linked antiglobulin test [81].

Sequencing of PCR-amplified band 3 cDNA from the original Wr(a+b–) propositus revealed a

Table 10.4 Frequency of Wr^a in predominantly white populations.

Population	No. tested	No. Wr(a+)	Wr^a frequency (%)	References
English	45 631	36	0.0008	[67,68]
English	5 253	2	0.0004	[69]
Scots	1 000	1	0.0010	[33]
Norwegians	5 138	0	0	[70]
Norwegians	3 140	2	0.0006	[70]
Swiss	3 753	2	0.0005	[71]
Italians	6 350	7	0.0011	[72]
Czechs	1 500	1	0.0007	[73]
Americans (Boston)	2 784	3	0.0011	[74]
Americans (New York)	5 000	5	0.0010	[75]
Americans (Ohio)	7 000	0	0	[76]

G1972A change in exon 16, predicting a Glu658Lys substitution within the fourth extracellular loop of band 3 [82] (Fig. 10.1). Three Wr(a–b+) individuals had the normal sequence (Glu658); seven Wr(a+b+) individuals were heterozygous for Glu658 and Lys658 codons.

Wr^a and Wr^b are resistant to treatment of red cells with trypsin, chymotrypsin, pronase, papain, and sialidase, and with the reducing agent AET [47,83]. Neither Wr^a nor Wr^b was detected on peripheral blood lymphocytes, granulocytes, or monocytes [84].

10.4.2 Association of band 3 with glycophorin A (GPA) and its importance in Wr^b expression

There is substantial evidence that band 3 and GPA are closely associated in the membrane. A monoclonal antibody to the cytoplasmic C-terminal domain of band 3 precipitated both band 3 and GPA [85], although most antibodies to either band 3 or GPA do not coprecipitate [2]. Binding of GPA antibodies to red cells significantly reduced mobility of band 3 [86–88]. GPA may facilitate the translocation of newly synthesized band 3 to the membrane [89]. GPA is not essential for band 3 expression at the cell surface, but in red cells deficient in GPA band 3 is imperfectly folded and moves slowly to the surface. In GPA-deficient cells the N-glycan on band 3 is of increased molecular weight and, despite normal quantities of band 3, anion transport is impaired (Sections 3.6.1 and 3.25). Red cells in mice with targeted inactivation of the band 3 gene ('knockout' mice) are deficient in both band 3 and

GPA, suggesting that band 3 plays a chaperone-like role and is essential for expression of GPA at the red cell surface [90]. This is not applicable to humans: GPA appears before band 3 on erythroid progenitor cells during human erythropoiesis [91,92]; a human erythroleukaemia cell line (K562) expresses GPA, but no band 3 [93,94]; and an infant with total band 3 deficiency has markedly reduced, but clearly present, GPA [95]. Red cells of transgenic mice expressing human GPA had reduced levels of mouse GPA, implying a competition between human and murine GPA for band 3 [96].

Despite a single amino acid substitution being the primary cause of the Wr^a/Wr^b dimorphism, Wr^b is not expressed in the absence of GPA. GPA-deficient, En(a–), red cells are Wr(a–b–) [97,98]. The only other Wr(a–b–) cells are those with some rare phenotypes involving hybrid glycophorins, which lack the part of GPA that reacts with antibodies called anti-En^{a}FR (Sections 3.6 and 3.11). Red cells of the two Wr(a+b–) patients demonstrated no abnormality in expression of the MNSsU or En^a antigens, of GPA, or of red cell sialic acid levels [99]. There was no abnormality in the sequence of *GYPA* cDNA from a Wr(a+b–) person [82].

Most monoclonal antibodies to GPA and band 3 do not coprecipitate both proteins, but monoclonal anti-Wr^b either precipitated GPA [100,101] or GPA together with band 3 [102,103]. Six sera containing red cell autoantibodies coprecipitated band 3 and GPA [104]. Three of the sera contained autoanti-Wr^b, but the other three sera contained no anti-Wr^b, suggesting that other epitopes may exist that depend on band 3 and GPA interaction. Dahr *et al.* [99] found that haemagglutination with alloanti-Wr[b] could be inhibited by purified fragments of GPA, but, like anti-En[a]FR, inhibitory activity was low and only detectable in the presence of lipid. One monoclonal anti-Wr[b] was inhibited by a synthetic peptide representing amino acid residues 65–70 of GPA; alloanti-Wr[b], autoanti-Wr[b], and two other monoclonal anti-Wr[b] were not inhibited [105]. Monoclonal anti-Wr[b] will not bind to human cell lines that do not express both GPA and band 3 [102]. The erythroleukaemia cell line K562 expresses GPA, but no band 3 or Wr[b], but transfection with band 3 cDNA induces Wr[b] expression [94]. During *ex vivo* erythropoiesis, Wr[b] appears at the cell surface at the same time as band 3, slightly after GPA [92]. Binding of antibodies to the extracellular domain of GPA causes immobilization of band 3, an effect that is significantly reduced in Wr(a+b–) cells [88].

Amino acid sequences of GPA and the hybrid glycophorin GP(B–A)Sch, which are associated with Wr[b] expression, were compared with those of GP(A–B)Hil and GP(B–A)Dantu, which are associated with the Wr(a–b–) phenotype. The results suggested that amino acid residues 55–68, an α-helical region close to the insertion of GPA into the membrane, might be important in Wr[b] expression [82,106]. Gln63Lys and Ala65Pro substitutions within GPA are both associated with abnormal Wr[b] expression (Section 3.16). Hybrid glycophorins expressing SAT, however, do not express Wr[b], despite having amino acids 1–70 or 1–71 derived from GPA, with a transmembrane domain derived from GPB (Section 3.11.3) [106]. It is likely therefore that the association between band 3 and GPA occurs between the single membrane spanning domain of GPA and the eighth membrane-spanning domain of band 3, and the extracellular regions adjacent to these domains.

Whether GPA is required for Wr[a] expression is not known. Attempts to identify any membrane component by immunoprecipitation with monoclonal anti-Wr[a] were unsuccessful [103].

10.4.3 Anti-Wr[a]

Anti-Wr[a] is a relatively common antibody. The reported incidence of anti-Wr[a] in the sera of normal donors varies in different studies: the highest frequency was 1 in 13 sera [76], but other studies have provided figures of between 1 in 56 and 1 in 100 [69,75,107]. The incidence increases dramatically in patients, postpartum women, and in people with other alloantibodies [69,75]. About one in three patients with autoimmune haemolytic anaemia has anti-Wr[a] [68,75]. Some anti-Wr[a] are directly agglutinating antibodies, but most require an antiglobulin test for detection. Of 44 anti-Wr[a], 19 (43%) were IgG, 16 (36%) were IgM, and nine (20%) were a mixture of IgG and IgM [107]. All nine anti-Wr[a] analysed for IgG isotype were IgG1 [108].

The first two anti-Wr[a], and a couple of other examples since, have caused severe HDN [66,109–111], although HDN caused by anti-Wr[a] remains a surprisingly rare event considering the frequency of the antibody [107]. Anti-Wr[a] has also been implicated in HTRs [71,112].

IgG1 mouse monoclonal anti-Wr[a] (BGU1-WR) was produced as a result of immunizing mice with Wr(a+) red cells [83].

10.4.4 Anti-Wr[b]

Alloanti-Wr[b] has been found in the sera of the two Wr(a+b–) patients [79,80], plus some Wr(a–b–) individuals with certain rare MNS phenotypes (Sections 3.6 and 3.11). There is little information regarding the clinical importance of alloanti-Wr[b]. An En(a–) patient with anti-Wr[b] and -En[a] suffered a mild delayed HTR after receiving six units of En(a+) blood [113] and red cells of a baby born to a mother with alloanti-Wr[b] gave a positive DAT, but transfusion was not required [114]. The result of a chemiluminescent functional assay suggested that an alloanti-Wr[b] would be likely to cause increased destruction of transfused Wr(b+) cells [115].

Anti-Wr[b] is a relatively common autoantibody specificity [116,117]. Issitt *et al.* [117] studied eluates from the DAT-positive red cells of 150 individuals: of 110 antibodies unrelated to Rh, 46 contained anti-Wr[b], four of them containing anti-Wr[b] alone. Thirty-four of the eluates containing anti-Wr[b] came from patients with autoimmune haemolytic anaemia. Two anti-Wr[b] autoantibodies in patients with DAT-positive red cells have been responsible for fatal intravascular haemolysis [118,119].

Many examples of murine monoclonal anti-Wr[b] [100,120–123] and one rhesus monoclonal anti-Wr[b] [123] have been reported.

10.5 Low frequency Diego antigens, DI5 to DI21

Diego was a simple system consisting of a pair of allelic antigens, Di[a] and Di[b], from 1967 until Wr[a] and Wr[b] joined the system in 1995. Since 1996, a further 17 antigens have joined the Diego system. These antigens are all of very low frequency (Table 10.5) and are associated with amino acid substitutions in or close to extracellular loops of band 3 (Table 10.6 and Fig. 10.1). All except KREP [144] previously belonged to the 700 Series of low frequency antigens (Chapter 27).

The low frequency antigens DI5 to DI21 (Table 10.1) were assigned to the Diego system following recognition of an association between antigen expression and a missense mutation in the band 3 gene [144,149–159]. In all cases the same methodology was adopted. Single strand conformation polymorphism (SSCP) analysis reveals differences in electrophoretic mobility that occur in single strands of PCR-amplified segments of DNA as a result of conformation changes caused by single nucleotide changes [161]. Exons 11–20 of *SLC4A1* encode the whole of the membrane domain of band 3. SSCP analysis was used to screen these exons for mutations in genomic DNA from individuals with low frequency red cell antigens. Indication of a mutation within an exon was followed by nucleotide sequencing.

In most cases at least two unrelated individuals with the low frequency antigen were shown to have the associated mutation. Only one Tr(a+) individual was available [153], so the assignment of Tr[a] to the Diego system remains provisional. The WARR mutation was found in a Native North American kindred, the only family containing WARR+ members [154], and the mutations associated with Vg[a] [150] and with KREP [144] were only identified in single families.

All the antigens are associated with a single amino acid substitution, apart from NFLD, in which two substitutions were found, and Sw[a], which represents two amino acids at the same position (Table 10.6). The substitutions are in the putative extracellular loops of band 3 (Fig. 10.1), with the exception of the substitution associated with Bp[a], which is in a membrane-spanning domain, but very close to loop 3 [150]. Bp[a] may therefore represent a conformational change in the third loop. Most of the amino acid changes are clustered on the third and fourth extracellular domains, but ELO and one of the NFLD substitutions are

on the first loop, Fr[a] is close to the second loop, and the Di[a]/Di[b] polymorphism is on loop 7. None of the positions of these amino acid changes challenges any of the models of protein topology in Fig. 10.1. There is no evidence that any of the substitutions has an effect on the function of the band 3 molecule or on binding of the red cell anion exchange inhibitor H_2DIDS (see Section 10.3.2). It is likely therefore that the third and fourth extracellular loops are not involved in anion exchange [150]. Most of the substituted amino acids are not well conserved in evolution, but Asn569, which is changed to lysine in the Bp[a]-associated substitution, is conserved in 12 anion exchanger homologues [150].

Adsorption of some sera containing anti-Wu, -NFLD, and -BOW with Wu+, NFLD+, or BOW+ cells will often remove all three antibodies [162]. BOW and NFLD represent different substitutions of Pro561, whereas Wu represents a substitution of Gly565 [144,150,156,157]. NFLD is associated with amino acid changes in the first and third extracellular loops [156]. The serological associations of NFLD with BOW and Wu suggest that Ala561 is most important in determining NFLD expression. Similar serological cross-reactivity occurs between Jn[a] and KREP, which represent different substitutions of Pro566 [144,158]. Some Sw(a+) red cells are SW1+, while others are SW1– [147,159]. Anti-Sw[a] appears to recognize changes associated with conversion of Arg646 to glutamine or tryptophan, whereas anti-SW1 is specific for the Arg646Trp substitution [159]. Hg[a] and Mo[a] represent different substitutions of Arg656 [150], but no serological association is reported.

The effects of proteases on low frequency Diego antigens are shown in Table 10.6. Band 3 has two chymotrypsin cleavage sites in the third extracellular loop, at Tyr553 and Tyr555. Consequently, the antigens in the third loop are mostly sensitive to α-chymotrypsin, whereas those in the fourth and seventh loop are resistant. This provides further evidence that Pro561Ala is the most important substitution in determining NFLD expression. There are two unexpected effects. One example of anti-ELO did not react with chymotrypsin-treated cells, though ELO is on the first loop. It is possible that the Arg432Trp substitution associated with ELO creates a new chymotrypsin site, giving rise to partial band 3 cleavage and loss of activity with one example of anti-ELO. Conformational changes to band 3 caused by protease digestion might explain why Bp[a], which is associated with an amino

Table 10.5 Other low frequency antigens of the Diego system and their frequencies in various populations.

Antigen			Population	No. tested	No. positive	Antigen frequency	References
DI5	Wd^a	Waldner	North American	4 000	0		[124]
			Norwegian	7 151	0		[125]
			African Hei//om	114	2*	0.0175	[126]
DI6	Rb^a	Redelberger	English	10 200	1	0.0001	[127]
DI7	WARR	Warrior	North American	8 275	1†		[128]
DI8	ELO		Canadian		958	0	[129]
			English	16 223	1	<0.0001	[129]
DI9	Wu	Wulfsberg	Norwegian	7 000	1	0.0001	[130]
			English	1 323	0		[130]
			Danish	2 021	4‡	0.0020	[131]
			Australian	16 472	4	0.0002	[132]
DI10	Bp^a	Bishop	English	75 000	1	<0.0001	[††]
			Norwegian	7 151	0		[125]
DI11	Mo^a	Moen	Norwegian	9 000	0		[133]
			Belgian	9 793	2	0.0002	[133]
DI12	Hg^a	Hughes	Welsh	5 434	2	0.0004	[134]
DI13	Vg^a	Van Vugt	Australian	17 209	1	<0.0001	[135]
DI14	Sw^a	Swann	English	55 410	9	0.0002	[67,68,136,††]
			English	17 661	1	<0.0001	[137]
••			Swiss	~7 000	3	~0.0004	[138]
			Canadian	5 000	3	0.0006	[139]
DI15	BOW	Bowyer	English	>55 000	0	<0.0001	[140]
DI16	NFLD	Newfoundland	North American	1 125	0		[141]
			Japanese	45 825	2	<0.0001	[142]
DI17	Jn^a	Nunhart	Norwegian	13 824	0	<0.0001	[125,131,143]
DI18	KREP						[144]
DI19§	Tr^a	Traversu	English	38 069	2	<0.0001	[††]
			Norwegian	9 500	0		[33]
DI20	Fr^a	Froese	Canadian	1 400	1**	0.0007	[145,146]
DI21	SW1						[147]

*Sisters. Only other Wd(a+) individuals have been Canadian Hutterites with the surname Waldner [124] and a black South African [126].
†Sister of WARR+ propositus.
‡Hov+. Later shown to be the same as Wu [148].
§Provisional assignment.
**Mennonite. Most Fr(a+) propositi have been found among Canadian Mennonites [145,146].
††TE Cleghorn, unpublished observations, 1962–67. Cited in [33].

Table 10.6 Effects of enzyme treatments and molecular basis of Diego system low frequency antigens (presented in order of associated amino acid substitutions from the N-terminus of band 3).

Antigen	Effects of enzymes*		Nucleotide change	Exon	Restriction enzymes†	Amino acid substitution	Loop‡	References
	Pap/tryp	Chym						
ELO	Resistant	Variable	C1294T	12	BstNI (MspI)	Arg432Trp	1	[149,150]
Fr^a			G1438A	13	(BsmAI)	Glu480Lys	2	[151,152]
Rb^a	Resistant	Variable	C1643T	14		Pro548Leu	3	[153]
Tr^a	Resistant	Sensitive	G1653C	14	(BbsI)	Lys551Asn	3	[153]
WARR	Resistant	Sensitive	C1655T	14	(BbsI)	Thr552Ile	3	[154]
Vg^a	Resistant	Sensitive	T1663C	14	DraIII	Tyr555His	3	[150]
Wd^a	Resistant	Sensitive	G1669A	14	MslI (MaeII)	Val557Met	3	[152,155]
BOW	Resistant	Sensitive	C1681T	14	(BanI)	Pro561Ser	3	[144,150, 156]
NFLD	Resistant	Sensitive	C1681G (A1287T)	14 (12)	HaeIII (BanI)	Pro561Ala (Glu429Asp)	3 (1)	[156]
Wu	Resistant	Sensitive	G1694C	14	(ApaI)	Gly565Ala	3	[150,157]
Jn^a	Resistant	Sensitive	C1696T	14	(ApaI) (HaeIII)	Pro566Ser	3	[158]
KREP	Resistant	Sensitive	C1696G	14	CfoI (Bsp1286I)	Pro566Ala	3	[144]
Bp^a	Sensitive	Sensitive	C1707A	14		Asn569Lys	3	[150]
Sw^a	Resistant	Resistant	G1937A or C1936T	16	(MspI)	Arg646Gln or Arg646Trp	4	[159]
SW1			C1936T	16	(MspI)	Arg646Trp	4	[159]
Hg^a	Resistant	Resistant	C1966T	16	(Cac8I)	Arg656Cys	4	[150]
Mo^a	Resistant	Resistant	G1967A	16		Arg656His	4	[150]
Wr^a	Resistant	Resistant	G1972A	16		Glu658Lys	4	[82]
Di^a	Resistant	Resistant	C2561T	19	(MspI) (NaeI)	Pro854Leu	7	[43]

*Pap/tryp, papain, ficin, and trypsin; Chym, α-chymotrypsin. Information mostly derived from Poole [160].
†Some restriction sites created (or destroyed) by the mutation.
‡Extracellular loop.

acid substitution in a transmembrane domain, close to the third extracellular loop, is sensitive to α-chymotrypsin, trypsin, and papain [150].

With the exception of anti-ELO, antibodies to the low frequency antigens from DI5 to DI21 have not been found to be clinically significant. A second ELO+ child of a woman with anti-ELO had mild HDN and her third ELO+ child had severe HDN, necessitating exchange transfusion [163,164]. The anti-ELO was IgG (mostly IgG3) and haemolytic IgM. Anti-Fr^a caused a positive DAT on cord red cells, but no other signs of HDN [165].

Some antisera contain antibodies to numerous red cell antigens of low frequency. These antibodies are produced with no obvious immunizing stimulus (see Chapter 27). Antibodies to all low frequency Diego antigens (with the possible exception of anti-Di^a) have been found in multispecific sera. Anti-ELO [163], -Sw^a, and -Fr^a [165] have also been produced as a result of immunization by antigen-positive red cells. No anti-Rb^a was found in five Rb(a–) mothers of Rb(a+) children [127], no anti-Wd^a was found in six Wd(a–) Hutterite mothers of a total of 30 Wd(a+) children [124], and no anti-NFLD was found in an NFLD– mother of three NFLD+ children [142].

10.6 Functional aspects of band 3

Over recent years it has become increasingly apparent that the function of red cells goes beyond transport of respiratory gases, yet the transport of oxygen to the tissues and of carbon dioxide (CO_2) back to the lungs are the primary red cell functions. Carbonic anhydrase, located in the red cell cytoplasm, hydrates CO_2 in the blood to bicarbonate (HCO_3^-), which is more soluble than CO_2. Band 3 acts as an anion exchanger, an antiporter that permits HCO_3^- to cross the membrane in exchange for Cl^- ions, preventing accumulation of HCO_3^- in the red cells. This facilitates transport of HCO_3^- in the plasma, greatly increasing the quantity of CO_2 that the blood can convey to the lungs [1–3]. Experiments involving coexpression of truncated band 3 fragments has provided evidence that integrity of the second extracellular loop of band 3 is necessary for transport activity [166]. None of the amino acid substitutions associated with blood group activity has been shown to have any functional significance. Only Fr^a is close to the second extracellular loop and Fr(a+) red cells had normal sulphate influx levels [152] (Section 10.5 and Fig. 10.1).

In addition to being a membrane transporter, band 3 has a structural function. The long N-terminal domain interacts with the red cell membrane skeleton (cytoskeleton), through the glycoproteins ankyrin, band 4.2, and band 4.1 [1]. The membrane skeleton, a lattice of glycoproteins beneath the red cell membrane, is very important in maintaining the shape and integrity of the red cells (see Section 18.7 for reviews). Many band 3 mutations result in abnormally shaped red cells. About 20% of cases of hereditary spherocytosis, a common, familial haemolytic anaemia characterized by small spheroid red cells, result from reduced levels of band 3 in the red cells caused by heterozygosity for a variety of mutations within the band 3 gene. Deficiency of the mutant protein from the red cell membrane is usually because of nonsense, frameshift, or splice site mutations, affecting mRNA stability, or missense mutations affecting protein stability [2,3] (see also Section 10.8). There is no evidence that any of the mutations responsible for the low frequency Diego system antigens affects red cell morphology.

Band 3 may also have a role in the removal of senescent red cells from the circulation. It has been proposed that the senescent cell antigen, which binds physiological IgG autoantibodies leading to phagocytosis of ageing cells, is a degradation product of band 3 [167].

Cryptic regions around external loops 3 and 7 of band 3, which only become exposed when the red cells

are infected with the malaria parasite *Plasmodium falciparum*, may be adhesive receptors, involved in the sequestration of infected red cells [168].

Band 3 is involved in expression of the Rh proteins and the Rh-associated glycoprotein (RhAG) and might enhance translocation of the whole Rh complex to the membrane or affect its conformation in the membrane. K562 erythroleukaemia cells transfected with both band 3 cDNA and Rh cDNA expressed substantially more Rh protein and RhAG than clones transfected with Rh cDNA alone [94,169].

Band 3 has very limited tissue distribution. In addition to erythroid cells, band 3 has only been detected in acid-secreting intercalated cells of the kidney collecting duct. The renal isoform of band 3 lacks the N-terminal 65 amino acid residues of erythroid band 3, probably as a result of transcription initiation from an alternative promoter region in intron 3. It has an important role in acid secretion by removing H^+ in the form of HCO_3^- ions [170]. Distal renal tubule acidosis (dRTA) is a condition associated with impaired acid secretion in the distal nephron and inability to acidify urine; symptoms include metabolic acidosis, hypokalaemia, nephrocalcinosis, kidney stones, and metabolic bone disease (reviewed in [171]). Heterozygosity for missense mutations in the region of the proposed sixth and seventh membrane-spanning domains and in the C-terminal domain of band 3 account for autosomal-dominant dRTA. Recessive dRTA is associated with homozygosity for missense mutations (Gly701Asp or Ala858Asp) or deletion of the codon for Val850 [172,173]. The reduction in anion transport associated with these mutations in transfected *Xenopus* oocytes is rescued, at least partially, by cotransfection with GPA cDNA [171–173], providing a possible explanation for the absence of any major erythroid defect associated with dRTA. Heterozygosity for these genes and for the transport-inactive band 3 gene associated with South-East Asian ovalocytosis (Section 10.8) also gives rise to dRTA [173].

10.7 Band 3 deficiency (Diego null phenotype)

Total deficiency of band 3 from the red cells has, until recently, generally been considered to be lethal. Although Diego null phenotype, as such, has not been reported, there is one description of a baby with total band 3 deficiency resulting from homozygosity for a band 3 mutation (Val488Met) [95]. The severely hydropic, anaemic baby was delivered by emergency caesarean section and resuscitated and kept alive by blood transfusion. A cord blood smear revealed dramatic erythroblastosis and poikilocytosis. The baby's red cells had no band 3, no band 4.2, and low levels of glycophorin A. At 3 months the baby developed dRTA. Absence of band 3 therefore is compatible with life but only with extreme medical intervention. Band 3-deficient mice, with targeted disruption of the band 3 gene, and cattle with a band 3 nonsense mutation, were able to survive, despite spherocytosis, haemolytic anaemia, and growth retardation [174–176].

10.8 South-East Asian ovalocytosis

A form of hereditary ovalocytosis, known as South-East Asian ovalocytosis (SAO), is relatively common in the southern Pacific region and confers protection against cerebral malaria in children (review in [2,3]). SAO results from heterozygosity for a band 3 gene with a 27-bp deletion, which encodes a variant protein (band 3 SAO) with a deletion of amino acids 400–408, the region of the protein at the boundary of the cytoplasmic N-terminal domain and the first membrane-spanning domain (Fig. 10.1). Band 3 SAO also has the Memphis I variant and is non-functional as an anion transporter. Despite its common occurrence, no person homozygous for this mutation has been found, supporting the assertion that homozygosity for any mutation that inactivates band 3 would normally be lethal.

Booth et al. [49] noticed that many red cell antigens were depressed on red cells of Melanesians with SAO. These antigens include Di^b and Wr^b, but also S, s, U, En^a, D, C, e, Kp^b, Jk^a, Jk^b, Xg^a, Sc1, LW, Ge2, Ge3, Ge4, I^T, and I^F [49,177]. Reduced binding to SAO cells was also detected with rodent monoclonal antibodies to extracellular epitopes on band 3 and with monoclonal anti-Wr^b [178]. Depression of antigens on band 3 in SAO may result from the disturbance of cooperative interactions between the membrane-spanning domains, important in maintaining structural integrity of band 3. Depression of antigens of the Rh membrane complex (RhD, RhCcEe, LW, SsU) could be a result of reduced translocation of the complex to the cell surface [169]. In addition there may be wider effects on other membrane proteins, caused by disruption of protein complexes involving band 3 and to an abnormal interaction between band 3 SAO (and dimers of band 3 and band 3 SAO) and the cytoskeleton [177,178].

References

1 Tanner MJA. Molecular and cellular biology of the erythrocyte anion exchanger (AE1). *Semin Hematol* 1993;30:34–57.
2 Tanner MJA. The structure and function of band 3 (AE1): recent developments (review). *Mol Mem Biol* 1997;14:155–65.
3 Bruce LJ, Tanner MJA. Erythroid band 3 variants and disease. *Baillière's Best Prac Res Clin Haematol* 1999;12:637–54.
4 Schofield AE, Martin PG, Spillet D, Tanner MJA. The structure of the human red blood cell anion exchanger (EPB3, AE1, Band 3) gene. *Blood* 1994;84:2000–12.
5 Tanner MJA, Martin PG, High S. The complete amino acid sequence of the human erythrocyte membrane anion-transport protein deduced from the cDNA sequence. *Biochem J* 1988;256:703–12.
6 Lux SE, John KM, Kopito RR, Lodish HF. Cloning and characterization of band 3, the human erythrocyte anion-exchange protein (AE1). *Proc Natl Acad Sci USA* 1989;86:9089–93.
7 Popov M, Tam LY, Jing L, Reithmeier RAF. Mapping the ends of transmembrane segments in a polytopic membrane protein: scanning N-glycosylation mutagenesis of extracytosolic loops in the anion exchanger, band 3. *J Biol Chem* 1997;272:18325–32.
8 Fujinaga J, Tang X-B, Casey JR. Topology of the membrane domain of human erythrocyte anion exchange protein, AE1. *J Biol Chem* 1999;274:6626–33.
9 Van Dort HM, Moriyama R, Low PS. Effect of band 3 subunit equilibrium on the kinetics and affinity of ankyrin binding to erythrocyte membrane vesicles. *J Biol Chem* 1998;273:14819–26.
10 Layrisse M, Arends T, Dominguez Sisico R. Nuevo grupo sanguíneo encontrado en descendientes de Indios. *Acta Med Venezolana* 1955;3:132–8.
11 Levine P, Robinson EA, Layrisse M, Arends T, Domingues Sisico R. The Diego blood factor. *Nature* 1956;177:40–1.
12 Thompson PR, Childers DM, Hatcher DE. Anti-Di^b: first and second examples. *Vox Sang* 1967;13:314–18.
13 Mourant AE, Kopec AC, Domaniewska-Sobczak K. *The Distribution of the Human Blood Groups and Other Polymorphisms*, 2nd edn. London: Oxford University Press, 1976.
14 Tills D, Kopec AC, Tills RE. *The Distribution of the Human Blood Groups and Other Polymorphisms* (Suppl. 1). Oxford: Oxford University Press, 1983.
15 Zafar M, Reid ME. Review: the Diego blood group system. *Immunohematology* 1993;9:35–40.

16 Cann HM, Van West B, Barnett CR. Genetics of Diego blood groups in Guatemalan Indians: use of antiserums to Diego a and Diego b antigens. *Science* 1968; **162**:1391–2.

17 Lewis M, Ayukawa H, Chown B, Levine P. The blood group antigen Diego in North American Indians and in Japanese. *Nature* 1956;**177**:1084.

18 Allen FH, Corcoran PA. Blood groups of the Penobscot Indians. *Am J Phys Anthrop* 1960;**18**:109–14.

19 Edwards-Moulds JM, Alperin JB. Studies of the Diego blood group among Mexican-Americans. *Transfusion* 1986;**26**:234–6.

20 Miyazaki T, Sato S, Kato T, Ikeda H. Human anti-Di^a monoclonal antibodies for mass screening. *Immunohematology* 2000;**16**:78–81.

21 Lin-Chu M, Broadberry RE, Chang FJ. The distribution of blood group antigens and alloantibodies among Chinese in Taiwan. *Transfusion* 1988;**28**:350–2.

22 Won CD, Shin HS, Kim SW, Swanson J, Matson GA. Distribution of hereditary blood factors among Koreans residing in Seoul, Korea. *Am J Phys Anthrop* 1960;**18**:115–24.

23 Layrisse M, Arends T. The 'Diego' blood factor distribution: genetic, clinical and anthropological significance. *Proc 6th Congr Int Soc Blood Transfus* 1958:114–6.

24 Riches RA, Laycock CM, Poole J. Anti-Di^a causing HDN in an English family: non-linkage of Diego and Colton genes is demonstrated [Abstract]. *20th Congr Int Soc Blood Transfus* 1988:299.

25 Kusnierz-Alejska G, Bochenek S. Haemolytic disease of the newborn due to anti-Di^a and incidence of the Di^a antigen in Poland. *Vox Sang* 1992;**62**:124–6.

26 Layrisse M, Arends T. The Diego blood factor in Negroid populations. *Nature* 1957;**179**:478–9.

27 Simmons RT. The apparent absence of the Diego (Di^a) and the Wright (Wr^a) blood group antigens in Australian Aborigines and in New Guineans. *Vox Sang* 1970;**19**:533–6.

28 Layrisse M, Arends T. The Diego blood factor in Chinese and Japanese. *Nature* 1956;**177**:1083–4.

29 Simmons RT, Albrey JA, Morgan JAG, Smith AJ. The Diego blood group: anti-Di^a and the Di(a+) blood group antigen found in Caucasians. *Med J Aust* 1968;**1**:406–7.

30 Graninger W. Anti-Di^a and the Di^a blood group: antigen found in an Austrian family. *Vox Sang* 1976;**31**:131–5.

31 Issitt PD, Wren MR, Rueda E, Maltz M. Red cell antigens in Hispanic blood donors. *Transfusion* 1987;**27**:117.

32 Lewis M, Kaita H, Chown B. The blood groups of a Japanese population. *Am J Hum Genet* 1957;**9**:274–83.

33 Race RR, Sanger R. *Blood Groups in Man*, 6th edn. Oxford: Blackwell Scientific Publications, 1975.

34 Levine P, Robinson EA. Some observations of the new human blood factor Di^a. *Blood* 1957;**12**:448–53.

35 Layrisse M, Sanger R, Race RR. The inheritance of the antigen Di^a: evidence for its independence of other

blood group systems. *Am J Hum Genet* 1959;**11**: 17–25.

36 Mueller TJ, Morrison M. Detection of a variant of protein 3, the major transmembrane protein of the human erythrocyte. *J Biol Chem* 1977;**252**:6573–6.

37 Yannoukakos D, Vasseur C, Driancourt C *et al.* Human erythrocyte band 3 polymorphism (band 3 Memphis): characterization of the structural modification (Lys 56→Glu) by protein chemistry methods. *Blood* 1991; **78**:1117–20.

38 Jarolim P, Rubin HL, Zhai S *et al.* Band 3 Memphis: a widespread polymorphism with abnormal electrophoretic mobility of erythrocyte band 3 protein caused by a substitution AAG→GAG (Lys→Glu) in codon 56. *Blood* 1992;**80**:1592–8.

39 Ranney HM, Rosenberg GH, Morrison M, Mueller TJ. Frequencies of band 3 variants of human red cell membranes in some different populations. *Br J Haematol* 1990;**75**:262–7.

40 Ideguchi H, Okubo K, Ishikawa A, Futata Y, Hamasaki N. Band 3-Memphis is associated with a lower transport rate of phosphoenolpyruvate. *Br J Haematol* 1992;**82**: 122–5.

41 Hsu L, Morrison M. A new variant of the anion transport protein in human erythrocytes. *Biochemistry* 1985; **24**:3086–90.

42 Spring FA, Bruce LJ, Anstee DJ, Tanner MJA. A red cell band 3 variant with altered stilbene disulphonate binding is associated with the Diego (Di^a) blood group antigen. *Biochem J* 1992;**288**:713–6.

43 Bruce LJ, Anstee DJ, Spring FA, Tanner MJA. Band 3 Memphis variant II: altered stilbene disulfonate binding and the Diego (Di^a) blood group antigen are associated with the human erythrocyte band 3 mutation Pro^{854}→Leu. *J Biol Chem* 1994;**269**:16155–8.

44 Salhany JM, Sloan RL, Schopfer LM. Characterization of the stilbenedisulphonate binding site on band 3 Memphis variant II (Pro-854→Leu). *Biochem J* 1996;**317**:509–14.

45 Castilho L, Rios M, Soares M, Menezes R, Costa FF. High frequency of the *DI*A* allele associated with the mutation Lys56Glu in Amazonian Indians [Abstract]. *Blood* 1999;**94**(Suppl.1):458a.

46 Jarolim P, Rubin HL, Moulds JM. Multiple molecular mechanisms resulting in the Di(a+b–) phenotype [Abstract]. *Transfusion* 1996;**36**(Suppl.):49S.

47 Daniels G. Effect of enzymes on and chemical modifications of high-frequency red cell antigens. *Immunohematology* 1992;**8**:53–7.

48 Biro V, Garratty G, Johnson CL, Marsh WL. Depressed blood group antigens on red cells from a Mexican donor. *Transfusion* 1983;**23**:65–6.

49 Booth PB, Serjeantson S, Woodfield DG, Amato D. Selective depression of blood group antigens associated with hereditary ovalocytosis among Melanesians. *Vox Sang* 1977;**32**:99–110.

50 Tatarsky J, Stroup M, Levine P, Ernoehazy WS. Another example of anti-Diego (Di^a). *Vox Sang* 1959;**4**:152–4.

51 Feller CW, Shenker L, Scott EP, Marsh WL. An anti-Diego^b (Di^b) antibody occurring during pregnancy. *Transfusion* 1970;**10**:279–80.

52 Nakajima H, Hayakawa Z, Ito H. A new example of anti-Di^b found in a Japanese woman. *Vox Sang* 1971;**20**:271–3.

53 Alves de Lima LM, Berthier ME *et al.* Characterization of an anti-Di^a antibody causing hemolytic disease in a newborn infant. *Transfusion* 1982;**22**:246–7.

54 Zupanska B, Brojer E, McIntosh J, Seyfried H, Howell P. Correlation of monocyte-monolayer assay results, number of erythrocyte-bound IgG molecules, and IgG subclass composition in the study of red cell alloantibodies other than D. *Vox Sang* 1990;**58**:276–80.

55 Hinckley ME, Huestis DW. An immediate hemolytic transfusion reaction apparently caused by anti-Di^a. *Rev Franc Transfus Immuno-Hémat* 1979;**22**:581–5.

56 Yasuda H, Ohto H, Yamaguchi O *et al.* Three episodes of delayed hemolytic transfusion reactions due to multiple red cell antibodies, anti-Di^a, anti-Jk^a and anti-E. *Transfus Sci* 2000;**23**:107–12.

57 Zago-Novaretti MC, Soares MOC, Dorlhiac-Llacer PE, Chamone DAF. Anti-Diego in multitransfused patients [Abstract]. *Rev Paulista Med* 1992;**110**(5):IH52.

58 Ishimori T, Fukumoto Y, Abe K *et al.* Rare Diego blood group phenotype Di(a+b–). I. Anti-Di^b causing hemolytic disease of the newborn. *Vox Sang* 1976;**31**:61–3.

59 Orlina AR, DiMauro J, Unger PJ. Hemolytic disease of the newborn due to anti-Di^b. *Am J Clin Pathol* 1979;**71**:713–4.

60 Uchikawa M, Shibata Y, Tohyama H *et al.* A case of hemolytic disease of the newborn due to anti-Di^b antibodies. *Vox Sang* 1982;**42**:91–2.

61 Habash J, Devenish A, Macdonald S, Garner S, Contreras M. A further example of anti-Di^b not causing haemolytic disease of the newborn. *Vox Sang* 1991;**61**:77.

62 Lin CK, Mak KH, Chan NK *et al.* Report on anti-Di^b encountered in two Hong Kong Chinese. *Immunohematology* 1997;**13**:17–19.

63 Issitt PD, Combs MR, Allen J, Melroy-Carawan H. Anti-Di^b as a red cell autoantibody. *Transfusion* 1996;**36**:802–4.

64 Daniels GL. *Blood group antigens of high frequency: a serological and genetic study.* PhD thesis, University of London, 1980.

65 Mollison PL, Engelfriet CP, Contreras M. *Blood Transfusion in Clinical Medicine,* 10th edn. Oxford: Blackwell Scientific Publications, 1997.

66 Holman CA. A new rare human blood-group antigen (Wr^a). *Lancet* 1953;**ii**:119.

67 Cleghorn TE. The frequency of the Wr^a, By and M^g blood group antigens in blood donors in the South of England. *Vox Sang* 1960;**5**:556–60.

68 Cleghorn TE. *The occurrence of certain rare blood group factors in Britain.* MD thesis, University of Sheffield, 1961.

69 Wallis JP, Hedley GP, Charlton D *et al.* The incidence of anti-Wr^a and Wr^a antigen in blood donors and hospital patients. *Transfus Med* 1996;**6**:361–4.

70 Kornstad L. Some observations on the Wright blood group system. *Vox Sang* 1961;**6**:129–35.

71 Metaxas MN, Metaxas-Bühler M. Studies on the Wright blood group system. *Vox Sang* 1963;**8**:707–16.

72 Liotta I, Purpura M, Dawes BJ, Giles CM. Some data on the low frequency antigens Wr^a and Bp^a. *Vox Sang* 1970;**19**:540–3.

73 Kout M. The incidence of the C^w, M^g and Wr^a agglutinogens in the population of Prague. *Vox Sang* 1962;**7**:242–4.

74 Walker ME, Tippett PA, Roper JM *et al.* Tests with some rare blood-group antibodies. *Vox Sang* 1961;**6**:357.

75 Greendyke RM, Banzhaf JC. Occurrence of anti-Wr^a in blood donors and in selected patient groups, with a note on the incidence of the Wr^a antigen. *Transfusion* 1977;**17**:621–4.

76 McGuire D, Funkhouser JW. A study of the Wright blood group system as found in a normal donor population [Abstract]. *Transfusion* 1967;**7**:385.

77 Lewis M, Kaita H, Chown B *et al.* A family with the rare red cell antigens Wr^a and 'super' Sd^a. *Vox Sang* 1973;**25**:336–40.

78 Lewis M, Kaita H, Philipps S, McAlpine PJ. The low-incidence red cell antigen Wr^a: genetic studies. *Transfusion* 1991;**31**:47–51.

79 Adams J, Broviac M, Brooks W, Johnson NR, Issitt PD. An antibody, in the serum of a Wr(a+) individual, reacting with an antigen of very high frequency. *Transfusion* 1971;**11**:290–1.

80 Dahr W, Schütt KH, Arndt-Hanser A *et al.* A novel phenotype within the Wright blood group collection [Abstract]. *Transfusion* 1992;**32**(Suppl.):55S.

81 Wren MR, Issitt PD. Evidence that Wr^a and Wr^b are antithetical. *Transfusion* 1988;**28**:113–8.

82 Bruce LJ, Ring SM, Anstee DJ *et al.* Changes in the blood group Wright antigens are associated with a mutation at amino acid 658 in human erythrocyte band 3: a site of interaction between band 3 and glycophorin A under certain conditions. *Blood* 1995;**85**:541–7.

83 Ring SM, Green CA, Swallow DM, Tippett P. Production of a murine monoclonal antibody to the low incidence red cell antigen Wr^a: characterization and comparison with human anti-Wr^a. *Vox Sang* 1994;**67**:222–5.

84 Ring SM. *An immunochemical investigation of the Wr^a and Wr^b blood group antigens.* PhD thesis, University of London, 1992.

85 Wainwright SD, Tanner MJA, Martin GEM, Yendle JE, Holmes C. Monoclonal antibodies to the membrane domain of the human erythrocyte anion transport protein.

Localization of the C-terminus of the protein to the cytoplasmic side of the red cell membrane and distribution of the protein in some human tissues. *Biochem J* 1989;258:211–20.

86 Nigg EA, Bron C, Giradet M, Cherry RJ. Band 3–glycophorin A association in erythrocyte membranes demonstrated by combining protein diffusion measurements with antibody-induced cross-linking. *Biochemistry* 1980;19:1887–93.

87 Che A, Cherry RJ. Loss of rotational mobility of band 3 proteins in human erythrocyte membranes induced by antibodies to glycophorin A. *Biophys J* 1995;68:1881–7.

88 Paulitschke M, Nash GB, Anstee DJ, Tanner MJA, Gratzer WB. Perturbation of red blood cell membrane rigidity by extracellular ligands. *Blood* 1995;86:342–8.

89 Groves JD, Tanner MJA. Glycophorin A facilitates the expression of human Band 3-mediated anion transport in *Xenopus* oocytes. *J Biol Chem* 1992;267:22163–70.

90 Hassoun H, Hanada T, Lutchman M *et al.* Complete deficiency of glycophorin A in red blood cells from mice with targeted inactivation of the band 3 (AE1) gene. *Blood* 1998;91:2146–51.

91 Southcott MJG, Tanner MJA, Anstee DJ. The expression of human blood group antigens during erythropoiesis in a cell culture system. *Blood* 1999;93:4425–35.

92 Daniels G, Green C. Expression of red cell surface antigens during erythropoiesis. *Vox Sang* 2000;78(Suppl.1):149–53.

93 Gahmberg CG, Andersson LC. K562: a human leukemia cell line with erythroid features. *Semin Hematol* 1981;18:72–7.

94 Beckman R, Smythe JS, Anstee DJ, Tanner MJA. Functional cell surface expression of band 3, the human red blood cell anion exchange protein (AE1), in K562 erythroleukemia cells: band 3 enhances the cell surface reactivity of Rh antigens. *Blood* 1998;92:4428–38.

95 Ribeiro ML, Alloisio N, Almeida H *et al.* Severe hereditary spherocytosis and distal renal tubular acidosis associated with total absence of band 3. *Blood* 2000;96:1602–4.

96 Auffray I, Marfatia S, de Jong K *et al.* Glycophorin A dimerization and band 3 interaction during erythroid membrane biogenesis: in vivo studies in human glycophorin A transgenic mice. *Blood* 2001;97:2872–8.

97 Issitt PD, Pavone BG, Goldfinger D, Zwicker H. An En(a–) red cell sample that types as Wr(a–b–). *Transfusion* 1975;15:353–5.

98 Issitt PD, Pavone BG, Wagstaff W, Goldfinger D. The phenotypes En(a–), Wr(a–b–), and En(a+), Wr(a+b–), and further studies on the Wright and En blood group systems. *Transfusion* 1976;16:396–407.

99 Dahr W, Wilkinson S, Issitt PD *et al.* High frequency antigens of human erythrocyte membrane sialoglyco-proteins. III. Studies on the En^{a}FR, Wr^b and Wr^a antigens. *Biol Chem Hoppe-Seyler* 1986;367:1033–45.

100 Ridgwell K, Tanner MJA, Anstee DJ. The Wr^b antigen, a receptor for *Plasmodium falciparum* malaria, is located on a helical region of the major membrane sialoglycoprotein of human red blood cells. *Biochem J* 1983;209:273–6.

101 Ridgwell K, Tanner MJA, Anstee DJ. The Wr^b antigen in St^a-positive and Dantu-positive human erythrocytes. *J Immunogenet* 1984;11:365–70.

102 Telen MJ, Chasis JA. Relationship of the human erythrocyte Wr^b antigen to an interaction between glycophorin A and band 3. *Blood* 1990;76:842–8.

103 Ring SM, Tippett P, Swallow DM. Comparative immunochemical analysis of Wr^a and Wr^b red cell antigens. *Vox Sang* 1994;67:226–30.

104 Leddy JP, Wilkinson SL, Kissel GE *et al.* Erythrocyte membrane proteins reactive with IgG (warm-reacting) anti-red blood cell autoantibodies. II. Antibodies coprecipitating band 3 and glycophorin A. *Blood* 1994;84:650–6.

105 Rearden A. Reactivity of monoclonal anti-Wr^b with a synthetic peptide. *Transfusion* 1989;29:187.

106 Huang C-H, Reid ME, Xie S-S, Blumenfeld OO. Human red blood cell Wright antigens: a genetic and evolutionary perspective on glycophorin A–band 3 interaction. *Blood* 1996;87:3942–7.

107 Lubenko A, Contreras M. The incidence of hemolytic disease of the newborn attributable to anti-Wr^a. *Transfusion* 1992;32:87–8.

108 Hardman JT, Beck ML. Hemagglutination in capillaries: Correlation with blood group specificity and IgG subclass. *Transfusion* 1981;21:343–6.

109 Wiener AS, Brancato GJ. Severe erythroblastosis fetalis caused by sensitization to a rare human agglutinogen. *Am J Hum Genet* 1953;5:350–5.

110 Daw E. Haemolytic disease of the newborn due to the Wright antigen. *J Obstet Gynaecol* 1971;78:377–8.

111 Jørgensen J, Jacobsen L. Erythroblastosis fetalis caused by anti-Wr^a (Wright). *Vox Sang* 1974;27:478–9.

112 van Loghem JJ, van der Hart M, Bok J, Brinkerink PC. Two further examples of the antibody anti-Wr^a (Wright). *Vox Sang* (old series) 1955;5:130–4.

113 Furuhjelm U, Nevanlinna HR, Pirkola A. A second Finnish En(a–) propositus with anti-En^a. *Vox Sang* 1973;24:545–9.

114 Langley JW, Issitt PD, Anstee DJ *et al.* Another individual (J.R.) whose red blood cells appear to carry a hybrid MNSs sialoglycoprotein. *Transfusion* 1981;21:15–24.

115 Poole J, Banks J, Kjeldsen-Kragh J *et al.* Second example of MiV/MiV phenotype with anti-Wr^b: a case study [Abstract]. *Transfus Med* 1997;7(Suppl.1):27.

116 Goldfinger D, Zwicker H, Belkin GA, Issitt PD. An autoantibody with anti-Wr^b specificity in a patient with warm autoimmune hemolytic anemia. *Transfusion* 1975;15:351–2.

117 Issitt PD, Pavone BG, Goldfinger D *et al*. Anti-Wr[b], and other autoantibodies responsible for positive direct antiglobulin tests in 150 individuals. *Br J Haematol* 1976;34:5–18.

118 Ainsworth BM, Fraser ID, Poole GD. Severe haemolytic anaemia due to anti-Wr[b] [Abstract]. *20th Congr Int Soc Blood Transfus*, 1988:82.

119 Dankbar DT, Pierce SR, Issitt PD, Gutgsell NS, Beck ML. Fatal intravascular hemolysis associated with auto anti-Wr[b] [Abstract]. *Transfusion* 1987;27:534.

120 Anstee DJ, Edwards PAW. Monoclonal antibodies to human erythrocytes. *Eur J Immunol* 1982;12:228–32.

121 Rouger P, Anstee D, Salmon C, eds. First International Workshop on Monoclonal Antibodies Against Human Red Blood Cell and Related Antigens. *Rev Franc Transfus Immuno-Hémat* 1988;31:261–364 (11 papers).

122 Gardner B, Parsons SF, Merry AH, Anstee DJ. Epitopes on sialoglycoprotein α: evidence for heterogeneity in the molecule. *Immunology* 1989;68:283–9.

123 Reid ME, Lisowska E, Blanchard D, eds. Third International Workshop on Monoclonal Antibodies Against Human Red Blood Cell and Related Antigens. *Transfus Clin Biol* 1997;4:57–96 (9 papers).

124 Lewis M, Kaita H. A 'new' low incidence 'Hutterite' blood group antigen Waldner (Wd[a]). *Am J Hum Genet* 1981;33:418–20.

125 Kornstad L. A rare blood group antigen, Ol[a] (Oldeide), associated with weak Rh antigens. *Vox Sang* 1986;50:235–9.

126 Moores P, Smart E, Marks M, Botha MC. Wd(a+) red blood cells in two sisters of a Hei//om Khoisan family in Namibia. *Hum Hered* 1990;40:257–61.

127 Contreras M, Stebbing B, Mallory DM *et al*. The Redelberger antigen Rb[a]. *Vox Sang* 1978;35:397–400.

128 Coghlan G, Crow M, Spruell P, Moulds M, Zelinski T. A 'new' low-incidence red cell antigen, WARR: Unique to native Americans? *Vox Sang* 1995;68:187–90.

129 Coghlan G, Green C, Lubenko A, Tippett P, Zelinski T. Low-incidence red cell antigen ELO (700.51): evidence for exclusion from thirteen blood group systems. *Vox Sang* 1993;64:240–3.

130 Kornstad L, Howell P, Jorgensen J, Larsen AMH, Wadsworth LD. The rare blood group antigen, Wu. *Vox Sang* 1976;31:337–43.

131 Kornstad L, Jerne D, Tippett P. The Haakestad antigen is identical with the Hov antigen. *Vox Sang* 1987;52:120–2.

132 Young S, Mallan M, Case J, Moulds J, Beal RW. Further examples of the Wulfsberg antigen. *Vox Sang* 1980;38:213–5.

133 Kornstad L, Brocteur J. A new, rare blood group antigen, Mo[a] (Moen) [Abstract]. *Joint Congr Int Soc Blood Transfus Am Assoc Blood Banks* 1972:58.

134 Rowe GP, Hammond W. A new low-frequency antigen, Hg[a] (Hughes). *Vox Sang* 1983;45:316–19.

135 Young S. Vg[a]: a new low incidence red cell antigen. *Vox Sang* 1981;41:48–9.

136 Cleghorn TE. A 'new' human blood group antigen, Sw[a]. *Nature* 1959;184:1324.

137 Contreras M, Lubenko A, Armitage S, Cleghorn T, Jenkins J. Frequency and inheritance of the Bx[a] (Box) antigen. *Vox Sang* 1980;39:225–8.

138 Metaxas MN, Metaxas-Buehler M. A Swiss family showing independent segregation of the Lutheran and Swann genes. *Vox Sang* 1976;31(Suppl.1):39–43.

139 Lewis M, Kaita H, Philipps S *et al*. The Swann phenotype 700:4,–41; genetic studies. *Vox Sang* 1988;54:184–187.

140 Chaves MA, Leak MR, Poole J, Giles CM. A new low-frequency antigen BOW (Bowyer). *Vox Sang* 1988;55:241–3.

141 Lewis M, Kaita H, Allderdice PW, Bergren M, McAlpine PJ. A 'new' low incidence red cell antigen, NFLD. *Hum Genet* 1984;67:270–1.

142 Okubo Y, Yamaguchi H, Seno T *et al*. The NFLD antigen in Japan. *Hum Hered* 1988;38:122–4.

143 Kornstad L, Kout M, Larsen AMH, Ørjasaeter H. A rare blood group antigen, Jn[a]. *Vox Sang* 1967;13:165–70.

144 Poole J, Bruce LJ, Hallewell H *et al*. Erythrocyte band 3 mutation Pro561→Ser gives rise to the BOW antigen and Pro566→Ala to a novel antigen KREP [Abstract]. *Transfus Med* 1998;8(Suppl.1):17.

145 Lewis M, Kaita H, McAlpine PJ, Fletcher J, Moulds JJ. A 'new' blood group antigen Fr[a]: incidence, inheritance and genetic linkage analysis. *Vox Sang* 1978;35:251–4.

146 Kaita H, Lewis M, McAlpine PJ. Exclusion of the red blood cell antigen Fr[a] from the Colton blood group system. *Transfusion* 1980;20:217.

147 Contreras M, Teesdale P, Moulds M *et al*. Sw[a]: a subdivision. *Vox Sang* 1987;52:115–19.

148 Moulds M, Kaita H, Kornstad L, Lubenko A. Evidence that the low-incidence antigens termed Wu (700.13) and Hov (700.38) are identical. *Vox Sang* 1992;62:53–4.

149 Zelinksi T, Punter F, McManus K, Coghlan G. The ELO blood group polymorphism is located in the putative first extracellular loop of human erythrocyte band 3. *Vox Sang* 1998;75:63–5.

150 Jarolim P, Rubin HL, Zakova D, Storry J, Reid ME. Characterization of seven low incidence blood group antigens carried by erythrocyte band 3 protein. *Blood* 1998;92:4836–43.

151 McManus K, Lupe K, Coghlan G, Zelinski T. An amino acid substitution in the putative second extracellular loop of RBC band 3 accounts for the Froese blood group polymorphism. *Transfusion* 2000;40:1246–9.

152 Jarolim P, Reid ME. Substitution 480Glu→Lys in erythroid band 3 underlies the Fr[a] blood group antigen and supports the existence of the second ectoplasmic loop of band 3 [Abstract]. *Blood* 2000;96:593a.

153 Jarolim P, Murray JL, Rubin HL, Smart E, Moulds JM. Blood group antigens Rb^a, Tr^a, and Wd^a are located in the third ectoplasmic loop of erythroid band 3. *Transfusion* 1997;37:607–15.

154 Jarolim P, Murray JL, Rubin HL, Coghlan G, Zelinski T. A Thr$_{552}$→Ile substitution in erythroid band 3 gives rise to the Warrior blood group antigen. *Transfusion* 1997;37:398–405.

155 Bruce LJ, Zelinski T, Ridgwell K, Tanner MJA. The low-incidence blood group antigen, Wd^a, is associated with the substitution Val$_{557}$→Met in human erythrocyte band 3 (*AE1*). *Vox Sang* 1996;71:118–20.

156 McManus K, Pongoski J, Coghlan G, Zelinski T. Amino acid substitutions in human erythroid protein, band 3 account for the low-incidence antigens NFLD and BOW. *Transfusion* 2000;40:325–9.

157 Zelinski T, McManus K, Punter F, Moulds M, Coghlan G. A Gly$_{565}$→Ala substitution in human erythrocyte band 3 accounts for the Wu blood group polymorphism. *Transfusion* 1998;38:745–8.

158 Poole J, Hallewell H, Bruce L *et al*. Identification of two new Jn(a+) individuals and assignment of Jn^a to erythrocyte band 3 [Abstract]. *Transfusion* 1997; 37(Suppl.):90S.

159 Zelinski T, Rusnak A, McManus K, Coghlan G. Distinctive Swann blood group genotypes: molecular investigations. *Vox Sang* 2000;79:215–18.

160 Poole J. Red cell antigens on band 3 and glycophorin A. *Blood Rev* 2000;14:31–43.

161 Orita M, Suzuki Y, Sekiya T, Hayashi K. Rapid and sensitive detection of point mutations and DNA polymorphisms using the polymerase chain reaction. *Genomics* 1989;5:874–9.

162 Kaita H, Lubenko A, Moulds M, Lewis M. A serologic relationship among the NFLD, BOW, and Wu red cell antigens. *Transfusion* 1992;32:845–7.

163 Ford DS, Stern DA, Hawksworth DN *et al*. Haemolytic disease of the newborn probably due to anti-ELO, an antibody to a low frequency red cell antigen. *Vox Sang* 1992;62:169–72.

164 Better PJ, Ford DS, Frascarelli A, Stern DA. Confirmation of anti-ELO as a cause of haemolytic disease of the newborn. *Vox Sang* 1993;65:70.

165 Harris PA, De la Vega MS, Clinton BA, Miller WV. Positive direct antiglobulin test due to anti-Fr^a in a newborn infant. *Transfusion* 1983;23:394–5.

166 Wang L, Groves JD, Mawby WJ, Tanner MJA. Complementation studies with co-expressed fragments of the human red cell anion transporter (band 3; AE1): the role of some exofacial loops in anion transport. *J Biol Chem* 1997;272:10631–8.

167 Kay MMB. Cellular and molecular biology of senescent cell antigen. In: G Garratty, ed. *Immunobiology of*

Transfusion Medicine. New York: Marcel Dekker, 1994: 173–98.

168 Oh SS, Chisti AH, Palek J, Liu S-C. Erythrocyte membrane alterations in *Plasmodium falciparum* malaria sequestration. *Curr Opin Hematol* 1997;4:148–54.

169 Beckmann R, Smythe JS, Anstee DJ, Tanner MJA. Coexpression of band 3 mutants and Rh polypeptides: differential effects of band 3 on the expression of the Rh complex containing D polypeptide and the Rh complex containing CcEe polypeptide. *Blood* 2001; 97:2496–505.

170 Kollert-Jöns A, Wagner S, Hübner S, Appelhans H, Drenckhahn D. Anion exchanger 1 in human kidney and oncocytoma differs from erythroid AE1 in its NH$_2$ terminus. *Am J Physiol* 1993;265:F813–21.

171 Bruce LJ, Unwin RJ, Wrong O, Tanner MJA. The association between familial distal renal tubular acidosis and mutations in the red cell anion exchanger (band 3, *AE1*) gene. *Biochem Cell Biol* 1998;76:723–8.

172 Tanphaichitr VS, Sumboonnanonda A, Ideguchi H *et al*. Novel AE1 mutations in recessive distal renal tubular acidosis: loss-of-function is rescued by glycophorin A. *J Clin Invest* 1998;102:2173–9.

173 Bruce LJ, Wrong O, Toye AM *et al*. Band 3 mutations, renal tubular acidosis and South East Asian ovalocytosis in Malaysia and Papua New Guinea: loss of up to 95% band 3 transport in red cells. *Biochem J* 2000;350:41–51.

174 Peters LL, Shivdasani RA, Lui SC *et al*. Anion exchanger 1 (band 3) is required to prevent erythrocyte membrane surface loss but not to form the membrane skeleton. *Cell* 1996;86:917–27.

175 Southgate CD, Chisti AH, Mitchell B, Yi SJ, Palek J. Targeted disruption of the murine erythroid band 3 gene results in spherocytosis and severe haemolytic anaemia despite a normal membrane skeleton. *Nature Genet* 1996;14:227–30.

176 Inaba M, Yawata A, Koshino I *et al*. Defective anion transport and marked spherocytosis and membrane instability caused by hereditary total deficiency of red cell band 3 in cattle due to a nonsense mutation. *J Clin Invest* 1996;97:1804–17.

177 Daniels GL, Johnson PH, Coetzer TL *et al*. Depressed Gerbich (glycophorin C/D) red cell antigens associated with Southeast Asian ovalocytosis (SAO) in a South African kindred. [Abstract]. *24th Congr Int Soc Blood Transfus, Makuhari, Japan*, 1996:110.

178 Smythe JS, Spring FA, Gardner B *et al*. Monoclonal antibodies recognizing epitopes on the extracellular face and intracellular N-terminus of the human erythrocyte anion transporter (band 3) and their applications to the analysis of South East Asian ovalocytes. *Blood* 1995;85:2929–36.

11 Yt blood group system

11.1 Introduction

Anti-Yt^a, a new antibody detecting an antigen of high frequency, was found during crossmatching and reported by Eaton *et al.* [1] in 1956. The antithetical antibody, anti-Yt^b, detects an antigen on red cells of about 8% of white people and was found 8 years later by Giles and Metaxas [2]. Yt, also known as the Cartwright system, remains a two-allele system (Table 11.1); an inherited Yt(a–b–) phenotype has not been found.

Yt^a and Yt^b represent an His353Asn amino acid substitution in acetylcholinesterase (AChE) on red cells. *YT* and *ACHE*, the gene encoding AChE, have independently been assigned to chromosome 7q22.1 (Chapter 32).

11.2 Yt antigens and red cell acetylcholinesterase

The complement-sensitive population of red cells (PNHIII) from patients with paroxysmal nocturnal haemoglobinuria (PNH) are deficient in glycoproteins which are anchored to the membrane by means of a glycophospholipid called glycosylphosphatidylinositol (GPI) (see Chapter 19). Telen *et al.* [3] demonstrated that most anti-Yt^a are non-reactive with PNHIII cells, but react with the relatively normal complement-insensitive population of cells (PNHI) from the same patient. Furthermore, in two PNH patients, the PNHI cells were Yt(b+), yet their PNHIII cells failed to react with anti-Yt^b. These results were interpreted as demonstrating that Yt^a and Yt^b are located on a GPI-linked glycoprotein.

In 1991, Spring *et al.* [4] demonstrated that Yt^a and Yt^b are on the GPI-linked red cell glycoprotein acetylcholinesterase (AChE). Immunoprecipitation with anti-Yt^a and -Yt^b isolated structures of apparent M_r 72 000 under reducing conditions and 160 000 under non-reducing conditions; structures of identical electrophoretic mobility were obtained by immunoprecipitation with monoclonal antibodies to AChE. The structures precipitated by anti-Yt^a and -Yt^b had AChE enzyme activity. Further proof that Yt antigens are on AChE was provided by a monoclonal antibody-specific immobilization of erythrocyte antigens (MAIEA) assay with alloanti-Yt^a and -Yt^b, and with monoclonal anti-AChE [5].

Red cell AChE is *N*-glycosylated: *N*-glycanase treatment of structures isolated with anti-Yt^a or -AChE reduced the apparent M_r from 72 000 to M_r 63 000 [4]. Estimates of 3000–5000 sites per red cell were obtained in quantitative analyses with monoclonal IgG anti-AChE, and estimates of 7000–10 000 sites were obtained with Fab fragments, suggesting that the enzyme exists in dimeric form in the red cell membrane [4].

AChE plays an essential part in neurotransmission. Acetylcholine is a neurotransmitter that permits the transmission of an electrical signal when released from a nerve terminal at a neuromuscular junction. AChE rapidly hydrolyses acetylcholine to terminate the signal. AChE exists in different tissues in a variety of forms, a result of post-translational modification and alternative splicing [6,7]. The function of red cell membrane-bound AChE is not known.

Partial human *ACHE* cDNA clones were obtained by screening a cDNA library constructed from fetal muscle and adult brain RNA with an oligonucleotide complementary to the amino acid sequence of a peptide derived from *Torpedo* AChE [8]. The complete gene encoding human AChE was cloned by screening a human genomic cosmid library with an oligonucleotide probe prepared by polymerase chain reaction (PCR) amplification of human DNA with primers corresponding to a conserved region of mouse AChE gene [7]. Three exons encode the signal peptide and N-terminal 535 amino acids; alternative splicing of the next exon results in structural divergence of the C-terminal domain so that a glycosylphosphatidyli-nositol (GPI) anchor may be attached in erythroid cells, but not in nervous tissue [7].

11.3 Yt^a and Yt^b

11.3.1 Frequency

Tests with the original anti-Yt^a on 1568 Oxford blood donors revealed five Yt(a–) samples, giving an incidence of Yt(a+) of 99.8% and a Yt^a gene frequency of 0.9559 [1,9] (Table 11.2). Giles *et al.* [9] found 8% of

Europeans to be Yt(b+), and the calculated gene frequencies fitted well with those obtained from the Oxford studies (Table 11.2). Genotype frequencies of Yt^a/Yt^a 0.8966, Yt^a/Yt^b 0.1006, and Yt^b/Yt^b 0.0028 calculated from the results of tests with anti-Yt^a and -Yt^b on 659 white Canadians (Table 11.2) correlated closely enough with the observed figures to suggest that no third allele is present [12].

Some other population studies are shown in Table 11.2. Tests with anti-Yt^a and -Yt^b on Israeli Arabs and Druse and on a variety of populations of Israeli Jews revealed a relatively high frequency of Yt^b [14]. None of 5000 Japanese were Yt(a–) and Yt^b has not been detected in relatively small samples of Japanese, Inuits, Thais, and Native Americans [15,16].

11.3.2 Inheritance and the molecular basis for the Yt polymorphism

The results of two large series of family studies are consistent with simple Mendelian inheritance of Yt^a and Yt^b in a codominant fashion, and absence of a silent allele [9,12].

Two single nucleotide changes in *ACHE* are associated with Yt^a/Yt^b polymorphism. One, C1057A in exon 2, encodes an His353Asn substitution; the other,

Table 11.1 Antigens of the Yt blood group system.

No.	Name	Relative frequency	Molecular basis
YT1	Yt^a	High	His353
YT2	Yt^b	Low	Asn353

Table 11.2 Population studies with anti-Yt^a and -Yt^b.

Population	No. tested	Phenotype frequencies		Gene frequencies		References
		Yt(a+)	Yt(b+)	Yt^a	Yt^b	
English	2568	0.998	nt	0.9559	0.0441	[1,9]
South Welsh	29802	0.999	nt	0.9761	0.0239	[10]
European	1399	nt	0.081	0.9587	0.0413	[9]
French	7510	0.997	0.081	0.958	0.042	[11]
White Canadians	659	1.000	0.106	0.9469	0.0531	[12]
African Americans	714	nt	0.084	0.9571	0.0429	[13]
Israeli Jews	2549	0.986	0.213	0.8845	0.1154	[14]
Israeli Arabs	85	0.976	0.235	0.8706	0.1294	[14]
Israeli Druse	77	0.974	0.260	0.8571	0.1429	[14]
Japanese	5000	1.000	nt			
	70*		0	1.0000	0.0000	[15]

*These 70 Japanese donors are also included in the 5000 tested with anti-Yt^a.
nt, not tested.

C1432T, is a silent mutation in exon 3 in the codon for Pro477 [17] (Table 11.1). A third single base polymorphism, in exon 5, did not correlate with Yt genotype and is not represented in the mature protein [17]. From a comparison of *Torpedo* AChE, the most studied form of the enzyme, the amino acid substitution at position 353 would be expected to be accessible to antibodies. The substitution has no effect on the catalytic activity of the enzyme [18].

11.3.3 Effects of enzymes and reducing agents

Yt^a is not affected by trypsin, but is destroyed by α-chymotrypsin treatment of the red cells; papain and ficin may also destroy the antigen, but this appears to depend on the anti-Yt^a used [1,19–22]. Yt^a is not sialidase-sensitive [21,22].

Yt^a and Yt^b are sensitive to disulphide bond reducing agents. Eight anti-Yt^a were non-reactive with red cells treated with $200\,mM$ dithiothreitol (DTT) [23]. Nine of 15 anti-Yt^a did not react with cells treated with 6% 2-aminoethylisothiouronium bromide (AET) and the other six sera showed reduced reactivity [24]. Yt^b, determined by two anti-Yt^b, was destroyed by $200\,mM$ DTT and $500\,mM$ 2-mercaptoethanol [25].

11.3.4 Development and distribution of Yt^a and Yt^b antigens

Yt antigens are present on red cells from cord blood samples. Yt^b appears to be fully developed at birth [26], but the strength of Yt^a on cord cells is weaker than that on red cells of adults [1,26,27]. Of 10 fetal red cell samples, taken at less than 32 weeks' gestation, eight did not react with anti-Yt^a and the other two reacted only very weakly [27].

AChE is present in nervous tissue and on erythroid cells [6], but little is known about the tissue distribution of Yt antigens. Yt^a was not detected by flow cytometry on lymphocytes, granulocytes, or monocytes [28].

11.4 Anti-Yt^a and -Yt^b

Despite the relatively low incidence of Yt(a–b+) phenotype, many examples of anti-Yt^a have been described [1,27,29–39]. Of 79 sera containing anti-Yt^a, 57 were monospecific and 22 contained a mixture of antibodies [39]. Yt^b appears to be a poor antigenic

stimulus as anti-Yt^b is rare and generally found in antibody mixtures; only a few examples are reported [2,9,26,40–42]. Anti-Yt^a and -Yt^b have been stimulated by pregnancy or transfusion; neither has been 'naturally occurring'.

Yt antibodies are mostly IgG and require an antiglobulin test to agglutinate red cells. Of those anti-Yt^a sera that could be subclassed, most contained IgG1 and often IgG4, some were solely IgG4, and none contained IgG3 [19,35,43]. Some anti-Yt^a bind complement [29], others do not [27,33].

Yt antibodies have not caused haemolytic disease of the newborn (HDN), despite several reports of women with anti-Yt^a having Yt(a+) children [13,27,29,30, 32,34], and one case of a woman with anti-Yt^b having a Yt(b+) child [26]. Anti-Yt^a is alleged to have been responsible for a fatal delayed haemolytic transfusion reaction (HTR) in a patient with sickle cell disease [44] and has been implicated in an immediate HTR [45]. However, many patients with anti-Yt^a have received multiple transfusions of Yt(a+) red cells with no ill effects [31,35,39]. Of 18 patients with anti-Yt^a who received Yt(a+) red cells, only three showed evidence of decreased red cell survival [39]. Survival studies with radiolabelled antigen-positive red cells have given widely variable results with Yt antibodies [27,30,31,33–35,38,46]; in a few cases it was predicted that incompatible red cells would be removed rapidly from the circulation [27,30,33]. Cellular assays have also given variable results, but none unequivocally predicted clinical significance [27,36, 39,42,43,45,46]. It appears therefore that each example of anti-Yt^a must be assessed independently. One example of anti-Yt^a appeared benign before transfusion of incompatible blood, but subsequently *in vivo* and *in vitro* assays gave indications of haemolytic potential [36].

Yt(a+) should be used for transfusion to patients with anti-Yt^a in emergency, when Yt(a–) red cells are not readily available. In most cases, it should be efficacious to use Yt(a+) red cells for patients with anti-Yt^a requiring elective surgery or regular transfusion, but a functional assay, such as a monocyte monolayer assay, should be performed first and at every subsequent event in an attempt to assess clinical significance of the antibody.

An apparent alloanti-Yt^a in a Yt(a+) patient led to speculation of an inherited Yt^a variant [47]. The antibody did not react with the patient's own cells or with those of his Yt(a+) father, but did react with his mother's red cells. The antibody appeared 9 days after transfusion of 5 units of blood and disappeared after a few months.

11.5 Transient Yt(a–b–) phenotype, anti-Yt^{ab}, and red cell AChE deficiency

In view of the vital role of AChE in neurotransmission, it is not surprising that no inherited null phenotype resulting from deletion or inactivating mutation of the *ACHE* gene has been found. A cardiac transplant candidate appeared to have the Yt(a–b–) phenotype, but some anti-Yt^a could be adsorbed and eluted from his cells [48]. His serum contained an antibody, anti-Yt^{ab}, which did not react with his own cells or with PNHIII cells, which lack GPI-linked proteins. Reduced 24-h *in vivo* survivals of radiolabelled Yt(a–b+) and Yt(a+b–) red cells suggested that only autologous red cells would be suitable for transfusion. Red cells of the patient contained about 10% of normal AChE and about 15% of normal AChE enzyme activity was detected [48]. Four months after the initial investigation, weak Yt^a activity was apparent by an antiglobulin test and red cell AChE content was 54–60% of normal.

References

1 Eaton BR, Morton JA, Pickles MM, White KE. A new antibody, anti-Yt^a, characterizing a blood group of high incidence. *Br J Haematol* 1956;2:333–41.

2 Giles CM, Metaxas MN. Identification of the predicted blood group antibody anti-Yt^b. *Nature* 1964;202: 1122–3.

3 Telen MJ, Rosse WF, Parker CJ, Moulds MK, Moulds JJ. Evidence that several high-frequency human blood group antigens reside on phosphatidylinositol-linked erythrocyte membrane proteins. *Blood* 1990;75: 1404–7.

4 Spring FA, Gardner B, Anstee DJ. Evidence that the antigens of the Yt blood group system are located on human erythrocyte acetylcholinesterase. *Blood* 1992;80: 2136–41.

5 Petty AC. Monoclonal antibody-specific immobilization of erythrocyte antigens (MAIEA): a new technique to selectively determine antigenic sites on red cell membranes. *J Immunol Methods* 1993;161:91–5.

6 Taylor P. The cholinesterases. *J Biol Chem* 1991;266: 4025–8.

7 Li Y, Camp S, Rachinsky TL, Getman D, Tayler P. Gene structure of mammalian acetylcholinesterase: alternative exons dictate tissue-specific expression. *J Biol Chem* 1991;266:23083–90.

8 Soreq H, Ben-Aziz R, Prody CA *et al.* Molecular cloning and construction of the coding region for human acetylcholinesterase reveals G+C-rich attenuating structure. *Proc Natl Acad Sci USA* 1990;87:9688–92.

9 Giles CM, Metaxas-Bühler M, Romanski Y, Metaxas MN. Studies on the Yt blood group system. *Vox Sang* 1967;13:171–80.

10 Gale SA, Rowe GP, Northfield FE. Application of a microtitre plate antiglobulin technique to determine the incidence of donors lacking high frequency antigens. *Vox Sang* 1988;54:172–3.

11 Salmon C, Cartron J-P, Rouger P. *The Human Blood Groups.* New York: Masson, 1984.

12 Lewis M, Kaita H, Philipps S *et al.* The Yt blood group system (ISBT, 011): genetic studies. *Vox Sang* 1987; 53:52–6.

13 Wurzel HA, Haesler WE. The Yt blood groups in American Negroes. *Vox Sang* 1968;15:304–5.

14 Levene C, Bar-Shany S, Manny N, Moulds JJ, Cohen T. The Yt blood groups in Israeli Jews, Arabs, and Druse. *Transfusion* 1987;27:471–4.

15 Nakajima H, Saito M, Murata S. The Yt blood group antigens in Japanese: the apparent absence of Yt^b. *J Anthrop Soc Nippon* 1980;88:455–6.

16 Mourant AE, Kopec AC, Domaniewska-Sobczak K. *The Distribution of the Human Blood Groups and Other Polymorphisms*, 2nd edn. London: Oxford University Press, 1976.

17 Bartels CF, Zelinski T, Lockridge O. Mutation at codon 322 in human acetylcholinesterase (ACHE) gene accounts for YT blood group polymorphism. *Am J Hum Genet* 1993;52:928–36.

18 Masson P, Froment M-T, Sorenson RC, Bartels CF, Lockridge O. Mutation His322Asn in human acetylcholinesterase does not alter electrophoretic and catalytic properties of the erythrocyte enzyme. *Blood* 1994;83:3003–5.

19 Vengelen-Tyler V, Morel PA. Serologic and IgG subclass characterization of Cartwright (Yt) and Gerbich (Ge) antibodies. *Transfusion* 1983;23:114–16.

20 Morton JA. Some observations on the action of blood-group antibodies on red cells treated with proteolytic enzymes. *Br J Haematol* 1962;8:134–47.

21 Rouger P, Dosda F, Girard M, Fouillade MT, Salmon C. Étude de la sensibilité de l'antigène Yt^a aux enzymes protéolytiques. *Rev Franc Transfus Immuno-Hémat* 1982;25:45–7.

22 Daniels G. Effect of enzymes on and chemical modifications of high-frequency red cell antigens. *Immunohematology* 1992;8:53–7.

23 Branch DR, Muensch HA, Sy Siok Hian AL, Petz LD. Disulfide bonds are a requirement for Kell and Cartwright (Yt^a) blood group antigen integrity. *Br J Haematol* 1983;54:573–8.

24 Levene C, Harel N. 2-Aminoethylisothiouronium-treated red cells and the Cartwright (Yt^a) antigen. *Transfusion* 1984;24:541.

25 Shulman IA, Nelson JM, Lam H-T. Loss of Yt^b antigen activity after treatment of red cells with either dithiothreitol or 2-mercaptoethanol. *Transfusion* 1986;26:214.

26 Ferguson SJ, Boyce F, Blajchman MA. Anti-Yt^b in pregnancy. *Transfusion* 1979;19:581–2.

27 Göbel U, Drescher KH, Pöttgen W, Lehr HJ. A second example of anti-Yt^a with rapid *in vivo* destruction of Yt(a+) red cells. *Vox Sang* 1974;27:171–5.

28 Dunstan RA. Status of major red cell blood group antigens on neutrophils, lymphocytes and monocytes. *Br J Haematol* 1986;62:301–9.

29 Bergvalds H, Stock A, McClure PD. A further example of anti-Yt^a. *Vox Sang* 1965;10:627–30.

30 Bettigole R, Harris JP, Tegoli J, Issitt PD. Rapid *in vivo* destruction of Yt(a+) red cells in a patient with anti-Yt^a. *Vox Sang* 1968;14:143–6.

31 Dobbs JV, Prutting DL, Adebahr ME, Allen FH, Alter AA. Clinical experience with three examples of anti-Yt^a. *Vox Sang* 1968;15:216–21.

32 Lavallée R, Lacombe M, Charron M, D'Angelo C. Un cas d'allo-immunisation fœto-maternelle due à un antigène de haute fréquence Yt^a. *Rev Franc Transfus Immuno-Hémat* 1970;13:71–6.

33 Ballas SK, Sherwood WC. Rapid *in vivo* destruction of Yt(a+) erythrocytes in a recipient with anti-Yt^a. *Transfusion* 1977;17:65–6.

34 Davey RJ, Simpkins SS. ^{51}Chromium survival of Yt(a+) red cells as a determinant of the *in vivo* significance of anti-Yt^a. *Transfusion* 1981;21:702–5.

35 Mohandas K, Spivack M, Delehanty CL. Management of patients with anti-Cartwright (Yt^a). *Transfusion* 1985;25:381–4.

36 AuBuchon JP, Brightman A, Anderson HJ, Kim B. An example of anti-Yt^a demonstrating a change in its clinical significance. *Vox Sang* 1988;55:171–5.

37 Hillyer CD, Hall JM, Tiegerman KO, Berkman EM. Case report and review: alloimmunization, delayed hemolytic transfusion reaction, and clinically significant anti-Yt^a in a patient with β-thalassemia/sickle cell anemia. *Immunohematology* 1991;7:102–6.

38 Nance SJ, Arndt P, Garratty G. Predicting the clinical significance of red cell alloantibodies using a monocyte monolayer assay. *Transfusion* 1987;27:449–52.

39 Eckrich RJ, Mallory DM, Sandler SG. Correlation of monocyte monolayer assays and posttransfusion survival of Yt(a+) red cells in patients with anti-Yt^a. *Immunohematology* 1995;11:81–4.

40 Ikin EW, Giles CM, Plaut G. A second example of anti-Yt^b. *Vox Sang* 1965;10:212–13.

41 Wurzel HA, Haesler W. Another example of anti-Yt^b. *Vox Sang* 1968;14:460–1.

42 Levy GJ, Selset G, McQuiston D *et al.* Clinical significance of anti-Yt^b: report of a case using a ^{51}Chromium red cell survival study. *Transfusion* 1988;28:265–7.

43 Pierce SR, Hardman JT, Hunt JS, Beck ML. Anti-Yt^a: characterization by IgG subclass composition and macrophage assay [Abstract]. *Transfusion* 1980;20:627–8.

44 Reed W, Walker P, Haddix T, Perkins HA. Fatal delayed hemolytic transfusion reaction (DHTR) due to anti-Yt^a in a patient with sickle cell disease (SCD) [Abstract]. *Transfusion* 1998;38:78S.

45 Hadley A, Wilkes A, Poole J, Arndt P, Garratty G. A chemiluminescence test for predicting the outcome of transfusing incompatible blood. *Transfus Med* 1999;9:337–42.

46 Kakaiya R, Sheahan E, Julleis J *et al.* ^{51}Chromium studies with an IgG1 anti-Yt^a. *Immunohematology* 1991;7:107.

47 Mazzi G, Raineri A, Santarossa L, De Roia D, Orazi BM. Presence of Yt^a antibody in a Yt(a+) patient. *Vox Sang* 1994;66:130–2.

48 Rao N, Whitsett CF, Oxendine SM, Telen MJ. Human erythrocyte acetylcholinesterase bears the Yt^a blood group antigen and is reduced or absent in the Yt(a–b–) phenotype. *Blood* 1993;81:815–19.

12 Xg blood group system

12.1 Introduction

The human sex chromosomes began to arouse the interest of blood groupers with the discovery in 1962 of an X-linked blood group locus, *XG*. Mann *et al.* [1] found an antibody, in the serum of a much transfused white man (Mr And.), detecting an antigen with a frequency that, unlike all previous blood groups, differed in males and females. Family studies confirmed the suspicion that expression of the antigen, named Xg^a (XG1), was controlled by an X-linked gene. No antigen antithetical to Xg^a has been found, so the allele of *Xg^a* (*XG 1*) is denoted *Xg* (*XG 0*).

CD99 (12E7), an antigen produced by *MIC2*, a gene on both X and Y chromosomes, is closely related to the Xg blood group [2]. Because Xg^a and CD99 are encoded by closely linked homologous genes, CD99 has become XG2 of the Xg system. Xg^a and CD99 have become invaluable tools in the study of X- and Y-linkage, X–Y pairing and recombination, X-inactivation, sex determination, X and Y aneuploidy, and various sex upsets, especially XX maleness.

12.2 Xg^a frequencies

The normal human chromosomal complement or karyotype is 46,XX in females and 46,XY in males. (Karyotypes are written with the total number of chromosomes first followed by the complement of sex chromosomes.) The *XG* gene resides on the X chromosome, but not on the Y chromosome. If a man has an *Xg^a* allele on his X chromosome his red cells are Xg(a+) and if he has an *Xg* allele they are Xg(a–). Homozygous *Xg^a/Xg^a* and heterozygous *Xg^a/Xg* women are Xg(a+); only homozygous *Xg/Xg* women are Xg(a–). Consequently, more women than men express Xg^a on their red cells.

Results of testing 6784 unrelated northern Europeans with anti-Xg^a were as follows: males, 66% Xg(a+) and 34% Xg(a–); females, 89% Xg(a+) and 11% Xg(a–) [3]. Phenotype, gene, and genotype frequencies are shown in Table 12.1. Gene frequencies were calculated by the formula of Haldane [4] (or see [5]). Results of other studies on a variety of ethnic groups are listed in Table 12.2. The incidence of *Xg^a* differs remarkably little between most of the populations studied.

12.3 Xg^a inheritance

Analysis of the Xg groups of 2540 northern European families with a total of 5824 children [3], together with many other families [25], including white Canadians [8], Sardinians [14], Israelis [15], and Japanese [21], proved that the *XG* locus is X-linked. With very few exceptions, Xg^a is inherited in a way expected of a character produced by an X-linked dominant gene. This expected pattern of inheritance is shown in Table 12.3.

Although the overwhelming majority of families with normal karyotypes fit the simple model presented in Table 12.3, there have been a few families that appear to break the rules of X-linked inheritance. According to these rules an Xg(a+) male must have received his Xg^a gene from his mother, yet 16 Xg(a+) sons of Xg(a–) mothers are recorded [3,8,25–27]. Race and Sanger [26] suggested that a small portion of the father's X chromosome, including the XG locus, may have been translocated onto his Y chromosome, this Y chromosome being transmitted to his sons. A more probable explanation also involves X–Y recombination, with Xg^a expression in the sons being regulated by a gene (XGR) derived from the paternal Y chromosome (Section 12.7.2). In one of the families, one of two Xg(a+) men with an Xg(a–) mother has an Xg(a–) son [26]. Xg(a+) men must have Xg(a+) daughters, who inherit their father's single X chromosome. Cases of Xg(a–) daughters with Xg(a+) fathers have been considered less significant violations of X-inheritance because of the difficulties involved in ruling out non-paternity [3,25].

12.4 Xgª antigen

12.4.1 Biochemistry of Xgª and effects of enzyme treatments

Xg^a is destroyed by treatment of the red cells with the proteases bromelin, ficin, papain, pronase, trypsin, and chymotrypsin [28,29]. Xg^a is not destroyed by sialidase.

By immunoblotting with alloanti-Xg^a, Herron and Smith [29] showed that Xg^a resides on a red cell mem-

Table 12.1 Phenotype, gene, and genotype frequencies calculated from results of tests with anti-Xgª on 6784 unrelated Northern Europeans [3].

		All	Males	Females
Phenotype	Xg(a+)	0.767	0.656	0.887
	Xg(a–)	0.233	0.344	0.113
Gene	Xg^a	0.659		
	Xg	0.341		
Genotype	Xg^a		0.659	
	Xg		0.341	
	Xg^a/Xg^a			0.434
	Xg^a/Xg			0.450
	Xg/Xg			0.116

Table 12.2 XG gene frequencies in various populations.

Population	No.	Xg^a	Xg	References
Northern European*	15716	0.66	0.34	[3,6–11]
Spaniards	636	0.59	0.41	[12]
Greeks	638	0.55	0.45	[13]
Sardinians	322	0.76	0.24	[14]
Israelis, non-Ashkenazi	201	0.68	0.32	[15]
White Brazilians	1078	0.74	0.26	[16]
Black New Yorkers and Jamaicans	219	0.55	0.45	[17]
Black Brazilians	827	0.57	0.43	[16]
Brazilian Mulattoes	786	0.62	0.38	[16]
Indians, Bombay	100	0.65	0.35	[18]
Indians, Singapore	91	0.57	0.43	[19]
Malays, Singapore	72	0.54	0.46	[19]
Thais	181	0.57	0.43	[20]
Japanese	529	0.68	0.32	[21]
Chinese, mainland	171	0.60	0.40	[7]
Chinese, Singapore	165	0.45	0.55	[19,22]
Chinese, Taiwan	178	0.53	0.47	[7]
Chinese, Hong Kong	1300	0.49	0.51	[23]
Taiwanese (Aboriginal)	164	0.38	0.62	[7]
Native Americans, Navajo	308	0.77	0.23	[7]
Australian Aborigines	352	0.79	0.21	[24]
New Guineans	263	0.85	0.15	[24]

*All the studies with people of Northern European extraction, which included people from North America, gave very similar gene frequencies.

Table 12.3 Phenotypes and genotypes of possible mating types and expected progeny.

Father		Mother		Sons		Daughters	
Xg(a+)	Xg^a	Xg(a+)	Xg^a/Xg^a	Xg(a+)	Xg^a	Xg(a+)	Xg^a/Xg^a
Xg(a+)	Xg^a	Xg(a+)	Xg^a/Xg	Xg(a+) Xg^a / Xg(a–) Xg		Xg(a+) Xg^a/Xg^a / Xg(a+) Xg^a/Xg	
Xg(a+)	Xg^a	Xg(a–)	Xg/Xg	Xg(a–)	Xg	Xg(a+)	Xg^a/Xg
Xg(a–)	Xg	Xg(a+)	Xg^a/Xg^a	Xg(a+)	Xg^a	Xg(a+)	Xg/Xg^a
Xg(a–)	Xg	Xg(a+)	Xg^a/Xg	Xg(a+) Xg^a / Xg(a–) Xg		Xg(a+) Xg/Xg^a / Xg(a–) Xg/Xg	
Xg(a–)	Xg	Xg(a–)	Xg/Xg	Xg(a–)	Xg	Xg(a–)	Xg/Xg

brane component, probably a sialoglycoprotein, of apparent M_r 22 500–28 000. Sialidase treatment of red cells reduced the apparent M_r of this structure by about 1500. Whether the Xg glycoprotein is associated with CD99 in the red cell membrane is controversial [30,31] (see Section 12.6).

The sequence of the *XG* gene (Section 12.8) predicts a 180 amino acid peptide with an extracellular N-terminal domain of about 142 residues, containing 16 potential O-glycosylation sites and no sites for *N*-glycosylation, a 20 residue transmembrane domain, and a 24 residue C-terminal cytoplasmic domain [32]. A putative 21 amino acid leader peptide is cleaved after membrane insertion.

12.4.2 Development and loss of Xgᵃ

Xgᵃ is developed at birth, but cord red cells may give weaker reactions than cells of adults [10,33]. Xgᵃ appears to develop quite late in fetal life: of 54 samples from fetuses between 6 and 20 weeks' gestation, only 19 were Xg(a+), a significantly lower Xgᵃ frequency than that found in adults [34]. The youngest Xg(a+) fetus was 12 weeks old.

Expression of Xgᵃ declines exponentially with red cell age, with an *in vivo* half-life of 47 days [35]. Between 5% and 10% of red cells from an Xg(a+) male lack Xgᵃ antigen [36]. During *in vitro* erythropoiesis, Xg glycoprotein appears on the erythroblasts after glycophorin A and band 3, but before the Rh proteins [37].

12.4.3 Dosage and site density

Xgᵃ is expressed equally strongly on the red cells of hemizygous males as on those of homozygous females,

but Xgᵃ expression on red cells of heterozygous females may be weaker [26]. About 5–10% of Xg(a+) females—all heterozygotes—have very weak expression of Xgᵃ. Weak Xgᵃ in males is very rare.

The number of Xgᵃ binding sites per Xg(a+) red cell was estimated to be about 9000 in one study [36], but only 159 in another [48].

12.4.4 Xgᵃ on other cells

In 1974 Fellous *et al.* [38] utilized a microcomplement fixation test to detect Xgᵃ on cultured fibroblasts from Xg(a+) donors and on human–rodent somatic cell hybrids. Xgᵃ cosegregated with a number of known X-linked characters confirming that Xgᵃ expression is controlled by an X-borne locus. The results also suggested that Xgᵃ on fibroblasts, like red cells, is not subject to X-inactivation (see Section 12.7.1). Alas, Fellous *et al.* were unable to repeat their feat of detecting Xgᵃ on cells other than red cells and neither, subsequently, could Hsu *et al.* [39].

XG gene transcripts were detected in fibroblasts [25], as well as in erythroid tissues and in heart, placenta, skeletal muscle, prostate, thyroid, spinal cord, and trachea [31]. Low levels of *XG* mRNA were also detected in some fetal tissues and in adult heart, lung, kidney, testis and some lymphoid cell lines [31,40].

12.5 Anti-Xgᵃ

The original anti-Xgᵃ was discovered by Mann *et al.* [1] in the serum of a multiply transfused man. Many more examples have since been identified [6,9,21,23,26,29,41–44]. Xgᵃ is apparently not very immunogenic yet, unlike other rare blood group antibodies, most sera containing anti-Xg^a are not 'contaminated' with other blood group antibodies. Twelve of the first 14 anti-Xg^a [26] and 11 of 13 anti-Xg^a found in Japanese volunteer donors [44] have been in men, somewhat surprising even considering the different frequencies of the Xg(a−) phenotype in men and women. In Hong Kong, four anti-Xg^a were identified in 325 serum samples referred for antibody investigation, and one anti-Xg^a was found in sera from 60 108 blood donors [23]; all five antibodies were in men. Anti-Xg^a often appear to be 'naturally occurring'. Although Xg^a antibodies occasionally agglutinate red cells directly, they are generally IgG, react by the antiglobulin method, and are often capable of fixing complement. One anti-Xg^a consisted of subclasses IgG1 and IgG2 [6].

Anti-Xg^a has never been held responsible for haemolytic disease of the newborn (HDN) or for a haemolytic transfusion reaction. One patient with anti-Xg^a received six units of Xg(a+) blood with no signs of a haemolytic reaction [41]. Repeated injections of small volumes of radiolabelled Xg(a+) red cells into a patient with anti-Xg^a survived normally [42]. Autoanti-Xg^a has been identified in a pregnant woman [43,45].

Murine monoclonal anti-Xg^a was produced by immunizing mice with a peptide corresponding to a segment from the N-terminal of the Xg glycoprotein [40].

12.6 CD99, a quantitative polymorphism related to Xg

In 1981 Goodfellow and Tippett [2] opened a new chapter in the Xg story when they observed that a monoclonal antibody to a determinant controlled by an X-borne gene (MIC2), was defining a red cell polymorphism related to the Xg blood group. The monoclonal antibody, called 12E7, was produced as a result of immunizing mice with human leukaemic T cells [46]. CD99, the antigen defined by the 12E7 antibody, is expressed on all human tissues tested [47], but on red cells, unlike other cells, the level of expression shows individual variation. By antiglobulin tests, radioimmunoassay, or flow cytometry, a quantitative polymorphism is observed and individuals can be subdivided into CD99 high and low expressors [2,48].

Testing of red cells from over 300 Europeans demonstrated the following association between Xg and CD99 [2]:

all Xg(a+) individuals are CD99 high expressors;

all Xg(a−) females are CD99 low expressors;

of Xg(a−) males about 68% are CD99 high expressors and 32% low expressors.

Goodfellow and Tippett [2] provided an innovative explanation for these data. They proposed a locus, YG, on the Y chromosome, which controls the level of expression of MIC2, the structural gene for CD99. YG would have two alleles, Yg^a and Yg. Individuals are CD99 high expressors if they have an Xg^a or Yg^a gene and CD99 low expressors if they have neither. Although family studies partially substantiated this theory [49], in light of information provided by some exceptional families Goodfellow et al. [50] modified the model to involve a locus on X and Y chromosomes, which regulates both Xg^a and CD99 red cell expression (described in Section 12.9). This putative regulator locus is called XGR.

Two examples of alloanti-CD99 have been found in healthy Japanese blood donors [51]. The antibodies gave the same pattern of reactions as monoclonal anti-CD99 with CD99 high and low expressor red cells. CD99 can therefore be considered a true blood group and has become XG2.

Like Xg^a, CD99 is located on a sialoglycoprotein. CD99 is destroyed by the proteases papain, pronase, trypsin, and chymotrypsin [47,52,53]. It is generally sialidase-resistant [47,52], but one exceptional CD99-like antibody did not react with sialidase-treated cells [53]. Immunoblotting of red cells, lymphocytes, various human cell lines, and human–rodent hybrid cells containing a human X or Y chromosome showed that CD99 is associated with a glycoprotein of approximate apparent M_r 32 000 [30,31,52–55]. Sialidase treatment of the cells resulted in a reduction in apparent M_r of the CD99 structure [30,31,52,55]. Immunoblotting of immunoprecipitates confirmed that CD99 and Xg^a are located on separate structures [31,31]. Partially purified CD99 glycoprotein inhibited anti-CD99 and anti-Xg^a [54]. In immunoprecipitation experiments, Petty and Tippett [30] found that alloanti-Xg^a coprecipitated Xg^a and CD99 glycoproteins, suggesting that these two homologous structures are associated in the membrane, possibly as a heterodimer. However, Fouchet et al. [31] were unable to repeat this result with a monoclonal antibody to the Xg glycoprotein. Cloning of MIC2 demonstrated that

CD99 is located on a protein of about 186 amino acids comprising an N-terminal signal peptide of 20 or 21 amino acids (cleaved after membrane insertion), about 100 extracellular residues, a hydrophobic transmembrane region, and a 36 amino acid cytoplasmic tail [56,57]. No difference in size or charge was detected between the X- and Y-encoded forms of the molecule [54].

There are an estimated 27 000 binding sites for anti-CD99 on lymphocytes, 4000 on platelets, and only 1000 on high expressor and 100 on low expressor red cells [52]. Reticulocytes from CD99 low expressors have lower levels of *MIC2* transcripts than those from CD99 high expressors [48].

12.7 X-chromosome inactivation and the pseudoautosomal region

12.7.1 X-chromosome inactivation

Normal mammalian somatic cells have two X chromosomes in the female, but only one in the male. As most X-borne genes do not have a homologue on the Y chromosome, the predicted difference in dosage of X-linked genes between male and female cells is compensated by a process called X-chromosome inactivation or Lyonization (reviews in [58,59]). In each somatic cell of an XX female only one of the X chromosomes is active, the other becoming permanently inactivated at an early stage in embryological development when a few million cells are formed. Whether the maternal or paternal X chromosome in any cell becomes inactivated is generally a matter of chance but, once inactivation has taken place, all descendants of that cell will have the same inactivated X chromosome. Female mammals are therefore mosaics of roughly equal numbers of cells with either the paternal or maternal X chromosome active. X-inactivation is a *cis* phenomenon, which spreads along the chromosome from an X-inactivation centre, where the gene *Xist* produces a large mRNA of 17 kb, which appears to coat the inactive X [59].

Originally it was thought likely that all X-borne genes were subject to inactivation, but it is now apparent that there are at least 20 genes on the X chromosome that escape inactivation (review in [60]). The first locus known to deviate from the rule of X-inactivation was *XG*. If *XG* were subject to inactivation, and assuming that Xgᵃ is a direct product of the *Xgᵃ* gene and

not manufactured outside the red cell, then heterozygous *Xgᵃ/Xg* women would be expected to have a mixed population of Xg(a+) and Xg(a−) red cells. No such mosaicism occurs. Natural chimeras have proven that mixtures of Xg(a+) and Xg(a−) red cells can be produced by the same marrow [26,61,62] and post-bone marrow transplant conversion from Xg(a−) to Xg(a+), and vice versa, provides further evidence that Xgᵃ production is restricted to the bone marrow [63].

MIC2, the structural gene for CD99, also escapes inactivation [64]. Hybrid cell lines containing only an inactivated human X chromosome expressed CD99 and the antigen was expressed at increasing levels in hybrid cells with multiple inactive X chromosomes.

When one of the X chromosomes in a female is structurally abnormal, for example when there is a substantial deletion of the long arm or an isochromosome of the short arm, the rules for random inactivation break down and there is preferential inactivation of the abnormal X. Although there can be no doubt that Xgᵃ is fully expressed on normal inactivated X chromosomes, there is evidence that *XG* is subject to inactivation on preferentially inactivated abnormal X chromosomes [65]. Xgᵃ cannot be detected on somatic cell hybrids, so this is very difficult to prove. The *XG* locus is on the short arm of the X chromosome. Thirteen of 20 propositi with deletions of the long arm or isochromosomes of the short arm of the X were Xg(a+) [66,67]. This frequency of Xgᵃ of 0.65 is very close to that for males and significantly different from the female distribution of 0.88, suggesting that only one *XG* gene is active in these women. *MIC2* is not inactivated on preferentially inactivated abnormal X chromosomes [64].

12.7.2 The pseudoautosomal region

During male meiosis it is important that the X and Y chromosomes segregate to separate spermatocytes. Consequently, like the autosomes, the X and Y chromosomes undergo pairing during the first meiotic division. However, this pairing only involves the telomeric regions of the short and long arms of each chromosome. Within the pairing regions genes are shared and recombination occurs. The pairing regions are called pseudoautosomal regions (PAR; PAR1 on the short arm and PAR2 on the long arm), because genes within these regions may not follow the rules of X-linked inheritance and could easily be mistaken for autosomally borne genes [68–71].

PAR1 has a recombination rate about 20 times the average rate for the genome. Some genes within PAR1 and very close to the telomere undergo 50% recombination and cannot be distinguished from autosomal genes on family evidence. *MIC2*, the structural gene for CD99, is pseudoautosomal, but situated very close to the pseudoautosomal boundary and only recombines with X- and Y-linked genes on the other side of the boundary in about 2% of male meioses [72]. Pseudoautosomal genes are on both X and Y chromosomes, so no dosage compensation is required and they do not participate in X-inactivation.

XG is not pseudoautosomal, but straddles the pseudoautosomal boundary on the X chromosome [32]. It is likely that on very rare occasions *XG* is involved in recombination with the Y, providing an explanation for the rare families in which Xg(a–) mothers have Xg(a+) sons [3,8,25–27] (Section 12.3).

12.8 *MIC2* and *XG* genes

CD99 is encoded by a gene at the *MIC2* locus. Human–rodent somatic cell genetics (see Section 32.2.3.3) has demonstrated that *MIC2* is located on both X and Y chromosomes [73–75]. Hybrid cells express CD99 when either X or Y is the only human chromosome retained [74]. *MIC2* cDNA was cloned by screening a cDNA expression library with a mixture of two monoclonal antibodies to CD99 epitopes

(12E7 and RFB-1) [56,76]. A cDNA probe was used to show that *MIC2* genes on the X and Y chromosomes are identical [76]. Somatic cell genetics [74] and *in situ* hybridization [77] have mapped *MIC2* to the tips of the short arms of the X and Y chromosomes, at Xpter→Xp22.32 and Ypter→Yp11.2 (Chapter 32).

Isolation of 95 kb of genomic DNA encompassing the entire *MIC2* gene revealed a 52 kb gene orientated toward the centromere and with its 5′ end 95 kb from the pseudoautosomal boundary (*PAB1X*) [78] (Fig. 12.1). The gene comprises 10 small exons: exon 1 encodes the leader peptide; exons 2–9 and 23 base pairs of exon 10 encode the CD99 protein (Table 12.4). No difference was detected between the organization of the X- and Y-borne alleles.

Genomic sequences between the 3′ end of *MIC2* and a CpG-rich region proximal to the pseudoautosomal boundary were used to isolate a 600-bp clone from a bone marrow cDNA library. This cDNA was, in turn, used to isolate an 820-bp transcript containing a 540-bp open reading frame capable of encoding a 180 amino acid polypeptide with a high level of homology with the CD99 protein, but not containing the sequence representing the CD99 epitope [32]. Mouse monoclonal and rabbit polyclonal antibodies raised to a 14 amino acid peptide synthesized to represent an N-terminal sequence of this cDNA, behaved as anti-Xg^a in haemagglutination tests and were shown to bind the same membrane structure as anti-Xg^a by an antibody-specific immobilization of antigens assay (a modification of MAIEA) [40]. The antibodies gave an identical

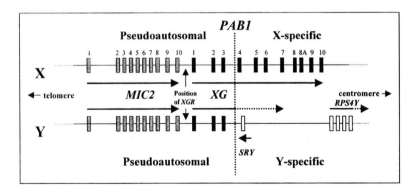

Fig. 12.1 A region of about 250 kb the X and Y chromosomes spanning the pseudoautosomal boundary (*PAB1*), showing the organization of *MIC2* and *XG* [32,79]. Both genes contain 10 exons on X, but only 3 exons of *XG* are on Y. *MIC2* and exons 1–3 of *XG* are pseudoautosomal; exons 4–10 of *XG* are X-specific. Exon 8A in *XG* was present in fibroblast RNA, but not erythroid RNA [25]. *SRY* and *RSP4Y* are Y-specific genes. The position of *XGR*, a proposed regulator of *XG* and *MIC2* expression on red cells [50], is shown between *MIC2* and *XG*.

Table 12.4 Organization of the *MIC2* and *XG* genes [25,32,78].

Exon	MIC2			XG		
	Exon size (bp)	Amino acids*	Intron size (kb)	Exon size (bp)	Amino acids*	Intron size (kb)
1	~244	1–23	23	246	1–21	12.5
2	33	23–34	3.2	42	21–35	3.3
3	48	34–50	2.4	24	35–43	8.3
4	45	50–65	0.6	63	43–64	7.0
5	69	65–88	1.0	63 (66)†	64–85	7.0
6	48	88–104	1.2	69	85–108	2.0
7	51	104–121	4.1	51	108–125	10.0
8A‡				45	(125–140)‡	
8	114	121–159	6.8	36	125–137 (140–152)	5.0
9	57	159–178	7.7	117	137–176 (152–191)	4.0
10	533	178–186		67 (244)	176–180 (191–195)	

*Amino acids encoded in CD99 by *MIC2* and in the major erythroid form of Xg protein (fibroblast form in parentheses) by *XG*.
†In a minority of *XG* cDNA clones an additional 3 bp, inserting a serine at position 86, appeared between exons 5 and 6 [25].
‡Exon 8A is present in fibroblast RNA, but not in erythroid RNA [25].

banding pattern to human anti-Xg[a] on immunoblots of red cell membranes. The *MIC2* homologue is therefore *XG*. Like *MIC2*, erythroid *XG* transcripts consist of 10 exons, with exon 1 encoding the leader peptide and exons 2–10 the native protein (Table 12.4). An additional exon, exon 8A, is present in transcripts from fibroblasts [25,32].

XG spans the pseudoautosomal boundary, *PAB1X*. Exons 1–3 are situated within the pseudoautosomal region (PAR1), whereas exons 4–10 are X-specific (Fig. 12.1). Exons 1–3 of *XG* are also present on the Y chromosome. Transcription from the *XG* promoter on Y results in a low abundance of transcripts that contain exons 1–3 of *XG* plus sequences from two downstream Y-linked genes, the gene for the testis-determining factor (*SRY*) and *RPS4Y*. The *SRY* sequence is in antisense configuration and most of these transcripts do not maintain an open reading frame [79]. *XGPY*, an expressed pseudogene of *XG* with a frameshift mutation in exon 5, is on the long arm of Y at Yq11.21 [79].

XG has two modes of inheritance: the 5′ end is subject to a recombination rate 20 times that of the genome average and is also involved in X/Y recombi-

nation; the 3′ end is only subject to X/X recombination, with an average recombination rate.

There is substantial amino acid sequence homology between CD99 and the Xg protein, with corresponding blocks of regions rich in acidic amino acids, basic amino acids, proline residues, and glycine residues [25]. The Asp61-Gly-Glu-Asn sequence of CD99 recognized by 12E7 antibody (anti-CD99) is in a region rich in acidic amino acids not present in the Xg protein.

Transfection of mouse fibroblastic cells with *XG* and/or *MIC2* cDNAs showed that Xg and CD99 proteins were expressed independently and at a similar level in single and double transfectants [31]. This suggests that the phenotypic association between Xg[a] and CD99 polymorphisms is regulated primarily at the transcriptional level and not through association of the glycoproteins in the membrane.

12.8.1 Xg polymorphism

Monoclonal antibodies to at least two separate epitopes on the Xg glycoprotein, human anti-Xg[a], and rabbit antibodies raised to a 14 amino acid peptide corresponding to an N-terminal sequence of the Xg polypeptide, all reacted with Xg(a+), but not Xg(a–), red cells [40]. This suggests that the Xg(a–) phenotype results from absence of the Xg glycoprotein from the red cell. Reverse-transcriptase polymerase chain reaction (PCR), with primers to exons 1 and 6 and 1 and 10 of *XG*, amplified fragments from Xg(a+) cord blood, but not Xg(a–) cord blood [25], indicating that substantially less RNA is produced by the *Xg* allele of *XG*, than by the *Xgᵃ* allele.

12.9 A model for explaining the association between the Xg and CD99 polymorphisms

When Goodfellow and Tippett [2] first recognized the unusual association between expression of Xgᵃ and CD99 on red cells, they proposed a hypothesis involving a gene (*YG*) on the Y chromosome. Both *XG* and *YG* regulate red cell expression of CD99 encoded by the structural gene *MIC2*. However, families demonstrating recombination between *MIC2* and *XG* and between *YG* and the X and Y chromosomes induced Goodfellow *et al.* [50] to modify their model.

In one family a normal 46,XX female had apparently received her father's *Xgᵃ* gene on one of her X chromosomes and yet a *MIC2* DNA probe showed that she had also received her father's Y chromosome pseudoautosomal region including his Y-borne *MIC2* gene. Recombination must have separated *MIC2* from the locus controlling expression of Xgᵃ.

Brothers receive the same Y chromosome from their father, yet seven of 172 Xg(a–) males did not have the same *YG* allele as their brother; that is, despite being Xg(a–), they differed in the level of their CD99 red cell expression [49]. In one family, part of which is shown in Fig. 12.2, all the males had the same Y chromosome, but not all the Xg(a–) males were CD99 high expressors; one (II-1) was a low expressor [50]. A *MIC2* RFLP showed that II-1 had inherited the same *MIC2* gene from his father as that received on an X chromosome by his two sisters (II-2 and II-4) and that he had inherited a different *MIC2* gene on a Y chromosome from his father from that received by his brother (II-3). Therefore, both *MIC2* and *YG* have been involved in an X–Y exchange, are pseudoautosomal on the Y chromosome, and are distal to the male sex-determining gene *SRY*.

In order to explain these phenomena Goodfellow *et al.* [50] proposed the existence of a regulator locus,

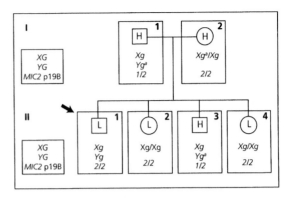

Fig. 12.2 Part of family showing *XG* and *YG* genotypes and *MIC2 Taq*I RFLP (p19B) genotypes, demonstrating recombination of *MIC2* and the gene determining CD99 red cell expression (*YG*) with the remainder of the sex chromosomes [50]. The father (I-1) has passed an X chromosome with a *MIC2* 2 allele to his two daughters (II-2 and II-4) and a Y chromosome with *MIC2* 1 and *Ygᵃ* (CD99 high expressor) alleles to one of his sons (II-3), but a Y chromosome with *MIC2* 2 and *Yg* (CD99 low expressor) alleles to his other son (II-1). H, CD99 high; L, CD99 low.

XGR, which controls *cis* expression of the structural loci *XG* and *MIC2* on the X chromosome and of *MIC2* on the Y chromosome. This gene is polymorphic. One allele (*XGRʰⁱᵍʰ*) induces Xgᵃ antigen expression from the *XG* locus and high CD99 expression from the *MIC2* locus; the other allele (*XGRˡᵒʷ*) prevents Xgᵃ expression and results in low level CD99 expression, probably by regulating transcription. All Xg(a+) individuals must have *XGRʰⁱᵍʰ* on at least one X chromosome and so they have high expression of CD99. Xg(a–) females must have *XGRˡᵒʷ* on both X chromosomes and therefore must have low expression of CD99. Xg(a–) males must have *XGRˡᵒʷ* on their X, but can have either *XGRʰⁱᵍʰ* or *XGRˡᵒʷ* on their Y, and so can have high or low expression of CD99 (Table 12.5). Although *XGR* is pseudoautosomal, it must be very close to the pseudoautosomal boundary (Fig. 12.1) as recombination resulting in Xgᵃ inheritance contravening the rules of X-linkage is extremely rare (Section 12.3).

This model, in which both Xgᵃ and CD99 expression on the red cells are controlled by the same gene (*XGR*), explains why the frequencies of Xgᵃ and CD99 high expression are so similar. It also provides an explanation for the families in which an Xg(a–) mother has an Xg(a+) son [3,8,25–27]. The son

Table 12.5 Effects of *High* and *Low* expression alleles of *XGR* on Xgª and CD99 red cell phenotypes.

	XGR allele		Phenotype	
Females	**X**	**X**		
	High	*High*	Xg(a+)	CD99 high
	High	*Low*	Xg(a+)	CD99 high
	Low	*Low*	Xg(a–)	CD99 low
Males	**X**	**Y**		
	High	*High*	Xg(a+)	CD99 high
	High	*Low*	Xg(a+)	CD99 high
	Low	*High*	Xg(a–)	CD99 high
	Low	*Low*	Xg(a–)	CD99 low

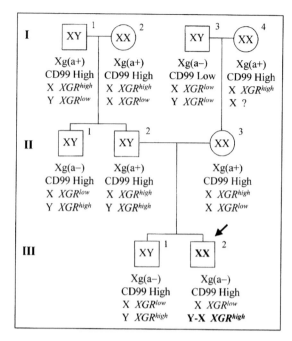

Fig. 12.3 Part of the family of an XX male demonstrating X–Y recombination [83], showing red cell Xg and CD99 phenotypes and suggested *XGR* genotypes. The XX male propositus (III-2) is Xg(a–) and must have received an X chromosome with an *XGR^low* allele from his mother (II-3) and an abnormal X chromosome from his father (II-2), which had lost its *XG* gene and gained *MIC2*, *XGR^high*, and the male sex determining gene by X–Y recombination. II-2 must have Y-borne *XGR^high* because his brother (II-1), who has the same Y chromosome, is Xg(a–) and CD99 high expressor.

receives his mother's *XG* gene on his X chromosome, but his father's Y-derived *XGR^high* allele on the same chromosome as a result of X–Y recombination between *XGR* and *XG*. It should be emphasized that this theory is conjectural, but it does provide a useful model for explaining the data.

12.10 XX males and sex chromosome aneuploidy

12.10.1 XX males

In order to maintain the chromosomal basis of sex determination, it is imperative that Y-borne genes outside the pseudoautosomal region are not normally involved in X–Y recombination, especially *SRY*, the gene controlling the testes determining factor. One occasion where this axiom appears to break down is in the rare case of XX males, sterile males with an apparently normal female karyotype. Approximately 1 in 20 000 men is 46,XX, yet is phenotypically and psychosexually male (reviews in [80,81]). Xg and CD99 have played an important part in determining the aetiology of this phenomenon.

In six families with informative Xg groups the XX male propositus had not received his father's *Xgª* gene, suggesting superficially that both X chromosomes were maternal in origin [26]. Ferguson-Smith [82] suggested that a small exchange of genetic material at the tips of the short arms of the X and Y chromosomes could result in a paternally derived X chromosome that has lost its *XG* locus and gained the Y-derived testis determining genes. This proposal is consistent

with the observed Xg distribution in XX males being much closer to that of XY males than to that of XX females [66,67]. A very informative family (Fig. 12.3) proved X–Y interchange as a cause of XX maleness [83]. The XX male propositus (III-2) is Xg(a–) and yet a CD99 high expressor, the first 46,XX person found with this phenotype. His Xg(a+) father (II-2) must have a *Ygª* gene (Y-borne *XGR^high*) as the father's brother (II-1), who must have the same Y chromosome, is Xg(a–) and a CD99 high expressor. The most probable explanation is that anomalous recombination between the X and Y chromosomes of the father of the propositus, outside the pseudoautosomal region, has produced an X chromosome in which part of the short arm, including the *XG* locus and pseudoautosomal region, has been replaced by part of the short arm of a Y chromosome, including the testis determining gene (*SRY*) and the pseudoautosomal region. The presence of Y chromosomal material in most XX males [designated Y(+)XX males] has been confirmed by the use of Y-specific DNA probes [84]. However, in a minority of XX males no Y-specific DNA was detected [84].

Occasionally XX males express a paternally derived *Xgᵃ* gene, suggesting that the X–Y recombination does not always involve the *XG* locus [26,81,85]. Evans *et al.* [85] were able to distinguish most XX males from XX females cytogenetically; in XX males the short arm of one X chromosome was significantly longer than that of the other X chromosome. Consequently, the X–Y interchange may involve an exchange of different amounts of genetic material, explaining how the recombinant chromosome could have both *XG* and *SRY* loci.

XX maleness can be explained by an exchange of genetic material between the X and Y chromosomes in about 80% of cases, but other, as yet undefined, mechanisms appear to be involved in the minority of examples of this form of sex reversal.

12.10.2 Sex chromosome aneuploidy

Aneuploidy is the term given to karyotypes in which the number of chromosomes is not a true multiple of the haploid number (23 in humans). Aneuploidies in which 1–5 X chromosomes are involved can be viable, presumably because in somatic cells only one X chromosome is active (Section 12.7.1). One or more Y chromosomes may also be involved. The Xg blood group provided a great deal of information about the non-disjunctions that have caused these chromosomal upsets, in some cases pinpointing the meiotic division at which non-disjunction occurred. A detailed account of the part played by Xg in our understanding of sex chromosome aneuploidy is given by Race and Sanger [26], with an update by Sanger *et al.* [67], and in the first edition of this book [5]. More recent evidence on the origin of the X chromosomes in sex chromosome aneuploidy has been elicited from studies with DNA probes [86].

12.11 Functional aspects and association with disease

Although the natural ligands are not known, CD99 appears to function as a receptor and adhesion mole-

cule. Engagement of certain monoclonal antibodies to CD99 induces apoptosis of thymocytes and mature T cells, possibly by a novel caspase-independent pathway [87,88]. On the other hand, CD99 also appears to have a role in T-cell activation. Cross-linking of CD99 on T cells by anti-CD99 enhanced T-cell proliferation and expression of CD25 (IL-2 receptor) and early markers of T-cell activation, CD69 and CD40L [89].

CD99 is involved in adhesion events. Certain monoclonal anti-CD99 block spontaneous T-cell rosette formation with sheep and human red cells [90]. Stimulation of CD99 with anti-CD99 induced homotypic aggregation of CD4⁺ CD8⁺ thymocytes and B lymphoblastoid cells [91,92]. The mechanism of CD99-induced aggregation may be different in thymocytes and B cells. A truncated isoform of CD99, which lacks most of the cytoplasmic domain as the result of alternative splicing of CD99 transcripts, may function in an opposite way to full-length CD99 by inhibiting CD99 induced homotypic aggregation of B cells [92].

High level expression of CD99 acts as a marker for Ewing's sarcoma and peripheral primitive neuroectodermal tumours (small round cell tumours of childhood and adolesence) [93]. Engagement of CD99 on Ewing tumour cells by a monoclonal anti-CD99 significantly inhibited growth, *in vivo* and *in vitro*, by delivering an apoptotic stimulus, providing a potential for therapeutic intervention [94].

Reduced expression of CD99 is a critical event in the development of Hodgkin's disease [95]. In addition, CD99-deficient cells in Hodgkin's disease have reduced expression of major histocompatability complex (MHC) class I molecules, which accumulate in the Golgi complex [96]. CD99 may be involved in post-Golgi trafficking by regulating transport to the surface membrane and this might provide an immunological escape mechanism for the malignant cells [96].

In contrast to CD99, almost nothing is known regarding the function of Xgᵃ. Structural homology between Xgᵃ and CD99 might suggest similar functions, but with so little known regarding the distribution of Xg glycoprotein on cells other than red cells, its function remains enigmatic.

12.12 Xgᵃ and CD99 in animals

Apart from humans, the only animals found to have Xgᵃ on their red cells are gibbons (*Hylobates lar lar*).

Fifty-two have been tested: 30% of males and 53% of females were Xg(a+), very suggestive of X-linkage. Other great apes (67 chimpanzees, two gorillas, 20 orang-utans, and five gibbons of the species *Hylobates pileatus*) as well as various monkeys (including 60 baboons), and a few non-primates, were all Xg(a–). CD99 was not detected on the red cells or peripheral blood lymphocytes of 10 gibbons, regardless of their Xg phenotype. CD99 was detected on red cells and fibroblasts of chimpanzees and gorillas, but not of orang-utans or any of the other mammals tested [26,97,98].

Genomic and cDNA analyses revealed *XG* and *MIC2* in non-human primates [25]. *XG* was also present in some other mammals and the position of *XG* at the pseudoautosomal boundary appears to be conserved in higher primates [25]. The chromosomal organization of the two homologous genes in tandem (Fig. 12.1) probably arose from a duplication event, which Ellis and Tippett [25] speculate occurred over 150 million years ago, before the mammalian radiation.

References

1 Mann JD, Cahan A, Gelb AG et al. A sex-linked blood group. *Lancet* 1962;i:8–10.

2 Goodfellow PN, Tippett P. A human quantitative polymorphism related to Xg blood groups. *Nature* 1981; 289:404–5.

3 Sanger R, Tippett P, Gavin J. The X-linked blood group system Xg: Tests on unrelated people and families of Northern European ancestry. *J Med Genet* 1971;8: 427–33.

4 Haldane JBS. Tests for sex-linked inheritance on population samples. *Ann Hum Genet* 1963;27:107–11.

5 Daniels G. *Human Blood Groups*. Oxford: Blackwell Science, 1995.

6 Devenish A, Burslem MF, Morris R, Contreras M. Serologic characteristics of a further example of anti-Xgª and the frequency of Xgª in North London blood donors. *Transfusion* 1986;26:426–7.

7 Dewey WJ, Mann JD. Xg blood group frequencies in some further populations. *J Med Genet* 1967;4:12–15.

8 Chown B, Lewis M, Kaita H. The Xg blood groups system: data on 294 white families, mainly Canadian. *Can J Genet Cytol* 1964;6:431–4.

9 Metaxas MN, Metaxas-Bühler M. An agglutinating example of anti-Xgª and Xgª frequencies in 558 Swiss blood donors. *Vox Sang* 1970;19:527–9.

10 Mayr WR. Das Blutfaktorensystem Xg. *Schweiz Med Wochenschr* 1969;99:1837–44.

11 Herbich J, Meinhart K, Szilvassy J. Verteilung 18 verschiedener Blutmerkmalsysteme bei 2440 Personen aus Wien und Umgebung. *Ärztl Lab* 1972;18:341–8.

12 Valls A. Los grupos sanguineos del sistema Xg en españoles. *Trab Inst Bernardino Sahagun Antrop Etnol* 1973;16:261–8.

13 Fraser GR, Steinberg AG, Defaranas B et al. Gene frequencies at loci determining blood-group and serum-protein polymorphisms in two villages in Northwestern Greece. *Am J Hum Genet* 1969;21:46–60.

14 Siniscalo M, Filippi G, Latte B et al. Failure to detect linkage between Xg and other X-borne loci in Sardinians. *Ann Hum Genet* 1966;29:231–52.

15 Adam A, Tippett P, Gavin J et al. The linkage relation of Xg to g-6-pd in Israelis: the evidence of a second series of families. *Ann Hum Genet* 1967;30:211–18.

16 Novaretti MC, Morganti L, Dorlhiac-Llacer PE, Chamone DAF. Xgª gene frequencies in Caucasian, Mulattoes and Black blood donors [Abstract]. *Blood* 1996;88(Suppl. 1):95B.

17 Gavin J, Tippett P, Sanger R, Race RR. The Xg blood groups of Negroes. *Nature* 1963;200:82–3. [In the 6th line of this paper there is a confused heading: it should be 'male' for the first two columns of figures and 'female' for the second two.]

18 Bhatia HM. Frequency of sex-linked blood group Xgª in Indians in Bombay: preliminary study. *Indian J Med Sci* 1963;17:491–2.

19 Saha N, Banerjee B. Xgª blood group in Chinese, Malays and Indians in Singapore. *Vox Sang* 1973;24:542–4.

20 Rantanaubol K, Ratanasirivanich P. Xg blood groups in Thais. *Nature* 1971;229:430.

21 Nakajima H, Murata S, Seno T. Three additional examples of anti-Xgª and Xg blood groups among the Japanese. *Transfusion* 1979;19:480–1.

22 Boon WH, Noades J, Gavin J, Race RR. Xg blood groups of Chinese. *Nature* 1964;204:1002.

23 Mak KH, Chua KM, Leong S, Devenish A. On the incidence of Xgª and anti-Xgª in Hong Kong Chinese. *Transfusion* 1993;33:443–4.

24 Simmons RT. X-linked blood groups, Xg, in Australian Aborigines and New Guineans. *Nature* 1970;227:1363.

25 Tippett P, Ellis N. The Xg blood group system: a review. *Transfus Med Rev* 1998;12:233–57.

26 Race RR, Sanger R. *Blood Groups in Man*, 6th edn. Oxford: Blackwell Scientific, 1975.

27 Sanger R, Race RR, Tippett P et al. Unexplained inheritance of the Xg groups in two families. *Lancet* 1964; i:955–6.

28 Habibi B, Tippett P, Lebesnerais M, Salmon C. Protease inactivation of the red cell antigen Xgª. *Vox Sang* 1979;36:367–8.

29 Herron R, Smith GA. Identification and immunochemical characterization of the human erythrocyte membrane glycoproteins that carry the Xgª antigen. *Biochem J* 1989;262:369–71.

30 Petty AC, Tippett P. Investigation of the biochemical relationship between the blood group antigens Xg^a and CD99 (12E7 antigen) on red cells. *Vox Sang* 1995; 69:231–5.

31 Fouchet C, Gane P, Huet M et al. A study of the coregulation and tissue specificity of *XG* and *MIC2* gene expression in eukaryotic cells. *Blood* 2000;95:1819–26.

32 Ellis NA, Ye T-Z, Patton S et al. Cloning of *PDBX*, an *MIC2*-related gene that spans the pseudoautosomal boundary on Xp. *Nat Genet* 1994;6:394–9.

33 Toivanen P, Hirvonen T. Fetal development of red cell antigens K, k, Lu^a, Lu^b, Fy^a, Fy^b, Vel and Xg^a. *Scand J Haematol* 1969;6:49–55.

34 Toivanen P, Hirvonen T. Antigens Duffy, Kell, Kidd, Lutheran and Xg^a on fetal red cells. *Vox Sang* 1973; 24:372–6.

35 Campana T, Szabo P, Piomelli S, Siniscalco M. The Xg^a antigen on red cells and fibroblasts. *Cytogenet Cell Genet* 1978;22:524–6.

36 Szabo P, Campana T, Siniscalco M. Radioimmune assay for the Xg(a) surface antigen at the individual red cell level. *Biochem Biophys Res Commun* 1977;78:655–62.

37 Daniels G, Green C. Expression of red cell surface antigens during erythropoiesis. *Vox Sang* 2000; 78(Suppl.1):149–53.

38 Fellous M, Bengtsson B, Finnegan D, Bodmer WF. Expression of the Xg^a antigen on cells in culture and its segregation in somatic cell hybrids. *Ann Hum Genet* 1974;37:421–30.

39 Hsu SH, Migeon BR, Bias WB. Unreliability of the microcomplement fixation method for Xg^a typing of culture fibroblasts. *Cytogenet Cell Genet* 1976;16:382–6.

40 Ellis NA, Tippett P, Petty A et al. *PBDX* is the *XG* blood group gene. *Nat Genet* 1994;8:285–9.

41 Cook IA, Polley MJ, Mollison PL. A second example of anti-Xg^a. *Lancet* 1963;i:857–9.

42 Sausais L, Krevans JR, Townes AS. Characteristics of a third example of anti-Xg^a [Abstract]. *Transfusion* 1964;4:312.

43 Yokoyama M, Eith DT, Bowman M. The first example of auto-anti-Xg^a. *Vox Sang* 1967;12:138–9.

44 Azar PM, Saji H, Yamanaka R, Hosoi T. Anti-Xg^a suspected of causing a transfusion reaction. *Transfusion* 1982;22:340–1.

45 Yokoyama M, McCoy JE. Further studies on auto anti-Xg^a antibody. *Vox Sang* 1967;13:15–17.

46 Levy R, Dilley J, Fox RI, Warnke R. A human thymus-leukemia antigen defined by hybridoma monoclonal antibodies. *Proc Natl Acad Sci USA* 1979;76:6552–6.

47 Goodfellow P. Expression of the 12E7 antigen is controlled independently by genes on the human X and Y chromosomes. *Differentiation* 1983;23:S35–9.

48 Fouchet C, Gane P, Cartron J-P, Lopez C. Quantitative analysis of XG blood group and CD99 antigens on human red cells. *Immunogenetics* 2000;51:688–94.

49 Tippett P, Shaw M-A, Green CA, Daniels GL. The 12E7 red cell quantitative polymorphism: control by the Y-borne locus, *Yg*. *Ann Hum Genet* 1986;50:339–47.

50 Goodfellow PJ, Pritchard C, Tippett P, Goodfellow PN. Recombination between the X and Y chromosomes: implications for the relationship between *MIC2*, *Xg* and *YG*. *Ann Hum Genet* 1987;51:161–7.

51 Uchikawa M, Tsuneyama H, Tadokoro K et al. An alloantibody to 12E7 antigen detected in 2 healthy donors [Abstract]. *Transfusion* 1995;35:23S.

52 Latron F, Blanchard D, Cartron J-P. Immunochemical characterization of the human blood cell membrane glycoprotein recognized by the monoclonal antibody 12E7. *Biochem J* 1987;247:757–64.

53 Daniels G, Tippett P. MAb 161: a monoclonal antibody detecting the 12E7 glycoprotein [Abstract]. *Proc 2nd Int Workshop Monoclonal Antibodies Against Human Red Blood Cells Related Antigens* 1990;127.

54 Banting GS, Pym B, Goodfellow PN. Biochemical analysis of an antigen produced by both human sex chromosomes. *EMBO J* 1985;4:1967–72.

55 Anstee DJ, Parsons SF, Mallinson G et al. Characterization of monoclonal antibodies against erythrocyte sialoglycoproteins by serological analysis, immunoblotting and flow cytometry. *Rev Franc Transfus Immuno-Hémat* 1988;31:317–32.

56 Goodfellow PN, Pym B, Pritchard C et al. MIC2: a human pseudoautosomal gene. *Phil Trans R Soc Lond B* 1988;322:145–54.

57 Banting GS, Pym B, Darling SM, Goodfellow PN. The *MIC2* gene product: epitope mapping and structural prediction analysis define an integral membrane protein. *Mol Immunol* 1989;26:181–8.

58 Lyon MF. X-chromosome inactivation and developmental patterns in mammals. *Biol Rev* 1972;47:1–35.

59 Lyon MF. X-chromosome inactivation. *Curr Biol* 1999;9:R235–7.

60 Davies K. The essence of inactivity. *Nature* 1991; 349:15–16.

61 Klinger R, Miggiano VC, Tippett P, Gavin J. Diabete mellito e nanismo ipofisario in chimera XX, XY. *Atti Acad Med Lomb* 1968;23:1392–6.

62 Ducos J, Marty Y, Sanger R, Race RR. Xg and X chromosome inactivation. *Lancet* 1971;ii:219–20.

63 Sparkes RS, Crist M, Sparkes MC. Evidence of autonomous red cell expression of Xg^a antigen in human bone marrow transplantation. *Vox Sang* 1984;46: 119–21.

64 Goodfellow P, Pym B, Mohandas T, Shapiro LJ. The cell surface antigen locus, *MIC2X*, escapes X-inactivation. *Am J Hum Genet* 1984;36:777–82.

65 Polani PE, Angell R, Giannelli F et al. Evidence that the *Xg* locus is inactivated in structurally abnormal X chromosomes. *Nature* 1970;227:613–16.

66 Sanger R, Tippett P, Gavin J. Xg groups and sex abnormalities in people of Northern European ancestry. *J Med Genet* 1971;8:417–26.

67 Sanger R, Tippett P, Gavin J, Teesdale P, Daniels GL. Xg groups and sex chromosome abnormalities in people of Northern European ancestry: an addendum. *J Med Genet* 1977;**14**:210–11.

68 Burgoyne PS. Genetic homology and crossing over in the X and Y chromosomes of mammals. *Hum Genet* 1982; **61**:85–90.

69 Burgoyne PS. Mammalian X and Y crossover. *Nature* 1986;**319**:258–9.

70 Ellis N, Goodfellow PN. The mammalian pseudoautosomal region. *Trends Genet* 1989;**5**:406–10.

71 Rappold GA. The pseudoautosomal regions of the human sex chromosomes. *Hum Genet* 1993;**92**:315–24.

72 Goodfellow PJ, Darling SM, Thomas NS, Goodfellow PN. A pseudoautosomal gene in man. *Science* 1986;**234**: 740–3.

73 Goodfellow P, Banting G, Levy R, Povey S, McMichael A. A human X-linked antigen defined by a monoclonal antibody. *Somat Cell Genet* 1980;**6**:777–87.

74 Goodfellow P, Banting G, Sheer D *et al.* Genetic evidence that a Y-linked gene in man is homologous to a gene on the X chromosome. *Nature* 1983;**302**:346–9.

75 Curry CJR, Magenis RE, Brown M *et al.* Inherited chondrodysplasia punctata due to a deletion of the terminal short arm of an X chromosome. *N Engl J Med* 1984; **311**:1010–5.

76 Darling SM, Banting GS, Pym B, Wolfe J, Goodfellow PN. Cloning an expressed gene shared by the human sex chromosomes. *Proc Natl Acad Sci USA* 1986;**83**:135–9.

77 Buckle V, Mondello C, Darling S, Craig IW, Goodfellow PN. Homologous expressed genes in the human sex chromosome pairing region. *Nature* 1985;**317**:739–41.

78 Smith MJ, Goodfellow PJ, Goodfellow PN. The genomic organization of the human autosomal gene *MIC2* and the detection of a related locus. *Hum Mol Genet* 1993;**2**: 417–22.

79 Weller PA, Critcher R, Goodfellow PN, German J, Ellis NA. The human Y chromosome homologue of *XG*. transcription of a naturally truncated gene. *Hum Mol Genet* 1995;**4**:859–68.

80 de la Chapelle A. The etiology of maleness in XX men. *Hum Genet* 1981;**58**:105–16.

81 de la Chapelle A, Savikurki H, Herva R *et al.* Aetiological studies in males with the karyotype 46,XX. In: *Aspects of Human Genetics*. Basel: Karger, 1984:25–42.

82 Ferguson-Smith MA. X-Y chromosomal interchange in the ætiology of true hermaphroditism and of XX Klinefelter's syndrome. *Lancet* 1966;**ii**:475–6.

83 de la Chapelle A, Tippett PA, Wetterstrand G, Page D. Genetic evidence of X–Y interchange in a human XX male. *Nature* 1984;**307**:170–1.

84 Petit C, de la Chapelle A, Levilliers J *et al.* An abnormal terminal X-Y interchange accounts for most but not all cases of human XX maleness. *Cell* 1987;**49**:595–602.

85 Evans HJ, Buckton KE, Spowart G, Carothers AD. Heteromorphic X chromosomes in 46,XX males: evidence for the involvement of XY interchange. *Hum Genet* 1979;**49**:11–31.

86 Jacobs PA, Hassold TJ. The origin of numerical chromosome abnormalities. *Adv Genet* 1995;**33**:101–33.

87 Bernard G, Breittmayer J-P, de Matteis M *et al.* Apoptosis of immature thymocytes mediated by E2/CD99. *J Immunol* 1997;**158**:2543–50.

88 Pettersen RD, Bernard G, Olafson MK, Pourtein M, Lie SO. CD99 signals caspase-independent T cell death. *J Immunol* 2001;**166**:4931–42.

89 Wingett D, Forcier K, Nielson CP. A role for CD99 in T cell activation. *Cell Immunol* 1999;**193**:17–23.

90 Bernard AF, Aubrit B, Raynal D, Pham D, Boumsell A. A T cell surface molecule different from CD2 is involved in spontaneous rosette formation with erythrocytes. *J Immunol* 1988;**140**:1802–7.

91 Bernard G, Zoccola D, Deckert M *et al.* The E2 molecule (CD99) specifically triggers homotypic aggregation of CD4⁺CD8⁺ thymocytes. *J Immunol* 1995;**154**:26–32.

92 Hahn J-H, Kim MK, Choi EY *et al.* CD99 (*MIC2*) regulates the LFA-1/ICAM-1-mediated adhesion of lymphocytes, and its gene encodes both positive and negative regulators of cellular adhesion. *J Immunol* 1997;**159**: 2250–8.

93 Ambros IM, Ambros PF, Strehl S *et al.* MIC2 is a specific marker for Ewing's sarcoma and peripheral primitive neuroectodermal tumors: evidence for a common histogenesis of Ewing's sarcoma and peripheral primitive neuroectodermal tumors from MIC2 expression and specific chromosome aberration. *Cancer* 1991;**67**:1886–93.

94 Scotlandi K, Baldini N, Cerisano V *et al.* CD99 engagement: an effective therapeutic strategy for Ewing tumors. *Cancer Res* 2000;**60**:5134–42.

95 Kim SH, Choi EY, Shin YK *et al.* Generation of cells with Hodgkin's and Reed–Sternberg phenotype through downregulation of CD99 (*Mic2*). *Blood* 1998;**92**: 4287–95.

96 Sohn HW, Shin YK, Lee I-S *et al.* CD99 regulates the transport of MHC Class I molecules from the Golgi complex to the cell surface. *J Immunol* 2001;**166**:787–94.

97 Gavin J, Noades J, Tippett P, Sanger R, Race RR. Blood group antigen Xgᵃ in gibbons. *Nature* 1964;**204**: 1322–3.

98 Shaw MA, Tippett P, Delhanty JDA, Andrews M, Goodfellow P. Expression of Xg and the 12E7 antigen in primates. *J Immunogenet* 1985;**12**:115–18.

13.1 Introduction

The Scianna system consists of a pair of antithetical antigens, the high and low incidence antigens Sc1 and Sc2, and an antigen of very high frequency, Sc3, absent only from cells of the null phenotype Sc:−1,−2,−3. Sc1 and Sc2 are located on a glycoprotein of about M_r 60 000.

The low incidence antigen Radin is biochemically related to Scianna, but is not proven to be part of the Scianna system. The Scianna and Radin loci are linked to *RH* on chromosome 1p (Chapter 32).

13.2 Sc1 and Sc2

In 1962, Schmidt *et al.* [1] identified an antibody in a white woman (Mrs N.S.) defining a new inherited antigen of very high frequency. They named the antigen Sm. The following year, Anderson *et al.* [2] described a new low incidence antigen, Bu^a. Lewis *et al.* [3] were quick to notice that the original Sm− cells were Bu(a+). Sm and Bu^a were renamed Sc1 and Sc2, respectively, following confirmation that they were the products of alleles [4,5].

In the family of Mrs N.S., red cells of the Sc:−1 propositus and those of her three Sc:−1 sibs were Sc:2, one of her Sc:1 sibs was Sc:2, and the other sib was Sc:−2. Sc:−1,2 red cells reacted more strongly than Sc:1,2 cells with anti-Sc2 [3]. Three consanguineous Sc:1,2 × Sc:1,2 matings from a large Mennonite family produced children with the following three phenotypes: three Sc:−1,2; 11 Sc:1,2; and seven Sc:1,−2 [4]. In the same pedigree were two Sc:1,−2 × Sc:−1,2 matings with a total of five Sc:1,2 children.

Testing of 269 000 South London blood donors with anti-Sc1 revealed one Sc:−1 individual [6], suggesting the following gene frequencies: *Sc1* 0.9981; and *Sc2* 0.0019. No Sc:−1 person was found as a result of testing red cells from 1600 North Americans [1,5] or 29 737 Welsh donors [7]. Frequency studies with anti-Sc2 are shown in Table 13.1. The variations reported among Canadians [2,5] could reflect the method of sampling. In tests with anti-Sc1 and -Sc2 on red cells from 1000 white Canadians, 983 were Sc:1,−2; 17 Sc:1,2; and none Sc:−1,2 [5]. The following gene and genotype frequencies were calculated:

Sc1 0.9915   *Sc1/Sc1* 0.9831
　　　　　　　Sc1/Sc2 0.0168
Sc2 0.0085   *Sc2/Sc2* 0.0001.

A combination of two sets of data from southern England provided a gene frequency for *Sc2* of 0.004 [8,9]. In Canada the frequency of *Sc2* is high amongst the Mennonite community, which may be responsible for the higher *Sc2* frequency in Canada than in northern Europe.

Sc1 is fully developed at birth [2]. Fluorescent flow cytometry demonstrated that Sc1 is not present on lymphocytes, granulocytes, or monocytes [15].

13.3 Sc3 and the Sc:−1,−2,−3 phenotype

The Sc:−1,−2 phenotype was found by McCreary *et al.* [16] in a patient from the Marshall Islands in the South Pacific (Micronesia). The patient's cousin was also Sc:−1,−2; her parents and other members of her family were Sc:1,−2. The serum of the propositus, who had been transfused 7 months previously, contained an antibody reactive with all cells save her own and those of her Sc:−1,−2 cousin. No similar antibody was detected in the serum of the cousin, despite four pregnancies.

A previously transfused white man with the Sc:−1,−2 phenotype had an antibody reactive with all cells except for his own and those of the Sc:−1,−2 Micronesians [17]. By adsorption studies with Sc:1,−2 and Sc:−1,2 cells, the antibody was shown not to be

Table 13.1 Frequency of Sc2 in various populations.

Population	No. tested	No. Sc:2	Sc2 frequency	References
Canadian donors	1000	1	0.0010	[1]
White Canadians	348	5*	0.0144	[2]
White Canadians	1000	17	0.0170	[5]
Londoners	1039	7	0.0067	[8]
Oxford donors	5306	41	0.0077	[9]
Warsaw donors	1025	9	0.0088	[8]
Berlin donors	2015	15	0.0074	[10]
Czech donors	2100	7	0.0033	[11]
Black Canadians	212	0		[12]
Manitoban Indians	100	0		[5]
Inuit	75	0		[5]
Japanese	4900	5	0.0005	[13]
Taiwanese	161	0		[14]

*Includes three Mennonites.

a mixture of anti-Sc1 and -Sc2, and was named anti-Sc3.

A third Sc:–1,–2 propositus with anti-Sc3, a previously transfused 4-year-old girl, was found in Papua New Guinea (Melanesia) [18]. Her mother was also Sc:–1,–2. Investigation of 29 other family members and villagers in her home area revealed six other Sc:–1,–2 individuals, two of whom were apparently not related to the patient.

Three antibodies to high incidence antigens found in previously transfused white men with Sc:1,–2 red cells failed to react with Sc:–1,–2 cells [19]. None of the antibodies reacted with autologous cells, but all three antibodies reacted with the red cells of the other two antibody makers and therefore have different specificities. One of the antibodies did not react with the red cells of an Sc:1,–2 sib of the antibody maker. Two of the antibodies reacted with 100 random red cell samples, the third with 8000 samples. Attempts at immunoblotting with these antibodies were unrewarding (G.L. Daniels, unpublished observations 1993). An antibody to a high frequency antigen detected, together with multiple Rh antibodies, in the serum of an Sc:1,–2 Senegalese patient, was non-reactive with Sc:–1,–2 cells and with cells of the patient's sib [20]. It is likely that these four antibodies detect high frequency determinants on the Scianna glycoprotein.

13.4 Antibodies

Scianna system antibodies are very uncommon. They react best by an antiglobulin test and do not fix complement. Directly agglutinating anti-Sc1 is known. No 'naturally occurring' Scianna alloantibody has been described.

The original anti-Sc2 was found in a transfused man; three of the donors were traced and red cells from one reacted with the antibody [2]. Four examples of anti-Sc2 were found among 14 anti-D sera produced by immunizing D– volunteers with D+ red cell samples, one of which was also Sc:2 [8]. Of 19 D– Sc:–2 individuals given at least two injections of D+ Sc:2 red cells, eight formed anti-D, but only one made anti-Sc2 [21].

No Scianna antibody has been incriminated in a transfusion reaction or in severe haemolytic disease of the newborn (HDN). IgG3 anti-Sc1 was responsible for a positive direct antiglobulin test (DAT) on a baby's red cells, but no treatment was required [6]. There is one report of anti-Sc2 causing mild HDN [22]. Survival studies with radiolabelled Sc:1,–2 cells suggested that the original anti-Sc3 may be clinically significant [16]. This antibody disappeared soon after its identification and was not restimulated by injection of Sc:1,–2 red cells. Anti-Sc3 in a Melanesian child could not be detected after splenectomy, even following transfusion of Sc:1,–2 blood [18]. One of the three Scianna-related antibodies described by Devine *et al.* [19] was reported to have caused a delayed haemolytic transfusion reaction.

Several examples of autoanti-Sc1 have been described [23–27]; two of them were in individuals whose red cells had weakened expression of Sc1 [24]. Two of the antibodies were only detectable in serum, not in plasma [23,27]. Autoimmune haemolytic anaemia in a young child caused by autoanti-Sc1 was resistant to steroid treatment, but did respond to splenectomy [25]. Two patients with anaemia, one with lymphoma and the other with Hodgkin's disease, had autoanti-Sc3 and depressed Sc1 and Sc3 red cell antigens [28]. Both antibodies reacted weakly with Sc:−1,2 cells compared to their reaction with Sc:1,−2 cells.

13.5 Biochemistry

13.5.1 Effects of enzymes and reducing agents

Treatment of Sc:1 red cells with the proteases papain, trypsin, and chymotrypsin did not affect their reactions with anti-Sc1 in haemagglutination tests; pronase and a mixture of trypsin and chymotrypsin reduced their reactivity [29]. Titrations of anti-Sc1 and -Sc2 with red cells treated with disulphide bond reducing agents showed that Sc1 and Sc2 are slightly weakened by 200 mM dithiothreitol (DTT) and substantially weakened by 6% 2-aminoethylisothiouronium bromide (AET) [30].

13.5.2 The Scianna glycoprotein

Spring et al. [30] demonstrated, by immunoblotting of red cell membranes with anti-Sc1 and -Sc2, that Scianna antigens are located on a glycoprotein of apparent M_r between 60 000 and 68 000. No bands were present if the red cells were treated with pronase or if the membranes were prepared in the presence of a thiol reducing agent, showing that one or more disulphide bonds are required for antigen integrity. Treatment of the red cells with endoglycosidase F, which cleaves N-glycans, caused only a slight reduction of binding by anti-Sc1 to the Scianna glycoprotein, but a complete loss of binding by anti-Sc2. It is possible that an amino acid substitution responsible for the Sc1/Sc2 polymorphism affects N-glycosylation of the molecule. Variation in sialic acid content of the N-glycans probably accounts for the diffuse nature of the bands representing the glycoprotein. Sialidase treatment of the cells had a small effect on the mobility of the glycoprotein, reducing the apparent M_r of the leading edge of the band by 500–1000, but also sharpening the band by reducing the M_r of the trailing edge by 3000. A proportion of the Scianna glycoprotein molecules may be attached to the cytoskeleton. The Scianna glycoprotein was also immunostained on protein blots by autoanti-Sc1 [25].

13.6 The Radin antigen (Rd)

There is strong immunochemical and genetic linkage evidence that the low incidence antigen Radin (Rd) belongs to the Scianna system. However, in the absence of proof, Rd maintains its autonomy as part of the 700 series of low incidence antigens with the number 700015.

Rausen et al. [31] identified the first five anti-Rd, all apparently stimulated through pregnancy. In the five families the Rd gene could be traced to Russian Jews, black people, northern Europeans, and a Native American. Rd frequencies are shown in Table 13.2. Rd is inherited as an autosomal dominant character [31,32,34].

Rd is well developed on cord cells [31]. It was unaffected by papain, ficin, and sialidase, destroyed by trypsin and chymotrypsin, and substantially weakened by AET (C.A. Green, unpublished observaions 1983).

Anti-Rd has been stimulated by pregnancy and

Table 13.2 Frequency of Rd in various populations.

Population	No. tested	No. Rd+	Rd frequency	References
Various ethnic groups	6773	0		[31]
New York Jews	562	3	0.0053	[31]
Danes	4933	24	0.0049	[32]
Canadians	770	3	0.0039	[33]
Manitoban Slavs	170	1	0.0059	[33]
Winnipeg donors	2864	9	0.0031	[33]

transfusion [31,32]. One example of apparently naturally occurring anti-Rd was found in an untransfused man [32]. Of 30 000 sera tested in Denmark, none contained anti-Rd [32]. The first five anti-Rd were all reported to have caused mild to moderate HDN, but only one baby required exchange transfusion [31].

The first suggestion that Rd might belong to the Scianna system came from the demonstration that the locus governing Rd is linked to *RH* and must be either at the *SC* locus or closely linked to it [33,35] (Chapter 32). Linkage to *RH* establishes that Rd cannot belong to any of the existing blood group systems except Scianna.

Spring [36] showed by immunoblotting that anti-Rd stained a broad band of apparent M_r about 60 000, which closely resembled the Scianna glycoprotein. There was a slight reduction in apparent M_r when sialidase-treated cells were used and some of the molecules were attached to the cytoskeleton. However, final proof that Sc1, Sc2, and Rd are on the same glycoprotein is lacking. Scianna glycoprotein isolated from Rd+ cells by immunoprecipitation with anti-Sc1, was not immunostained by anti-Rd on a protein blot. A person with the Rd+ Sc:1,2 phenotype has been found [35] so, if Rd is on the Scianna glycoprotein, then Rd is not at the same position as Sc1 and Sc2.

Red cells of the four Sc:1,–2 individuals lacking high incidence Scianna-related antigens described in Section 13.3 were Rd– [20] (P. Spruell, personal communication 1997), so Rd is not antithetical to any of these antigens.

References

1 Schmidt RP, Griffitts JJ, Northman FF. A new antibody, anti-Sm, reacting with a high incidence antigen. *Transfusion* 1962;2:338–40.

2 Anderson C, Hunter J, Zipursky A, Lewis M, Chown B. An antibody defining a new blood group antigen, Buª. *Transfusion* 1963;3:30–3.

3 Lewis M, Chown B, Schmidt RP, Griffitts JJ. A possible relationship between the blood group antigens Sm and Buª. *Am J Hum Genet* 1964;16:254–5.

4 Lewis M, Chown B, Kaita H. On the blood group antigens Buª and Sm. *Transfusion* 1967;7:92–4.

5 Lewis M, Kaita H, Chown B. Scianna blood group system. *Vox Sang* 1974;27:261–4.

6 Kaye T, Williams EM, Garner SF, Leak MR, Lumley H. Anti-Sc1 in pregnancy. *Transfusion* 1990;30:439–40.

7 Gale SA, Rowe GP, Northfield FE. Application of a microtitre plate antiglobulin technique to determine the incidence of donors lacking high frequency antigens. *Vox Sang* 1988;54:172–3.

8 Seyfried H, Frankowska K, Giles CM. Further examples of anti-Buª found in immunized donors. *Vox Sang* 1966; 11:512–16.

9 Noades JE, Corney G, Cook PJL *et al.* The Scianna blood group lies distal to uridine monophosphate kinase on chromosome 1p. *Ann Hum Genet* 1979;43:121–32.

10 Fünfhausen G, Gremplewski K. Die Verteilung des Blutgruppenantigens Buª in Berlin. *Z Ärztl Fortbild Qualitatssich* 1967;61:769.

11 Calkovská Z. Mitteilung über zwei weitere Familien mit einem Vorkommen von Buª. *Folia Haematol* 1974; 101:661–6.

12 Lewis M, Chown B, Kaita H, Philipps S. Further observations on the blood group antigen Buª. *Am J Hum Genet* 1964;16:256–60.

13 Nagao N, Tomita T, Okubo Y, Yamaguchi H. Low frequency antigen, Doª, Coᵇ, Sc2, in Japanese [Abstract]. *24th Congr Int Soc Blood Transfus* 1996;145.

14 Yung CH, Chow MP, Hu HY, Mou LL, Lyou JY, Lee TD. Blood group phenotypes in Taiwan. *Transfusion* 1989; 29:233–5.

15 Dunstan RA. Status of major red cell blood group antigens on neutrophils, lymphocytes and monocytes. *Br J Haematol* 1986;62:301–9.

16 McCreary J, Vogler AL, Sabo B, Eckstein EG, Smith TR. Another minus–minus phenotype: Bu(a–)Sm–. Two examples in one family [Abstract]. *Transfusion* 1973; 13:350.

17 Nason SG, Vengelen-Tyler V, Cohen N, Best M, Quirk J. A high incidence antibody (anti-Sc3) in the serum of a Sc:–1,–2 patient. *Transfusion* 1980;20:531–5.

18 Woodfield DG, Giles C, Poole J, Oraka R, Tolanu T. A further null phenotype (Sc–1–2) in Papua New Guinea [Abstract]. *19th Congr Int Soc Blood Transfus* 1986;651.

19 Devine P, Dawson FE, Motschman TL *et al.* Serologic evidence that Scianna null (Sc:–1,–2) red cells lack multiple high-frequency antigens. *Transfusion* 1988;28:346–9.

20 Banks J, Poole J, Ligthart PC, Saez M. A complex serological investigation involving antibodies to two high frequency antigens [Abstract]. *Transfus Med* 1998; 8(Suppl.1):28 and personal communication.

21 Mollison PL, Engelfriet CP, Contreras M. *Blood Transfusion in Clinical Medicine*, 10th edn. Oxford: Blackwell Science, 1997.

22 DeMarco M, Uhl L, Fields L *et al.* Hemolytic disease of the newborn due to the Scianna antibody, anti-Sc2. *Transfusion* 1995;35:58–60.

23 Tregellas WM, Holub MP, Moulds JJ, Lacey PA. An example of autoanti-Sc1 demonstrable in serum but not in plasma [Abstract]. *Transfusion* 1979;19:650.

24 McDowell MA, Stocker I, Nance S, Garratty G. Auto anti-Sc1 associated with autoimmune hemolytic anemia [Abstract]. *Transfusion* 1986;26:578.

25 Owen I, Chowdhury V, Reid ME *et al.* Autoimmune

hemolytic anemia associated with anti-Sc1. *Transfusion* 1992;**32**:173–6.

26 Issitt PD, Anstee DJ. *Applied Blood Group Serology*, 4th edn. Durham, Montgomery Scientific Publication, 1998.

27 Pierce SR, Orr DL, Brown PJ, Tillman G. A serum-reactive/plasma-nonreactive antibody with Scianna specificity [Abstract]. *Transfusion* 1998;**38**:36S.

28 Peloquin P, Moulds M, Keenan J, Kennedy M. Anti-Sc3 as an apparent autoantibody in two patients [Abstract]. *Transfusion* 1989;**29**:49S.

29 Daniels G. Effect of enzymes on and chemical modifications of high-frequency red cell antigens. *Immunohematology* 1992;**8**:53–7.

30 Spring FA, Herron R, Rowe G. An erythrocyte glycoprotein of apparent M_r 60 000 expresses the Sc1 and Sc2 antigens. *Vox Sang* 1990;**58**:122–5.

31 Rausen AR, Rosenfield RE, Alter AA *et al*. A 'new' infrequent red cell antigen, Rd (Radin). *Transfusion* 1967;**7**:336–42.

32 Lundsgaard A, Jensen KG. Two new examples of anti-Rd: a preliminary report on the frequency of the Rd (Radin) antigen in the Danish population. *Vox Sang* 1968;**14**:452–7.

33 Lewis M, Kaita H. Genetic linkage between the Radin and Rh blood group loci. *Vox Sang* 1979;**37**:286–9.

34 Race RR, Sanger R. *Blood Groups in Man*, 6th edn. Oxford: Blackwell Scientific Publications, 1975.

35 Lewis M, Kaita H, Philipps S *et al*. The position of the Radin blood group locus in relation to other chromosome 1 loci. *Ann Hum Genet* 1980;**44**:179–84.

36 Spring FA. Characterization of blood-group-active erythrocyte membrane glycoproteins with human antisera. *Transfus Med* 1993;**3**:167–78.

14 Dombrock blood group system

14.1 Introduction

Prior to 1992, Dombrock remained a simple, polymorphic blood group system with two antigens, Do^a (DO1) and Do^b (DO2), the products of alleles. The discovery by Banks et al. [1] that red cells of the rare phenotype Gy(a–) Hy– Jo(a–) were also Do(a–b–) led to Gy^a becoming DO3 and the phenotypically and biochemically related antigens Hy and Jo^a becoming DO4 and DO5 (Table 14.1). Table 14.2 shows the known Dombrock phenotypes. Antigens of the Dombrock system are located on a glycosylphosphatidylinositol (GPI)-linked glycoprotein, a member of the ADP-ribosyltransferase family, Asn265Asp representing the Do^a/Do^b polymorphism.

DO is located on chromosome 12p13.2–12.1 (see Chapter 32).

14.2 Biochemistry and molecular genetics of the Dombrock glycoprotein

Dombrock system antigens are on a glycoprotein that is anchored to the red cell membrane through GPI. Membrane proteins of this type are described in Chapter 19. PNHIII red cells, the complement-sensitive population of red cells from patients with paroxysmal nocturnal haemoglobinuria (PNH), lack GPI-linked proteins. PNHIII cells are deficient in the five Dombrock system antigens, whereas these antigens are expressed on the normal population of cells (PNHI) from the same patient [2–4].

Spring and Reid [2] demonstrated, by immuno-blotting under non-reducing conditions, that Gy^a and Hy are on membrane glycoproteins of apparent M_r 46 750–57 500. Cross-immunoprecipitation and immunoblotting experiments showed that Do^a, Gy^a, Hy, and Jo^a are on the same protein [1–3]. Treatment of intact cells with endoglycosidase F reduced the M_r of the glycoprotein by about 11 000, showing

that it is N-glycosylated; there is no substantial O-glycosylation. The glycoprotein, isolated by immuno-precipitation, migrates faster on sodium dodecyl sulphate polyacrylamide gel electrophoresis (SDS PAGE) under reducing conditions (M_r 45 000–54 000) and intact disulphide bonds are required for full expression of Gy^a and Hy. A putative dimer was also detected by immunoprecipitation [2].

By screening a database of approximately 5000 expressed sequence tags (ESTs) derived from differentiating erythroid cells for genes localized to chromosome 12p and encoding a GPI-anchor motif, Gubin et al. [5] identified a candidate for the DO gene (which they called DOK1). Stable transfection of a K562 erythroleukaemic cell line with the candidate DO open reading frame led to expression of Do^a, Gy^a, Hy, and Jo^a at the cell surface [5]. DO spans 14 kb and contains three exons encoding a protein of 314 amino acids with five putative N-glycosylation sites and six cysteine residues (including one in the signal peptide). Exon 1 encodes residues 1–45, including a 44 amino acid signal peptide, exon 2 encodes residues 49–285, and exon 3 encodes residues 286–314, including a 17 amino acid GPI-anchor motif.

14.3 Dombrock antigens

14.3.1 Do^a and Do^b (DO1 and DO2)

In 1965, Swanson et al. [6] identified an antibody in the serum of Mrs Dombrock, which defined a new antigen (Do^a) on the red cells of 64% of Europeans. The gene controlling this antigen was soon shown to be distinct from most other blood group loci [6,7]. Not until 1973 was the antithetical antibody, anti-Do^b, identified by Molthan et al. [8].

There are only limited frequency studies concerning Dombrock. Almost all data have been derived from investigations with anti-Do^a alone. Most of the informa-

Table 14.1 Antigens of the Dombrock system.

Number	Name	Frequency (%)	Comments
DO1	Do^a	66*	Antithetical to Do^b (DO2). Asn265
DO2	Do^b	82*	Antithetical to Do^a (DO1). Asp265
DO3	Gy^a	>99	Absent from Dombrock null cells
DO4	Hy	>99	Absence associated with weakened Do^b (DO2) and Gy^a (DO3), and with Gly108Val and Leu300Val
DO5	Jo^a	>99	Absent from all Hy– (DO:–4) cells

*Northern Europeans; Do^b calculated from gene frequencies.

tion is summarized in Table 14.3. From the northern European gene frequencies [9] the following genotype frequencies have been calculated: Do^a/Do^a 0.1764; Do^a/Do^b 0.4872; and Do^b/Do^b 0.3364 (assuming Do^b is the only allele of Do^a). The frequency of Do^a is somewhat lower in black people than in white people, and substantially lower in Mongoloid people (Table 14.3).

Many families have been tested with anti-Do^a. These include 201 northern European families (573 children) [9], 76 Israeli families (224 children) [9], 148 Canadian families (470 children) [10], and 79 Japanese families (159 children) [11]. In all, Do^a behaved as an autosomal dominant character and the frequencies of the various mating types and of Do(a+) and Do(a–) children fitted reasonably well with those expected from the gene frequencies. A small number of families from other ethnic groups also conformed to this simple pattern of inheritance [9].

Tests on over 100 individuals have shown that the DNA polymorphism is associated with an A793G

Table 14.2 Known Dombrock system phenotypes and their approximate frequencies.

Do^a	Do^b	Gy^a	Hy	Jo^a	Frequencies	
					White people (%)	Black people (%)
+	–	+	+	+	18	11
+	+	+	+	+	49	44
–	+	+	+	+	33	45
–	–	–	–	–	Rare	0
–	w	w	–	–	0	Rare
w	vw	+	w	–	0	Rare

w, weakened expression of antigen; vw, very weak expression of antigen.

Table 14.3 Incidence of Do^a and calculated frequencies of Do^a and Do^b genes in various populations.

Population	Total tested	No. Do(a+)	Do^a frequency	Gene frequencies		References
				Do^a	Do^b	
Northern Europeans	755	501	0.6636	0.4200	0.5800	[6,7,9]
White North Americans	700	446	0.6371	0.3976	0.6024	[10]
White Americans	391	250	0.6394	0.3995	0.6005	[11]
African Americans	161	89	0.5528	0.3313	0.6687	[11]
African Americans	76	34	0.4474	0.2566	0.7434	[9]
Japanese	760	179	0.2355	0.1257	0.8743	[12,13]
Thais	423	57	0.1348	0.0698	0.9302	[14]

Do^b gene frequency assumes that Do^b is the only allele of Do^a.

transition in exon 2 of *DO* [5,15]. *Do*^{a} encodes Asn265; *Do*^{b} encodes Asp265. Two silent nucleotide changes, at positions Tyr126 and Leu208, may also be associated with the Do^a/Do^b polymorphism [5].

14.3.2 Gy^a (DO3) and the Dombrock null phenotype

An American family of Czech origin, in which four of seven children from a second cousin mating lacked a new public antigen Gy^a, was described by Swanson *et al.* [16] in 1967. The propositus and her sister had anti-Gy^a in their sera; the propositus was in her fifth pregnancy and her sister had two children. A second family, also of Czech descent, contained two Gy(a–) sisters, both of whom had been pregnant and both of whom had anti-Gy^a in their sera [17]. Six more Gy(a–) individuals were found in an English family, possibly of Romany stock [18]. The four multiparous sisters had anti-Gy^a, whereas their two Gy(a–) brothers did not. Six Gy(a–) propositi have been found in Japanese; all were female and all were ascertained through the presence of anti-Gy^a [19]. A Gy(a–) Hong Kong Chinese man with anti-Gy^a had probably been transfused 40 years previously [20].

No Gy(a–) individual was found among 9350 Japanese blood donors [19] or 10 145 Americans, including 75 African Americans and 611 Native Americans [16]. Gy(a–) has not been found in people of African origin.

Gy(a–) is inherited as a recessive character. Several families are known with more than one Gy(a–) sib, in which both parents are Gy(a+) [16,18,19,21]. In most cases the parents were consanguineous [16,19,21].

Gy(a–) red cells also lack the high incidence antigens Hy and Jo^a [22,23]. The discovery that eight unrelated Gy(a–) individuals had the previously unknown phenotype Do(a–b–) led to Gy^a, Hy, and Jo^a becoming part of the Dombrock system and the Gy(a–) phenotype being recognized as a Dombrock null phenotype [1].

Three unrelated Gy(a–) individuals had a mutation in the invariant splice site of intron 1 of *DO* [24]. The *DO* transcript appears to lack exon 2. The mutation creates an *Alu*I restriction site.

14.3.3 Hy (DO4)

The first anti-Hy, identified in the serum of an African American woman at the delivery of her third child, was very briefly reported by Schmidt *et al.* [25]. Other examples of anti-Hy followed [22,26,27]; all were made by Hy– black propositi, most of whom had Hy– sibs.

Moulds *et al.* [22] recognized a phenotypic relationship between Hy and Gy^a. Hy– black people have weakened Gy^a antigen, whereas Hy– people of European or Japanese origin are also Gy(a–) (Table 14.2). If immunized, Gy(a–) Hy– individuals make anti-Gy^a, whereas Gy(a+^{w}) Hy– individuals make anti-Hy. Anti-Gy^a does not contain separable anti-Hy: three adsorptions of anti-Gy^a with Gy(a+^{w}) Hy– cells removed all antibody, while an eluate from the adsorbing cells behaved as the original serum [22]. All of 15 Gy(a+^{w}) Hy– individuals were Do(a–) and had weak expression of Do^b [1].

Screening with anti-Gy^a, diluted so that it would not react with Gy(a+^{w}) Hy– cells, revealed no negative among 4530 white North Americans, 735 Czechs, 683 white South African, 846 black North Americans, 1023 black South Africans, 633 South African Asian Indians, or 1679 Pima Native Americans [22]. Two of 597 Apache were Gy(a+^{w}) Hy– [22]; the only individuals reported who are not of African origin, although some racial admixture was suspected.

In seven individuals, the Gy(a+^{w}) Hy– phenotype was associated with G232T encoding Gly108Val, in exon 2 of a *Do*^{b} allele (encoding Asp265) [28]. In most of these samples there was also a C898G mutation in exon 3 encoding a Leu300Val substitution in the GPI-anchor motif, which could be responsible for the reduced expression of Gy^a and Do^b.

14.3.4 Jo^a (DO5)

Anti-Jo^a (Joseph) was first reported by Jensen *et al.* [29] when cells and sera of two African American patients with antibodies to high incidence antigens were found to be mutually compatible. A third example was found in an African American sickle cell disease patient with a Jo(a–) brother [30]. All three makers of anti-Jo^a had been transfused and two had also been pregnant. Antibodies found in the sera of five African American women and initially called anti-Jc^a [23] were later shown to be anti-Jo^a [31]. Red cells from 3000 New Yorkers, mostly white, and from 7689 African Americans were tested with anti-Jo^a: none was Jo(a–) [29].

Laird-Fryer *et al.* [23] found that all Hy– red cells,

whether Gy(a–) Hy– or Gy(a+^{w}) Hy–, were Jo(a–). All makers of anti-Jo^a were Gy(a+) Hy+ Jo(a–) [23,32,33]. There is some degree of weakening of Hy antigen on Gy(a+) Hy+ Jo(a–) cells compared with Gy(a+) Hy+ Jo(a+) cells [3]. Four of 20 Jo(a–) samples were Hy– [32]. Five of six Jo(a–) individuals, all black, had weak Do^a and barely detectable Do^b; the other, an Hispanic, was Do(a+b–) with weak Do^a [1] (Table 14.2).

14.3.5 Development and distribution of Dombrock antigens

Do^a, Do^b, and Jo^a are fully expressed on cord red cells [6,8,23,29]. In contrast, it is reported that Gy^a and Hy are expressed only weakly on cord cells [18,22].

DO was not expressed before 4 days of culture of peripheral blood nuclear cells in the presence of erythropoietin [5]. *DO* mRNA was detected in spleen, lymph node, bone marrow and fetal liver, but not in thymus or peripheral blood leucocytes [5].

14.3.6 Effects of enzymes and reducing agents

Dombrock system antigens are resistant to papain or ficin treatment of red cells, and an antiglobulin test with papain- or ficin-treated cells is often the optimal method for using Dombrock reagents, especially anti-Do^a and -Do^b. Dombrock system antigens are sensitive to trypsin, chymotrypsin, and pronase, which either destroy the antigens or cause a marked reduction in their expression [1–3]. Sialidase treatment has no effect. The antigens are also sensitive to the action of the reducing agents AET and DTT [1–3,33].

14.4 Dombrock system antibodies

14.4.1 Anti-Do^a and -Do^b

Since the original discoveries [6,8], other examples of anti-Do^a [34–41] and -Do^b [41–45] have been reported and many more are known. Examples of anti-Do^a and -Do^b occur in approximately equal numbers suggesting that Do^a and Do^b do not differ markedly in immunogenicity, considering their similar frequencies. Anti-Do^a and -Do^b usually occur in sera containing mixtures of multiple antibodies to red cell antigens, although examples of pure anti-Do^a [37,40] and -Do^b [45] have been identified. No 'naturally occurring' Dombrock antibody is reported, but one anti-Do^a

was produced in a woman during her first Do(a+) pregnancy [36].

Anti-Do^a and -Do^b generally react by an antiglobulin test, working best with papain- or ficin-treated cells. They are usually IgG and unable to fix complement [11,37,42].

Dombrock antibodies have not been implicated in haemolytic disease of the newborn (HDN), although anti-Do^a have caused positive direct antiglobulin reactions with neonatal red cells [36,37,40]. Anti-Do^a [38,39,41] and -Do^b [41,43–45] have been responsible for acute and delayed haemolytic transfusion reactions, and may be a particular complication of transfusion in sickle cell disease [41]. *In vivo* red cell survival studies and *in vitro* monocyte monolayer assays confirm that anti-Do^a and -Do^b can cause accelerated red cell destruction [11,45]. However, in one case of anti-Do^a survival was normal and subsequent transfusion of incompatible blood produced no adverse reaction [46]. Detection of anti-Do^a and -Do^b in antibody mixtures has often been delayed because these haemolytic antibodies are easily mistaken for clinically insignificant red cell alloantibodies or autoantibodies, or for HLA antibodies [38,39,41,44].

14.4.2 Anti-Gy^a (-DO3), -Hy (-DO4), and -Jo^a (-DO5)

Gy^a appears to be very immunogenic as virtually all reported Gy(a–) women who have been pregnant have anti-Gy^a in their serum [16–18,22]. An elderly man, who had never been transfused, had transient anti-Gy^a, which disappeared after 3 months [47]. Unlike most Gy(a–) cells, his red cells could adsorb and elute anti-Hy, leading to the suggestion that this patient may have had an acquired Gy(a–) phenotype [48]. Apart from this one case, there is no reported example of 'naturally occurring' anti-Gy^a, -Hy, or -Jo^a.

Anti-Gy^a, -Hy, and -Jo^a are usually IgG, react best by an antiglobulin test, and do not fix complement [16,18,22,26,27,29,30,33,47,49]. One anti-Gy^a also contained some IgA and bound complement as determined by a two-stage antiglobulin test [18]. One anti-Hy, which directly agglutinated Hy+ cells, was IgM plus IgG [49].

Like anti-Do^a and -Do^b, the other Dombrock system antibodies have never been implicated in HDN, despite numerous opportunities. One anti-Hy has been responsible for a haemolytic transfusion reaction in a man who received 2 units of Hy+ blood [26]. A man with anti-Gy^a tolerated 10 units of Gy(a+) blood with no adverse effect [20]. The patient with transient anti-Gy^a showed normal *in vivo* survival of Gy(a+) cells [47]. Anti-Hy was responsible for shortened *in vivo* red cell survival [27] and anti-Jo^a in a sickle cell patient caused significant removal of radiolabelled Jo(a+) cells compared with Jo(a–) cells [50].

A murine monoclonal antibody (5B10) bound to all red cells, but only very weakly to those of the Gy(a–) (Dombrock null) phenotype [51].

14.5 Functional aspects

Exon 2 of *DO* contains a motif characteristic of a family of adenosine diphosphate (ADP)-ribosyltransferases [5], which catalyse the transfer of ADP-ribose from nicotinamide adenine dinucleotide (NAD$^+$) to a protein substrate [52]. The Dombrock glycoprotein could have a role in modification of proteins at the red cell surface and might be involved in NAD$^+$ clearance of the serum [5].

The product of the *Do^b* allele contains an Arg-Gly-Asp motif, characteristic of adhesion molecules involved in cellular interaction [5]. However, this motif is disrupted in the product of *Do^a*, where it becomes Arg-Gly-Asn.

References

1 Banks JA, Hemming N, Poole J. Evidence that the Gy^a, Hy and Jo^a antigens belong to the Dombrock blood group system. *Vox Sang* 1995;68:177–82.

2 Spring FA, Reid ME. Evidence that the human blood group antigens Gy^a and Hy are carried on a novel glycosylphosphatidylinositol-linked erythrocyte membrane glycoprotein. *Vox Sang* 1991;60:53–9.

3 Spring FA, Reid ME, Nicholson G. Evidence for expression of the Jo^a blood group antigen on the Gy^a/Hy-active glycoprotein. *Vox Sang* 1994;66:72–7.

4 Telen MJ, Rosse WF, Parker CJ, Moulds MK, Moulds JJ. Evidence that several high-frequency human blood group antigens reside on phosphatidylinositol-linked erythrocyte membrane proteins. *Blood* 1990;75:1404–7.

5 Gubin AN, Njoroge JM, Wojda U *et al.* Identification of the Dombrock blood group glycoprotein as a polymorphic member of the ADP-ribosyltransferase gene family. *Blood* 2000;96:2621–7.

6 Swanson J, Polesky HF, Tippett P, Sanger R. A 'new' blood group antigen, Do^a. *Nature* 1965;206:313.

7 Tippett P, Sanger R, Swanson J, Polesky HF. The Dombrock blood group system. *Proc 10th Congr Europ Soc Haematol* 1965;II:1443–6.

8 Molthan L, Crawford MN, Tippett P. Enlargement of the Dombrock blood group system: the finding of anti-Do^b. *Vox Sang* 1973;24:382–4.

9 Tippett P. Genetics of the Dombrock blood group system. *J Med Genet* 1967;4:7–11.

10 Lewis M, Kaita H, Giblett ER, Anderson JE. Genetic linkage analysis of the Dombrock (*Do*) blood group locus. *Cytogenet Cell Genet* 1978;22:313–18.

11 Polesky HF, Swanson JL. Studies on the distribution of the blood group antigen Do^a (Dombrock) and the characteristics of anti-Do^a. *Transfusion* 1966;6:268–70.

12 Nakajima H, Skradski K, Moulds JJ. Do^a (Dombrock) blood group antigen in the Japanese. *Vox Sang* 1979; 36:103–4.

13 Nakajima H, Moulds JJ. Do^a (Dombrock) blood group antigen in the Japanese: tests on further population and family samples. *Vox Sang* 1980;38:294–6.

14 Chandanayingyong D, Sasaki TT, Greenwalt TJ. Blood groups of the Thais. *Transfusion* 1967;7:269–76.

15 Rios M, Hue-Roye K, Lee AH *et al.* DNA analysis for the Dombrock polymorphism. *Transfusion* 2001;41:1143–6.

16 Swanson J, Zweber M, Polesky HF. A new public antigenic determinant Gy^a (Gregory). *Transfusion* 1967; 7:304–6.

17 Race RR, Sanger R. *Blood Groups in Man*, 6th edn. Oxford: Blackwell Scientific Publications, 1975.

18 Clark MJ, Poole J, Barnes RM, Miller JF, Smith DS. Study of the Gregory blood group in an English family. *Vox Sang* 1975;29:301–5.

19 Okubo Y, Nagao N, Tomita T, Yamaguchi H, Moulds JJ. The first examples of the Gy(a–), Hy– phenotype and anti-Gy^a found in Japan. *Transfusion* 1986;26:214–5 and personal communication.

20 Mak KH, Lin CK, Ford DS, Cheng G, Yuen C. The first example of anti-Gy^a detected in Hong Kong. *Immunohematology* 1995;11:20–1.

21 Massaquoi JM. Two further examples of anti-Gy^a. *Transfusion* 1975;15:150–1.

22 Moulds JJ, Polesky HF, Reid M, Ellisor SS. Observations on the Gy^a and Hy antigens and the antibodies that define them. *Transfusion* 1975;15:270–4.

23 Laird-Fryer B, Moulds MK, Moulds JJ, Johnson MH, Mallory DM. Subdivision of the Gy^a–Hy phenotypes [Abstract]. *Transfusion* 1981;21:633.

24 Rios M, Hue-Roye K, Miller JL, Reid ME. Molecular basis associated with the Dombrock null phenotype [Abstract]. *Blood* 2000;96:452a.

25 Schmidt RP, Frank S, Baugh M. New antibodies to high incidence antigenic determinants (anti-So, anti-El, anti-Hy and anti-Dp) [Abstract]. *Transfusion* 1967;7:386.

26 Beattie KM, Castillo S. A case report of a hemolytic trans-

fusion reaction caused by anti-Holley. *Transfusion* 1975; 15:476–80.

27 Hsu TCS, Jagathambal K, Sabo BH, Sawitsky A. Anti-Holley (Hy): characterization of another example. *Transfusion* 1975;15:604–7.

28 Rios M, Hue-Roye K, Øyen R, Reid ME. Molecular basis of the Gy(a+ʷ) Hy– phenotype [Abstract]. *Transfus Clin Biol* 2001;8(Suppl.1):14S.

29 Jensen L, Scott EP, Marsh WL et al. Anti-Joᵃ: an antibody defining a high-frequency erythrocyte antigen. *Transfusion* 1972;12:322–4.

30 Morel P, Myers M, Marsh WL, Bergren M. The third example of anti-Joᵃ: inheritance of the Joᵃ red cell antigen [Abstract]. *Transfusion* 1976;16:531.

31 Weaver T, Lacey P, Carty L. Evidence that Joᵃ and Jcᵃ are synonymous [Abstract]. *Transfusion* 1986;26: 561.

32 Weaver T, Kavitsky D, Carty L et al. An association between the Joᵃ and Hy phenotypes [Abstract]. *Transfusion* 1984;24:426.

33 Brown D. Reactivity of anti-Joᵃ with Hy– red cells [Abstract]. *Transfusion* 1985;25:462.

34 Webb AJ, Lockyer JW, Tovey GH. The second example of anti-Doᵃ. *Vox Sang* 1966;11:637–9.

35 Williams CH, Crawford MN. The third example of anti-Doᵃ. *Transfusion* 1966;6:310.

36 Polesky HF, Swanson J, Smith R. Anti-Doᵃ stimulated by pregnancy. *Vox Sang* 1968;14:465–6.

37 Moulds J, Futrell E, Fortez P, McDonald C. Anti-Doᵃ: further clinical and serological observations [Abstract]. *Transfusion* 1978;18:375.

38 Kruskall MS, Greene MJ, Strycharz DM, Getman EM, Cawley A. Acute hemolytic transfusion reaction due to anti-Dombrockᵃ (Doᵃ) [Abstract]. *Transfusion* 1986;26:545.

39 Judd WJ, Steiner EA. Multiple hemolytic transfusion reactions caused by anti-Doᵃ. *Transfusion* 1991;31:477–8.

40 Roxby DJ, Paris JM, Stern DA, Young SG. Pure anti-Doᵃ stimulated by pregnancy. *Vox Sang* 1994;66:49–50.

41 Strupp A, Cash K, Uehlinger J. Difficulties in identifying antibodies in the Dombrock blood group system in multiply alloimmunized patients. *Transfusion* 1998;38: 1022–5.

42 Yvart J, Cartron J, Fouillade MT et al. Un nouvel exemple d'anti-Doᵇ. *Rev Franc Transfus Immuno-Hémat* 1977;20:395–400.

43 Moheng MC, McCarthy P, Pierce SR. Anti-Doᵇ implicated as the cause of a delayed hemolytic transfusion reaction. *Transfusion* 1985;25:44–6.

44 Halverson G, Shanahan E, Santiago I et al. The first reported case of anti-Doᵇ causing an acute hemolytic transfusion reaction. *Vox Sang* 1994;66:206–9.

45 Shirey RS, Boyd JS, King KE et al. Assessment of the clinical significance of anti-Doᵇ. *Transfusion* 1998;38: 1026–9.

46 Gudino M, Kranwinkel R, Lenart S, Harrison L. Successful transfusion of Dombrock [Do(a+)] red blood cells to a patient with anti-Do(a) [Abstract]. *Transfusion* 1986;26:546.

47 Ellisor SS, Reid ME, Avoy DR, Toy PTCY, Mecoli J. Transient anti-Gyᵃ in an untransfused man: serologic characteristics and cell survival study. *Transfusion* 1982; 22:166–8.

48 Reid ME, Ellisor SS, Sabo B. Absorption and elution of anti-Hy from one of four Gy(a–) human red blood cell samples. *Transfusion* 1982;22:528–9.

49 Barrett VJ, O'Brien MM, Moulds JJ et al. Anti-Holley detected in a primary immune repsonse. *Immunohematology* 1996;12:62–5.

50 Viggiano E, Jacobson G, Zurbito F. A Chromium⁵¹ survival study on a patient with anti-'Joᵃ/Jcᵃ' [Abstract]. *Transfusion* 1985;25:446.

51 Rao N, Udani M, Nelson J, Reid ME, Telen MJ. Investigations using a novel monoclonal antibody to the glycosylphosphatidylinositol-anchored protein that carries Gregory, Holley, and Dombrock blood group antigens. *Transfusion* 1995;35:459–64.

52 Koch-Nolte F, Haag F. Mono(ADP-ribosyl)transferases and related enzymes in animal tissues: emerging gene families. *Adv Exp Med Biol* 1997;419:1–13.

15 Colton blood group system

15.1 Introduction

Colton is a relatively simple blood group system. It consists of a single polymorphism, with high and low incidence alleles represented by Co^a and Co^b antigens, respectively. A third antigen, Co3, is present on all cells save those of the null phenotype, Co(a–b–) (Table 15.1).

The *CO* locus is on chromosome 7p (Chapter 32) and the Co(a–b–) phenotype is sometimes associated with acquired chromosome 7 monosomy. The Colton antigens are located on aquaporin-1, a water channel-forming protein. An amino acid substitution accounts for the Colton polymorphism (Table 15.1).

15.2 The Colton glycoprotein, aquaporin-1, and the gene that encodes it

Aquaporin-1 (AQP1), an integral protein of red cell and kidney membranes, is a member of the aquaporin family of water channels (reviewed in [1,2]). Aquaporins are part of the major intrinsic protein (MIP) superfamily of transmembrane channel proteins of animals, plants, and bacteria (reviewed in [3]). AQP1 is of M_r 28000 in its unglycosylated form and 40000–60000 in its glycosylated form. There are between 120000 and 160000 molecules per red cell, arranged as tetramers, with each tetramer containing one glycosylated molecule [4]. Polymerase chain reaction (PCR) amplification of human fetal liver cDNA template with degenerate oligonucleotide primers representing the amino acid sequence of the N-terminal region of AQP1 provided a probe for isolation of *AQP1* cDNA from a human bone marrow cDNA library. The sequence of the 807 bp open reading frame predicts a 269 amino acid polypeptide, which spans the membrane six times and has cytoplasmic N- and C-termini [5] (Fig. 15.1). The two halves of AQP1 are sequence-related and each has three membrane-spanning domains and each has a loop, one extracellular (E in Fig. 15.1) and one cytoplasmic (B), containing the Asn-Pro-Ala (NPA) motif characteristic of the MIP family. In accordance with several structural models these two NPA motifs may interact within the membrane to form a single aqueous channel spanning the bilayer [6–8]. The first extracellular loop may be *N*-glycosylated, the oligosaccharide resembling the *N*-glycan of band 3 and expressing ABH activity [9].

The 17 kb *AQP1* gene consists of four exons encoding amino acids 1–128, 129–183, 184–210, and 211–269, and has been localized, by *in situ* hybridization, to chromosome 7p14 [10]. The *AQP1* promoter contained TATA and CCAAT boxes, SP1, AP1, AP2, and E-box elements, and erythroid-specific CACCC and Kruppel-like (CACCCA) elements [11].

Localization of *AQP1* to the same region of chromosome 7 as CO (Chapter 32) led to the discovery that the Colton antigens are on AQP1. Smith *et al.* [9] found that AQP1 could be selectively precipitated with anti-Co^a and -Co^b from red cells of the appropriate Colton phenotypes. Anti-Co3 precipitated AQP1 from Co(a+b–) and Co(a–b+) cells.

15.3 Co^a and Co^b (CO1 and CO2)

In 1967, Heistö *et al.* [12] gave the name anti-Co^a to three antibodies defining a new inherited public antigen. Three years later Giles *et al.* [13] identified the antithetical antibody, anti-Co^b, and a new blood group polymorphism was born.

From seven separate studies with anti-Co^a on a total of 13460 white donors from northern Europe [12,14,15], the USA [15], and Canada [16,17], 27 were Co(a–), giving a frequency for Co^a of 99.8%.

Table 15.1 Antigens of the Colton system.

No.	Name	Relative frequency	Comments
CO1	Co^a	High	Allelic to Co^b (CO2), Ala45
CO2	Co^b	Low	Allelic to Co^a (CO1), Val45
CO3	Co3	High	Absent from Co(a–b–) cells

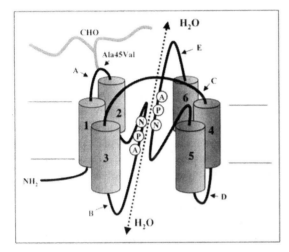

Fig. 15.1 Three-dimensional model for AQP1 in the plasma membrane [1,2,6–8]. The six membrane-spanning domains are shown as cylinders and numbered from the N-terminus. A, C, and E represent the three extracellular loops; B and D, two cytoplasmic loops. B and E are extended loops that pass into the membrane to form a pore through which water molecules pass. NPA represents the Asn-Pro-Ala motifs in loops E and B. The N- and C-terminal domains are attached to the cytoplasmic ends of the first and sixth membrane-spanning domains, although the C-terminus is not visible. CHO, N-glycan at Asn42. Ala45Val, site of Colton polymorphism.

From five series of tests with anti-Co^b on 5186 white donors from England [13], Canada [17], Australia [18,19], and New Zealand [18], 443 (8.5%) were Co(b+). Gene and genotype frequencies calculated from these data (assuming that Co^a and Co^b are the only alleles present) are shown in Table 15.2; those calculated from the results of tests with anti-Co^a correlate remarkably well with those derived from tests with anti-Co^b. Very few studies are reported on other ethnic

Table 15.2 Antigen, gene, and genotype frequencies in white people, determined from tests with anti-Co^a [12–17] and -Co^b [13,17–19].

		With anti-Co^a	With anti-Co^b
Antigens	Co^a	0.998	
	Co^b		0.085
Genes	Co^a	0.955	0.956
	Co^b	0.045	0.044
Genotypes	Co^a/Co^a	0.912	0.914
	Co^a/Co^b	0.086	0.084
	Co^b/Co^b	0.002	0.002

groups. Of 1706 African Americans, all were Co(a+) [15]. The following Co^b frequencies were obtained: 4.6% in Miami Hispanics (799 tested) [20]; 2% in Cree Indians (100 tested) [21]; 0.58% in Japanese (2244 tested) [22].

The gene frequencies in Table 15.2 provide very strong evidence that Co^a and Co^b are codominant and that any third allele at that locus must be very rare. This has been confirmed by family investigations [12,15,17]. Apparent parental exclusions based on Colton phenotypes in two families may be explained by the presence of a rare silent allele, Co [23,24]. Support for this comes from single dose scores in titrations with anti-Co^a and -Co3 (Section 15.4).

The Colton polymorphism is associated with a C134T change in exon 1, the Co^a allele encoding alanine at position 45 and the Co^b allele encoding valine [9]. This is on the first extracellular loop of AQP1 (loop A), close to the site of N-glycosylation (Asn42) (Fig. 15.1). Altered glycosylation may prevent expression of Colton antigens; Xenopus oocytes expressing human AQP1 do not bind anti-Co^a [9]. A PfiMI restriction site is created by the Co^b allele.

Co^a and Co^b are resistant to denaturation by the proteases papain, trypsin, chymotrypsin, and pronase, by sialidase, and by the disulphide bond reducing agent 2-aminoethylisothiouronium bromide (AET).

Co^a was not detected by flow cytometry on lymphocytes, monocytes, or granulocytes [25].

15.4 Co3 and the Co(a–b–) phenotype

In 1974 Rogers et al. [26] identified the awaited

Colton null phenotype, Co(a–b–), in a French-Canadian woman and two of her four sibs. Her parents and other two sibs were Co(a+b–). The serum of the propositus contained an antibody, anti-Co3, which reacted with all cells except those of the Co(a–b–) phenotype and could not be separated into anti-Coᵃ and -Coᵇ components by adsorption and elution. Five other unrelated Co(a–b–) Co:–3 individuals are reported, all ascertained through the presence of anti-Co3 and all of European extraction [27–31]. One had a Co(a–b–) Co:–3 brother with anti-Co3 [27]. No negative was found as a result of testing 40 000 donors (29 000 North Americans, 9000 Australians, 2000 Finns) with anti-Co3 [30].

Molecular genetical analyses have been performed on four Co(a–b–) Co:–3 propositi and each has a different background.

1 Homozygosity for a deletion encompassing most or all of exon 1 [32].

2 Homozygosity for a single base insertion at nucleotide 307 (exon 1), initiating a reading frameshift after Gly104, in the third membrane-spanning domain [32]. The mutations in cases 1 and 2 would result in no production of a substantial proportion of the protein. Consequently, no AQP1 would be expected in the red cell membrane, and none was detected by immunoblotting [32].

3 Homozygosity for C614A in exon 3, encoding Asn192Lys [31]. This substitution converts the Asn-Pro-Ala motif in the third extracellular loop (E in Fig. 15.1) to Lys-Pro-Ala. It is predicted that such a change in this important motif would result in failure of the protein to reach the membrane [31]. The two children of the propositus were Co(a+b–) and heterozygous at codon 192.

4 Homozygosity for C113T in exon 1, encoding Pro38Leu [32]. Trace amounts of apparently normal AQP1 were detected on immunoblots of red cell membranes probed with monoclonal anti-AQP1 and the red cells reacted weakly with an extremely potent (titre 32 000) anti-Co3 [30]. Protein instability brought about by the amino acid substitution probably accounts for the low level of AQP1 in the membranes of this woman. *Xenopus* oocytes transfected with *AQP1* cDNA containing the Pro38Leu mutation had osmotic water permeabilities higher than those transfected with no *AQP1* cDNA, but substantially lower than those transfected with normal *AQP1* cDNA [32].

Red cells of propositus 1 (above) had normal morphology, haematocrit, and haemoglobin levels, but a slightly reduced life span *in vivo* [33].

Red cells of a child with a unique form of congenital dyserythropoietic anaemia (CDA), but no AQP1 mutation, had less than 10% of normal AQP1 levels and were Co(a–b–), but reacted normally with potent anti-Co3 [34,35]. The patient's red cells were also CD44-deficient, In(a–b–), AnWj–, and had weak LWᵃᵇ (see Chapter 21) and very low osmotic water permeability. Red cells with other forms of CDA have normal Colton antigens. The parents and sister of the patient were Co(a+b–).

Like Coᵃ and Coᵇ, Co3 is resistant to protease, sialidase, and AET treatment of red cells.

15.5 Colton antigens and monosomy 7

Monosomy 7 of the bone marrow, the loss of one chromosome 7 from haemopoietic stem cells, is a rare chromosomal abnormality associated with acute myeloid leukaemia and preleukaemic dysmyelopoietic syndromes. Monosomy 7 is often associated with Co(a–b–) Co:–3 phenotype or with weakening of Coᵃ and Co3 [36–38]. Of 35 monosomy 7 patients, eight had either Co(a–b–) Co:–3 or Co(a+ʷb–) Co3-weak red cells [38]. None of these eight had been recently transfused, whereas transfused red cells were present in the circulation of 21 of the remaining 27 Co(a+b–) patients. Either weakness of Colton antigens cannot be detected in the presence of transfused cells or transfusion confers some beneficial effect on the expression of Colton antigens [38].

CO is located on chromosome 7 (Chapter 32). Zelinski *et al.* [39] suggested that absence of Colton antigens in some monosomy 7 patients results from loss of one allele because of the monosomy and altered expression of the product of the other allele brought about by the concomitant haematological disorder.

15.6 Colton antibodies

15.6.1 Anti-Coᵃ

Many examples of anti-Coᵃ have been identified. Like anti-Coᵇ and -Co3, they are generally IgG and react best by the antiglobulin test, especially if protease-treated cells are used, although an agglutinating IgM anti-Coᵃ has been reported [40].

Anti-Coᵃ has caused severe haemolytic disease of

the newborn (HDN) [41] and has been implicated in single cases of acute [42] and delayed haemolytic transfusion reactions [43]. An *in vivo* survival study with radiolabelled Co(a+b–) red cells suggested that compatible blood should be provided for patients with anti-Co^a [40].

Anti-Co^a in a Co(a+b+) patient, shown to have the Co^a/Co^b phenotype by genomic analysis, was considered either to detect a partial Co^a antigen or to be an autoantibody [44]. Considering the role of AQP1 in the kidney (Section 15.7), autoanti-Co^a might provide an explanation for the patient's chronic renal insufficiency.

15.6.2 Anti-Co^b

Anti-Co^b, a relatively rare antibody, was not detected in sera from 1430 transfused and non-transfused patients, or in sera from seven patients known to have been transfused with Co(a–) blood [12]. Anti-Co^b is often found in sera containing other blood group antibodies.

Complement binding anti-Co^b was responsible for an acute haemolytic reaction in a patient transfused with Co(a+b+) blood [45]. A mild delayed transfusion reaction has also been attributed to anti-Co^b [46]. *In vivo* survival studies demonstrated accelerated destruction of radiolabelled Co(b+) cells in patients with anti-Co^b [47,48]. Co^b is fully developed at birth [49], but there is no report of serious HDN caused by anti-Co^b.

15.6.3 Anti-Co3

Anti-Co3 has caused severe HDN requiring neonatal transfusion with maternal blood [29,30]. Transfusion of Co(a+b–) blood to a patient with anti-Co3 resulted in a mild haemolytic reaction, but no renal impairment [31]. A very high titred anti-Co3 consisted of IgG1, IgG3, and some IgG2, was complement binding, and was haemolytic *in vitro* [30].

A 'mimicking autoanti-Co3' in a non-Hodgkin's lymphoma patient with Co(a–b–) Co:3 red cells directly agglutinated most red cells, but a papain antiglobulin test was required to demonstrate reactivity with the patient's own cells and with Co(a–b–) Co:–3 cells [50].

15.6.4 An antibody reactive only when Co^a and Co^b are both present

An antibody produced by a Co(a+b–) patient reacted with an antiglobulin test with 12 examples of Co(a+b+) red cells, but not with eight examples of Co(a–b+) or many examples of Co(a+b–) cells [51]. In Co^a/Co^b heterozygotes, it is feasible that binding of this antibody is dependent on the conformational effects of interactions between valine and alanine at position 45 of different molecules within AQP1 tetramers of the red cell membrane.

15.7 Functional aspects

AQP1 functions to form channels in the plasma membrane that enhance osmotically driven water transport. According to the model of Murata *et al.* [7], the extended loops B and E in Fig. 15.1 form a channel through the membrane with a pore diameter of about 3 Å, only slightly larger than the 2.8 Å diameter of a water molecule. Interaction with the asparagine residues of the Asn-Pro-Ala motifs enhances transfer of water molecules, while preventing H$^+$ transport [7]. In addition to red cells, AQP1 is strongly expressed in the proximal convoluted tubules and descending thin limbs of the kidney and has also been detected in various other epithelia and endothelia. AQP1 has a role in reabsorption of water from the glomerular filtrate in the proximal tubule and thin descending loop of Henle [1,2]. AQP1 may also enable red cells to rehydrate rapidly after their shrinkage in the hypertonic environment of the renal medulla [52]. This would act in concert with the urea transporter, which also serves to reduce cell shrinkage in the renal medulla by enhancing the permeability of the red cell to urea (Section 9.6). Red cell AQP1 might also play a part in CO$_2$ transport in the peripheral blood. *Xenopus* oocytes expressing AQP1 demonstrated significantly increased CO$_2$ permeability in the presence of carbonic anhydrase, compared with oocytes not expressing AQP1 [53]. However, no difference was detected between CO$_2$ permeability of red cells from wild-type and AQP1 knockout mice [54]. AQP1 has been detected in several other organs and tissues: lung, where it may be involved in maintaining water balance; brain, where it could play a part in regulation of cerebospinal fluid; and eye, where it might have a role in secretion and uptake of the aqueous humour [1,2].

401

Three Co(a–b–) propositi had about an 80% reduction in red cell osmotic water permeabilities and no AQP1 from renal tubules could be detected by immunoblot analysis of their urinary sediment [32], yet no health defect appeared to be associated with the AQP1 deficiency (see Section 15.4). AQP1-null mice were grossly normal, but became severely dehydrated and lethargic compared with control mice after water deprivation for 36 h [55]. It is therefore likely that AQP1 in the thin descending limb of Henle is required for the production of concentrated urine during times of water shortage [56]. AQP1 function in renal tubules may be shared with other members of the aquaporin family, possibly AQP2, absence of which results in a rare form of nephrogenic diabetes insipidus [1,2]; in red cells the function may be shared with AQP3, which probably functions mainly as a water and glycerol channel [57].

References

1 Agre P, Bonhivers M, Borgnia MJ. The aquaporins, blueprints for cellular plumbing systems. *J Biol Chem* 1998;273:14659–62.

2 Borgnia M, Nielsen S, Engel A, Agre P. Cellular and molecular biology of the aquaporin water channels. *Annu Rev Biochem* 1999;68:425–58.

3 Park JH, Saier MH Jr. Phylogenetic characterization of the MIP family of transmembrane channel proteins. *J Membr Biol* 1996;153:171–80.

4 Denker BM, Smith BL, Kuhajda FP, Agre P. Identification, purification, and partial characterization of a novel M_r 28 000 integral membrane protein from erythrocytes and renal tubules. *J Biol Chem* 1988;263:15634–42.

5 Preston GM, Agre P. Isolation of the cDNA for erythrocyte integral membrane protein of 28 kilodaltons: member of an ancient channel family. *Proc Natl Acad Sci USA* 1991;88:11110–14.

6 Jung JS, Preston GM, Smith BL, Giggino WB, Agre P. Molecular structure of the water channel through aquaporin CHIP: the hourglass model. *J Biol Chem* 1994; 269:14648–54.

7 Murata K, Mitsuoka K, Hirai T *et al.* Structural determinants of water permeation through aquaporin-1. *Nature* 2000;407:599–605.

8 de Groot BL, Heymann JB, Engel A *et al.* The fold of aquaporin 1. *J Mol Biol* 2000;300:987–94.

9 Smith BL, Preston GM, Spring F, Anstee DJ, Agre P. Human red cell Aquaporin CHIP. I. Molecular characterization of ABH and Colton blood group antigens. *J Clin Invest* 1994;94:1043–9.

10 Moon C, Preston GM, Griffin CA, Jabs EW, Agre P. The human Aquaporin-CHIP gene: structure, organization, and chromosomal localization. *J Biol Chem* 1993; 268:15772–8.

11 Umenishi F, Verkman AS. Isolation of the human aquaporin-1 promoter and functional characterization in human erythroleukemia cell lines. *Genomics* 1998; 47:341–9.

12 Heistö H, van der Hart M, Madsen G *et al.* Three examples of new red cell antibody, anti-Coª. *Vox Sang* 1967;12:18–24.

13 Giles CM, Darnborough J, Aspinall P, Fletton MW. Identification of the first example of anti-Coᵇ. *Br J Haematol* 1970;19:267–9.

14 Smith DS, Stratton F, Howell P, Riches R. An example of anti-Coª found in pregnancy. *Vox Sang* 1970;18:62–6.

15 Race RR, Sanger R. *Blood Groups in Man*, 6th edn. Oxford: Blackwell Scientific Publications, 1975.

16 Wray E, Simpson S. A further example of anti-Coª and two informative families with Co(a–) members. *Vox Sang* 1968;14:130–2.

17 Lewis M, Kaita H, Chown B, Giblett ER, Anderson J. Colton blood groups in Canadian Caucasians: frequencies, inheritance and linkage analysis. *Vox Sang* 1977; 32:208–13.

18 Case J. A pure example of anti-Coᵇ and frequency of the Coᵇ antigen in New Zealand and Australian blood donors. *Vox Sang* 1971;21:447–50.

19 Brackenridge CJ, Case J, Sheehy AJ. Distributions, sex and age effects, and joint associations between phenotypes of 14 genetic systems in an Australian population sample. *Hum Hered* 1975;25:520–9.

20 Issitt PD, Wren MR, Rueda E, Maltz M. Red cell antigens in Hispanic blood donors. *Transfusion* 1987;27:117.

21 Lucciola L, Kaita H, Anderson J, Emery S. The blood groups and red cell enzymes of a sample of Cree Indians. *Can J Genet Cytol* 1974;16:691–5.

22 Nagao N, Tomita T, Okubo Y, Yamaguchi H. Low frequency antigen, Doª, Coᵇ, Sc2, in Japanese [Abstract]. *24th Congr Int Soc Blood Transfus* 1996: 145.

23 Moulds JJ, Dykes D, Polesky HF. A silent allele in the Colton blood group system [Abstract]. *Transfusion* 1974;14:508.

24 Swanson JL, Eckman JR. Co(a–b+ᵂ) phenotype in a patient with paroxysmal nocturnal hemoglobinuria: association with unusual Colton phenotypes in other family members [Abstract]. *Transfusion* 1978;18:376.

25 Dunstan RA. Status of major red cell blood group antigens on neutrophils, lymphocytes and monocytes. *Br J Haematol* 1986;62:301–9.

26 Rogers MJ, Stiles PA, Wright J. A new minus–minus phenotype: three Co(a–b–) individuals in one family [Abstract]. *Transfusion* 1974;14:508.

27 Fuhrmann U, Kloppenburg W, Krüger H-W. Entibindung einer Schwangeren mit einem seltenen Phänotyp im Colton-Blutgruppensytem. *Geburtsh Frauenheilk* 1979;39:66–7.

28 Theuriere M, de la Camara C, DiNapoli J, Øyen R. Case

report of the rare Co(a–b–) phenotype. *Immunohematology* 1985;2:16–17.

29 Savona-Ventura C, Grech ES, Zieba A. Anti-Co3 and severe hemolytic disease of the newborn. *Obstet Gynecol* 1989;73:870–2.

30 Lacey PA, Robinson J, Collins ML *et al*. Studies on the blood of a Co(a–b–) proposita and her family. *Transfusion* 1987;27:268–71.

31 Chrétien S, Cartron JP, de Figueiredo M. A single mutation inside the MPA motif of aquaporin-1 found in a Colton-null phenotype. *Blood* 1999;93:4021–3.

32 Preston GM, Smith BL, Zeidel ML, Moulds JJ, Agre P. Mutations in aquaporin-1 in phenotypically normal humans without functional CHIP water channels. *Science* 1994;265:1585–7.

33 Mathai JC, Mori S, Smith BL *et al*. Functional analysis of aquaporin-1 deficient red cells: the Colton-null phenotype. *J Biol Chem* 1996;271:1309–13.

34 Parsons SF, Jones J, Anstee DJ *et al*. A novel form of congenital dyserythropoietic anemia associated with deficiency of erythroid CD44 and a unique blood group phenotype [In (a–b–), Co(a–b–)]. *Blood* 1994;83:860–8.

35 Agre P, Smith BL, Baumgarten R *et al*. Human red cell Aquaporin CHIP. II. Expression during normal fetal development and in a novel form of congenital dyserythropoietic anemia. *J Clin Invest* 1994;94:1050–8.

36 de la Chapelle A, Vuopio P, Sanger R, Teesdale P. Monosomy-7 and the Colton blood-groups. *Lancet* 1975; ii:817.

37 Boetius G, Hustinx TWJ, Smits APT *et al*. Monosomy 7 in two patients with a myeloproliferative disorder. *Br J Haematol* 1977;37:101–9.

38 Pasquali F, Bernasconi P, Casalone R *et al*. Pathogenetic significance of 'pure' monosomy 7 in myeloproliferative disorders: analysis of 14 cases. *Hum Genet* 1982; 62:40–51.

39 Zelinski T, Kaita H, Gilson T *et al*. Linkage between the Colton blood group locus and *ASSP11* on chromosome 7. *Genomics* 1990;6:623–5.

40 Kurtz SR, Kuszaj T, Ouellet R, Valeri CR. Survival of homozygous Co^a (Colton) red cells in a patient with anti-Co^a. *Vox Sang* 1982;43:28–30.

41 Simpson WKH. Anti-Co^a and severe haemolytic disease of the newborn. *S Afr Med J* 1973;47:1302–4.

42 Covin RB, Evans KS, Olshock R, Thompson HW. Acute hemolytic transfusion reaction caused by anti-Co^a. *Immunohematology* 2001;17:45–9.

43 Kitzke HM, Julius H, Delaney M, Studnicka L, Landmark J. Anti-Co^a implicated in delayed hemolytic transfusion reaction [Abstract]. *Transfusion* 1982; 22:407.

44 Leo A, Cartron JP, Strittmatter M, Rowe G, Roelcke D. Case report: anti-Co^a in a Co-(a+)-typed patient with chronic renal insufficiency. *Beitr Infusionsther Transfusionsmed* 1997;34:185–9.

45 Lee EL, Bennett C. Anti-Co^b causing acute hemolytic transfusion reaction. *Transfusion* 1982;22:159–60.

46 Squires JE, Larison PJ, Charles WT, Milner PF. A delayed hemolytic transfusion reaction due to anti-Co^b. *Transfusion* 1985;25:137–9.

47 Dzik WH, Blank J. Accelerated destruction of radiolabeled red cells due to anti-Colton^b. *Transfusion* 1986;26:246–8.

48 Hoffmann JJML, Overbeeke MAM. Characteristics of anti-Co^b *in vitro* and *in vivo*: a case study. *Immunohematology* 1996;12:11–13.

49 Henke J, Basler M, Baur MP. Further data on the development of red blood cell antigens Lu^a, Lu^b, and Co^b. *Forensic Sci Int* 1982; 20: 233–6.

50 Moulds M, Strohm P, McDowell MA, Moulds J. Autoantibody mimicking alloantibody in the Colton blood group system [Abstract]. *Transfusion* 1988;28:36S.

51 Campbell G, Williams E, Skidmore I, Poole J. A novel Colton-related antibody reacting only with Co(a+b+) cells [Abstract]. *Transfus Med* 1999;9(Suppl.1):30.

52 Smith BL, Baumgarten R, Nielsen S *et al*. Concurrent expression of erythroid and renal aquaporin CHIP and appearance of water channel activity in perinatal rats. *J Clin Invest* 1993;92:2035–41.

53 Nakhoul NL, Davis BA, Romero MF, Boron WF. Effect of expressing the water channel aquaporin-1 on the CO_2 permeability of *Xenopus* oocytes. *Am J Physiol* 1998; 274:C543–8.

54 Yang B, Fukuda N, van Hoek A *et al*. Carbon dioxide permeability of aquaporin-1 measured in erythrocytes and lung of aquaporin-1 null mice and in reconstituted proteoliposomes. *J Biol Chem* 2000;275:2686–92.

55 Ma T, Yang B, Gillespie A *et al*. Severly impaired urinary concentrating ability in transgenic mice lacking aquaporin-1 water channels. *J Biol Chem* 1998; 273:4296–9.

56 Chou C-L, Knepper MA, van Hoek AN *et al*. Reduced water permeability and altered ultrastructure in thin descending limb of Henle in aquaporin-1 null mice. *J Clin Invest* 1999;103:491–6.

57 Roudier N, Verbavatz J-M, Maurel C, Ripoche P, Tacnet F. Evidence for the presence of aquaporin-3 in human red blood cells. *J Biol Chem* 1998;273:8407–12.

16 LW blood group system

16.1 Introduction and history

A phenotypic relationship between LW and the Rh antigen D delayed recognition of LW as an independent blood group system for at least 20 years, until 1963. Only in 1982 was LW resolved into a three-antigen system (Table 16.1).

The first anti-LW, described by Landsteiner and Wiener [1] in 1940, was called anti-Rhesus and resulted from immunizing rabbits, and later guinea pigs, with blood from the monkey *Macacus rhesus*. This antibody appeared to be of the same specificity as a human alloantibody described, but not named, by Levine and Stetson [2] in 1939. Both human and animal antibodies were called anti-Rh.

As early as 1942, Fisk and Foord [3] demonstrated that guinea pig anti-Rh differed from human anti-Rh (later called anti-D) when they observed that red cells from all neonates, whether Rh-positive (D+) or Rh-negative (D–) as defined by the human anti-Rh, were positive with guinea pig anti-Rh. In 1952, Murray and Clark [4] produced anti-Rh by immunizing guinea pigs with either Rh-positive or Rh-negative adult human red cells, or with heat extracts from those cells. Levine *et al*. [5,6] repeated and confirmed this work and also showed that animal anti-Rh agglutinated D+ cells with the D antigen 'blocked' by non-agglutinating anti-D; effective blocking was demonstrated by the failure of these cells to be agglutinated by human anti-D. Furthermore, adsorption–elution tests demonstrated that the animal anti-'D-like', as it was now called, bound to D– cells, although it only agglutinated D+ cells.

Two D+ women made alloantibodies that appeared to be anti-D, but which behaved atypically because they were easily adsorbed by D– cells and therefore resembled animal 'D-like' antibodies [7]. The red cells of these women did not react with guinea pig anti-Rh, even by adsorption–elution [8]. As the name Rh was firmly established in the literature and in common usage for the clinically important CDE groups, Levine *et al*. [8] suggested that the antigen defined by the animal and rare human 'D-like' antibodies be called LW in honour of Landsteiner and Wiener.

Although LW and D are different antigens, they are phenotypically related. D+ cells of adults express LW more strongly than D– cells, so anti-LW is easily mistaken for anti-D unless adsorption tests are done or rare D+ LW– cells are used. Rh_{null} cells, which lack all Rh antigens, also lack LW [8].

To distinguish the different LW+ phenotypes of D+ and D– cells, Levine and Cellano [9] named the former LW_1 and the latter LW_2. Swanson *et al*. [10] observed that red cells of LW– people with anti-LW in their serum [11,12] were not always mutually compatible. To accommodate this, numbering of LW phenotypes was extended [13]: LW– red cells (with normal Rh antigens) were divided into LW_3 and LW_4. LW_3 red cells did not react with anti-LW made by LW_3 individuals, but did react with anti-LW made by LW_4 individuals, whereas LW_4 cells did not react with any LW antibodies.

A further complication is transient LW– phenotype [14]. This non-inherited phenotype, called acquired LW–, is often indistinguishable from LW_3 or LW_4 (Section 16.6).

A new low incidence antigen, Nea, present in 5–6% of the Finnish population [15], was found to have a phenotypic relationship with D similar to that of LW [16]. Sistonen and Tippett [17] observed that anti-Nea

Table 16.1 Antigens of the LW system.

Number	Name	Relative frequency	Comments
LW5	LW^a	High	Antithetical to LW6 (LW^b); Gln70
LW6	LW^b	Low	Antithetical to LW5 (LW^a); Arg70
LW7	LW^{ab}	High	

LW1 to LW4 are obsolete as they were previously used as phenotype designations.

and anti-LW made by LW$_3$ individuals were detecting the products of alleles. This led to the renaming of the LW system antigens: the antigen detected by the anti-LW of LW$_3$ individuals became LW^a; Ne^a became LW^b; LW$_4$ phenotype became LW(a–b–); and the antigen detected by the anti-LW of LW$_4$ individuals became LW^{ab} (Table 16.2).

The LW^a, LW^b, LW^{ab} notation will be used in this chapter wherever possible, although this is sometimes difficult as many publications predate the discovery of anti-LW^b and it is not always possible to decide whether 'anti-LW' were really anti-LW^a or anti-LW^{ab}. In the International Society for Blood Transfusion (ISBT) notation, use of the numbers LW1 to LW4 has been avoided to prevent confusion with the old phenotype designations (Table 16.1).

LW antigens reside on a red cell membrane glycoprotein of about M_r 40 000 named CD242 or ICAM-4, an intercellular adhesion molecule (Section 16.8). The LW^a/LW^b polymorphism is associated with a Gln70Arg substitution (Section 16.3.2).

The *LW* locus is located on chromosome 19p13.3 (Chapter 32).

16.2 The LW glycoprotein (ICAM-4) and the gene that encodes it

Immunochemical analyses with alloanti-LW^{ab} (Mrs Big. serum) and monoclonal anti-LW^{ab} demonstrated that LW antigens are located on a red cell membrane component of about M_r 40 000 [18–21]. A broad band representing M_r 37 000–47 000 obtained by immunoblotting with monoclonal anti-LW^{ab} under non-reducing conditions was 'sharpened' to M_r 36 000–43 000 when sialidase-treated ghosts were used, suggesting that the size range is because of heterogeneity of sialylation [18]. LW glycoprotein is *O*- and *N*-glycosylated. Its M_r was reduced by 2000 and 17 000 following treatment with *O*-glycanase and *N*-glycanase, respectively [21]. The presence of ethylenediaminetetra-acetic acid (EDTA) inhibits expression of LW^a, LW^b, and LW^{ab} on red cells [19]. Antigen expression could be restored to normal by Mg^{2+} ions, but not by Mn^{2+} or Ca^{2+}.

Comparison of the LW glycoprotein with Rh protein by two-dimensional chymotryptic iodopeptide mapping dispelled any possibility that the LW glycoprotein is a glycosylated form of an Rh protein or that Rh polypeptide is a precursor of LW glycoprotein [21,22]. An M_r 31 000 Rh protein appeared to be co-precipitated with LW glycoprotein and so these structures may be associated within the membrane as part of a non-covalently bonded functional complex, the Rh cluster.

Bailly *et al.* [23] obtained partial amino acid sequences from LW glycoprotein purified by immunoaffinity with monoclonal anti-LW^{ab} (BS46).

Table 16.2 LW phenotypes and genotypes.

Old notation		Current notation		Reactions with anti-		
Phenotype		Phenotype	Genotype	LW^a	LW^b	LW^{ab}
LW+	LW$_1$ or LW$_2$	LW(a+b–)	*LW^a/LW^a* or *LW^a/LW*	+	–	+
		LW(a+b+)	*LW^a/LW^b*	+	+	+
LW–	LW$_3$	LW(a–b+)	*LW^b/LW^b* or *LW^b/LW*	–	+	+
LW–	LW$_4$	LW(a–b–)	*LW/LW*	–	–	–
Rh$_{null}$	LW$_0$	LW(a–b–)		–	–	–

Oligonucleotide primers based on these sequences were designed and the polymerase chain reaction (PCR) amplification product was used to screen a human bone marrow cDNA library. The nucleotide sequence of an isolated cDNA clone predicted a polypeptide of M_r 26 500. A rabbit antibody raised to a synthetic peptide with a sequence corresponding to the 15 N-terminal amino acids reacted with the purified LW glycoprotein on immunoblots and agglutinated, in an antiglobulin test, all red cells tested apart from those with the LW(a–b–) phenotype. D+ cells were more strongly agglutinated than D– cells. LW(a–b+) D+ cells reacted only weakly. The original LW sequence [23] contained errors involving three bases affecting the sequence of 16 amino acids in the signal peptide [24].

LW cDNA encodes a 271 amino acid protein with a 30 residue signal peptide, a 208 amino acid N-terminal extracellular domain, a 21 amino acid hydrophobic membrane spanning domain, and a 12 amino acid C-terminal cytoplasmic domain [23]. There are potential N-glycosylation sites at Asn38, Asn48, Asn160, and Asn193 (counting from the N-terminus of the mature protein [23]). Typical N-glycosylation at all four sites would produce a glycoprotein of M_r 38 000–46 000. The proposed presence of three disulphide bonds at three pairs of cysteine residues (Cys39–Cys83, Cys123–Cys180, Cys43–Cys87) is supported by the sensitivity of LW antigens to thiol-reducing agents.

The LW glycoprotein is a member of the immunoglobulin superfamily (IgSF), with two I-set IgSF domains (Fig. 16.1) (see Section 6.2.2). It is structurally related to the intercellular adhesion molecule ICAM-2, and to the first two IgSF domains of ICAM-1 and ICAM-3. Three-dimensional models of LW glycoprotein have been built, based on the crystal structure of ICAM-2 [25,26]. The potential function of LW glycoprotein, also known as ICAM-4, is discussed in Section 16.8.

The 2.65 kb LW gene is organized into three exons [27] (Fig. 16.1). Exon 1 encodes the 5′ untranslated sequence (96 bp), the signal peptide, and the first IgSF domain. Exon 1 is separated by a 129-bp intron from exon 2, which encodes the second IgSF domain and is separated by a 147-bp intron from exon 3, which encodes the transmembrane domain, the cytoplasmic tail, and 3′ untranslated sequence. The promoter region has no TATA or CAAT box, but includes potential binding sites for transcription factors, including

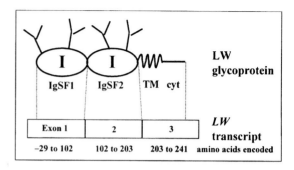

Fig. 16.1 Diagrammatic representation of the LW glycoprotein (ICAM-4) showing the two extracellular I-set IgSF domains, each with two N-glycans, the transmembrane domain (TM), and the cytoplasmic tail (cyt). Also shown is the relationship of the protein structure to the three exons of the LW gene.

those involved in erythroid and megakaryocytic expression [27]. LW has not been detected on megakaryocytes.

16.3 LW^a and LW^b (LW5 and LW6)

16.3.1 Frequency

In most populations, LW^a and LW^b are antigens of very high and low frequency, respectively. Polymorphism of LW was first observed in the Finnish population [15,17]. The highest frequency of LW^b has been found in Baltic Latvians and Lithuanians, and LW^b appears to be a Baltic marker, its presence in other populations being an indicator of the degree of Baltic genetic influence [28] (Table 16.3).

The calculated gene, genotype, and phenotype frequencies for the Finnish population are as follows.

LW^a	0.971	LW^a/LW^a	LW(a+b–)	0.9429
		LW^a/LW^b	LW(a+b+)	0.0563
LW^b	0.029	LW^b/LW^b	LW(a–b+)	0.0008

16.3.2 Inheritance LW^a and LW^b and the molecular basis of the LW polymorphism

Prior to the identification of anti-LW^b, all LW(a–) propositi with normal Rh groups were ascertained through their antibody (for LW reviews at this time, see [7,13,29]). The inherited LW(a–) phenotype could only be distinguished from the acquired phenotype by family studies. Family studies have confirmed that

Table 16.3 Frequency of the LW^b allele in various populations [28].

Population	No. tested	LW^b frequency
Latvians	677	0.059
Lithuanians	829	0.057
Estonians*	800	0.040
Finns	6270	0.029
Russians (Vologda area)	383	0.022
Poles (Poland and USA)	747	0.020
Swedes (Gotland)	199	0.010
Swedes* (Lund)	395	0.003
Hungarians (Budapest)	421	0.004
Swiss*	502	0.001
Belgians (Liège)	211	0
Japanese (Osaka)	500	0
African Somali	1020	0

*Tested for LW^b only.

LW^a and LW^b are codominant alleles [15,30]. Before the relationship of LW and Ne^a was appreciated, the genes responsible for their production had been shown to be independent of the *RH* complex locus [8,10,11,15,31,32], and this was confirmed by the Finnish family studies [30].

The LW^a/LW^b polymorphism is associated with an A308G base change in exon 1 of *LW*, encoding a Gln70Arg substitution in the first IgSF domain of the LW glycoprotein [24]. This was confirmed by detection of LW^a and LW^b on COS-7 simian cells transiently transfected with LW^a and LW^b cDNA, respectively. The LW^b allele lacks a *Pvu*I restriction site. Monoclonal anti-LW^{ab} bound more strongly to COS-7 cells transfected with LW^a cDNA, than with those transfected with LW^b cDNA [24].

16.4 LW(a–b–) and LW^{ab} (LW7)

Inherited LW(a–b–) phenotype is exceedingly rare. Of 10 552 Canadians tested with anti-LW^{ab}, none was negative [12]. The original propositus, a white Canadian antenatal patient (Mrs Big.) with anti-LW^{ab}, had an LW(a–b–) brother [12,17]. Red cells of her three children reacted with her anti-LW^{ab}, but the cells of two of them reacted only weakly. The LW-null phenotype of Mrs Big. results from homozygosity for a 10-

bp deletion in exon 1 (codons 86–89) of an LW^a gene, which introduces a premature stop codon and encodes a truncated protein lacking transmembrane and cytoplasmic domains [27].

The only other propositus was a previously transfused patient from Papua New Guinea, also ascertained through anti-LW^{ab} [33]. He had an LW(a–b–) sister. His LW(a+b–) son had normal LW^a and LW^{ab} red cell antigens, whereas red cells of his LW(a+b–) daughter had weak expression of LW^a and LW^{ab}.

16.5 LW expression and effects of enzymes and reducing agents

16.5.1 Phenotypic relationship to D

Stronger reactions with D+ than D– cells have been noted for many anti-LW^a and -LW^{ab} [9,11,12,31]. For some sera this difference is so great that the antibody could be misidentified as anti-D. Inconsistency in the ability of LW antibodies to distinguish D+ from D– cells may reflect different ratios of IgM : IgG (see Section 16.7.1.2). Estimation of antigen site density with monoclonal anti-LW^{ab} gave the following results: D+ adult, 4400; D– adult, 2835; D+ cord, 5150; D– cord, 3620 [18].

It has been reported that the strength of expression of LW on D+ red cells is not influenced by the CcEe antigens or by D zygosity [34]. However, Gibbs [35] showed that the strength of LW reflected D antigen strength: DcE/DcE cells had more D and LW than DcE/dce, which had more than DCe/dce cells. Red cells with weak D (D^u) gave similar strength reactions to D– cells in titrations of anti-LW^a [34]. LW^b has a similar relationship with D [16], but because LW^b is a low incidence antigen anti-LW^b would never be mistaken for anti-D.

16.5.2 Development of LW

LW is expressed strongly on the red cells of neonates. Animal anti-LW react more strongly with red cells from cord blood samples, both D+ and D–, than with those of adults; human anti-LW do not always make this distinction so clearly [34]. The strength of LW antigens, as judged by guinea pig anti-LW, decreases from birth until the adult level is reached at about 5 years of age [34]. During erythropoiesis *in vitro* LW appears either at the erythroid colony-forming unit

(CFU-E) stage [36] or later at the proerythroblast stage [37].

16.5.3 Dosage effects

Some effect of gene dosage was observed by Sistonen *et al.* [30]: 722 of 10 014 LW(a+) red cell samples from Finns gave weak reactions with anti-LW^a and were subsequently tested with anti-LW^b; 374 of these were LW(b+). From the gene frequencies only 41 of 722 LW(a+) Finns would be expected to be LW(b+) if they had not been partially selected by gene dosage. The strength of the D antigen is far more important than *LW^a* and *LW^b* zygosity in determining the strength of LW^a and LW^b antigens.

16.5.4 Effects of enzymes and reducing agents

LW^a, LW^b, and LW^{ab} are unaffected by treatment of intact cells with the proteases papain, ficin, trypsin, or chymotrypsin, but are destroyed by pronase [38]. Treatment of intact red cells with sialidase has no affect on their reaction with anti-LW^a or anti-LW^{ab} [39]. The disulphide bond-reducing agents dithiothreitol (DTT) and 2-aminoethylisothiouronium bromide (AET) either destroy or greatly reduce LW^a and LW^{ab} activity on red cells [39,40].

16.6 Acquired LW-negative phenotypes and transient anti-LW

The expression of LW on red cells can be affected by non-genetic factors. The acquired LW-negative phenotype is associated with loss of LW^a and, possibly, LW^{ab} and LW^b, and is generally found through the presence of anti-LW^a or -LW^{ab} in the patient's serum. Both antigen loss and antibody production may be temporary.

The first and fullest description of this phenomenon is the report by Giles and Lundsgaard [14] of transient anti-LW in the serum of a D– woman during her first pregnancy. Just before delivery her serum contained anti-C+D and -LW, and her cells were considered LW–, although they gave a weakly positive direct antiglobulin test (DAT). A year after delivery her red cells were LW+ and her anti-LW had disappeared. Chown *et al.* [41] suggested that transient production of anti-LW may not be very rare when they reported three more examples, two in pregnant D– women and one in a transfused D+ patient. They proposed that the

red cells had genuinely lost their LW antigens and that the phenotype did not result from blocking of antigen sites by anti-LW.

Eleven of 18 D– men immunized with D+ red cells transiently produced an antibody resembling anti-LW, suggesting that anti-LW may be an antecedent in the immune response leading to production of anti-D [41]. Three months after transplantation of a D+ boy with bone marrow from his D– sister, anti-LW and anti-D were present, presumably resulting from a primary response of transplanted lymphocytes [42]. After 2 years the anti-LW had disappeared and very weak anti-D remained.

The expression of LW on red cells may be depressed during some diseases and re-expressed at normal strength in remission. Several similar examples are known in patients with lymphoma, leukaemia, sarcoma, and other forms of malignancy [29,43–45]. Such patients, found because of anti-LW^a or -LW^{ab} in their sera, often die without regaining normal strength LW antigens. Two cycles of relapse associated with LW(a–) phenotype and production of anti-LW^a, followed by regaining of LW^a antigen and disappearance of antibody during chemotherapy-induced remission, occurred in a Japanese patient with malignant lymphoma [45]. Occasionally, transient LW-negative phenotype occurs in the absence of malignancy, apparent immunological disorder, or pregnancy [46,47].

Red cells of most people with an acquired LW(a–b–) phenotype are, as expected, non-reactive with anti-LW^{ab}. Occasionally, however, acquired LW(a–) red cells react with anti-LW^{ab}, suggesting that either conformational changes in the LW glycoprotein are involved or a truncated protein, possibly lacking the first IgSF domain, is present.

There appears to be a reciprocal relationship between the amount of LW antigen expressed on red cells and the broadness of the specificity of the anti-LW in the serum [41]. Red cells of some LW(a–b–) patients are LW^{ab}+ and their transient antibodies behave as anti-LW^a; others are LW^{ab}-negative and they make anti-LW^{ab}. Many transient 'anti-LW' cannot be fitted neatly into anti-LW^a or anti-LW^{ab} specificity, presumably reflecting an intermediate stage.

An LW(a–) LW^{ab}+ patient with anti-LW^a in his serum when first tested, later became LW^{ab}– during terminal illness [30]. Two brothers and two daughters of the patient were LW(a–) LW^{ab}+. (The patient was married to his cousin.) Subsequently, available family members were tested with anti-LW^b: one brother and both daughters were LW(b+). The patient's cells recovered from frozen storage were LW(b−) by direct testing, but adsorbed anti-LW^b, suggesting that LW^b may be lost with the other LW antigens.

16.7 LW antibodies

16.7.1 Alloantibodies

16.7.1.1 Anti-LW^a

Alloanti-LW^a are found in the sera of immunized LW(a−b+) individuals. Unless the red cells of the antibody maker are tested with anti-LW^b, other LW(a−) individuals are present in the family, or the antibody maker is shown to be LW^b/LW^b by genomic testing, it is almost impossible to distinguish true alloanti-LW^a from that associated with an acquired LW(a−) phenotype. Most examples of alloanti-LW^a have probably been stimulated by transfusion; one is attributed solely to pregnancy [29], another to immunization of a male volunteer for production of anti-D [48].

16.7.1.2 Anti-LW^{ab}

There are only two examples of alloanti-LW^{ab}, the antibodies of the only two propositi known to have an inherited LW(a−b−) phenotype [12,33]. The first propositus (Mrs Big.) had been pregnant three times, but never transfused. Initially, the anti-LW^{ab} was very potent, reacting much more strongly with D+ (1 : 32 000) than with D− cells (about 1 : 1000). When the antibody decreased in titre it no longer distinguished D+ from D− cells [12]. Perrault [49] separated the serum into IgM and IgG components and found that the fractions with greatest amount of IgM were most efficient in distinguishing D+ from D− cells.

16.7.1.3 Anti-LW^b

Several anti-LW^b have been found in Finland [50]. Although the original anti-LW^b serum did not contain any other irregular antibodies, other reagents have contained additional antibodies such as anti-K, -Kp^a, and -Ul^a. All the Finnish makers of anti-LW^b were D+, suffered from chronic haematological disease, and were multitransfused [50].

16.7.1.4 Transient antibodies

Transient antibodies should probably be considered autoantibodies because they are produced by genetically LW+ individuals. Although red cells of people with transient LW antibodies often give a positive DAT, in some cases the red cells have an acquired LW− phenotype and the anti-LW behaves as an alloantibody (Section 16.6). These antibodies are difficult to distinguish from true alloantibodies and, from a transfusion point of view, are generally managed in the same way. True alloantibodies, transient antibodies, and those of undetermined status will be considered together for clinical significance.

16.7.1.5 Clinical significance

No LW antibody has been responsible for a transfusion reaction or for haemolytic disease of the newborn (HDN). Many patients with anti-LW^a or -LW^{ab} have been successfully transfused with crossmatch-incompatible D− red cells [43,45–47,51,52] and the very potent anti-LW^{ab} of Mrs Big. caused no more than minimal evidence of HDN in her D− third baby [12].

LW antibodies are mostly IgG, with IgG1 the main component [46,48,51]. One anti-LW^a was IgM and IgG [11] and another was inactive by an antiglobulin test and was probably IgM [32]. In most patients with anti-LW^a or -LW^{ab}, where *in vitro* phagocytosis assays or *in vivo* red cell survival studies have been carried out, the results predicted that transfusion with D− cells would be efficacious [45,46,48,51,52]. Exceptions were two examples of IgG3 anti-LW^{ab} [44,53]. In one only 53% of radiolabelled D− LW+ red cells remained 1 h after injection into the patient and both antibodies produced high scores in mononuclear phagocyte assays. *In vivo* red cell survival tests in a patient with potent anti-LW^b resulted in a rapid elimination of radiolabelled LW(b+) (D type not specified) cells, with a half-life of 2–5 h [15]. An occasional LW antibody might have the potential to be haemolytic, but this has not been demonstrated *in vivo*.

16.7.2 Autoantibodies

16.7.2.1 Cold autoanti-LW

In screening 45 000 blood samples, Perrault [49] found 10 examples of autoanti-LW. Most of the antibody makers were healthy blood donors or were pregnant, although one had ulcerative colitis and the other a buccal tumour. The antibodies were not associated with any increased red cell destruction. These antibodies could only be detected by a low-ionic strength polybrene method in an AutoAnalyser at temperatures below 37°C; they were not detectable by manual techniques.

16.7.2.2 Autoimmune haemolytic anaemia

Levine [54] suggested that anti-LW is the most frequent antibody in cases of autoimmune haemolytic anaemia (AIHA) with a positive DAT. Celano and Levine [55] used LW(a–b+) cells to adsorb eluates from red cells of six AIHA patients and found anti-LW^a in all six; one eluate contained only anti-LW. Vos *et al.* [56], using LW(a–b–) LW^{ab}– cells, found that six of eight eluates from red cells of patients with warm AIHA contained anti-LW, although never as the sole antibody.

16.7.3 Animal antibodies

Anti-LW was first made in rabbits [1] and later, more successfully, in guinea pigs. Anti-LW has been stimulated in these animals by injections of red cells from rhesus monkeys (*Macaca mulatta*), from baboons, and from D+ or D– humans [1–6,9,34,57–59]. Heat extracts of human D+ and D– cells also stimulate anti-LW [4–6].

Guinea pig and rabbit anti-LW failed to react with LW(a–b+) cells, so behaved as anti-LW^a. There is no evidence that anti-LW^{ab} has been produced by these animals because there is no reported study with both LW(a–b+) and LW(a–b–) cells.

LW(a–b+) and LW(a–b–) (Mrs Big.) red cells are able to stimulate anti-LW in guinea pigs [56,57]. Only Rh$_{null}$ cells have failed to elicit any such response in animals [54,57,60]. The response to red cells of Mrs Big. is surprising. Considering the nature of the mutation responsible for her LW-null phenotype, no LW glycoprotein would be expected to be present in her red cell membranes (Section 16.4).

16.7.4 Monoclonal anti-LW^{ab}

Of four monoclonal antibodies identified as anti-LW^{ab}, three (IgG1) were derived from mice immunized with human red cells (BS46, BS56, BS87) [61,62], and one (IgM) from a mouse immunized with rhesus monkey red cells (NIM-M8) [63]. The four antibodies reacted with all cells except those of LW(a–b–) and Rh$_{null}$ phenotypes; LW(a–b+) cells gave strongly positive reactions with three of the antibodies, but BS87 only reacted with papain treated LW(a–b+) cells [62]. Three of the reagents reacted much more strongly with D+ cells than with D– cells [61,62]. Binding of the murine anti-LW^{ab} to red cells could be totally blocked by human anti-LW^{ab} and partially blocked by human anti-LW^a; anti-D did not inhibit the reaction [61]. Domain-deletion experiments suggested that the epitopes for the three IgG antibodies are on the first IgSF domain [25]. Five other monoclonal antibodies to the LW glycoprotein, five binding to domain 1 and one to domain 2, were produced by immunizing mice with a recombinant chimeric protein consisting of the two IgSF domains of LW and the Fc fragment of IgG1 [64].

16.8 Functional aspects

ICAMs are intercellular adhesion molecules, a group of five related structures belonging to the IgSF (see Section 6.2.2) [65,66]. The N-terminal domain of ICAM-4, the LW glycoprotein (CD242), is an I-set IgSF domain that shares about 30% sequence identity with that of the other ICAMs [23]. ICAM-2 (CD102), like ICAM-4, has two IgSF domains; ICAM-1 (CD54) and ICAM-3 (CD50) each have five IgSF domains; ICAM-5 has nine domains [66].

ICAMs are ligands for integrins, adhesion molecules consisting of heterodimers for various α and β transmembrane subunits. Eighteen different α subunits combine with eight different β subunits to form over 20 different integrins [67]. ICAMs bind the CD11a/CD18 ($\alpha_L\beta_2$) integrin LFA-1 (lymphocyte function-related antigen-1), which is present on lymphocytes, granulocytes, monocytes, and macrophages [66]. However, there is some controversy over which integrins function as ligands for ICAM-4 [25,26,66,68]. Although this could be because of the different experimental techniques used by different research teams, it might also reflect promiscuity in ICAM-4 ligand binding.

Despite the absence of a conserved sequence motif considered critical for LFA-1 binding and present in ICAM-1, -2, -3, and -5, the Paris group [25,68] found that ICAM-4 is a ligand for LFA-1 and also for the

CD11b/CD18 integrin Mac1 ($\alpha_M\beta_2$), a ligand for ICAM-1. Binding of leucocyte cell lines, including monocytes, B, T, NK, and THP-1 cells, to immobilized ICAM-4 isolated from red cells was blocked by anti-CD18 and binding to T cells was also blocked by anti-CD11a [68]. Transfected mouse fibroblasts expressing human LFA-1 or Mac1 adhered to an immobilized recombinant ICAM-4-Fc construct [25]. This adhesion could be blocked by monoclonal anti-CD11a, -CD11b, -CD18, and -LW[ab]. Results of domain-deletion experiments suggest that LFA-1 binds the first IgSF domain of ICAM-4, whereas Mac1 binding requires both domains. Immobilized LFA-1 and Mac1 integrins bound red cells, which do not have ICAM-1, -2, or -3 [68].

The Bristol group [26,66] found that ICAM-4 is a ligand for the integrin very late antigen-4 (VLA-4, CD49d/CD29, $\alpha_4\beta_1$) on haemopoietic cells and for α_v (CD51) integrins (predominantly $\alpha_v\beta_1$ and $\alpha_v\beta_5$) on non-haemopoietic cells. This was demonstrated by immobilizing a recombinant ICAM-4-Fc fusion protein, containing both ICAM-4 IgSF domains, and inhibiting adhesion of haemopoietic and non-haemopoietic cell lines with peptides and monoclonal antibodies. Site-directed mutagenesis revealed that neither of the putative binding motifs in the first IgSF domain is critical for integrin binding, so a novel integrin-binding mechanism must be involved.

Although the other ICAMs are adhesion molecules of lymphocytes, granulocytes, and monocytes, and may be more widely expressed, it appears that ICAM-4 (LW) is restricted to erythroid cells and, possibly, placenta [66]. LW transcripts were only detected in erythroblasts and fetal liver, and not in a B lymphocytic cell line [69] (although there is one report of LW[ab] expression on subsets of B and T lymphocytes [63]). During erythropoiesis in vitro, LW appears either at the CFU-E stage [36] or later at the proerythroblast stage [37]. An important phase in erythropoiesis is the clustering of erythroblasts around bone marrow macrophages to form erythroblastic islands. The erythroblast can then extrude its nucleus, which is ingested by the macrophage. Adhesive interactions between ICAM-4 and VLA-4 on adjacent erythroblasts and between ICAM-4 on erythroblasts and α_v integrins on macrophages may assist in the stability of these erythroblastic islands [26,66]. Binding of red cells to macrophages in the spleen through adhesive interactions involving ICAM-4 could also play a part in the removal of senescent red cells [66]. However, the functional importance of LW must be considered in light of the absence of any obvious pathology associated with ICAM-4 absence in the inherited LW(a–b–) phenotype and in Rh$_{null}$.

Like the Lutheran glycoprotein, expression of ICAM-4 may be elevated on sickle red cells and antibodies to ICAM-4 partially inhibit adhesion of sickle red cells to activated endothelium [66]. Interactions between ICAM-4 on red cells and α_v integrins on the endothelial cells of vessel walls may be involved in the microvascular occlusions that produce the painful crises of sickle cell disease.

16.9 LW antigens in animals

Summarizing work with animal anti-LW from several laboratories shows that LW antigen has been detected on red cells of all primate species tested, including chimpanzee, gorilla, orang-utan, baboon, and a variety of other species of monkey [1,6,58,70,71]. LW has not been found on the red cells of any of the non-primate species tested: rabbit, mouse, rat, sheep, goat, horse, and cattle.

References

1 Landsteiner K, Wiener AS. An agglutinable factor in human blood recognized by immune sera for rhesus blood. *Proc Soc Exp Biol NY* 1940;**43**:223.

2 Levine P, Stetson RE. An unusual case of intragroup agglutination. *J Am Med Assoc* 1939;**113**:126–7.

3 Fisk RT, Foord AG. Observations on the Rh agglutinogen of human blood. *Am J Clin Pathol* 1942;**12**:545–52.

4 Murray J, Clark EC. Production of anti-Rh in guinea pigs from human erythrocyte extracts. *Nature* 1952;**169**:886–7.

5 Levine P, Celano M, Fenichel R, Singher H. A 'D'-like antigen in rhesus red blood cells and in Rh-positive and Rh-negative red cells. *Science* 1961;**133**:332–3.

6 Levine P, Celano M, Fenichel R, Pollack W, Singher H. A 'D-like' antigen in rhesus monkey, human Rh positive and human Rh negative red blood cells. *J Immunol* 1961;**87**:747–52.

7 Race RR, Sanger R. *Blood Groups in Man*, 6th edn. Oxford: Blackwell Scientific Publications, 1975.

8 Levine P, Celano MJ, Wallace J, Sanger R. A human 'D-like' antibody. *Nature* 1963;**198**:596–7.

9 Levine P, Celano MJ. Agglutinating specificity of LW factor in guinea pig and rabbit anti-Rh serums. *Science* 1967;**156**:1744–6.

10 Swanson JL, Azar M, Miller J, McCullough JJ. Evidence

for heterogeneity of LW antigen revealed in a family study. *Transfusion* 1974;**14**:470–4.

11 Swanson J, Matson GA. Third example of a human 'D-like' antibody or anti-LW. *Transfusion* 1964;**4**:257–61.

12 deVeber LL, Clark GW, Hunking M, Stroup M. Maternal anti-LW. *Transfusion* 1971;**11**:33–5.

13 Beck ML. The LW system: a review and current concepts. In: *A Seminar on Recent Advances in Immunohematology.* Arlington: American Association of Blood Banks, 1973:83–100.

14 Giles CM, Lundsgaard A. A complex serological investigation involving LW. *Vox Sang* 1967;**13**:406–16.

15 Sistonen P, Nevanlinna HR, Virtaranta-Knowles K *et al.* Ne^a, a new blood group antigen in Finland. *Vox Sang* 1981;**40**:352–7.

16 Sistonen P. A phenotypic association between the blood group antigen Ne^a and the Rh antigen D. *Med Biol* 1981;**59**:230–3.

17 Sistonen P, Tippett P. A 'new' allele giving further insight into the LW blood group system. *Vox Sang* 1982; **42**:252–5.

18 Mallinson G, Martin PG, Anstee DJ *et al.* Identification and partial characterization of the human erythrocyte membrane component(s) that express the antigens of the LW blood-group system. *Biochem J* 1986; **234**:649–52.

19 Bloy C, Hermand P, Blanchard D *et al.* Surface orientation and antigen properties of Rh and LW polypeptides of the human erythrocyte membrane. *J Biol Chem* 1990;**265**:21482–7.

20 Moore S. Identification of red cell membrane components associated with rhesus blood group antigen expression. In: J-P Cartron, C Rouger, C Salmon, eds. *Red Cell Membrane Glycoconjugates and Related Genetic Markers.* Paris: Librairie Arnette, 1983:97–106.

21 Bloy C, Blanchard D, Hermand P *et al.* Properites of the blood group LW glycoprotein and preliminary comparison with Rh proteins. *Mol Immunol* 1989;**26**: 1013–19.

22 Bloy C, Hermand P, Cherif-Zahar B, Sonneborn HH, Cartron J-P. Comparative analysis by two-dimensional iodopeptide mapping of the RhD protein and LW glycoprotein. *Blood* 1990;**75**:2245–9.

23 Bailly P, Hermand P, Callebaut I *et al.* The LW blood group glycoprotein is homologous to intercellular adhesion molecules. *Proc Natl Acad Sci USA* 1994; **91**:5306–10.

24 Hermand P, Gane P, Mattei MG *et al.* Molecular basis and expression of the LW^a/LW^b blood group polymorphism. *Blood* 1995;**86**:1590–4.

25 Hermand P, Huet M, Callebaut I *et al.* Binding sites of leukocyte β_2 integrins (LFA-1, Mac-1) on the human ICAM-4/LW blood group proteins. *J Biol Chem* 2000;**275**:26002–10.

26 Spring FA, Parsons SF, Ortlepp S *et al.* Intercellular adhesion molecule-4 binds α_4β_1 and α_V-family integrins

through novel integrin-binding mechanisms. *Blood* 2001;**98**:458–66.

27 Hermand P, Le Pennec PY, Rouger P, Cartron J-P, Bailly P. Characterization of the gene encoding the human LW blood group protein in LW+ and LW– phenotypes. *Blood* 1996;**87**:2962–7.

28 Sistonen P, Virtaranta-Knowles K, Denisova R *et al.* The LW^b blood group as a marker of prehistoric Baltic migrations and admixture. *Hum Hered* 1999; **49**:154–8.

29 Giles CM. The LW blood group: a review. *Immunol Commun* 1980;**9**:225–42.

30 Sistonen P, Green CA, Lomas CG, Tippett P. Genetic polymorphism of the LW blood group system. *Ann Hum Genet* 1983;**47**:277–84.

31 White JC, Rolih S, Wilkinson SL, Hatcher BJ, Issitt PD. A new example of anti-LW and further studies on heterogeneity of the system. *Transfusion* 1975;**15**:368–72.

32 Tippett P. *Serological study of the inheritance of unusual Rh and other blood group phenotypes.* PhD thesis, University of London, 1963.

33 Poole J, Ford D, Tozer R *et al.* A case of LW(a–b–) in Papua New Guinea [Abstract]. *24th Congr Int Soc Blood Transfus,* 1996:144.

34 Swanson J, Polesky HF, Matson GA. The LW antigen of adult and infant erythrocytes. *Vox Sang* 1965;**10**:560–6.

35 Gibbs MB. The quantitative relationship of the Rh-like (LW) and D antigens of human erythrocytes. *Nature* 1966;**210**:642–3.

36 Southcott MJG, Tanner MJA, Anstee DJ. The expression of human blood group antigens during erythropoiesis in a cell culture system. *Blood* 1999; **93**:4425–35.

37 Bony V, Gane P, Bailly P, Cartron J-P. Time-course expression of polypeptides carrying blood group antigens during human erythroid differentiation. *Br J Haematol* 1999;**107**:263–74.

38 Lomas CG, Tippett P. Use of enzymes in distinguishing anti-LW^a and anti-LW^ab from anti-D. *Med Lab Sci* 1985;**42**:88–9.

39 Daniels G. Effect of enzymes on and chemical modifications of high-frequency red cell antigens. *Immunohematology* 1992;**8**:53–7.

40 Konigshaus GJ, Holland TI. The effect of dithiothreitol on the LW antigen. *Transfusion* 1984;**24**:536–7.

41 Chown B, Kaita H, Lowen B, Lewis M. Transient production of anti-LW by LW-positive people. *Transfusion* 1971;**11**:220–2.

42 Swanson J, Scofield T, Krivit W *et al.* Donor-derived LW, Rh and M antibodies in post BMT chimera [Abstract]. *Joint Congr Int Soc Blood Transfus and Am Ass Blood Banks,* 1990:34.

43 Perkins HA, McIlroy M, Swanson J, Kadin M. Transient LW-negative red blood cells and anti-LW in a patient with Hodgkin's disease. *Vox Sang* 1977;**33**:299–303.

44 Villalba R, Ceballos P, Fornés G, Eisman M, Gómez Villagrán JL. Clinically significant anti-LW^{ab} by monocyte monolayer assay. *Vox Sang* 1995;**68**:66–7.

45 Komatsu F, Kajiwara M. Transient depression of LW^a antigen with coincident production of anti-LW^{ab} repeated in relapses of malignant lymphoma. *Transfus Med* 1996;**6**:139–43.

46 Reid ME, O'Day TM, Toy PTCY, Carlson T. Anti-LW in a transient LW(a–b–) individual: serologic characteristics and clinical significance. *J Med Technol* 1986; **3**:117–19.

47 Devenish A. An example of anti-LW^a in a 10-month-old infant. *Immunohematology* 1994;**10**:127–9.

48 Napier JAF, Rowe GP. Transfusion significance of LW^a allo-antibodies. *Vox Sang* 1987;**53**:228–30.

49 Perrault R. 'Cold' IgG autologous anti-LW: an immunological comparison with immune anti-LW. *Vox Sang* 1973;**24**:150–64.

50 Sistonen P. *The LW (Landsteiner–Wiener) blood group system: elucidation of the genetics of the LW blood group based on the finding of a 'new' blood group antigen.* PhD thesis, University of Helsinki, 1984.

51 Cummings E, Pisciotto P, Roth G. Normal survival of Rh$_0$(D) negative, LW(a+) red cells in a patient with allo-anti LW^a. *Vox Sang* 1984;**46**:286–90.

52 Chaplin H, Hunter VL, Rosche ME, Shirey RS. Long-term *in vivo* survival of Rh(D)-negative donor red cells in a patient with anti-LW. *Transfusion* 1985;**25**:39–43.

53 Herron R, Bell A, Poole J *et al.* Reduced survival of isotope-labelled Rh(D)-negative donor red cells in a patient with anti-LW^{ab}. *Vox Sang* 1986;**51**:314–17.

54 Levine P. Rh and LW blood factors. *Int Convoc Immunol, Buffalo NY, 1968.* Basel: Karger 1969, 140–3.

55 Celano MJ, Levine P. Anti-LW specificity in autoimmune acquired hemolytic anemia. *Transfusion* 1967;**7**:265–8.

56 Vos GH, Petz LD, Garratty G, Fudenberg HH. Autoantibodies in acquired hemolytic anemia with special reference to the LW system. *Blood* 1973;**42**:445–53.

57 Polesky HF, Swanson J, Olson C. Guinea pig antibodies to ? Rh-Hr precursor. Proc 11th Congr Int Soc Blood Transfus, 1966. *Bibl Haemat* 1968;**29**(1):384–7.

58 Wiener AS, Moor-Jankowski J, Brancato GJ. LW factor. *Haematologia* 1969;**3**:385–93.

59 Wiener AS, Socha WW, Gordon EB. Fractionation of human anti-Rh$_0$ sera by absorption with red cells of apes. *Haematologia* 1971;**5**:227–40.

60 Levine P, Celano MJ, Vos GH, Morrison J. The first human blood, –––/–––, which lacks the 'D-like' antigen. *Nature* 1962;**194**:304–5.

61 Sonneborn H-H, Uthemann H, Tills D *et al.* Monoclonal anti-LW^{ab}. *Biotest Bull* 1984;**2**:145–8.

62 Sonneborn H-H, Ernst M, Voak D. A new monoclonal anti-LW (BS 87) [Abstract]. *Vox Sang* 1994;**67** (Suppl.2):114.

63 Oliveira OLP, Thomas DB, Lomas CG, Tippett P. Restricted expression of LW antigen on subsets of human B and T lymphocytes. *J Immunogenet* 1984;**11**:297–303.

64 Blanchard D, Hermand P, Petit-Le Roux Y, Cartron JP, Bailly P. Preparation of monoclonal antibodies directed against the ICAM-4/LW blood group protein [Abstract]. *Vox Sang* 2000;**78**(Suppl.1):P024.

65 Wang J, Springer TA. Structural specializations of immunoglobulin superfamily members for adhesion to integrins and viruses. *Immunol Rev* 1998;**163**: 197–215.

66 Parsons SF, Spring FA, Chasis JA, Anstee DJ. Erythroid cell adhesion molecules Lutheran and LW in health and disease. *Baillière's Best Prac Clin Haematol* 1999; **12**:729–45.

67 Hynes RO. Integrins: versatility, modulation and signaling in cell adhesion. *Cell* 1992;**69**:11–25.

68 Bailly P, Tontti E, Hermand P, Cartron J-P, Gahmberg CG. The red cell LW blood group protein is an intercellular adhesion molecule which binds to CD11/CD18 leukocyte integrins. *Eur J Immunol* 1995;**25**:3316–20.

69 Hermand P, Gane P, Lucien N, Cartron JP, Bailly P. Erythrocyte restricted expression of the LW blood group antigens [Abstract]. *Transfus Clin Biol* 1996;**3**:52S.

70 Levine P, Celano MJ. Presence of 'D-like' antigens on various monkey red blood cells. *Nature* 1962; **193**:184–5.

71 Shaw M-A. Monoclonal anti-LW^{ab} and anti-D reagents recognize a number of different epitopes: use of red cells of non-human primates. *J Immunogenet* 1986; **13**:377–86.

17 Chido/Rodgers blood group system

17.1 Introduction

Chido and Rodgers antigens are not located on intrinsic red cell structures, but on the fourth component of complement (C4), which becomes bound to the red cells from the plasma. As Chido/Rodgers antigens are readily detected on red cells by conventional blood grouping methods and were considered to be blood group antigens before the association with C4 was disclosed, they have been adopted as the seventeenth blood group system. Currently, nine Chido/Rodgers antigens have been defined [1]: Ch1 to Ch6, Rg1, and Rg2 have frequencies greater than 90%; W.H. has an incidence of about 15%. A complex relationship exists between these nine determinants and polymorphic variation of the C4 α-chain.

In Section 17.2, anti-Ch and -Rg will be considered as simple monospecific antibodies, and their complexities are discussed in Section 17.5.

17.2 Basic serology

Antibodies to a relatively high frequency antigen, called anti-Chido (anti-Ch) by Harris et al. [2], were described as 'nebulous' because antigen strength was variable and difficulty in distinguishing weakly positive from negatively reacting red cells could not be resolved by adsorption experiments. All seven of the original anti-Ch sera were found in multiply transfused patients; in six of them no other atypical antibody was detected [2]. Middleton and Crookston [3] found that the reaction of anti-Ch with Ch+ red cells was inhibited by plasma from Ch+, but not Ch–, individuals. Furthermore, plasma of people with weak Ch expression on their red cells was as effective in inhibition tests as plasma from strongly Ch+ individuals.

Inhibition techniques therefore are more effective than testing of red cells for phenotype determination. Ch– red cells can be converted to Ch+ by incubation in Ch+ plasma [4,5]. About 97% of white donors are Ch+ [3,6]. The gene controlling Ch production is inherited as an autosomal dominant character and the locus is strongly linked to *HLA* [7].

When Longster and Giles [8] described anti-Rg (Rodgers), the resemblance to anti-Ch was patent: the antibody reacted with red cells of about 97% of white people, strength of red cell Rg expression was variable, and the reaction with Rg+ red cells was specifically inhibited by Rg+ plasma. The high frequencies of both Ch and Rg precluded an allelic relationship, yet the excessive rarity of the Ch– Rg– phenotype suggested a genetical association. The locus controlling Rg expression is also very tightly linked to *HLA*, with strong association between Rg– and HLA-B8 [9,10]. The gene producing Rg antigen is inherited in an autosomal dominant fashion [8,9].

About 2.5% of Rg+ plasmas were partially effective in inhibiting anti-Rg and initially appeared to represent a quantitative variant [8]. Partial inhibition of anti-Ch and -Rg was later shown to be caused by some Ch/Rg antisera containing antibodies to more than one determinant [6,11–15]. This polyspecificity became the basis of much of the complexity described in Section 17.5.

Reliable results can be obtained by testing red cells with anti-Ch or -Rg if a suitable technique is used [16,17]. Ch and Rg antigens are expressed less strongly on cord cells than on red cells of adults, although cord and adult plasma are equally effective at inhibiting Ch/Rg antibodies [3,18,19]. The effect of enzymes on Ch and Rg antigens will be described in Section 17.3.

17.3 Ch and Rg antigens are located on C4

C4 is the fourth component of complement, involved in the classical pathway of complement activation. Activation of C1 by binding to IgG or IgM molecules, usually on a cell surface, results in the cleavage of C4 into a small fragment, C4a, and a large fragment, C4b. C4b immediately becomes covalently bonded to the cell surface because of the breaking of an intramolecular thioester bond, a rare type of bond involving the side chains of cysteine and glutamine. When broken, the thioester bond generates a very reactive carbonyl group, which can couple instantaneously to a membrane-bound macromolecule. C4b can then bind C2. The activated C4b,2a complex cleaves C3 and brings about a cascade reaction involving C5–9 and culminating in the puncturing of the cell membrane.

The product of the C4 gene is a pro-C4 molecule, a single polypeptide chain of M_r 200 000, which is subsequently cleaved into α (95 000), β (75 000), and γ (30 000) chains. These three polypeptides are glycosylated and linked together by disulphide bonds (Fig. 17.1). The α-chain occupies most of the molecular surface and is responsible for most of the biological activities of the molecule. C4b represents the whole molecule minus a short N-terminal fragment, C4a. Degradation of membrane-bound C4b, primarily by factor I, releases most of the molecule and leaves C4d covalently bound to the membrane. A similar effect is produced by trypsin treatment of membrane-bound C4b (reviews on complement and C4 in [20,21]).

Structural polymorphism of C4 was first recognized by electrophoresis [22]. Most studies of the C4 polymorphism have employed the technique of immunofixation electrophoresis, in which plasma proteins are separated in agarose gels and the C4 visualized by layering the gel with rabbit antihuman C4 followed by Coomassie brilliant blue protein stain, which reveals the bound antibody. By this method C4 of most people appeared to fall into one of three patterns:

1 four rapidly migrating bands (C4A);
2 four slowly migrating bands (C4B); or
3 both sets of bands together [23,24] (Fig. 17.2).

On the basis of family data, O'Neill *et al.* [24,25] suggested that C4A and C4B were not the products of codominant alleles, but represented genes at two very closely linked loci, *C4A* and *C4B*, with common silent alleles at each locus. People who only have the faster migrating bands are homozygous for the silent allele at the *C4B* locus (*C4B*Q0*, quantity zero) and those who only have the slower bands are homozygous for a silent gene at the *C4A* locus (*C4A*Q0*). People with both sets of bands have at least one active allele at each locus. The excessive rarity of C4 deficiency because of homozygosity for silent alleles at both loci was explained by a high level of linkage disequilibrium between the two loci, so that the haplotype *C4A*Q0 B*Q0* very seldom occurs. For those wishing to read the original papers, it should be pointed out that O'Neill *et al.* [24,25] used the notation C4F (fast) and C4S (slow) for C4A (acidic) and C4B (basic), respectively.

Concurrently with formulating their two-locus theory, O'Neill *et al.* [25] showed that the Ch and Rg antigens are associated with C4. Ch+ Rg+ plasma has both C4A and C4B isotypes, Ch+ Rg– plasma has only C4B, and Ch– Rg+ plasma has only C4A (Fig. 17.2). Ch and Rg antigens therefore appeared to be located on the products of the *C4B* and *C4A* loci, respectively. C4-deficient plasma lacked both Ch and Rg activity, whether the C4-deficient plasma was obtained from rare C4-deficient individuals [25–28] or was produced by removal of C4 from normal plasma by goat anti-C4 on an affinity column [25]. (Apparent Ch/Rg activity of red cells in C4 deficient individuals with Ch– Rg– plasma [26,28,29] could have been because of the presence of contaminating HLA antibodies in the

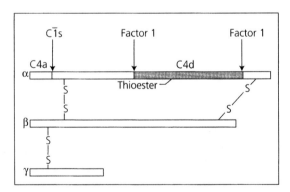

Fig. 17.1 The C4 molecule, showing the three polypeptide chains linked by disulphide bonds, the C4a fragment, which is cleaved by the action of C1s, the site of the thioester bond, which causes the molecule to become covalently bonded to a cell surface, and the C4d region, which carries the Ch and Rg determinants and remains bound to the cell after cleavage of the remainder of the molecule by factor I. After [20].

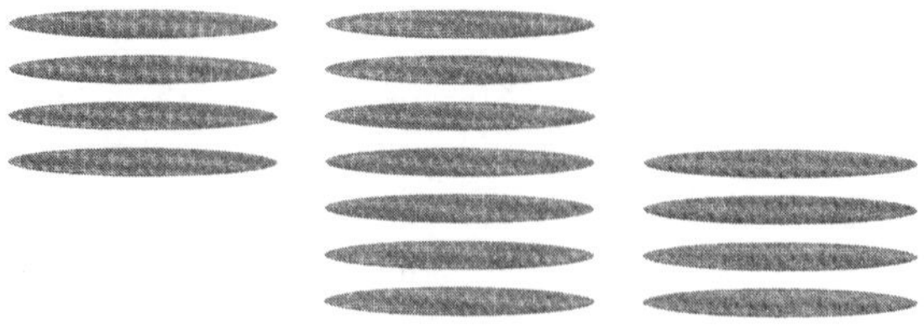

Phenotype	**C4A**		**C4AB**		**C4B**	
	Rg+	Ch–	Rg+	Ch+	Rg–	Ch+
Locus	*C4A*	*C4B*	*C4A*	*C4B*	*C4A*	*C4B*
Possible genotypes	*A/A*	*Q0/Q0*	*A/A* *A/A* *A/Q0* *A/Q0*	*B/B* *B/Q0* *B/B* *B/Q0*	*Q0/Q0*	*B/B*

Fig. 17.2 The common C4 electrophoretic patterns showing C4 and Ch/Rg phenotypes, and suggested C4 genotypes [25]. The extremely rare *C4A*Q0 B*Q0* haplotype is not included.

Ch/Rg reagents [28].) Red cells coated with C4 *in vitro* are directly agglutinated by anti-Ch and -Rg; antibodies that would normally require antihuman globulin to agglutinate the same red cells when uncoated [30]. C4-coated red cells acquire the Ch/Rg phenotype of the serum donor. Ch and Rg determinants on C4-coated red cells are relatively resistant to trypsin cleavage and must reside on the C4d fragment remaining bound to the red cell after trypsin cleavage of C4b [30]. Ch/Rg activity of uncoated red cells probably results from low level adsorption of C4 *in vivo*, either via the classical pathway or by spontaneous cleavage of the thioester [31]. The two-locus theory of O'Neill *et al.* for genetic control of C4 and of Ch/Rg expression has been confirmed, but the situation has become very complex. Some of these complexities will be described in Sections 17.4 and 17.5.

The usual technique for coating red cells with C4 for serological purposes involves dropping freshly drawn citrated blood into a low ionic-strength 10% sucrose solution [30,32]. These red cells are coated with C4 and C3 and are useful either for Ch/Rg typing by direct agglutination with appropriate antibodies or as indicator cells in Ch/Rg plasma inhibition tests. If red cells coated with C4 from another person are required, washed cells are mixed with the required fresh plasma (ABO compatible) and added to the sucrose solution. Trypsin treatment of cells coated with C4 and C3 cleaves the C3 and C4b leaving C4d coated cells. Red cells can also be coated with C4 *in vitro* or *in vivo* by complement fixing IgM antibodies [30].

Serological tests suggest that Ch and Rg antigens on native 'uncoated' red cells, but not on cells coated with C4 by the 10% sucrose method, are denatured by the proteases trypsin, chymotrypsin, papain, ficin, and pronase [3,8,18,19,30]. By counting red cell bound C4d molecules with a radiolabelled monoclonal anti-C4d, Giles *et al.* [33] showed that trypsin treatment reduces the number of detectable C4d molecules by about 50%. This reduces the number of C4d molecules on native cells, but not on coated cells, to a level below the threshold required for detection by agglutination tests with anti-Ch and -Rg. Ch and Rg antigens on native and coated cells are resistant to removal by chloroquine or sulphydryl reagents, evidence that the small quantities of C4d on native red cells are covalently bound. C4 binding to red cells appears to be dependent on sialic acid. Sialidase treatment of red cells coated *in vitro* with C4 had no affect on Ch/Rg expression, but native cells treated with sialidase could no longer be C4 coated by the 10% sucrose method [34]. Red cells of the En(a–) and M^k phenotypes, which lack the major red cell sialic acid-rich glycoprotein, glycophorin A (GPA, Section 3.6), had weakened expression of Ch, and some examples also reacted weakly with anti-Rg [35].

There are four basic serological methods for determining Ch/Rg phenotypes:

1 testing of the subject's red cells with anti-Ch and -Rg;

2 inhibition of anti-Ch and -Rg with the subject's plasma;

3 testing of the subject's red cells coated with C4 from their own plasma; and

4 testing of homologous red cells coated with the subject's C4.

17.4 Further complexities of C4

17.4.1 The complex polymorphisms of C4

Following the detection of two structural loci for C4 [24,25] and improved methods of electrophoretic separation of desialylated C4 proteins, a host of C4 variants were recognized and a variety of different notations used [36–39]. In 1983 Mauff and 21 other authors [40] representing all of the major laboratories working on C4 genetics agreed upon a single nomenclature for C4, which has subsequently been modified [41–43]. As the 1983 nomenclature is used in most publications on the complexities of C4 and Ch/Rg, that nomenclature is used in this chapter. The protein products of *C4A* generally have the most acidic (anodal) migration on agarose gel electrophoresis and the products of *C4B* generally have the more basic (cathodal) migration. The C4 variants or allotypes are numbered, the most common being *C4A 3* and *C4B 1*. Their genes are designated *C4A*3* and *C4B*1*, respectively. C4A Q0 and C4B Q0 represent unexpressed allotypes. There are at least 24 alleles at the *C4A* locus and 27 at the *C4B* locus, including a silent allele, *C4A*Q0* and *C4B*Q0*, at each [43]. In white people there are four *C4A* and three *C4B* alleles occurring with frequencies greater than 1% and producing variants with different electrophoretic mobilities: *C4A*2*, *C4A*3*, *C4A*4*, *C4A*6*, *C4B*1*, *C4B*2*, and *C4B*3*.

How are the products of the *C4A* and *C4B* genes distinguished? This is far from straightforward, although a variety of techniques is available.

17.4.1.1 Agarose gel immunofixation electrophoresis of desialylated plasma

This method is briefly described in Section 17.3. Although most C4A proteins migrate anodally with respect to C4B proteins, there is some overlap, preventing precise definition by this method alone.

17.4.1.2 SDS polyacrylamide gel electrophoresis

The α-chains of C4A and C4B differ by M_r 2000, as determined by SDS PAGE [44–46]: C4A 96 000; C4B 94 000. This is ascertained most effectively by immunoblotting with anti-C4, anti-Ch, or anti-Rg [45,46]. The difference in apparent M_r is probably caused by differences in configuration. Other differences in banding patterns may also be detected by immunoblotting [47].

17.4.1.3 Functional assays

C4B is significantly more active than C4A in haemolytic overlay experiments [37]. Agarose gels containing separated plasma components are examined for haemolysis after being overlaid with red cells sensitized with a complement-fixing antibody and C4-deficient serum to provide all of the other complement components. C4A binds more effectively than C4B to amino acid, whereas C4B binds more effectively to hydroxyl groups [48].

17.4.1.4 Ch and Rg typing

In most cases, C4A expresses Rg and C4B expresses Ch. Exceptions to this rule represent 'reversed antigenicity' [46,49]. For example, C4A 1 reacts with anti-Ch but not anti-Rg; C4B 5 (now called C4B 45) reacts with anti-Rg and with only some anti-Ch. The complexities of Ch and Rg are described in Section 17.5.

17.4.2 Molecular genetics of C4

C4A is 22 kb long and consists of 41 exons; *C4B* is 22 or 16 kb long, the shorter gene resulting from the loss of a 6.8-kb intron [50,51]. Both coding and noncoding regions of *C4A* and *C4B* are highly conserved. There is over 99% identity between the DNA nucleotide sequences of the two genes and between the amino acid sequences of the two proteins [52]. Eight amino acid changes within a region of the C4d fragment of the α-chain, close to the thioester bond, account for differences between isotypes (C4A and C4B) and allotypes (variants of these proteins) [52–55]. Four amino acid residues encoded by exon 26 determine isotype: the sequence for residues 1101–1106 of the pro-C4 molecule is *Pro-Cys*-Pro-Val-*Leu-Asp* in C4A and *Leu-Ser*-Pro-Val-*Ile-His* in C4B. *C4A* and *C4B* are distinguished by an *N1aIV* restriction fragment-length polymorphism (RFLP) [56]. Amino acid substitutions at positions 1054, 1157, 1188, and

1191, encoded by exons 25 and 28, account for the C4 allotypes and the various Ch and Rg determinants (Table 17.1). A detailed structural model to explain the location of Ch/Rg antigenic determinants and their correlation with the C4A and C4B isotypes [57] is described in Section 17.5.

Other complications occur that affect the C4 haplotype. Duplicated C4 genes appear to be quite common [13,39,59–61]: C4A*3 A*2 and C4B*2 B*1 both have frequencies close to 1% in Caucasians. There is also a high incidence of null alleles, about half of which result from a 28-kb DNA deletion [62,63]. Carroll et al. [62] have proposed that gene duplications and deletions may have arisen by gene misalignment and unequal crossing-over, as shown in Fig. 17.3. C4A*Q0 also results from a 2-bp insertion in exon 29 generating a stop codon in exon 30 [64]. Alternatively, a C4B gene may appear to be absent because it has been changed to an identical copy of its neighbouring C4A homologue by a process of gene conversion [65,66]. Intragenic unequal crossing-over, resulting in C4A/B hybrid genes, could explain reversed antigenicity—C4A variants that express Ch determinants and C4B variants that express Rg [46,67] (mechanisms of unequal crossing-over and gene conversion are discussed in Section 3.10). RFLP analysis of 76 haplotypes revealed that 58 had two C4 genes, 12 had one C4 gene, and six had three C4 genes [68].

C4B is flanked by the steroid 21-hydroxylase (cytochrome P450) gene CYP21B and C4A by its pseudogene CYP21A (Fig. 17.3). These loci are closely linked on chromosome 6 in the class III region of the major histocompatibility complex (Chapter 32).

17.5 Further complexities of Chido and Rodgers

Detection by plasma inhibition methods of three Rodgers phenotypes, Rg+ , Rg–, and Rg partial inhibitor [8], and of four Chido phenotypes, Ch+, Ch–, and two types of Ch partial inhibitor [6,11], led Giles [6,14,15] to isolate two Rodgers and three Chido antibodies. Anti-Rg1, -Rg2, -Ch1, -Ch2, and -Ch3 define antigens of relatively high incidence. Rg+ plasmas are Rg:1,2; Rg– are Rg:–1,–2; and Rg partial inhibitors are Rg:1,–2. Rg:–1,2 has not been found and if the model of Yu et al. [57] is correct (see below) does not exist. Ch+ plasmas are Ch:1,2,3, Ch– are Ch:–1,–2,–3, and the two types of Ch partial inhibitors are

Table 17.1 Sequence analysis of different C4 allotypes of known antigenic status (from [57,58]).

Allotype	Amino acid residues from N-terminus								Ch/Rg expression								
	1054	1101	1102	1105	1106	1157	1188	1191	Rg1	Rg2	Ch1	Ch2	Ch3	Ch4	Ch5	Ch6	WH
C4A 3	Asp	Pro	Cys	Leu	Asp	Asn	Val	Leu	+	+	–	–	–	–	–	–	
C4A 1	Gly	Pro	Cys	Leu	Asp	Ser	Ala	Arg	–	–	+	–	+	–	+	+	
C4B 3	Gly	Leu	Ser	Ile	His	Ser	Ala	Arg	[–]	–	+	+	+	–	+	+	
C4B 1	Gly	Leu	Ser	Ile	His	Asn	Ala	Arg	[–]	–	+	+	–	+	+	–*	
C4B 2	Asp	Leu	Ser	Ile	His	Ser	Ala	Arg	[+]	–	+	–	+	+	–	–*	
C4B 5†	Asp	Leu	Ser	Ile	His	Ser	Val	Leu	+	–	–	–	–	+	–	+	+

* Assumed phenotype.
† Now called C4B 45 [42].

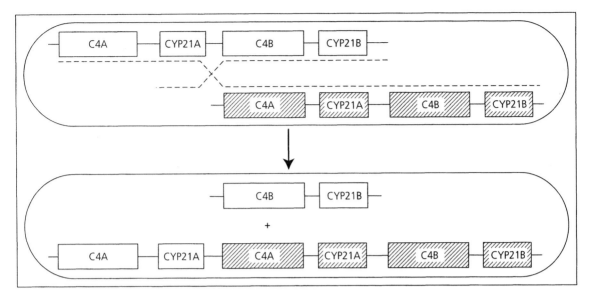

Fig. 17.3 Model demonstrating gene misalignment and unequal crossing-over between homologous chromosomes resulting in deletion of *C4A* and *CYP21* on one chromosome and duplication of *C4A* and *CYP21A* on the other [62].

Table 17.2 Ch (1–3) and Rg phenotypes and frequencies in English (309 tested) and Japanese (89 tested) donors [1,6,70].

Phenotype	English (%)	Japanese (%)
Rg:1,2	95	100
Rg:1,–2	3	0
Rg:–1,–2	2	0
Ch:1,2,3	88	75
Ch:1,–2,3	5	24
Ch:1,2,–3	3	0
Ch:–1,–2,–3	4	1
Ch:–1,2,–3	Very rare	
Ch:1,–2,–3	Very rare	

Ch:1,–2,3 and Ch:1,2,–3. Ch:–1,2,–3 and Ch:1,–2,–3 are extremely rare variants [61,69]; Ch:–1,2,3 and Ch:–1,–2,3 have not been detected and may not exist [57]. The frequencies of these phenotypes are shown in Table 17.2. All C4 molecules express either Rg1 or Ch1; no C4 molecule expresses both. Ch1, Ch2, and Ch3 can be detected on uncoated red cells [19].

Ch and Rg phenotypes do not correlate with specific C4 allotypes in a straightforward manner (Table 17.3), although a few generalizations can be made [67]. Of the partial inhibitor phenotypes, Rg:1,–2 is

found predominantly with the haplotype *C4A*3 A*2 B*Q0*, there is a strong association between Ch:1,–2,3 and *C4B*2*, and Ch:1,2,–3 is most frequently associated with *C4A*6 B*1*, but also with *C4A*3 B*1*.

Further complexities arose with the detection by Giles [72] of another three high frequency Ch determinants, Ch4, Ch5 and Ch6. Antibodies to these specificities can only be reliably detected by testing polyspecific anti-Ch reagents with Ch:–1,–2,–3 red cells coated with C4 of various allotypes, especially those of reversed Ch/Rg antigenicity. Ch4 was detected on all C4B allotypes and Ch4 is not produced by any haplotypes with *C4B*Q0*, including *C4A*1 B*Q0*, which produces Ch1 and Ch3 in the absence of Rg1 and Rg2. Ch5 associates with Ch2 on C4B; Ch2 is only present on C4B, but Ch5 is also detected on C4A 1. Ch6 is associated with Ch3 on C4B, but, unlike Ch3, Ch6 is always detected on Rg:1,–2 C4 allotypes.

Another Ch/Rg antibody, W.H., was identified in the serum of a multiply transfused man, which also contained anti-Ch1 and -Ch4 [58]. W.H. expression is associated with allotypes producing Ch6 and Rg1 in the absence of Rg2 [58,73].

All Rg antisera contain anti-Rg1 and anti-Rg2 [14,15]; with very rare exceptions [74] all Ch antisera contain anti-Ch1, which is often the only specificity [14,15]. The approximate frequencies with which

Table 17.3 Nine antigenic determinants and one hypothetical determinant (Rg3) in 16 combinations predicted by Yu *et al.* [57] and Giles and Jones [58], 13 of which have been detected (from Giles [71]). The 1983 allotype nomenclature is used.

No.	Rg1	Rg2	(Rg3)*	Ch1	Ch2	Ch3	Ch4	Ch5	Ch6	WH	C4 isotype	Associated C4 allotype(s)
1	+	+†	+	−	+	−	+	+	−	−	B	B3
2	+	+	+	−	−	−	−	+	−	−	A	A3
3	+	+	+	−	−	−	+	−	−	−	B	B5
4	+	+	+	−	−	−	−	−	−	−	A	A1‡ A2 A3 A4 A5 A6
5	+	−†	−	−	+	−	+	+	+	+	(B)	Not found
6	+	−	−	−	−	−	+	+	+	+	A	A3 A(3,2)§
7	+	−†	−	−	−	−	+	−	+	+	B	B5
8	+	−	−	−	−	−	−	+	+	+	A	A3
9	−	−†	+	+	+	−	+	+	−	−	B	B1 B3
10	−	−†	+	+	−	−	−	+	−	−	(A)	Not found
11	−	−†	+	+	−	−	+	−	−	−	(B)	Not found
12	−	−†	+	+	−	−	−	−	−	−	A	A1‡
13	−	−	−	+	+	+	+	+	+	−	B	B1 B3
14	−	−	−	+	−	+	−	+	+	−	A	A1‡
15	−	−	−	+	−	+	+	−	+	−	B	B2 B3 B5 B6
16	−	−†	−	+	−	+	−	−	+	−	A	A1‡

*Hypothetical determinant.
†Predicted Rg phenotype not detected by haemagglutination inhibition.
‡C4 A1 is a heterogeneous electrophoretic group of allotypes.
§Duplicated C4A haplotypes.

each of the other specificities have been found in anti-Ch reagents are as follows: anti-Ch2, 25%; anti-Ch3, 10%; anti-Ch4, 75%; anti-Ch5, 16%; and two examples each of anti-Ch6 and W.H. antibody [1]. Rg antibodies are only found in Rg:−1,−2 individuals. Ch antibodies are usually found in people with the Ch:−1,−2,−3,−4,−5,−6 phenotype, but a few exceptions are reported: anti-Ch2 plus -Ch5 in a Ch:1,−2,3,4,−5,6 person [74]; anti-Ch2 plus -Ch4 in a Ch:1,−2,3,−4,5,6 person [75]; anti-Ch1 in a Ch:−1,−2,−3,−4,5,6 person [76]; and anti-Ch1, -Ch3, and -Ch4 in a Ch:−1,−2,−3,−4,5 person [76]. Serum of a Ch– Rg– C4-deficient patient contained an antibody to C4d not recognizable as any Ch or Rg antibody, although traces of anti-Ch and -Rg may also have been present [28].

From serological data on the two Rg and six Ch determinants, and from derived amino acid sequences of several C4 allotypes, Yu *et al.* [57] devised a model to explain Ch/Rg antigenicity. The model is represented in the diagram in Fig. 17.4 and in some of the data presented in Table 17.1. The model involves the concept of sequential epitopes and conformational epitopes. Expression of a sequential epitope is dependent on one

or more amino acid residues within a single sequence of a few residues. Conformational epitopes are more dependent on the shape of the molecule and require the presence of more than one sequential epitope. Ch1 and Ch6 are sequential epitopes: Ch1 requires Ala1188 and Arg1191; Ch6 requires Ser1157. Ch3, a conformational epitope, requires the presence of both Ch1 and Ch6. Ch4 and Ch5 are sequential epitopes: Ch4 requires Leu1101, Ser1102, Ile1105, and His1106 (defining the C4B isotype); Ch5 requires Gly1054. The conformational epitope Ch2 requires the presence of both Ch4 and Ch5. Rg1, a sequential epitope, requires Val1188 and Leu1191. Rg2, a conformational epitope, requires the expression of Rg1 and Asn1157. Asn1157 was assumed to represent a sequential epitope called Rg3, although no anti-Rg3 has been found. W.H. represents a conformational epitope expressed when valine and leucine occupy 1188 and 1191, respectively (Rg1) and when Ser1157 (Ch6) is present [58]. A study of 325 families supported the extended model without exception [71]. The model allows for the 16 possible combinations shown in Tables 17.3, 13 of which have been recognized.

In addition to anti-Rg1 and -Rg2, two of 10 Rg anti-

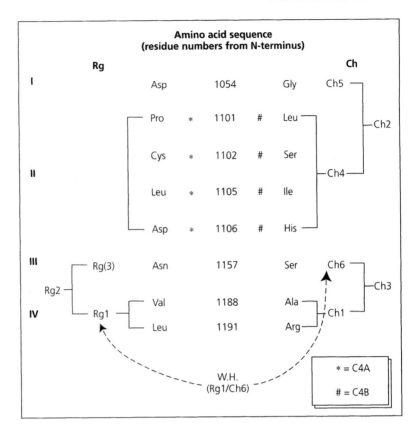

Fig. 17.4 A structural model for the location of Ch/Rg determinants on C4 [57,71]. Ch1, Ch4, Ch5, Ch6, and Rg1 represent sequential epitopes; Ch2, Ch3, Rg2, and W.H. represent conformational epitopes involving two sequential epitopes; Rg(3) represents a hypothetical sequential epitope.

sera contained an antibody specific for an epitope on the β-chain of C4 [77]. The antibody could not be separated from anti-Rg2 and a strong, but incomplete, association exists between Rg2 and the β-chain epitope.

C4 genes producing Ch1 or Rg1 determinants can be distinguished by an *EcoO* 109 RFLP, regardless of C4A or C4B isotype [56]. A polymerase chain reaction (PCR)-based method combining isotype- and allele-specific amplification with sequence-specific primers enables the prediction of all Ch and Rg determinants [78,79]. This has led to the proposal of a new four-digit nomenclature for C4 allotypes, in which the first two digits represent the protein allotype as defined by immunofixation agarose gel electrophoresis and the second two digits represent the genotypic combination of Ch/Rg epitopes [79].

17.6 ISBT terminology

According to the International Society of Blood Transfusion (ISBT) terminology, Chido/Rodgers is system 17 and has the symbol CH/RG. Antigens Ch1 to Ch6 are CH/RG1 to CH/RG6, WH is CH/RG7, Rg1 is CH/RG11, and Rg2 is CH/RG12. Numbers CH/RG8 to CH/RG10 are available for additional Ch antigens.

17.7 Chido/Rodgers antibodies

Details of the specificities of Ch and Rg antibodies are described in Section 17.5.

17.7.1 Clinical significance

Ch/Rg antibodies are IgG, mostly IgG2 and IgG4 [80]; they are not considered clinically significant from the red cell transfusion aspect. Ch/Rg antibodies have not caused any obvious signs of haemolytic transfusion reactions and radiolabelled Ch+ cells transfused to patients with anti-Ch survive normally [2,81–86]. However, anti-Ch and -Rg have been implicated in severe anaphylactic reactions following infusion of fresh frozen plasma, plasma fraction, or platelet concentrates containing plasma [87–89], although these events are exceptional.

421

17.7.2 Monoclonal antibodies

A number of murine monoclonal antibodies to epitopes on C4d have been produced. Their specificities are close to anti-Ch1, -Rg1, and -Ch3 [90–92].

17.8 Associations with disease

C4 deficiency and its associated Ch/Rg-null phenotype are accompanied by the autoimmune disease systemic lupus erythematosus (SLE) in all but four of 18 published cases [93]. This association may result from ineffective dissolution and removal of immune aggregates in the absence of C4 [20].

There is a significantly greater susceptibility to SLE in individuals with a *C4A* gene deletion (*C4A*Q0*) than in the general population [94–97]. It is not surprising therefore that symptoms of SLE have been diagnosed in substantially more Rg– individuals, mostly homozygous for *C4A*Q0*, than Rg+ people [98]. *C4A*Q0* has also been associated with several other autoimmune diseases, including Graves' disease and rheumatoid arthritis [93].

References

1 Giles CM. Antigenic determinants of human C4, Rodgers and Chido. *Exp Clin Immunogenet* 1988;5:99–114.
2 Harris JP, Tegoli J, Swanson J et al. A nebulous antibody responsible for cross-matching difficulties (Chido). *Vox Sang* 1967;12:140–2.
3 Middleton J, Crookston MC. Chido-substance in plasma. *Vox Sang* 1972;23:256–61.
4 Molthan L. The Chido antigen: some developments [Abstract]. *Joint Mtg Am Assoc Blood Banks and Int Soc Haematol* 1972:57.
5 Swanson JL. Laboratory problems associated with leukocyte antibodies. In: *A Seminar on Recent Advances in Immunohematology*. Arlington: American Association of Blood Banks 1973, 121–55.
6 Giles CM. A new genetic variant for Chido. *Vox Sang* 1984;46:149–56.
7 Middleton J, Crookston MC, Falk JA et al. Linkage of Chido, HL-A. *Tissue Antigens* 1974;4:366–73.
8 Longster G, Giles CM. A new antibody specificity, anti-Rg^a, reacting with a red cell and serum antigen. *Vox Sang* 1976;30:175–80.
9 Giles CM, Gedde-Dahl T, Robson EB et al. Rg^a (Rodgers) and the HLA region: linkage and associations. *Tissue Antigens* 1976;8:143–9.
10 James J, Stiles P, Boyce F, Wright J. The HL-A type of Rg(a–) individuals. *Vox Sang* 1976;30:214–16.
11 Nordhagen R, Olaisen B, Teisberg P, Gedde-Dahl T. Association between the electrophoretically-determined *C4M* haplotype product and partial inhibition of anti-Ch^a. *J Immunogenet* 1980;7:301–6.
12 Nordhagen R, Olaisen B, Teisberg P, Gedde-Dahl T. Heterogeneity of the Chido and Rodgers antigens. *Proc 9 Int Tagung Gesellschafr Forens Blutgruppenkunde* 1981: 507–517.
13 Nordhagen R, Olaisen B, Teisberg P, Gedde-Dahl T, Thorsby E. C4 haplotype products and partial inhibition of anti-Rodgers sera. *J Immunogenet* 1981;8:485–91.
14 Giles CM. 'Partial inhibition' of anti-Rg and anti-Ch reagents. I. Assessment for Rg/Ch typing by inhibition. *Vox Sang* 1985;48:160–6.
15 Giles CM. 'Partial inhibition' of anti-Rg and anti-Ch reagents. II. Demonstration of separable antibodies for different determinants. *Vox Sang* 1985;48:167–73.
16 Rittner Ch, Tippett P, Giles CM et al. An international reference typing for Ch and Rg determinants on rare human C4 allotypes. *Vox Sang* 1984;46:224–34.
17 Lomas CG, Green CA, Atkins C, Daniels GL, Tippett P. A simple method for Ch and Rg testing. *Med Lab Sci* 1983;40:65–6.
18 Nordhagen R, Heier Larsen AM, Beckers D. Chido, Rodgers and C4: *in vivo* and *in vitro* coating of red blood cells, grouping and antibody detection. *Vox Sang* 1979; 37:170–8.
19 Atkins CJ. *Chido and Rodgers: a serological study of their variations on the red cell and in plasma*. MSc thesis, Brunel University, 1985.
20 Porter RR. Complement polymorphism, the major histocompatibility complex and associated diseases: a speculation. *Mol Biol Med* 1983;1:161–8.
21 Law SKA, Reid KBM. *Complement*, 2nd edn. Oxford: IRL Press, 1995.
22 Rosenfeld SI, Ruddy S, Austen KF. Structural polymorphism of the fourth component of human complement. *J Clin Invest* 1969;48:2283–92.
23 Teisberg P, Åkesson I, Olaisen B, Gedde-Dahl T, Thorsby E. Genetic polymorphism of C4 in man and localisation of a structural C4 locus to the HLA gene complex of chromosome 6. *Nature* 1976;264:253–4.
24 O'Neill GJ, Yang SY, Dupont B. Two *HLA*-linked loci controlling the fourth component of complement. *Proc Natl Acad Sci USA* 1978;75:5165–9.
25 O'Neill GJ, Yang SY, Tegoli J, Berger R, Dupont B. Chido and Rodgers blood groups are distinct antigenic components of human complement C4. *Nature* 1978; 273:668–70.
26 O'Neill GJ. The genetic control of Chido and Rodgers blood group substances. *Semin Hematol* 1981;18:32–8.
27 Crookston MC, Tilley CA. Antigens acquired from plasma by red cells and lymphocytes: ABH, Lewis, and C4 (Chido and Rodgers). In: C Salmon, ed. *Blood Groups and Other Red Cell Surface Markers in Health and Disease*. New York: Masson, 1982:111–23.

28 Giles CM, Swanson JL. Anti-C4 in the serum of a transfused C4-deficient patient with systemic lupus erythematosus. *Vox Sang* 1984;46:291–9.

29 O'Neill GJ, Berger R, Ballow M, Yunis EJ, Dupont B. Chido, Rodgers and C4 deficiency. *Transplant Proc* 1979;11:1941–3.

30 Tilley CA, Romans DG, Crookston MC. Localisation of Chido and Rodgers determinants to the C4d fragment of human C4. *Nature* 1978;276:713–5.

31 Atkinson JP, Chan AC, Karp DR *et al.* Origin of the fourth component of complement related Chido and Rodgers blood group antigens. *Complement* 1988; 5:65–76.

32 Giles CM. Antigens in plasma. In: *A Seminar on Antigens on Blood Cells and Body Fluids.* Arlington: American Association of Blood Banks, 1980:33–49.

33 Giles CM, Davies KA, Walport MJ. *In vivo* and *in vitro* binding of C4 molecules on red cells: a correlation of numbers of molecules and agglutination. *Transfusion* 1991;31:222–8.

34 Wilfert K, Atkins CJ, Tippett P. Ch and Rg antigens on sialidase treated red cells [Abstract]. *Transfus Med* 1991;1(Suppl.2):57.

35 Tippett P, Storry JR, Walker PS, Okubo Y, Reid ME. Glycophorin A-deficient red cells may have a weak expression of C4-bound Ch and Rg antigens. *Immunohematology* 1996;12:4–7.

36 Olaisen B, Teisberg P, Jonassen R, Gedde-Dahl T. The C4 system: formal and population genetics. *Hum Genet* 1979;50:187–92.

37 Awdeh ZL, Alper CA. Inherited structural polymorphism of the fourth component of human complement. *Proc Natl Acad Sci USA* 1980;77:3576–80.

38 Mauff G, Bender K, Giles CM *et al.* Human C4 polymorphism: pedigree analysis of qualitative, quantitative, and functional parameters as a basis for phenotype interpretations. *Hum Genet* 1984;65:362–72.

39 Bruun-Petersen G, Lamm LU, Jacobsen BK, Kristensen T. Genetics of complement C4: two homoduplication haplotypes *C4S C4S* and *C4F C4F* in a family. *Hum Genet* 1982;61:36–8.

40 Mauff G, Alper CA, Awdeh Z *et al.* Statement on the nomenclature of human C4 allotypes. *Immunobiology* 1983;164:184–91.

41 Mauff G, Alper CA, Dawkins R *et al.* C4 nomenclature statement (1990). *Complement Inflamm* 1990;7:261–8.

42 WHO-IUIS Nomenclature Sub-Committee. Revised nomenclature for human complement component C4. *Eur J Immunogenet* 1993;20:301–5.

43 Mauff G, Luther B, Schneider PM *et al.* Reference report for complement component C4. *Exp Clin Immunogenet* 1998;15:249–60.

44 Lundwall Å, Hellman U, Eggersten G, Sjöquist J. Isolation of tryptic fragments of human C4 expressing Chido and Rodgers antigens. *Mol Immunol* 1982;19:1655–65.

45 Roos MH, Mollenhauer E, Démant P, Rittner C. A molecular basis for the two locus model of human complement component C4. *Nature* 1982;298:854–6.

46 Roos MH, Giles CM, Demant P, Mollenhauer E, Rittner C. Rodgers (Rg) and Chido (Ch) determinants of human C4: characterization of two C4 B5 subtypes, one of which contains Rg and Ch determinants. *J Immunol* 1984;133:2634–40.

47 Giles CM, Robson T. Immunoblotting human C4 bound to human erythrocytes *in vivo* and *in vitro. Clin Exp Immunol* 1991;84:263–9.

48 Dodds AW, Law S-KA, Porter RR. The purification and properties of some less common allotypes of the fourth component of human complement. *Immunogenetics* 1986;24:279–85.

49 Rittner C, Giles CM, Roos MH, Démant P, Mollenhauer E. Genetics of human C4 polymorphism: detection and segregation of rare and duplicated haplotypes. *Immunogenetics* 1984;19:321–33.

50 Carroll MC, Alper CA. Polymorphism and molecular genetics of human C4. *Br Med Bull* 1987;43:50–65.

51 Yu CY. The complete exon–intron structure of a human complement component *C4A* gene: DNA sequences, polymorphism, and linkage to the 21-hydroxylase gene. *J Immunol* 1991;146:1057–66.

52 Belt KT, Carroll MC, Porter RR. The structural basis of the multiple forms of human complement component C4. *Cell* 1984;36:907–14.

53 Hellman U, Eggertsen G, Lundwall Å, Engström Å, Sjöquist J. Primary sequence differences between Chido and Rodgers variants of tryptic C4d of the human complement system. *FEBS Lett* 1984;170:254–8.

54 Belt KT, Yu CY, Carroll MC, Porter RR. Polymorphism of human complement component C4. *Immunogenetics* 1985;21:173–80.

55 Yu CY, Belt KT, Giles CM, Campbell RD, Porter RR. Structural basis of the polymorphism of human complement components C4A and C4B: gene size, reactivity and antigenicity. *EMBO J* 1986;5:2873–81.

56 Yu CY, Campbell RD. Definitive RFLPs to distinguish between human complement C4A/C4B isotypes and the major Rodgers/Chido determinants: application to the study of *C4* null alleles. *Immunogenetics* 1987; 25:383–90.

57 Yu CY, Campbell RD, Porter RR. A structural model for the location of the Rodgers and the Chido antigenic determinants and their correlation with the human complement component C4A/C4B isotypes. *Immunogenetics* 1988;27:399–405.

58 Giles CM, Jones JW. A new antigenic determinant for C4 of relatively low frequency. *Immunogenetics* 1987; 26:392–4.

59 Raum D, Awdeh Z, Andersen J *et al.* Human C4 haplotypes with duplicated C4A or C4B. *Am J Hum Genet* 1984;36:72–9.

60 Carroll MC, Belt T, Palsdottir A, Porter RR. Structure

and organization of the *C4* genes. *Phil Trans R Soc London B* 1984;**306**:379–88.

61 Giles CM, Uring-Lambert B, Boksch W *et al*. The study of a French family with two duplicated C4A haplotypes. *Hum Genet* 1987;**77**:359–65.

62 Carroll MC, Palsdottir A, Belt KT, Porter RR. Deletion of complement C4 and steroid 21-hydroxylase genes in the HLA class III region. *EMBO J* 1985;**4**:2547–52.

63 Schneider PM, Carroll MC, Alper CA *et al*. Polymorphism of the human complement C4 and steroid 21-hydroxylase genes: restriction fragment length polymorphisms revealing structural deletions, homoduplications, and size variants. *J Clin Invest* 1986;**78**:650–7.

64 Barba G, Rittner C, Schneider PM. Genetic basis of human complement C4A deficiency: detection of a point mutation leading to nonexpression. *J Clin Invest* 1993; **91**:1681–6.

65 Palsdottir A, Arnason A, Fossdal R, Jensson O. Gene organization of haplotypes expressing two different C4A allotypes. *Hum Genet* 1987;**76**:220–4.

66 Braun L, Schneider PM, Giles CM, Bertrams J, Rittner C. Null alleles of human complement C4: evidence for pseudogenes at the *C4A* locus and for gene conversion at the *C4B* locus. *J Exp Med* 1990;**171**:129–40.

67 Giles CM, Batchelor JR, Dodi IA *et al*. C4 and *HLA* haplotypes associated with partial inhibition of anti-Rg and anti-Ch. *J Immunogenet* 1984;**11**:305–17.

68 Teisberg P, Jonassen R, Mevåg B, Gedde-Dahl T, Olaisen B. Restriction fragment length polymorphisms of the complement component C4 loci on chromosome 6: studies with emphasis on the determination of gene number. *Ann Hum Genet* 1988;**52**:77–84.

69 Skanes VM, Larsen B, Giles CM. C4B3 allotype with a novel Ch phenotype. *Immunogenet* 1985;**22**:609–16.

70 Giles CM, Tokunaga K, Zhang WJ *et al*. The antigenic determinants, Rg/Ch/WH, expressed by Japanese C4 allotypes. *J Immunogenet* 1988;**15**:267–75.

71 Giles CM, Uring-Lambert B, Goetz J *et al*. Antigenic determinants expressed by human C4 allotypes: a study of 325 families provides evidence for the structural antigenic model. *Immunogenetics* 1988;**27**:442–8.

72 Giles CM. Three Chido determinants detected on the B5Rg+ allotype of human C4: their expression in Ch-typed donors and families. *Hum Immunol* 1987; **18**:111–22.

73 Moulds JM, Roberts SL, Wells TD. DNA sequence analysis of the C4 antigen WH: evidence for two mechanisms of expression. *Immunogenetics* 1996;**44**:104–7.

74 Giles CM, Hoffman M, Moulds M, Harris M, Dalmasso A. Allo-anti-Chido in a Ch-positive patient. *Vox Sang* 1987;**52**:129–33.

75 Fisher B, Laycock C, Poole J, Powell H. A new allo anti-Ch specificity in a patient with a rare Ch positive phenotype [Abstract]. *Transfus Med* 1993;**3**(Suppl.1):84.

76 Poole J, Moulds JM, Fisher B *et al*. Two Ch+ individuals with allo anti-Ch [Abstract]. *Transfusion* 1996;**36**:55S.

77 Robson T, Heard RNS, Giles CM. An epitope on C4 β light (L) chains detected by human anti-Rg: its relationship with β chain polymorphism and MHC associations. *Immunogenetics* 1989;**30**:344–9.

78 Barba GMR, Braun-Heimer L, Rittner C, Schneider PM. A new PCR-based typing of the Rodgers and Chido antigenic determinants of the fourth component of human complement. *Eur J Immunogenet* 1994;**21**:325–39.

79 Schneider PM, Stradman-Bellinghausen B, Rittner C. Genetic polymorphism of the fourth component of human complement: Population study and proposal for a revised nomenclature based on genomic PCR typing of Rodgers and Chido determinants. *Eur J Immunogenet* 1996; **23**:335–44.

80 Szymanski IO, Huff SR, Delsignore R. An autoanalyzer test to determine immunoglobulin class and IgG subclass of blood group antibodies. *Transfusion* 1982;**22**:90–5.

81 Middleton JI. Anti-Chido: a crossmatching problem. *Can J Med Technol* 1972;**34**:41–62.

82 Moore HC, Issitt PD, Pavone BG. Successful transfusion of Chido-positive blood to two patients with anti-Chido. *Transfusion* 1975;**15**:266–9.

83 Tilley CA, Crookston MC, Haddad SA, Shumak KH. Red blood cell survival studies in patients with anti-Ch^a, anti-Yk^a, anti-Ge, and anti-Vel. *Transfusion* 1977; **17**:169–72.

84 Silvergleid AJ, Wells RF, Hafleigh EB *et al*. Compatibility test using ^{51}Chromium-labeled red blood cells in crossmatch positive patients. *Transfusion* 1978;**18**:8–14.

85 Nordhagen R, Aas M. Survival studies of ^{51}Cr Ch(a+) red blood cells in a patient with anti-Ch^a, and massive transfusion of incompatible blood. *Vox Sang* 1979;**37**: 179–81.

86 Strohm PL, Molthan L. Successful transfusion results using Rg(a+) blood in four patients with anti-Rg^a. *Vox Sang* 1983;**45**:48–52.

87 Lambin P, Le Pennec PY, Hauptmann G *et al*. Adverse transfusion reactions associated with a precipitating anti-C4 antibody of anti-Rodgers specificity. *Vox Sang* 1984;**47**:242–9.

88 Westhoff CM, Sipherd BD, Wylie DE, Toalson LD. Severe anaphylactic reactions following transfusions of platelets to a patient with anti-Ch. *Transfusion* 1992;**32**: 576–9.

89 Wibaut B, Mannessier L, Horbez C *et al*. Anaphylactic reactions associated with anti-Chido antibody following platelet transfusions. *Vox Sang* 1995;**69**:150–1.

90 Giles CM, Ford DS. A monoclonal anti-C4d that demonstrates a specificity related to anti-Ch. *Transfusion* 1986;**26**:370–4.

91 Giles CM, Fielder AHL, Lord DK, Robson T, O'Neill GJ. Two monoclonal anti-C4d reagents react with epitopes closely related to Rg:1 and Ch:1. *Immunogenetics* 1987;**26**:309–12.

92 Chrispeels J, Grabbe J, Stradmann B *et al*. Rapid purification of the fourth component of human complement and

production of C4-specific monoclonal antibodies including isotype-specific ones [Abstract]. *Complement* 1987;**4**:142.

93 Moulds JM. Association of blood group antigens with immunologically important proteins. In: G Garratty, ed. *Immunobiology of Transfusion Medicine*. New York: Dekker, 1994: 273–97.

94 Fielder AHL, Walport MJ, Batchelor JR *et al.* Family study of the major histocompatibility complex in patients with systemic lupus erythematosus: importance of null alleles of C4A and C4B in determining disease susceptibility. *Br Med J* 1983;**286**:425–8.

95 Reveille JD, Arnett FC, Wilson RW, Bias WB, McLean RH. Null alleles of the fourth component of complement and HLA haplotypes in familial systemic lupus erythematosus. *Immunogenetics* 1985;**21**:299–311.

96 Dunckley H, Gatenby PA, Hawkins B, Naito S, Serjeantson SW. Deficiency of C4A is a genetic determinant of systemic lupus erythematosus in three ethnic groups. *J Immunogenet* 1987;**14**:209–18.

97 Fan Q, Uring-Lambert B, Weill B *et al.* Complement component C4 deficiencies and gene alterations in patients with systemic lupus erythematosus. *Eur J Immunogenet* 1993;**20**:11–21.

98 Edwards-Moulds J, Arnett FC, Moulds JJ. Increased incidence of Rodgers negative individuals observed in systemic lupus erythematosus patients [Abstract]. *Transfusion* 1989;**29**:16S.

18

Gerbich blood group system

18.1 Introduction

The Gerbich system consists of seven antigens, three of very high frequency and four of low frequency (Table 18.1). They are located on either or both of the red cell membrane sialoglycoproteins, glycophorin C (GPC, CD236C) and glycophorin D (GPD), or on closely related glycoproteins. GPD is a truncate version of GPC. GPC and GPD are produced by the same gene, *GYPC*, as a result of initiation of mRNA translation at two sites. *GYPC* consists of four exons.

There are three rare phenotypes in which the red cells lack one or more of the three high frequency Gerbich antigens. Ge:–2,3,4 (Yus phenotype) and Ge:–2,–3,4 (Gerbich phenotype) result from deletions of *GYPC* exon 2 and exon 3, respectively. Ge:–2,–3,–4 (Leach or Ge-null phenotype) is usually caused by a deletion of exons 3 and 4, although a single nucleotide deletion was involved in one case. The low frequency antigens Wb, An^a, and Dh^a all result from point mutations in *GYPC*; Ls^a arises from a duplication of *GYPC* exon 3.

GYPC is located on chromosome 2q14–q21 (Chapter 32).

18.2 Glycophorin C (GPC) and glycophorin D (GPD), and *GYPC*, the gene that encodes them

18.2.1 Red cell membrane sialoglycoproteins

Glycophorin is a name given to several sialic acid-rich glycoproteins of the red cell membrane that are detected after sodium dodecyl sulphate polyacrylamide gel electrophoresis (SDS PAGE) by periodic acid–Schiff (PAS) staining. The major sialoglycoproteins are glycophorin A (GPA) and glycophorin B (GPB), homologous structures carrying the antigens of the MNS system (Chapter 3). The minor sialoglycoproteins, glycophorin C (GPC) and glycophorin D (GPD), are another pair of homologous structures, which represent about 6% and 1% of PAS staining material, respectively [1]. GPC and GPD carry the Gerbich system antigens. There is no genetical relationship between glycophorins A and B and glycophorins C and D, as they are produced by independent genes on different chromosomes.

A number of synonyms have been used for GPC (CD236C, β-sialoglycoprotein, component D, PAS–2′) and GPD (γ-sialoglycoprotein, component E) (see Table 3.5).

18.2.2 GPC and GPD

The apparent M_r of GPC and GPD on SDS PAGE is 40 000 and 30 000, respectively (reviews in [2–4]). By the use of Fab fragments of monoclonal antibodies, the number of molecules per red cell has been estimated as 143 000 for GPC and 225 000 for GPC plus GPD [5].

The first 47 amino acid residues of GPC were determined by manual sequencing [6]. Colin *et al.* [7] used a mixture of 32 synthetic oligonucleotides, each of which represented the sequence of amino acid residues 19–23 of GPC, as radioactive hybridization probes in order to isolate *GYPC* cDNA from a human reticulocyte cDNA library. From the cloned cDNA the amino acid sequence of GPC shown in Fig. 18.1 was deduced.

GPC has three domains: a glycosylated N-terminal extracellular domain (residues 1–57) containing one N-linked oligosaccharide at Asn8 and sites for 12 O-linked oligosaccharides; a hydrophobic membrane-spanning domain (58–81); and a C-terminal cytoplasmic domain (82–128) [7,8]. The cytoplasmic domain of GPC interacts with the red cell membrane skeleton (Section 18.7). An N-terminal signal peptide is often associated with transmembrane glycoproteins, including GPA and GPB, and cleaved from the mature protein. No such signal peptide is encoded by *GYPC* [8].

The N-terminus of GPD is blocked and only partial amino acid sequences have been determined [9]. For reasons discussed below (Section 18.2.3), GPD is almost certainly a truncate version of GPC, lacking the N-terminal 21 amino acid residues of GPC and identical to residues 22–128 of GPC. This is consistent with the following details:

1 GPD has no *N*-glycosylation;

2 GPD lacks epitopes present on the N-terminal domain of GPC [10];

3 Ge3 antigen, which represents a region around amino acid residues 40–50 of GPC, is also present on GPD [11] (Section 18.3.2.2); and

4 antigenic determinants detected by monoclonal and polyclonal antibodies produced in animals are present on the cytoplasmic domains of both GPC and GPD [9,12,13] (see Fig. 18.3).

18.2.3 GPC and GPD are encoded by the same gene

Despite the high level of homology between GPC and GPD, no homologous gene could be detected in genomic DNA using *GYPC* cDNA as a probe. This led to proposals that a separate GPD gene does not exist and that GPC and GPD are both produced by *GYPC*

Table 18.1 Antigens of the Gerbich system.

No.	Name	Relative frequency	Associated glycophorin
GE2	Ge2	High	GPD N-terminal region
GE3	Ge3	High	GPC amino acids 42–50 and GPD 21–29
GE4	Ge4	High	GPC N-terminal region
GE5	Webb	Low	GPC Asn*8Ser
GE6	Ls^a	Low	GPC and GPD from gene with duplicated exon 3
GE7	An^a	Low	GPD Ala2Ser
GE8	Dh^a	Low	GPC Leu14Phe

N-glycosylated.
Obsolete: GE1.

```
              * * *  ◆  *          *        |  * ***    * * *            *
NH₂  MWSTRSPNST AWPLSLEPDP GMASASTTMH TTTIAEPDPG MSGWPDGRME
GPC  1                     |22                                      50
GPD                        |1                                       29

     TSTPTIMDIV VIAGVIAAVA IVLVSLLFVM LRYMYRHKGT YHTNEAKGTE
GPC  51                                                     100
GPD  30                                                      79

     FAESADAALQ GDPALQDAGD SSRKEYFI  COOH
GPC  101                           128
GPD   80                           107
```

Fig. 18.1 Amino acid sequence of GPC and GPD (see Table 3.6 for code). * Probable sites of O-glycosylation. ◆; Site of N-glycosylation; T, trypsin cleavage site. Underlined sequence represents the membrane-spanning domain. Double underlined are RHK and YFI tripeptides, binding motifs for protein 4.1R and p55, respectively.

427

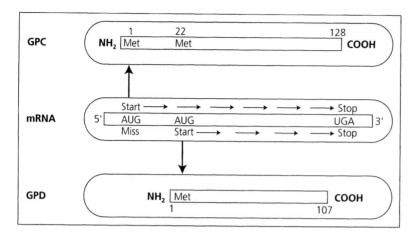

Fig. 18.2 Production of GPC and GPD from a single gene by a process of leaky initiation of mRNA translation. When translation commences at the first AUG start codon a 128 amino acid GPC polypeptide is produced (above). If the first AUG codon is missed, then translation may commence at a second AUG site and a shorter 107-residue GPD polypeptide is produced (below).

[14,15]. As suggested by Tanner *et al.* [15], this occurs as a result of initiation of translation of *GYPC* mRNA at two different sites, to produce two polypeptides.

The process of protein synthesis, in which the nucleotide sequence of mRNA is translated into an amino acid sequence, commences at an AUG codon (a methionine codon, ATG in DNA), although a 10-nucleotide consensus sequence including the AUG codon is also important for effective initiation of translation. Newly processed polypeptides have methionine at their N-terminus, although this is usually cleaved from the mature protein. The RNA sequence around the start codon for GPC (CCAGGAAUGU) does not conform closely with the consensus start sequence (CC(A/G)CCAUGG) found in eukaryote transcripts; the sequence around a downstream AUG triplet (CCGGGGAUGG), the codon for Met22 of GPC, is a closer fit to the consensus sequence [15]. A process referred to as 'leaky initiation of translation' occurs in which the initiation site at the codon for Met1 of GPC is sometimes missed during the scanning of *GYPC* mRNA. Scanning continues along the mRNA until the second initiation site at Met22 is reached, where translation begins to produce GPD, a shorter molecule comprising amino acid residues 22–128 of GPC (Fig. 18.2). *GYPC* cDNA transfected into COS-7 cells produced GPC and GPD, cDNA with a deletion of ATG at position 1 produced only GPD, cDNA with an ATG to ACG mutation at position 22 produced only GPC, and cDNA with ATG to ACG mutations at positions 1 and 22 produced neither glycoprotein [16]. A mutation at nucleotide 4 (ATG T to ATG G), creating a more consensus motif around the first ATG codon, resulted in a

doubling of expression of GPC compared with GPD [16].

18.2.4 Organization of *GYPC*

The 13.5 kb *GYPC* gene is organized into four exons (Table 18.2) [11,17]. Exons 1–3 encode the extracellular domain of GPC, exon 4 the membrane-spanning and cytoplasmic domains. Exons 2 and 3 show a high level of homology, probably arising from exon duplication, although exon 3 contains an insert of 27 nucleotides not present in exon 2, encoding amino acid residues 42–50 of GPC. The intronic flanking regions of exons 2 and 3 demonstrate an even higher level of homology than do the coding regions.

The upstream promoter region *GYPC* contains the ubiquitous *cis*-acting elements, CACC, TATA, and SP1, plus three erythroid-specific GATA-1 binding sites and a binding site for a novel erythroid–megakaryocyte-specific factor, NF-E6 [18,19].

18.3 The high frequency antigens Ge2, Ge3, and Ge4, and the Gerbich-negative phenotypes

18.3.1 Serological history

Gerbich began as a simple, inherited blood group antigen of very high frequency. In 1960 Rosenfield *et al.* [20] described antibodies of apparently identical specificity in three women (including Mrs Gerbich); the families of two of these women showed the antigen

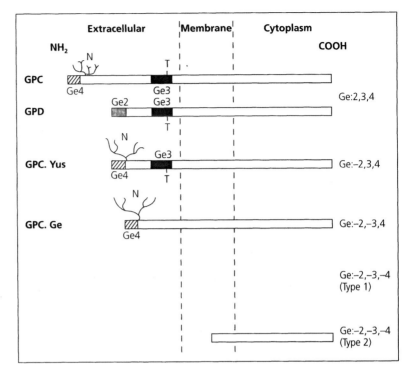

Fig. 18.3 Diagram representing GPC, GPD, and related structures characteristic of Gerbich-negative phenotypes. Ge:2,3,4 cells have both GPC and GPD; Ge:–2,3,4 and Ge:–2,–3,4 cells have GPCYus and GPCGe, respectively, but no GPC or GPD. In most Ge:–2,–3,–4 (Leach phenotype) cells, no GPC, GPD, or related molecule is present (Type 1), but in one example a GPC/D C-terminal fragment was detected (Type 2). T, trypsin cleavage site at Arg48.

Table 18.2 Organization of *GYPC*.

Exon	Amino acid residues		Characteristics
	GPC	GPD	
1	1–16		N-terminus and part of extracellular domain of GPC; *N*-glycan; Ge4
2	17–35	1–14	GPC Met22 (translation initiation site for GPD); part of extracellular domain of GPC and GPD including N-terminus of GPD; Ge2 on GPD
3	36–63	15–42	Part of extracellular domain of GPC and GPD; Ge3 on GPC and GPD; trypsin cleavage site on GPC and GPD
4	64–128	43–107	Membrane-spanning and cytoplasmic domains of GPC and GPD

to be an inherited character. The simplicity of the Gerbich system was short lived. By 1961, there were two types of anti-Gerbich and two Gerbich-negative phenotypes. Cleghorn [21] and Barnes and Lewis [22] found that the red cells of Mrs Yus, a Turkish Cypriot woman, failed to react with two of the original anti-Gerbich sera, but did react with the other, the antibody of Mrs Gerbich herself. The serum of Mrs Yus contained an antibody that reacted with all cells tested apart from her own and those of the original three Gerbich-negatives. Adsorption of Mrs Gerbich's serum with Mrs Yus's cells removed all antibody. Although the Yus type is not strictly Gerbich-negative, as the cells react with the antibody of Mrs Gerbich, it is generally considered Gerbich-negative because the cells fail to react with the majority of antibodies made by Gerbich-negative people [23]. Both Gerbich-negative phenotypes are exceedingly rare in most populations.

Further complexities of the Gerbich system arose from studies of the Melanesians of Papua New Guinea. Not only was Gerbich found to be polymor-

Table 18.3 Gerbich-negative phenotypes.

Ge:-2,3,4	Yus phenotype
Ge:-2,-3,4	Gerbich phenotype
Ge:-2,-3,-4	Leach phenotype

phic among some populations of the north-east coast of New Guinea [24,25], but Booth and McLoughlin [25] found yet another Gerbich-related antibody in a Ge+ Melanesian. This antibody failed to react with Gerbich-negative cells of Gerbich and Yus types, but also did not react with red cells of up to 15% of Ge+ Melanesians. Thus it now appeared that there were at least three types of anti-Gerbich and, in addition to the common Ge+ phenotype and two Gerbich-negative phenotypes, a rare Gerbich phenotype present in some Melanesians. Booth and McLoughlin [25] proposed a numerical notation for Gerbich phenotypes, shown in modified form in Table 18.3. Red cells of the Melanesian phenotype (Ge:-1,2,3) and the two examples of anti-Ge1 [25,26] have not been widely used and are not available for further study. Consequently, Ge1 now appears to be obsolete and the Melanesian phenotype is omitted from Table 18.3.

Some monoclonal antibodies were shown to be related to the Gerbich system because they agglutinated all red cells except those of the Ge:-2,-3 (Gerbich) and Ge:-2,3 (Yus) phenotypes, although they reacted with these cells by an antiglobulin test [27,28]. Anstee *et al.* [28,29] found that red cells of two unrelated Ge:-2,-3 women failed to react with the Gerbich-related monoclonal antibodies by any technique. This new Gerbich-negative phenotype was called the Leach phenotype. An alloantibody in the serum of a Leach phenotype patient [30] behaved in a very similar manner to the monoclonal antibodies and became anti-Ge4. Leach phenotype red cells are Ge:-2,-3,-4; all other red cells have Ge4 (Table 18.3).

18.3.2 High frequency antigens Ge2, Ge3, and Ge4

18.3.2.1 Ge2

Anti-Ge2 is the most common Gerbich alloantibody. It is the antibody characteristic of the Ge:-2,3,4 phenotype, but is also the most frequently encountered antibody in the Ge:-2,-3,4 and Ge:-2,-3,-4 phenotypes.

Of 17 antibodies from Ge:-2,-3 people, only four were anti-Ge3, the other 13 were anti-Ge2 [23]; of the six Leach phenotype individuals with antibody, four had anti-Ge2, one anti-Ge3, and one anti-Ge4 [28,30–33]. Anti-Ge2 has also been called anti-Ge1,2 [25].

Immunoblotting with numerous examples of alloanti-Ge2 demonstrated that the Ge2 antigen is located on GPD, but not on GPC [12,34] (Fig. 18.3). It is on the N-terminal tryptic peptide of GPD (residues 1–27) [34]. Treatment of intact red cells with trypsin or papain destroys Ge2; chymotrypsin and pronase do not [23]. About 50% of anti-Ge2 show a reduction in strength of reaction with sialidase treated cells [23].

As GPC and GPD are encoded by the same gene and GPD is a shorter version of GPC, then GPD cannot have any amino acid sequence that is not present in GPC. Ge2 is usually at the N-terminus of GPD. Anti-Ge2 might recognize an amino acid sequence only when it is in the conformation of the N-terminus of GPD and not when it is an internal sequence within GPC. Alternatively, the Ge2 determinant could involve the free amino group of GPD and the adjacent amino acid sequence. Some anti-Ge2 do not react with red cells after acetylation of membrane proteins with acetic anhydride, suggesting that a free amino group is involved in the epitope detected by those antibodies [35]. Anti-Ge2 probably represents a heterogeneous collection of antibodies that react with epitopes at the N-terminal region of GPD.

18.3.2.2 Ge3

Anti-Ge3 has been found in immunized Ge:-2,-3,4 and Ge:-2,-3,-4 individuals, but is far less common than anti-Ge2 [23,31]. It has been called anti-Ge1,2,3 [25], but adsorption of anti-Ge3 with Ge:-2,3,4 cells removes all antibody; no anti-Ge2 remains [21]; (likewise, no anti-Ge1 remained after adsorption with Ge:-1,2,3 cells [24,25]).

Like Ge2, Ge3 is destroyed by trypsin, but not by chymotrypsin or pronase [23]. Unlike Ge2, Ge3 is resistant to treatment of intact red cells with papain [23,36]. Consequently, papain-treated cells can be used for distinguishing anti-Ge2 and -Ge3 in the absence of the very rare Ge:-2,3,4 cells.

Immunoblotting with human alloantibodies and with rodent monoclonal antibodies showed that Ge3 is present on both GPC and GPD [5,12,34,37,38] (Fig.

18.3). Alloanti-Ge3 eluted from either GPC or GPD on an immunoblot detected both GPC and GPD on a separate immunoblot, showing that anti-Ge3 is a single antibody to an antigen common to both proteins [12].

Ge3 is encoded by exon 3 of *GYPC*. Ge3 is missing in those rare phenotypes resulting from deletion of exon 3, but not from those resulting from a deletion of exon 2 (Section 18.3.3). Exon 2 and exon 3 are very similar apart from a 27 nucleotide insert in exon 3, representing amino acids 42–50 of GPC (21–29 of GPD) (Section 18.2.4), so Ge3 must be in this region. This accords with earlier evidence obtained by haemagglutination inhibition with fragments of GPC [34].

18.3.2.3 Ge4

The only example of alloanti-Ge4 was identified in the serum of a woman with the Ge:–2,–3,–4, Leach phenotype [30]. Anti-Ge4 was also found in the serum of a patient with a transient GPC deficiency [39]. Numerous monoclonal antibodies have been produced that behave serologically as anti-Ge4 [5,10,27–29, 40,41].

Ge4 is usually situated near the N-terminus of GPC and therefore is not on GPD [10,28,29,39] (Fig. 18.3). Detailed analyses of monoclonal antibodies specific for GPC have shown that some require the amino group of Met1 of GPC for binding, whereas others detect other epitopes within the first 21 amino acids of GPC, but not involving Met1 [10,38]. Most required normal O-glycosylation of the GPC for effective binding. Ge4 is destroyed by trypsin and papain treatment of the red cells.

18.3.3 Gerbich-negative phenotypes

Outside Papua New Guinea, Gerbich-negative phenotypes are very rare. Screening of over 44 000 blood samples from white populations with anti-Ge2 or -Ge3 produced only one Gerbich-negative (Table 18.4). Many Gerbich-negative individuals have been studied, ascertained through their antibodies [20–22,28,31–33,39,42,44,45,47–50].

18.3.3.1 Ge:–2,3,4 (Yus phenotype)

Ge:–2,3 appears to be rarer than Ge:–2,–3, but this may reflect different propensities to making antibody [23,49]. Ge:–2,3 has been found in white people (including Arabs, a Turkish Cypriot, and a Middle Eastern Jew) and in black people (including Ethiopian Jews); it has not been found in Papua New Guinea. Family studies demonstrate that Ge:–2,3 phenotype is inherited [20,21,51].

SDS PAGE followed by staining for sialoglycoproteins or by immunoblotting with antibodies to GPC and GPD shows that Ge:–2,3,4 red cells contain no GPC or GPD. However, there is a GPC-like structure (GPCYus), represented on SDS gels by a broad, diffusely staining band of apparent M_r 32 500–36 500, situated between the positions for GPC and GPD

Table 18.4 Frequency studies performed by testing red cells of random individuals with Gerbich antibodies.

Antibody	Population tested		No. tested	No. negative	References
Anti-Ge2	English, Danes, New Zealanders, Californians		28 331	0	[20,21,42,43]
Anti-Ge3	New Yorkers*		11 000	0	[20]
Anti-Ge3	French		5 912	1	[43,44]
		Total	45 243	1	
Anti-Ge2	Melanesians of Papua New Guinea				[25]
	Sepik region		748	182	
	Morobe region		1 014	517	
	Highlands		1 348	1	
Anti-Ge2	Japanese		22 000	0	[45]
Unknown	Thais		4 253	1	[46]

*Including at least 1500 black people and 100 Asians, mostly Chinese.

[12,28,52]. This structure carries Ge4 and Ge3 [12,28] (Fig. 18.3). In red cell membranes from *GYPC/GYPC.Yus* heterozygotes, GPC, GPD, and GPCYus are present [51].

Analysis of genomic DNA and cDNA showed that Ge:–2,3,4 individuals are homozygous for a *GYPC* gene (*GYPC.Yus*) in which the second exon is deleted [11,53,54] (Fig. 18.3). The protein product is a GPC-like molecule (GPCYus) lacking amino acid residues 17–35, with no loss of Ge4 or Ge3 (Fig. 18.3). The sec-ond translation initiation site (Met22) is lost, so no GPD is formed and therefore no Ge2 is expressed.

Ge:–2,3,4 may also result from heterozygosity for *GYPC.Yus* and *GYPC.Ge* [57,58]. Five of 10 Ge:–2,3 propositi were found to have both GPCYus and GPCGe [57].

18.3.3.2 Ge:–2,–3,4 (Gerbich phenotype)

This is the typical Gerbich-negative phenotype, the

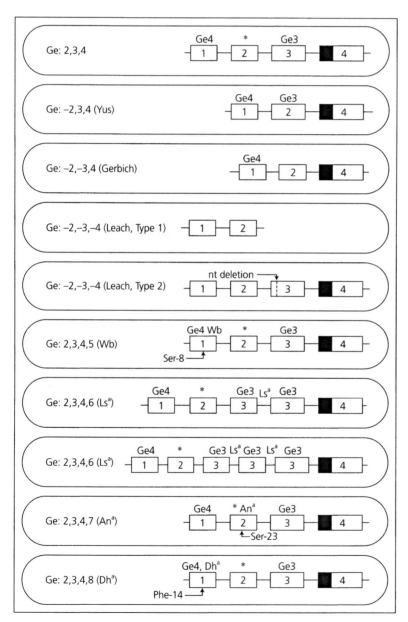

Fig. 18.4 The genomic organization of *GYPC* and variants of *GYPC* responsible for rare Gerbich phenotypes. The boxes represent exons and the shaded area in exon 4 represents the region encoding the membrane-spanning domain. *Second translation start codon (Met22). *GYPC* genes with duplication, triplication, and quadruplication of exon 2 do not result in any qualitative change to the Gerbich phenotype [55,56] and are not shown.

probable phenotype of Mrs Gerbich, although her cells were never tested with anti-Ge4. Ge:–2,–3 is polymorphic in certain regions of Papua New Guinea [25] (Table 18.4). Ge:–2,–3 is rare in all other populations tested, but has been found among people of European and African origin, Native Americans, Japanese, and Polynesians. Family studies demonstrated that Ge:–2,–3 phenotype is inherited [20,44,45,47,51,59].

Like the Ge:–2,3,4 phenotype, Ge:–2,–3,4 cells have no GPC or GPD, but have a diffusely staining abnormal GPC-like structure (GPCGe) of mobility between that of GPC and GPD [12,28,52]. The apparent M_r of GPCGe is 30 500–34 500, slightly less than that of GPCYus. GPCGe carries Ge4, but no Ge3 [12,28] (Fig. 18.3). GPCGe is trypsin-resistant, unlike GPC, GPD, and GPCYus [28]. Consequently, GPC monoclonal antibodies (anti-Ge4) agglutinate trypsin-treated red cells of the Ge:–2,–3,4 phenotype, or cells of individuals heterozygous for the gene responsible for Ge:–2,–3,4, but not trypsin-treated cells of any other Gerbich phenotype.

Ge:–2,–3,4 results from a GYPC gene (GYPC.Ge) with a deletion of exon 3 [11,17,53,58,60] (Fig. 18.4), encoding a GPC-like structure (GPCGe) lacking amino acid residues 36–63 of GPC. GPCGe is slightly smaller than GPCYus because exon 3 is larger than exon 2 owing to a 27-nucleotide insert. Loss of exon 3 also explains absence of Ge3 and of the trypsin cleavage site at Arg48 (Fig. 18.3). However, it does not explain the absence of GPD and therefore of Ge2. Colin et al. [17] suggested that a GPD molecule lacking most of its extracellular domain might not be transported to the membrane or might be unstable and rapidly degraded. GPCGe and GPCYus carry N-glycans with variable numbers of repeating lactosamine units, explaining their diffuse appearance on electrophoresis gels [12]. They may also have altered O-glycosylation [61].

It is probable that GYPC genes with deletions of exon 2 or exon 3 arose from an intragenic unequal crossing-over, an event that would have simultaneously produced genes with duplications of exons 2 or 3 [11,17] (see Fig. 18.5). This topic is returned to in the section on Ls^a (Section 18.4.2).

18.3.3.3 Ge:–2,–3,–4 (Leach phenotype)

The Leach phenotype is the null phenotype of the Gerbich system. Ge:–2,–3,–4 red cells do not react with any Gerbich antibodies or related monoclonal antibodies. Six propositi with the Ge:–2,–3,–4 phenotype have been reported, all white English or North Americans [28,30–33]. Two families have demonstrated inheritance of the Ge:–2,–3,–4 phenotype [31,32]. Ge:–2,–3,–4 red cells are totally devoid of GPC and GPD [11,12,28,31,32] (Fig. 18.3).

Ge:–2,–3,–4 has at least two genetic backgrounds. Southern analysis and polymerase chain reaction (PCR) amplification of genomic DNA from five unrelated Ge:–2,–3,–4 individuals demonstrated a deletion of exons 3 and 4 of GYPC [11,54,62,63] (Fig. 18.4). Surprisingly, mRNA derived from this deleted gene was detected in reticulocytes from Ge:–2,–3,–4 individuals, despite the gene lacking the normal polyadenylation signal [63]. If any protein were produced by this gene, it would lack the membrane-spanning and cytoplasmic domains and could not be inserted into the membrane. In one other Ge:–2,–3,–4 individual [30], GYPC was apparently complete, but sequencing of exon 3 revealed a single nucleotide deletion within codon 45 resulting in a frameshift and premature generation of a stop codon at codon 56 [62] (Fig. 18.4). Consequently, it was predicted that most of exon 3 and all of exon 4 would not be translated and so viable GPC could not be produced. An M_r 12 000 component was detected, however, which bound a monoclonal antibody to an epitope on the cytoplasmic domains of GPC and GPD and appeared to represent the C-terminal domain of GPC/D [64] (Fig. 18.3). This led to speculation that translation is reinitiated at an alternative start sequence overlapping the premature stop codon.

GPC and GPD are associated with the membrane skeleton, probably acting as a link between the membrane and the skeletal proteins (Section 18.7). One characteristic of the Ge:–2,–3,–4 phenotype is elliptocytosis [12,28,29,31,32]. Between 20% and 61% of the red cells of five Ge:–2,–3,–4 phenotype individuals were classed as elliptocytes [31]. Two Ge:–2,–3,–4 brothers had a long-standing history of mild anaemia [33]. Ge:–2,–3,–4 phenotype membranes have reduced mechanical stability [65,66] and may be released into the circulation as normal discocytes, but become distorted when exposed to shear stress and elongation [67]. Elliptocytes were present in a patient with a temporary reduction in red cell membrane GPC content and normal GPD content, but were not present when her GPC levels returned to normal [39].

Ge:−2,−3,4 and Ge:−2,3,4 cells show no sign of ellipto-cytosis [28] and have normal membrane stability [66], despite GPC and GPD deficiency, presumably because of the presence of the GPC-like molecules, GPCGe and GPCYus, in these cells.

18.3.3.4 An unusual Gerbich phenotype resulting from a single base change in *GYPC*

Red cells of a patient with apparent anti-Ge2 reacted with 20 alloanti-Ge2, one autoanti-Ge2, four alloanti-Ge3, and one alloanti-Ge4, but did not react with one alloanti-Ge2, one autoanti-Ge3, and one autoanti-Ge4. Her antibody did not react with her own cells or with those of four of her eight sibs. Immunoblotting of her red cell membranes revealed GPC, GPD, and GPCGe. Molecular genetical analyses showed that she is heterozygous for two rare genes at the *GYPC* locus:
1 *GYPC.Ge* (*GYPC* with a deletion of exon 3); and
2 *GYPC* with an A173T base change in exon 3, encoding Asp58Val in GPC (Asp37Val in GPD) in the region of the insertion of these molecules into the membrane.

The antibody of the propositus, which immunostained GPC on blots of normal red cell membranes, appears to react with GPC with Asp58, but not with Val58. It is unclear why this antibody did not react with GPD or with GPCYus, both of which have aspartic acid at the position equivalent to amino acid 58 of GPC [68].

18.3.3.5 Association with the Kell blood group system

Several reports link the Ge:−2,−3 phenotype with a depression of Kell system antigens, although the effect is variable [23,28,30,31,44,45]. The phenomenon may affect all high frequency Kell antigens and K, if present [44]. Alternatively, K11 antigen may be the only antigen to show weakness [23]. Nine of 11 Ge:−2,−3 samples showed different degrees of weakening of Kell system antigens, whereas none of six Ge:−2,3 samples showed any such Kell depression [23]. At least four Ge:−2,−3,−4 propositi have depression of Kell system antigens [28,30,31].

The genes controlling the Gerbich and Kell systems are independent and located on separate chromosomes. Although the biochemistry and molecular genetics of Gerbich and Kell are well understood, nothing is known about the biochemical nature of their association.

A possible association between Gerbich and the Vel antigen is described in Section 28.2.2.

18.4 Low frequency Gerbich antigens

Four antigens belonging to the Gerbich system have a low frequency in all populations tested. These antigens were all assigned to the Gerbich system through biochemical evidence. No individual homozygous for any of the rare genes responsible for these low incidence antigens has been found, so it must be remembered that in all cases studied a normal *GYPC* gene producing normal GPC and GPD is present.

18.4.1 Wb (GE5)

Wb (Webb) is an inherited low frequency red cell antigen first described by Simmons and Albrey [69] in 1963 (Table 18.5). The original anti-Wb was found in ABO grouping serum [69]; no further example was found in 2000 Australian sera [69], but three examples were detected in 7544 British sera [43,70]. Wb is sensitive to trypsin and sialidase treatment, but resistant to chymotrypsin treatment [65,78,79].

The Wb+ phenotype is associated with a reduced level of normal GPC and with the presence of an abnormal GPC (GPCWb), with an apparent M_r about 3000 lower than that of GPC [78,79]. Treatment of Wb− red cells with endoglycosidase F, which cleaves *N*-linked oligosaccharide chains from glycoproteins, results in a reduction in the apparent M_r of GPC to a similar level to that of GPCWb; treatment of Wb+ cells with endoglycosidase F has no effect on GPCWb.

Amplification and sequencing of exon 1 of *GYPC* from Wb+ individuals revealed an A23G point mutation encoding an Asn8Ser substitution in GPC [53,80] (Fig. 18.4). Asn8 is *N*-glycosylated in GPC and this loss of *N*-glycosylation explains the reduced M_r of GPCWb. Whether Ser8 of GPCWb is *O*-glycosylated has not been determined.

18.4.2 Lsª (GE6)

Lsª (Lewis II) [43] is the same as Rlª [74,81] and is polymorphic in Finns and people of African origin, but rare in other populations (Table 18.5). The original anti-Lsª was found in an anti-B reagent; other exam-

Table 18.5 Frequencies of low frequency Gerbich antigens.

Antigen	Population	No. tested	No. positive	Antigen frequency	References
Wb GE5	White Australians	3 550	2	0.0006	[69]
	English	15 815	3	0.0002	[43]
	Welsh	10 117	8	0.0008	[70]
	Japanese	3 470	0		[71,72]
Lsᵃ GE6	Finnish	1 113	18	0.0162	[43,73]
	Norwegians	7 151	8	0.0011	[74]
	African Americans	110	1	0.0091	[43]
	Black West Indians	878	9	0.0103	[43]
	West Africans	81	2	0.0204	[43]
	Japanese	200 000	8	<0.0001	[75]
	English	5 887	0		[43]
Anᵃ GE7	Finnish	10 000	6	0.0006	[76]
	Swedish	3 266	2	0.0006	[76]
Dhᵃ GE8	Danish	2 493	0		[77]

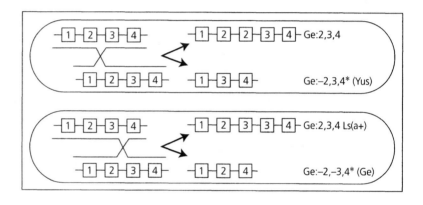

Fig. 18.5 Diagram showing two intragenic unequal crossing-over events resulting in four abnormal *GYPC* genes, two with exon deletions and two with exon duplications. A duplication of exon 3 is associated with Lsᵃ antigen. *The Gerbich-negative phenotypes only occur when there is homozygosity for the aberrant gene (or heterozygosity for two aberrant genes).

ples were found in sera containing multiple antibodies to low frequency antigens [74] and during pretransfusion crossmatching [82]. Anti-Lsᵃ was associated with haemolytic disease of the newborn (HDN) necessitating exchange transfusion, but not proven to be the cause [83]. One anti-Lsᵃ was found by screening over 4000 normal sera from Europeans [43,73] and 19 examples were found in 44 000 Japanese donor sera [75]. Lsᵃ is trypsin-sensitive, but resistant to ficin and sialidase [84].

Lsᵃ became associated with Gerbich when Macdonald *et al.* [84] found that Ls(a+) red cells had, in addition to normal GPC and GPD, abnormal GPC and GPD molecules, each with an apparent M_r 5500 greater than its normal counterpart. Both abnormal

structures immunostained very strongly with anti-Ge3. GPCLsᵃ also bound monoclonal anti-Ge4 and GPDLsᵃ bound anti-Ge2. *GYPC* from Ls(a+) individuals has a duplication of exon 3 (Fig. 18.4) [11,85]. The presence of an extra exon 3 explains why GPCLsᵃ and GPDLsᵃ are of increased size and have strongly expressed Ge3 antigens.

Intragenic crossing-over has been suggested as a mechanism to explain the origin of the *GYPC* exon 2 and 3 deletions responsible for the Ge:–2,3,4 and Ge:–2,–3,4 phenotypes, respectively [11,17] (Section 18.3.3). Each unequal crossing-over event would also generate *GYPC* with a duplication of either exon 2 or 3 (Fig. 18.5). The junction of two contiguous exons 3 would produce a unique amino acid sequence, probably representing the Ls^a antigen. A synthetic peptide (TPTIMDIVVIA-EPDPG) representing the last 11 amino acids encoded by the 3′ end of exon 3 followed by the first five amino acids encoded by the 5′ end of exon 3 inhibited anti-Ls^a [86]. A junction of two contiguous exons 2 does not encode a unique sequence and so no associated low frequency antigen would be expected.

A monoclonal antibody (CBC-96) to an epitope on GPC agglutinated Ls(a+) cells at a significantly higher dilution than that required to agglutinate cells of common Gerbich phenotype, presumably because the epitope is more exposed on the extended molecule [56]. Uchikawa *et al.* used an appropriate dilution of this antibody to screen red cells of 200 000 Japanese donors. Of the 60 samples strongly agglutinated, eight were Ls(a+) [75]. One of these eight samples had enhanced Ls^a expression and had GPC and GPD molecules (GPCKS and GPDKS) with an apparent M_r 6000 greater than GPCLs^a and GPDLs^a, resulting from a triplication of *GYPC* exon 3 [56] (Fig. 18.4). Forty samples (0.02%) had *GYPC* with a duplication of exon 2, the putative result of the unequal crossing-over event responsible for the exon 2 deletion of the Ge:−2,3,4 phenotype (Fig. 18.5), and six (0.003%) had a quadruplication of exon 2 [55,56]. As predicted [11], no low frequency antigen associated with GPC and GPD molecules containing multiple products of exon 2 of *GYPC* was found, as this does not create a unique amino acid sequence.

18.4.3 An^a (GE7)

An^a (Ahonen), originally described by Furuhjelm *et al.* [76], was found in about 0.06% of Finns and Swedes (Table 18.5). Anti-An^a has been found in about 1 in 1000 normal sera and does not appear to require red cell stimulation [76]. An^a is destroyed by trypsin, papain, and sialidase [35].

Immunoblotting of An(a+) red cell membranes and of GPC and GPD isolated from An(a+) red cells showed that An^a is located on GPD, but not on GPC [35]. Analysis of *GYPC* cDNA from two An(a+) individuals revealed a G67T nucleotide change in exon 2, which predicts an alanine to serine substitution at position 23 of GPC and at position 2 of GPD [35]. This raises the question, why is An^a only expressed on GPD when the amino acid substitution occurs in both GPC and GPD? An^a does not appear to involve the free

amino group at the N-terminus of GPD as acetylation of red cell surface proteins does not affect An^a expression [35]. Consequently, Daniels *et al.* [35] suggested that anti-An^a recognizes a conformational difference in the N-terminal region of GPD resulting from the amino acid substitution, which is not apparent when the same substitution occurs within the GPC chain. Titrations of anti-Ge2 sera with An(a+) and An(a−) red cells suggested that some anti-Ge2 do not react with GPDAn^a, although the results were not conclusive [35].

18.4.4 Dh^a (GE8)

The first anti-Dh^a (Duch) was an IgM 'naturally occurring' antibody found when the serum reacted with the red cells of a Danish blood donor during pretransfusion compatibility testing [77] (Table 18.5). Identification of anti-Dh^a in sera of two blood donors led to the discovery of an English family with eight Dh(a+) members in three generations [87]. Treatment of intact red cells with trypsin, papain, ficin, pronase, or sialidase destroys Dh^a; chymotrypsin does not [77,87].

Spring [88] demonstrated by immunoblotting of Dh(a+) red cell membranes and GPC isolated from those cells that Dh^a is located on GPC, but not on GPD. PCR analysis of cDNA from two Dh(a+) sibs revealed a C40T nucleotide change in exon 1 of *GYPC*, encoding a Leu14Phe substitution [89]. Dh^a is not present on GPD, as codon 14 is 5′ of the GPD translation-initiation site. Dh^a is not affected by endoglycosidase F treatment of the cells and so is not dependent on the presence of the N-glycan at Asn8 [88]. Dh^a on red cells is sialidase-sensitive, suggesting the necessity for normal O-glycosylation of GPC, but anti-Dh^a was specifically inhibited by a synthetic peptide representing amino acid residues 8–21 of GPCDh^a (NSTAWPF-SLEPNPG) [86].

18.5 Gerbich antibodies

18.5.1 Alloantibodies

Gerbich antibodies are usually stimulated by pregnancy or transfusion, but some are apparently 'naturally occurring' [25,42,43,45,58]. Eighty-nine (13%) of 664 sera from Gerbich-negative Melanesians had Gerbich antibodies and the frequency of anti-Gerbich was about the same in men as in women [25]. Some

Gerbich antibodies may be IgM [90,91], but the majority are IgG, mostly IgG1 [91].

Gerbich antibodies have been eluted from direct antiglobulin test (DAT)-positive cord red cells [20,48–50,92], but no case of serious HDN has been described, despite one of the antibodies being IgG3 and giving a strongly positive result in a monocyte phagocytosis assay [92]. A Ge:−2,−3,4 patient with a Gerbich antibody became jaundiced after transfusion of 3 units of incompatible blood and showed indications of poor survival of the transfused red cells [93]. Another patient with anti-Ge2 received 16 units of incompatible red cells over 3 weeks with no clinical evidence of haemolysis [94]. Results of *in vivo* survival studies with a few Gerbich antibodies have suggested potential clinical significance [95–97].

A weak antibody suggested some association between the Gerbich and Rh systems [98]. The antibody reacted with all red cells tested except nine of 10 Gerbich-negative samples and Rh_{null}, D−−, and cells with some other variant Rh phenotypes.

18.5.2 Autoantibodies

There are four reports of Gerbich autoantibodies causing severe autoimmune haemolytic anaemia: three resembled anti-Ge2 [99–101], the other resembled anti-Ge3 [102]. One was IgA [100], another IgM [101]. Gerbich-positive red cells of a patient with anti-Ge2 in his serum gave a negative DAT, but anti-Ge2 could be eluted [103]. Immunoblotting with this antibody and with another Ge2-like autoantibody showed that they bound to GPC, but not GPD and therefore differed from most alloanti-Ge2 [103,104]. Both patients had reduced expression of target antigen on their cells. Autoanti-Ge3 behaved like alloanti-Ge3 on immunoblots by binding to GPC and GPD [104].

An antibody resembling anti-Ge4 in a Ge:2,3,4 patient with aplastic anaemia and with elliptocytes in her peripheral blood did not cause autoimmune haemolysis [39,105]. The antibody bound GPC, GPCGe, and GPCYus, but did not bind GPD [39]. The patient's red cells had a substantially reduced content of GPC, but normal GPD. Two years later, antibody was no longer present in the patient's serum, the GPC content of her red cell membranes had returned to normal, no elliptocytes were present, and the antibody from an earlier sample reacted with her red cells [39].

18.5.3 Monoclonal antibodies

Many monoclonal antibodies associated with Gerbich define epitopes close to the N-terminus of GPC and behave serologically as anti-Ge4 [5,10,27–29,38,40, 41,55,106,107] (see Section 18.3.2.3). The epitopes of most include Met1 of GPC, but some involve amino acids 16–23 [55,107]. Several rodent monoclonal anti-Ge3 have been produced [5,37,38]. Rodent monoclonal antibodies behaving serologically as anti-Ge2 bound GPC [61,107] or GPC and GPD (one to amino acids 36–39, another to 31–40) [107,108]. One of the monoclonal anti-Ge2 immunostained GPCGe on a protein blot, but did not react with Ge:−2,−3,4 red cells [108]. An IgM monoclonal anti-Ge2 defined an epitope involving amino acids 15–22 (SLEPDPGM) on GPC, yet did not react with GPCGe, possibly because of altered O-glycosylation [61]. This antibody cross-reacted with an epitope (amino acids 22–27, EDPDIP) on the cytoplasmic N-terminal domain of band 3.

18.6 Development and distribution of Gerbich antigens

Ge2 and Ge3 are well developed at birth [20]. Gerbich antigen (type unspecified) was detected in 19 fetuses aged 17.5–28 weeks [43]. During erythropoiesis, GPC and GPD are present on erythroid cells at an early stage of differentiation, though glycosylation may not be complete [106]. GPC, detected by a monoclonal antibody (BRIC4) to a glycosylation-dependent epitope, was strongly expressed on 84% of CD34+ cells derived from cord blood [109].

GPC and GPD are not erythroid-specific, although the level of expression and the degree of glycosylation of the proteins may differ in erythroid and non-erythroid cells. Initiation of transcription of *GYPC* probably occurs at different sites in erythroid and non-erythroid cells [18]. GPC has been detected on T-lymphocytes and, weakly, on B-lymphocytes and platelets; GPC was not detected on granulocytes or platelets [18,106]. *GYPC* mRNA was detected in human erythroblasts, erythroleukaemic cell lines, and fetal liver, but not in adult liver [7], and in human kidney [8]. In order to avoid any effect of differential glycosylation, a monoclonal antibody (BGRL-100) to the cytoplasmic C-terminal domain of GPC and GPD was used to immunostain human tissues [13]. Immunostaining was apparent on fetal liver (mostly on cells of erythroid lineage), sinusoids of adult liver, kidney glomeruli, and neural cells in the brain.

18.7 Functional aspects — association of GPC and GPD with the membrane skeleton

The shape and flexibility of red cells is maintained by a submembranous matrix containing three major proteins: spectrin, actin, and protein 4.1R (reviews in [110–112]). Transmembrane protein band 3 (anion exchanger) is linked to the cytoskeleton through ankyrin, protein 4.2, and 4.1R, representing the major site of attachment of the skeletal network to the membrane (Section 10.6). GPC and GPD serve a similar function [113–121]. Protein 4.1R links GPC and GPD to the spectrin–actin network, with the phosphoprotein p55 functioning to stabilize the interaction. The Arg-His-Lys tripeptide at positions 86–88 of GPC bind to a sequence within the M_r 30 000 domain of 4.1R encoded by exon 8 of the 4.1R gene; the tripeptide Tyr-Phe-Ile at the C-terminus of GPC binds to the PDZ domain of p55; and the D5 domain of p55 binds to a sequence encoded by exon 10 of the 4.1R gene [116–121] (Fig. 18.6). Protein 4.1 also binds calmodulin and increased levels of Ca^{2+} decreases affinity of 4.1R interactions with p55 and GPC [121]. Protein 4.1R therefore plays an important part in regulating the GPC–4.1R–p55 ternary complex.

There are about 200 000 molecules of 4.1R per red cell [10], about the same as the total number of GPC and GPD molecules [5]. Patients with hereditary elliptocytosis caused by 4.1R deficiency have a 70–90% reduction of GPC and GPD, are p55 deficient, and have complete elliptocytosis [115,122–124]. GPC- and GPD-deficient Ge:–2,–3,–4 red cells have about 25% reduction in 4.1R and about 98% reduction in p55 [115]. Protein 4.1R reassociates with red cell membranes of common phenotype stripped of skeletal proteins, but not with stripped Ge:–2,–3,–4 membranes [116].

The functions of the extracellular domains of GPC and GPD are unknown. Like GPA and GPB, an important function of these heavily sialylated structures could be to contribute to the glycocalyx (see Section 3.25). Although one of the major functions of the glycocalyx is to act as a barrier to invasion by pathologic microorganisms, GPC and GPD, like GPA and GPB,

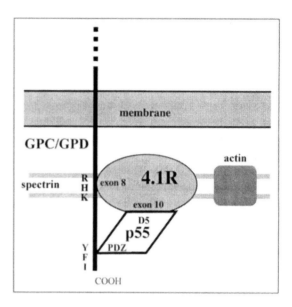

Fig. 18.6 Model of the GPC–4.1R–p55 ternary complex linking the red cell membrane to the spectrin–actin matrix. An Arg-His-Lys (RHK) tripeptide of the cytoplasmic domain of GPC (or GPD) interacts with protein 4.1R; a Tyr-Phe-Ile (YF1) tripeptide of GPC interacts with p55; and 4.1R interacts with p55.

are red cell receptors for influenza A and B viruses [125].

The level of invasion of Ge:–2,–3,–4 red cells by the malaria parasite *Plasmodium falciparum* was only 57% of that of Gerbich-positive cells [126], although Ge:–2,–3,4 cells were invaded normally [127]. BAEBL, a member of the *Plasmodium* receptor family for red cell invasion, did not bind to sialidase- or trypsin-treated red cells and had reduced binding to Ge:–2,–3,4 and Ge:–2,3,4 cells (Ge:–2,–3,–4 cells were not available) [127]. BAEBL has homology to EBA-175, the *P. falciparum* receptor specific for GPA (see Section 3.23.1), but bound normally to GPA-deficient, En(a–) red cells. If there is any selective advantage of Gerbich-negative phenotype in areas where *P. falciparum* malaria is endemic, this might provide an explanation for the high incidence of Ge:–2,–3,4 in Papua New Guinea.

References

1 Furthmayr H. Glycophorins A, B, C: a family of sialoglycoproteins — isolation and preliminary characterization of trypsin derived peptides. *J Supramolec Struct* 1978;9:79–95.

2 Reid ME. Biochemistry and molecular cloning analysis of human red cell sialoglycoproteins that carry Gerbich blood group antigens. In: P Unger, B Laird-Fryer, eds. *Blood Group Systems: MN and Gerbich*. Arlington: American Association of Blood Banks, 1989:73–103.

3 Colin Y, Le Van Kim C. Gerbich blood groups minor glycophorins. In: J-P Cartron, P Rouger, eds. *Blood Cell Biochemistry*, Vol. 6. *Molecular Basis of Major Human Blood Group Antigens*. New York: Plenum Press, 1995:331–50.

4 King M-J. Structure, polymorphisms and biological role of glycophorins A, B, C and D. In: M-J King, ed. *Consequences of Genetic Polymorphisms and Variations*. London: Imperial College Press, 2000:149–92.

5 Smythe J, Gardner B, Anstee DJ. Quantitation of the number of molecules of glycophorins C and D on normal red blood cells using radioiodinated Fab fragments of monoclonal antibodies. *Blood* 1994;83:1668–72.

6 Dahr W, Beyreuther K, Kordowicz M, Krüger J. N-terminal amino acid sequence of sialoglycoprotein D (glycophorin C) from human erythrocyte membranes. *Eur J Biochem* 1982;125:57–62.

7 Colin Y, Rahuel C, London J *et al.* Isolation of cDNA clones and complete amino acid sequence of human erythrocyte glycophorin C. *J Biol Chem* 1986;261:229–33.

8 High S, Tanner MJA. Human erythrocyte membrane sialoglycoprotein β: the cDNA sequence suggests the absence of a cleaved N-terminal signal sequence. *Biochem J* 1987;243:277–80.

9 El-Maliki B, Blanchard D, Dahr W, Beyreuther K, Cartron J-P. Structural homology between glycophorins C and D of human erythrocytes. *Eur J Biochem* 1989;183:639–43.

10 Dahr W, Blanchard D, Kiedrowski S *et al.* High-frequency antigens of human erythrocyte membrane sialoglycoproteins. VI. Monoclonal antibodies reacting with the N-terminal domain of glycophorin C. *Biol Chem Hoppe-Seyler* 1989;370:849–54.

11 High S, Tanner MJA, Macdonald EB, Anstee DJ. Rearrangements of the red-cell membrane glycophorin C (sialoglycoprotein β) gene: a further study of alterations in the glycophorin C gene. *Biochem J* 1989;262:47–54.

12 Reid ME, Anstee DJ, Tanner MJA, Ridgwell K, Nurse GT. Structural relationships between human erythrocyte sialoglycoproteins β and γ and abnormal sialoglycoproteins found in certain rare human erythrocyte variants lacking the Gerbich blood-group antigen(s). *Biochem J* 1987;244:123–8.

13 King M-J, Holmes CH, Mushens RE *et al.* Reactivity with erythroid and non-erythroid tissues of a murine monoclonal antibody to a synthetic peptide having amino acid sequence common to cytoplasmic domain of human glycophorins C and D. *Br J Haematol* 1995;89:440–8.

14 Le Van Kim C, Colin Y, Blanchard D *et al.* Gerbich blood

group deficiency of the Ge:–1,–2,–3 and Ge:–1,–2,3 types: immunochemical study and genomic analysis with cDNA probes. *Eur J Biochem* 1987;165:571–9.

15 Tanner MJA, High S, Martin PG, Anstee DJ, Judson PA, Jones TJ. Genetic variants of human red-cell membrane sialoglycoprotein β: study of the alterations occurring in the sialoglycoprotein-β gene. *Biochem J* 1988;250:407–14.

16 Le Van Kim C, Piller V, Cartron J-P, Colin Y. Glycophorins C and D are generated by the use of alternative translation initiation sites. *Blood* 1996;88:2364–5.

17 Colin Y, Le Van Kim C, Tsapis A *et al.* Human erythrocyte glycophorin C: gene structure and rearrangement in genetic variants. *J Biol Chem* 1989;264:3773–80.

18 Le Van Kim C, Colin Y, Mitjavila M-T *et al.* Structure of the promoter region and tissue specificity of the human glycophorin C gene. *J Biol Chem* 1989;264:20407–14.

19 Colin Y, Joulin V, Le Van Kim C, Roméo P-H, Cartron J-P. Characterization of a new erythroid/megakaryocyte-specific nuclear factor that binds the promoter of the housekeeping human glycophorin C gene. *J Biol Chem* 1990;265:16729–32.

20 Rosenfield RE, Haber GV, Kissmeyer-Nielsen F *et al.* Ge, a very common red-cell antigen. *Br J Haematol* 1960;6:344–9.

21 Cleghorn TE. *The occurrence of certain rare blood group factors in Britain.* MD thesis, University of Sheffield, 1961.

22 Barnes R, Lewis TLT. A rare antibody (anti-Ge) causing hæmolytic disease of the newborn. *Lancet* 1961;ii:1285–6.

23 Daniels GL. Studies on Gerbich negative phenotypes and Gerbich antibodies [Abstract]. *Transfusion* 1982;22:405.

24 Booth PB, Albrey JA, Whittaker J, Sanger R. Gerbich blood group system: a useful genetic marker in certain Melanesians of Papua and New Guinea. *Nature* 1970; 228:462.

25 Booth PB, McLoughlin K. The Gerbich blood group system, especially in Melanesians. *Vox Sang* 1972;22:73–84.

26 Macgregor A, Booth PB. A second example of anti-Ge1, and some observations on Gerbich subgroups. *Vox Sang* 1973;25:474–8.

27 Daniels GL, Banting G, Goodfellow P. A monoclonal antibody related to the human blood group Gerbich. *J Immunogenet* 1983;10:103–5.

28 Anstee DJ, Ridgwell K, Tanner MJA, Daniels GL, Parsons SF. Individuals lacking the Gerbich blood-group antigen have alterations in the human erythrocyte membrane sialoglycoproteins β and γ. *Biochem J* 1984;221:97–104.

29 Anstee DJ, Parsons SF, Ridgwell K *et al.* Two individuals with elliptocytic red cells apparently lack three minor erythrocyte membrane sialoglycoproteins. *Biochem J* 1984;218:615–19.

30 McShane K, Chung A. A novel human alloantibody in the Gerbich system. *Vox Sang* 1989;**57**:205–9.

31 Daniels GL, Shaw M-A, Judson PA *et al*. A family demonstrating inheritance of the Leach phenotype: a Gerbich-negative phenotype associated with elliptocytosis. *Vox Sang* 1986;**50**:117–21.

32 Reid ME, Martynewycz MA, Wolford FE, Crawford MN, Miller LH. Leach type Ge– red cells and elliptocytosis. *Transfusion* 1987;**27**:213–14.

33 Rountree J, Chen J, Moulds MK *et al*. A second family demonstrating inheritance of the Leach phenotype [Abstract]. *Transfusion* 1989;**29**:15S.

34 Dahr W, Kiedrowski S, Blanchard D *et al*. High frequency antigens of human erythrocyte membrane sialoglycoproteins. V. Characterization of the Gerbich blood group antigens: Ge2 and Ge3. *Biol Chem Hoppe-Seyler* 1987;**368**:1375–83.

35 Daniels G, King M-J, Avent ND *et al*. A point mutation in the *GYPC* gene results in the expression of the blood group An^a antigen on glycophorin D but not glycophorin C: further evidence that glycophorin D is a product of the *GYPC* gene. *Blood* 1993;**10**:3198–203.

36 Mohammed MT, O'Day T, Sugasawara E. Gerbich (Ge) antibody classification using enzyme-treated red cells. *Transfusion* 1986;**26**:120.

37 Loirat MJ, Gourbil A, Frioux Y, Muller JY, Blanchard D. A murine monoclonal antibody directed against the Gerbich 3 blood group antigen. *Vox Sang* 1992;**62**:45–8.

38 Loirat MJ, Dahr W, Muller JY, Blanchard D. Characterization of new monoclonal antibodies directed against glycophorins C and D. *Transfus Med* 1994;**4**:147–55.

39 Daniels GL, Reid ME, Anstee DJ, Beattie KM, Judd WJ. Transient reduction in erythrocyte membrane sialoglycoprotein β associated with the presence of elliptocytes. *Br J Haematol* 1988;**70**:477–81.

40 Anderson SE, McKenzie JL, McLoughlin K, Beard MEJ, Hart DNJ. The inheritance of abnormal sialoglycoproteins found in a Gerbich-negative individual. *Pathology* 1986;**18**:407–12.

41 Telen MJ, Scearce RM, Haynes BF. Human erythrocyte antigens. III. Characterization of a panel of murine monoclonal antibodies that react with human erythrocyte and erythroid precursor membranes. *Vox Sang* 1987;**52**:236–43.

42 McLoughlin K, Rogers J. Anti-Ge^a in an untransfused New Zealand male. *Vox Sang* 1970;**19**:94–6.

43 Race RR, Sanger R. *Blood Groups in Man*, 6th edn. Oxford: Blackwell Scientific Publications 1975.

44 Muller A, André-Liardet J, Garretta M, Brocteur J, Moullec J. Observations sur un anticorps rare: l'anti-Gerbich. *Rev Franc Transfus* 1973;**16**:251–7.

45 Okubo Y, Yamaguchi H, Seno T *et al*. The rare red cell phenotype Gerbich negative in Japanese. *Transfusion* 1984;**24**:274–5.

46 Chandanayingyong D, Bejrachandra S, Metaseta P, Pongsataporn S. Further study of Rh, Kell, Duffy, P, MN, Lewis and Gerbich blood groups of the Thais. *SE Asia J Trop Med Public Health* 1979;**10**:209–11.

47 Nunn HD, Giles CM, Seidl S. Anti-Ge, as a transfusion problem. *Vox Sang* 1967;**13**:23–6.

48 Peddle LJ, Josephson JE, Lawton A. Auto-donation in the management of placenta previa and erythroblastosis in a pregnancy complicated by Gerbich iso-immunization. *Vox Sang* 1970;**18**:547–50.

49 Reid M, Rector D, Danneskiold T. Anti-Gerbich: a case report. *Immunohematology* 1984;**1**(2):7–8.

50 Sacks DA, Johnson CS, Platt LD. Isoimmunization in pregnancy to Gerbich antigen. *Am J Perinatol* 1985;**2**:208–10.

51 Reid ME, Sullivan C, Taylor M, Anstee DJ. Inheritance of human-erythrocyte Gerbich blood group antigens. *Am J Hum Genet* 1987;**41**:1117–23.

52 Dahr W, Moulds J, Baumeister G *et al*. Altered membrane sialoglycoproteins in human erythrocytes lacking the Gerbich blood group antigens. *Biol Chem Hoppe-Seyler* 1985;**366**:201–11.

53 Chang S, Reid ME, Conboy J, Kan YW, Mohandas N. Molecular characterization of erythrocyte glycophorin C variants. *Blood* 1991;**77**:644–8.

54 Johnson P, Daniels G. A mutation analysis on *GYPC*, the gene encoding the Gerbich blood group antigens. *Transfus Med* 1997;**7**:239–44.

55 Uchikawa M, Tsuneyama H, Onodera T, Murata S, Juji T. A new high-molecular-weight glycophorin C variant with duplication of exon 2 in the glycophorin C gene. *Transfus Med* 1997;**7**:305–9.

56 Uchikawa M. Rare blood group variants in Japanese. *10th Regional Congr Int Soc Blood Transfus Western Pacific Region*, 1999:198–201.

57 Moulds M, Dahr W, Kiedrowski S *et al*. Serological and biochemical studies on variants within the Gerbich blood group system [Abstract]. *Transfusion* 1987;**27**:533.

58 Loirat MJ, Pineau-Vincent F, Schiffer C, Muller JY, Blanchard D. Inheritance of abnormal glycophorin C of the Gerbich and Yussef type in a French family. *Vox Sang* 1996;**70**:92–6.

59 Reid ME, Poole J, Liew YW, Pinder L. A Polynesian family showing co-dominant inheritance of normal glycophorin C and the Gerbich variant form of glycophorin C. *Immunohematology* 1992;**8**:29–32.

60 Serjeantson SW, White BS, Bhatia K, Trent RJ. A 3.5 kb deletion in the glycophorin C gene accounts for the Gerbich-negative blood group in Melanesians. *Immunol Cell Biol* 1994;**72**:23–7.

61 Loirat MJ, Czerwinski M, Duk M, Blanchard D. The murine monoclonal antibody NaM26–4C6 identifies a common structure on band 3 and glycophorin C. *Transfus Med* 1999;**9**:69–79.

62 Telen MJ, Le Van Kim C, Chung A, Cartron J-P, Colin Y.

Molecular basis for elliptocytosis associated with glycophorin C and D deficiency in the Leach phenotype. *Blood* 1991;78:1603–6.

63 Winardi R, Reid M, Conboy J, Mohandas N. Molecular analysis of glycophorin C deficiency in human erythrocytes. *Blood* 1993;81:2799–803.

64 Pinder JC, Chung A, Reid ME, Gratzer WB. Membrane attachment sites for the membrane cytoskeletal protein 4.1 of the red blood cell. *Blood* 1993;82:3482–8.

65 Reid ME, Chasis JA, Mohandas N. Identification of a functional role for human erythrocyte sialoglycoproteins β and γ. *Blood* 1987;69:1068–72.

66 Reid ME, Anstee DJ, Jensen RH, Mohandas N. Normal membrane function of abnormal β-related erythrocyte sialoglycoproteins. *Br J Haematol* 1987;67:467–72.

67 Nash GB, Parmar J, Reid ME. Effects of deficiencies of glycophorins C and D on the physical properties of the red cell. *Br J Haematol* 1990;76:282–7.

68 King M-J, Kosanke J, Reid ME *et al*. Co-presence of a point mutation and a deletion of exon 3 in the glycophorin C gene and concomitant production of a Gerbich-related antibody. *Transfusion* 1997;37:1027–34.

69 Simmons RT, Albrey JA. A 'new' blood group antigen Webb (Wb) of low frequency found in two Australian families. *Med J Aust* 1963;i:8–10.

70 Bloomfield L, Rowe GP, Green C. The Webb (Wb) antigen in South Wales donors. *Hum Hered* 1986;36:352–6.

71 Ikemoto S, Nakajima H, Furuhata T. The Webb (Wb) blood antigen among the Japanese. *Proc Jpn Acad* 1964;40:432–3.

72 Nakajima H, Ikemoto S, Tokunaga E, Furuhata T. Further investigation of the Webb (Wb) blood antigen among the Japanese. *Proc Jpn Acad* 1965;41:86–7.

73 Cleghorn TE, Contreras M, Bull W. The occurrence of the red cell antigen Ls^a in Finns [Abstract]. *14th Congr Int Soc Blood Transfus*, 1975:47.

74 Kornstad L. A rare blood group antigen, Rl^a (Rosenlund). *Immunol Commun* 1981;10:199–207.

75 Onodera T, Tsuneyama H, Uchikawa M *et al*. Ls^a (GE6) positive red cells in Japanese [Abstract]. *24th Congr Int Soc Blood Transfus*, 1996:145.

76 Furuhjelm U, Nevanlinna HR, Gavin J, Sanger R. A rare blood group antigen An^a (Ahonen). *J Med Genet* 1972;9:385–91.

77 Jorgensen J, Drachmann O, Gavin J. Duch, Dh^a: a low frequency red cell antigen. *Hum Hered* 1982;32:73–5.

78 Reid ME, Shaw M-A, Rowe G, Anstee DJ, Tanner MJA. Abnormal minor human erythrocyte membrane sialoglycoprotein (β) in association with the rare blood-group antigen Webb (Wb). *Biochem J* 1985;232:289–91.

79 Macdonald EB, Gerns LM. An unusual sialoglycoprotein associated with the Webb-positive phenotype. *Vox Sang* 1986;50:112–16.

80 Telen MJ, Le Van Kim C, Guizzo ML, Cartron J-P, Colin Y. Erythrocyte Webb-type glycophorin C variant lacks N-glycosylation due to an asparagine to serine substitution. *Am J Hematol* 1991;37:51–2.

81 Kornstad L, Green CA, Sistonen P, Daniels GL. Evidence that the low-incidence red cell antigens Rl^a and Ls^a are identical. *Immunohematology* 1996;12:8–10.

82 Clark AL, Dorman SA. Anti-Ls^a: case study of an antibody to a low-incidence antigen. *Transfusion* 1986;26:368–9.

83 Sistonen P. Some notions on clinical significance of anti-Ls^a and independence of Ls from Colton, Kell and Lewis blood group loci [Abstract]. *19th Congr Int Soc Blood Transfus* 1986:652.

84 Macdonald EB, Condon J, Ford D, Fisher B, Gerns LM. Abnormal beta and gamma sialoglycoprotein associated with the low-frequency antigen Ls^a. *Vox Sang* 1990;58:300–4.

85 Reid ME, Mawby W, King M-J, Sistonen P. Duplication of exon 3 in the glycophorin C gene gives rise to the Ls^a antigen. *Transfusion* 1994;34:966–9.

86 Storry JR, Reid ME, Mawby W. Synthetic peptide inhibition of antibodies to low prevalence antigens of the Gerbich blood group system [Abstract]. *Transfusion* 1994;34:24S.

87 Spring F, Poole J, Liew YW, Poole G, Banks J. The low incidence antigen Dh^a: serological and immunochemical studies [Abstract]. *Transfus Med* 1990;1(Suppl.1):66.

88 Spring FA. Immunochemical characterisation of the low-incidence antigen, Dh^a. *Vox Sang* 1991;61:65–8.

89 King MJ, Avent ND, Mallinson G, Reid ME. Point mutation in the glycophorin C gene results in the expression of the blood group antigen Dh^a. *Vox Sang* 1992;63:56–8.

90 Tilley CA, Crookston MC, Haddad SA, Shumak KH. Red blood cell survival studies in patients with anti-Ch^a, anti-Yk^a, anti-Ge, and anti-Vel. *Transfusion* 1977;17:169–72.

91 Vengelen-Tyler V, Morel PA. Serologic and IgG subclass characterization of Cartwright (Yt) and Gerbich (Ge) antibodies. *Transfusion* 1983;23:114–16.

92 Miller R, Volny M, Unger P, Shapiro A. A mild case of hemolytic disease of the newborn due to anti-Ge2,3 subclass IgG3 [Abstract]. *Transfusion* 1996;36:25S.

93 Smart EA, Reddy V, Smith L, Baxter L. Clinically significant anti-Ge detected in a South African patient [Abstract]. *24th Congr Int Soc Blood Transfus*, 1996:73.

94 Mochizuki T, Tauxe WN, Ramsey G. *In vivo* crossmatch by Chromium-51 urinary excretion from labeled erythrocytes: a case of anti-Gerbich. *J Nucl Med* 1990;31:2042–5.

95 DiNapoli J, Gingras A, Diggs E, Alicea-Tossas E, Kessler L. Survival of Ge+ red cells in a patient with anti-Ge1,2: data from ^51Cr, flow cytometric, IgG subclass, and

monocyte erythrophagocytosis assays [Abstract]. *Transfusion* 1986;26:545.

96 Nance SJ, Arndt P, Garratty G. Predicting the clinical significance of red cell alloantibodies using a monocyte monolayer assay. *Transfusion* 1987;27:449–52.

97 Pearson HA, Richards VL, Wylie BR *et al.* Assessment of clinical significance of anti-Ge in an untransfused man. *Transfusion* 1991;31:257–9.

98 Issitt PD, Gutgsell NS, Bonds SB, Wallas CH. An antibody that suggests an association between the Rh and Gerbich antigen-bearing red cell membrane components [Abstract]. *Transfusion* 1988;28:20S.

99 Reynolds MV, Vengelen-Tyler V, Morel PA. Autoimmune hemolytic anemia associated with autoanti-Ge. *Vox Sang* 1981;41:61–7.

100 Göttsche B, Salama A, Mueller-Eckhardt C. Autoimmune hemolytic anemia associated with an IgA autoanti-Gerbich. *Vox Sang* 1990;58:211–14.

101 Sererat T, Veidt D, Arndt PA, Garratty G. Warm autoimmune hemolytic anemia associated with an IgM autoanti-Ge. *Immunohematology* 1998;14:26–9.

102 Shulman IA, Vengelen-Tyler V, Thompson JC, Nelson JM, Chen DCT. Autoanti-Ge associated with severe autoimmune hemolytic anemia. *Vox Sang* 1990;59:232–4.

103 Poole J, Reid ME, Banks J *et al.* Serological and immunochemical specificity of a human autoanti-Gerbich-like antibody. *Vox Sang* 1990;58:287–91.

104 Reid ME, Vengelen-Tyler V, Shulman I, Reynolds MV. Immunochemical specificity of autoanti-Gerbich from two patients with autoimmune haemolytic anaemia and concomitant alteration in the red cell membrane sialoglycoprotein β. *Br J Haematol* 1988;69:61–6.

105 Beattie KM, Sigmund KE. A Ge-like autoantibody in the serum of a patient receiving gold therapy for rheumatoid arthritis. *Transfusion* 1987;27:54–7.

106 Villeval J-L, Le Van Kim C, Bettaieb A *et al.* Early expression of glycophorin C during normal and leukemic human erythroid differentiation. *Cancer Res* 1989;49:2626–32.

107 Reid E, Lisowska E, Blanchard D. Coordinator's report: glycophorin/band 3 and associated antigens. *Transfus Clin Biol* 1997;4:57–64.

108 Janvier D, Veaux S, Benbunan M. New murine monoclonal antibodies directed against glycophorins C and D, have anti-Ge2 specificity. *Vox Sang* 1998;74:101–5.

109 Daniels G, Green C. Expression of red cell surface antigens during erythropoiesis. *Vox Sang* 2000; 78(Suppl.1):149–53.

110 Bennett V. The spectrin–actin junction of erythrocyte membrane skeletons. *Biochim Biophys Acta* 1989; 988:107–21.

111 Palek J, Lambert S. Genetics of the red cell membrane skeleton. *Semin Hematol* 1990;27:290–332.

112 Mohandas N, Chasis JA. Red blood cell deformability, membrane material properties and shape: regulation by transmembrane, skeletal and cytosolic proteins and lipids. *Semin Hematol* 1993;30:171–92.

113 Owens JW, Mueller TJ, Morrison M. A minor sialoglycoprotein of the human erythrocyte membrane. *Arch Biochem Biophys* 1980;204:247–54.

114 Mueller TJ, Morrison M. Glyconnectin (PAS 2), a membrane attachment site for the human erythrocyte cytoskeleton. In: WC Krukeberg, WC Eaton, GJ Brewer, eds. *Erythrocyte Membranes 2: Recent Clinical and Experimental Advances.* New York: AR Liss, 1981: 95–112.

115 Alloisio N, Venezia ND, Rana A *et al.* Evidence that red blood cell protein p55 may participate in the skeleton-membrane linkage that involves protein 4.1 and glycophorin C. *Blood* 1993;82:1323–7.

116 Hemming NJ, Anstee DJ, Mawby WJ, Reid ME, Tanner MJA. Localization of the protein 4.1-binding site on human erythrocyte glycophorins C and D. *Biochem J* 1994;299:191–6.

117 Marfatia SM, Lue RA, Branton D, Chisti AH. *In vitro* binding studies suggest a membrane-associated complex between erythroid p55, protein 4.1, and glycophorin C. *J Biol Chem* 1994;269:8631–4.

118 Hemming NJ, Anstee DJ, Staricoff MA, Tanner MJA, Mohandas N. Identification of the membrane attachment sites for protein 4.1 in the human erythrocyte. *J Biol Chem* 1995;270:5360–6.

119 Marfatia SM, Lue RA, Branton D, Chishti AH. Identification of the protein 4.1 binding interface on glycophorin C and p55, a homologue of the *Drosophila discs-large* tumor suppressor protein. *J Biol Chem* 1995;270:715–19.

120 Marfatia SM, Morais-Chabral JH, Kim AC, Byron O, Chisti AH. The PDZ domain of human erythrocyte p55 mediates its binding to the cytoplasmic carboxyl terminus of glycophorin C: analysis of the binding interface by *in vitro* mutagenesis. *J Biol Chem* 1997;272:24191–7.

121 Nunomura W, Takakuwa Y, Parra M, Conboy J, Mohandas N. Regulation of protein 4.1R, 55, and glycophorin C ternary complex in human erythrocyte membrane. *J Biol Chem* 2000;275:24540–6.

122 Alloisio N, Morlé L, Bachir D *et al.* Red cell membrane sialoglycoprotein β in homozygous and heterozygous 4.1(−) hereditary elliptocytosis. *Biochim Biophys Acta* 1985;816:57–62.

123 Sondag D, Alloisio N, Blanchard D *et al.* Gerbich reactivity in 4.1(−) hereditary elliptocytosis and protein 4.1 level in blood group Gerbich deficiency. *Br J Haematol* 1987;65:43–50.

124 Reid ME, Takakuwa Y, Conboy J, Tchernia G, Mohandas N. Glycophorin C content of human erythrocyte membrane is regulated by protein 4.1. *Blood* 1990;75:2229–34.

125 Ohyama K, Endo T, Ohkuma S, Yamakawa T. Isolation and influenza virus receptor activity of glycophorins B,

C and D from human erythrocyte membranes. *Biochim Biophys Acta* 1993;**1148**:133–8.

126 Pasvol G, Anstee D, Tanner MJA. Glycophorin C and the invasion of red cells by *Plasmodium falciparum*. *Lancet* 1984;i:907–8.

127 Mayer DCG, Kaneko O, Hudson-Taylor DE, Reid ME, Miller LH. Characterization of a *Plasmodium falciparum* erythrocyte-binding protein paralogous to EBA-175. *Proc Natl Acad Sci USA* 2001;**98**:5222–7.

19 Cromer blood group system

19.1 Introduction

Cromer system antigens are located on the complement regulatory glycoprotein decay-accelerating factor (DAF or CD55), which is attached to the red cell membrane by a glycosylphosphatidylinositol (GPI) anchor. The system includes 10 antigens (Table 19.1): seven of very high frequency; three of low frequency. All are absent from red cells of the Cromer-null phenotype called the Inab phenotype, an inherited DAF deficiency. Cells lacking the Cromer system antigen Dr^a express the other high frequency Cromer antigens weakly. Complement-sensitive red cells from patients with paroxysmal nocturnal haemoglobinuria (PNH) are deficient in DAF and other GPI-linked proteins and do not express Cromer system antigens. The molecular bases for all Cromer system phenotypes are known (Table 19.1).

DAF (*CD55*) is part of the regulator of complement activation cluster on chromosome 1q32, which contains several genes encoding related glycoproteins (Chapter 32).

19.2 Decay-accelerating factor and the Cromer system

19.2.1 DAF (CD55)

DAF is an intrinsic membrane glycoprotein of red cells, granulocytes, platelets, and lymphocytes, and is widely distributed throughout the body (reviewed in [1]). It is also present in soluble form in body fluids including plasma and urine. DAF functions to regulate complement activity (Section 19.5).

DAF is part of a family of glycoproteins anchored to cell membranes by means of a glycophospholipid called glycosylphosphatidylinositol (GPI) (reviewed in [2–4]). The typical structure of a GPI anchor is shown in Fig. 19.1. Examples of other GPI-linked red cell membrane glycoproteins are described briefly in Sections 19.5 and 19.7. The complement-sensitive red cell population (PNHIII) from patients with the rare, acquired, haemolytic disease PNH are deficient in all GPI-linked proteins [5] (see Section 19.5).

Oligonucleotide probes based on the N-terminal amino acid sequence of DAF were used to isolate *DAF* cDNA from libraries derived from HeLa epithelial cell line and HL-60 promyelocytic leukaemia cell line [6,7]. The cDNA sequence predicted a 347 amino acid protein preceded by a 34 amino acid N-terminal leader peptide sequence. The DAF polypeptide has four regions of marked homology of about 60 amino acid residues each called complement control protein repeats (CCPs) or short consensus repeats (SCRs), followed by a 70 amino acid serine/threonine-rich O-glycosylated domain, and a hydrophobic stretch of 24 amino acids (Fig. 19.2). A minor form of *DAF* cDNA contained a 118-nucleotide *Alu* insert, produced as a result of alternative splicing [6]. The M_r 70 000 red cell membrane form of DAF possesses multiple, highly sialylated, O-glycans in the serine/threonine-rich region and a single N-linked oligosaccharide between the first two CCPs [8]. Each CCP domain contains four cysteine residues and is maintained in a folded conformation by two disulphide bonds. In a three-dimensional model of DAF based on the structure of factor H, a functionally homologous protein, each CCP domain of DAF consists of five β strands and the four CCPs are arranged in a helical fashion [9].

Table 19.1 Antigens of the Cromer system.

No.	Name	Relative frequency	Comments	Molecular basis*
CROM1	Cr^a	High		Ala193 (Pro)
CROM2	Tc^a	High	Antithetical to Tc^b and Tc^c	Arg18 (Leu or Pro)
CROM3	Tc^b	Low	Antithetical to Tc^a and Tc^c	Leu18 (Arg or Pro)
CROM4	Tc^c	Low	Antithetical to Tc^a and Tc^b	Pro18 (Arg or Leu)
CROM5	Dr^a	High	All antigens weak in Dr(a–)	Ser165 (Leu)
CROM6	Es^a	High		Ile46 (Asn)
CROM7	IFC	High	Absent from Inab phenotype cells	(Inactivating mutations)
CROM8	WES^a	Low	Antithetical to WES^b	Arg48 (leu)
CROM9	WES^b	High	Antithetical to WES^a	Leu48 (Arg)
CROM10	UMC	High		Thr216 (Met)

* Shown in parentheses are the amino acids associated with an antigen negative phenotype.

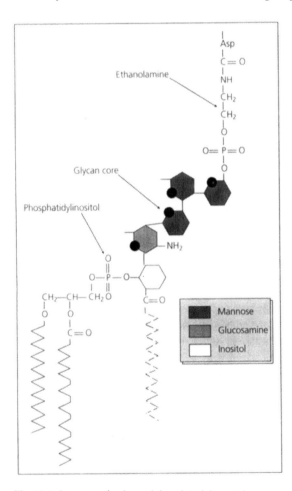

Fig. 19.1 Structure of a glycosylphosphatidylinositol anchor. The protein is linked through ethanolamine to a glycan core, attached to phosphatidylinositol, which is embedded in the cell membrane. Three fatty acids are present in red cells. Redrawn from [3].

The *DAF* gene spans about 40 kb and is organized into 11 exons [10] (Table 19.2).

19.2.2 Cromer system antigens are located on DAF

In 1987, Spring *et al.* [11] showed that two murine monoclonal antibodies, considered Cromer-related because they did not react with Inab phenotype cells and reacted only very weakly with Dr(a–) cells, stained on red cell membrane immunoblots a sialoglycoprotein of apparent M_r 70 000. This structure was subsequently shown to be DAF [12,13]. Immunoblotting with human alloantibodies has demonstrated that the Cromer system antigens Cr^a, Tc^a, Dr^a, IFC, WES^a, WES^b, and UMC are all carried on DAF [11–15]. Further confirmation that DAF is the Cromer antigen has come from monoclonal antibody-specific immobilization of erythrocyte antigens (MAIEA) assay [16,17], binding assays and haemagglutination-inhibition tests with recombinant DAF constructs [18–20], and association of mutations in the *DAF* gene variant Cromer phenotypes [18,21–26] (Table 19.1).

Red cells of the Cromer-null (Inab) phenotype have no more than minimal activity with murine monoclonal and rabbit anti-DAF [12,13,27,28]. PNHIII cells, which are deficient in DAF, did not react with antibodies to high frequency Cromer system antigens [12,13].

19.3 Inab, the Cromer-null phenotype, and anti-IFC (-CROM7)

The Inab phenotype, a Cromer-null phenotype in

Table 19.2 Organization of the *DAF* gene.

Exon	Size (bp)	3′ intron size (kb)	Amino acids*	Region of DAF encoded	Antigens encoded
1		0.5	−34−−1	5′ untranslated; signal peptide	
2	186	2.3	−1–62	CCP-1	Tc^a/Tc^b/Tc^c, Es^a, WES^a/WES^b
3	192	0.9	62–126	CCP-2	
4	100	1.0	126–159	CCP-3$_A$	
5	86	4.3	159–188	CCP-3$_B$	Dr^a
6	189	5.4	188–251	CCP-4	Cr^a, UMC
7	126	0.6	251–293	Ser/Thr rich$_A$	
8	81	1.9	293–320	Ser/Thr rich$_B$	
9	21	1.2	320–327	Ser/Thr rich$_C$	
10	118	19.8	(327–366)	*Alu* (alternatively spliced)	
11	956		327–347	Hydrophobic; 3′ untranslated	

*Residue 1 is first amino acid of mature protein.

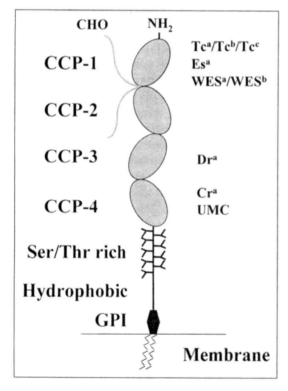

Fig. 19.2 Diagrammatic representation of the DAF glycoprotein showing the four short consensus repeats (CCPs), the O-glycosylated serine/threonine-rich region, the hydrophobic region, and the glycosylphosphatidylinositol (GPI) anchor inserted into the cell membrane. Also shown are the locations of the Cromer system antigens on the four CCPs.

which the red cells lack all Cromer system antigens, is very rare. Only five unrelated Inab phenotype individuals have been reported: three Japanese [24,25,29], a Jewish American [30], and a white American woman of Italian descent, whose brother also had the Inab phenotype [31]. Red cells of two individuals originally considered to have the Inab phenotype [32,33] were subsequently shown to have low levels of DAF [22]; one of them had the Dr(a−) phenotype (Section 19.4.3). A black patient with anti-IFC had a transient Inab phenotype [34]. One year after the original diagnosis, his red cells expressed DAF and he had a normal Cromer phenotype.

Sequencing of genomic DNA and of cDNA derived from the original Inab phenotype propositus demonstrated a nonsense mutation in codon 53 of *DAF* exon 2: TGG, a tryptophan codon, to TGA, a stop codon [22]. Translation of *DAF* mRNA in this individual could not proceed beyond amino acid residue 53 within the first CCP domain. The mutation created a *Bcl*I restriction site. Another Japanese propositus was also homozygous for the same mutation; his parents were heterozygous for the mutation [25]. The third Japanese Inab propositus had a different mutation; a C1579A transversion 24 bp upstream of the 3′ end of exon 2 created a novel splice site (TGGTCAGA to TG-gtaaga), giving rise to a 26-bp deletion in the mRNA and resulting a reading frameshift and a translation stop codon immediately downstream of the mutation [24]. Consequently, translation would be terminated at the codon for the first amino acid of CCP-2. The point mutation, but no deletion, was detected in genomic DNA. The mutation causes the loss of a *Mbo*I site.

Sera from four of the Inab phenotype propositi contained anti-IFC, an antibody reacting with all red cells apart from those of the Inab phenotype [25,29–31]. Haemagglutination-inhibition experiments with soluble–recombinant constructs representing different segments of DAF showed that anti-IFC comprises a mixture of antibodies to each of the four CCPs [25]. An antibody with all the characteristics of anti-IFC was found in the serum of a 12-year-old African American boy [25,35]. His red cells were never tested with Cromer system antibodies, but it is likely that he had the Inab phenotype. Anti-IFC in a patient with transient Inab phenotype disappeared when the red cells returned to normal [34].

Three of the five Inab propositi, plus the African American boy who probably had the Inab phenotype, had intestinal disorders including protein-losing enteropathy [29,35], Crohn's disease [30], and blood capillary angioma of the small intestine [25]. DAF is present on the epithelial surface of intestinal mucosa [36], but any suggestion of an association between DAF-deficiency and intestinal disease is offset by the absence of any such disorder in one of the Japanese propositi [24] or in an 86-year-old Inab phenotype woman and her 70-year-old brother [31].

19.4 Cromer system antigens and antibodies

19.4.1 Cr^a (CROM1)

In 1965 McCormick *et al.* [37] described an antibody in the serum of a African American antenatal patient, Mrs Cromer, which reacted with red cells of more than 4000 African American donors, but not with her own cells or with those of two of her sibs. The antibody, mistakenly thought to be antithetical to anti-Go^a [37], was later named anti-Cr^a by Stroup and McCreary [38] who also recognized a possible serological association with the antibody now called anti-Tc^a. Many more examples have been found [35,38–43]; all are in black people, with the exception of one Spanish American [39]. Cr^a is inherited as a Mendelian dominant character [37–39]. Two of 8858 black Detroit donors were Cr(a–) [44].

DAF cDNA deletion-mutants lacking the regions encoding each of the four CCPs were used to transfect Chinese hamster ovary (CHO) cells [45]. Anti-Cr^a reacted on immunoblots with lysates from these transfected cells with the single exception of those transfected with the cDNA lacking the region encoding CCP-4 [18]. Sequencing of genomic DNA from three Cr(a–) individuals revealed a G679C change encoding an Ala193Pro substitution in CCP-4 [18] (Tables 19.1 and 19.2).

19.4.2 Tc^a (CROM2), Tc^b (CROM3), Tc^c (CROM4), and Tc^{a}Tc^b

Two antibodies of identical specificity, shown to be related to anti-Cr^a through common absence from Inab phenotype cells [29], were named anti-Tc^a when a third example was described [46]. One Tc(a–) individual was found as a result of testing red cells from 950 African American donors with anti-Tc^a; none was found from testing 5000 white donors or 5000 Japanese [46].

Anti-Tc^b, an antibody in a serum also containing anti-Go^a, reacted with red cells of about 6% of African Americans; no white Tc(b+) person has been found [47]. All Tc(a–) black people are Tc(b+) and family studies showed that *Tc^a* and *Tc^b* are alleles [47]. From the results of testing 350 African American donors with anti-Tc^b the following gene and genotype frequencies were calculated [47]: *Tc^a* 0.97, *Tc^b* 0.03; *Tc^a/Tc^a* 0.941, *Tc^a/Tc^b* 0.058, *Tc^b/Tc^b* 0.001.

Red cells of a Tc(a–b–) white woman and her sister, neither of whom had the Inab phenotype, were found to have a low frequency antigen, which was subsequently named Tc^c [48]. Both parents and three of four other sibs were Tc(a+b–c+). Six months after the delivery of a Tc(a+) child, the serum of the Tc(a–b–c+) propositus contained an antibody that represents inseparable anti-Tc^{a}Tc^b; it reacted with neither her own cells nor with those of her Tc(a–b–c+) sister, but did react with Tc(a–b+c–) and Tc(a+b–c–) cells [48]. A second example of anti-Tc^{a}Tc^b has been found in a Tc(a–b–) white woman [49].

Analysis of cells transfected with *DAF* cDNA deletion-mutant constructs showed that Tc^a is on CCP-1 of DAF. G to T and G to C transversions at nucleotide 155, encoding Arg18Leu and Arg18Pro substitutions, are responsible for Tc^b and Tc^c expression, respectively [18,23,26] (Tables 19.1 and 19.2). The *Tc^b*

mutation creates a *Stu*I restriction site and both Tc^b and Tc^c mutations destroy an *Rsa*I site.

19.4.3 Drᵃ (CROM5)

At least three Dr(a–) propositi, all Uzbekistani Jews, have been found in Israel through the presence of anti-Drᵃ in their sera [50–52]. One of the four sibs of the original Dr(a–) propositus was also Dr(a–) [50]; in the second family the propositus had no Dr(a–) sib, but three of her four children were Dr(a–) [51]; in the third family three of the four sibs of the propositus were Dr(a–) [52]. Other examples of Dr(a–) with anti-Drᵃ have been identified in an Uzbekistani Jew [53], a Russian woman [22,32], and a Japanese blood donor [25]. Another Dr(a–) Japanese donor did not have anti-Drᵃ [54].

In addition to lacking Drᵃ, Dr(a–) red cells have weak expression of all other high frequency Cromer system antigens as they have only 40% of normal expression of cell surface DAF [21]. Immunoblotting revealed no gross alteration in Dr(a–) DAF, but did confirm the quantitative difference [21,55]. In one case, Dr(a–) phenotype was originally mistaken for the Inab phenotype [22,32].

Lublin *et al.* [21,22] sequenced polymerase chain reaction (PCR)-amplified genomic DNA from four unrelated Dr(a–) individuals and demonstrated in each a C596T transition in exon 5 of *DAF* encoding a Ser165Leu substitution within CCP-3 (Tables 19.1 and 19.2). This mutation results in the loss of a *Taq*I restriction site. Sequencing of cDNA derived from Dr(a–) individuals revealed two *DAF* transcripts: a minor one encoding full length DAF with the Ser165Leu substitution and a more abundant form having a 44-nucleotide deletion, which introduces a reading frameshift and the generation of a premature stop codon six codons downstream from the deletion. Any polypeptide produced by the major transcript would consist of an N-terminal leader sequence plus 165 amino acid residues representing the first two and a half CCPs of DAF, but lacking the remainder of the molecule, including the GPI anchor [22]. Only DAF encoded by the minor transcript is present at the cell surface, explaining the low levels of DAF and weak expression of the Cromer antigens. The two transcripts are probably the products of alternative splicing. The C to T mutation responsible for the loss of Drᵃ creates a cryptic splice site 44 nucleotides upstream of intron 4

so that 44 nucleotides of exon 3 are spliced-out of the majority of the mRNA molecules together with intron 4. Restriction analyses with *Taq*I suggested that the two Japanese Dr(a–) propositi have the same mutation [25,32].

Chinese hamster ovary cell lines were transfected with either the wild-type, *Drᵃ DAF* cDNA or with *DAF* cDNA representing the variant allele. The latter was created by site-directed *in vitro* mutagenesis to introduce the C596T change (and without the 44-nucleotide deletion). The allele-specific transfectants were tested for Drᵃ expression on membrane-bound DAF by flow cytometry and for secreted Drᵃ by haemagglutination-inhibition. The results confirmed that the single amino acid substitution was responsible for loss of Drᵃ antigen expression [21].

19.4.4 WESᵃ (CROM8) and WESᵇ (CROM9)

WESᵃ is a low frequency antigen detected on the red cells of 61 of 10 982 (0.56%) Finns [56], two of 1610 (0.12%) white Americans [57], seven of 1460 (0.48%) African Americans [57], and five of 245 (2.04%) black North Londoners [58]. WESᵃ was not found among 210 Belgians, 747 Poles, 1073 Hungarians, 707 Latvians, 500 Japanese, or 1026 Somalis [55].

Only two examples of antibodies to the high frequency antigen WESᵇ are known, both found in the sera of black women with WES(a+) red cells [58,59]. Anti-WESᵇ gave higher titration scores with WES(a–) red cells than with WES(a+) red cells [58]. The only other known WESᵃ homozygote was a Finnish woman with six WES(a+) and no WES(a–) children [58].

Tests of transfected cells expressing DAF constructs comprising single CCPs suggested that WESᵇ is situated on CCP-1 [19]. Amplification and sequencing of *DAF* exon 2 from WES(a+b–) and WES(a–b+) individuals revealed that the WESᵇ/WESᵃ polymorphism results from a T245G change, which encodes a Leu48Arg substitution [26] (Tables 19.1 and 19.2). The *WESᵃ* allele lacks an *Afl*II restriction site that is present in *WESᵇ*. In a MAIEA assay, two murine monoclonal antibodies to epitopes on CCP-1 blocked binding of anti-Tcᵃ, whereas a third did not. The opposite result was obtained with the same monoclonal antibodies and anti-WESᵇ, suggesting that Tcᵃ and WESᵇ are on opposing faces of CCP-1 [17]. These results support the molecular model of Kuttner-Kondo *et al.* [9].

19.4.5 Es^a (CROM6)

Only two examples of anti-Es^a and two Es(a−) propositi are known:
1 a woman of Mexican descent with two Es(a−) and one Es(a+) sibs, and whose parents were first cousins [60]; and
2 an African American man [61].

None of 3400 random donors was Es(a−). Anti-WES^b reacts slightly less strongly with Es(a−) cells than with Es(a+) cells, whereas two examples of WES(a+b−) cells reacted only very weakly with anti-Es^a, requiring adsorption–elution tests for detection [58].

MAIEA analysis suggested that Es^a is on CCP-1 of DAF [16]. Sequencing of DAF exon 2 from the African American Es(a−) propositus revealed homozygosity for a T239A transversion, encoding an Ile46Asn substitution in CCP-1 [26] (Tables 19.1 and 19.2). This amino acid substitution is very close to Leu48Arg, responsible for the WES^b/WES^a polymorphism, explaining the serological interaction between Es^a and WES^b.

19.4.6 UMC (CROM10)

The only known UMC− propositus is a Japanese blood donor detected during screening for donor antibodies in northern Japan [14]. One of her three sibs was also UMC−. None of 45 610 Japanese donors was UMC−.

Anti-UMC was shown to detect a determinant on CCP-4 of DAF by haemagglutination-inhibition tests with soluble-recombinant DAF constructs lacking different CCPs [20]. The UMC− propositus was then shown to be homozygous for a C749T transition in exon 6 of DAF encoding a Thr216Met substitution [26] (Tables 19.1 and 19.2).

19.4.7 Other serological characteristics of Cromer system antigens

Cromer system antigens are readily destroyed by treatment of the red cells with α-chymotrypsin, but not by trypsin, papain, ficin, or sialidase, and in this way are easily distinguished from virtually all other blood group antigens. Treatment of intact red cells with the sulphydryl-reducing agents 2-aminoethylisothiouronium bromide (AET) and dithiothreitol (DTT) results in only slight weakening of the Cromer antigens. This

is surprising, considering that each CCP domain is maintained in its folded configuration by two disulphide bonds (Section 19.2.1).

Haemagglutination-inhibition has demonstrated that Cromer system antigens are present in serum of individuals with the corresponding antigen on their red cells [31,46,51,56,58,62]. Anti-Cr^a, -Tc^a, -Dr^a, -IFC, and -UMC were inhibited by concentrated urine from individuals with antigen-positive red cells [14,15].

Anti-Cr^a can be readily removed from sera by adsorption with platelet concentrates [63,64].

19.4.8 Clinical significance of Cromer system antibodies

Cromer system antibodies are mostly IgG [35], although IgM anti-Cr^a is reported [43]. IgG1 generally predominates, but Cromer system antibodies of all four subclasses have been reported [43,52,53,56, 61,65–68].

Cromer system antibodies are not usually not considered clinically significant and there are many reports of successful transfusion of incompatible red cells to patients with anti-Cr^a [39,42,68,69] and one with anti-Tc^a [98]. Yet anti-Cr^a [68] and -Tc^a [70] have been blamed for clinical transfusion reactions, with the anti-Tc^a destroying six units of Tc(a+) red cells, three of them within a day of transfusion. Conclusions from in vivo red cell survival studies and in vitro functional assays with Cromer system antibodies have varied, some suggesting that the antibodies are of no clinical importance [39–43,49,52,53,63,67–69], others predicting reduced survival of transfused incompatible red cells [30,35,46,53,61,64,66–68,70, 71]. Only 38% of radiolabelled IFC+ red cells survived 24 h after injection into an Inab phenotype man with anti-IFC [30] and another example of anti-IFC removed all IFC+ cells within 15 min of injection [35]. Anti-Tc^a comprising IgG1, IgG2, and IgG4 gave results in the monocyte monolayer assay (MMA) suggestive of clinical significance; 2 years later the serum contained only IgG2 and IgG4, and the MMA and in vivo red cell survival tests suggested that incompatible transfusion would be well tolerated [67]. Transplantation of a Dr(a+) kidney into a Dr(a−) patient with IgG2 plus IgG4 anti-Dr^a was successful, with good graft function and no increase in titre of the antibody [52].

Despite the indications that Cromer system antibodies often have the potential to be haemolytic, these antibodies are never responsible for clinical signs of haemolytic disease of the newborn (HDN). DAF is present on placental trophoblast epithelial cells derived from the fetus [72]. During the course of two consecutive pregnancies, anti-Cr^a titre decreased from 128 or 512 to <4 [63]. In other cases, strongly reactive anti-Cr^a, -Dr^a, and -WES^b became undetectable in the maternal plasma during the second and third trimesters of pregnancy, only to reappear shortly after parturition [53,59]. It is likely therefore that maternal Cromer system antibodies become absorbed by the placenta, protecting the fetus from the antibodies.

19.4.9 Monoclonal antibodies

Numerous rodent monoclonal antibodies to DAF have been produced, defining epitopes on each of the four CCPs [11,20,45,73]. They generally behave like anti-IFC as they do not react with red cells of the Inab phenotype and react only very weakly with Dr(a–) cells. One monoclonal antibody to an epitope on CCP-1 gave weaker reactions than normal with Tc(a–b+c–) cells and even weaker reactions with Tc(a–b–c+) cells [73].

19.5 Functional aspects of DAF and CD59 — GPI-linked complement-regulatory proteins

DAF protects cells from complement-mediated damage by inhibiting the amplification stage of complement activation. DAF inhibits association and accelerates dissociation of C4b2a and C3bBb, the C3 convertases of the classical and alternative pathways, respectively. The second, third, and fourth, but not the first, CCPs of DAF appear to be important in regulating C3 convertase activity [45]. DAF has a wide distribution in the body. It is present on granulocytes, monocytes, and lymphocytes [1], and on many epithelial cells, including placental trophoblast epithelium, where it might have a role in protecting the fetus from maternal complement-mediated attack [72] (see Section 19.4.8).

CD59, also known as the membrane inhibitor of reactive lysis (MIRL), is a complement-regulatory glycoprotein of the Ly-6 superfamily. It inhibits complement-mediated haemolysis by binding to C8 and C9 and preventing assembly of the membrane-at-

tack complex. CD59 is present on red cells, but does not have blood group activity. It has an apparent M_r of around 18 000 and is glycosylated at Asn18. The CD59 gene has been cloned and sequenced and is situated on chromosome 11. Like DAF, CD59 is attached to the red cell membrane by a GPI anchor (for reviews on CD59 see [3,4,74]). Several murine monoclonal antibodies have been used to analyse CD59 glycoprotein on red cells [73,75].

Paroxysmal nocturnal haemoglobinuria, a disease characterized by intravascular haemolysis, is caused by multifarious somatic mutations in PIG-A, an X-linked gene essential for the biosynthesis of the GPI anchor of the GPI-linked proteins of haemopoietic cells [4,76,77]. The affected red cells in PNH patients (PNHIII cells) are deficient in all GPI-linked proteins [5], including DAF and CD59, and can be lysed, in vitro, by acidified human serum, a process that involves the activation of the alternative complement pathway. Despite DAF deficiency, red cells of the Inab phenotype show no evidence of haemolysis and none of the six individuals with this phenotype had any symptoms of haematological disease [24,25,27,28]. Unlike PNH cells, Inab phenotype cells are not lysed by acidified serum or by cobra venom and they are no more than slightly more susceptible to lysis than normal cells in standard complement-mediated lysis tests, such as lysis in the presence of cold antibody or sucrose [27,28]. DATs on Inab phenotype cells with antibodies to human complement components demonstrated that there is no accumulation of C3 fragments on Inab phenotype cells, as might have been expected in the absence of a C3 convertase inhibitor [27,28]. When CD59 has been inactivated by the addition of monoclonal anti-CD59, however, Inab phenotype red cells are haemolysed by acidified human serum [25,33]. In a reactive lysis assay, coating red cells with either anti-CD55 or -CD59 induced lysis, anti-CD59 having the more pronounced effect [78]. These results suggest that DAF and CD59 share the role of protecting red cells from the activity of autologous complement. CD59 appears more effective than DAF in this respect: a patient with red cell CD59 deficiency resulting from homozygosity for single base deletion within the CD59 gene, but with normal levels of DAF and other GPI-linked glycoproteins, had a mild PNH-like haemolytic anaemia [79,80]. In a complement-mediated lysis sensitivity (CLS) test, the following scores (in CLS units) were obtained: DAF-deficient (Inab) red cells, 4.6; CD59-deficient red cells, 11.7; DAF- and CD59-deficient (PNHIII) red cells, 47.6 [81]. CD59 may also have the dubious function of protecting red cells infected with *Plasmodium falciparum* from complement-mediated destruction [82].

DAF may also be involved in cellular interaction. It is a ligand for CD97, a seven-span transmembrane receptor of T and B cells [83].

19.6 DAF as a receptor for pathogenic microorganisms

Like globoside, the P antigen (Section 4.11.1), DAF is exploited as an attachment site on epithelial cells for strains of *Escherichia coli* associated with urinary tract infection, cystitis, and protracted diarrhoea [84]. Fimbriae from 075X-positive *E. coli* agglutinated red cells *in vitro*, with the exception of those with the Inab and Dr(a–) phenotypes [85]. The 075X and other fimbria-like adhesins that bind to Dr^a are referred to as Dr adhesins. *E. coli* and purified Dr adhesins-bound Chinese hamster ovary (CHO) cells transfected with normal *DAF* cDNA, but not untransfected cells or cells transfected with *DAF* cDNA encoding the Ser165Leu substitution associated with the Dr(a–) phenotype [86]. Immunofluorescence assays with Dr adhesin isolated from a recombinant bacterial strain showed that its ligand (DAF expressing Dr^a) is widely distributed on the surface of epithelial cells [87]. Renal tubular basement membrane, Bowman's capsule, and renal transitional epithelium showed the highest level of fluorescence.

DAF is a ligand for many picornaviruses, which includes echoviruses and coxsackieviruses [88]. Some echoviruses are capable of agglutinating red cells [89]. Binding of echovirus 7 to CHO cells transfected with *DAF* cDNA deletion mutants showed a requirement of CCP-2, -3, and -4 [90]. Monoclonal antibody to CCP-3 blocked attachment of echoviruses to susceptible cells [90,91].

19.7 Other GPI-linked proteins on red cells

Several other GPI-linked proteins are present on red cells. Some carry blood group antigens and are described in the relevant chapters: Yt antigens on acetylcholinesterase (Chapter 11); Dombrock glycoprotein (Chapter 14); JMH (CDw108) (Chapter 24); and Emm antigen (Chapter 28). Mentioned below are three other GPI-linked proteins, detected on red cells by monoclonal antibodies, but not associated with any blood group antigen.

LFA-3 (CD58) has wide tissue distribution and is present in the red cell membrane, but is not known to be associated with any blood group. Most LFA-3 molecules in the red cell membrane are GPI anchored, although a minority population have transmembrane and cytoplasmic domains. LFA-3 functions as a cell adhesion molecule and is involved in T cell activation through binding to CD2, but the function of LFA-3 on red cells is unknown (reviewed in [92,93]).

C8-binding protein is another red cell membrane protein reported to have complement regulatory activity [94]. It is absent from PNH red cells and therefore is probably GPI-linked [95].

The prion protein, PrP^C, is a GPI-linked glycoprotein widely distributed on cells of different tissues, including mononuclear leucocytes and platelets in the blood. A conformational isoform of PrP^C, called PrP^{Sc}, is responsible for transmissible spongiform encephalopathies, such as Creutzfeldt–Jakob disease (CJD) and variant CJD (review in [96]). PrP^C is present, at relatively low levels, on normal red cells, but not on PNHIII cells [97].

References

1 Lublin DM, Atkinson JP. Decay-accelerating factor: biochemistry, molecular biology, and function. *Annu Rev Immunol* 1989;7:35–58.

2 Low MG, Saltiel AR. Structural and functional roles of glycosyl-phosphatidylinositol in membranes. *Science* 1988;239:268–75.

3 Telen MJ. Erythrocyte blood group antigens associated with phosphatidylinositol glycan-linked proteins. In: G Garratty, ed. *Immunobiology of Transfusion Medicine*. New York: Dekker, 1994:97–110.

4 Rosse WF, Ware RE. The molecular basis of paroxysmal nocturnal hemoglobinuria. *Blood* 1995;86:3277–86.

5 Nicholson-Weller A, March JP, Rosenfield SI, Austen KF. Affected erythrocytes of patients with paroxysmal nocturnal hemoglobinuria are deficient in the complement regulatory protein, decay accelerating factor. *Proc Natl Acad Sci USA* 1983;80:5066–70.

6 Caras IW, Davitz MA, Rhee L *et al.* Cloning of decay-accelerating factor suggests novel use of splicing to generate two proteins. *Nature* 1987;325:545–9.

7 Medof ME, Lublin DM, Holers VM *et al.* Cloning and characterization of cDNAs encoding the complete sequence of decay-accelerating factor of human complement. *Proc Natl Acad Sci USA* 1987;84:2007–11.

451

8 Lublin DM, Krsek-Staples J, Pangburn MK, Atkinson JP. Biosynthesis and glycosylation of the human complement regulatory protein decay-accelerating factor. *J Immunol* 1986;**137**:1629–35.

9 Kuttner-Kondo L, Medof ME, Brodbeck W, Shoham M. Molecular modeling and mechanism of action of human decay-accelerating factor. *Protein Eng* 1996;**9**:1143–9.

10 Post TW, Arce MA, Liszewski MK *et al.* Structure of the gene for human complement protein decay accelerating factor. *J Immunol* 1990;**144**:740–4.

11 Spring FA, Judson PA, Daniels GL *et al.* A human cell-surface glycoprotein that carries Cromer-related blood group antigens on erythrocytes and is also expressed on leucocytes and platelets. *Immunology* 1987;**62**:307–13.

12 Telen MJ, Hall SE, Green AM, Moulds JJ, Rosse WF. Identification of human erythrocyte blood group antigens on decay accelerating factor (DAF) and an erythrocyte phenotype negative for DAF. *J Exp Med* 1988;**167**:93–8.

13 Parsons SF, Spring FA, Merry AH *et al.* Evidence that Cromer-related blood group antigens are carried on decay accelerating factor (DAF) suggests that the Inab phenotype is a novel form of DAF deficiency [Abstract]. *20th Congr Int Soc Blood Transfus*, 1988:116.

14 Daniels GL, Okubo Y, Yamaguchi H, Seno T, Ikuta M. UMC, another Cromer-related blood group antigen. *Transfusion* 1989;**29**:794–7.

15 Daniels G. Cromer-related antigens: blood group determinants on decay-accelerating factor. *Vox Sang* 1989;**56**:205–11.

16 Petty AC, Daniels GL, Anstee DJ, Tippett PA. Use of the MAIEA technique to confirm the relationship between the Cromer antigens and decay-accelerating factor and to assign provisionally antigens to the short-consensus repeats. *Vox Sang* 1993;**65**:309–15.

17 Petty AC, Green CA, Daniels GL. The monoclonal antibody-specific immobilisation of erythrocyte antigens assay (MAIEA) in the investigation of human red cell antigens and their associated membrane proteins. *Transfus Med* 1997;**7**:179–88.

18 Telen MJ, Rao N, Udani M *et al.* Molecular mapping of the Cromer blood group Cr^a and Tc^a epitopes of decay accelerating factor: toward the use of recombinant antigens in immunohematology. *Blood* 1994;**84**:3205–11.

19 Telen MJ, Rao N, Lublin DM. Location of WES^b on decay-accelerating factor. *Transfusion* 1995;**35**:278.

20 Daniels GL, Green CA, Powell RM, Ward T. Hemagglutination-inhibition of Cromer blood group antibodies with soluble recombinant decay-accelerating factor. *Transfusion* 1998;**38**:332–6.

21 Lublin DM, Thompson ES, Green AM, Levene C, Telen MJ. Dr(a−) polymorphism of decay accelerating factor: biochemical, functional, and molecular characterization and production of allele-specific transfectants. *J Clin Invest* 1991;**87**:1945–52.

22 Lublin DM, Mallinson G, Poole J *et al.* Molecular basis

of reduced or absent expression of decay-accelerating factor in Cromer blood group phenotypes. *Blood* 1994;**84**:1276–82.

23 Udani MN, Anderson N, Rao N, Telen MJ. Identification of the *Tc^b* allele of the Cromer blood group gene by PCR and RFLP analysis. *Immunohematology* 1995; **11**:1–4.

24 Wang L, Uchikawa M, Tsuneyama H *et al.* Molecular cloning and characterization of decay-accelerating factor deficiency in Cromer blood group Inab phenotype. *Blood* 1998;**91**:680–4.

25 Daniels GL, Green CA, Mallinson G *et al.* Decay-accelerating factor (CD55) deficiency in Japanese. *Transfus Med* 1998;**8**:141–7.

26 Lublin DM, Kompelli S, Storry JR, Reid ME. Molecular basis of Cromer blood group antigens. *Transfusion* 2000;**40**:208–13.

27 Telen MJ, Green AM. The Inab phenotype: characterization of the membrane protein and complement regulatory defect. *Blood* 1989;**74**:437–41.

28 Merry AH, Rawlinson VI, Uchikawa M, Daha MR, Sim RB. Studies on the sensitivity to complement-mediated lysis of erythrocytes (Inab phenotype) with a deficiency of DAF (decay accelerating factor). *Br J Haematol* 1989;**73**:248–53.

29 Daniels GL, Tohyama H, Uchikawa M. A possible null phenotype in the Cromer blood group complex. *Transfusion* 1982;**22**:362–3.

30 Walthers L, Salem M, Tessel J, Laird-Fryer B, Moulds JJ. The Inab phenotype: another example found [Abstract]. *Transfusion* 1983;**23**:423.

31 Lin RC, Herman J, Henry L, Daniels GL. A family showing inheritance of the Inab phenotype. *Transfusion* 1988;**28**:427–9.

32 Reid ME, Mallinson G, Sim RB *et al.* Biochemical studies on red blood cells from a patient with the Inab phenotype (decay-accelerating factor deficiency). *Blood* 1991;**78**: 3291–7.

33 Holguin MH, Martin CB, Bernshaw NJ, Parker CJ. Analysis of the effects of activation of the alternative pathway of complement on erythrocytes with an isolated deficiency of decay accelerating factor. *J Immunol* 1992;**148**:498–502.

34 Matthes TW, Poole J, Nagy M *et al.* First example of the Inab phenotype in a black individual [Abstract]. *Blood* 2000;**96**:108b–9b and personal communication.

35 Daniels GL. *Blood group antigens of high frequency: a serological and genetical study.* PhD thesis, University of London, 1980.

36 Medof ME, Walter EI, Rutgers JL, Knowles DM, Nussenzweig V. Identification of the complement decay-accelerating factor (DAF) on epithelium and glandular cells and in body fluids. *J Exp Med* 1987;**165**:848–64.

37 McCormick EE, Francis BJ, Gelb AB. A new antibody apparently defining an allele of Go^a [Abstract]. *18th Ann Mtg Am Ass Blood Banks*, 1965.

38 Stroup M, McCreary J. Cr^a, another high frequency blood group factor [Abstract]. *Transfusion* 1975;**15**:522 and personal communication.

39 Smith KJ, Coonce LS, South SF, Troup GM. Anti-Cr^a: family study and survival of chromium-labeled incompatible red cells in a Spanish-American patient. *Transfusion* 1983;**23**:167–9.

40 Ross DG, McCall L. Transfusion significance of anti-Cr^a. *Transfusion* 1985;**25**:84.

41 Leatherbarrow MB, Ellisor SS, Collins PA *et al*. Assessing the clinical significance of anti-Cr^a and anti-M in a chronically transfused sickle cell patient. *Immunohematology* 1988;**4**:71–4.

42 Whitsett CF, Oxendine SM. Survival studies with another example of anti-Cr^a. *Transfusion* 1991;**31**:782–3.

43 Dickson AC, Guest C, Jordon M, Banks J, Kumpel BM. Case report: anti-Cr^a in pregnancy. *Immunohaematology* 1995;**11**:14–17.

44 Winkler MM, Hamilton JR. Previously tested donors eliminated to determine rare phenotype frequencies [Abstract]. *Joint Congr Int Soc Blood Transfus and Am Ass Blood Banks*, 1990:158.

45 Coyne KE, Hall SE, Thompson ES *et al*. Mapping of epitopes, glycosylation sites, and complement regulatory domains in human decay accelerating factor. *J Immunol* 1992;**149**:2906–13.

46 Laird-Fryer B, Dukes CV, Lawson J *et al*. Tc^a: a high-frequency blood group antigen. *Transfusion* 1983;**23**:124–7.

47 Lacey PA, Block UT, Laird-Fryer BJ *et al*. Anti-Tc^b, an antibody that defines a red cell antigen antithetical to Tc^a. *Transfusion* 1985;**25**:373–6.

48 Law J, Judge A, Covert P *et al*. A new low frequency factor proposed to be the product of an allele to Tc^a [Abstract]. *Transfusion* 1982;**22**:413.

49 Bell JA, Johnson ST, Moulds M *et al*. Clinical significance of anti-Tc^ab in the second example of a Tc(a–b–) individual [Abstract]. *Transfusion* 1989;**29**:17S.

50 Levene C, Harel N, Lavie G *et al*. A 'new' phenotype confirming a relationship between Cr^a and Tc^a. *Transfusion* 1984;**24**:13–15.

51 Levene C, Harel N, Kende G *et al*. A second Dr(a–) proposita with anti-Dr^a and a family with Dr(a–) in two generations. *Transfusion* 1987;**27**:64–5.

52 Nakache R, Levene C, Sela R, Kaufman S, Shapira Z. Dr^a (Cromer-related blood group antigen)-incompatible renal transplantation. *Vox Sang* 1998;**74**:106–8.

53 Reid ME, Chandrasekaran V, Sausais L, Jeannot P, Bullock R. Disappearance of antibodies to Cromer blood group system antigens during mid pregnancy. *Vox Sang* 1996;**71**:48–50.

54 Uchikawa M, Tsuneyama H, Wang L *et al*. Rare Cromer blood group phenotypes detected in Japanese [Abstract]. *24th Congr Int Soc Blood Transfus*, 1996: 143.

55 Daniels G, Levene C. Immunoblotting of Dr(a–) cells with antibodies to Cromer-related antigens. *Vox Sang* 1990;**59**:127–8.

56 Sistonen P, Nevanlinna HR, Virtaranta-Knowles K *et al*. WES, a 'new' infrequent blood group antigen in Finns. *Vox Sang* 1987;**52**:111–14.

57 Copeland TR, Smith JH, Wheeling RM, Rudolph MG. The incidence of WES^a in 3072 donors in the United States. *Immunohematology* 1991;**7**:76–7.

58 Daniels GL, Green CA, Darr FW, Anderson H, Sistonen P. A 'new' Cromer-related high frequency antigen probably antithetical to WES. *Vox Sang* 1987;**53**:235–8.

59 Poole J, Banks J, Chatfield C *et al*. Disappearance of the Cromer antibody anti-WES^b during pregnancy [Abstract]. *Transfus Med* 1998;**8**(Suppl.1):16.

60 Tregellas WM. Description of a new blood group antigen, Es^a [Abstract]. *18th Congr Int Soc Blood Transfus*, 1984:163.

61 Reid ME, Marfoe RA, Mueller AL *et al*. A second example of anti-Es^a, an antibody to a high incidence Cromer antigen. *Immunohematology* 1996;**12**:112–14.

62 Daniels GL. Characteristics of Cromer related antibodies [Abstract]. *Transfusion* 1983;**23**:410.

63 Sacks DA, Garratty G. Isoimmunization to Cromer antigen in pregnancy. *Am J Obstet Gynecol* 1989;**161**: 928–9.

64 Judd WJ, Steiner EA, Miske V. Adsorption of anti-Cr^a by human platelet concentrates. *Transfusion* 1991;**31**: 286.

65 Reid ME, Ellisor SS, Dean WD. Elution of anti-Cr^a: superiority of the digitonin-acid elution method. *Transfusion* 1985;**25**:172–3.

66 McSwain B, Robins C. A clinically significant anti-Cr^a. *Transfusion* 1988;**28**:289–90.

67 Anderson G, Gray LS, Mintz PD. Red cell survival studies in a patient with anti-Tc^a. *Am J Clin Pathol* 1991;**95**:87–90.

68 Byrne PC, Eckrich RJ, Malamut DC, Mallory DM, Sandler SG. Use of the monocyte monolayer assay (MMA) to predict the clinical significance of anti-Cr^a [Abstract]. *Transfusion* 1995;**35**:61S.

69 Chapman RL, Hare V, Oglesby BL. Successful repeated transfusions of Cr(a+) blood to a patient with anti-Cr^a [Abstract]. *Transfusion* 1992;**32**:23S.

70 Kowalski MA, Pierce SR, Edwards RL *et al*. Hemolytic transfusion reaction due to anti-Tc^a. *Transfusion* 1999;**39**:948–50.

71 Gorman MI, Glidden HM. Another example of anti-Tc^a. *Transfusion* 1981;**21**:579.

72 Holmes CH, Simpson KL, Wainwright SD *et al*. Preferential expression of the complement regulatory protein decay accelerating factor at the fetomaternal interface during pregnancy. *J Immunol* 1990;**144**:3099–105.

73 Moulds JM, Blanchard D, Daniels G *et al*. Coordinator's report: complement regulatory proteins. *Transfus Clin Biol* 1997;**4**:117–9. [See following four papers, pp. 121–34.]

453

74 Lachmann PJ. The control of homologous lysis. *Immunol Today* 1991;**12**:312–15.

75 Fletcher A, Bryant JA, Gardner B *et al*. New monoclonal antibodies in CD59: use for the analysis of peripheral blood cells from paroxysmal nocturnal haemoglobinuria (PNH) patients and for the quantitation of CD59 on normal and decay accelerating factor (DAF)-deficient erythrocytes. *Immunology* 1992;**75**:507–12.

76 Takeda J, Miyata T, Kawagoe K *et al* Deficiency of the GPI anchor caused by somatic mutation of the PIG-A gene in paroxysmal nocturnal hemoglobinuria. *Cell* 1994;**73**:703–11.

77 Bessler M, Schaefer A, Keller P. Paroxysmal nocturnal hemoglobinuria: insights from recent advances in molecular biology. *Transfus Med Rev* 2001;**15**:255–67.

78 Yuan FF, Bryant JA, Fletcher A. Protease-modified erythrocytes: CD55 and CD59 deficient PNH-like cells. *Immunol Cell Biol* 1995;**73**:66–72.

79 Yamashina M, Ueda E, Kinoshita T *et al*. Inherited complete deficiency of 20-kilodalton homologous restriction factor (CD59) as a cause of paroxysmal nocturnal hemoglobinuria. *N Engl J Med* 1990;**323**:1184–9.

80 Motoyama N, Okada N, Yamashina M, Okada H. Paroxysmal nocturnal hemoglobinuria due to hereditary nucleotide deletion in the HRF20 (CD59) gene. *Eur J Immunol* 1992;**22**:2669–73.

81 Shichishima T, Saitoh Y, Terasawa T *et al*. Complement sensitivity of erythrocytes in a patient with inherited complete deficiency of CD59 or with the Inab phenotype. *Br J Haematol* 1999;**104**:303–6.

82 Wiesner J, Jomaa H, Wilhelm M *et al*. Host cell factor CD59 restricts complement lysis of *Plamodium falciparum*-infected erythrocytes. *Eur J Immunol* 1997;**27**: 2708–13.

83 Hamann J, Vogel B, van Schijndel GMW, van Lier RAW. The seven-span transmembrane receptor CD97 has a cellular ligand (CD55, DAF). *J Exp Med* 1996;**184**:1185–9.

84 Moulds JM, Nowicki S, Moulds JJ, Nowicki BJ. Human blood groups: incidental receptors for viruses and bacteria. *Transfusion* 1996;**36**:362–4.

85 Nowicki B, Moulds J, Hull R, Hull S. A hemagglutinin of uropathogenic *Escherichia coli* recognizes the Dr blood group antigen. *Infect Immun* 1988;**56**:1057–60.

86 Nowicki B, Hart A, Coyne KE, Lublin DM, Nowicki S. Short consensus repeat-3 domain of recombinant decay-accelerating factor is recognized by *Escherichia coli* re-

combinant Dr adhesin in a model of a cell–cell interaction. *J Exp Med* 1993;**178**:2115–21.

87 Nowicki B, Truong L, Moulds J, Hull R. Presence of the Dr receptor in normal human tissues and its possible role in the pathogenesis of ascending urinary tract infection. *Am J Pathol* 1988;**133**:1–4.

88 Evans DJ, Almond JW. Cell receptors for picornaviruses as determinants of cell tropism and pathogenesis. *Trends Microbiol* 1998;**6**:198–202.

89 Goldfield M, Srihongse S, Fox JP. Hemagglutinins associated with certain enteric viruses. *Proc Soc Exp Biol Med* 1957; **96**: 788–91.

90 Clarkson NA, Kaufman R, Lublin DM *et al*. Characterization of the echovirus 7 receptor: domains of CD55 critical for virus binding. *J Virol* 1995;**69**:5497–501.

91 Bergelson JM, Chan M, Solomon KR *et al*. Decay-accelerating factor (CD55), a glycosylphosphatidylinositol-anchored complement regulatory protein, is a receptor for several echoviruses. *Proc Natl Acad Sci USA* 1994;**91**:6245–8.

92 Springer TA, Dustin ML, Kishimoto TK, Marlin SD. The lymphocyte function-associated LFA-1, CD2, and LFA-3 molecules: cell adhesion receptors of the immune system. *Annu Rev Immunol* 1987;**5**:223–52.

93 Anstee DJ, Spring FA. Red cell membrane glycoproteins with a broad tissue distribution. *Transfus Med Rev* 1989;**3**:13–23.

94 Schönermark S, Rauterberg EW, Shin ML *et al*. Homologous species restriction in lysis of human erythrocytes: a membrane-derived protein with C8-binding capacity functions as an inhibitor. *J Immunol* 1986;**136**: 1772–6.

95 Hänsch GM, Schönermark S, Roelcke D. Paroxysmal nocturnal hemoglobinuria type III: lack of an erythrocyte membrane protein restricting the lysis by C5b-9. *J Clin Invest* 1987;**80**:7–12.

96 Prusiner SB. Prions. *Proc Natl Acad Sci USA* 1998;**95**:13363–83.

97 Mallinson G, Spring FA, Houldsworth S *et al*. Normal prion protein is expressed on the surface of human red blood cells [Abstract]. *Transfus Med* 2000;**10**(Suppl.1): 17.

98 Hoffer J, Zurbito F, Reid ME *et al*. Laboratory assessment of *in-vivo* survival of crossmatch incompatible blood in a patient with anti-Tcᵃ [Abstract]. *Transfusion* 1994;**34**:20S.

20 Knops blood group system and the Cost antigens

20.1 Introduction

The Knops system consists of three pairs of antithetical antigens, plus Yk^a (Table 20.1). These antigens are defined by clinically insignificant antibodies that are notoriously difficult to identify. They are all located on complement receptor 1 (CR1, CD35), a member of the complement control protein superfamily. The McC^a/McC^b and Sl^a/Vil polymorphisms are associated with amino acid substitutions in CR1 (Table 20.1). The Helgeson phenotype appears, by conventional serological methods, to be a Knops-null phenotype, although very low levels of CR1 are present on the red cells.

CR1 (CD35) is part of the Regulators of Complement Activity gene cluster on chromosome 1q32.

Cs^a is an antigen of moderately high frequency, serologically related to Yk^a. Cs^a does not appear to be on CR1, so Cs^a and its antithetical antigen, Cs^b, comprise the Cost collection (collection 205, Table 20.1 and Section 20.8).

20.2 Complement receptor 1 (CR1) and the Knops system

20.2.1 CR1 (CD35)

CR1 is a glycoprotein of about M_r 200 000 present on red cells, granulocytes, monocytes, B-lymphocytes, a subset of T cells, glomerular podocytes, and follicular-dendritic cells in lymph nodes (reviews on CR1 in [1–3]). A soluble form of CR1 (sCR1) is present in plasma. The primary structure of the CR1 polypeptide has been elucidated from the cDNA sequence [4–6].

The most common allotype of CR1 (CR1*1) consists of 2039 amino acids, which include a 41 amino acid N-terminal signal peptide (cleaved from the mature protein), a 1930 amino acid extracellular domain, a 25 amino acid transmembrane region, and a 43 amino acid cytoplasmic domain. Like some other complement regulatory proteins, including decay-accelerating factor (DAF, Chapter 19), the extracellular domain is organized into a number of regions of amino acid sequence homology, each comprising about 60 residues, called complement control protein repeats (CCPs) or short consensus repeats (SCRs). The extracellular domain of the CR1*1 allotype consists of 30 CCPs (Fig. 20.1). Each CCP domain contains four cysteine residues and is maintained in a folded conformation by two disulphide bonds. Further homology divides the N-terminal 28 CCPs into four regions called long homologous repeats (LHRs), each comprising seven CCPs.

Four allotypes of CR1 of different molecular weight have been identified: the common CR1*1 allotype (previously known as CR1-A, M_r 190 000 under non-reducing conditions); the less common CR1*2 allotype (CR1-B, M_r 220 000); and the rare CR1*3 (CR1-C, M_r 160 000) and CR1*4 (CR1-D, M_r 250 000) allotypes [1,7]. These allotypes differ in the numbers of LHRs making up the extracellular domain and may have arisen as a result of intragenic unequal crossing-over [8]. The number of CR1 molecules per red cell differs considerably from person to person, varying from 20 to over 800 [9]. This red cell quantitative polymorphism is independent of the size polymorphism and is associated with a CR1 *Hind*III restriction fragment-length polymorphism (RFLP) in white peo-

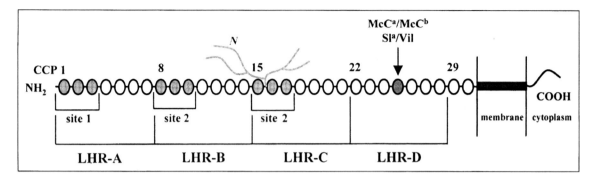

Fig. 20.1 Diagrammatic representation of the most common allotype of CR1 (CR1*1), showing the 30 complement control protein repeats (CCP), the four long homologous repeats (LHR), one of the 6–8 N-linked oligosaccharides (N), the transmembrane region, and the cytoplasmic domain, the active sites (site 1 and the duplicated site 2), and the position of the McC and Sl polymorphisms.

Table 20.1 Antigens of the Knops system and Cost collection.

Number	Name	Comments
Knops system		
KN1	Kn^a	Antithetical to Kn^b (KN2)
KN2	Kn^b	Antithetical to Kn^a (KN1)
KN3	McC^a	Lys1590. Antithetical to McC^b (KN6)
KN4	Sl^a	Arg1601. Antithetical to Vil (KN7)
KN5	Yk^a	
KN6	McC^b	Glu1590. Antithetical to McC^a (KN3)
KN7	Vil	Gly1601. Antithetical to Sl^a (KN4)
Cost collection		
COST1	Cs^a	Antithetical to Cs^b (COST2)
COST2	Cs^b	Antithetical to Cs^a (COST1)

ple, but not in African Americans (for review on CR1 polymorphisms see [3]).

There are 25 potential sites for N-glycosylation [5], but the approximate 25 000 reduction in M_r of CR1 treated with endoglycosidase F suggests 6–8 N-glycans per molecule [1]. CR1 is not O-glycosylated [10].

The 133–160 kb *CR1* gene is organized into 39 exons (*CR1*1* allele) or 47 exons (*CR1*2*). Each LHR is represented by eight exons. In each LHR, CCPs 1, 5, and 7 are encoded by one exon each; CCPs 2 and 6 by two exons each; and CCPs 3 and 4 by a single exon [8,11] (Table 20.2). The major transcription start site is probably 111 bp upstream of the translation-initiating ATG codon [8].

20.2.2 Knops system antigens are located on CR1

In 1991, Rao *et al.* [12] and Moulds *et al.* [13] independently demonstrated that Knops system antigens are situated on CR1. Immunoprecipitation of radiolabelled red cell membrane proteins with anti-Kn^a, -McC^a, -Sl^a, -Yk^a, and several other antibodies with related specificities produced bands on sodium dodecyl sulphate (SDS) polyacrylamide gels identical to those produced by precipitation with monoclonal anti-CR1. Furthermore, after immunoprecipitation with monoclonal anti-CR1, affinity purified CR1 could be detected on immunoblots with human anti-Kn/McC serum [12]. When two CR1 allotypes (1 and 2) were present, two bands were generally detected with the monoclonal and human antibodies [12,13]. However, in one individual apparently heterozygous for *Yk^a*, two bands, representing allotypes CR1*1 and CR1*2, were detected with the monoclonal anti-CR1, but only the band representing the CR1*1 allotype was detected after precipitation by human anti-Yk^a [9]. The location of Kn^a, McC^a, Sl^a, and Yk^a on CR1 was confirmed by neutralization of the corresponding antibodies with soluble, recombinant CR1 [14] and with monoclonal anti-CR1, by the monoclonal antibody-specific immobilization of erythrocyte antigens (MAIEA) assay [15]. Furthermore, the McC^a/McC^b and Sl^a/Vil

Table 20.2 Domains of CR1 encoded by the 39 exons of *CR1*1*.

LHR-A		LHR-B		LHR-C		LHR-D			
Exon	CCP	Exon	CCP	Exon	CCP	Exon	CCP	Exon	Domain
2	1	10	8	18	15	26	22	34	29
3	2a	11	9a	19	16a	27	23a	35	30
4	2b	12	9b	20	16b	28	23b	36	TMa
5	3,4	13	10,11	21	17,18	29	24,25	37	TMb
6	5	14	12	22	19	30	26	38	cyto
7	6a	15	13a	23	20a	31	27a	39	3' UT
8	6b	16	13b	24	20b	32	27b		
9	7	17	14	25	21	33	28		

Exon 1 encodes the leader peptide.
CCP, complement control protein domain; cyto, cytoplasmic domain; LHR, long homologous repeat; TM, trans-membrane domain; UT, untranslated.

polymorphisms are associated with single nucleotide polymorphisms in *CR1* [16] (Section 20.4). In contrast, the immunochemical methods described above all gave negative results with anti-Cs^a, suggesting that Cs^a is not on CR1 [13–15].

In 1973, Swanson [17] reported that Yk^a was present in plasma, as detected by haemagglutination inhibition, and on leucocytes, as detected by adsorption tests. Although these experiments could not be repeated elsewhere [18], the known distribution of CR1 (Section 20.2.1) gives credibility to Swanson's findings.

20.3 Helgeson, a null phenotype in the Knops system?

The major serological characteristic that led to the Knops, McCoy, and Sl^a antigens being ranked together has been their apparent absence from the red cells of one of the discoverers of Kn^a, Margaret Helgeson (M.H.), and from other red cells of the same phenotype [19–23]. The apparent absence of Yk^a from these cells was demonstrated later [9]. In fact, Helgeson phenotype cells do not represent a true Knops-null phenotype because they express very low levels of Knops antigens [9,12,13], and may even be agglutinated in antiglobulin tests by the most potent examples of Knops antibodies [9]. Consequently, Helgeson phenotype, unlike null phenotypes in other systems, is not associated with an antibody to a generic Knops system antigen. The Helgeson phenotype has an incidence of about 1% in African and white Americans [22,23].

Red cells of the Helgeson phenotype have a very low number of CR1 molecules per red cell, approximating 10% of normal [9,12,13]. Knops antigens could be detected on CR1 of Helgeson phenotype cells by immunoprecipitation, flow cytometry, or MAIEA [12,13,15]. Levels of CR1 were normal on red cells of individuals who lacked only one of the Knops system antigens and who had made the corresponding antibody [13]. Expression of Knops antigens, as detected by an antiglobulin test, correlates strongly with the number of CR1 molecules per red cell. Cells with between 20 and 100 CR1 molecules are negative with Knops antibodies by the antiglobulin test (Helgeson phenotype), cells with 100–150 molecules are weak or negative depending on the antibody used, and cells with more than 200 molecules are generally positive with all antibodies tested [9]. It is likely that the Helgeson phenotype and other weaknesses of Knops antigens result from inherited low copy number of CR1, whereas absence of single antigens in individuals who may make the corresponding antibody is caused by mutations within the *CR1* gene.

20.4 Antigens of the Knops system

20.4.1 Kn^a and Kn^b (KN1 and KN2)

Kn^a, the original Knops antigen, was first reported in 1970 by Helgeson et al. [19]. Kn^a has an incidence of about 98–99% (Table 20.3). The three Kn(a–) sibs described in the original paper [19] were later shown to have the Helgeson phenotype.

An antibody in a serum containing anti-Kp^a, which reacted with red cells of 4.2% of Kp(a–) Australian blood donors (Table 20.3), reacted with virtually all Kn(a–) McC(a+) red cell samples, but with no Kn(a–) McC(a–) samples [24]. Consequently, Mallan et al. [24] suggested that the serum contained anti-Kn^b, an antibody antithetical to anti-Kn^a. No other example of anti-Kn^b has been reported. Anti-Kn^b does not react with the red cells of black people, including Kn(a–) McC(a+) individuals, so Kn^a may have different alleles in black and in white people [25,26].

20.4.2 McC^a and McC^b (KN3 and KN6)

McC^a (McCoy) was identified and shown to be associated with Kn^a by Molthan and Moulds [20]. Although Kn^a and McC^a have frequencies well in excess of 90%, 53% of McC(a–) individuals were also Kn(a–). The frequency of Mc(a–) is 1–2% in white Americans, but varies between 3 and 10% in different surveys of African Americans (Table 20.4) and West Africans [20,22,26].

As anti-Kn^b appears to be antithetical to anti-Kn^a in white people, so anti-McC^b is antithetical to anti-McC^a in black people [16,17,25]: 45.3% of black donors are McC(b+) (Table 20.4), which includes all Kn(a+) McC(a–), but no Kn(a–) McC(a–) individuals.

No McC(b+) white person has been found. Family studies show that McC^a and McC^b are inherited, apparently as the products of codominant alleles [20,26]. Gene frequencies in West Africans are McC^a 0.72, McC^b 0.28.

The McC^a/McC^b polymorphism is associated with an A4795G change in exon 29 of CR1, encoding a Lys1590Glu substitution in CCP 25 in LHR-D of CR1 (Fig. 20.1) [16]. Discrepancies between phenotype and genotype in about 6% of samples were accounted for mainly by genes encoding low CR1 copy number. Recombinant soluble CR1 (sCR1) containing Lys1590 inhibited anti-McC^a, but not anti-McC^b, whereas sCR1 containing Glu1590 inhibited anti-McC^b, but not anti-McC^a.

20.4.3 Sl^a and Vil (KN4 and KN7)

Sl^a (Swain–Langley), an antigen of high incidence in white people, but of distinctly lower frequency in black people (Table 20.3), was described in 1980 by Lacey et al. [21] and Molthan [23] (who called it McC^c). All McC(a–) black people are Sl(a–), whether they are Kn(a–) or Kn(a+), but 45% of Kn(a+) McC(a+) African Americans are also Sl(a–). All Kn(a–) McC(a–) white people are also Sl(a–), but only 1% of Kn(a+) McC(a+) white people were Sl(a–) and all four

Table 20.3 Frequencies of Knops antigens.

Antigen	Population	No. tested	No. positive	Antigen frequency	References
Kn^a	Americans	2071	2067	0.9981	[19]
	White Americans	2482	2431	0.9795	[22]
	African Americans	894	883	0.9877	[22]
Kn^b	Australians	166	7	0.0422	[24]
	Americans	63	3	0.0476	[24]
McC^a	White Americans	3860	3802	0.9850	[20,22]
	African Americans	645	624	0.9674	[20]
	African Americans	894	837	0.9362	[22]
McC^b	African Americans	371	168	0.4528	[25]
Sl^a	White Americans	111	110	0.9910	[21]
	African Americans	109	66	0.6055	[21]
	White Americans	722	705	0.9765	[23]
	African Americans	371	191	0.5148	[23]
Yk^a	White Americans	2889	2598	0.8993	[22]
	African Americans	1117	1098	0.9830	[22]

Kn(a+) McC(a–) individuals found in testing 722 white donors were Sl(a+). Sl(a–) has a frequency of around 70% in West Africans [26].

An antibody, anti-Vil, appeared to be antithetical to anti-Sl^a when testing red cells from black people, but no Vil+ white person was found [21].

The Sl^a/Vil polymorphism is associated with A4828G in exon 29 of *CR1*, encoding an Arg1601Gly substitution in CCP 25 of CR1 [16]. Discrepancies between Sl^a/Vil phenotype and genotype in about 12% of samples were accounted for mainly by genes encoding low CR1 copy number. Soluble CR1 containing Arg1601 inhibited anti-Sl^a, but not anti-Vil, except when the sCR1 also contains Glu1590 (McC^b), when anti-Sl^a was not inhibited. This is probably caused by the change from a positively charged lysine to a negatively charged glutamic acid at position 1590 affecting the conformation of the Sl^a epitope around position 1601 [16]. McC(a–) Sl(a+) phenotype is not found in black people [16,23,25]. Soluble CR1 containing Gly1601 inhibited anti-Vil, but not anti-Sl^a.

Many other antibodies have been found that do not react with Kn(a–) McC(a–) (Helgeson phenotype) red cells, but which differ from those described above. These antibodies are often referred to as anti-Kn/McC.

20.4.4 Yk^a (KN5)

The original anti-Yk^a (York) was initially thought to be anti-Cs^a because it failed to react with two Cs(a–) samples. The cells of Mrs York, however, were Cs(a+), so Yk^a was described by Molthan and Giles [18] as a new antigen related to Cs^a.

Yk^a is inherited as a Mendelian dominant character [18]. The frequency of the *Yk^a* gene, calculated from the data shown in Table 20.3, is 0.6826 in white Americans and 0.8696 in African Americans. There may be some heterogeneity in the specificity of Yk^a antibodies [27].

The incidence of the Cs(a–) Yk(a–) phenotype in white Americans is 0.0163 [22]. If there was no association between Cs^a and Yk^a, the expected phenotype frequency would be 0.0048, about three times less than that observed. Cs(a–) Yk(a–) has an incidence of 0.0035 in African Americans [22], about 17 times that expected assuming no association. Two family studies indicated that the genes for Cs^a and Yk^a segregate

independently [18], but doubt was subsequently cast on this when one of the families was retested [22].

When Molthan and Moulds [20] reported McC^a they found that 37% of McC(a–) white people were Yk(a–) and 29% Cs(a–); 2.2% of McC(a–) black people were Yk(a–) and 17% were Cs(a–). These figures differ substantially from those expected if no relationship between McC^a, Yk^a, and Cs^a existed; 100 times more McC(a–) donors were Yk(a–) Cs(a–) Kn(a–) than would be predicted from the frequencies of these antigens. Although the original Helgeson phenotype cells (M.H.) are Yk(a–) Cs(a–), three other examples were Yk(a–) Cs(a+) [9].

20.4.5 Some other serological characteristics of Knops antigens

20.4.5.1 Antigen strength

Knops antigens show a variation in strength between individuals, which cannot readily be correlated with dosage resulting from zygosity [18,20,22], but does correlate with red cell CR1 levels [9]. A reduction in expression of Knops antigens often appears to occur with red cell storage, but this could not be demonstrated conclusively in controlled tests with Knops antibodies against freshly bled red cells and cells stored for 35 days [28]. CR1 density per red cell decreases with cell ageing, possibly because of protease cleavage of the protein near its stalk [3].

Daniels *et al.* [29] found that strength of the Knops antigens is also affected by presence of an *In(Lu)* gene (see Chapter 6). In(Lu) Lu$_{null}$ cells gave lower mean titration scores with anti-Kn^a, -McC^a, -Yk^a, and -Sl^a, and with anti-Cs^a, than did Lu(a–b+) or Lu(a+b+) cells from members of the same family. This effect of *In(Lu)* could not be confirmed in a later study, by comparison of In(Lu) cells with unrelated donors of common Lutheran phenotype [30].

Knops antigens are generally well expressed on red cells from cord samples. Two babies of McC(a–) mothers with high titre anti-McC^a were also McC(a–) at birth, but became McC(a+) within their first year of life [31]. Maternal anti-McC^a may have been responsible for impaired McC^a antigen expression *in utero*.

20.4.5.2 Effects of enzymes and reducing agents

Knops system antigens are generally resistant to

treatment of the red cells with ficin and papain [20–22,32,33], although this may depend on the antibody and method of enzyme treatment used. Two of 33 anti-McC^a failed to react with ficin-treated McC(a+) cells [22]. One weak example of anti-Yk^a did not react with ficin-treated cells initially, but after the patient was transfused with seven units of Yk(a+) blood the more avid anti-Yk^a reacted strongly with ficinized cells [22]. Kn^a, McC^a, and Yk^a are destroyed by trypsin and chymotrypsin treatment of the cells, which helps to distinguish them from Cs^a [33].

Kn^a, McC^a, and Yk^a are destroyed, or at least weakened, by the disulphide bond reducing agents 2-aminoethylisothiouronium bromide (AET) and dithiothreitol (DTT), also distinguishing them from Cs^a [33–35].

20.5 Knops system antibodies

20.5.1 Antibody characteristics

The term 'high-titre low-avidity' (HTLA) has been used for many years to describe antibodies to a variety of antigens, including those of the Knops system. Although most of these antibodies react at high dilution despite their low avidity, some examples do not share these characteristics and the HTLA label is of little value.

Knops antibodies are generally troublesome to work with. This is partly because of the variation in antigen strength, but also because it is difficult to adsorb the antibodies to completion or to obtain active eluates from weak antigen-positive cells. Consequently, it is almost impossible to distinguish antigen-negative cells from weakly positive cells, especially when stored or 'travelled' red cells are used.

Knops antibodies are generally IgG; they react by an antiglobulin test and do not bind complement [22,36]. There is little information regarding IgG subclass: one Knops system antibody was IgG4 [37]; another contained IgG1, IgG3, and IgG4, as well as IgA [38]. There is only one report of an apparently 'naturally occurring' Knops system antibody; anti-Kn^a in a woman who denied previous pregnancy or transfusion [39]. Of 602 blood donors lacking one or more of the Knops antigens or Cs^a, none had made a corresponding antibody [22]. Most people with one or more Knops antibodies have been transfused, but there are a few examples of anti-Kn^a, -McC^a, and

-Yk^a stimulated by pregnancy alone [22,38,40]. About 50% of sera with Knops antibodies or anti-Cs^a also contained antibodies to other red cell antigens [22].

20.5.2 Clinical significance

Knops antibodies are clinically benign, apart from the danger of masking the presence of more dangerous antibodies that are commonly present in the same serum. Knops antibodies should be ignored when selecting blood for transfusion. There are numerous accounts of patients with one of these antibodies being transfused with no ill effects [18–20,37,39,41–45]. Radiolabelled incompatible red cells in patients with Knops antibodies show either normal or only slightly reduced survival [37–39,41,44,46,47], and *in vitro* phagocytosis assays often give very low scores [37,39]. *In vitro* functional assays involving monocytes may, however, give false positive results with Knops antibodies, because these antibodies can bind red cells to monocytes via CR1 rather than the Fc receptor, FcγR1 [45].

There is no report of haemolytic disease of the newborn (HDN) caused by a Knops antibody, despite numerous opportunities [31,40,48]. CR1 expression on red cells is reduced during pregnancy, reaching its nadir in the third trimester and returning to normal within 48 h postpartum [49].

20.6 Functional aspects of CR1, a complement-regulating protein

The major function of red cell CR1 is to bind and process C3b/C4b coated immune complexes and to transport them to the liver and spleen for removal from the circulation. CR1 has decay accelerating activity (DAA) for C3 and C5 convertases of the classical and alternative pathways and acts as a cofactor for the factor I-mediated cleavage of C3b and C4b (reviewed in [1,50]). In the common allotype of CR1 (Fig. 20.1), most of the cofactor activity for C3b and C4b resides in CCPs 8–10 (site 2) and is duplicated in the nearly identical CCPs 15–17 [51]. DAA for C3 convertases resides in CCPs 1–3 (site 1), whereas DAA for C5 convertases requires both sites 1 and 2 [52]. CR1 also enhances phagocytosis of C3b and C4b coated particles by neutrophils and monocytes.

In vivo and *in vitro* haemolysis of PNHIII red cells, which have CR1 but are deficient in DAF and CD59

Table 20.4 Cs^a frequencies.

Population	No. tested	No. Cs(a+)	Cs^a frequency	References
Northern Europeans	363	354	0.9752	[32]
Black Africans and Americans	53	51	0.9623	[32]
White Americans	2028	1931	0.9522	[22]
African Americans	894	883	0.9877	[22]
Yk(a–) white Americans	96	84	0.8750	[18]
Yk(a–) African Americans	13	12	0.9231	[18]

(Chapter 19), suggests that CR1 plays a minor part in protection of red cells from complement-mediated lysis. CR1 appears to represent a privileged site on red cells for IgG binding, as relatively large quantities of IgG may be bound to CR1 without subsequent lysis or phagocytosis of the red cells [53]. This may explain why Knops system antibodies do not significantly reduce the survival of transfused incompatible red cells (Section 20.5.2).

20.7 Associations of CR1 with malaria and other pathogens

Red cells infected with selected cultures of the malarial parasite *Plasmodium falciparum* form rosettes with other infected red cells and with uninfected red cells. Rowe *et al.* [54] showed that infected cells do not form rosettes with uninfected red cells that have very low levels of CR1 (Helgeson phenotype) and that there is substantially reduced rosetting with Sl(a–) cells, compared with Sl(a+) cells. Furthermore, compared with Sl(a+) cells, Helgeson phenotype red cells and other cells with the Sl(a–) phenotype showed reduced levels of binding to COS-7 cells transfected with the *P. falciparum var* gene expressing PfEMP1, the parasite ligand involved in rosetting. Sl(a–) is present in about 70% of West Africans, 40–50% of African Americans, but in only about 2% of white Americans (Section 20.4.3). Rosetting is associated with severe disease by clogging the microvasculature of vital organs including the brain, so it is feasible that the Sl(a–) phenotype has a selective advantage in areas where *P. falciparum* malaria is endemic. The regions of CR1 required for formation of *P. falciparum* rosettes have been localized to the areas of LHR-B and -C that act as binding sites for activated C3b (Fig. 20.1) [55]. These

are remote from the site of the Sl^a polymorphism in LHR-D.

Leishmanioses are insect-transmitted diseases caused by protozoa of the genus *Leishmania*, which live in mononuclear phagocytes. On entering the human bloodstream, the promastigotes become coated with natural anti-*Leishmania* antibodies, which activate complement. C3 coating the surface of the pathogen then serves as a ligand for CR1 on the surface of monocytes, and the parasite is ingested by conventional phagocytosis [56]. The bacteria *Legionella pneumophila*, *Mycobacterium leprae*, and *M. tuberculosis* utilize similar mechanisms involving CR1 for invading phagocytes [57].

20.8 The Cost collection: Cs^a and Cs^b (COST1 and COST2)

When Giles *et al.* [32] described three patients with antibodies reactive with the red cells of 98% of northern Europeans, they named this antibody anti-Cs^a after two of the original patients, Mrs Co. and Mrs St. Numerous family studies have shown that Cs^a is inherited as a dominant character and that it is not part of the ABO, MNS, Rh, Kell, Duffy, Kidd, Yt, or Scianna systems, is probably not part of P and Lewis, and that there is a possible association between Cs^a and Do^a [32,58]. Table 20.4 shows the results of frequency studies with anti-Cs^a.

Anti-Cs^a share many characteristics with Knops system antibodies (Section 20.5) and are difficult to work with, primarily because of the variability in expression of the Cs^a antigen. Like Knops system antibodies, anti-Cs^a are of no significance clinically. A patient with anti-Cs^a was successfully transfused with 11 units of Cs(a+) blood and *in vivo* survival of radiolabelled

Cs(a+) cells in patients with anti-Cs^a have been close to normal [59].

An antibody in a multiply transfused woman with a weak Cs^a antigen was named anti-Cs^b by Molthan and Paradis [60]. Fifty-six of 59 Cs(a–) samples were Cs(b+); the remaining three were Cs(a–b–), suggesting the presence of a third allele. The existence of a third allele was supported by a family study. Fifty-five (31%) of 175 Cs(a+) samples were Cs(b+).

Despite phenotypic associations with the Knops system antigens, especially Yk^a (see Section 20.4.4), Cs^a and Cs^b are not included in the Knops system for the following reasons:

1 Cs^a could not be shown to be on CR1 [13,15];

2 Cs^a was easily detected on three of four Helgeson phenotype samples [9]; and

3 Cs^a is resistant to treatment of red cells with trypsin, chymotrypsin, and AET [33].

The nature of the association between Cs^a and the Knops system remains obscure.

References

1 Ahearn JM, Fearon DT. Structure and function of the complement receptors, CR1 (CD35) and CR2 (CD21). *Adv Immunol* 1989;46:183–219.

2 Hourcade D, Holers VM, Atkinson JP. The regulators of complement activation (RCA) gene cluster. *Adv Immunol* 1989;45:381–416.

3 Cohen JHM, Atkinson JP, Klickstein LB *et al.* The C3b/C4b receptor (CR1, CD35) on erythrocytes: methods for study of polymorphisms. *Mol Immunol* 1999;36:819–25.

4 Klickstein LB, Wong WW, Smith JA *et al.* Human C3b/C4b receptor (CR1): demonstration of long homologous repeating domains that are composed of the short consensus repeats characteristic of C3/C4 binding proteins. *J Exp Med* 1987;165:1095–112.

5 Klickstein LB, Bartow TJ, Miletic V *et al.* Identification of distinct C3b and C4b recognition sites in the human C3b/C4b receptor (CR1, CD35) by deletion mutagenesis. *J Exp Med* 1988;168:1699–717.

6 Hourcade D, Miesner DR, Atkinson JP, Holers VM. Identification of an alternative polyadenylation site in the human C3b/C4b receptor (complement receptor type 1) transcriptional unit and prediction of a secreted form of complement receptor type 1. *J Exp Med* 1988;168:1255–70.

7 Moulds JM, Brai M, Cohen J *et al.* Reference typing report for complement receptor 1 (CR1). *Exp Clin Immunogenet* 1998;15:291–4.

8 Vik DP, Wong WW. Structure of the gene for the F allele of complement receptor type 1 and sequence of the coding region unique to the S allele. *J Immunol* 1993;151:6214–24.

9 Moulds JM, Moulds JJ, Brown M, Atkinson JP. Antiglobulin testing for CR1-related (Knops/MCoy/Swain–Langley/York) blood group antigens: negative and weak reactions are caused by variable expression of CR1. *Vox Sang* 1992;62:230–5.

10 Lublin DM, Griffith RC, Atkinson JP. Influence of glycosylation on allelic and cell-specific M_r variation, receptor processing, and ligand binding of the human complement C3b/C4b receptor. *J Biol Chem* 1986;261:5736–44.

11 Wong WW, Cahill JM, Rosen MD *et al.* Structure of the human CR1 gene: molecular basis of the structural and quantitative polymorphisms and identification of a new CR1-like allele. *J Exp Med* 1989;169:847–63.

12 Rao N, Ferguson DJ, Lee S-F, Telen MJ. Identification of human erythrocyte blood group antigens on the C3b/C4b receptor. *J Immunol* 1991;146:3502–7.

13 Moulds JM, Nickells MW, Moulds JJ, Brown MC, Atkinson JP. The C3b/C4b receptor is recognized by the Knops, McCoy, Swain–Langley, and York blood group antisera. *J Exp Med* 1991;173:1159–63.

14 Moulds JM, Rowe JM. Neutralization of Knops system antibodies using soluble complement receptor 1. *Transfusion* 1996;36:517–20.

15 Petty AC, Green CA, Poole J, Daniels GL. Analysis of Knops blood group antigens on CR1 (CD35) by the MAIEA test and by immunoblotting. *Transfus Med* 1997;7:55–62.

16 Moulds JM, Zimmerman PA, Doumbo OK *et al.* Molecular identification of Knops blood group polymorphisms found in long homologous region D of complement receptor 1. *Blood* 2001;97:2879–85.

17 Swanson JL. Laboratory problems associated with leukocyte antibodies. In: *A Seminar on Recent Advances in Immunohematology*. Arlington: American Association of Blood Banks, 1973:121–55.

18 Molthan L, Giles CM. A new antigen, Yk^a (York), and its relationship to Cs^a (Cost). *Vox Sang* 1975;29:145–53.

19 Helgeson M, Swanson J, Polesky HF. Knops–Helgeson (Kn^a), a high-frequency erythrocyte antigen. *Transfusion* 1970;10:137–8.

20 Molthan L, Moulds J. A new antigen, McC^a (McCoy), and its relationship to Kn^a (Knops). *Transfusion* 1978;18:566–8.

21 Lacey P, Laird-Fryer B, Block U *et al.* A new high incidence blood group factor, Sl^a; and its hypothetical allele [Abstract]. *Transfusion* 1980;20:632.

22 Molthan L. The serology of the York–Cost–McCoy–Knops red blood cell system. *Am J Med Technol* 1983;49:49–55.

23 Molthan L. Expansion of the York, Cost, McCoy, Knops blood group system: the new McCoy antigens McC^c and McC^d. *Med Lab Sci* 1983;40:113–21.

24 Mallan MT, Grimm W, Hindley L *et al.* The Hall serum:

detecting Kn[b], the antithetical allele to Kn[a] [Abstract]. *Transfusion* 1980;20:630–1.

25 Molthan L. The status of the McCoy/Knops antigens. *Med Lab Sci* 1983;40:59–63.

26 Moulds JM, Kassambara L, Middleton JJ *et al*. Identification of complement receptor 1 (CR1) polymorphisms in West Africa. *Genes Immun* 2000;1:325–9.

27 Rolih SD. High-titer, low-avidity (HTLA) antibodies and antigens: a review. *Transfus Med Rev* 1989;3:128–39.

28 Moulds JM, Brown LL, Brukheimer E. Loss of Knops blood group systems antigens from stored blood. *Immunohematology* 1995;11:46–50.

29 Daniels GL, Shaw MA, Lomas CG, Leak MR, Tippett P. The effect of *In(Lu)* on some high-frequency antigens. *Transfusion* 1986;26:171–2.

30 Moulds JM, Shah C. Complement receptor 1 red cell expression is not controlled by the *In(Lu)* gene. *Transfusion* 1999;39:751–5.

31 Ferguson SJ, Blajchman MA, Guzewski H, Taylor CR, Moulds J. Alloantibody-induced impaired neonatal expression of a red blood cell antigen associated with maternal alloimmunization. *Vox Sang* 1982;43:82–6.

32 Giles CM, Huth MC, Wilson TE, Lewis HBM, Grove GEB. Three examples of a new antibody, anti-Cs[a], which reacts with 98% of red cell samples. *Vox Sang* 1965;10:405–15.

33 Daniels G. Effect of enzymes on and chemical modifications of high-frequency red cell antigens. *Immunohematology* 1992;8:53–7.

34 Moulds JJ, Moulds MK. Inactivation of Kell blood group antigens by 2-aminoethylisothiouronium bromide. *Transfusion* 1983;23:274–5.

35 Toy EM. Inactivation of high-incidence antigens on red blood cells by dithiothreitol. *Immunohematology* 1986;2:57–9.

36 Moulds MK. Serological investigation and clinical significance of high-titer, low-avidity (HTLA) antibodies. *Am J Med Technol* 1981;47:789–95.

37 Ballas SK, Viggiano E, Draper EK. Survival of Kn(a+) McC(a+) red cells in a patient with anti-'Kn[a]/McC[a]'. *Transfusion* 1984;24:22–4.

38 Ghandhi JG, Moulds JJ, Szymanski IO. Shortened long-term survival of incompatible red cells in a patient with anti-McCoy-like antibody: immunoglobulin characteristics of this antibody. *Transfusion* 1984;24:16–18.

39 Baldwin ML, Ness PM, Barrasso C *et al*. *In vivo* studies of the long-term ^{51}Cr red cell survival of serologically incompatible red cell units. *Transfusion* 1985;25:34–8.

40 Molthan L. Biological significance of the York, Cost, McCoy and Knops alloantibodies. *Rev Franc Transfus Immuno-Hémat* 1982;25:127–47.

41 Wells RF, Korn G, Hafleigh B, Grumet FC. Characterization of three new apparently related high frequency antigens. *Tranfusion* 1976;16:427–33.

42 Ryden SE. Successful transfusion of a patient with anti-Yk[a]. *Transfusion* 1981;26:130–1.

43 Harpool DR. Anti-Sl[a]: lack of effect on transfused Sl(a–) red cells. *Transfusion* 1983;23:402–3.

44 Lau PYL, Jewlachow V, Leahy MF. Successful transfusion of Yk[a]-positive red cells in a patient with anti-Yk[a]. *Vox Sang* 1993;64:254–5.

45 Hadley A, Wilkes A, Poole J, Arndt P, Garratty G. A chemiluminescence test for predicting the outcome of transfusing incompatible blood. *Transfus Med* 1999;9:337–42.

46 Tilley CA, Crookston MC, Haddad SA, Shumak KH. Red blood cell survival studies in patients with anti-Ch[a], anti-Yk[a], anti-Ge, and anti-Vel. *Transfusion* 1977;17:169–72.

47 Schanfield MS, Stevens JO, Bauman D. The detection of clinically significant erythrocyte alloantibodies using a human mononuclear phagocyte assay. *Transfusion* 1981;21:571–6.

48 Eska P, Rosche ME, Grindon AJ. Uneventful delivery of patient with antibody in Knops group. *Transfusion* 1976;16:190–1.

49 Imrie HJ, McGonigle TP, Liu DTY, Jones DRE. Reduction in erythrocyte complement receptor 1 (CR1, CD35) and decay accelerating factor (DAF, CD55) during normal pregnancy. *J Reprod Immunol* 1996;31:221–7.

50 Law SKA, Reid KBM. *Complement*, 2nd edn. Oxford: IRL Press, 1995.

51 Krych M, Clemenza L, Howdeshell D *et al*. Analysis of the functional domains of complement receptor type 1 (C3b/C4b receptor; CR1) by substitution mutagenesis. *J Biol Chem* 1994;269:13273–8.

52 Krych-Goldberg M, Hauhart R, Subramanian VB *et al*. Decay accelerating activity of complement receptor type 1 (CD35): two active sites are required for dissociating C5 convertases. *J Biol Chem* 1999;274:31160–8.

53 Reinagel ML, Gezen M, Ferguson PJ *et al*. The primate erythrocyte complement receptor (CR1) as a privileged site: binding of immunoglobulin G to erythrocyte CR1 does not target erythrocytes for phagocytosis. *Blood* 1997;89:1068–77.

54 Rowe JA, Moulds JM, Newbold CI, Miller LH. *P. falciparum* rosetting mediated by a parasite-variant erythrocyte membrane protein and complement-receptor 1. *Nature* 1997;388:292–5.

55 Rowe JA, Rogerson SJ, Raza A *et al*. Mapping of the region of complement receptor (CR) 1 required for *Plasmodium falciparum* rosetting and demonstration of the importance of CR1 in rosetting in field isolates. *J Immunol* 2000;165:6341–6.

56 Dominguez M, Toraño A. Immune adherence-mediated opsonophagocytosis: the mechanism of *Leishmania* infection. *J Exp Med* 1999;189:25–35.

57 Cooper NR. Complement evasion strategies of microorganisms. *Immunol Today* 1991;12:327–31.

58 Giles CM. Serologically difficult red cell antibodies with special reference to Chido and Rodgers blood groups. In: JF Mohn, RW Plunkett, RK Cunningham, RM Lambert,

eds. *Human Blood Groups, 5th Int Convoc Immunol, Buffalo NY.* Basel: Karger, 1977:268–76.

59 Shore GM, Steane EA. Survival of incompatible red cells in a patient with anti-Cs[a] and three other patients with antibodies to high-frequency red cell antigens [Abstract]. *Transfusion* 1978;18:387–8.

60 Molthan L, Paradis DJ. Anti-Cs[b]: the finding of the antibody antithetical to anti-Cs[a]. *Med Lab Sci* 1987;44:94–6.

21 Indian blood group system and the AnWj antigen

21.1 Introduction

Indian is a polymorphism in people from the Indian subcontinent and Arabs. In^a and In^b are of low and high incidence, respectively. They are located on CD44, a ubiquitous glycoprotein with a variety of functions, mostly associated with its ability to bind hyaluronan, a component of the extracellular matrix. The In^b/In^a polymorphism results from an Arg46Pro substitution.

The gene encoding CD44 is on chromosome 11 at 11p13 (Chapter 32).

The high frequency antigen AnWj (901009) has not been assigned to the Indian system, but is either located on an isoform of CD44 or is closely associated with it.

21.2 CD44 and the Indian antigens

21.2.1 CD44

CD44 is a 'cluster of differentiation' that includes a host of monoclonal antibodies to epitopes on glycoproteins present on cells of many tissues, including red cells [1]. The CD44 glycoprotein has also been called *In(Lu)*-related p80, p85, Hermes antigen, and lymphocyte homing associated cell adhesion molecule (H-CAM).

Immunoprecipitation and immunoblotting experiments with CD44 monoclonal antibodies revealed a major red cell membrane component of apparent M_r 80 000 [2–4]. This component was only detected when immunoblotting was performed under non-reducing conditions, confirming the importance of intact disulphide bonds in the integrity of most CD44 epitopes. Immunoblotting of endoglycosidase-F treated red cells, which revealed a substantial reduction in appar-

ent M_r of the 80 000 component, demonstrated that the molecule is a glycoprotein containing N-linked oligosaccharides, which are not essential to antigen activity [2,5]. There are an estimated 6000–10 000 copies of CD44 per red cell [6].

The *CD44* gene spans 50 kb of DNA and consists of 20 exons [7,8]. CD44 exists as multiple isoforms, arising partly from alternative splicing of at least 10 of the 20 exons during processing of the *CD44* transcript (Fig. 21.1) and partly from variation in glycosylation [7,8]. CD44H (haemopoietic), the standard form of the molecule, is the CD44 isoform present on red cells and leucocytes. It consists of a 248 amino acid N-terminal extracellular domain, which contains products of none of the alternatively spliced exons, a 21 amino acid membrane-spanning domain, and a 72 amino acid C-terminal cytoplasmic tail [9–11]. The extracellular domain can be divided into two regions:
1 a membrane proximal region containing sites for O-glycosylation and chondroitin sulphate linkage, and
2 a distal region, folded into a globular domain through disulphide bonding of its six cysteine residues, containing a region homologous to cartilage link protein and five of the six potential N-glycosylation sites (Fig. 21.2). The extensive glycosylation and addition of the glycosaminoglycan chondroitin, has led to CD44 being described as a proteoglycan. The cytoplasmic domain may interact with the membrane skeleton [2] and there is evidence that CD44 can bind band 4.1 or ankyrin, *in vitro* [12].

21.2.2 Indian antigens are located on CD44

Spring *et al.* [2] showed that In^a and In^b are carried on the CD44 glycoprotein. Immunoblotting of membranes from antigen-positive cells under non-

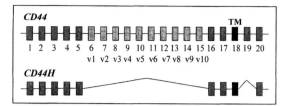

Fig. 21.1 Organization of *CD44* showing the 20 exons, including the 10 alternatively spliced exons, v1–10, within the region encoding the extracellular domain (exons 1–17) and the exon encoding the transmembrane domain (TM, exon 18). The lower figure shows the exons encoding the haemopoietic form of CD44, CD44H.

reducing conditions with purified human anti-In^a and -In^b revealed an M_r 80 000 component of identical mobility to CD44; no such component was detected in membranes from In(a–b+) and In(a+b–) cells, respectively. CD44 glycoprotein isolated from human red cell membranes by immunoprecipitation with monoclonal anti-CD44 reacted with anti-In^b on an immunoblot [2]. Anti-In^b was shown, by radioimmunoassay, to bind CD44 glycoprotein isolated from human red cells and leucocytes [2,13] and positive results were obtained in monoclonal antibody-specific immobilization of erythrocyte antigens (MAIEA) assays performed with human alloanti-In^b and mouse monoclonal anti-CD44 [14,15].

21.3 In^a and In^b (IN1 and IN2)

In 1973, a new antigen present on red cells of about 3% of Indians from Bombay was named In^a by Badakere *et al.* [16,17]. Two years later, Giles [18] found that an antibody to a public antigen, Salis, was antithetical to anti-In^a and the antibody became anti-In^b.

21.3.1 Frequencies and inheritance

Of 1749 Bombay Indians, 51 (3%) were In(a+) [17]. This gives a frequency for the In^a allele of 0.0147, and the following genotype frequencies can be deduced: In^a/In^a 0.0002; In^a/In^b 0.0290; In^b/In^b 0.9708. A higher frequency of In^a was found in some Arabs: 59 of 557 (10.6%) Iranians and 29 of 246 (11.8%) Arabs in Bombay were In(a+) [19]. In^a is virtually unknown in

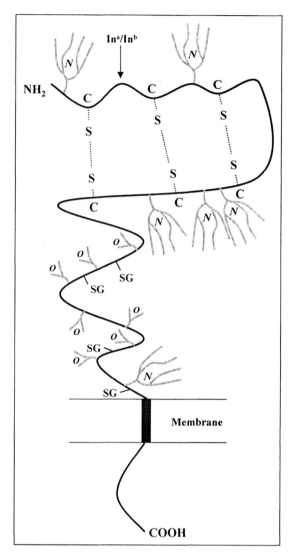

Fig. 21.2 Model of CD44H. The extracellular domain consists of two regions: a membrane-proximal region containing one *N*-glycosylation site (*N*), several *O*-glycosylation sites (*O*), and several Ser-Gly chondroitin sulphate linkage sites (SG); and a distal region containing five *N*-glycosylation sites and six cysteine residues (C), which suggests the presence of three disulphide bonds (S–S). The position of the amino acid substitution responsible for the In^a/In^b polymorphism is shown.

other populations. Two of 700 Indian blood donors were In(b–) [20], far in excess of the number expected from the calculated genotype frequencies given above. Of 251 members of the Asian immigrant population of northern England, two were In(a+b–), eight were

In(a+b+), and 241 were In(a–b+); again an excess of In(a+b–) [21].

From the limited number of families reported, In^a and In^b appear to be inherited as codominant autosomal alleles [17,18,22]. A silent allele could explain the presence of In(a+b–) in two generations of one family [22].

Red cells of a girl with a novel form of congenital dyserythropoietic anaemia and gross deficiency of red cell CD44 were In(a–b–); they were also Co(a–b–), AnWj–, and weak for LW^{ab} [23]. The girl's parents and sister were In(a–b+), providing no information on whether her unique phenotype is inherited.

21.3.2 Molecular basis for the Indian polymorphism

The In^a/In^b polymorphism results from a single base change in exon 2 of *CD44* encoding an amino acid substitution: the common allele, In^b, has G252 and encodes Arg46; In^a has C252 and encodes Pro46 [24] (see [9] for numbering). Jurkat human leukaemia cell line was transfected with *CD44* cDNA constructs from In^b or In^a alleles, or from the In^b allele with a G252C change introduced by site-directed mutagenesis. All three types of transfectant produced CD44 protein, but only cells transfected with the cDNA with wild-type In^b sequence expressed In^b. Other changes detected in some In(a+b–) individuals (T322C, silent; T370C, silent; A441C, Tyr109Ser; A831G, Glu239Gly) do not appear to affect expression of the Indian antigens.

21.3.3 Antigen characteristics

In^a and In^b are protease-sensitive. Both antigens are destroyed by papain, pronase, trypsin, and chymotrypsin [17,18,21,22,25–27], but are resistant to treatment of red cells with sialidase [27, C.A. Green and G.L. Daniels, unpublished observations]. In^a and In^b are destroyed by the disulphide bond-reducing agents 2-aminoethylisothiouronium bromide (AET) and dithiothreitol (DTT) [20,22,27,28,29]. Higher concentrations of the reducing agents than generally used for treating red cells may be required to destroy antigen expression. Reactivity of most CD44 antibodies with red cells is destroyed, or partially destroyed, by treatment of the cells with proteases and with AET and DTT [2,3,5,6,30], although trypsin-, chy-

motrypsin-, and AET-resistant epitopes exist [6]. CD44 is not affected by sialidase treatment of the red cells.

In(a–b+) and In(a+b+) red cells could be distinguished by titration with anti-In^b [20]. Red cells from cord samples and from pregnant women show reduced expression of In^a [25,26]. From results of an indirect immunoradiometric assay, red cells of neonates were estimated to have about 25% of the adult number of In^a antigen sites [26]. Red cells of pregnant women have about 38% of the normal adult number, the number of sites returning to normal 3–6 months after delivery [26]. No weakness of In^b was detected on cord red cell samples by serological titration [21].

CD44 is present in serum [30,31] and In^b can be detected in serum by haemagglutination inhibition (T. Kaye, personal communication, 1978).

21.4 Effect of *In(Lu)* on CD44 and In^b

Telen *et al.* [5,30] demonstrated by flow cytometry that a CD44 monoclonal antibody (A3D8) showed markedly reduced levels of binding with red cells of individuals with *In(Lu)*, the dominant inhibitor of the Lutheran system and of some other red cell antigens (see Section 6.4). One example of Lu_{null} In(Lu) cells bound between 25% and 39% of the quantity of anti-CD44 bound by normal cells [5]. Reduced binding was not seen with Lu_{null} cells of recessive and X-linked types, and the recessive Lu_{null} may even have had enhanced binding of CD44 antibodies [32]. With some CD44 antibodies the reduced binding to In(Lu) cells can also be detected by conventional serological techniques [2,4,33]. Normal human sera reduced binding of anti-CD44 to red cells by 67% in inhibition experiments, whereas serum from an Lu_{null} In(Lu) individual reduced binding by only 33% [30].

Immunoprecipitation and immunoblotting of membranes from In(Lu) cells revealed only a trace of CD44 [2–4,6], whereas recessive and X-linked Lu_{null} cells had normal, or even slightly enhanced, CD44 expression [32,34].

Anti-In^b has a reduced titre with Lu_{null} In(Lu) cells, compared with cells of normal Lutheran type and with Lu_{null} cells of the recessive and X-linked types [2,22]. A band of markedly reduced intensity was seen with membranes from In(Lu) cells blotted with anti-In^b [2].

21.5 Indian antibodies

Indian antigens appear to be good immunogens. Thirty of 39 In(a–) donors immunized for anti-D production with D+ In(a+) red cells made anti-In^a [25]. Anti-In^a has also been produced in response to transfusion of a unit of In(a+) blood [35]. One anti-In^b was produced in an untransfused woman during her first pregnancy [22]. Anti-In^a and -In^b often agglutinate antigen-positive red cells directly, although the strength of reaction is generally enhanced by antiglobulin [18,21,25].

Radiolabelled In(a+) red cells were eliminated from the circulation of two individuals with anti-In^a within 20 min, suggesting potential for a transfusion reaction [25]. There is one case of anti-In^b causing an immediate haemolytic transfusion reaction after infusion of 50 mL of incompatible blood [20]. Reduced *in vivo* survival of In(b+) cells in a patient an anti-In^b was observed at 24 h [22]. Neither anti-In^a nor -In^b has been implicated in haemolytic disease of the newborn (HDN). In(b+) cord cells from babies born to mothers with IgG1 anti-In^b do not usually give a positive direct antiglobulin test (DAT) and anti-In^b cannot usually be detected in the infants' sera [21,22,36]. In one case with maternal anti-In^b of high titre, red cells of the baby did give a positive DAT and anti-In^b could be eluted from them [37]. However, there was no sign of HDN and Garner and Devenish [37] postulate that binding of anti-In^b to CD44 on fetal monocytes and macrophages could have a blocking effect on FcγR1.

Numerous murine monoclonal antibodies to non-polymorphic epitopes on CD44 (examples in [38]) and one macaque monoclonal antibody [39] have been produced. One murine monoclonal antibody with In^b specificity (LO-Leu-A) has been identified [38].

21.6 Functional aspects of CD44

CD44 proteoglycan, once called the human brain-granulocyte-T lymphocyte antigen [40], is a ubiquitous structure: very few types of tissues or cells lack CD44. It is present on circulating red cells, B and T lymphocytes, granulocytes, and monocytes [2,4,30,40], and on thymus, central nervous system white matter, epidermis, skeletal muscle, and epithelium from stomach, intestine, liver, bladder, lung, and breast [1,6,41].

Many functions have been attributed to CD44, the functions being regulated by the inclusion of the products of the various alternatively spliced exons (Fig. 21.1). Functions of CD44 include the following: adhesion of leucocytes to endothelial cells, stromal cells, and the extracellular matrix (ECM); participation in T and B cell activation in response to immunological stimuli; lymphocyte–endothelial cell interactions involved in the localization of lymphocytes to the site of inflammation; modelling of the ECM during wound healing and embryonic development. CD44 has also been implicated in tumour metastasis (reviewed in [1,42,43]). Most of these interactions involve binding of CD44 to hyaluronan, a high molecular weight glycoaminoglycan that is a major component of the ECM and is also present on cell surfaces. CD44 also binds collagen, fibronectin, and laminin, proteins of the ECM that fill the spaces between cells. CD44 appears to have a regulatory role in normal haemopoiesis (reviewed in [44]). Hyaluronan binding by CD44 may be involved in adhesion of haemopoietic progenitors, including erythroid burst-forming units (BFU-E), to the bone marrow stroma, during haemopoiesis [44,45]. A patient with red cell CD44 deficiency, but normal levels of CD44 on leucocytes, had a unique form of congenital dyserythropoietic anaemia [23].

CD44 contains three copies of a putative hyaluronan binding motif, BX$_7$B (B=arginine or lysine; X$_7$= seven non-acidic amino acids), present in proteins that bind hyaluronan [46]. Experiments involving site-directed mutagenesis identified several amino acid residues that were considered important in the binding of CD44 to hyaluronan, one of which was Arg46 (the second B of a BX$_7$B hyaluronan-binding motif). Mutating Arg46 to Gly in CD44 constructs abolished hyaluronan binding [46]. In(a+b–) phenotype results from homozygosity for *CD44* alleles encoding Pro46 (Section 21.3.2), yet the In^a Arg46Pro substitution does not reduce hyaluronan binding to intact CD44H *in vitro* [24]. A combined modelling and mutagenesis study has subsequently suggested that Arg41, Tyr42, Arg78, and Tyr79 are critical for hyaluronan binding, and Lys68, Asn100, Asn101, and Tyr105 support binding [47].

21.7 AnWj (901009)

Anti-Anton, an antibody to a high frequency antigen in the serum of a pregnant woman, was first mentioned by Boorman and Tippett (unpublished observations,

1972, cited in [48]) and a second example was described in 1980 [49]. Both antibodies failed to react with In(Lu) Lu_{null} cells and with cord cells. The notation Lu15 was set aside for Anton, but was shown to be inappropriate when anti-Anton was found to react with recessive Lu_{null} cells [50].

Anti-Wj, an autoantibody reported in 1983 by Marsh *et al.* [51], reacted with red cells from 415 random donors and three recessive Lu_{null} individuals, but failed to react with 14 examples of In(Lu) red cells and with cord cells. Some binding of anti-Wj to In(Lu) cells could be demonstrated by adsorption and elution.

In 1985 Poole and Giles [52] suggested that even though anti-Anton were alloantibodies and anti-Wj was an autoantibody they may be detecting the same determinant. Red cells of a patient with Hodgkin's disease had a temporary acquired loss of Wj; they were negative with four examples of anti-Wj autoantibodies and were also negative with anti-Anton [53]. The serum of the patient contained an antibody described as alloanti-Wj. At remission, 6 months later, the antibody had disappeared and the patient's cells were Wj+ and Anton+. It is now accepted that anti-Anton and -Wj have the same specificity and the name AnWj (901009) has been given to the antigen they define. LU15 (005015) is now obsolete.

21.7.1 AnWj antigen

21.7.1.1 Inheritance and frequency

The rare AnWj– phenotype is usually acquired and may be transient, but in 1991 Poole *et al.* [54] showed that it could also be inherited. Two of seven sibs of an AnWj– Arab woman with anti-AnWj were AnWj–. The consanguineous parents and the six children of the propositus were AnWj+, suggesting that the AnWj– phenotype in this family results from homozygosity of a rare recessive gene. The family study demonstrated that AnWj is not controlled by *LU*, or by *ABO*, *MNS*, *RH*, *KEL*, *FY*, *JK*, *XG*, or *XK*.

Anti-AnWj screening of red cells from 2400 American donors revealed three Lu_{null} In(Lu) samples, but no AnWj– red cells with normal Lutheran antigens [55].

21.7.1.2 AnWj and the Lu_{null} phenotype

Like In^b and several other red cell antigens outside the Lutheran system, AnWj is expressed only very weakly on red cells of individuals with the dominant gene *In(Lu)* (see Chapter 6). Usually no AnWj antigen can be detected on these Lu_{null} cells by direct testing, but anti-AnWj can be adsorbed and eluted from In(Lu) cells [54]. Lu_{null} cells of the recessive and X-linked types have normal AnWj expression [50,56].

AnWj differs from Lutheran and Indian system antigens in being resistant to trypsin, chymotrypsin, and the disulphide bond-reducing agent AET.

21.7.1.3 Development of AnWj antigen

Analysis of red cells from 36 infants revealed that the age at which conversion from AnWj– to AnWj+ takes place varies from infant to infant, but occurs between the ages of 3 and 46 days and requires less than 1 day to complete [57]. This rapid, 'all or nothing' phenomenon is unexpected as the red cells in the circulation are not all produced at the same time and no evidence could be found for a conversion factor in the serum [57]. Whatever causes the change from AnWj– to AnWj+ in infants might be reversible on rare occasions, as the adult AnWj– phenotype with concurrent presence of anti-AnWj has been found to be transient in several patients and in a healthy individual [53,57–59].

21.7.1.4 AnWj as a receptor for *Haemophilus influenzae*

Although the bacterium *Haemophilus influenzae* is a commensal of the throat of most healthy people, it may also cause respiratory tract infections and, more seriously, is a major cause of bacterial meningitis in young children. Some strains of *H. influenzae* express fimbriae (short, thread-like processes attached to the cell walls), which are probably involved in adherence to nasopharyngeal epithelial cells.

Fimbriae-bearing strains of *H. influenzae* isolated from patients with invasive disease and respiratory tract infections agglutinated most red cell samples from adults, including recessive Lu_{null} cells, but did not agglutinate cord cells, In(Lu) cells, or AnWj– red cells of both acquired and inherited types [60,61]. Anti-AnWj inhibited agglutination of AnWj+ red cells by the bacteria.

H. influenzae bound to buccal epithelial cells, including those from one individual with transient

AnWj– red cells, two with *In(Lu)* genes, and several neonates, but did not bind to buccal epithelial cells from three AnWj– members of the Arab family with inherited AnWj– phenotype [61,62]. Adherence of *H. influenzae* to epithelial cells was not inhibited by anti-AnWj [62]. Although the receptors for *H. influenzae* adherence on red cells and epithelial cells may not be identical, they appear to have a common genetic basis.

21.7.2 Anti-AnWj

21.7.2.1 Human antibodies

Anti-AnWj may be autoantibodies, apparent alloantibodies in individuals with an acquired AnWj– phenotype, or true alloantibodies. The propositus and her AnWj– sister in the only family with more than one AnWj– member had anti-AnWj. Neither had been transfused, but both had been pregnant; their AnWj– brother, who had not been transfused, did not have anti-AnWj [54]. It is a little surprising that anti-AnWj can be stimulated by pregnancy considering the very low level of AnWj antigen on neonatal red cells.

Anti-AnWj has been incriminated in severe haemolytic transfusion reactions [59,63]. This haemolytic potential has been supported by *in vivo* red cell survival studies [63–65]. In a patient with autoanti-AnWj and depressed red cell AnWj expression, radiolabelled autologous red cells survived normally, but AnWj+ allogeneic cells had reduced survival [66]. If available, In(Lu) Lu$_{null}$ cells are most suitable for transfusing patients with anti-AnWj. There was no indication of HDN in any of the children of a mother with anti-AnWj [54].

21.7.2.2 Monoclonal anti-AnWj

Two monoclonal antibodies (H86 and M447) produced from mice immunized with human T-cell lines derived from patients with acute lymphocytic leukaemia have AnWj specificity [67]. These antibodies reacted with all red cells by an antiglobulin test, except cord cells, In(Lu) cells, and cells of AnWj– phenotype. Reactions with AnWj+ cells showed substantial variation in strength.

21.7.3 AnWj may be located on CD44 glycoprotein

In(a–b–) red cells of the patient with a novel form of congenital dyserythopoietic anaemia and a gross deficiency of red cell CD44 were AnWj– [23]. Positive results were obtained with MAIEA analyses performed with either anti-CD44 or -AnWj murine monoclonal antibodies and anti-In^b or -AnWj human antibodies [14]. The CD44-negative human leukaemia cell line, Jurkat, transfected with *CD44* cDNA reacted with human and mouse monoclonal anti-AnWj [68]. Immunoblotting with anti-AnWj revealed an M_r 80 000 component in normal red cells and in Chinese hamster ovary cells (CHO) and murine erythroleukaemia (MEL) cells transfected with *CD44* cDNA, but not in non-transfected CHO or MEL cells, or in In(Lu) red cells [68]. The anti-AnWj also bound an M_r 200 000 structure in red cells and transfected CHO cells. Telen *et al.* [68] suggest that AnWj antigen is located on a trypsin-resistant region of an isoform of CD44 that is not present on red cells of the newborn. AnWj might also be on the M_r 200 000 chondroitinated isoform of CD44.

References

1 Barclay AN, Brown MH, Law SKA *et al. The Leucocyte Antigen Facts Book*, 2nd edn. London: Academic Press, 1997.

2 Spring FA, Dalchau R, Daniels GL *et al.* The In^a and In^b blood group antigens are located on a glycoprotein of 80 000 MW (the CDw44 glycoprotein) whose expression is influenced by the *In(Lu)* gene. *Immunology* 1988;64:37–43.

3 Telen MJ, Palker TJ, Haynes BF. Human erythrocyte antigens. II. The *In(Lu)* gene regulates expression of an antigen on an 80-kilodalton protein of human erythrocytes. *Blood* 1984;64:599–606.

4 Telen MJ, Shehata H, Haynes BF. Human medullary thymocyte p80 antigen and *In(Lu)*-related p80 antigen reside on the same protein. *Hum Immunol* 1986;17:311–24.

5 Telen MJ, Rogers I, Letarte M. Further characterization of erythrocyte p80 and the membrane protein defect of *In(Lu)* Lu(a–b–) erythrocytes. *Blood* 1987;70:1475–81.

6 Anstee DJ, Gardner B, Spring FA *et al.* New monoclonal antibodies in CD44 and CD58: their use to quantify CD44 and CD58 on normal human erythrocytes and to compare the distribution of CD44 and CD58 in human tissues. *Immunology* 1991;74:197–205.

7 Screaton GR, Bell MV, Jackson DG *et al.* Genomic struc-

ture of DNA encoding the lymphocyte homing receptor CD44 reveals at least 12 alternatively spliced exons. *Proc Natl Acad Sci USA* 1992;89:12160–4.

8 Tölg C, Hofmann M, Herrlich P, Ponta H. Splicing choice from ten variant exons establishes CD44 variability. *Nucl Acid Res* 1993;21:1225–9.

9 Stamenkovic I, Amiot M, Pesando JM, Seed B. A lymphocyte molecule implicated in lymph node homing is a member of the cartilage link protein family. *Cell* 1989;56: 1057–62.

10 Goldstein LA, Zhou DFH, Picker LJ et al. A human lymphocyte homing receptor, the Hermes antigen, is related to cartilage proteoglycan core and link proteins. *Cell* 1989;56:1063–72.

11 Harn H-J, Isola N, Cooper DL. The multispecific cell adhesion molecule CD44 is represented in reticulocyte cDNA. *Biochem Biophys Res Commun* 1991;178: 1127–34.

12 Nunomura W, Takakuwa Y, Tokimitsu R et al. Regulation of CD44-protein 4.1 interaction by Ca^{2+} and calmodulin: implications for modulation of CD44–ankyrin interaction. *J Biol Chem* 1997;272: 30322–8.

13 Telen MJ, Ferguson DJ. Relationship of In^b antigen to other antigens on *In(Lu)*-related p80. *Vox Sang* 1990;58:118–21.

14 Rao N, Udani M, Telen MJ. Demonstration by monoclonal antibody immobilization of erythrocyte antigens and dot blot that both the In and AnWj blood group antigens reside on CD44 [Abstract]. *Transfusion* 1994;34:25S.

15 Petty AC, Green CA, Daniels GL. The monoclonal antibody-specific immobilization of erythrocyte antigens assay (MAIEA) in the investigation of human red-cell antigens and their associated membrane proteins. *Transfus Med* 1997;7:179–88.

16 Badakere SS, Joshi SR, Bhatia HM et al. Evidence for a new blood group antigen in the Indian population (a preliminary report). *Indian J Med Res* 1973;61:563.

17 Badakere SS, Parab BB, Bhatia HM. Further observations on the In^a (Indian) antigen in Indian populations. *Vox Sang* 1974;26:400–3.

18 Giles CM. Antithetical relationship of anti-In^a with the Salis antibody. *Vox Sang* 1975;29:73–6.

19 Badakere SS, Vasantha K, Bhatia HM et al. High frequency of In^a antigen among Iranians and Arabs. *Hum Hered* 1980;30:262–3.

20 Joshi SR. Immediate haemolytic transfusion reaction due to anti-In^b. *Vox Sang* 1992;63:232–3.

21 Longster GH, Robinson EAE. Four further examples of anti-In^b detected during pregnancy. *Clin Lab Haematol* 1981;3:351–6.

22 Ferguson DJ, Gaal HD. Some observations on the In^b antigen and evidence that anti-In^b causes accelerated destruction of radiolabeled red cells. *Transfusion* 1988;28:479–82.

23 Parsons SF, Jones J, Anstee DJ et al. A novel form of congenital dyserythropoietic anemia associated with deficiency of erythroid CD44 and a unique blood group phenotype [In(a–b–) Co(a–b–)]. *Blood* 1994;83: 860–8.

24 Telen MJ, Udani M, Washington MK et al. A blood group-related polymorphism of CD44 abolishes a hyalouronan-binding consensus sequence without preventing hyalouronan binding. *J Biol Chem* 1996; 271:7147–53.

25 Bhatia HM, Badakere SS, Mokashi SA, Parab BB. Studies on the blood group antigen In^a. *Immunol Commun* 1980;9:203–15.

26 Dumasia AN, Gupte SC. Quantitation of In^a blood group antigens. *Indian J Med Res B* 1990;92:50–3.

27 Daniels G. Effect of enzymes on and chemical modifications of high-frequency red cell antigens. *Immunohematology* 1992;8:53–7.

28 Joshi SR, Bhatia HM. Effect of 2-aminoethyl isothiouroniumbromide on In^a/In^b blood group antigens. *Indian J Med Res* 1987;85:420–1.

29 Dahr W, Krüger J. Solubilization of various blood group antigens by the detergent Triton X-100. *Forensic Sci Int* 1983;23:49–50.

30 Telen MJ, Eisenbarth GS, Haynes BF. Human erythrocyte antigens: regulation of expression of a novel erythrocyte surface antigen by the inhibitor Lutheran *In(Lu)* gene. *J Clin Invest* 1983;71:1878–86.

31 Lucas MG, Green AM, Telen MJ. Characterization of the serum *In(Lu)*-related antigen: identification of a serum protein related to erythrocyte p80. *Blood* 1989; 73:596–600.

32 Telen MJ, Green AM. Human red cell antigens. V. Expression of *In(Lu)*-related p80 antigens by recessive-type Lu(a–b–) red cells. *Transfusion* 1988;28:430–4.

33 Daniels G. Lutheran related antibodies. *Rev Franc Transfus Immuno-Hémat* 1988;31:447–52.

34 Judson PA, Spring FA, Parsons SF, Anstee DJ, Mallinson G. Report on group 8 (Lutheran) antibodies. *Rev Franc Transfus Immuno-Hémat* 1988;31:433–40.

35 Joshi SR, Gupta D, Choudhury RK, Choudhury N. Transfusion-induced anti-In^a following a single-unit transfusion. *Transfusion* 1993;33:444.

36 Sosler SD, Saporito C, Perkins JT, Unger PJ, Orlina AR. The clinical and serologic behavior of another example of anti-In^b. *Transfusion* 1989;29:465.

37 Garner SF, Devenish A. Do monocyte ADCC assays accurately predict the severity of hemolytic disease of the newborn caused by antibodies to high-frequency antigens? *Immunohematology* 1996;12:20–6.

38 Stoll M, Dalchau R, Schmidt RE. Cluster report: CD44. In: W Knapp, B Dörken, WR Gilks et al., eds. *Leukocyte Typing IV*. Oxford: Oxford University Press, 1989:619–22.

39 Blancher A, Øyen R, Tossas E, Reid ME, Roubinet F. A macaque monoclonal antibody anti-CD44: a useful

471

reagent for identifying the dominant type Lu(a–b–). *Immunohematology* 1999;**15**:82.

40 Dalchau R, Kirkley J, Fabre JW. Monoclonal antibody to a human brain-granulocyte-T lymphocyte antigen probably homologous to the W 3/13 antigen of the rat. *Eur J Immunol* 1980;**10**:745–9.

41 Flanagan BF, Dalchau R, Allen AK, Daar AS, Fabre JW. Chemical composition and tissue distribution of the human CDw44 glycoprotein. *Immunology* 1989;**67**: 167–75.

42 Borland G, Ross JA, Guy K. Forms and functions of CD44. *Immunology* 1998;**93**:139–48.

43 Bajorath J. Molecular organization, structural features, and ligand binding characteristics of CD44, a highly variable cell surface glycoprotein with multiple functions. *Proteins* 2000;**39**:103–11.

44 Chan JY-H, Watt SM. Adhesion receptors on haematopoietic progenitor cells. *Br J Haematol* 2001; **112**:541–57.

45 Oostendorp RAJ, Spitzer E, Brandl M, Eaves CJ, Dörmer P. Evidence for differences in the mechanisms by which antibodies against CD44 promote adhesion of erythroid and granulopoietic progenitors to marrow stromal cells. *Br J Haematol* 1998;**101**:436–45.

46 Yang B, Yang BL, Savani RC, Turley EA. Identification of a common hyaluronan binding motif in the hyaluronan binding proteins RHAMM, CD44 and link protein. *EMBO J* 1994;**13**:286–96.

47 Bajorath J, Greenfield B, Munro SB, Day AJ, Aruffo A. Identification of CD44 residues important for hyaluronan binding and delineation of the binding site. *J Biol Chem* 1998;**273**:338–43.

48 Race RR, Sanger R. *Blood Groups in Man*, 6th edn. Oxford: Blackwell Scientific Publications, 1975.

49 Daniels GL. *Blood group antigens of high frequency: a serological and genetical study*. PhD thesis, University of London, 1980.

50 Poole J, Giles CM. Observations on the Anton antigen and antibody. *Vox Sang* 1982;**43**:220–2.

51 Marsh WL, Brown PJ, DiNapoli J *et al*. Anti-Wj: an autoantibody that defines a high-incidence antigen modified by the *In(Lu)* gene. *Transfusion* 1983;**23**:128–30.

52 Poole J, Giles C. Anton and Wj, are they related? *Transfusion* 1985;**25**:443.

53 Mannessier L, Rouger P, Johnson CL, Mueller KA, Marsh WL. Acquired loss of red-cell Wj antigen in a patient with Hodgkin's disease. *Vox Sang* 1986;**50**: 240–4.

54 Poole J, Levene C, Bennett M *et al*. A family showing inheritance of the Anton blood group antigen AnWj and independence of AnWj from Lutheran. *Transfus Med* 1991;**1**:245–51.

55 Lukasavage T. Donor screening with anti-AnWj. *Immunohematology* 1993;**9**:112.

56 Norman PC, Tippett P, Beal RW. An Lu(a–b–) phenotype caused by an X-linked recessive gene. *Vox Sang* 1986;**51**:49–52.

57 Poole J, Van Alphen L. *Haemophilus influenzae* receptor and the AnWj antigen. *Transfusion* 1988;**28**:289.

58 Harris T, Steiert S, Marsh WL, Berman LB. A Wj-negative patient with anti-Wj. *Transfusion* 1986;**26**:117.

59 Magrin G, Harrison C. One hour ^{51}Cr survival in a patient with anti-AnWj [Abstract]. *20th Congr Int Soc Blood Transfus*, 1988:228.

60 van Alphen L, Poole J, Overbeeke M. The Anton blood group antigen is the erythrocyte receptor for *Haemophilus influenzae*. *FEMS Microbiol Lett* 1986; **37**:69–71.

61 van Alphen L, Levene C, Geelan-van den Broek L *et al*. Combined inheritance of epithelial and erythrocyte receptors for *Haemophilus influenzae*. *Infect Immun* 1990;**58**:3807–9.

62 van Alphen L, Poole J, Geelen L, Zanen HC. The erythrocyte and epithelial cell receptors for *Haemophilus influenzae* are expressed independently. *Infect Immun* 1987;**55**:2355–8.

63 de Man AJM, van Dijk BA, Daniels GL. An example of anti-AnWj causing haemolytic transfusion reaction. *Vox Sang* 1992;**63**:238.

64 Harrison CR, Heinz R, Chaudhuri TK. Clinical management of a patient with anti-Anton [Abstract]. *Transfusion* 1985;**25**:463.

65 Davis K, Lucchesi G, Lyle B, Bradley P. A further example of anti AnWj in an individual of common Lutheran phenotype [Abstract]. *Joint Congr Int Soc Blood Transfus and Am Assoc Blood Banks* 1990:153.

66 Whitsett CF, Hare VW, Oxendine SM, Pierce JA. Autologous and allogeneic red cell survival studies in the presence of autoanti-AnWj. *Transfusion* 1993;**33**:845–7.

67 Knowles RW, Bai Y, Lomas C, Green C, Tippett P. Two monoclonal antibodies detecting high frequency antigens absent from red cells of the dominant type of Lu(a–b–) Lu:–3. *J Immunogenet* 1982;**9**:353–7.

68 Telen MJ, Rao N, Udani M, Liao H-X, Haynes BF. Relationship of the AnWj blood group antigen to expression of CD44 [Abstract]. *Transfusion* 1993;**33**:48S.

22 Ok blood group system

22.1 Introduction

The very high frequency antigen Okᵃ (OK1) is the only antigen of the Ok system. Okᵃ is located on the immunoglobulin superfamily molecule CD147. The rare Ok(a–) phenotype results from a Glu92Lys substitution.

BSG, the gene encoding Okᵃ, is located on chromosome 19pter–p13.2 (Chapter 32).

22.2 Okᵃ (OK1)

The producer of the original anti-Okᵃ (Mrs S.Ko.G.), reported by Morel and Hamilton [1] in 1979, came from a small Japanese island. Her parents were consanguineous and two of her three sibs were also Ok(a–). No other Ok(a–) individual was found as a result of testing red cells from 400 other people from Mrs S.Ko.G.'s home island, 870 donors from other parts of Japan, 3976 American blood donors of Oriental appearance, 9053 white Americans, 1570 African Americans, and 1378 Mexican Americans [1]. A total of eight families with Ok(a–) individuals are known, all Japanese [2].

Okᵃ is not affected by treatment of intact cells with the proteases trypsin, chymotrypsin, papain, or pronase, with sialidase, or with the disulphide bond-reducing agent 2-aminoethylisothiouronium bromide (AET).

22.3 Anti-Okᵃ

22.3.1 Alloanti-Okᵃ

Mrs S.Ko.G. had not been pregnant, but had been transfused at least once [1]. Her Ok(a–) sister had five children, at least two of whom were Ok(a+), but had not made anti-Okᵃ. Three hours after injection of radiolabelled Ok(a+) red cells, only 10% remained in the circulation of Mrs S.Ko.G. [1]. A mononuclear phagocyte assay with anti-Okᵃ gave similar values to those obtained with antibodies known to have caused significant shortening of red cell survival [1].

Only one other alloanti-Okᵃ is known (H. Yamaguchi and Y. Okuba, personal communication, 1983).

22.3.2 Monoclonal anti-Okᵃ

TRA-1-85 is an IgG1 monoclonal antibody produced from spleen cells of a mouse immunized with human teratocarcinoma cell line [3]. The antibody reacted, by an antiglobulin test, with all red cells tested except those of three Ok(a–) propositi. It also reacted, by radioimmunoassay, with leucocytes from Ok(a+) individuals, but not with those from an Ok(a–) person.

Numerous other monoclonal antibodies to CD147 have been produced [4–7], but none is reported to have Okᵃ specificity.

22.4 CD147, the Ok glycoprotein, and the molecular basis of Ok(a–)

Immunoblotting of membranes from Ok(a+) red cells with murine monoclonal or human anti-Okᵃ showed that Okᵃ is situated on a glycoprotein ranging in apparent M_r 35000–68000 [3]. To purify the Ok glycoprotein, Spring *et al.* [2] used a monoclonal antibody (MA103 [4]), which defines an epitope on the Ok glycoprotein, yet reacts with Ok(a–) red cells. The N-terminal 30 amino acids were found to be identical to those of a glycoprotein called M6 [5]. M6, also known as EMMPRIN, basigin (mouse), OX-47 (rat), and neurothelin (chicken), now has the cluster of differentiation designation CD147 [8]. Mouse NS-0 cells transfected with *CD147* cDNA expressed Ok^a, except when the cDNA was from an Ok(a–) individual [2].

Human *CD147* cDNA was isolated both by screening a human cDNA library with a fragment of mouse basigin cDNA [9] and by expression cloning of cDNA derived from human T cell and B cell libraries [5]. CD147 is a single chain transmembrane molecule with a signal peptide of 18 amino acids, an N-terminal extracellular domain of 187 amino acids, a 24 amino acid membrane-spanning domain, which contains a single charge glutamic acid residue and a leucine zipper, and a 40 residue cytoplasmic domain. It is a member of the immunoglobulin superfamily (IgSF) of adhesion molecules and receptors (see Chapters 6 and 16) and the extracellular domain is organized into one C2 set and one V set IgSF domains (Fig. 22.1) [5,10]. Three *N*-glycans, one on the C2 set domain and two on the V set domain, comprise about 50% of the mass of the glycoprotein.

The *CD147* consists of 10.8 kb organized into eight exons (Fig. 22.1) [11]. Approximately 95 kb of the 5′ flanking sequence contained three SP1 and two AP2 sites, but no TATA or CAAT box [11].

CD147 cDNA from three Ok(a–) individuals contained a G274A mutation in exon 3, which encodes a Glu92Lys substitution in the N-terminal C2-set IgSF domain [2] (nucleotide and amino acid numbering from ATG/Met1 [10]). Because Ok(a–) results from homozygosity for a missense mutation, the finding of anti-Ok^b in Japan would not be unexpected.

22.5 Tissue distribution and function of CD147

In addition to red cells, CD147 is present on all leucocytes and human leukaemic cell lines and has been detected on all human cells examined, although some tissues show differentiation-related expression [2–5]. Early haemopoietic progenitors express Ok^a strongly, but the level of expression decreases during erythroid development [12].

Highly conserved sequence homologies within the cytoplasmic and transmembrane domains suggest that CD147 could be a component of a signal transduction complex. CD147 appears to be a leucocyte activation-associated glycoprotein, as expression on leucocytes is strongly up-regulated upon cell activation [5]. Binding of monoclonal antibodies that mimic the natural ligand of CD147 induced homotypic aggregation of a monocytic cell line (U937) through activation of the LFA-1/ICAM-1 intercellular adhesion pathway [7]. CD147 on tumour cells induces production of collagenase and other extracellular matrix metalloproteinases (MMP) and may be involved in tumour invasion and metastasis [10]. In healthy tissue, CD147 may function in embryonic development or wound healing by causing dermal fibroblasts to increase their MMP production, thus facilitating tissue remodelling [10]. CD147 is a cell surface receptor for extracellular cyclophilin A (CyPA), a protein that becomes incorporated into the virions of HIV-1 and significantly enhances an early step of cellular HIV-1 infection. CD147 appears to be a cofactor that mediates activity of virus-associated CyPA and is required for efficient infection by HIV-1 [13].

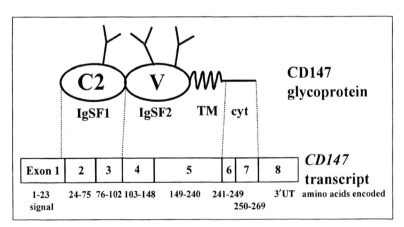

CD147 glycoprotein

IgSF1 IgSF2 TM cyt

| Exon 1 | 2 | 3 | 4 | 5 | 6 | 7 | 8 |

1-23   24-75 76-102 103-148 149-240 241-249   3′UT amino acids encoded
signal   250-269

CD147 transcript

Fig. 22.1 Diagrammatic representation of the CD147 glycoprotein showing the C2 and V set IgSF domains with one and two *N*-glycans, respectively, the transmembrane domain (TM), and the cytoplasmic tail (cyt). Also shown is the relationship of the protein structure to the eight exons of the *CD147* gene, including a 23 amino acid signal peptide.

On red cells, CD147 appears to interact specifically with two members of the monocarboxylate transporter (MCT) family, MCT1 and MCT4, which transport monocarboxylates, such as lactate and pyruvate, across the plasma membrane [14]. CD147 may be required for proper translocation of the MCTs to the plasma membrane. In mice, masking of CD147 by F(ab')$_2$ fragments of monoclonal anti-CD147 disrupts the migration of red cells out of the spleen, inducing splenomegaly, anaemia and, consequently, erythropoietin-mediated erythropoiesis [15]. CD147 may therefore have an important role in the recirculation of mature red cells from the spleen into the general circulation.

References

1 Morel PA, Hamilton HB. Ok^a: an erythrocytic antigen of high frequency. *Vox Sang* 1979;**36**:182–5.
2 Spring FA, Homes CH, Simpson KL *et al.* The Ok^a blood group antigen is a marker for the M6 leukocyte activation antigen, the human homolog of OX-47 antigen, basigin and neurothelin, an immunoglobulin superfamily molecule that is widely expressed in human cells and tissues. *Eur J Immunol* 1997;**27**:891–7.
3 Williams BP, Daniels GL, Pym B *et al.* Biochemical and genetic analysis of the Ok^a blood group antigen. *Immunogenetics* 1988;**27**:322–9.
4 Mattes MJ, Cairncross JG, Old LJ, Lloyd KO. Monoclonal antibodies to three widely distributed human cell surface antigens. *Hybridoma* 1983;**2**:253–64.
5 Kasinrerk W, Fiebiger E, Stefanová I *et al.* Human leukocyte activation antigen M6, a member of the Ig superfamily, is the species homologue of rat OX-47, mouse basigin, and chicken HT7 molecule. *J Immunol* 1992;**149**: 847–54.
6 Stockinger H, Ebel T, Hansmann C *et al.* CD147 (neurothelin/basigin) workshop panel report. *Leucocyte Typing VI.* Y Kishimoto, H Kikutani, AE Von Dem Borne et al., eds. New York: Garland, 1998:760–3.
7 Kasinrerk W, Tokrasinwit N, Phunpae P. CD147 monoclonal antibodies induce homotypic cell aggregation of monocytic cell line U937 LFA-1/ICAM-1 pathway. *Immunology* 1999;**96**:184–92.
8 Staffler G, Stockinger H. CD 147. *J Biol Regul Homeost Agents* 2000;**14**:327–30.
9 Miyauchi T, Masuzawa Y, Muramatsu T. The basigin group of the immunoglobulin superfamily: complete conservation of a segment in and around transmembrane domains of human and mouse basigin and chicken HT7 antigen. *J Biochem* 1991;**110**:770–4.
10 Biswas C, Zhang Y, DeCastro R *et al.* The human tumor cell-derived collagenase stimulatory factor (renamed EMMPRIN) is a member of the immunoglobulin superfamily. *Cancer Res* 1995;**55**:434–9.
11 Guo H, Majmudar G, Jensen TC *et al.* Characterization of the gene for human EMMPRIN, a tumor cell surface inducer of matrix metalloproteinases. *Gene* 1998; **220**:99–108.
12 Bony V, Gane P, Bailly P, Cartron J-P. Time-course expression of polypeptides carrying blood group antigens during human erythroid differentiation. *Br J Haematol* 1999;**107**:263–74.
13 Pushkarsky T, Zybarth G, Dubrovsky L *et al.* CD147 facilitates HIV-1 infection by interacting with virus-associated cyclophilin A. *Proc Natl Acad Sci USA* 2001;**98**:6360–5.
14 Halestrap AP, Price NT. The proton-linked monocarboxylate transporter (MCT) family: structure, function, and regulation. *Biochem J* 1999;**343**:281–99.
15 Coste I, Gauchat J-F, Wilson A *et al.* Unavailability of CD147 leads to selective erythrocyte trapping in the spleen. *Blood* 2001;**97**:3984–8.

23 RAPH blood group system

23.1 Introduction

MER2 (RAPH1), described by Daniels *et al.* [1] in 1987, was the first new independent red cell surface polymorphism to be defined by monoclonal antibodies. MER2 is also recognized by four human alloantibodies [2] and is the sole antigen of the blood group system named RAPH after the original example of alloanti-MER2.

MER2 is encoded by a gene on the tip of the short arm of chromosome 11 at 11p15 [1] (Chapter 32).

23.2 The MER2 red cell polymorphism and the MER2 antigen (RAPH1)

MER2 monoclonal antibodies react with red cells by an indirect antiglobulin test with anti-mouse IgG. The strength of reaction varies between red cell samples [1]. Of 1016 English blood donors, 92% were MER2+ and 8% MER2–, giving gene frequencies of about 0.72 for *MER2+* and 0.28 for *MER2–*. Analysis of 103 northern European families with a total of 294 children confirmed that MER2 is inherited as a Mendelian dominant character.

Titration scores with anti-MER2 on red cells of members of a large Sardinian family demonstrated that the dominant inhibitor gene *In(Lu)* exerted a slight depressing effect on MER2 expression (see Section 6.4.4.5). Scores for nine family members with *In(Lu)* (Lu$_{null}$) varied from 0 to 15 with a mean of 6, whereas scores for 12 members without *In(Lu)* [Lu(a–b+)] varied from 12 to 21 with a mean of 16.

MER2 is resistant to papain and sialidase treatment of red cells, but is destroyed by trypsin, chymotrypsin, pronase, and the disulphide-bond reducing agent 2-aminoethylisothiouronium bromide (AET). Immunoprecipitation with anti-MER2 and sodium dodecyl sulphate polyacrylamide gel electrophoresis (SDS

PAGE) revealed a band of apparent M_r 40 000[3]. MER2 is expressed on CD34+ cells, but there is a dramatic decrease in expression during *ex vivo* erythropoiesis [3].

CD44 glycoprotein, which carries the In^a and In^b blood group antigens, is also produced by a gene on the short arm of chromosome 11 and suppressed by *In(Lu)* (Chapter 21). MER2 is not located on CD44. CD44 monoclonal antibodies react as strongly with MER2– cells as with MER2+ cells and the genes coding for CD44 and MER2 are at different positions on the short arm of chromosome 11 (Chapter 32). A glycoprotein homologous to CD44 called LYVE-1 or HAR [4,5] and encoded by a gene on chromosome 11p15 is a candidate for the MER2 antigen, although the tissue distribution of this hyaluronan receptor makes identity unlikely.

23.3 MER2 antibodies

23.3.1 Monoclonal anti-MER2

The monoclonal antibodies 1D12 and 2F7 were produced from splenocytes of a mouse immunized with human small cell carcinoma line [1]. The antibodies were found as a result of screening, by a complement-dependent cytotoxicity test, with a human × hamster hybrid cell line containing chromosome 11 as its only human chromosome. Blocking experiments demonstrated that both antibodies detect epitopes on the same cell surface antigen [1].

23.3.2 Human alloanti-MER2

In 1988, Daniels *et al.* [2] described three examples of human anti-MER2, all made by Jews originating from India and living in Israel. Two were sibs and the third was unrelated. All had renal failure requiring dialysis and regular blood transfusion. In two cases the antibodies were detected before commencement of dialysis and before the patients had been transfused. All three antibodies react by the antiglobulin test with anti-human IgG.

In tests on red cells from 138 blood donors of selected MER2 phenotype, there was almost complete concordance (with only three exceptions) between the results obtained with monoclonal anti-MER2 and with the human antibodies. Those exceptions, positive reactions with the human sera on three MER2– red cell samples, were probably caused by the presence of anti-HLA-B7 (anti-Bgᵃ) in all three sera. Two of the human antibodies completely blocked, and one partially blocked, the reaction of monoclonal anti-MER2 with MER2+ red cells, implying that the MER2 epitope is either identical to, or very close to, the antigen detected by the human antibodies.

The two sibs with anti-MER2 have received numerous transfusions of crossmatch incompatible blood over a number of years with apparently no ill effects or indications of reduced red cell survival.

One other example of alloanti-MER2 has been identified in a healthy blood donor, a Turkish woman who had never been transfused but had been pregnant twice [6].

23.4 Is anti-MER2 production associated with kidney disease?

Despite about 8% of Europeans being MER2–, only four examples of alloanti-MER2 have been found [2,6]. Three of these antibodies were from patients on renal dialysis as a result of kidney failure, all from the same small ethnic group, Indian Jews living in Israel [2]. It is possible that most people who lack MER2 from their red cells still have the antigen on other cells,

explaining the extreme rarity of anti-MER2, but that in some Indian Jews a mutation or even a small chromosomal deletion could mean that the MER2 antigen is totally absent, thus explaining their ability to make anti-MER2. If MER2, or possibly the product of a very closely linked gene deleted together with MER2, were essential for effective kidney function, then their absence might explain the kidney failure in three of the four people known to have made anti-MER2. This is all pure conjecture, but future investigations into the presence of MER2 in tissues other than blood, especially renal tissue, may shed some light on the biological significance of the MER2 antigen.

References

1 Daniels GL, Tippett P, Palmer DK *et al.* MER2: a red cell polymorphism defined by monoclonal antibodies. *Vox Sang* 1987;52:107–10.
2 Daniels GL, Levene C, Berrebi A *et al.* Human alloantibodies detecting a red cell antigen apparently identical to MER2. *Vox Sang* 1988;55:161–4.
3 Lucien N, Bony V, Gane P *et al.* MER2 expression on hematopoietic cells and during erythroid differentiation further characterization of MER2 antigen the product of the RAPH blood group system [Abstract]. *Transfus Clin Biol* 2001;8(Suppl.1):14S.
4 Banerji S, Ni J, Wang S-X *et al.* LYVE-1, a new homologue of the CD44 glycoprotein, is a lymph-specific receptor for hyaluronan. *J Cell Biol* 1999;144:789–801.
5 Winkelmann JC, Basu S. HAR: a novel homolog of CD44 and putative hyaluronic acid receptor encoded by a gene on human chromosome 11p15 [Abstract]. *Blood* 1998;92(Suppl.1):586A.
6 Verhoeven G, Schaap RC, Champagne K, Poole J, Overbeeke M. The first allo-anti MER2 found in a healthy female blood donor. *Vox Sang* 1998;74(Suppl.1):Abstract 1439.

24 JMH blood group system

24.1 Introduction

The very high frequency antigen JMH (JMH1) is the only antigen of the John Milton Hagen (JMH) system. JMH– is usually an acquired phenotype, although it was inherited as a dominant character in one family; inherited variants of JMH are known. The JMH antigen is the semaphorin CDw108.

SEMA7A, the gene encoding CDw108, is located on chromosome 15q23–24 (Chapter 32).

24.2 JMH (JMH1)

Before Sabo et al. [1] coined the term anti-JMH in 1978, a variety of different names had been used in reference laboratories for a collection of antibodies found predominantly, but not exclusively, in elderly patients. In most cases JMH– is probably an acquired phenotype. In many patients with anti-JMH, JMH may not have been totally lost as the red cells give a weakly positive direct antiglobulin test (DAT), and in some cases anti-JMH may be eluted [2]. JMH– can also be a transient phenomenon: two JMH– children with different chromosomal disorders later became JMH+ [3]. JMH is usually expressed very weakly on the red cells of neonates, achieving full strength during the first few years of life. JMH is destroyed by proteases (papain, trypsin, chymotrypsin) and by the disulphide bond-reducing agent 2-aminoethylisothiouronium bromide (AET). JMH is not affected by sialidase.

In the only family in which the JMH– phenotype has been shown to be inherited, JMH– appeared in three generations, so autosomal dominant inheritance of the JMH– phenotype is likely [4]. None of the JMH– members of the family had anti-JMH and their red cells did not give a positive DAT.

A few individuals have alloantibodies to high frequency antigens that do not react with JMH– cells, yet their red cells are JMH+ (Table 24.1). These very rare phenotypes appear to be inherited in an autosomal recessive manner. The JMH-like antibodies differ from anti-JMH because they do not react with the antibody makers' own JMH+ cells or with the JMH+ cells of some of their sibs. Where tested, red cells and antibodies of these individuals are not mutually compatible, indicating that several different JMH variants exist [5–7]. Two sibs with an unusual form of congenital dyserythropoietic anaemia had markedly reduced expression of JMH [10].

24.3 Anti-JMH

24.3.1 Human antibodies

Most JMH– patients have been ascertained through anti-JMH in their serum. Often they have no history of transfusion or pregnancy [3,5,11]. JMH antibodies are usually predominantly IgG4, although IgG1 and IgG2 may also be present [11–13] and an IgG3 anti-JMH has been described [14].

There are numerous cases where patients with anti-JMH have been transfused with JMH+ blood with no adverse effects [1,2,11,13]. One such patient received 20 units of JMH+ blood in 10 months, with the expected haemoglobin rise [13]. Radiolabelled JMH+ red cells often survive normally in patients with anti-JMH [1,2,13], but there are reports of slightly accelerated clearance of JMH+ cells [15] and of anti-JMH giving positive results in monocyte functional assays [14,15]. An IgG1 JMH-like alloantibody in a JMH+ man gave a strongly positive result in a monocyte monolayer assay and in an in vivo study only 46% of ^{51}Cr-labelled JMH+ cells survived after 24 h [6].

Most women with anti-JMH have been beyond child-bearing age, so very little is known about the effect of this antibody in pregnancy. A 26-year-old antenatal patient was found to have anti-JMH and the

Table 24.1 Reactions of anti-JMH and JMH-related alloantibodies and monoclonal antibody (MAb) [5–9].

| Red cells | Anti-JMH | JMH-related alloantibodies | | | | MAb |
		RM	VG	GP	DW	H8
JMH+	+	+	+	+	+	+
JMH–	–*	–	–	–/+^{w}	–	–
RM and sibs	+	–	–	nt	nt	–
VG and sibs	+	+	–	nt	nt	+
GP and sib	–/+^{w}	+	nt	–	nt	+^{w}
DW and sibs	–/+^{w}	+	nt	nt	–	+

* JMH– red cells often give a weak direct antiglobulin reaction with JMH– cells.
+^{w}, Weakly positive reaction; –/+^{w}, negative with some cells, weakly positive with others.

resulting twins were both JMH– (M. Contreras and G.L. Daniels, unpublished observations, 1984). When retested 10 months later, one twin had normal JMH expression and the other had very weak JMH.

24.3.2 Monoclonal antibodies

Monoclonal antibodies of the CDw108 cluster of differentiation may also be considered anti-JMH [16] (Section 24.3). A monoclonal antibody (H8), produced from a mouse immunized with a human lymphoid cell line derived from a patient with acute lymphocytic leukaemia, appeared to have the same specificity as one of the JMH-like antibodies produced by a JMH+ person (R.M.). H8 reacted with neither JMH– red cells nor with the cells of R.M. [8,9]. (Table 24.1). H8 blocked the reaction of human anti-JMH and related antibodies with JMH+ cells [9].

24.4 JMH glycoprotein is the semaphorin CDw108

Immunoblotting and immunoprecipitation techniques with human anti-JMH and with the monoclonal JMH-related antibody (H8) showed that JMH is located on a structure of apparent M_r 76 000 in JMH+ red cells, but not in JMH– cells [17]. This structure is a glycosylphosphatidylinositol (GPI)-linked protein (see Chapter 19); it is cleaved from the red cell by phosphatidylinositol-specific phospholipase C and is not present on the complement-sensitive population of red cells (PNHIII) of patients with paroxysmal nocturnal haemoglobinuria [17,18]. Mudad *et al.* [16]

subsequently demonstrated by immunochemical techniques that the JMH glycoprotein is CDw108. JMH– cells lacked CDw108.

In 1999, Yamada *et al.* [19] isolated CDw108 glycoprotein by immunoprecipitation and obtained a partial amino acid sequence. They used this sequence to clone cDNA containing a 1998-bp open reading frame from a library generated from a leukaemic T cell line. Transfection experiments confirmed that this transcript encodes CDw108. CDw108 is the same as Sema7A (H-Sema-L), a member of the semaphorin family of glycoproteins. The *SEMA7A* gene had been cloned in 1998 by screening human cDNA libraries with sequences derived from human expressed sequence tags (EST) identified by comparison with a herpes viral semaphorin [20]. Nascent CDw108/Sema7A is a 666 amino acid polypeptide, which includes a 46 amino acid signal peptide and a 19 amino acid GPI anchor motif. The mature protein consists of a 500 amino acid sema domain, containing four N-glycosylation and six myristoylation sites, and a 70 amino acid immunoglobulin-like domain of the C2 set, containing one N-glycosylation site (Fig. 24.1) [19,20]. The protein contains 19 cysteine residues, so some disulphide bonding is likely; JMH expression is destroyed by disulphide bond-reducing agents.

SEMA7A consists of at least 13 exons [20].

The function of CDw108 on red cells is not known. Secreted and membrane-bound proteins of the semaphorin family are known to function as signals, guiding axons in developing nervous tissue. Semaphorins and their receptors may also be involved in control of cellular functions, most likely in cell–cell repulsion

479

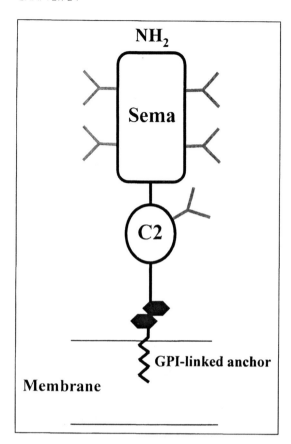

Fig. 24.1 Diagram of CDw108 (Sema7A), showing the large, N-terminal sema domain, the C2-set Ig-like domain, and the GPI-linked anchor. Y, N-glycan.

[21]. CDw108 is preferentially expressed on activated lymphocytes and contains an Arg-Gly-Asp (267–269) cell attachment motif common in adhesion molecules. High expression of *SEMA7A* mRNA was found in placenta, testis, and spleen, and low expression in the brain and thymus [19,20].

In vivo loss of JMH in the acquired JMH– red cell phenotype could be caused by the action of a cellular protease [22]. Incubation of red cells at 37°C for 45 min results in the release into the supernatant of a JMH-active protein of apparent M_r 67 000. This release is abolished by the addition of protease inhibitors. Release of the 67 000 structure from isolated red cell membranes only occurs when the cytoplasmic contents of red cells is added or when neutrophils are present [22]. It is likely that the inherited absence of

JMH-like epitopes (Table 24.1) results from mutations within the CDw108 gene.

References

1 Sabo B, Moulds J, McCreary J, Anti JMH: another high titer-low avidity antibody against a high frequency antigen [Abstract]. *Transfusion* 1978;**18**:387.

2 Whitsett CF, Moulds M, Pierce JA, Hare V. Anti-JMH identified in serum and in eluate from red cells of a JMH-negative man. *Transfusion* 1983;**23**:344–5.

3 Daniels GL. *Blood group antigens of high frequency: a serological and genetical study.* PhD thesis, University of London, 1980.

4 Kollmar M, South SF, Tregellas WM. Evidence of a genetic mechanism for the production of the JMH negative phenotype [Abstract]. *Transfusion* 1981;**21**:612.

5 Moulds JJ, Levene C, Zimmerman S. Serological evidence for heterogeneity among antibodies compatible with JMH-negative red cells [Abstract]. *17th Congr Int Soc Blood Transfus,* 1982:287.

6 Mudad R, Rao N, Issitt PD *et al.* JMH variants: serologic, clinical, and biochemical analysis in two cases. *Transfusion* 1995;**35**:925–30.

7 Issitt PD, Anstee DJ. *Applied Blood Group Serology,* 4th edn. Durham: Montgomery Scientific Publications, 1998.

8 Daniels GL, Knowles RW. A monoclonal antibody to the high frequency red cell antigen JMH. *J Immunogenet* 1982; **9**:57–9.

9 Daniels GL, Knowles RW. Further analysis of the monoclonal antibody H8 demonstrating a JMH-related specificity. *J Immunogenet* 1983;**10**:257–8.

10 Bobolis KA, Lande WM, Telen MJ. Markedly weakened expression of JMH in a kindred with congenital hemolytic anemia [Abstract]. *Transfusion* 1991;**31**:46S.

11 Baldwin ML, Ness PM, Barrasso C *et al. In vivo* studies of the long term ^{51}Cr red cell survival of serologically incompatible red cell units. *Transfusion* 1985;**25**:34–8.

12 Pope J, Lubenko A, Lai WYY. A survey of the IgG subclasses of antibodies to high frequency red cell antigens [Abstract]. *Transfus Med* 1991;**1**(Suppl.2):58.

13 Tregellas WM, Pierce SR, Hardman JT, Beck ML, Anti JMH: IgG subclass composition and clinical significance [Abstract]. *Transfusion* 1980;**20**:628.

14 Geisland J, Corgan M, Hillard B. An example of anti-JMH with characteristics of a clinically significant antibody. *Immunohematology* 1990;**6**:9–11.

15 Hadley A, Wilkes A, Poole J, Arndt P, Garratty G. A chemiluminescence test for predicting the outcome of transfusing incompatible blood. *Transfus Med* 1999; **9**:337–42.

16 Mudad R, Rao N, Angelisova P, Horejsi V, Telen MJ.

Evidence that CDw108 membrane protein bears the JMH blood group antigen. *Transfusion* 1995;35:566–70.

17 Bobolis KA, Moulds JJ, Telen MJ. Isolation of the JMH antigen on a novel phosphatidylinositol-linked human membrane protein. *Blood* 1992;79:1574–81.

18 Telen MJ, Rosse WF, Parker CJ, Moulds MK, Moulds JJ. Evidence that several high-frequency human blood group antigens reside on phosphatidylinositol-linked erythrocyte membrane proteins. *Blood* 1990;75:1404–7.

19 Yamada A, Kubo K, Takeshita T *et al*. Molecular cloning of a glycosylphosphatidylinositol-anchored molecule CDw108. *J Immunol* 1999;162:4094–100.

20 Lange C, Liehr T, Goen M *et al*. New eukaryotic semaphorins with close homology to semaphorins of DNA viruses. *Genomics* 1998;51:340–50.

21 Tamagnone L, Comoglio PM. Signalling by semaphorin receptors: cell guidance and beyond. *Trends Cell Biol* 2000;10:377–83.

22 Bobolis KA, Telen MJ. Biochemical study of possible mechanisms of acquired loss of JMH antigen expression [Abstract]. *Transfusion* 1991;31:46S.

25.1 Introduction

The subject of cold agglutination, as defined by Roelcke [1], involves, 'the occurrence and reaction of autoantibodies, reacting optimally in the cold (0°C) with red blood cells'. These autoantibodies are termed cold agglutinins. Low titre cold agglutinins are present in the sera of all adults. The most prevalent of these autoantibodies is a heterogeneous assembly of specificities called anti-I; antibodies that react with the red cells of almost all adults, but do not react, or at best react only weakly, with the red cells of neonates. Anti-I are generally weak, but potent examples may be found as autoantibodies in patients with cold haemagglutinin disease (CHAD) or following *Mycoplasma pneumoniae* infection. In a rare inherited phenotype called adult i the red cells express very little I antigen. Alloanti-I is generally present in sera of i adults.

The i antigen has a reciprocal relationship with I. It is expressed only very weakly on the cells of most adults, but strongly on fetal, neonatal, and adult i red cells. Anti-i cold agglutinins may be haemolytic and are often present in sera of patients with infectious mononucleosis.

I and i determinants are carbohydrate structures carried on glycolipids and glycoproteins. They are internal structures of ABH-active oligosaccharides. The i-active structure is a linear chain of repeating *N*-acetyllactosamine units and is the precursor of the branched I-active structures. In normal development i antigen is converted to I antigen by the branching of i-active linear oligosaccharide chains, catalysed by a $\beta 1,6$-*N*-acetylglucosaminyltransferase, the product of the *I* gene.

Ii antigens comprise Collection 207 of the International Society of Blood Transfusion (ISBT) terminology (Chapter 1). I is I1 (207001) and i is I2 (207002).

Although most cold agglutinins are Ii antibodies, many other specificities are known that detect determinants on carbohydrate structures of membrane glycoproteins and glycolipids (Section 25.9).

25.2 Ii antigens

25.2.1 I antigen (I1)

Wiener *et al.* [2] were the first to give the name I to an antigen of variable strength detected by an autoantibody of very high titre, although many examples of anti-I must have been studied previously. Red cells of a few people reacted only very weakly with anti-I and this weak-I phenotype was designated i. Further studies with this antibody, and with other examples identified since, have shown that I antigen strength varies from person to person and titration scores follow a normal distribution curve [3,4].

Reports of more anti-I soon followed and most reacted only very weakly with cord red cell samples [5,6]. Marsh *et al.* [7] subdivided I antigen: I^D (developed) is the I antigen on most adult cells, but not cord or adult i cells; I^F (fetal) is the I antigen expressed on all human red cells including cord and adult i cells. I^D therefore has a reciprocal relationship with i. It is important to remember that most anti-I are autoantibodies, generally monoclonal and highly heterogeneous, so any subdivision of I is an oversimplification (see Section 25.4.1).

Treatment of red cells with proteases or with sialidase generally enhances expression of Ii antigens. The number of I antigen sites per red cell has been estimated at between 32 000 and 500 000 [8–10].

25.2.2 i Antigen (I2)

When Marsh and Jenkins [11] and Marsh [12] found two cold agglutinating antibodies that behaved in an opposite manner to anti-I—reacting strongly with cord cells and adult i cells, but only very weakly with normal adult cells—they named the antibodies anti-i. Some potent anti-i react quite strongly with adult cells, but their titre may be 1000 times higher with cord cells. Adult i cells generally have higher expression of i than cord cells. The number of i antigen sites has been estimated to be between 20000 and 65000 on cord cells and between 30000 and 70000 on adult i cells [10].

Expression of i is depressed on red cells of adults with an *In(Lu)* gene, a dominant inhibitor of Lutheran and various other red cell antigens (Chapter 6).

25.2.3 I^T antigen

I^T is the name given by Booth *et al.* [13] to an antigen detected by cold agglutinins present in the sera of a high proportion of Melanesians and expressed strongly on cord cells, weakly on normal adult cells, and weaker still on adult i cells. The 'T' stands for 'transition' as I^T was assumed to represent a developing I antigen at the transition from I to i [13]. The high I^T activity on red cells from fetuses ranging in age from 11 to 16 weeks does not support this hypothesis [14]. The very weak I^T antigens of about 15% of Melanesians from the coastal region of Papua is associated with ovalocytosis, in which oval-shaped red cells have weakened expression of a variety of blood group antigens, including I^T [15,16]. South-East Asian ovalocytosis, a hereditary condition common in Papua New Guinea, results from a deletion within the band 3 gene (Section 10.8).

25.3 Adult i and other rare phenotypes

25.3.1 Serology of adult i

Red cells of the rare adult i phenotype are rich in i antigen, but have very low levels of I. Two basic types of adult i have been identified: i_1 mostly in white people and i_2 found in black people and occasionally in white people [5,6,11,12]. Cells of the i_1 phenotype have less I and more i than i_2 cells. Anti-I from i_1 individuals can be adsorbed by i_2, but not i_1, cells. Some descriptions of adult i phenotypes are found in [17–22].

25.3.2 Frequency of adult i

Table 25.1 shows results of several population studies carried out by screening with anti-I.

Only two i adults, one white and one black, were found by screening 2.5 million serum samples from American donors for the presence of anti-I [26]. In another study, eight i adults were found as a result of testing sera of 22700 pregnant women (0.035%) for anti-I, but only four were found among 135100 nonpregnant patients (0.003%) [27]. These figures suggest that I depression may be a transient phenotype in pregnancy.

Table 25.1 Frequency of adult i phenotype in various populations determined by testing red cells with anti-I.

| Population | No. tested | Adult i | | References |
		No.	Frequency (%)	
England, London	17000	0		[5]
Scotland, Glasgow	6000	2*	0.03	[4]
France	10090	1	0.01	[23]
USA, New York	22000	5†	0.02	[2]
African Americans, Detroit	8552	1	0.01	[24]
Japan	1017	0		[19]
Taiwan	562	0		[25]

*Both white i_2: one American, one Scottish.
†Four black, one white.

25.3.3 Inheritance of adult i

Numerous family studies have shown that adult i is inherited as a recessive character. *I* and *i* behave as alleles, with *i* recessive to *I*. Race and Sanger [4] were disturbed by an excess of i sibs of i propositi. In Japan, seven of 31 i adults had consanguineous parents [28]. In some families with adult i members, red cells of obligate heterozygotes have reduced I and enhanced i compared with cells from unrelated controls (a phenotype that has been called I_{int}) [12]. For descriptions of Ii family studies see references [4,6,12,17–22, 25,26,28–32].

I almost certainly encodes a transferase enzyme, which employs i antigen as a substrate to produce I antigen (Section 25.4).

25.3.4 Association between adult i and congenital cataracts

In 1972, Yamaguchi *et al.* [20] reported four adult i propositi with a total of four i and seven I sibs. All eight adult i individuals had congenital cataracts; all seven I individuals had normal vision. These families suggested the possibility of close linkage between the *I* locus and the locus for congenital cataract. In Japan, adult i phenotype is almost invariably accompanied by cataracts [28,31]. Of 31 Japanese adult i donors and patients, 29 suffered impaired vision from cataracts, and in the 11 families studied there was no recombination between Ii phenotype and cataracts [28]. Two of 92 Chinese in Taiwan with congenital cataracts had the adult i phenotype and two Chinese families supported the recessive inheritance of i adult with congenital cataracts [25,33]. In people of European origin, adult i phenotype is not generally accompanied by congenital cataract, but the association has been reported in two families [26,32].

The nature of the association between Ii and congenital cataracts in Orientals, and in some Europeans is unknown. In two Taiwanese families, the adult i phenotype and congenital cataracts were associated with missense mutations encoding Gly348Glu and Arg383His substitutions in the gene encoding the I branching enzyme (*GCNT2*), which abolish enzyme activity (Section 25.4.2). In a third family, *GCNT2* was deleted [33].

25.3.5 Other rare phenotypes

Red cells of seven of 5864 healthy blood donors in Bombay (0.1%) reacted very weakly with anti-I, but did not react with anti-i [34]. The I antigen on these red cells was either weaker or of about the same strength as that on cord cells and there was much lower expression of I^T than on normal adult i cells. Analysis of two large three-generation families showed the rare phenotype to be inherited, although the mode of inheritance appeared to be complex, depending partly on ABO group [34,35]. All individuals with the unusual phenotype were group A_1 or A_1B.

Similar phenotypes with depressed expression of both I and i have been found outside India in A_1, B and O individuals [36,37].

25.4 Biochemistry and molecular genetics

25.4.1 Structure of I and i

Ii antigens are carbohydrates and present on the interior structures of the complex oligosaccharides that carry ABH and Lewis antigens, so this section should be read in conjunction with Sections 2.2 and 2.3. Like the ABH-active structures, Ii determinants on red cell membranes are detected on three major classes of macromolecules:

1 N-linked oligosaccharides of glycoproteins, especially band 3 and band 4.5;
2 simple glycolipids; and
3 complex glycolipids (polyglycosylceramides).

Ii determinants are either accessible or present as partially or totally masked antigens. They are not only detected on red cells, but on many other cell types and in various body secretions (Section 25.5). Recommended reviews on Ii biochemistry are found in [1,38–41] and some important papers on I and i biochemistry in [42–56].

I and i antigens are based entirely on Type 2, Galβ1→4GlcNAc, chains. They may be concealed in ABH-active oligosaccharides and revealed by the stepwise removal of terminal monosaccharides by chemical degradation [43,44]. Anti-i detect linear structures, prevalent on fetal cells. The basic i structure is an unbranched polylactosamine comprising at least two N-acetyllactosamine units:

Galβ1→4GlcNAcβ1→3Galβ1→4GlcNAc→R.

Paragloboside, which has a single lactosamine unit, is not i active; hexasaccharides of three lactosamine units are generally better inhibitors of anti-i than the tetrasaccharide shown above [50,56].

I antigen activity is associated with the branched structure:

Galβ1→4GlcNAcβ1
                    3
                        Galβ1→4GlcNAc→R
                    6
Galβ1→4GlcNAcβ1

There are relatively few of these branched structures present on the glycolipids and glycoproteins of fetal cells because most branching occurs soon after birth [46]. Highly branched polyglycosylceramide molecules, not present in the membranes of fetal or neonatal cells, have a high level of I activity. Ii-active oligosaccharide chains on glycoproteins are generally more complex and linked through *N*-acetylglucosamine to asparagine. Some examples of i- and I-active glycolipids are shown in Table 25.2.

Much of the chemistry of Ii antigens has been worked out with the aid of numerous monoclonal autoantibodies, which differ in their fine specificities. Although no two anti-I appear to be identical they can be subdivided into three general categories [51]:

1 those recognizing the Galβ1→4GlcNAcβ1→6 branch (typified by the antibodies Ma. and Woj.);
2 those recognizing the Galβ1→4GlcNAcβ1→3 sequence with branching (Step.); and
3 those requiring both branches for activity (Phi.).

The basic i and I structures are usually further glycosylated. Ii antibodies vary in their ability to combine with determinants that have additional glycosylation. Terminal galactose residues may be fucosylated by H-transferase to produce an H-active structure which, in turn, may act as an acceptor substrate for A- and B-transferases to catalyse the addition of *N*-acetylgalactosamine and galactose, respectively (Section 2.3). In red cells of the rare O_h (Bombay) phenotype, in which terminal fucosylation of Ii-active oligosaccharides does not occur because of the absence of H-fucosyltransferase, I antigen expression is enhanced (Section 2.13.6). Destruction of H antigen by treatment of red cells with α1,2-fucosidase from *Aspergillus niger* also elevates I expression [57]. Alternatively, the terminal galactose of Ii-active oligosaccharides may be sialylated. This prevents fucosylation and subsequent conversion to A- and B-active structures. These sialylated structures have moderate I or i activity, which is enhanced by sialidase treatment. Furthermore, in the I-active structure, sialylation of the terminal galactose of one branch may prevent fucosylation of the terminal galactose of the other branch, enhancing I activity [38,39,54,58].

Little is known about the biochemistry of I^T, but Issitt [59] has suggested that I^T might be more closely related to Lud (Section 25.9) than I or i and may be on Type 1 chains rather than Type 2 chains.

25.4.2 Biosynthesis of i and I

The biosynthesis of i requires the sequential action of

Table 25.2 Some examples of i- and I-active glycolipids.

i   Galβ1→4GlcNAcβ1→3Galβ1→4GlcNAcβ1→3Galβ1→4Glc→Cer

I   Galβ1→4GlcNAcβ1
                    3
                        Galβ1→4GlcNAcβ1→3Galβ1→4Glc→Cer
                    6
Galβ1→4GlcNAcβ1

I   Galβ1→4GlcNAcβ1
                    3
                        Galβ1→4GlcNAcβ1
                    6   3
Galβ1→4GlcNAcβ1   Galβ1→4GlcNAcβ1→3Galβ1→3Glc→Cer
                                    6
                    Galβ1→4GlcNAcβ1

β1,3-N-acetylglucosaminyltransferase and β1,4-galactosyltransferase. The i antigen is transformed into an I-active structure by the I branching enzyme, a β1,6-N-acetylglucosaminyltransferase [38,39,54,58].

Chinese hamster ovary (CHO) cells usually express i, but no I. Bierhuizen *et al.* [60] used a gene transfer procedure (similar to that described in Section 2.3.1.1 for isolation of an α1,2-fucosyltransferase gene) in order to clone cDNA encoding a β1,6-N-acetylglucosaminyltransferase from a cDNA expression library derived from human teratocarcinoma cells, which express large quantities of I-active branched structures. Following primary and secondary transfection, CHO cells expressing I antigen were isolated by panning with anti-I (Ma). The cloned cDNA contained an open reading frame and hydropathy analysis predicted a type II transmembrane protein with topology characteristic of a glycosyltransferase (Section 2.3). I activity of CHO cells transfected with the cloned cDNA appeared to result from branching of i-active N-acetyllactosamine chains at GlcNAcβ1→6Gal linkages, so the cloned gene probably encodes the I-branching enzyme, a β1,6-N-acetylglucosaminyltranferase (IGnT). The complete sequence encoding IGnT is divided over three exons and sequences upstream of the transcription site have promoter activity and contain TATA-like sequences [61].

The amino acid sequence of IGnT showed substantial homology with another β1,6-N-acetylglucosaminyltransferase (C2GnT), which catalyses the addition of N-acetylglucosamine to Galβ1→3GalNAc, but not to Galβ1→4GalNAc, forming the core 2 O-glycan branch. *In situ* hybridization revealed that both genes are located on chromosome 9q21 [60]. The genes encoding these β1,6-N-acetylglucosaminyltransferases, and a closely related pseudogene, probably arose by gene duplication and subsequent divergence [61,62].

The I-branching enzyme is presumably of low activity in fetal cells, explaining the deficiency of branched oligosaccharide chains and consequent low I and high i activity. Simple unbranched oligosaccharides predominate on red cells from i adults [63], because no active branching enzyme is present owing to mutation or deletion of the *GCNT2* gene [33] (Section 25.3.4). Presence of normal quantities of I antigen in saliva, milk, and plasma of i adults (Section 25.5.1) suggests that different I-branching enzymes may be responsible for I antigen synthesis in different tissues (compare

α1,2-fucosyltransferases in red cell membranes and in secretions, Section 2.3.1).

25.5 Distribution of Ii antigens

Clausen and Hakomori [41] refer to I and i as histo-blood group antigens because, like ABH, Ii antigens are not restricted to red blood cells, but are found on the surface of most human cells and on soluble glycoproteins in various body fluids.

25.5.1 Body fluids

25.5.1.1 Saliva

I antigen can be detected in saliva by haemagglutination inhibition, but with only rare examples of anti-I [29,64,65]. A high titred autoanti-I was inhibited to a varying extent by all 181 salivas tested, with no correlation between degree of inhibition and the presence of ABH or Lewis substances [65]. However, with anti-I Sti. the concentration of I substance in saliva is a function of ABH secretor status, non-secretors having much greater quantities of salivary I substance than secretors [66,67]. This result is not surprising as non-secretor salivas lack the H-transferase responsible for fucosylation of the I-active structures. Saliva from an adult i ABH non-secretor contained a normal quantity of I substance [67], suggesting that the branched oligosaccharide chains, virtually absent from the red cells of i adults, may be present in their body fluids.

There appears to be some i antigen present in human saliva, which can be detected by a minority of anti-i [29,68].

25.5.1.2 Milk

I is present in human milk in greater quantities than in saliva and most anti-I are inhibited to some extent by milk [22,64,69]. Milk from an adult i woman contained as much I substance as milk from I controls and her milk inhibited her own anti-I [22]. Milk from four I women contained anti-I (or anti-HI) and I substance [69].

The presence of i in human milk is more difficult to detect [22,29]. Certainly, milk from an i adult contained no more i substance than that from an I control [22].

25.5.1.3 Plasma

I antigen is generally difficult to detect in plasma by haemagglutination inhibition [29,65], but Rouger *et al.* [70] found an anti-I serum that was inhibited by all 39 plasmas tested. The average level of I antigen in plasma from neonates was 25% of that in plasma from adults [70]. Plasma from an adult i person contained a normal amount of I antigen, but plasma from an individual with I–i– red cells had a reduced quantity of plasma I antigen [67]. Unlike saliva, there is no relationship between I concentration in plasma and ABH secretor status [66,67,70].

Haemagglutination by anti-i is inhibited by serum or plasma from most adults and from cord blood samples [29,68,70,71]. An i-active glycoprotein, with no detectable I, A, B, or H activity, was isolated from serum on an anti-i affinity column [71].

25.5.1.4 Other body fluids

I and i antigens have been detected in amniotic fluid, urine, and ovarian cyst fluid [29,72,73].

25.5.2 Other blood cells

I and i are present on lymphocytes from cord and adult blood [74,75]. Anti-I and -i are potent cold lymphocytotoxins, effective at killing B and T lymphocytes [74,76,77]. Anti-i monoclonal antibodies were specific for subsets of B lymphocytes and for most pre-B cells in adult bone marrow [78]. Anti-I and -i are also cytotoxic for peripheral blood monocytes and macrophages, and about 25% of granulocytes [79,80]; they are equally effective at killing granulocytes obtained from either maternal or cord blood samples [79]. Platelets tested with anti-I by flow cytometry produced a broad distribution curve, with the majority of platelets having a low density of I antigens compared with A and B antigens [81].

25.5.3 Other tissues

The gastrointestinal mucosae and the mucins they secrete have been studied in detail for Ii antigens, especially with anti-I (Ma), which detects the structure Galβ1→4GlcNAcβ1→6. This I (Ma) structure is detected in gastrointestinal glycoproteins from ABH non-secretors, but not those from secretors, where it is concealed by the ABH immunodominant monosaccharides [82,83].

The i antigen is a characteristic of dividing cells present on a variety of cell types including lymphoblasts, fibroblasts, erythroblasts, and thymocytes [84].

The erythroleukaemia cell lines K562 and HEL express i antigen strongly, suggesting that these cells are undifferentiated [85,86]. A small population of K562 cells expressed I, but no I was detected on HEL cells [85]. The i of K562 cells was converted to I when sodium butyrate, but not hemin, was used to induce the cells to differentiate [86].

25.5.4 Other animal species

Wiener *et al.* [87] tested red cells from over 160 different animal species and found that the distribution of Ii antigens cuts across taxonomic lines. Red cells of most adult primates, including chimpanzees and various monkeys, resemble human neonatal and adult i cells by lacking I^D and expressing i [7,87–89]. In tests on red cells of various non-primate species (cat, dog, guinea pig), there was no evidence of a developmental change of i to I [89].

25.6 Ontogenesis and oncogenesis

Ii antigens represent developmental antigens on red cells and in many other tissues. The conversion from i to I occurs as a result of branching of the carbohydrate chains of glycoproteins and glycolipids, catalysed by a β1,6-*N*-acetylglucosaminyltransferase (Section 25.4). In red cells, and probably most other tissues, conversion begins around the time of birth. Fetal and neonatal red cells have very little I antigen expression and very few branched chains. The increase in I strength and concomitant reduction in i antigen expression reaches adult levels at the age of between 6 and 18 months [12,90] and coincides with the branching process of oligosaccharide chains [46]. High expression of i antigen is also a characteristic of immature and less differentiated adult cells [41]. Conversion from i to I is part of a continual process of erythroid differentiation; circulating 'young' red cells have higher i expression than 'old' cells [91]. The i antigen is detected in the germinating layer of squamous epithelium, such as that from the intestine, whereas branching of the oligosaccharides occurs in the more differentiated cell layers and i is no longer present [92].

I and i often demonstrate altered expression on neoplastic cells and may be considered oncodevelopmental antigens (reviewed in [40,93,94]). These changes probably result from incomplete biosynthesis of ABH determinants or by a block in the oligosaccharide chain branching process. In the words of Watanabe and Hakomori [46], 'the process of ontogenesis of a blood group carbohydrate chain occurs as step-by-step elongation and arborization, and that blocking of such a development of a carbohydrate chain occurs in the process of oncogenesis'.

25.7 Ii antibodies

25.7.1 Anti-I

25.7.1.1 Autoanti-I

The original anti-I was an autoantibody responsible for haemolytic anaemia [2] as were most subsequent examples of high titred anti-I agglutinins [3,95,96]. Potent cold reactive antibodies responsible for CHAD are usually of I specificity. These antibodies are generally monoclonal, accounting for the heterogeneity of their specificity. They are usually IgMκ, but IgMλ and IgG autoanti-I occur [1]. A detailed description of CHAD is beyond the scope of this book and recommended reviews are in [1,75,97–99]. These antibodies directly agglutinate I-positive red cells at 4°C with varying thermal amplitude, but are generally inactive above 30°C. In CHAD, the presence of high titre serum IgG anti-IgMκ light chain correlates with low titre of I/i cold agglutinin, probably the result of B cell suppression [100].

By the use of rabbit antibodies raised against purified cold agglutinins, anti-I and -i IgM molecules were shown to share a set of idiotypes, distinct from those shared by anti-Pr agglutinins and from that of anti-I (Ma), known to have an unusual I specificity [101]. A rat monoclonal antibody, 9G4, recognizes a cross-reacting idiotypic determinant present on virtually all pathogenic anti-I and -i cold agglutinins and specifically inhibits haemagglutination by these antibodies [102,103]; it does not generally react with cold agglutinins of other specificities (anti-Pr, etc.) [104]. The epitope recognized by 9G4 is on an IgM heavy chain variable region derived from a single highly conserved common gene segment V4-34 (previously called V_H4-21) [78,105–107]. Although all non-pathogenic mon-

oclonal, naturally occurring anti-i also appear to be V4-34 encoded antibodies [108], this is not the case for non-pathogenic anti-I where V_H3 genes are often involved [109]. A majority of IgM Rh antibodies also have the V4-34 encoded heavy chain segment. In addition to their Rh specificity, these antibodies always have cold agglutinin activity directed against I/i antigens [110,111].

Transient, polyclonal, or oligoclonal autoanti-I may arise from infection, most typically by *Mycoplasma pneumoniae* [1,97]. At least 50% of patients with pneumonia induced by *M. pneumoniae* produce high titred cold agglutinins during the 3 weeks after the onset of respiratory symptoms [1]. It is likely that the pathogen modifies a sialylated I-active receptor making it immunogenic and that antibody is then produced to the modified structure [112–114]. Sialylated I determinants are recognized by anti-Sia-lb2 (anti-Gd) and anti-Sia-b1 (anti-Fl) cold agglutinins (Section 25.9) and these antibodies occur together with anti-I in the majority of cases of *M. pneumoniae*-induced cold agglutinin production [115,116]. Most people have weak cold-reactive autoanti-I in their serum [117].

25.7.1.2 Alloanti-I

Anti-I of fairly high titre is usually present in the sera of i adults [4]. Although adult i red cells are not totally devoid of I antigen, the anti-I can be referred to as alloanti-I as it does not react with autologous cells. These antibodies are almost invariably IgM and usually only active at low temperatures. Rare examples may be haemolytic and have a thermal range up to 37°C [22].

Less than 1% of radiolabelled I+ red cells survived 15 min after injection into an i adult with anti-I, a clear indication that his antibody had the potential to provoke a dangerous transfusion reaction [118]. A previous study in an adult i patient suggested a less extreme destruction of injected I-positive cells by anti-I [17].

Analysis by adsorption and elution of 22 sera containing cold agglutinins that could not be clearly defined as anti-I or -i revealed that all contained a separable mixture of both antibodies [119].

25.7.1.3 Anti-I lectin

Lectin prepared from the gonads of *Aplysia depilans*, a

marine mollusc (sea slug), behaved serologically as anti-I [120]. All other lectins resembling anti-I have specificities dependent on the presence of ABH or P antigens [120] (Section 25.7.5).

25.7.2 Anti-i

Alloanti-i has not been identified. The first three examples of autoanti-i were from patients with reticulosis, one of whom died with autoimmune haemolytic anaemia [4–6]; a fourth example was in a patient with myeloid leukaemia [96]. Anti-i is a rare alternative to anti-I in CHAD [97]. Anti-i are heterogeneous in specificity [10,44,84,121]. They appear to be exclusively V4-34-encoded IgM antibodies [108].

Anti-i is often found in the serum of patients with infectious mononucleosis and occasionally causes haemolysis. Estimates of the proportion of infectious mononucleosis patients with anti-i vary between 8% and 90%, but only very few develop haemolytic complications [88,122–124]. These antibodies may be IgM [88,124–128] or, in some cases, may be IgG anti-i combined with IgM anti-IgG [123,128]. One of the IgM anti-i behaved like a Donath–Landsteiner antibody (haemolysis following incubation of red cells in serum at 4°C and subsequent warming to 37°C) [127], as did an IgG anti-i detected in a patient with chronic paroxysmal cold haemoglobinuria [129].

The presence of anti-i is associated with immunodeficiency. Autoanti-i activity was detected in 50% of patients with Wiskott–Aldrich syndrome, a rare X-linked recessive immunodeficiency [78], and in 64% of patients with AIDS [130]. Infection with Epstein–Barr virus, the pathogen associated with infectious mononucleosis, is endemic in AIDS.

Maternal IgG autoanti-i can cross the placenta and has resulted in positive direct antiglobulin reactions on cord cells and mild neonatal jaundice [131,132]. Acute intravascular haemolysis in a patient with anti-i followed infusion of 2 units of blood deemed compatible by an immediate spin crossmatch technique [133].

Monoclonal anti-i was produced *in vitro* by a heterohybridoma of mouse myeloma and human lymphocytes from lymph nodes of a lung cancer patient [92], and by heterohybridomas and lymphoblastoid cell lines derived from splenocytes of a Wiskott–Aldrich syndrome patient [78].

25.7.3 Anti-I^T

Anti-I^T defines an antigen expressed strongly on cord cells, weakly on most adult cells, and very weakly on adult i cells (Section 25.2.3). Cold agglutinins were detected in 76% of Melanesians from Papua New Guinea; of the six analysed in detail, one was anti-I and five were anti-I^T [13]. Anti-I^T was found in 84% of Yanomama Indians of Venezuela [134].

The first four examples of anti-I^T in white people were all IgG and all in patients with Hodgkin's disease [14,135]. Three of these antibodies were considered haemolytic and responsible for autoimmune haemolytic anaemia [14]. Six other examples of IgG autoanti-I^T were not apparently clinically significant as judged by response to incompatible transfusion and *in vitro* survival studies [136,137]; none was from a patient with Hodgkin's disease. IgM anti-I^T can cause haemolytic anaemia [138,139].

25.7.4 Anti-j

Cold agglutinins in two patients, which agglutinated adult and cord red cells, behaved as anti-Ii and were named anti-j by Roelcke *et al.* [140]. These antibodies reacted with protease- and sialidase-treated red cells, but not with cells treated with endo-β-galactosidase, which cleaves Type 2 oligosaccharide chains. The antibodies were inhibited by linear (i) and branched (I) Type 2 structures. The two anti-j were unusual cold agglutinins as they were IgMλ molecules; they resembled most pathogenic anti-I and -i by expressing the 9G4 idiotype, a characteristic of antibodies encoded by a gene utilizing a V4-34 sequence.

25.7.5 Ii antibodies and the H, ABO, and P groups

Considering the heterogeneity of Ii antibodies and the close biochemical association between Ii and the H, A, and B antigens, it is of no surprise that some antibodies appear to show a preference for I determinants with attached H, A, or B immunodominant monosaccharides. The most abundant of these antibodies is anti-HI, which does not react, or at least reacts only very weakly, with I-positive cells of the rare H-deficient phenotypes. These antibodies are described in Section 2.15.8. Some anti-I resemble anti-HI by giving stronger reactions with O or A_2 cells than with A_1

red cells [5,96,141]. Anti-Hi has also been reported [142]. Some anti-I react more strongly with A or B or A and B cells than with O cells. These antibodies have been called anti-AI (or -A$_1$I) [6,141,143,144], -BI [143,145–147], and -(A+B)I [148]. Anti-HILe^b (or -ILe^{b}H) agglutinated only O or A$_2$, I-positive, Le(a–b+) cells [149,150].

P1 antibodies that do not agglutinate P1+ cord or P1+ adult i red cells are called anti-IP1 [151]. An antibody reacting only weakly with cord and adult i cells, and not at all with p cells, was named anti-IP [152]. Anti-I^{T}P was responsible for fatal autoimmune haemolytic anaemia [153].

25.8 Ii antigens and disease

Red cells of patients with dyserythropoietic conditions often have elevated expression of i [80,154–157]. These conditions include thalassaemia, sickle cell disease, congenital dyserythropoietic anaemia II (HEMPAS), Diamond–Blackfan syndrome, myeloblastic erythropoiesis, sideroblastic erythropoiesis, refractory anaemia, paroxysmal nocturnal haemoglobinuria (PNH), and acute leukaemias. Red cells with increased i antigen also appear in the circulation of people subjected to repeated phlebotomy [158]. I expression is not generally decreased in these conditions [155]. When red cell production is inadequate to meet demands, the proliferative stress on the erythroid precursors results in shortened maturation time before the red cell precursors appear in the peripheral blood. This could account, at least in part, for enhanced i expression [154,155,158]. In PNH, elevation of i was detected on affected (CD59-negative) and unaffected (CD59-positive) populations of cells, suggesting that enhanced i expression is a non-specific affect of haemopoietic stress [157].

As mentioned in Section 25.5.2, i antigen is detected on lymphocytes from adults and from cord samples [74]. In chronic lymphocytic leukaemia there is a reduction in lymphocyte i expression, as detected by some anti-i [159]. In acute lymphoid leukaemia, blast cells have as much i antigen as normal lymphocytes; in acute myeloid leukaemia, blast cells have much less i antigen [160]. Lymphoblasts can be distinguished from myeloblasts by their i expression in undifferentiated acute leukaemia and in chronic myeloid leukaemia in blast-cell crisis [161].

25.9 Other cold agglutinins

In addition to anti-I and -i, cold agglutinins of numerous other specificities have been defined, mostly by Roelcke et al. (for reviews see [1,59,162]). These antibodies and some characteristics of the determinants they define are listed in Table 25.3. All comply with the definition of cold agglutinins: autoantibodies to red cell antigens that react optimally in the cold (0°C) [1]. Apart from anti-j, they are usually IgMκ monoclonal antibodies.

The most abundant cold agglutinins, after anti-I and -i, are the Pr antibodies. These detect protease-labile determinants on the O-linked sialotetrasaccharides and sialotrisaccharides of red cell sialoglycoproteins found predominantly on glycophorins A and B. These glycoproteins also carry blood group M, N, S, and s antigens and so Pr is described in Chapter 3 (Section 3.6.4). Pr antibodies are heterogeneous and have been subdivided. Anti-Pr$_1$, -Pr$_2$, and -Pr$_3$ are distinguished from each other by the effects of certain chemical modifications of their determinants [1]. Anti-Pr$_1$ and -Pr$_3$ are further subdivided by their reactions with animal cells: anti-Pr$_{1h}$ and -Pr$_{3h}$ react exclusively with human red cells; anti-Pr$_{1d}$ and anti-Pr$_{3d}$ agglutinate human and dog red cells [1]. Anti-Sa, like anti-Pr$_2$, detects an antigen present on glycophorin A and also on some gangliosides [178,179]. A few anti-Pr and -Sa are IgAκ [164,180]. Pr antibodies may be associated with rubella infection [181]. An IgGλ anti-Pr$_1$ caused severe haemolysis in a child after infection with the rubella virus [181].

Anti-Sia-lb (anti-sialo-linear-branched, formerly anti-Gd) represents a heterogeneous collection of antibodies detecting protease-resistant, sialidase-sensitive antigens located on gangliosides and created by the α2,3-sialylation of I- and i-active structures (branched and linear) on glycolipids [1,165,168]. Anti-Sia-lb1 (anti-Gd$_1$) require only a terminal sialic acid residue for activity (NeuNAcα2,3–); anti-Sia-lb2 (anti-Gd$_2$) also require subterminal galactose (NeuAcα2→3Galβ1–) [166]. Sia-lb antibodies also bind sialyl-Le^a (sLe^a) and sialyl-Le^x (sLe^x) structures (see Table 2.3) expressed on nucleated cells and in soluble cancer-related mucins [182].

Sia-b1 (Fl) antigen is located on glycolipids with sialylated branched structures, whereas Sia-l1 (Vo) and Li are probably α2,3-sialylated linear structures on glycolipids [114,167–170,183].

Table 25.3 Antigens defined by cold agglutinins, showing reactions of the antibodies with adult (Ad), cord (Cd), adult i (i ad), papain- (Pap) and sialidase-treated (Sial) red cells.

Antigen	Ad	Cd	i ad	Pap	Sial	Comments	References
I	+	w	w	+	+	Branched; glycoproteins and glycolipids	See text
i	w	+	+	+	+	Linear; glycoproteins and glycolipids	See text
I^T	w	+	w	+	+		See text
j	+	+	+	+	+	Linear and branched; glycoproteins and glycolipids	[140]
Pr$_{1-3}$	+	+	+	0	0	O-glycans of glycophorins	*
Pr$_a$	+	+	+	0	+		*
Sa	+	+	+	w	0	O-glycans of glycophorins and gangliosides	[163,164]*
Sia-lb1 (Gd$_1$)	+	+	+	+	0	Sialylated linear and branched; glycolipids	[165,166]
Sia-lb2 (Gd$_2$)	+	+	+	+	0	Sialylated linear and branched; glycolipids	[165,166]
Sia-b1 (Fl)	+	w	w	+	0	Sialylated branched; glycolipids	[167,168]
Sia-l1 (Vo)	w	+	+	+	w	Sialylated linear; glycolipids	[168,169]
Li	w	+	+	+	0	Sialylated linear; glycolipids	[168,170]
Lud	+	w	+	w	0		[171]
Me	+	+		+	+	Enhanced by human milk	[172]
Om	+	+		+	+	Not enhanced by human milk	[173]
Ju	+	+		w	w		[174]
IgM^{WOO}	0	0	0	0	+	Type 1 chain	[175]
Rx	+	w	+	+	+	pH optimum 6.5; previously Sd^x	[176,177]

*See Section 3.6.4.

+, Strong agglutination; w, relatively weak agglutination compared with +; 0, no agglutination.

Very little is known about the biochemistry of the Lud, Om, Me, and Ju antigens. Anti-Lud recognizes α2,3-sialylated Type 1 chain sequences [1,183]. Activity of the unfortunately named anti-Me, which is not related to anti-M^e of the MNS system, is enhanced by preheated human milk, but not by individual milk sugars [172]. Anti-Om activity is slightly reduced by human milk [173], which distinguishes it from anti-Me. Anti-Me and -Om may resemble anti-j [140]. The cold agglutinin IgM^{WOO}, which agglutinates sialidase-treated cells, but not untreated cells, recognizes the Type 1 chain Galβ1→3GlcNAcβ1→3Galβ1→4Glc/GlcNAc [175]. Anti-Rx was originally named anti-Sd^x because it appeared to be inhibited by Sd(a+) but not Sd(a–) urine [176,184]. This was shown to be a non-specific effect, probably resulting from the extreme pH dependency of the antibody [177].

References

1 Roelcke D. Cold agglutination. *Transfus Med Rev* 1989;3:140–66.

2 Wiener AS, Unger LJ, Cohen L, Feldman J. Type-specific cold auto-antibodies as a cause of acquired hemolytic anemia and hemolytic transfusion reactions: biologic test with bovine red cells. *Ann Intern Med* 1956;44:221–40.

3 Crookston JH, Dacie JV, Rossi V. Differences in the agglutinability of human red cells by the high-titre cold antibodies of acquired haemolytic anaemia. *Br J Haematol* 1956;2:321–31.

4 Race RR, Sanger R. *Blood Groups in Man*, 6th edn. Oxford: Blackwell Scientific Publications, 1975.

5 Jenkins WJ, Marsh WL, Noades J *et al*. The I antigen and antibody. *Vox Sang* 1960;5:97–106.

6 Tippett P, Noades J, Sanger R *et al*. Further studies of the I antigen and antibody. *Vox Sang* 1960;5:107–21.

7 Marsh WL, Nichols ME, Reid ME. The definition of two I antigen components. *Vox Sang* 1971;20:209–17.

8 Evans RS, Turner E, Bingham M. Studies with radio-iodinated cold agglutinins of 10 patients. *Am J Med* 1965;38:378–95.

9 Olesen H. Thermodynamics of the cold agglutinin reaction. *Scand J Clin Lab Invest* 1966;18:1–15.

10 Doinel C, Ropars C, Salmon C. Quantitative and thermodynamic measurements on I and i antigens of human red blood cells. *Immunology* 1976;30:289–97.

11 Marsh WL, Jenkins WJ. Anti-i: a new cold antibody. *Nature* 1960;188:753.

12 Marsh WL. Anti-i: a cold antibody defining the Ii relationship in human red cells. *Br J Haematol* 1961;7:200–9.

13 Booth PB, Jenkins WJ, Marsh WL. Anti I^T: a new antibody of the I blood-group system occurring in certain Melanesian sera. *Br J Haematol* 1966;12:341–4.

14 Garratty G, Petz LD, Wallerstein RO, Fudenberg HH. Autoimmune hemolytic anemia in Hodgkin's disease associated with anti-I^T. *Transfusion* 1974;14:226–31. [See letter in *Transfusion* 1974;14:630.]

15 Booth PB. The occurrence of weak I^T red cell antigen among Melanesians. *Vox Sang* 1972;22:64–72.

16 Booth PB, Serjeantson S, Woodfield DG, Amato D. Selective depression of blood group antigens associated with hereditary ovalocytosis among Melanesians. *Vox Sang* 1977;32:99–110.

17 Claflin AJ. Three members of one family with the phenotype i; one with an anti-I antibody. *Transfusion* 1963;3:216–19.

18 Jakobowicz R, Simmons RT. The identification of anti-I agglutinins in human serum: an atypical antibody which simulates a non-specific cold agglutinin. *Med J Aust* 1964;1:194–5.

19 Yamaguchi H, Okubo Y, Tomita T, Yamano H, Tanaka M. A rare i (I-negative) phenotype blood found in Japanese families. *Proc Jpn Acad* 1970;46:889–92.

20 Yamaguchi H, Okubo Y, Tanaka M. A note on possible close linkage between the Ii blood locus and a congenital cataract locus. *Proc Jpn Acad* 1972;48:625–8.

21 Dzierzkowa-Borodej W, Kazmierczak Z, Ziemniak J. The antigens of Ii blood group system in a further case of i$_2$ (Bi$_2$) adult person. *Arch Immunol Ther Exp* 1972;20:851–9.

22 Marsh WL, Jensen L, Decary F, Colledge K. Water-soluble I blood group substance in the secretions of i adults. *Transfusion* 1972;12:222–6.

23 Ducos J, Ruffie J, Colombies P, Marty Y, Ohayon E. I antigen in leukaemic patients. *Nature* 1965;208:1329–30.

24 Winkler MM, Hamilton JR. Previously tested donors eliminated to determine rare phenotype frequencies [Abstract]. *Joint Congr Int Soc Blood Transfus and Am Ass Blood Banks*, 1990:158.

25 Lin-Chu M, Broadberry RE, Okubo Y, Tanaka M. The i phenotype and congenital cataracts among Chinese in Taiwan. *Transfusion* 1991;31:676–7.

26 Page PL, Langevin S, Petersen RA, Kruskall MS. Reduced association between the Ii blood group and congenital cataracts in white patients. *Am J Clin Pathol* 1987;87:101–2.

27 Godwin DJ, Combs MR, Telen MJ, Issitt PD. Increased incidence of the i phenotype in pregnancy [Abstract]. *Joint Congr Int Soc Blood Transfus and Am Ass Blood Banks*, 1990:155.

28 Okubo Y, Yamaguchi H. I-negative phenotype and cataract [Abstract]. *19th Congr Int Soc Blood Transfus*, 1986:147.

29 Burnie K. Ii antigens and antibodies. *Can J Med Technol* 1973;35:5–26.

30 Signal T, Booth PB. A New Zealand family with i members. *Vox Sang* 1976;30:391–5.

31 Ogata H, Okubo Y, Akabane T. Phenotype i associated with congenital cataract in Japanese. *Transfusion* 1979;19:166–8.

32 Macdonald EB, Douglas R, Harden PA. A Caucasian family with the i phenotype and congenital cataracts. *Vox Sang* 1983;44:322–5.

33 Yu L-C, Twu Y-C, Chang C-Y, Lin M. Molecular basis of the adult i phenotype and the gene responsible for the expression of the human blood group I antigen. *Blood* 2001;98:3840–5.

34 Joshi SR, Bhatia HM. A new red cell phenotype I–i–: red cells lacking both I and i antigens. *Vox Sang* 1979;36:34–8.

35 Joshi SR, Bhatia HM. I–i– phenotype in a large kindred Indian family. *Vox Sang* 1984;46:157–60.

36 Jorgensen JR. A new phenotype in the Ii blood group system. *Vox Sang* 1968;15:171–6.

37 Dzierzkowa-Borodej W, Lisowska E, Leskiewicz A, Leszczak L. An unusual expression of Ii antigens in erythrocytes of a healthy adult person. *Vox Sang* 1974;27:57–66.

38 Feizi T. The blood group Ii system: a carbohydrate antigen system defined by naturally monoclonal or oligoclonal autoantibodies of man. *Immunol Commun* 1981;10:127–56.

39 Hakomori S. Blood group ABH and Ii antigens of human erythrocytes: chemistry, polymorphism, and their developmental change. *Semin Hematol* 1981;18:39–62.

40 Feizi T. Demonstration by monoclonal antibodies that carbohydrate structures of glycoproteins and glycolipids are onco-developmental antigens. *Nature* 1985;314:53–7.

41 Clausen H, Hakomori S. ABH and related histo-blood group antigens: immunochemical differences in carrier isotypes and their distribution. *Vox Sang* 1989;56:1–20.

42 Feizi T, Kabat EA, Vicari G, Anderson B, Marsh WL. Immunochemical studies on blood groups. XLVII. The I antigen complex-precursors in the A, B, H, Le^a and Le^b blood group system-hemagglutination-inhibition studies. *J Exp Med* 1971;133:39–52.

43 Feizi T, Kabat EA, Vicari G, Anderson B, Marsh WL. Immunochemical studies on blood groups. XLIX. The I antigen complex: specificity differences among anti-I sera revealed by quantitative precipitin studies; partial structure of the I determinant specific for one anti-I serum. *J Immunol* 1971;106:1578–92.

44 Feizi T, Kabat EA. Immunochemical studies on blood groups. LIV. Classification of anti-I and anti-i sera into groups based on reactivity patterns with various antigens related to the blood group A, B, H, Le^a, Le^b and precursor substances. *J Exp Med* 1972;135:1247–58.

45 Ebert W, Roelcke D, Weicker H. The I antigen of human red cell membrane. *Eur J Biochem* 1975;53: 505–15.

46 Watanabe K, Hakomori S-I. Status of blood group carbohydrate chains in ontogenesis and in oncogenesis. *J Exp Med* 1976;144:644–53.

47 Gardas A. Studies on the I-blood-group-active sites on macro-glycolipids from human erythocytes. *Eur J Biochem* 1976;68:185–91.

48 Feizi T, Childs RA, Hakomori S-I, Powell ME. Blood-group-Ii-active gangliosides of human erythrocyte membranes. *Biochem J* 1978;173:245–54.

49 Childs RA, Feizi T, Fukuda M, Hakomori S-I. Blood-group-I activity associated with Band 3, the major intrinsic membrane protein of human erythrocytes. *Biochem J* 1978;173:333–6.

50 Niemann H, Watanabe K, Hakomori S, Childs RA, Feizi T. Blood group i and I activities of 'lacto-N-norhexaosylceramide' and its analogues: the structural requirements for i-specificities. *Biochem Biophys Res Commun* 1978;81:1286–93.

51 Feizi T, Childs RA, Watanabe K, Hakomori SI. Three types of blood group I specificity among monoclonal anti-I autoantibodies revealed by analogues of a branched erythrocyte glycolipid. *J Exp Med* 1979;149:975–80.

52 Watanabe K, Hakomoi S, Childs RA, Feizi T. Characterization of a blood group I-active ganglioside: structural requirements for I and i specificities. *J Biol Chem* 1979;254:3221–8.

53 Fukuda M, Fukuda MN, Hakomori S. Developmental change and genetic defect in the carbohydrate structure of band 3 glycoprotein of human erythrocyte membrane. *J Biol Chem* 1979;254:3700–3.

54 Koscielak J, Zdebska E, Wilczynska Z, Miller-Podraza H, Dzierzkowa-Borodej W. Immunochemistry of Ii-active glycosphingolipids of erythrocytes. *Eur J Biochem* 1979;96:331–7.

55 Okada Y, Kannagi R, Levery SB, Hakomori S-I. Glycolipid antigens with blood group I and i specificities from human adult and umbilical cord erythrocytes. *J Immunol* 1984;133:835–42.

56 Gooi HC, Veyrières A, Alais J et al. Further studies of the specificities of monoclonal anti-i and anti-I antibodies using chemically synthesized, linear oligosaccharides of the poly-N-acetyllactosamine series. *Mol Immunol* 1984;21:1099–104.

57 Doinel C, Ropars C, Rufin JM. I and H activities of human red blood cells treated with an 1,2-α-L-fucosidase from *Aspergillus niger*. *Rev Franc Transfus Immuno-Hémat* 1980;23:259–69.

58 Piller F, Cartron J-P, Maranduba A et al. Biosynthesis of blood group I antigens. Identification of a UDP-GlcNAc:GlcNAcβ1–3Gal(-R)β1–6(GlcNAc to Gal) N-acetylglucosaminyltransferase in hog gastric mucosa. *J Biol Chem* 1984;259:13385–90.

59 Issitt PD. Cold-reactive autoantibodies outside the I and P blood groups. In: JM Moulds, LL Woods, eds. *Blood Groups: P, I, Sd^a and Pr*. Arlington: American Association of Blood Banks, 1991: 73–112.

60 Bierhuizen MFA, Mattei M-G, Fukuda M. Expression of the developmental I antigen by a cloned human cDNA encoding a member of a β-1,6-N-acetylglucosaminyltransferase gene family. *Genes Dev* 1993;7:468–78.

61 Bierhuizen MFA, Maemura K, Kudo S, Fukuda M. Genomic organization of core 2 and branching β-1,6-N-acetylglucosaminyltransferases: implication for evolution of the β-1,6-N-acetylglucosaminyltransferase gene family. *Glycobiology* 1995;5:417–25.

62 Bierhuizen MFA, Maemura K, Fukuda M. Isolation and characterization of a pseudogene related to human core 2 β-1,6-N-acetylglucosaminyltransferase. *Glycocon J* 1995;12:857–64.

63 Fukuda MN, Fukuda M, Hakomori S. Cell surface modification by endo-β-galactosidase: change of blood group activities and release of oligosaccharides from glycoproteins and glycosphingolipids of human erythrocytes. *J Biol Chem* 1979;254:5458–65.

64 Marsh WL, Nichols ME, Allen FH. Inhibition of anti-I sera by human milk. *Vox Sang* 1970;18:149–54.

65 Dzierzkowa-Borodej W, Seyfried H, Nichols M, Reid M, Marsh WL. The recognition of water-soluble I blood group substance. *Vox Sang* 1970;18:222–34.

66 Rouger P, Juszczak G, Doinel C, Salmon C. Relationship between I and H antigens. I. A study of the plasma and saliva of a normal population. *Transfusion* 1980; 20:536–9.

67 Rouger P, Juszczak G, Doinel C et al. Relationship between I and H antigens. II. Study of the H and I deficient phenotypes. *Immunol Commun* 1980;9:161–72.

68 de Boissezon J-F, Marty Y, Ducos J, Abbal M. Présence constante d'une substance inhibitrice de l'anticorps anti-i dans le sérum humain normal. *CR Acad Sci Paris* 1970;271:1448–51.

69 Dzierzkowa-Borodej W, Osinska M. Anti-I antibodies in human milk. *Arch Immunol Ther Exp* 1971; 19:609–12.

70 Rouger P, Riveau D, Salmon C. Detection of the H and I blood group antigens in normal plasma: a comparison with A and i antigens. *Vox Sang* 1979;37:78–83.

71 Cooper AG, Brown MC. Serum i antigen: a new human blood-group glycoprotein. *Biochem Biophys Res Commun* 1973;55:297–304.

72 Cooper AG. Soluble blood group I substance in human amniotic fluid. *Nature* 1970;227:508–9.

73 Feizi T, Cederqvist LL, Childs R. The blood group I and i antigens of amniotic fluid. I. Association of I and i antigens with blood group A, B and H antigens. *Br J Haematol* 1975;30:489–97.

74 Shumak KH, Rachkewich RA, Crookston MC,

Crookston JH. Antigens of the Ii system on lympho-cytes. *Nature New Biol* 1971;231:148–9.

75 Pruzanski W, Shumak KH. Biologic activity of cold-reacting autoantibodies. *N Engl J Med* 1977;297:583–9.

76 Shumak KH, Rachkewich RA, Greaves MF. I and i anti-gens on normal human T and B lymphocytes and on lymphocytes from patients with chronic lymphocytic leukemia. *Clin Immunol Immunopathol* 1975;4:241–7.

77 Pruzanski W, Farid N, Keystone E, Armstrong M, Greaves MF. The influence of homogeneous cold agglu-tinins on human B and T lymphocytes. *Clin Immunol Immunpathol* 1975;4:248–57.

78 Grillot-Courvalin C, Brouet J-C, Piller F *et al.* An anti-B cell autoantibody from Wiskott–Aldrich syndrome which recognises i blood group specificity on normal human B cells. *Eur J Immunol* 1992;22:1781–8.

79 Pruzanski W, Farid N, Keystone E, Armstrong M. The influence of homogeneous cold agglutinins on poly-morphonuclear and mononuclear phagocytes. *Clin Immunol Immunpathol* 1975;4:277–85.

80 Pruzanski W, Delmage KJ. Cytoxic and cytolytic activi-ty of homogeneous cold agglutinins on peripheral blood monocytes. *Clin Immunol Immunpathol* 1977;7: 130–8.

81 Dunstan RA, Simpson MB. Heterogeneous distribution of antigens on human platelets demonstrated by fluores-cence flow cytometry. *Br J Haematol* 1985;61:603–9.

82 Picard J, Edward DW, Feizi T. Changes in the expression of the blood group A, B, H, Le^a and Le^b antigens and the blood group precursor associated I (MA) antigen in glycoprotein-rich extracts of gastric carcinomas. *J Clin Lab Immunol* 1978;1:119–28.

83 Picard JK, Feizi T. Peanut lectin and anti-Ii antibodies reveal structural differences among human gastrointes-tinal glycoproteins. *Mol Immunol* 1983;20:1215–20.

84 Thomas DB. The i antigen complex: a new specificity unique to dividing human cells. *Eur J Immunol* 1974;4:819–24.

85 Kannagi R, Papayannopoulou T, Nakamoto B *et al.* Carbohydrate antigen profiles of human erythr-oleukemia cell lines HEL and K562. *Blood* 1983;62:1230–41.

86 Testa U, Henri A, Bettaieb A *et al.* Regulation of i- and I-antigen expression in the K562 cell line. *Cancer Res* 1982;42:4694–700.

87 Wiener AS, Moor-Jankowski J, Gordon EB, Davis J. The blood factors I and i in primates including man, and in lower species. *Am J Phys Anthrop* 1965;23:389–96.

88 Jenkins WJ, Koster HG, Marsh WL, Carter RL. Infec-tious mononucleosis: an unsuspected source of anti-i. *Br J Haematol* 1965;11:480–3.

89 Chiewsilp P, Colledge KI, Marsh WL. Water soluble I blood group substance in the secretions of rhesus monkeys. *Vox Sang* 1971;21:30–6.

90 Pawlak Z, Lopez M. Développement des antigènes ABH et Ii chez les enfants de 0 à 16 ans. *Rev Franc Transfus Immuno-Hémat* 1979;22:253–63.

91 Testa U, Rochant H, Henri A *et al.* Change in i-antigen expression of erythrocytes during *in vivo* aging. *Rev Franc Transfus Immuno-Hémat* 1981;24:299–305.

92 Hirohashi S, Clausen H, Nudelman E *et al.* A human monoclonal antibody directed to blood group i antigen: heterohybridoma between human lymphocytes from regional lymph nodes of a lung cancer patient and mouse myeloma. *J Immunol* 1986;136:4163–8.

93 Feizi T. The I and i antigens on certain normal and pathologic tissues. *Rev Franc Transfus Immuno-Hémat* 1978;21:165–74.

94 Hakomori S. Histo-blood group antigens as tumor-associated carbohydrate antigens and ligands for cell adhesion. In: J-P Cartron, P Rouger, eds. *Blood Cell Biochemistry*, Vol. 6. New York: Plenum Press, 1995: 421–43.

95 Weiner W, Shinton NK, Gray IR. Antibody of blood-group specificity in simple ('cold') haemolytic anaemias. *J Clin Pathol* 1960;13:232–6.

96 van Loghem JJ, van der Hart M, Veenhoven-van Riesz E *et al.* Cold auto-agglutinins and haemolysins of anti-I and anti-i specificity. *Vox Sang* 1962;7:214–21.

97 Mollison PL, Engelfriet CP, Contreras M. *Blood Transfusion in Clinical Medicine*, 10th edn. Oxford: Blackwell Science, 1997.

98 Pruzanski W, Shumak KH. Biologic activity of cold-re-acting autoantibodies. *N Engl J Med* 1977;297:538–42.

99 Feizi T. The monoclonal antibodies of cold agglutinin syndrome: properties of the monoclonal autoanti-bodies. *Med Biol* 1980;58:300–2.

100 Terness P, Navolan D, Opelz G, Roelcke D. Inverse as-sociation between IgG–anti-κ and antierythrocyte autoantibodies in patients with cold agglutination. *Blood* 1999;94:4343–6.

101 Feizi T, Kunkel HG, Roelcke D. Cross idiotypic speci-ficity among cold agglutinins in relation to combining activity for blood group-related antigens. *Clin Exp Im-munol* 1974;18:283–93.

102 Stevenson FK, Wrightham M, Glennie MJ *et al.* Anti-bodies to shared idiotypes as agents for analysis and therapy for human B cell tumors. *Blood* 1986;68: 430–6.

103 Stevenson FK, Smith GJ, North J, Hamblin TJ, Glennie MJ. Identification of normal B-cell counterparts of neo-plastic cells which secrete cold agglutinins of anti-I and anti-i specificity. *Br J Haematol* 1989;72:9–15.

104 Smith G, Spellerberg M, Boulton F, Roelcke D, Stevenson F. The immunoglobulin V_H gene, V_H4-21, specifically encodes autoanti-red cell antibodies against the I or i antigens. *Vox Sang* 1995;68:231–5.

105 Leoni J, Ghiso J, Goñi F, Frangione B. The primary structure of the Fab fragment of protein KAU, a mono-clonal immunoglobulin M cold agglutinin. *J Biol Chem* 1991;266:2836–42.

106 Pascual V, Victor K, Lelsz D *et al*. Nucleotide sequence analysis of the V regions of two IgM cold agglutinins: evidence that the V_H4-21 gene segment is responsible for the major cross-reactive idiotype. *J Immunol* 1991;**146**:4385–91.

107 Silberstein LE, Jefferies LC, Goldman J *et al*. Variable region gene analysis of pathologic human autoantibodies to the related i and I red blood cell antigens. *Blood* 1991;**78**:2372–86.

108 Schutte MEM, van Es JH, Silberstein LE, Logtenberg T. V_H4.21-encoded natural autoantibodies with anti-i specificity mirror those associated with cold hemagglutinin disease. *J Immunol* 1993;**151**:6569–76.

109 Jefferies LC, Carchidi CM, Silberstein LE. Naturally occurring anti-i/I cold agglutinins may be encoded by different V_H3 genes as well as the V_H4.21 gene segment. *J Clin Invest* 1993;**92**:2821–33.

110 Thorpe SJ, Boult CE, Stevenson FK *et al*. Cold agglutinin activity is common among human monoclonal IgM Rh system antibodies using the V_{4-34} heavy chain variable segment. *Transfusion* 1997;**37**:1111–16.

111 Thorpe SJ, Turner CE, Stevenson FK *et al*. Human monoclonal antibodies encoded by the V4–34 gene segment show cold agglutinin activity and variable multireactivity which correlates with the predicted charge of the heavy-chain variable region. *Immunology* 1998; **93**:129–36.

112 Feizi T, Taylor-Robinson D. Cold agglutinin anti-I and *Mycoplasma pneumoniae*. *Immunology* 1967;**13**: 405–9.

113 Loomes LM, Uemura K, Childs RA *et al*. Erythrocyte receptors for *Mycoplasma pneumoniae* are sialylated oligosaccharides of Ii antigen type. *Nature* 1984; **307**:560–3.

114 Loomes LM, Uemura K-I, Feizi T. Interaction of *Mycoplasma pneumoniae* with erythrocyte glycolipids of I and i antigen types. *Infect Immun* 1985;**47**:15–20.

115 König AL, Kreft H, Hengge U, Braun RW, Roelcke D. Coexisting anti-I and anti-Fl/Gd cold agglutinins in infections by *Mycoplasma pneumoniae*. *Vox Sang* 1988;**55**:176–80.

116 Roelcke D, Kreft H, Northoff H, Gallasch E. Sia-b1 and I antigens recognized by *Mycoplasma pneumoniae*-induced human cold agglutinins. *Transfusion* 1991; **31**:627–30.

117 Issitt PD, Jackson VA. Useful modifications and variations of technics in work on I system antibodies. *Vox Sang* 1968;**15**:152–3.

118 Chaplin H, Hunter VL, Malecek AC, Kilzer P, Rosche ME. Clinically significant allo-anti-I in an I-negative patient with massive hemorrhage. *Transfusion* 1986; **26**:57–61.

119 Jackson VA, Issitt PD, Francis BJ, Garris ML, Sanders CW. The simultaneous presence of anti-I and anti-i in sera. *Vox Sang* 1968;**15**:133–41.

120 Gilboa-Garber N, Sudakevitz D, Levene C. A comparison of *Aplysia* lectin anti-I specificity with human anti-I and several other I-detecting lectins. *Transfusion* 1999;**39**:1060–4.

121 Dzierzkowa-Borodej W, Voak D. Subtypes of i demonstrated by the use of atypical Ii cell types and inhibition studies. *Br J Haematol* 1979;**41**:105–13.

122 Rosenfield RE, Schmidt PJ, Calvo R, McGinniss MH. Anti-i, a frequent cold agglutinin in infectious mononucleosis. *Vox Sang* 1965;**10**:631–4.

123 Capra JD, Dowlin P, Cook S, Kunkel HG. An incomplete cold-reactive γG antibody with I specificity in infectious mononucleosis. *Vox Sang* 1969;**16**:10–17.

124 Hossaini AA. Anti-i in infectious mononucleosis. *Am J Clin Pathol* 1970;**53**:198–203.

125 Troxel DB, Innella F, Cohen RJ. Infectious mononucleosis complicated by hemolytic anemia due to anti-i. *Am J Clin Pathol* 1966;**46**:625–31.

126 Wilkinson LS, Petz LD, Garratty G. Reappraisal of the role of anti-i in haemolytic anaemia in infectious mononucleosis. *Br J Haematol* 1973;**25**:715–22.

127 Burkart PT, Hsu TCS. IgM cold-warm hemolysins in infectious mononucleosis. *Transfusion* 1979;**19**:535–8.

128 Gronemeyer P, Chaplin H, Ghazarian V, Tuscany F, Wilner GD. Hemolytic anemia complicating infectious mononucleosis due to the interaction of an IgG cold anti-i and an IgM cold rheumatoid factor. *Transfusion* 1981;**21**:715–18.

129 Shirey RS, Park K, Ness PM *et al*. An anti-i biphasic hemolysin in chronic paroxysmal cold hemoglobinuria. *Transfusion* 1986;**26**:62–4.

130 McGinniss MH, Macher AM, Rook AH, Alter HJ. Red cell autoantibodies in patients with acquired immune deficiency syndrome. *Transfusion* 1986;**26**:405–9.

131 Gerbal A, Lavallée R, Ropars C *et al*. Sensibilisation des hématies d'un nouveau-né par un auto-anticorps anti-i d'origine maternelle de nature IgG. *Nouv Rev Franc Hémat* 1971;**11**:689–700.

132 Branch DR. Detection of complement (C3d) coated cells in a newborn due to maternal anti-i. *Transfusion* 1979;**19**:348–9.

133 Judd WJ, Steiner EA, Abruzzo LV *et al*. Anti-i causing acute hemolysis following a negative immediate-spin crossmatch. *Transfusion* 1992;**32**:572–5.

134 Layrisse Z, Layrisse M. High incidence cold autoagglutinins of anti-I^T specificity in Yanomama Indians of Venezuela. *Vox Sang* 1968;**14**:369–82.

135 Garratty G, Haffleigh B, Dalziel J, Petz LD. An IgG anti-I^T detected in a Caucasian American. *Transfusion* 1972;**12**:325–9.

136 Silvergleid AJ, Wells RF, Hafleigh EB *et al*. Compability test using ^{51}Chromium-labeled red blood cells in crossmatch positive patients. *Transfusion* 1978;**18**:8–14.

137 Hafleigh EB, Wells RF, Grumet FC. Nonhemolytic IgG anti I^T. *Transfusion* 1978;**18**:592–7.

138 Schmidt PJ, McCurdy P, Havell T, Jenkins A, McGinniss

M. An anti-I^T of clinical significance [Abstract]. *Transfusion* 1974;**14**:507.

139 Postoway N, Capon S, Smith L, Rosenbaum D, Garratty G. Cold agglutinin syndrome caused by anti-I^T [Abstract]. *Joint Congr Int Soc Blood Transfus and Am Ass Blood Banks*, 1990:85.

140 Roelcke D, Kreft H, Hack H, Stevenson FK. Anti-j: human cold agglutinins recognizing linear (i) and branched (I) Type 2 chains. *Vox Sang* 1994;**67**:216–21.

141 Gold ER. Observations on the specificity of anti-O and anti-A$_1$ sera. *Vox Sang* 1964;**9**:153–9.

142 Bird GWG, Wingham J. Erythrocyte autoantibody with unusual specificity. *Vox Sang* 1977;**32**:280–2.

143 Salmon C, Homberg JC, Liberge G, Delarue F. Autoanticorps a spécificités multiples, anti-HI, anti-AI, anti-BI, dans certains éluats d'anémie hémolytique. *Rev Franc Etud Clin Biol* 1965;**10**:522–5.

144 Baumgarten A, Curtain CC. A high frequency of cold agglutinins of anti-IA specificity in a New Guinea Highland population. *Vox Sang* 1970;**18**:21–6.

145 Tegoli J, Harris JP, Issitt PD, Sanders CW. Anti-IB, an expected 'new' antibody detecting a joint product of the I and B genes. *Vox Sang* 1967;**13**:144–57.

146 Drachmann O. An autoaggressive anti-BI(O) antibody. *Vox Sang* 1968;**14**:185–93.

147 Morel P, Garratty G, Willbanks E. Another example of anti-IB. *Vox Sang* 1975;**29**:231–3.

148 Doinel C, Ropars C, Salmon C. Anti-I(A+B): an autoantibody detecting an antigenic determinant of I and a common part to A and B. *Vox Sang* 1974;**27**:515–23.

149 Tegoli J, Cortez M, Jensen L, Marsh WL. A new antibody, anti-ILe^{b}H, specific for a determinant formed by the combined action of the I, Le, Se and H gene products. *Vox Sang* 1971;**21**:397–404.

150 Branch D, Powers T. A second example of anti-ILe^{b}H. *Transfusion* 1979;**19**:353.

151 Issitt PD, Tegoli J, Jackson V, Sanders CW, Allen FH. Anti IP$_1$: antibodies that show an association between the I and P blood group systems. *Vox Sang* 1968;**14**:1–8.

152 Allen FH, Marsh WL, Jensen L, Fink J. Anti IP: an antibody defining another product of interaction between the genes of the I and P blood group systems. *Vox Sang* 1974;**27**:442–6.

153 Ramos RR, Curtis BR, Eby CS, Ratkin GA, Chaplin H. Fatal outcome in a patient with autoimmune hemolytic anemia associated with an IgM bithermic anti-I^{T}P. *Transfusion* 1994;**34**:427–31.

154 Giblett ER, Cutbush Crookston M. Agglutinability of red cells by anti-i in patients with thalassæmia major and other hæmatological disorders. *Nature* 1964;**201**:1138–9.

155 Crookson MC. Anomalous ABO, H and Ii phenotypes in disease. In: G Garratty, ed. *Blood Group Antigens and Disease*. Arlington: American Association of Blood Banks, 1983:67–84.

156 Reid ME, Bird GWG. Associations between human red cell blood group antigens and disease. *Transfus Med Rev* 1990;**4**:47–55.

157 Navenot J-M, Muller J-Y, Blanchard D. Expression of blood group i antigen and fetal hemoglobin in paroxysmal nocturnal hemoglobinuria. *Transfusion* 1997;**37**:291–7.

158 Hillman RS, Giblett ER. Red cell membrane alteration associated with 'marrow stress'. *J Clin Invest* 1965;**44**:1730–6.

159 Shumak KH, Beldotti LE, Rachkewich RA. Diagnosis of haematological disease using anti-i. I. Disorders with lymphocytosis. *Br J Haematol* 1979;**41**:399–405.

160 Shumak KH, Rachkewich RA, Beldotti LE. Diagnosis of haematological disease using anti-i. II. Distinction between acute myeloblastic and acute lymphoblastic leukaemia. *Br J Haematol* 1979;**41**:407–411.

161 Shumak KH, Baker MA, Taub RN, Coleman MS and the Toronto Leukemia Study Group. Myeloblastic and lymphoblastic markers in acute undiffentiated leukemia and chronic myelogenous leukemia in blast crisis. *Cancer Res* 1980;**40**:4048–52.

162 Roelcke D. Sialic acid-dependent red blood cell antigens. In: G Garratty, ed. *Immunobiology of Transfusion Medicine*. New York: Dekker, 1994:69–95.

163 Roelcke D, Pruzanski W, Ebert W et al. A new human monoclonal cold agglutinin Sa recognizing terminal N-acetylneuraminyl groups on the cell surface. *Blood* 1980;**55**:677–81.

164 Pereira A, Mazzara R, Escoda L et al. Anti-Sa cold agglutinin of IgA class requiring plasma exchange-therapy as early manifestation multiple myeloma. *Ann Hematol* 1993;**66**:315–18.

165 Roelcke D, Riesen W, Geisen HP, Ebert W. Serological identification of the new cold agglutinin specificity anti-Gd. *Vox Sang* 1977;**33**:304–6.

166 Roelcke D, Brossmer R. Different fine specificities of human monoclonal anti-Gd cold agglutinins. *Prot Biol Fluids* 1984;**31**:1075–8.

167 Roelcke D. A further cold agglutinin, Fl, recognizing a N-acetylneuraminic acid-determined antigen. *Vox Sang* 1981;**41**:98–101.

168 Roelcke D, Hengge U, Kirschfink M. Neolacto (Type-2 chain)-sialoautoantigens recognized by human cold agglutinins. *Vox Sang* 1990;**59**:235–9.

169 Roelcke D, Kreft H, Pfister A-M. Cold agglutinin Vo: an IgMλ monoclonal human antibody recognizing a sialic acid determined antigen fully expressed on newborn erythrocytes. *Vox Sang* 1984;**47**:236–41.

170 Roelcke D. Li cold agglutinin: a further antibody recognizing sialic acid-dependent antigens fully expressed on newborn erythrocytes. *Vox Sang* 1985;**48**:181–3.

171 Roelcke D. The Lud cold agglutinin: a further antibody recognizing N-acetylneuraminic acid-determined antigens not fully expressed at birth. *Vox Sang* 1981;**41**:316–18.

172 Salama A, Pralle H, Mueller-Eckhardt C. A new red

blood cell cold autoantibody (anti-Me). *Vox Sang* 1985;49:277–84.

173 Kajii E, Ikemoto S. A cold agglutinin: Om. *Vox Sang* 1989;56:104–6.

174 Göttsche B, Salama A, Mueller-Eckhardt C. Autoimmune hemolytic anemia caused by a cold agglutinin with a new specificity (anti-Ju). *Transfusion* 1990; 30:261–2.

175 Picard JK, Loveday D, Feizi T. Evidence for sialylated Type 1 blood group chains on human erythrocyte membranes revealed by agglutination of neuraminidase-treated erythrocytes with Walenström's macroglobulin IgM[WOO] and hybridoma antibody FC 10.2. *Vox Sang* 1985;48:26–33.

176 Marsh WL, Johnson CL, Øyen R *et al.* Anti-Sd[x]: a 'new' auto-agglutinin related to the Sd[a] blood group. *Transfusion* 1980;20:1–8.

177 Bass LS, Rao AH, Goldstein J, Marsh WL. The Sd[x] antigen and antibody: biochemical studies on the inhibitory property of human urine. *Vox Sang* 1983;44:191–6.

178 Dahr W, Lichthardt D, Roelcke D. Studies of the receptor sites of the monoclonal anti-Pr and -Sa cold agglutinins. *Prot Biol Fluids* 1981;29:365–8.

179 Uemura K, Roelcke D, Nagai Y, Feizi T. The reactivities of human erythrocyte autoantibodies anti-Pr$_2$, anti-Gd, Fl and Sa with gangliosides in a chromatogram binding assay. *Biochem J* 1984;219:865–74.

180 Roelcke D, Hack H, Kreft H *et al.* IgA cold agglutinins recognize Pr and Sa antigens expressed on glycophorins. *Transfusion* 1993;33:472–5.

181 König AL, Schabel A, Sugg U, Brand U, Roelcke D. Autoimmune hemolytic anemia caused by IgGλ-monotypic cold agglutinins of anti-Pr specificity after rubella infection. *Transfusion* 2001;41:488–92.

182 Gallart T, Roelcke D, Blay M *et al.* Anti-Sia-lb (anti-Gd) cold agglutinins bind the domain NeuNAcα2–3Gal in sialyl Lewis[x], sialyl Lewis[a], and related carbohydrates on nucleated cells and in soluble cancer-associated mucins. *Blood* 1997;90:1576–87.

183 Roelcke D, Hack H, Kreft H, Gross HJ. α2,3-Specific desialylation of human red cells: effect on the autoantigens of the Pr, Sa and Sia-l1, b1, lb1 series. *Vox Sang* 1998;74:109–12.

184 Marsh WL, Johnson CL, Dinapoli J *et al.* Immune hemolytic anemia caused by auto anti-Sd[x]: a report on six cases [Abstract]. *Transfusion* 1980;20:647.

26 Er antigens

26.1 Introduction

Er^a and Er^b are high and low frequency antigens, respectively, and are probably the products of alleles. They constitute collection 208 of the International Society of Blood Transfusion (ISBT) terminology, the Er collection: Er^a is ER1 (208001); Er^b is ER2 (208002).

26.2 Er^a and Er^b (ER1 and ER2)

26.2.1 Inheritance and frequencies

Families of two of the original three Er(a−) propositi described by Daniels *et al.* [1] in 1982 showed Er(a−) to be an inherited character. One of the families (Rod.), however, had Er(a−) members in two generations suggesting that inheritance might not be straightforward. In 1988, Hamilton *et al.* [2] described an antibody to a low frequency antigen, named Er^b, that reacted with five of six Er(a−) red cell samples. Analysis of the Rod. family with anti-Er^b showed that the presence of Er(a−) in two generations resulted from an Er(a−b+)× Er(a+b+) mating [2]. *Er^a* and *Er^b* therefore appear to be inherited regularly as codominant alleles. One Er(a−) sample was Er(b−), as were the Er(a+) cells of the daughter of an Er(a−b+) mother, suggesting the presence of a third allele [2]. An antibody in an Er(a−b−) patient with consanguineous parents reacted with all red cells tested, including Er(a−) cells, and may be anti-Er^{ab} [3].

Family studies have shown that Er is not part of the ABO, MNS, P, Duffy, Kidd, or Dombrock systems [1,2,4].

True Er(a−) phenotype has only been found in people of European origin ([1,5–7] and several other unpublished examples), although an abnormal Er(a−) phenotype was identified in a Japanese family [4] (Section 26.2.3). No Er(a−) individual was found by tests on red cells from 63 762 mostly white [1,5,8] and 13 521 Japanese [4] blood donors.

Four of 605 random white donors were Er(b+) and the frequency of the *Er^b* allele is calculated as 0.0033 [2]. If the existence of a third allele is disregarded, the *Er^a* allele has a frequency of 0.9967 and Er(a−) would only be expected in about 1 in 100 000 white people.

26.2.2 Antigen characteristics

Er^a is fully expressed on cord cells and is not sensitive to the treatment of red cells with proteases (trypsin, chymotrypsin, papain, ficin, pronase), sialidase, or the disulphide-bond reducing agent 2-aminoethylisothiouronium bromide (AET) [1,9,10]. Incubation of red cells in low pH ethylenediaminetetra-acetic acid (EDTA) glycine buffers, often used in antibody elution tests, resulted in loss of the Er^a antigen. There was total antigen loss at pH 2.0, partial loss at pH 2.5, and no apparent loss at pH 3.0 [9].

Er^b is resistant to treatment of red cells with ficin, papain, or dithiothreitol (DTT) [2].

26.2.3 Serological complexities

Red cells of a Japanese woman and two of her sibs were negative with five anti-Er^a (including the original), but reacted with three others [4]. Positive and negative results were confirmed by adsorption techniques. The serum of the propositus, who had been transfused twice and pregnant three times, contained an antibody that resembled anti-Er^a: it reacted with all cells except Er(a−b+) cells and those of the propositus and two of her sibs.

A number of antibodies to high incidence antigens

react weakly with Er(a–) cells. Cross-testing of red cells and sera presents a highly complex pattern of reactions and results have not always concurred between different laboratories (G.L. Daniels, J. Poole and P. Lacey, unpublished observations).

26.3 Antibodies

All the recorded producers of anti-Er^a had been transfused; most had also been pregnant [1,4–7]. The antibodies are IgG and do not fix complement [1,4,5]. In two patients with anti-Er^a, Er(a+) red cells gave a positive direct antiglobulin test (DAT) after transfusion, but there were no signs of haemolysis [1,5]. Monocyte phagocytosis assays and *in vivo* red cell survival studies provided additional evidence that these antibodies are not clinically significant [1,5]. Red cells of two babies born to women with anti-Er^a gave positive DATs, but neither had any other signs of haemolytic disease of the newborn (HDN).

The producer of the only known anti-Er^b had been pregnant five times, but never transfused; two of her three children were Er(b+) [2]. Red cells of her second Er(b+) baby gave a positive DAT, but no treatment for HDN was required. Unfortunately, very little of the antibody remains and anti-Er^b is not generally available.

References

1 Daniels GL, Judd WJ, Moore BPL *et al*. A 'new' high frequency antigen Er^a. *Transfusion* 1982;22:189–93.
2 Hamilton JR, Beattie KM, Walker RH, Hartrick MB. *Er^b*, an allele to *Er^a*, and evidence for a third allele, *Er*. *Transfusion* 1988;28:268–71.
3 Arriaga F, Garratty G, Poole J, Marty ML. A novel antibody against antigens of the Er system: anti-Er^{ab}. *Vox Sang* 2000;78(Suppl.1):abstract P154.
4 Naoki K, Okuma S, Uchiyama E *et al*. Er(a–) red cell phenotype in Japan. *Transfusion* 1991;31:572–3.
5 Thompson HW, Skradski KJ, Thoreson JR, Polesky HF. Survival of Er(a+) red cells in a patient with allo-anti-Er^a. *Transfusion* 1985;25:140–1.
6 Lylloff K, Georgsen J, Grunnet N, Jersild C. On the inheritance of the Er^a red cell antigen. *Transfusion* 1987;27:118.
7 Rowe GP. On the inheritance of Er and the frequency of Er^a. *Transfusion* 1988;28:87–8.
8 Gale SA, Rowe GP, Northfield FE. Application of a microtitre plate antiglobulin technique to determine the incidence of donors lacking high frequency antigens. *Vox Sang* 1988;54:172–3.
9 Liew YW, Uchikawa M. Loss of Er^a antigen in very low pH buffers. *Transfusion* 1987;27:442–3.
10 Daniels G. Effect of enzymes on and chemical modifications of high-frequency red cell antigens. *Immunohematology* 1992;8:53–7.

27 Low frequency antigens

27.1 Antigens

Many red cell antigens have been identified that occur only very rarely in most populations and have not been shown to belong to any of the existing blood group systems or collections. Some have only been found in a solitary family. In the numerical notation, low frequency antigens (LFAs) make up the 700 series. The criteria for joining this series of antigens are as follows:
1 the antigen must have a frequency of less than 1%;
2 it must be an inherited character;
3 it must not be part of an existing blood group system or be related closely enough to another antigen to merit collection status;
4 it must have been shown to be serologically distinct from all other antigens of low frequency; and
5 antibody and red cells carrying the antigen must be available, so that further examples can be identified.

Race, Sanger and Cleghorn [1] defined 'private' antigens as having an incidence of less than one in 400 (0.25%). All the antigens currently in the 700 series are private antigens according to this definition.

LFAs of the 700 series are listed in Table 27.1. Many numbers have become obsolete, either because the corresponding antigens have been elevated to blood group systems or collections, or because they have become extinct, as a result of antibody or antigen-positive red cells being unavailable. Since 1996, 16 of the 700 series antigens have joined the Diego system (Chapter 10). Frequencies of LFAs are shown in Table 27.2.

When recombination is demonstrated between the gene controlling an LFA and that for a blood group system, the LFA is considered not part of that system. None of the 700 series antigens has been shown to be independent of all blood group systems. The LFAs and the systems they have been excluded from were tabulated in the first edition of this book [27]. As this information has not changed, the table is not duplicated here.

Table 27.1 Low frequency antigens: the 700 series.

Number	Name	Symbol	References
700002	Batty	By	[2]
700003	Christiansen	Chr^a	[3]
700005	Biles	Bi	[4]
700006	Box	Bx^a	[5,6]
700015	Radin	Rd	Chapter 13
700017	Torkildsen	To^a	[7]
700018	Peters	Pt^a	[8]
700019	Reid	Re^a	[9]
700021	Jensen	Je^a	[10]
700023	Hey	Hey	[11]
700028	Livesay	Li^a	[12]
700039	Milne		[13]
700040	Rasmussen	RASM	[14]
700043	Oldeide	Ol^a	[15]
700044		JFV	[16]
700045	Katagiri	Kg	[17]
700047	Jones	JONES	[18]
700049		HJK	[19]
700050		HOFM	[20]
700052		SARA	[21]
700053		LOCR	[22]
700054		REIT	*
		SHIN	[23]

*J.R. Hamilton and G. Coghlan, unpublished observations, 1993.

27.2 Antibodies

Frequencies and some characteristics of antibodies to LFAs are shown in Table 27.3. Like most other blood group antibodies, antibodies to some LFAs arise from immunization caused by pregnancy or transfusion; a few have been responsible for haemolytic disease of the newborn (HDN) (Section 27.3.5). In most cases, however, the antibodies arise as a result of no known stimulus and are often found together with other anti-

Table 27.2 Frequencies of low frequency antigens.

Antigen 700		Population	No. tested	No. positive	Antigen frequency	References
002	By	English	31 522	2	0.0001	[24]
003	Chr^a	Danish	500	1	0.0020	[3]
005	Bi	American	1 110	0		[4]
006	Bx^a	English	24 106	2	<0.0001	[1,5,6]
015	Rd					Chapter 13
017	To^a	Norwegian	6 461	1	0.0002	[7]
018	Pt^a	New Zealand	14 500	0	<0.0001	[8]
		Norwegian	21 825	0	<0.0001	[8,15]
		English	10 200	1	0.0001	[25]
019	Re^a	Canadian	>10 000	0	<0.0001	[9]
		English	6 635	1	0.0002	[26]
		Welsh	4 770	0		[26]
021	Je^a	Danish	>1 000	0		[10]
023	Hey	French	8 127	2	0.0002	[11]
039	Milne	New Zealand	2 643	0		[13]
040	RASM	North American	9 541	0		[14]
043	Ol^a	Norwegian	7 151	1	0.0001	[15]
044	JFV	German	1 014	0		[16]
045	Kg	Japanese	600	0		[17]
047	JONES	White	16 746	1	<0.0001	[18]
050	HOFM	Dutch	926	0		[20]
053	LOCR	North American	1 826	1	0.0005	[22]
054	REIT	Canadian	4 086	0		*
	SHIN	Japanese	3 000	1	0.0003	[23]

* J.R. Hamilton and G. Coghlan, unpublished observations, 1993.

bodies to LFAs. Some sera contain numerous antibodies to LFAs. Serum samples from the same donor taken at different times may contain different specificities and the antibodies often react by different methods. Occasionally, sera containing an 'immune' antibody to an LFA also contain apparently 'naturally occurring' antibodies to other LFAs. As an example, the serum of a healthy blood donor, Mrs Tillett, contained the following antibodies to red cell antigens of low frequency: anti-Pt^a, -M^g (MNS11), -Vw (MNS12), -Ri^a (MNS16), -Hut (MNS19), -Dantu (MNS25), -Or (MNS31), -Go^a (RH30), -Rh32, -Evans (RH37), -Wr^a (DI3), -Wd^a (DI5), -Rb^a (DI6), -ELO (DI8), -Bp^a (DI10), -Mo^a (DI11), -Vg^a (DI13), -BOW (DI15), -NFLD (DI16), -Jn^a (DI17), -Tr^a (DI19), -Ls^a (GE6), and eight unpublished specificities.

Antibodies to LFAs usually come to light for one of the following reasons:
1 the antibody causes HDN;
2 a single red cell sample reacts with a patient's serum during compatibility testing;
3 a serum blood grouping reagent contains a contaminating antibody to an LFA that gives an unexpected reaction during red cell phenotyping;
4 an antibody is detected when sera are screened with antigen positive red cells; or
5 an additional specificity is found in a serum known to contain one or more antibodies to LFAs when it is tested against cells of rare phenotype.

When red cells react with a serum known to contain a certain antibody to an LFA, the assumption cannot be made that those red cells carry that specific LFA,

Table 27.3 Frequencies and characteristics of antibodies to low frequency antigens.

Antibody Anti-700	Antibody frequency[1]	Immune	Present in multispecific sera[2]	References
002 By	1/7987 0/2000	Yes[3]	Yes	[1,2,28]
003 Chr[a]			No	[3]
005 Bi		Yes[3]	No	[4]
006 Bx[a]	0/8000 1/23 081	[4]	Yes	[1,5,6]
017 To[a]	66/5704 ~48/300		No	[7,29,30]
018 Pt[a]			Yes	[8,25,31]
019 Re[a]	0/2358	Yes[3]	No	[9,26]
021 Je[a]	1/>100 000		No	[10]
023 Hey	0/3060	Yes[5]	Yes	[11,32]
028 Li[a]		Yes	No	[12]*
039 Milne	58/1242	[6]	Yes	[13]
040 RASM	0/543	Yes[3]	No	[14]
043 Ol[a]			Yes	[15]
044 JFV	0/534	Yes[3]	No	[16]
045 Kg		Yes[3]	No	[17]
047 JONES	0/2000	Yes[3]	Yes	[18]
049 HJK		Yes[3]	No	[19]
050 HOFM		Yes[3]	No	[20]
052 SARA	1/3150		Yes	[21]
053 LOCR		Yes[3]	No	[22]
054 REIT		Yes[3]		†
SHIN	0/19 380[7]	[8]	Yes	[23]

*C.A. Green, Y.W. Liew and T. Kaye, personal communication, 1984.

†J.R. Hamilton and G. Coghlan, unpublished observations, 1993.

[1]The number of sera found to contain the antibody in the total number of sera from random blood donors tested. Where more than one survey is reported, the results are shown separately.

[2]Sera containing several or many antibodies to LFAs.

[3]See Section 27.3.5 for notes on clinical significance.

[4]No anti-Bx[a] in three Bx(a–) mothers of Bx(a+) children [6].

[5]Hey– woman who had two Hey+ pregnancies and produced anti-Hey; there were no signs of HDN. Her Hey– daughter had one Hey+ pregnancy and did not produce anti-Hey. No anti-Hey in four Hey– recipients of Hey+ blood [32].

[6]No anti-Milne in two Milne– mothers of Milne+ children [13].

[7]One anti-SHIN found in sera from 1662 Japanese hospital patients [23].

[8]No anti-SHIN in two SHIN– mothers of SHIN+ children [23].

because the serum may contain more antibodies than those previously known to be present. Consequently, cross-adsorption–elution tests must be carried out for confirmation. However, this cross-adsorption method is not infallible, as antibodies of related, but different, specificities might be removed together from a serum by adsorption with red cells apparently expressing only one of the antigens.

27.3 Additional information on some of the antigens and antibodies

27.3.1 Rd (700015)

Genetical and biochemical evidence strongly support Rd being part of an expanded Scianna system. Rd is described in Chapter 13.

27.3.2 Ptª (700018)

Many examples of anti-Ptª have been found, all in sera containing other 'naturally occurring' antibodies to LFAs [8,25,31]. Herron *et al.* [33] used anti-Ptª in immunoblotting experiments with red cell membranes prepared under non-reducing conditions to show that Ptª is located on a membrane component of apparent M_r 31 600. This structure might be associated with the membrane skeleton.

27.3.3 Liª (700028)

There is a suggestion in one family of linkage between the gene controlling Liª and the *LU* locus. If an untested husband is assumed to be Lu(a–), then the lod score is 2.709 at a recombination fraction of 0.0, very close to statistical significance; if the father were Lu(a+) the score is 1.204 [12]. Immunoblotting of Li(a+) cells in order to determine whether Liª is on the Lutheran glycoproteins revealed no bands.

27.3.4 Low frequency antigens associated with Rh: Olª (700043), HOFM (700050), and LOCR (700053)

Members of a three-generation Norwegian family are the only Ol(a+) individuals known [15]. Ol(a+) red cells have depressed expression of Rh antigens, especially C, E, and, to a lesser extent, D. Yet recombination between the genes controlling Olª and Rh means that Olª does not belong to the Rh system. The possibility that Olª is located on the Rh-associated glycoprotein (Section 5.5.7) needs to be investigated.

HOFM is associated with depressed C antigen in the only family in which it has been detected [20] and LOCR is transmitted with *dce* and altered expression of c in two of three families studied [22]. Family studies do not provide statistically significant evidence

that either antigen belongs to the Rh system (see Section 5.17.1).

27.3.5 Clinical significance of antibodies to low frequency antigens

Most antibodies to LFAs of the 700 series do not appear to be clinically significant. Severe HDN in the HJK+ baby of a mother with anti-HJK (700049) was treated by three intrauterine transfusions [19]. Anti-Kg (700045) and anti-REIT (700054) were also responsible for HDN requiring exchange transfusion [17, J.R. Hamilton and G. Coghlan, unpublished observations, 1993]; HDN caused by anti-JFV (700044) [16] and by anti-JONES (700047) [18] was treated by phototherapy and blood transfusion. Antibodies to the Rh-associated antigens HOFM (700050) and LOCR (700053) both caused mild HDN [20,22]. Anti-Bi (700005) may also have been responsible for HDN [4]. Anti-By (700002), -Reª (700019), and -RASM (700040) caused a positive DAT on cord red cells, but no other signs of HDN [2,9,14,26].

LFAs do not create a major transfusion problem. However, a potentially dangerous antibody to an LFA could remain undetected if a full crossmatch is not performed. Presence of an unrecognized anti-LFA in a blood grouping reagent can also prove hazardous.

References

1 Race RR, Sanger R, Cleghorn TE. *Blood Groups in Man*, 6th edn. Oxford: Blackwell Scientific Publications, 1975.
2 Simmons RT, Were SOM. A 'new' family blood group antigen and antibody (By) of rare occurrence. *Med J Aust* 1955;ii:55–9.
3 Kissmeyer-Nielsen F. A new rare blood-group antigen, Chrª. *Vox Sang* (old series) 1955;5:102–3.
4 Wadlington WB, Moore WH, Hartmann RC. Maternal sensitization due to Bi. A presumed 'new, private' red cell antigen. *Am J Dis Child* 1961;101:623–30.
5 Jenkins WJ, Marsh WL. Autoimmune hæmolytic anæmia. *Lancet* 1961;ii:16–18.
6 Contreras M, Lubenko A, Armitage S, Cleghorn T, Jenkins J. Frequency and inheritance of the Bxª (Box) antigen. *Vox Sang* 1980;39:225–8.
7 Kornstad L, Øyen R, Cleghorn TE. A new rare blood group antigen Toª (Torkildsen) and an unsolved factor Skjelbred. *Vox Sang* 1968;14:363–8.
8 Pinder LB, Staveley JM, Douglas R, Kornstad L. Ptª: a new private antigen. *Vox Sang* 1969;17:303–5.

9 Guévin R-M, Taliano V, Fiset D, Bérubé P, Kaita H. L'antigène Reid, un nouvel antigène privé. *Rev Franc Transfus* 1971;**14**:455–9.

10 Skov F. A new rare blood group antigen, Je^a. *Vox Sang* 1972;**23**:461–3.

11 Yvart J, Gerbal A, Salmon C. A new 'private' antigen: Hey. *Vox Sang* 1974;**26**:41–4.

12 Riches RA, Laycock CM. A new low frequency antigen Li^a (Livesey). *Vox Sang* 1980;**38**:305–9.

13 Pinder LB, Farr DE, Woodfield DG. Milne, a new low-frequency antigen. *Vox Sang* 1984;**47**:290–2.

14 Brown A, Plantos M, Moore BPL, Jones T. RASM, a 'new' low-frequency blood group antigen. *Vox Sang* 1986;**51**:133–5.

15 Kornstad L. A rare blood group antigen, Ol^a (Oldeide), associated with weak Rh antigens. *Vox Sang* 1986;**50**:235–9.

16 Kluge A, Roelcke D, Tanton E *et al*. Two examples of a new low-frequency red cell antigen, JFV. *Vox Sang* 1988;**55**:44–7.

17 Ichikawa Y, Sato C, McCreary J, Lubenko A. Kg, a new low-frequency red cell antigen responsible for hemolytic disease of the newborn. *Vox Sang* 1989;**56**:98–100.

18 Reid M, Fischer ML, Green C *et al*. A private red cell antigen, Jones, causing haemolytic disease of the newborn. *Vox Sang* 1989;**57**:77–80.

19 Rouse D, Weiner C, Williamson R. Immune hydrops fetalis attributable to anti-HJK. *Obstet Gynecol* 1990;**76**:988–90.

20 Hoffmann JJML, Overbeeke MAM, Kaita H, Loomans AAH. A new, low-incidence red cell antigen (HOFM), associated with depressed C antigen. *Vox Sang* 1990;**59**:240–3.

21 Stern DA, Hawksworth DN, Watt JM, Ford DS. A new low-frequency red cell antigen, 'SARAH'. *Vox Sang* 1994;**67**:64–7.

22 Coghlan G, McCreary J, Underwood V, Zelinski T. A 'new' low-incidence red cell antigen, LOCR, associated with altered expression of Rh antigens. *Transfusion* 1994;**34**:492–5.

23 Nakajima H, Satoh H, Komatsu F *et al*. SHIN, a low frequency red cell antigen, found in two Japanese blood donors. *Hum Hered* 1993;**43**:69–73.

24 Cleghorn TE. The frequency of the Wr^a, By and M^g blood group antigens in blood donors in the South of England. *Vox Sang* 1960;**5**:556–60.

25 Contreras M, Stebbing B, Armitage SE, Lubenko A. Further data on the Pt^a antigen. *Vox Sang* 1978;**35**: 181–3.

26 Rowe GP, Bowell P. Two further examples of the low-frequency antigen Re^a (Reid). *Vox Sang* 1985;**49**:400–2.

27 Daniels G. *Human Blood Groups*. Oxford: Blackwell Science, 1995:634.

28 Jakobowicz R, Albrey JA, McCulloch WJ, Simmons RT. A further example of anti-By (Batty) in the serum of a woman whose red cells are of the A$_x$(A$_o$) subgroup of group A. *Med J Aust* 1960;**ii**:294–6.

29 Crossland JD, Kornstad L, Giles CM. Third example of the blood group antigen To^a. *Vox Sang* 1974;**26**:280–2.

30 Gralnick MA, Sherwood GK, De Peralta F, Schmidt PJ. Torkildsen: experience with the low-incidence antigen in the United States [Abstract]. *Prog 24th Ann Mtg Am Ass Blood Banks*, 1971:105–6.

31 Young DJ, Smith DS. A further example of the low frequency antigen Pt^a. *Clin Lab Haematol* 1983;**5**:307–12.

32 Strohm PL. The Hey antigen and antibody: a second family study and the first example of an IgG anti-Hey. *Vox Sang* 1982;**43**:31–4.

33 Herron R, Smith GA, Young D, Smith DS. Partial characterisation of the human erythrocyte antigen Pt^a. *Vox Sang* 1989;**56**:112–16.

28 High frequency antigens

28.1 Introduction

High frequency antigens (HFAs) were originally classified together in the 900 series of antigens, equivalent to the 700 series for low frequency antigens. When the collections were introduced into the blood group terminology in 1990, the 900 series was decimated and was consequently abandoned and replaced by the 901 series. A red cell antigen may belong to the 901 series if it fits the following criteria:

1 it must have a frequency greater than 90% (although all antigens discussed in this chapter have frequencies in excess of 99% in most populations and so can be described as 'public' antigens);

2 it must be inherited;

3 it must not be eligible to join a blood group system, form a new system, or be so closely related to another antigen as to merit collection status; and

4 it must have been shown to be serologically distinct from all other antigens of high frequency.

The 901 series currently contains 11 antigens (Table 28.1). These include Sd^a, which has a frequency of about 91% and is described in Chapter 29. It also includes AnWj (901009) and Duclos (901013) which, because of biochemical associations, are described in the chapters on the Indian (Section 21.7) and Rh (Section 5.5.7.1) systems, respectively. Results of some frequency studies are shown in Table 28.2. Table 28.3 shows a few characteristics of the antigens.

The HFAs and the blood group systems they have been excluded from were tabulated in the first edition of this book [33]. As this information has not changed, the table is not duplicated here.

Antibodies to HFAs are a transfusion hazard as compatible blood is often very difficult to obtain. Anti-Vel (901001) and -Lan (901002) have both caused severe haemolytic transfusion reactions. With the exception of MAM (901016), none of the antibodies described in this chapter has been implicated in haemolytic disease of the newborn (HDN) requiring more radical treatment than phototherapy.

In addition to the HFAs described below, numerous others exist that have not been reported. Most reference laboratories have a large assortment of sera called 'antibodies to unidentified public antigens'.

28.2 Vel (901001)

When Sussman and Miller [1] described anti-Vel in 1952, Vel became the first reported public antigen that was not part of an established blood group system. Anti-Vel is a dangerous antibody that has been responsible for haemolytic transfusion reactions (Section 28.2.3).

28.2.1 Frequency and inheritance

Some of the largest studies of testing random donors with anti-Vel are shown in Table 28.2. The Vel– phenotype was found to have an incidence of about 1 in 3000 in predominantly white English blood donors [11–13], with the following gene frequencies: Vel^+ 0.9821; Vel^- 0.0179. There are no reports of studies on large numbers of donors from other ethnic groups. Vel could be polymorphic in some populations: four of 328 Thais [35] and two of 160 Chilcotin Indians from Canada [36] were Vel–.

In the families of 11 Vel– propositi the sib count, excluding propositi, approached very closely 3 : 1 for Vel+ : Vel–, the ratio expected if the Vel– phenotype results from homozygosity for a recessive allele [11]. A sib count of 20 Vel+ and 16 Vel– was obtained from 17

Table 28.1 High frequency antigens: the 901 series.

Number	Name	Symbol	References
901001		Vel	[1]
901002	Langereis	Lan	[2]
901003	August	At^a	[3]
901005		Jr^a	[4]
901008		Emm	[5]
901009	Anton	AnWj	Chapter 21
901012	Sid	Sd^a	Chapter 29
901013	Duclos		Chapter 5
901014		PEL	[6]
901015		ABTI	[7]
901016		MAM	[8]

Obsolete: 901004 Jo^a is now DO5; 901006 Ok^a is OK1; 901007 JMH is JMH1; 901010 Wr^b is DI4; 901011 is RAPH1.

Swedish families with Vel– propositi, but this excess of Vel– might be explained by inbreeding in one family and the possibility of one untested parent being Vel– [12]. In six families that demonstrate that Vel does not belong to the P system an excess of Vel-negatives were P_2, with a probability of significance of about $1:70$. This supports earlier speculations of an association between Vel and P [12]. In two families Vel– occurred in two generations [16,17] and in one family in three generations [37].

28.2.2 Vel antigen

The strength of Vel antigen shows a great deal of individual variation and in some people expression is very

Table 28.2 Frequencies of high frequency antigens in various populations.

Antigen 901	Population	No. tested	No. negative	Antigen frequency	References
001 Vel	American	21 000	8	0.9996	[1,9,10]
	British	99 637	25	0.9997	[11–14]
	French	10 000	4	0.9996	[15]
	Australian	5 000	2	0.9996	[16]
	Finnish	18 920	0	>0.9999	[17]
	Swedish	91 605	52	0.9994	[12]
	Norwegian	5 009	4	0.9992	[17]
002 Lan	American	6 653	1	0.9998	[18–22]
	British	28 992	0	>0.9999	[14,23]
	Dutch	4 000	1	0.9997	[2]
	Japanese	15 000	0	>0.9999	[24]
	Black South African*	6 000	4	0.9993	[25]
003 At^a	American†	9 600	0		[3,19]
	African American	14 251	1	0.9999	[26,27]
005 Jr^a	Japanese	19 298	5	0.9997	[28]
	Japanese	28 744	19	0.9993	[29]
	Japanese, Osaka	994	2	0.9980	[30]
	Japanese, Niigata	460	8	0.9826	[31]
	American	9 545	0		[17,32]
	English	1 200	0		‡
	Asian	1 041	0		[17]
008 Emm	English	730	0		[5]
015 ABTI	Israeli Jews	509	0		[7]
	Israeli Arabs	121	0		[7]
GIL	American	23 251	0	>0.9999	[34]
	African American	2 841	0		[34]

*Including donors of mixed ethnic origin.
†Including about 2200 African Americans [3].
‡M Contreras, personal communication, 1982.

Table 28.3 Effects of treatment of red cells with enzymes and 2-aminoethylisothiouronium bromide (AET) on high frequency antigens (HFAs), and the expression of HFAs on red cells from cord samples.

Antigen 901	Tryp	Chym	Pap	Sial	AET	Cord
001 Vel	+	+	+	+	+	weak
002 Lan	+	+	+	+	+	+
003 Atª	+	+	+	+	+	+
005 Jrª	+	+	+	+	+	+
008 Emm	+	+	+	+	+	+
009 AnWj	+	+	+	+	+	−
013 Duclos*	+	weak	+	+	+	+
014 PEL	+	+	+	+	+	+
015 ABTI	+	+	+	+	+	+
016 MAM	+	+	+	+	+	+
GIL	+	+	+	+	+	weak

Chym, chymotrypsin; Pap, papain; Sial, sialidase; Tryp, trypsin.
+, Antigen present; −, antigen not present.
*Duclos-like antigen detected by monoclonal antibody MB-2D10.

weak. It is advisable to use a two-stage complement addition antiglobulin test to confirm a negative result with anti-Vel on red cells of individuals who have not produced anti-Vel. In population studies where apparent negatives were not checked in this way it is likely that donors with very weak Vel antigens have been mistyped as Vel−. Proposals for subdivisions of Vel based on qualitative variations [38] were subsequently dismissed as resulting from purely quantitative variations [39].

Vel is generally expressed less strongly on cord red cells than on those of adults [10,17,40]. Vel has been detected on fetal red cells as early as 12 weeks' gestation [41]. A patient who was Vel− when first tested developed a Vel antigen of normal strength during pregnancy; this Vel antigen persisted for at least 6 months after delivery [12].

Serological associations have been found between Vel and some other antigens of high frequency. Three of 14 anti-Vel failed to react with four Ge:−2,−3,4 samples, but did react with single examples of Ge:−2,3,4 and Ge:−2,−3,−4 cells [42]. Six of eight Vel− samples were weakly reactive and one was non-reactive with anti-ABTI [7] (Section 28.11).

Vel is not destroyed by proteases (Table 28.3); on the contrary, treatment of cells with papain or ficin enhances detection of weak Vel antigens.

Vel was not detected on lymphocytes, granulocytes, or monocytes by fluorescence flow cytometry [43].

28.2.3 Anti-Vel

Vel alloantibodies are never 'naturally occurring' and most producers of anti-Vel have been transfused; yet Vel antibodies are predominantly IgM and fix complement. Some anti-Vel haemolyse Vel+ cells [9–11,13,15,44–47]. This lytic characteristic is destroyed by heating the serum to 56°C; in some sera it returns with addition of fresh complement [9,10,45], in others it does not [10,11,15]. One anti-Vel was IgG1, another contained IgG1 and IgG3 [48].

Anti-Vel is a dangerous antibody. The first anti-Vel and other examples since have caused severe immediate haemolytic transfusion reactions [1,15,37,47,49]. Furthermore, anti-Vel may be missed in compatibility testing if inappropriate techniques are used [46,47]. Only 3% of radiolabelled Vel+ cells survived 1 h after injection into a patient with IgG anti-Vel [50]. However, in some cases patients with weak anti-Vel have been successfully transfused with Vel+ red cells [39,51].

Anti-Vel has not been implicated in a serious case of HDN, although several examples of anti-Vel have been found in pregnant women [1,16,40,52,53]. The lack of HDN is probably because most anti-Vel are predominantly IgM and Vel antigen is usually expressed weakly on neonatal red cells, especially in babies heterozygous for the Vel+ gene. In one case in which the anti-Vel was IgG1 plus IgG3, cord red cells gave a positive direct antiglobulin test (DAT), anti-Vel could be eluted from the cells, and the baby was treated by phototherapy [52].

There are four reports of autoanti-Vel [13,49, 54,55]. Two were responsible for autoimmune haemolytic anaemia [49,55], although in one case, a 9-week-old infant, the red cells gave a negative DAT [49]. The other two autoanti-Vel did not appear to destroy autologous red cells as determined by *in vivo* survival studies [13,54].

28.3 Lan (901002)

A severe haemolytic transfusion reaction resulted in the identification of a new public antigen, Lan [2]. The patient, Mr Lan, had a Lan– brother. Two other public antigens, Gn^a and So, were later shown to be the same as Lan [18,19,56].

28.3.1 Frequency and inheritance

Screening of red cells from almost 40 000 blood donors from the USA, UK, and the Netherlands (mostly white) revealed only two Lan-negatives (Table 28.2), an incidence of about 1 in 20 000 and an estimated frequency for the *Lan$^+$* gene of 0.9929. Four of 6000 South African donors of black and mixed ethnic origin were Lan– [25]. Anti-Lan has been identified in two African Americans [57,58] and three Japanese [24].

The Lan– phenotype results from homozygosity for a rare recessive gene. In the five families of Lan–propositi in which both parents were tested, all were Lan+; none of 25 children in these families with a Lan–parent was Lan– [2,18,19,21–24, A. Gerbal and G.L. Daniels, unpublished observations, 1975]. In one family, from a very small region in the Krakow province of Poland, the Lan– phenotype appears in two generations: the propositus has two Lan– sibs and a Lan– nephew [18].

A quantitative variant, in which Lan is expressed very weakly, has also been shown to be inherited [59]. Red cells with this Lan-weak phenotype can easily be mistaken for Lan–. Five of 15 apparent Lan– samples were subsequently shown to have weak Lan on testing with more potent reagents [60].

28.3.2 Anti-Lan

The first two examples of anti-Lan were identified

within a couple of weeks of uneventful transfusions [2,20]. However, anti-Lan may be stimulated by pregnancy alone [18,19,24,61]. There is no report of 'naturally occurring' alloanti-Lan; none of the Lan–sibs of Lan– propositi has anti-Lan.

Lan alloantibodies are mostly IgG1 and IgG3, although IgG2 and IgG4 may also be present [24,48,62,63]. Some anti-Lan fix complement [2,23,24,64], others do not [20,24].

The original anti-Lan was responsible for an immediate haemolytic transfusion reaction characterized by fever and chills [2]. The potential of other examples of anti-Lan to cause red cell destruction has been demonstrated by *in vivo* red cell survival studies and *in vitro* functional assays [64–67]. Addition of a source of fresh complement is often required in order to obtain a positive result with anti-Lan in a monocyte monolayer assay [64,66,67].

Anti-Lan has not been implicated in serious HDN. In three cases cord red cells gave a positive DAT, but in only two of these was anti-Lan detected in an eluate [22,23,61]. Two of the babies required phototherapy treatment [22,61] and one of them (whose red cells were also coated with anti-c and -Jk^a) received a transfusion of Lan+ red cells [61].

The only reported autoanti-Lan was in a patient with mild haemolytic anaemia [65]. Her red cells appeared to have depressed Lan expression and gave a weakly positive DAT.

28.4 At^a (August, 901003)

The first anti-At^a was described by Applewhaite *et al.* [3] in 1967 and six more examples were reported in 1973 [68]. Another public antigen, El [19], was later shown to be the same as At^a [69].

28.4.1 Frequency and inheritance

All At(a–) propositi, 14 of whom have been reported [3,19,26,68,70–73], are black. Of about 16 450 African Americans tested, only one was At(a–) [26,27,70] (Table 28.2). With one exception [26], all known At(a–) individuals have been ascertained through anti-At^a in the serum of the propositus.

Of the published families, nine At(a–) propositi had five At(a–) sibs and 16 At(a+) sibs, and all 11 children with an At(a–) parent were At(a+) [3,19,68,71–73]. This excludes one family in which an At(a–) propositus appears to have an At(a–) sib and an At(a–) mother, but in which the true relationship of these family members is uncertain [68]. The figures suggest that At(a–) results from homozygosity of a recessive gene.

28.4.2 Anti-At^a

Anti-At^a may be stimulated by transfusion or pregnancy. No example of 'naturally occurring' anti-At^a is known. At^a antibodies are mostly IgG, reacting by an antiglobulin test, but one example also contained some IgM, which directly agglutinated At(a+) red cells [68]. One anti-At^a was IgG1, another consisted of IgG1, IgG3, and IgG4 [48].

One anti-At^a caused an immediate haemolytic transfusion reaction with chills and nausea during a red cell survival study [72] and another a severe delayed haemolytic transfusion reaction after transfusion of multiple units of At(a+) red cells [73]. At^a antibodies facilitate rapid destruction of ^{51}Cr-labelled At(a+) red cells *in vivo* and give positive results in *in vitro* functional assays [71,72,74]. The 12 women reported to have made anti-At^a had a total of 70 pregnancies. One of the babies had moderately severe HDN, which required treatment by phototherapy [70].

28.5 Jr^a (901005)

The first five examples of anti-Jr^a were described briefly in 1970 by Stroup and MacIlroy [4], who were able to test the families of four of the propositi and found a total of seven Jr(a–) sibs, none of whom had made anti-Jr^a.

28.5.1 Frequency, ethnic distribution, and inheritance

Jr(a–) is much less rare in Japanese than in most other populations (Table 28.2). Frequencies vary greatly in different regions of Japan [29] with an incidence of Jr(a–) of around 1 in 60 in the Niigata region of northwest Japan [31]. Jr(a–) has been found in people of northern European extraction [32,75], in the Gypsy population of Slovakia [76], in Bedouin Arabs [77], and in a Mexican [78]. These were all found through the presence of anti-Jr^a; no non-Japanese Jr(a–) has been found by screening with anti-Jr^a.

There are few reports of family studies involving Jr(a–) propositi. Of 51 sibs of Jr(a–) propositi, 10 were Jr(a–) and 41 were Jr(a+), suggesting that Jr(a–) results from homozygosity for a recessive gene [17].

28.5.2 Anti-Jr^a

Anti-Jr^a may be stimulated by transfusion [76,79] or by pregnancy [28,30,32,75–78,80–82], and has been detected in untransfused Jr(a–) women during their first pregnancy [81,82]. IgM anti-Jr^a was found in the sera of two Jr(a–) brothers who had not been transfused (S. Armitage, personal communication, 1979). Most anti-Jr^a are IgG and those that have been subclassed were IgG1, sometimes together with IgG3 [63,77,81,82]. Anti-Jr^a may fix complement [28,78].

Anti-Jr^a has been responsible for a positive DAT on cord cells from which anti-Jr^a could be eluted [28,78,81,82]. Anti-Jr^a may have caused neonatal jaundice, although no treatment other than phototherapy has been required [28,80,81]. Hyperbilirubinaemia in the baby of a woman with high titre anti-Jr^a was attributed to prematurity [32].

A patient with anti-Jr^a developed rigors after transfusion of 150 mL of crossmatch incompatible blood [83]. In another patient with anti-Jr^a, transfused with 3 units of Jr(a+) blood, there was a sharp increase in titre of her antibody and anti-Jr^a could be eluted from transfused red cells for 35 days, but there was no sign of a haemolytic transfusion reaction apart from a gradual disappearance of Jr(a+) red cells from the circulation [82]. Injection of radiolabelled Jr(a+) red cells into a patient with anti-Jr^a resulted in moderate destruction of the cells with no Jr(a+) cells remaining after 24 h [75].

An IgG3 human monoclonal anti-Jr^a was produced by a heterohybridoma derived from mouse myeloma cells and Epstein–Barr virus (EBV)-transformed lymphocytes from a blood donor with anti-Jr^a [29].

28.6 Emm (901008)

Four propositi whose red cells lacked the high frequency antigen Emm were described by Daniels *et al.* [5]: a Frenchman born in Madagascar, a white American, a Pakistani, and a French Canadian. All had anti-Emm in their sera, as did the Emm– brother of the Canadian. Four of the five examples of anti-Emm were produced by men and were apparently 'naturally occurring'; one of the antibodies was IgM, the other four were IgG. Two further examples of anti-Emm in untransfused Emm– males have been identified [84].

Emm antigen is probably a glycosylphosphatidylinositol (GPI)-linked protein. PNHIII red cells from a paroxysmal nocturnal haemoglobinuria patient were Emm–, while the PNHI cells were Emm+ (see Chapter 19) [84,85].

28.7 AnWj (901009)

AnWj is a high frequency antigen that is expressed only very weakly on the red cells of individuals with an *In(Lu)* gene (Section 6.4.4.4). Evidence exists that AnWj is closely associated with CD44 glycoprotein, the membrane structure that carries antigens of the Indian system, so AnWj is described in Section 21.7.

28.8 Duclos (901013)

Duclos antigen, defined by a single alloantibody, is dependent on the presence of Rh antigens and of U antigen of the MNS system; that is, anti-Duclos reacts with all cells except those Rh_{null} cells that are U-negative. Duclos appears to be located on the Rh-associated glycoprotein and is described in Section 5.5.7.1.

28.9 PEL (901014)

The first two PEL– propositi with anti-PEL were French Canadian women [6]. The second PEL– propositus had three PEL– sibs. Two other examples of antibodies to high frequency antigens that did not react with PEL– cells were found in the propositi of French Canadian families, but the red cells of these propositi and their compatible sibs reacted very weakly with anti-PEL. This weak reaction required adsorption tests for detection. The PEL-like antibodies in these two propositi were provisionally named anti-MTP [6]. Of the 18 sibs of propositi with anti-PEL (or anti-MTP), red cells of six were compatible with the serum of the propositus.

All four producers of anti-PEL (or anti-MTP) had been transfused and three had also been pregnant. Red cells of the baby of the original PEL– propositus gave a negative DAT and there was no sign of HDN. Radiolabelled PEL+ cells survived normally in the other propositus with anti-PEL, but only 74% survived after 24 h in one of the patients with anti-MTP [6].

28.10 ABTI (901015)

The only three examples of anti-ABTI were present in multiparous women from an inbred Israeli Arab family [7]. None had been transfused and there was no evidence of HDN in any of their children. Three other members of the family were also ABTI–. No other example of ABTI– was found from testing Israeli blood donors (Table 28.2) or from 70 blood samples from a health clinic in the Arab village in which the propositus lived. The possibility of an association between ABTI and Vel is discussed in Section 28.2.2. Anti-ABTI reacted by an antiglobulin test with anti-IgG. The original anti-ABTI was IgG1 plus IgG3.

28.11 MAM (901016)

Two MAM– propositi, ascertained through the presence of anti-MAM in their sera during their third pregnancy, were described by Montgomery *et al.* [8]. One propositus was of partial Irish and Cherokee descent, the other was Arabic. The second propositus had a MAM– sister, who had been pregnant once and also had anti-MAM. The MAM– sisters are first cousins once removed. A third MAM– propositus with anti-MAM was also found during her third pregnancy [86]. None of the MAM– women had a history of transfusion.

Anti-MAM is a clinically significant antibody. The third baby of the second propositus had severe HDN, requiring intrauterine transfusion. Red cells of the third babies of the other two propositi gave a positive DAT, but there was no HDN. The baby of the first propositus was thrombocytopenic, which could have been caused by anti-MAM, but was probably because of anti-HPA-1a, which was also present in the mother. Two of the anti-MAM contained IgG1 and IgG3, and one also had IgG2 [8]. Monocyte monolayer assays suggested that anti-MAM has the potential to shorten substantially survival of transfused MAM+ red cells [8].

Immunoblotting of red cell membranes with anti-MAM revealed a diffuse band of apparent M_r 23 000–80 000, with a discrete band at M_r 18 000. MAM is present on lymphocytes, granulocytes, monocytes, and probably platelets from peripheral blood, and on the majority of leukaemia, fibroblast, embryonic kidney, and endothelial cell lines, but not on an epithelial cell line [8].

28.12 GIL

Five examples of anti-GIL have been identified, all in white women who had been pregnant at least twice [34]. GIL has not joined the 901 series as it has not been shown to be an inherited character. No GIL–individual has been found by screening with anti-GIL (Table 28.2). Red cells of two of the babies of mothers with anti-GIL gave a positive DAT, but there were no clinical symptoms of HDN. Anti-GIL may have been responsible for a haemolytic transfusion reaction and results of monocyte monolayer assays with two anti-GIL suggested a potential to cause accelerated destruction of transfused GIL+ red cells.

References

1 Sussman LN, Miller EB. Un nouveau facteur sanguin 'Vel'. *Rev Hémat* 1952;7:368–71.

2 van der Hart M, Moes M, VD Veer M, van Loghem JJ. Ho and Lan: two new blood group antigens. Paper read at *VIIIth Europ Cong Haem*, 1961.

3 Applewhaite F, Ginsberg V, Gerena J, Cunningham CA, Gavin J. A very frequent red cell antigen, At^a. *Vox Sang* 1967;13:444–5.

4 Stroup M, MacIlroy M. Jr. Five examples of an antibody defining an antigen of high frequency in the Caucasian population [Abstract]. *Prog 23rd Ann Mtg Am Ass Blood Banks*, 1970:86.

5 Daniels GL, Taliano V, Klein MT, McCreary J. Emm: a red cell antigen of very high frequency. *Transfusion* 1987;27:319–21.

6 Daniels GL, Simard H, Goldman M *et al.* PEL, a 'new' high-frequency red cell surface antigen. *Vox Sang* 1996;70:31–3.

7 Schechter Y, Chezar J, Levene C *et al.* ABTI (901015), a new red cell antigen of high frequency [Abstract]. *Transfusion* 1996;36:25S.

8 Montgomery WM, Jr, Nance SJ, Donnelly SF *et al.* MAM: a 'new' high-incidence antigen found on multiple cell lines. *Transfusion* 2000;40:1132–9.

9 Levine P, Robinson EA, Herrington LB, Sussman LN. Second example of the antibody for the high-incidence blood factor Vel. *Am J Clin Pathol* 1955;25:751–4.

10 Sussman LN. Current status of the Vel blood group system. *Transfusion* 1962;2:163–71.

11 Cleghorn TE. *The occurrence of certain rare blood group factors in Britain.* MD thesis, University of Sheffield, 1961.

12 Cedergren B, Giles CM, Ikin EW. The Vel blood group in Northern Sweden. *Vox Sang* 1976;31:344–55.

13 Herron R, Hyde RD, Hillier SJ. The second example of an anti-Vel auto-antibody. *Vox Sang* 1979;36:179–81.

14 Gale SA, Rowe GP, Northfield FE. Application of a microtitre plate antiglobulin technique to determine the incidence of donors lacking high frequency antigens. *Vox Sang* 1988;54:172–3.

15 Battaglini PF, Ranque J, Bridonneau C, Salmon C, Nicoli RM. Etude du facteur VEL dans la population marseillaise à propos d'un cas d'immunisation anti-VEL. *Proc 10th Cong Int Soc Blood Transfus*, 1964:309–11.

16 Albrey JA, McCulloch WJ, Simmons RT. Inheritance of the Vel blood group in three families. *Med J Aust* 1965; 2:662–5.

17 Race RR, Sanger R. *Blood Groups in Man*, 6th edn. Oxford: Blackwell Scientific Publications, 1975.

18 Fox JA, Taswell HF. Anti-Gn^a, a new antibody reacting with a high-incidence erythrocytic antigen. *Transfusion* 1969;9:265–9.

19 Frank S, Schmidt RP, Baugh M. Three new antibodies to high-incidence antigenic determinants (anti-El, anti-Dp, and anti-So). *Transfusion* 1970;10:254–7.

20 Grindon AJ, McGinniss MH, Issitt PD, Reihart JK, Allen FH. A second example of anti-Lan. *Vox Sang* 1968;15: 293–6.

21 Clancey M, Bonds S, van Eys J. A new example of anti-Lan and two families with Lan-negative members. *Transfusion* 1972;12:106–8.

22 Page PL. Hemolytic disease of the newborn due to anti-Lan. *Transfusion* 1983;23:256–7.

23 Smith DS, Stratton F, Johnson T *et al.* Haemolytic disease of the newborn caused by anti-Lan antibody. *Br Med J* 1969;3:90–2.

24 Okubo Y, Yamaguchi H, Seno T *et al.* The rare red cell phenotype Lan negative in Japanese. *Transfusion* 1984;24:534–5.

25 Smart EA, Reddy V, Fogg P. Anti-Lan and the rare Lan-negative phenotype in South Africa. *Vox Sang* 1998;74(Suppl.1):abstract 1433.

26 Winkler MM, Hamilton JR. Previously tested donors eliminated to determine rare phenotype frequencies [Abstract]. *Joint Cong Int Soc Blood Transfus and Am Ass Blood Banks*, 1990:158.

27 Vengelen-Tyler V. Efficient use of scarce sera in screening thousands of donors [Abstract]. *Transfusion* 1985; 25:476.

28 Nakajima H, Ito K. An example of anti-Jr^a causing hemolytic disease of the newborn and frequency of Jr^a antigen in the Japanese population. *Vox Sang* 1978;35:265–7.

29 Miyazaki T, Kwon KW, Yamamoto K *et al.* A human monoclonal antibody to high-frequency red cell antigen Jr^a. *Vox Sang* 1994;66:51–4.

30 Yamaguchi H, Okubo Y, Seno T *et al.* A rare phenotype blood Jr(a–) occurring in two successive generations of a Japanese family. *Proc Jpn Acad* 1976;52:521–3.

31 Yamada K, Nagashima S, Kishi M *et al.* [Abstract]. *24th Ann Mtg Jpn Soc Blood Transfus*, 1976: 50 (in Japanese). Cited in [30].

32 Tritchler JE. An example of anti-Jrᵃ. *Transfusion* 1977;**17**:177–8.

33 Daniels G. *Human Blood Groups.* Oxford: Blackwell Science, 1995: 645.

34 Daniels GL, DeLong EN, Hare V *et al.* GIL: a red cell antigen of very high frequency. *Immunohematology* 1998;**14**:49–52.

35 Chandanayingyong D, Sasaki TT, Greenwalt TJ. Blood groups of the Thais. *Transfusion* 1967;**7**:269–76.

36 Alfred BM, Stout TD, Lee M, Birkbeck J, Petrakis NL. Blood groups, phosphoglucomutase, and cerumen types of the Anaham (Chilcotin) Indians. *Am J Phys Anthrop* 1970;**32**:329–38.

37 Levine P, White JA, Stroup M. Seven Veᵃ (Vel) negative members in three generations of a family. *Transfusion* 1961;**1**:111–15.

38 Issitt PD, Øyen R, Reihart JK *et al.* Anti-Vel2, a new antibody showing heterogeneity of Vel system antibodies. *Vox Sang* 1968;**15**:125–32.

39 Issitt PD, Anstee DJ. *Applied Blood Group Serology,* 4th edn. Durham: Montgomery Scientific Publications, 1998.

40 Drachmann O, Lundsgaard A. Prenatal assessment of blood group antibodies against 'public' antigens: an example of anti-Ve (Vel) in pregnancy. *Scand J Haematol* 1970;**7**:27–42.

41 Toivanen P, Hirvonen T. Fetal development of red cell antigens K, k, Luᵃ, Luᵇ, Fyᵃ, Fyᵇ, Vel and Xgᵃ. *Scand J Haematol* 1969;**6**:49–55.

42 Issitt P, Combs M, Carawan H *et al.* Phenotypic association between Ge and Vel [Abstract]. *Transfusion* 1994;**34**:60S.

43 Dunstan RA. Status of major red cell blood group antigens on neutrophils, lymphocytes and monocytes. *Br J Haematol* 1986;**62**:301–9.

44 Wiener AS, Gordon EB, Unger LJ. Sensitization to the very high frequency blood factor Vel, with observations on the occurrence of the very rare Vel-negative type among siblings. *Bull Jew Hosp Brooklyn* 1961;**3**:46–51.

45 Bradish EB, Shields WF. Another example of anti-Vel. *Am J Clin Pathol* 1959;**31**:104–6.

46 Storry JR, Mallory DM. Misidentification of anti-Vel due to inappropriate use of techniques [Abstract]. *Transfusion* 1993;**33**:17S.

47 Neppert J, Bartz L, Clasen C. Unsatisfactory detection of an *in vivo* haemolytic anti-Vel by the gel test. *Vox Sang* 1998;**75**:70–1.

48 Garratty G, Arndt P, Nance P. IgG subclass of blood group alloantibodies to high frequency antigens [Abstract]. *Transfusion* 1996;**36**:50S.

49 Becton DL, Kinney TR. An infant girl with severe autoimmune hemolytic anemia: apparent anti-Vel specificity. *Vox Sang* 1986;**51**:108–11.

50 Tilley CA, Crookston MC, Haddad SA, Shumak KH. Red blood cell survival studies in patients with anti-Chᵃ, anti-Ykᵃ, anti-Ge, and anti-Vel. *Transfusion* 1977;**17**:169–72

51 Davey RJ, Procter JL. Elimination of a requirement for Vel-negative red blood cells and successful transfusion following chromium-51 survival study. *Immunohematology* 1995;**11**:39–42.

52 Williams CK, Williams B, Pearson J, Steane SM, Steane EA. An example of anti-Vel causing mild hemolytic disease of the newborn [Abstract]. *Transfusion* 1985;**25**:462.

53 Stiller RJ, Lardas O, Haynes de Regt R. Vel isoimmunization in pregnancy. *Am J Obstet Gynecol* 1990;**162**:1071–2.

54 Szalóky A, van der Hart M. An auto-antibody anti-Vel. *Vox Sang* 1971;**20**:376–7.

55 Ferrer Z, Cornwall S, Berger R *et al.* A third example of haemolytic auto-anti-Vel. *Rev Franc Transfus Immuno-Hémat* 1984;**27**:639–44.

56 Nesbitt R. The red cell antigen Gnᵃ [Abstract]. *Transfusion* 1979;**19**:354.

57 Sturgeon JK, Ames TL, Howard SD, Waxman DA, Danielson CF. Report of an anti-Lan in an African American [Abstract]. *Transfusion* 2000;**40**:115S.

58 Ferraro ML, Trich MB, Smith JF. The rare red cell phenotype, Lan–, in an African-American [Abstract]. *Transfusion* 2000;**40**:121S–2S.

59 Poole J, Rowe GP, Leak M. Weak expression of high frequency antigens and their significance in transfusion practice [Abstract]. *20th Cong Int Soc Blood Transfus*, 1988:303.

60 Storry JR, Øyen R. Variation in Lan expression. *Transfusion* 1999;**39**:109–10.

61 Shertz WT, Carty L, Wolford F. Hemolytic disease of the newborn caused by anti-Lan, anti-Jkᵃ, and anti-c. *Transfusion* 1987;**27**:117.

62 Vengelen-Tyler V, Morel PA. The relationship of anti-Lan and -Jrᵃ 'HTLA' antibodies [Abstract]. *Transfusion* 1981;**21**:603.

63 Pope J, Lubenko A, Lai WYY. A survey of the IgG subclasses of antibodies to high frequency red cell antigens [Abstract]. *Transfus Med* 1991;**1**(Suppl.2): 58.

64 Judd WJ, Oberman HA, Silenieks A, Steiner EA. Clinical significance of anti-Lan. *Transfusion* 1984;**24**:181.

65 Dzik W, Blank J, Getman E *et al.* Hemolytic anemia and RBC destruction due to auto anti-Lan [Abstract]. *Transfusion* 1985;**25**:462.

66 Nance SJ, Arndt P, Garratty G. Predicting the clinical significance of red cell alloantibodies using a monocyte monolayer assay. *Transfusion* 1987;**27**:449–52.

67 Nance SJ, Arndt PA, Garratty G. The effect of fresh normal serum on monocyte monolayer assay reactivity. *Transfusion* 1988;**28**:398–9.

68 Gellerman MM, McCreary J, Yedinak E, Stroup M. Six additional examples of anti-Atᵃ. *Transfusion* 1973; **13**:225–30.

69 Brown A, Harris P, Daniels GL *et al*. At^a (August) and El (Eldr) are synonymous. *Transfusion* 1983;**44**:123–5.

70 Culver PL, Brubaker DB, Sheldon RE, Martin M, Richter CA. Anti-At^a causing mild hemolytic disease of the newborn. *Transfusion* 1987;**27**:468–70.

71 Sweeney JD, Holme S, McCall L *et al*. At(a–) phenotype: description of a family and reduced survival of At(a+) red cells in a proposita with anti-At^a. *Transfusion* 1995;**35**:63–7.

72 Ramsey G, Sherman LA, Zimmer AM *et al*. Clinical significance of anti-At^a. *Vox Sang* 1995;**69**:135–7.

73 Cash K, Brown T, Sausais L, Uehlinger J, Reed LJ. Severe delayed hemolytic transfusion reaction secondary to anti-At^a. *Transfusion* 1999;**39**:834–7.

74 Hadley A, Wilkes A, Poole J, Arndt P, Garratty G. A chemiluminescence test for predicting the outcome of transfusing incompatible blood. *Transfus Med* 1999;**9**:337–42.

75 Kendall AG. Clinical importance of the rare erythrocyte antibody anti-Jr^a. *Transfusion* 1976;**16**:646–7.

76 Pisacka M, Prosicka M, Kralova M *et al*. Six cases of anti-Jr(a) antibody detected in one year: a probable relation with gipsy ethnic minority from central Slovakia. *Vox Sang* 2000;**78** (Suppl.1):abstract P146.

77 Levene C, Sela R, Dvilansky A, Yermiahu T, Daniels G. The Jr(a–) phenotype and anti-Jr^a in two Beduin Arab women in Israel. *Transfusion* 1986;**26**:119–20.

78 Vedo M, Reid ME. Anti-Jr^a in a Mexican American. *Transfusion* 1978;**18**:569.

79 Verska JJ, Larson NL. Autologous transfusion in cardiac surgery: a case report of a patient with a rare antibody. *Transfusion* 1973;**13**:219–20.

80 Orrick LR, Golde SH. Jr^a mediated hemolytic disease of the newborn infant. *Am J Obstet Gynecol* 1980;**137**:135–6.

81 Toy P, Reid M, Lewis T, Ellisor S, Avoy DR. Does anti-Jr^a cause hemolytic disease of the newborn? *Vox Sang* 1981;**41**:40–4.

82 Bacon J, Sherrin D, Wright RG. Case report: anti-Jr^a. *Transfusion* 1986;**26**:543–4.

83 Jowitt S, Powell H, Shwe KH, Love EM. Transfusion reaction due to anti-Jr^a [Abstract]. *Transfus Med* 1994;**4**(Suppl.1):49.

84 Reid ME, Øyen R, Sausais L *et al*. Two additional examples of anti-Emm [Abstract]. *Transfusion* 1998;**38**:101S.

85 Telen MJ, Rosse WF, Parker CJ, Moulds MK, Moulds JJ. Evidence that several high-frequency human blood group antigens reside on phosphatidylinositol-linked erythrocyte membrane proteins. *Blood* 1990;**75**:1404–7.

86 Denomme GA, Fernandes BJ, Lauzon D, Montgomery WM Jr, Moulds MK. First example of maternal–fetal incompatibility due to anti-MAM with an absence of thrombocytopenia [Abstract]. *Transfusion* 2000;**40**:28S.

29.1 Introduction

Numerous antibodies of identical specificity were studied in several laboratories for at least 10 years before Macvie et al. [1] and Renton et al. [2] simultaneously reported the specificity in 1967 and named it anti-Sd^a. The delay in reporting this specificity was because of difficulties in distinguishing between negative and weakly positive reactions. Sd^a shows considerable individual variation in strength of expression. A 'mixed field' reaction, with small agglutinates among a sea of unagglutinated cells, is a characteristic of reactions with anti-Sd^a. If the unagglutinated cells are separated and retested with anti-Sd^a, a 'mixed field' picture is again apparent [2]. About 91% of white people have Sd(a+) red cells and so Sid qualifies for inclusion in the 901 series of high frequency antigens and has the number 901011. As Sid differs so significantly, both in frequency and characteristics, from the other 901 series antigens, it has been given a separate chapter.

29.2 Sd^a and Cad

29.2.1 Variation in strength of Sd^a: the Sd(a++) or Cad phenotype

The strength of expression of Sd^a on Sd(a+) cells varies from barely recognizable to extremely strong. In haemagglutination tests with a strong anti-Sd^a, about 1% of individuals have strong agglutination with big clumps of cells; about 80% have moderate sized agglutinates consisting of 10–20 cells; about 10% have only occasional tiny agglutinates; and about 9% have no agglutination [1]. Weak examples of anti-Sd^a react with only a few Sd(a+) samples and may be mistaken for antibodies to a low frequency antigen.

In 1968, Cazal et al. [3] described a new private anti-

gen, Cad, in a Mauritian family. Cells of the Cad+ members were polyagglutinable and, despite being group O or B, were agglutinated by Dolichos biflorus seed extract, a lectin that generally only agglutinates A$_1$ cells (Chapter 2). After demonstrating that red cells with very strong Sd^a expression are also agglutinated by Dolichos lectin and that Cad cells are very strongly Sd(a+), Sanger et al. [4] concluded that Cad represents the high end of a continuous curve of Sd^a antigen strength. There is considerable variation in agglutination strength with Dolichos and with human anti-Sd^a of these 'super-Sid' or Sd(a++) cells between individuals and within families [5–11]. Cazal et al. [6,11] proposed the terms Cad1, Cad2, Cad3, and Cad4 to describe different Sd(a++) Dolichos-positive phenotypes, with Cad1 the strongest polyagglutinable type. As Cad probably represents the expression of an extra strong Sd^a gene, the term Sd(a++) will be used here to describe all phenotypes in which the red cells have sufficiently strong Sd^a to be agglutinated by Dolichos lectin. The term Cad will be restricted to describe the rare phenotype of members of the Cad family, still probably the strongest Sd(a++) cells encountered.

Sd(a++) cells of the Cad family are polyagglutinable [3]; that is, they are agglutinated by most human sera. Although other Sd(a++) cells are generally polyagglutinable, this is usually less obvious as selected sera and sensitive methods are required to detect the agglutination [9,10]. Sd(a++) polyagglutination differs from all other forms of polyagglutination (Chapter 31).

Race and Sanger [5] suggested that weak anti-Sd^a is present in the sera of most people and is responsible for the polyagglutination of Sd(a++) cells. Polyagglutinable Sd(a++) cells are not agglutinated by sera from people with Sd(a++) cells and adsorption experiments showed that the ability of red cells to remove the 'polyagglutinating' antibody from sera was proportional to the strength of their Sd^a antigen [5]. Furthermore, the stronger the Sd^a antigen on Sd(a++) cells, the greater the number of 'normal' sera that would agglutinate them [12].

29.2.2 Sd^a in body fluids and other tissues

Sd^a can be detected, by haemagglutination inhibition, in the saliva of individuals with Sd(a+) red cells [1,13], with greater quantities present in neonatal than adult saliva [13]. Sd^a can also be detected in human serum and milk, but by far the greatest abundance is found in meconium and urine [13]. Inhibition of anti-Sd^a with urine is considered the most reliable method of determining Sd^a phenotype. Incubation of Sd(a–) red cells in plasma from Sd(a+) or Sd(a++) persons does not render them agglutinable with anti-Sd^a [1,5].

Sd^a has been found, in variable quantities, in the urine of 12 species of mammals [13]. Guinea pig urine is an extremely concentrated source of Sd^a and a useful tool in blood group antibody identification. No Sd^a substance has been detected in birds [13].

Of the human tissues, kidney is a very rich source of Sd^a [13], with activity localized to the distal convoluted tubules and collecting ducts [14]. Morgan *et al.* [15] suggested that it may be advantageous to consider Sd^a compatibility when selecting donor kidneys for allograft. Sd^a is also present in colon and stomach [16,17], but was not detected in small intestine, muscle, liver, spleen, or brain [16].

29.2.3 Frequency and inheritance

The frequency of Sd^a, as determined by testing red cells, is about 90%. Three surveys gave the following results: 290 English blood donors, 91.4% Sd(a+) [1]; 131 English donors, 91.0% Sd(a+) [2]; 1307 Italian donors, 89.3% Sd(a+) [18]. A higher incidence of Sd(a+) is obtained when urine is tested by haemagglutination inhibition. Sd^a was detected in the urine of 96.1% of English blood donors [13] and 93.4% of north Italians [18]. The gene and genotype frequencies in English donors determined by urine inhibition are: *Sd^a* 0.8030; *Sd* 0.1970; *Sd^a/Sd^a* 0.6448; *Sd^a/Sd* 0.3164; *Sd/Sd* 0.0388.

Sd(a++) is very rare in Europeans, but may be less infrequent in the Far East. Table 29.1 shows some frequency determinations on group O and B donors tested with *Dolichos* lectin. These frequencies are somewhat arbitrary as they are partly dependent on the potency of the lectin preparation used.

Tests with anti-Sd^a on 55 families with a total of 168 children demonstrated that Sd^a is inherited as a dominant character [1]. Sd(a++), as detected by *Dolichos* lectin, is also inherited in a dominant manner [3,5–8,10–12,21]. Family studies have shown that Sd^a is not part of the ABO, MNS, P1, Rh, Lutheran, Kell, Duffy, Kidd, Xg, Dombrock, or XK systems [1,5,8,10]. One Canadian family provided a suggestion of linkage between the genes for Sd(a++) and Wr^a (*SLC4A1* or *DI*), with six non-recombinants and no recombinant, providing a lod score of 1.806 at a recombination fraction (θ) of zero [8].

29.2.4 Sd^a in babies and pregnant women

Red cells of fetuses and newborn infants are Sd(a–) and become Sd(a+) about 10 weeks postnatally [1,2,16]. Red cells of the son of an Sd(a++) father were nonreactive with *Dolichos* lectin at birth, but were agglutinated by the lectin 6 months later [10]. Saliva, urine, and meconium from neonates generally contain abundant Sd^a substance [13].

An increased frequency of Sd(a–) red cell phenotype is found among pregnant women [1,16,22]. Spitalnik *et al.* [22] found that 22% of women in the first trimester of pregnancy and 36% at term were Sd(a–), whereas Pickles and Morton [16] found that 75% of women at term and about 25% 6 weeks postpartum had Sd(a–) red cells. Sd^a is present in the urine of most Sd(a–) pregnant women [13].

29.3 Sid antibodies and lectins

29.3.1 Anti-Sd^a

Anti-Sd^a is disclosed in the sera of about 1% of donor sera when Sd(a+) cells are used for detection [1,2]. The incidence of anti-Sd^a is increased when Sd(a++) cells are used [22], and the exceptionally strong Sd(a++) Cad cells are agglutinated by most sera. Sd^a antibodies are usually IgM and active at 20°C [1,2,16], although IgG anti-Sd^a has been identified [22,23].

Anti-Sd^a are not generally considered a transfusion hazard [1,16,22,24], although transfusion of Sd(a+) cells to patients with anti-Sd^a may evoke a significant increase in IgG antibody titre [22]. Most survival studies with ^{51}Cr-labelled cells in patients with anti-Sd^a

Table 29.1 Frequencies of Sd(a++) in various populations as detected by different preparations of *Dolichos biflorus* lectin.

Population	No. tested	No. positive	Frequency	References
French, Montpellier	250 000	0		[3]
French (four centres)	78 526	56	0.0007	[10]
Canadian, Winnipeg	1 425	2	0.0014	[8]
Canadian, Toronto	2 191	1	0.0005	[5]
Japanese	51 420	15	0.0003	[7]
Hong Kong Chinese	36 037	110	0.0031	[19]
Thai	14 261	37	0.0026	[12,20]

have shown insignificant reduction in red cell survival, even when Sd(a++) cells were used [25,26]. A couple of haemolytic reactions, allegedly caused by transfusion of Sd(a++) cells to a patient with IgM anti-Sd^a, are reported [25,26].

29.3.2 Lectins and other non-human sources of anti-Sd^a

Dolichos biflorus, a lectin specific for terminal *N*-acetylgalactosamine, agglutinates A$_1$, Tn-positive, and Sd(a++) cells [27]. These reactions can be inhibited by *N*-acetylgalactosamine [4]. Adsorption and elution experiments show that a single lectin in *Dolichos* extracts is responsible for the agglutination of A$_1$, Tn, and Sd(a++) cells [5,28]. Sd(a++) cells express more determinants than A$_1$ or Tn cells, so an apparently specific anti-Sd(a++) can be produced by dilution of the lectin or by partial adsorption with A$_1$ or Tn cells. Further adsorptions with these cells, or adsorption with Sd(a++) cells, removes all activity.

The seed lectins *Salvia horminum*, *S. farinacea*, and *Leonurus cardiaca* [29–31], and the snail lectins *Helix pomatia* and *H. aspersa* [6,32–35] agglutinate Sd(a++) cells. These reactions are inhibited by *N*-acetylgalactosamine [29,31,33,34]. Sd(a++) and Tn specificity in the *Salvia* lectins can be separated by adsorption [29] and *L. cardiaca* contains very little Tn activity, which can easily be eliminated by dilution [31]. The anti-A$_1$ lectins *Phaseolus lunatus* and *P. limensis* do not agglutinate even the strongest of Sd(a++) cells [32–34].

Chicken serum contains a 'naturally occurring' antibody reactive with Sd(a++) cells [36]. After immunization of a chicken with Sd(a++) cells, the serum agglutinated Sd(a++) cells and also reacted with all Sd(a+) cells by an antiglobulin test [5,36]. Separable anti-Tn and an antibody that agglutinates Sd(a++)

cells were identified in the serum of the non-poisonous snake *Python sebae* [37].

29.4 Biochemistry

Studies with lectins described above strongly suggested that Sd^a expression is dependent on an oligosaccharide structure with *N*-acetylgalactosamine at its non-reducing end. *Dolichos biflorus* lectin was thought to be specific for *N*-acetylgalactosamine in the α-linked position [33,34], so it was somewhat surprising when the terminal non-reducing sugar for Sd^a-active glycoprotein turned out to be *N*-acetyl-D-galactosamine in β-linkage with galactose [38].

29.4.1 Sd^a in urine

In 1970 Morton and Terry [39] partially separated Sd^a-active material from human urine by ethanol precipitation. Ten years later, Soh *et al.* [40] showed that Sd^a activity is associated with Tamm–Horsfall protein (THP), the most abundant glycoprotein in urine [41]. This macromolecule of apparent M_r 78 000 is secreted by the kidney and is composed of 70% protein and 30% carbohydrate, the latter predominantly in the form of *N*-glycans [42]. Seven of the eight potential *N*-glycosylation sites are glycosylated [43]. Uromodulin, a glycoform of THP in which the O-glycans are radically modified, is present only in the urine of pregnant women and is a potent inhibitor of antigen-induced T cell proliferation [44].

Sd(a+) THP contains between 1% and 2% *N*-acetylgalactosamine, whereas that from Sd(a−) individuals contains virtually none; no difference in the amino acid composition of THP from Sd(a+) and Sd(a−) individuals could be detected [15,40]. Sd^a-active THP was precipitated by *Dolichos* and *Helix pomatia* lectins and by human anti-Sd[a] [15,45]. A pentasaccharide isolated from Sd[a]-active THP is shown in Table 29.2b [46,47]. This pentasaccharide strongly inhibited the reactivity of anti-Sd[a] with Sd(a+) cells and of *Dolichos* lectin with Sd(a++) cells. The pentasaccharide was not present on THP from Sd(a–) urine, whereas its presumed precursor, a tetrasaccharide lacking *N*-acetylgalactosamine (Table 29.2a), was present on both Sd[a]-active and -inactive glycoproteins [48]. Tetrasaccharides prepared by the cleavage of *N*-acetylgalactosamine or sialic acid residues from the Sd[a]-active pentasaccharides were without Sd[a] activity

[49]. A mucin of apparent M_r 340 000 and high *N*-acetylgalactosamine content, which inhibited anti-Sd[a] as effectively as THP, was isolated by affinity chromatography with *H. pomatia* lectin [50]. So at least two substances in human urine carry the Sd[a] determinant.

THP in urine is a key anti-adherence factor for *Escherichia coli*, the principal cause of urinary tract infection. THP binds specifically to type 1 fimbriated *E. coli*, coating the adhesins and preventing adherence of the pathogen to urothelial receptors [51].

Table 29.2 Some structures associated with different Sd[a] phenotypes (for abbreviations see Table 2.4).

Tetrasaccharide and pentasaccharide isolated from THP
(a) Sd(a–) and Sd(a+)

$$
\begin{array}{l}
\text{Gal}\beta1{\rightarrow}4\text{GlcNAc}\beta1{\rightarrow}3\text{Gal} \\
\quad\quad 3 \\
\quad\quad \uparrow \\
\text{NeuAc}\alpha2
\end{array}
$$

(b) Sd(a+)

$$
\begin{array}{l}
\text{GalNAc}\beta1{\rightarrow}4\text{Gal}\beta1{\rightarrow}4\text{GlcNAc}\beta1{\rightarrow}3\text{Gal} \\
\quad\quad\quad\quad\quad\quad 3 \\
\quad\quad\quad\quad\quad\quad \uparrow \\
\quad\quad\quad \text{NeuAc}\alpha2
\end{array}
$$

Tetrasaccharide and pentasaccharide from glycophorin A
(c) Sd(a–), Sd(a+), and Sd(a++)

$$
\begin{array}{l}
\text{Gal}\beta1{\rightarrow}3\text{GalNAc—Ser/Thr} \\
\quad\quad 3 \quad\quad\quad 6 \\
\quad\quad \uparrow \quad\quad\quad\; \uparrow \\
\text{NeuAc}\alpha2 \;\; \text{NeuAc}\alpha2
\end{array}
$$

(d) Sd(a++)

$$
\begin{array}{l}
\text{GalNAc}\beta1{\rightarrow}4\text{Gal}\beta1{\rightarrow}3\text{GalNAc—Ser/Thr} \\
\quad\quad\quad\quad\quad\quad 3 \quad\quad\quad 6 \\
\quad\quad\quad\quad\quad\quad \uparrow \quad\quad\quad\; \uparrow \\
\quad\quad\quad\quad\quad \text{NeuAc}\alpha2 \;\; \text{NeuAc}\alpha2
\end{array}
$$

Sialosylparagloboside and Sd[a] ganglioside
(e) Sd(a–), Sd(a+), and Sd(a++)

$$
\begin{array}{l}
\text{Gal}\beta1{\rightarrow}4\text{GlcNAc}\beta1{\rightarrow}3\text{Gal}\beta1{\rightarrow}4\text{Glc—Cer} \\
\quad\quad 3 \\
\quad\quad \uparrow \\
\text{NeuAc}\alpha2
\end{array}
$$

(f) Sd(a+) and Sd(a++)

$$
\begin{array}{l}
\text{GalNAc}\beta1{\rightarrow}4\text{Gal}\beta1{\rightarrow}4\text{GlcNAc}\beta1{\rightarrow}3\text{Gal}\beta1{\rightarrow}4\text{Glc—Cer} \\
\quad\quad\quad\quad\quad\quad 3 \\
\quad\quad\quad\quad\quad\quad \uparrow \\
\quad\quad\quad \text{NeuAc}\alpha2
\end{array}
$$

29.4.2 Sdᵃ on red cells

Most biochemical analysis of Sdᵃ on red cells has been carried out on the Sd(a++) cells of members of the Cad family, which have exceptionally high levels of Sdᵃ activity. Sodium dodecyl sulphate polyacrylamide gel electrophoresis (SDS PAGE) revealed that glycophorin A (GPA) and glycophorin B (GPB) from Cad red cells have an increase in apparent M_r of 3000 and 2000, respectively, compared with normal red cells [52]. This is caused by the addition of a β-linked N-acetylgalactosamine residue to most of the disialotetrasaccharides characteristic of these glycoproteins [53] (Tables 29.2c and d, and Chapter 3). The resulting pentasaccharide (Table 29.2d) inhibited *Dolichos* lectin and anti-Sdᵃ, and the altered GPA molecules bound to the lectin in affinity columns [52–54]. Red cells from the original Cad propositus had approximately 12 pentasaccharides per GPA molecule, cells from two other Sd(a++) individuals had 2–3 pentasaccharides per GPA molecule, and Sd(a+) and Sd(a–) cells had no pentasaccharides [55]. Increased apparent M_r of decay accelerating factor (CD55) in Cad cells was also assumed to be because of the presence of additional N-acetylgalactosamine residues [56].

Thin layer chromatography of Cad red cell membranes demonstrated an unusual profile characterized by reduction in the content of sialosylparagloboside (Table 29.2e), the major ganglioside in normal cells, and the presence of a new ganglioside of lower mobility [57]. The unusual ganglioside, which binds *H. pomatia* lectin and inhibits anti-Sdᵃ, represents sialosylparagloboside with an additional terminal β-N-acetylgalactosamine residue (Table 29.2f) [57,58]. The structure of the terminal pentasaccharide of this ganglioside is identical to that of Sdᵃ-active THP shown in Table 29.2b [58]. Small quantities of this ganglioside were detected in membranes from Sd(a+), but not Sd(a–) red cells, and might represent the major Sdᵃ-active structure in Sd(a+) cells [57].

29.4.3 The Sdᵃ glycosyltransferase

The product of the *Sdᵃ* gene is most probably a β1,4-N-acetylgalactosaminyltransferase that catalyses the transfer of N-acetylgalactosamine in β-linkage from a nucleotide carrier to an appropriate tetrasaccharide acceptor substrate molecule. Such enzymes have been detected in human urine from Sd(a+) but not Sd(a–)

individuals [48,59], in human kidney [60], in human large intestine [61], and in guinea pig kidney [62,63]. Sd(a–) THP was the best acceptor for the human urine enzyme, but the disialotetrasaccharides of GPA were also suitable acceptors [59]. Preparations from human kidney catalysed the transfer of N-acetylgalactosamine to sialosylparagloboside, but not to native GPA, although tryptic peptides of GPA were good acceptor substrates [57,60] For more details see [64].

A segment of cDNA encoding the Sdᵃ-transferase has been obtained from the total RNA fraction of human gastric mucosa, by reverse transcriptase polymerase chain reaction (PCR) with primers representing the murine β1,4-N-acetylgalactosaminyltransferase cDNA sequence [65].

27.5 Malaria

Sd(a++) cells of the Cad family are relatively resistant to invasion by the malarial parasite *Plasmodium falciparum* [66] (see Section 3.23.1). Sialic acid on glycophorin molecules is required by *P. falciparum* merozoites for invasion of the red cells. Cartron *et al.* [66] propose that this sialic acid is not available on the O-glycans of Cad cells as a result of chemical interaction with the acetyl group of the extra N-acetylgalactosamine residues.

References

1 Macvie SI, Morton JA, Pickles MM. The reactions and inheritance of a new blood group antigen, Sdᵃ. *Vox Sang* 1967;**13**:485–92.

2 Renton PH, Howell P, Ikin EW, Giles CM, Goldsmith KLG. Anti-Sdᵃ, a new blood group antibody. *Vox Sang* 1967;**13**:493–501.

3 Cazal P, Monis M, Caubel J, Brives J. Polyagglutinabilité héréditaire dominant: antigène privé (Cad) correspondant à un anticorps public et à une lectine de *Dolichos biflorus*. *Rev Franc Transfus Immuno-Hémat* 1968;**11**:209–21.

4 Sanger R, Gavin J, Tippett P, Teesdale P, Eldon K. Plant agglutinin for another human blood-group. *Lancet* 1971;i:1130.

5 Race RR, Sanger R. *Blood Groups in Man*, 6th edn. Oxford: Blackwell Scientific Publications, 1975.

6 Cazal P, Monis M, Bizot M. Les antigènes Cad et leurs rapports avec les antigènes A. *Rev Franc Transfus* 1971;**14**:321–34.

7 Yamaguchi H, Okubo Y, Ogawa Y, Tanaka M. Japanese families with group O and B red cells agglutinable by *Dolichos biflorus* extract. *Vox Sang* 1973;**25**:361–9.

8 Lewis M, Kaita H, Chown B *et al.* A family with the rare red cell antigens Wr^a and 'super' Sd^a. *Vox Sang* 1973;**25**:336–40.

9 Lopez M, Gerbal A, Bony V, Salmon C. Cad antigen: comparative study of 50 samples. *Vox Sang* 1975;**28**:305–13.

10 Gerbal A, Lopez M, Chassaigne M *et al.* L'antigène Cad dans la population française. *Rev Franc Transfus Immuno-Hémat* 1976;**14**:415–29.

11 Cazal P, Monis M, Bizot M. Les antigènes Cad en 1976. *Rev Franc Transfus Immuno-Hémat* 1977;**20**:165–73.

12 Sringarm S, Chiewsilp P, Tubrod J. Cad receptor in Thai blood donors. *Vox Sang* 1974;**26**:462–6.

13 Morton JA, Pickles MM, Terry AM. The Sd^a blood group antigen in tissues and body fluids. *Vox Sang* 1970;**19**:472–82.

14 Morton JA, Pickles MM, Vanhegan RI. The Sd^a antigen in the human kidney and colon. *Immunol Invest* 1988;**17**:217–24.

15 Morgan WTJ, Soh CPC, Donald ASR, Watkins WM. Observations on the blood group Sd^a activity of Tamm & Horsfall urinary glycoprotein. *Rev Franc Transfus Immuno-Hémat* 1981;**24**:37–51.

16 Pickles MM, Morton JA. The Sd^a blood group. In: *Human Blood Groups, 5th Int Convoc Immunol, Buffalo NY.* Basel: Karger 1977, 277–86.

17 Piller F, Cartron J-P, Tuppy H. Increase of blood group A and loss of blood group Sd^a activity in the mucus from human neoplastic colon. *Rev Franc Transfus Immuno-Hémat* 1980;**23**:599–611.

18 Conte R, Serafini-Cessi F. Comparison between the erythrocyte and urinary Sd^a antigen distribution in a large number of individuals from Emilia-Romagna, a region of northern Italy. *Transfus Med* 1991;**1**:47–9.

19 Mak KH, Leong S, Chan NK. Incidence of Cad antigen among Chinese donors in Hong Kong [Abstract]. *20th Congr Int Soc Blood Transfus*, 1988:303.

20 Sringarm S, Chupungart C, Giles CM. The use of *Ulex europaeus* and *Dolichos biflorus* extracts in routine ABO grouping of blood donors in Thailand: some unexpected findings. *Vox Sang* 1972;**23**:537–45.

21 Lopez M, Gerbal A, Girard-Debord M, Salmon C. Trois sujets A$_{end}$ Cad dans une famille française. *Rev Franc Transfus Immuno-Hémat* 1977;**20**:457–66.

22 Spitalnik S, Cox MT, Spennacchio J, Guenther R, Blumberg N. The serology of Sd^a effects of transfusion and pregnancy. *Vox Sang* 1982;**42**:308–12.

23 Silvergleid AJ, Wells RF, Hafleigh EB *et al.* Compatibility test using ^{51}chromium-labeled red blood cells in crossmatch positive patients. *Transfusion* 1978;**18**:8–14.

24 Colledge KI, Kaplan HS, Marsh WL. Massive transfusion of Sd(a+) blood to a recipient with anti-Sd^a, without clinical complication [Abstract]. *Transfusion* 1973;**13**:340.

25 Peetermans ME, Cole-Dergent J. Haemolytic transfu-sion reaction due to anti-Sd^a. *Vox Sang* 1970;**18**:67–70.

26 Reznicek MJ, Cordle DG, Strauss RG. A hemolytic reaction implicating Sd^a antibody missed by immediate spin crossmatch. *Vox Sang* 1992;**62**:173–5.

27 Bird GWG. Lectins in immunohematology. *Transfus Med Rev* 1989;**3**:55–62.

28 Bird GWG, Wingham J. Cad (super Sd^a) in a British family with Eastern connections: a note on the specificity of the *Dolichos biflorus* lectin. *J Immunogenet* 1976;**3**:297–302.

29 Bird GWG, Wingham J. Haemagglutinins from *Salvia*. *Vox Sang* 1974;**26**:163–6.

30 Moore BPL, Marsh S. Identification of strong Sd(a+) and Sd(a++) red cells by hemagglutinins from *Salvia horminum*. *Transfusion* 1975;**15**:132–4.

31 Bird GWG, Wingham J. Anti-Cad lectin from the seeds of *Leonurus cardiaca*. *Clin Lab Haematol* 1979;**1**:57–9.

32 Myllylä G, Furuhjelm U, Nordling S *et al.* Persistent mixed field polyagglutinability: electrokinetic and serological aspects. *Vox Sang* 1971;**20**:7–23.

33 Bird GWG, Wingham J. Some serological properties of the Cad receptor. *Vox Sang* 1971;**20**:55–61.

34 Uhlenbruck G, Sprenger I, Heggen M, Leseney AM. Diagnosis of the 'Cad' blood group with agglutinins from snails and plants. *Z Immun-Forsch* 1971;**141**: 290–1.

35 Bizot M. Comportement de quelques extraits de gastéropodes terrestres vis-à-vis des substances de spécificité Sd^a. *Rev Franc Transfus* 1972;**15**:371–5.

36 Bizot M, Cayla J-P. Hétéro-anticorps anti-Cad du poulet. *Rev Franc Transfus* 1972;**15**:195–202.

37 Lockyer WJ, Gold ER, Bird GWG. Anti-Tn and anti-Cad in the serum of the non-poisonous snake *Python sebae*. *Med Lab Sci* 1977;**34**:311–17.

38 Donald ASR, Soh CPC, Watkins WM, Morgan WTJ. N-acetyl-D-galactosaminyl-β-(1→4)-D-galactose: a terminal non-reducing structure in human blood group Sd^a-active Tamm–Horsfall urinary glycoprotein. *Biochem Biophys Res Commun* 1982;**104**:58–65.

39 Morton JA, Terry AM. The Sd^a blood group antigen. Biochemical properties of urinary Sd^a. *Vox Sang* 1970;**19**:151–61.

40 Soh CPC, Morgan WTJ, Watkins WM, Donald ASR. The relationship between the N-acetylgalactosamine content and the blood group Sd^a activity of Tamm and Horsfall urinary glycoprotein. *Biochem Biophys Res Commun* 1980;**93**:1132–9.

41 Kokot F, Dulawa J. Tamm–Horsfall protein updated. *Nephron* 2000;**85**:97–102.

42 Fletcher AP. The Tamm and Horsfall glycoprotein. In: A Gottschalk, ed. *Glycoproteins: Their Composition, Structure, and Function*, 2nd edn. Amsterdam: Elsevier, 1972:892–908.

43 van Rooijen JJM, Voskamp AF, Kamerling JP, Vliegenthart FG. Glycosylation sites and site-specific

glycosylation in human Tamm–Horsfall glycoprotein. *Glycobiology* 1999;**9**:21–30.

44 Easton RL, Patankari MS, Clark GF, Morris HR, Dell A. Pregnancy-associated changes in the glycosylation of Tamm–Horsfall glycoprotein. *J Biol Chem* 2000;**275**:21928–38.

45 Serafini-Cessi F, Conte R. Precipitin reaction between Sd^a-active human Tamm–Horsfall glycoprotein and anti-Sd^a serum. *Vox Sang* 1982;**42**:141–4.

46 Donald ASR, Yates AD, Soh CPC, Morgan WTJ, Watkins WM. A blood group Sd^a-active pentasaccharide isolated from Tamm–Horsfall urinary glycoprotein. *Biochem Biophys Res Commun* 1983;**115**: 625–31.

47 Donald ASR, Feeney J. Oligosaccharides obtained from a blood-group-Sd^{a+} Tamm–Horsfall glycoprotein. *Biochem J* 1986;**236**:821–8.

48 Donald ASR, Soh CPC, Yates AD *et al.* Structure, biosynthesis and genetics of the Sd^a antigen. *Biochem Soc Trans* 1987;**15**:606–8.

49 Donald ASR, Yates AD, Soh CPC, Morgan WTJ, Watkins WM. The human blood-group-Sd^a determinant: a terminal non-reducing carbohydrate structure in N-linked and mucin-type glycoproteins. *Biochem Soc Trans* 1984;**12**:596–9.

50 Cartron J-P, Kornprobst M, Lemonnier M *et al.* Isolation from human urines of a mucin with blood group Sd^a activity. *Biochem Biophys Res Commun* 1982;**106**:331–7.

51 Pak J, Pu Y, Zhang Z-T, Hasty DL, Wu X-R. Tamm–Horsfall protein binds to type 1 fimbriated *Escherichia coli* and prevents *E. coli* from binding to uroplakin Ia and Ib receptors. *J Biol Chem* 2001; **276**:9924–30.

52 Cartron J-P, Blanchard D. Association of human erythrocyte membrane glycoproteins with blood-group Cad specificity. *Biochem J* 1982;**207**:497–504.

53 Blanchard D, Cartron J-P, Fournet B *et al.* Primary structure of the oligosaccharide determinant of blood group Cad specificity. *J Biol Chem* 1983;**258**:7691–5.

54 Herkt F, Parente JP, Leroy Y *et al.* Structure determination of oligosaccharides isolated from Cad erythrocyte membranes by permethylation analysis and 500-MHz ^{1}H-NMR spectroscopy. *Eur J Biochem* 1985;**146**: 125–9.

55 Blanchard D, Capon C, Leroy Y, Cartron J-P, Fournet B. Comparative study of glycophorin A derived O-glycans from human Cad, Sd(a+) and Sd(a–) erythrocytes. *Biochem J* 1985;**232**:813–18.

56 Spring FA, Judson PA, Daniels GL *et al.* A human cell-surface glycoprotein that carries Cromer-related blood group antigens on erythrocytes and is also expressed on leucocytes and platelets. *Immunology* 1987;**62**: 307–13.

57 Blanchard D, Piller F, Gillard B, Marcus D, Cartron J-P. Identification of a novel ganglioside on erythrocytes with blood group Cad specificity. *J Biol Chem* 1985;**260**:7813–6.

58 Gillard BK, Blanchard D, Bouhours J-F *et al.* Structure of a ganglioside with Cad blood group antigen activity. *Biochemistry* 1988;**27**:4601–6.

59 Serafini-Cessi F, Malagolini N, Dall'Olio F. Characterization and partial purification of β-N-acetylgalactosaminyltransferase from urine of Sd^{a+} individuals. *Arch Biochem Biophys* 1988;**266**:573–82.

60 Piller F, Blanchard D, Huet M, Cartron J-P. Identification of a α-NeuAc-(2→3)-β-D-galactopyranosyl N-acetyl-β-D-galactosaminyltransferase in human kidney. *Carbohydr Res* 1986;**149**:171–84.

61 Malagolini N, Dall'Olio F, Di Stefano G *et al.* Expression of UDP-GalNAc: NeuAcα2,3Galβ-R β1,4(GalNAc to Gal) N–acetylgalactosaminyltransferase involved in the synthesis of Sd^a antigen in human large intestine and colorectal carcinomas. *Cancer Res* 1989;**49**:6466– 6470.

62 Serafini-Cessi F, Dall'Olio F. Guinea-pig kidney β-N-acetylgalactosaminyltransferase towards Tamm–Horsfall glycoprotein: requirement of sialic acid in the acceptor for transferase activity. *Biochem J* 1983;**215**:483–9.

63 Soh CPC, Donald ASR, Feeney J, Morgan WTJ, Watkins WM. Enzymic synthesis, chemical characterisation and Sd^a activity of GalNAcβ1–4[NeuAcα2–3]Galβ1–4GlcNAc and GalNAcβ1–4[NeuAcα2–3]Galβ1–4Glc. *Glycocon J* 1989;**6**: 319–32.

64 Watkins WM. Sd^a and Cad antigens. In: J-P Cartron, P Rouger, eds. *Blood Cell Biochemistry*, Vol. 6. New York: Plenum Press, 1995:351–75.

65 Dohi T, Yuyama Y, Natori Y *et al.* Detection of N-acetylgalactosaminyltransferase mRNA which determines expression of Sd^a blood group carbohydrate structure in human gastrointestinal mucosa and cancer. *Int J Cancer* 1996;**67**:626–31.

66 Cartron J-P, Prou O, Luilier M, Soulier JP. Susceptibility to invasion by *Plasmodium falciparum* of some human erythrocytes carrying rare blood group antigens. *Br J Haematol* 1983;**55**:639–47.

30 Human leukocyte associated (HLA) Class I antigens on red cells

Class I products of the genes of the major histocompatibility complex (MHC), *HLA-A*, *-B*, and *-C*, were initially detected on leucocytes but have since been shown to be present on virtually all nucleated cells. Their primary function is the presentation of foreign antigens to cytotoxic T cells. The very highly polymorphic MHC is located on chromosome 6p21. (For a more detailed description see Roitt [1] or any textbook on immunology.) Mature human red blood cells are not nucleated and do not generally have easily detectable HLA antigens. On occasion, however, certain HLA antigens are expressed strongly enough on red cells to be detected by conventional blood grouping techniques. Because red cells are unsuitable for HLA phenotyping, HLA is not considered a blood group system and HLA antibodies that react with red cells (often called Bg antibodies) are generally regarded by blood group serologists as unwelcome contaminants of antisera.

The discovery that HLA antigens can be expressed on red cells came when Morton *et al.* [2,3] showed that an assortment of rather indeterminate and troublesome blood group antigens on red cells, called the Bg (Bennett–Goodspeed) antigens [4–6], were strongly related to the HLA antigens on white cells. Bg[a] showed almost complete concordance with HLA-B7 [2], Bg[b] correlated with HLA-B17, and Bg[c] with HLA-A28 [3]. Bg(c+) red cells may also react with anti-HLA-A2, which is known to cross-react with HLA-28 [7,8], and many other cross-reactions occur. Other HLA antigens have been detected on red cells: HLA-A10 and -B8 are often quite strongly expressed [3,9] and HLA-A9, -B12, and -B15 may also be detected [10]. HLA expression on red cells is always weaker than on white cells [3,9]. Many individuals never express HLA on their red cells, even though their lymphocytes carry an appropriate antigen [11]. HLA expression on red cells varies substantially between individuals of the same HLA phenotype and within an individual over a period of time [9]. Red cells may be positive for a particular HLA antigen for months or years and then become negative for that antigen for a similar period [11].

HLA antigen strength on red cells does not appear to be inherited in a conventional manner and an HLA antigen may be detected on the red cells of a person, but not on those of either parent [2,6,12,13]. Much of the work on HLA expression of red cells was carried out on an AutoAnalyser [6–10,13–17] or by an albumin antiglobulin test read in capillaries [18,19]. Radioimmunoassay and flow cytometry revealed that red cells of about 50% of blood donors bound monoclonal antibodies directed at monomorphic determinants on HLA class I molecules [20]. Individuals with HLA-B7 on their lymphocytes always express measurable red cell HLA antigens [20,21]. Red cell-reactive antibodies were detected in all sera containing cytotoxic anti-HLA-B7 [15].

It has been estimated that the number of HLA sites on red cells is in the range of 40–550, compared with 100 000 on T lymphocytes [22]. This explains why it is very difficult to remove haemagglutinating HLA antibodies from sera by adsorbing with red cells when they are readily removed by white cells [2,3,14,15].

Red cells of people with HLA-B7 have significantly more HLA Class I molecules on their red cells than those without HLA-B7 [22]. Marked increase in red cell HLA expression is also associated with systemic lupus erythematosus (SLE) and, to a lesser extent, rheumatoid arthritis [23]. The mean numbers of HLA Class I molecules per red cell are estimated as follows: B7-negative, 66; B7-positive, 260; B7-negative SLE patients, 302; B7-positive SLE patients, 666 [22]. HLA-B7 patients with infectious mononucleosis have greatly increased expression of the HLA-B7 on their red cells, which sometimes takes years to return to normal [24]. Certain red cell HLA antigens are elevated in patients with leukaemia and a variety of other haematological diseases [25]. Strong expression of red cell HLA in healthy subjects is rare, but has been reported [12,17].

Class I MHC molecules are heterodimers consisting of an M_r 45 000 α-chain with three extracellular domains, $α_1$, $α_2$, and $α_3$, non-covalently associated with an M_r 11 000 polypeptide, $β_2$-microglobulin

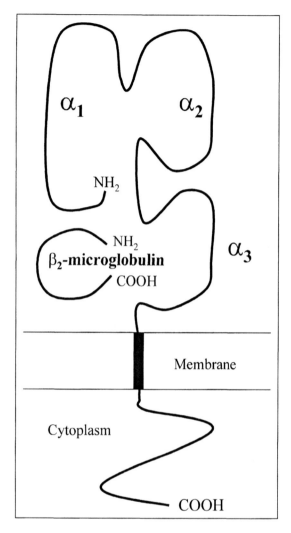

Fig. 30.1 Diagrammatic representation of Class I MHC glycoprotein, showing the larger α-chain with its α_1, α_2, and α_3 extracellular domains, and the smaller non-covalently associated β_2-microglobulin.

(Fig. 30.1). HLA antigenic determinants reside on the α_1 and α_2 domains. β_2-microglobulin is not encoded by the MHC on chromosome 6, but by a gene on chromosome 15. Immunoblotting of red cells with monoclonal antibodies to Class I α-chain and to β_2-microglobulin gave bands of apparent M_r 45 000 and 11 000, respectively, suggesting that red cell HLA antigens are carried on structures similar or identical to those on nucleated cells [26].

Red cell-reactive HLA antibodies are inhibited by plasma from individuals with the corresponding anti-

gens on their white cells [9,27]. This, together with the finding that red cell HLA activity is destroyed by treatment of the cells with chloroquine, led to a proposal that HLA antigens might be adsorbed onto the red cell surface from the plasma rather than being intrinsic red cell antigens [28]. However, there is a weight of evidence against this, supporting the thesis that HLA antigens on red cells represent remnants of those antigens present in greater quantity on nucleated red cell precursors [29,30]. Treatment of red cells with chloroquine only removes the β_2-microglobulin; the α-chain remains intact and loss of antigenic expression is probably a result of configurational changes [31]. Some HLA activity returns if chloroquine-treated cells are incubated in purified β_2-microglobulin [31]. Furthermore, the number of HLA Class I molecules on red cells decreases with ageing of those cells, the opposite of what would be expected if the antigens were acquired from the plasma [22]. The level of expression of HLA Class I and β_2-microglobulin is reduced during erythroid differentiation [32]. Red cell HLA antigens are not destroyed by treatment of the red cells with papain, ficin, pronase, trypsin, chymotrypsin, or with the sulphydryl-reducing agents 2-aminoethylisothiouronium bromide (AET) and dithiothreitol (DTT) [9,31]. Many of the HLA α-chains in plasma are of M_r 39 000, differing from those on red cells because they lack the hydrophobic transmembrane domain [33].

HLA antibodies have not been implicated in haemolytic disease of the newborn. In one patient, a haemolytic transfusion reaction was blamed on anti-HLA-A2 and -B7, but the evidence was inconclusive [34]. There have been reports of increased destruction of radiolabelled red cells by HLA antibodies, although this appears to affect only a minority of red cells in the circulation [12,16,35]. HLA antibodies reactive with red cells are often a nuisance in antibody investigations, but the difficulties can be reduced by stripping the HLA antigens from the red cells with chloroquine [28] or ethylenediaminetetra-acetic acid (EDTA)/glycine-HCl [36].

References

1 Roitt IM. *Essential Immunology*, 9th edn. Oxford: Blackwell Science 1997.
2 Morton JA, Pickles MM, Sutton L. The correlation of the Bg^a blood group with the HL-A7 leucocyte group: demonstration of antigenic sites on red cells and leucocytes. *Vox Sang* 1969;17:536–47.

3 Morton JA, Pickles MM, Sutton L, Skov F. Identification of further antigens on red cells and lymphocytes: association of Bg^b with W17 (Te57) and Bg^c with W28 (Da15,Ba*). *Vox Sang* 1971;**21**:141–53.

4 Buchanan DI, Afaganis A. The Bennett–Goodspeed–Sturgeon or 'Donna' red cell antigen and antibody. *Vox Sang* 1963;**8**:213–18.

5 Chown B, Lewis M, Kaita H. The Bennett–Goodspeed antigen or antigens. *Vox Sang* 1963;**8**:281–8.

6 Seaman MJ, Benson R, Jones MN, Morton JA, Pickles MM. The reactions of the Bennett–Goodspeed group of antibodies tested with the AutoAnalyzer. *Br J Haematol* 1967;**13**:464–73.

7 Nordhagen R, Ørjasæter H. Association between HL-A and red cell antigens: an AutoAnalyzer study. *Vox Sang* 1974;**26**:97–106.

8 Nordhagen R. Association between HLA and red cell antigens. VIII. Haemagglutinins in another series of cytotoxic anti-HLA-A2 sera. *Vox Sang* 1978;**35**:375–7.

9 Nordhagen R. Association between HLA and red cell antigens. V. A further study of the nature and behaviour of the HLA antigens on red blood cells and their corresponding haemagglutinins. *Vox Sang* 1978;**35**: 49–57.

10 Nordhagen R. Association between HLA and red cell antigens. IV. Further studies of haemagglutinins in cytotoxic HLA antisera. *Vox Sang* 1977;**32**:82–9.

11 Crawford MN. *HLA and the red cell*. Monograph, Accugenics: 1983.

12 van der Hart M, Szaloky A, van den Berg-Loonen EM, Englefriet CP, van Loghem JJ. Présence d'antigènes HL-A sur les hématies d'un donneur normal. *Nouv Rev Franc Hémat* 1974;**14**:555–63.

13 Nordhagen R. Association between HLA and red cell antigens. VI. Family Studies. *Vox Sang* 1978;**35**:58–64.

14 Nordhagen R. Association between HL-A and red cell antigens. II. Absorption and titration analyses. *Vox Sang* 1974;**27**:124–33.

15 Nordhagen R. Association between HL-A and red cell antigens. III. Studies of haemagglutinins in cytotoxic anti-HL-A7 and anti-HL-A5 related sera. *Vox Sang* 1975;**29**:23–35.

16 Nordhagen R, Aas M. Association between HLA and red cell antigens. VII. Survival studies of incompatible red blood cells in a patient with HLA-associated haemagglutinins. *Vox Sang* 1978;**35**:319–23.

17 Nordhagen R. HLA antigens on red blood cells: two donors with extraordinarily strong reactivity. *Vox Sang* 1979;**37**:209–15.

18 Crawford MN, Pollack MS. Confirmation of Bg-HLA relationships by antiglobulin microcytotoxicity testing. *Transfusion* 1978;**18**:731–3.

19 Crawford MN, Schroeder ML. Bg^a and Bg^b correlations with HLA antigens by capillary tube technique. *Transfusion* 1980;**20**:594–6.

20 Rivera R, Scornik JC. HLA antigens on red cells. Implications for achieving low HLA antigen content in blood transfusions. *Transfusion* 1986;**26**:375–81.

21 Salama A, Mueller-Eckhardt G, Strauss B-E, Mueller-Eckhardt C. HLA-B7 on human red blood cells: improved detection by a radioactive anti-IgG test. *Tissue Antigens* 1982;**19**:183–8.

22 Botto M, So AK-L, Giles CM, Mason PD, Walport MJ. HLA class I expression on erythrocytes and platelets from patients with systemic lupus erythematosus, rheumatoid arthritis and from normal subjects. *Br J Haematol* 1990;**75**:106–11.

23 Giles CM, Walport MJ, David J, Darke C. Expression of MHC Class 1 determinants on erythrocytes of SLE patients. *Clin Exp Immunol* 1987;**69**:368–74.

24 Morton JA, Pickles MM, Darley JH. Increase in strength of red cell Bg^a antigen following infectious mononucleosis. *Vox Sang* 1977;**32**:27–37.

25 Morton JA, Pickles MM, Turner JE, Cullen PR. Changes in red cell Bg antigens in haematological disease. *Immunol Commun* 1980;**9**:173–90.

26 Giles CM, Botto M, King MJ. A study of HLA (Bg) on red cells and platelets by immunoblotting with monoclonal antibodies. *Transfusion* 1990;**30**:126–32.

27 Swanson JL. Laboratory problems associated with leukocyte antibodies. In: *A Seminar on Recent Advances in Immunohematology*. Arlington: American Association of Blood Banks, 1973: 121–55.

28 Swanson JL, Sastamoinen R. Chloroquine stripping of HLA A,B antigens from red cells. *Transfusion* 1985;**25**:439–40.

29 Harris R, Zervas JD. Reticulocyte HLA-antigens. *Nature* 1969;**221**:1062–3.

30 Brown G, Biberfeld P, Christensson B, Mason DY. The distribution of HLA on human lymphoid, bone marrow and peripheral blood cells. *Eur J Immunol* 1979;**9**:272–5.

31 Giles CM, Darke C, Rowe GP, Botto M. HLA Class 1 (Bg) antigens on red cells of SLE patients: a serological study with polyclonal and monoclonal antibodies. *Vox Sang* 1989;**56**:254–61.

32 Daniels G, Green C. Expression of red cell surface antigens during erythropoiesis. *Vox Sang* 2000;**78**(Suppl.1):149–53.

33 Krangel MS. Two forms of HLA Class I molecules in human plasma. *Hum Immunol* 1987;**20**:155–65.

34 Latoni GE, Benson K, Leparc GF, Agosti S. Hemolytic transfusion reaction due to autoantibodies with HLA specificity [Abstract]. *Transfusion* 1999;**39**:42S.

35 Panzer S, Mueller-Eckhardt G, Salama A *et al.* The clinical significance of HLA antigens on red cells: survival studies in HLA-sensitized individuals. *Transfusion* 1984;**24**:486–9.

36 Champagne K, Spruell P, Chen J, Voll L, Schlanser G. EDTA/glycine-acid versus chloroquine diphosphate treatment for stripping Bg antigens from red blood cells. *Immunohematology* 1999;**15**:66–8.

Polyagglutination and cryptantigens

31.1 Introduction

Polyagglutination was defined by Bird [1] as, 'The agglutination of red cells, irrespective of blood group, by many sera, the abnormality being a property of the red cells and not the sera.' Microbial polyagglutination generally results from the effect of bacterial or viral glycosidases revealing concealed antigenic determinants, called cryptantigens. These enzymes catalyse the cleavage of terminal monosaccharides or acetyl groups from the oligosaccharide chains of membrane glycoproteins or glycolipids. Polyagglutination occurs because of the presence of IgM antibodies against these cryptantigens present in the serum of most people; sera from those individuals with polyagglutinable red cells usually lack the corresponding antibody. Somatic mutation resulting in incomplete biosynthesis of oligosaccharides may lead to a more persistent expression of cryptantigen. Another type of polyagglutination arises from the inheritance of very rare antigens, which are detected by antibodies in most adult human sera. A classification of polyagglutination is provided in Table 31.1.

Lectins, non-immunoglobulin extracts from plants and occasionally animals, have proved invaluable in the identification and classification of cryptantigens and polyagglutination. Some of the most useful lectins are listed in Table 31.2 (for reviews on polyagglutination see [1,11–19]).

31.2 Acquired polyagglutination and the cryptantigens involved

31.2.1 Microbial polyagglutination

Microbial polyagglutination is associated with septicaemia, bowel or respiratory tract infections, wound infections, and conditions such as tumours or obstruc-

tions that compromise the integrity of the bowel wall and permit entry of microbial enzymes into the blood [12,16]. Occasionally microbial polyagglutination is detected in apparently healthy individuals, presumably because of subclinical infection or an undetected intestinal lesion [14]. Before microbial enzymes can modify red cell membrane structures they must be present in sufficient quantity to neutralize plasma enzyme inhibitors [12]. Cryptantigens are quite commonly detectable with lectins, but not with human sera, on the red cells of patients with various infections, sometimes before the infection has been diagnosed [12]. Microbial polyagglutination is usually transient, with the polyagglutinability of the cells diminishing as infection abates.

Red cells may also become polyagglutinable *in vitro*, either as a result of bacterial contamination of blood samples or by the use of enzymes isolated from microorganisms.

31.2.1.1 T polyagglutination

The Hübener–Thomsen–Friedenreich phenomenon [20] or T activation of red cells results from microbial sialidases catalysing the cleavage of sialic acid residues from the O-linked disialotetrasaccharides of the major red cell sialoglycoproteins, glycophorins A and B, and from other glycoproteins and glycolipids. The T determinant is basically terminal D-galactose in β1,3 linkage with N-acetylgalactosamine (Table 31.3 and see Chapter 3). T exposure causes depression of M and N antigens [17] and the reduction in cell surface charge makes T-active cells agglutinable by *Glycine soja* lectin [8]. Sialidases from bacteria such as *Clostridium perfringens*, *Vibrio cholerae*, and pneumococci, and from the influenza virus, have all been responsible for *in vivo* T cryptantigen exposure. T activation is more common in infants than in adults and is particularly associated with paediatric intestinal disorders [21,22]. Bird [13] has listed many of the published examples of T transformation.

In 1964, Bird [2] found that extracts of peanuts, *Arachis hypogaea*, made a powerful anti-T lectin. The term 'peanut-positive polyagglutination' now refers to the exposure of any of five cryptantigens, T, Tk, Th, Tx, or Tr, that bind *Arachis hypogaea* lectin (Table 31.2). Red cells of 52 (0.5%) of 9672 hospital patients were agglutinated by *Arachis hypogaea* lectin, but in only one patient were the cells polyagglutinable [23]. Monoclonal antibodies with T specificity have been produced following the immunization of rodents with desialylated red cells [24–26] or with synthetic glyco-conjugates [27,28]. Some monoclonal anti-Le^a cross-react with T-activated Le(a–) red cells [29].

T polyagglutination is occasionally accompanied by haemolysis [30]. Whether this is caused by complement fixing anti-T in the patient's serum or by an effect of the associated infection is unclear. Haemolytic uraemic syndrome in children following pneumococcal infection may be caused by the effect of bacterial sialidase; T activation of red cells, platelets, and renal glomeruli could be responsible for the characteristic symptoms of haemolytic anaemia, thrombocytopenia, and renal failure [31,32]. Transfusion of plasma or whole blood containing anti-T has been implicated as a cause of severe haemolytic reactions in infants with necrotizing enterocolitis and T-activated red cells, although this complication is rare [30,33].

Leucocytes and platelets of individuals with T-polyagglutinable red cells also express T antigen [34].

31.2.1.2 Th polyagglutination

Th polyagglutination, first reported by Bird *et al.* [35] in 1978, is distinguished from T polyagglutination by the use of lectins (Table 31.2) and probably represents a weak expression or early stage of T activation [36]. Sialidase from *Corynebacterium aquaticum* is responsible for Th activation [36]. Sialidases from *Vibrio cholerae*, when used under conditions of particularly mild hydrolysis, will also produce Th activity *in vitro*. Release of sialic acid below a critical quantity (20 μg per 10^{10} red cells) leads to Th activity, whereas libera-

Table 31.1 Classification of polyagglutination.

Acquired
Microbial
Cryptantigens uncovered by microbial enzymes
 T, Tk, Th, Tx, Acquired B
Adsorption of bacteria or bacterial products onto cell surface
Non-microbial (persistent)
Biosynthetic blockage caused by somatic mutation
 Tn, ?Th

Inherited
Sd(a++) (Cad), HEMPAS, NOR, Hyde Park

Undetermined
VA, Tr

Table 31.2 Reactions of lectins with cryptantigens and with Sd(a++) and Hyde Park polyagglutinable cells.

Lectins	T	Th	Tk	Tx	Tn	Sd(a++)	Hyde Park	Tr	Reference
Arachis hypogaea	+	+	+	+	–	–	w	+	[2]
Vicia hyrcanica	+	+	+		–	–	+		[3]
Vicia cretica	+	+	–	–	–	–	w		[4]
Vicia villosa	+	–	–	–	+	+	+	+	[5]
Griffonia simplicifolia (GSII)	–	–	+	–	–	–	+	+	[6]
Medicago disciformis	+	+	–	–	–		+		[7]
Dolichos biflorus (B and O only)	–	–	–	–	+	+	–	–	[8]
Salvia sclarea	–	–	–	–	+	–	–	+	[9]
Salvia horminum	–	–	–	–	+	+	w	+	[9]
Leonurus cardiaca	w	–	–	–	–	+	–		[10]
Glycine soja	+	–	–	–	+	+	+/–		[8]

w, weak agglutination.
+/–, reactive with strong examples only.

tion of greater quantities of sialic acid results in T polyagglutinability [36]. It is possible that Th activity represents the removal of only one sialic acid residue from the tetrasaccharide shown in Table 31.3, exposing terminal galactose, but not the T disaccharide (Galβ1→3GalNAc).

Red cells from 22 of 200 cord samples were Th activated (but not polyagglutinable); in six of these the mother's red cells were also Th active [37]. A patient with Th polyagglutination and peritonitis from a perforated colonic tumour died as a result of severe intravascular haemolysis [38].

It is possible that a persistent form of Th polyagglutination resulting from incomplete biosynthesis also occurs. Persistent Th activation in the absence of infection was identified in five of seven children with congenital hypoplastic anaemia [39], and in a patient with myelodysplasia whose red cells were also Tn active [40].

31.2.1.3 Tk polyagglutination

Tk polyagglutination [41] is most readily distinguished from T polyagglutination by the use of GSII, a Tk-specific lectin isolated from the seeds of *Griffonia simplicifolia* (previously *Bandeiraea simplicifolia*) [6]. Expression of Tk is enhanced by papain treatment and Tk-activated cells are not sialic acid-deficient [41]. *Vicia hyrcanica* seeds contain separable T- and Tk-specific lectins [3]. Monoclonal anti-Tk has been produced by immunizing mice with endo-β-galactosidase-modified red cells [42].

Tk polyagglutination is usually associated with

Table 31.3 O-linked oligosaccharides of sialoglycoproteins from normal red cells and from T- and Tn-activated cells. See Table 2.4 for abbreviations.

Normal	NeuAcα2→3Galβ1→3GalNAc—Ser/Thr
	6
	↑
	NeuAcα2
T	Galβ1→3GalNAc—Ser/Thr
Tn	GalNAc—Ser/Thr
Sialyl-Tn	GalNAc—Ser/Thr
	6
	↑
	NeuAcα2

Bacteroides fragilis infection [43], but *Serratia marcescens*, *Candida albicans*, and *Aspergillus niger* have also been responsible [14,15]. Endo- and exo-β-galactosidases secreted by these pathogens cleave oligosaccharides at Galβ1→4GlcNAc linkages on ABH and Ii active blood group substances (Tables 2.3, 2.5, and 25.2) exposing terminal N-acetylglucosamine residues, the Tk receptor [44–46]. Tk-transformed red cells may have reduced expression of ABH and Ii antigens [47,48]. GSII lectin is inhibited by N-acetylglucosamine [6,49] and monoclonal anti-Tk was adsorbed by GlcNAcβ1→3Galβ1→4Glcβ–R coupled to silica beads [42]. Endo-β-galactosidases from *B. fragilis*, *Escherichia freundii*, and *Flavobacterium keratolycus* have been used to produce Tk-activated red cells *in vitro* [42,46,50].

Tk polyagglutination is often associated with acquired B polyagglutination (Section 31.2.1.5).

31.2.1.4 Tx cryptantigen

Tx was identified by Bird *et al.* [51] on the red cells of children with pneumococcal infections and could be produced, *in vitro*, by the action on red cells of culture supernatant from pneumococci derived from these patients. Tx is distinguished from T by *Vicia cretica* lectin (Table 31.2). Tx is only slightly weakened by papain treatment [51]. A persistent form of Tx polyagglutination was detected over a period of 5 years in a woman with myelodysplastic syndrome and no symptoms of infection [52].

31.2.1.5 Acquired B

Acquired B phenomenon is described in detail in Section 2.14.1. It is caused by microbial deacetylases converting N-acetylgalactosamine of an A determinant to galactosamine, which resembles galactose closely enough for the cells to be agglutinated by some anti-B reagents. Acquired B is usually associated with a unique polyagglutination, but is often also associated with Tk, and occasionally T or Th, polyagglutination.

31.2.2 Non-microbial polyagglutination

31.2.2.1 Tn polyagglutination

In Tn polyagglutination, otherwise known as persistent mixed-field polyagglutination, only a proportion of the red cells are polyagglutinable [53,54]: between 30% and 90% are agglutinated by anti-Tn, the remainder are Tn-negative [11]. Like T, Tn is located on O-linked oligosaccharides of red cell glycoproteins, chiefly glycophorins A and B [55]. The Tn determinant is N-acetylgalactosamine attached to serine or threonine (Table 31.3) [55–57]. The N-acetylgalactosamine residue is sometimes sialylated, to form sialyl-Tn (Table 31.3) [58].

Tn is exposed because of defective oligosaccharide biosynthesis resulting from somatic mutation [59,60], not by degradation of the oligosaccharide by microbial enzymes. Tn is the biosynthetic precursor of T, which is a precursor of the disialotetrasaccharide typical of red cell sialoglycoproteins (Table 31.3). In Tn-polyagglutinable cells, conversion of the Tn monosaccharide to the T disaccharide does not occur because of deficiency of T transferase, a β-3-D-galactosyltransferase [61,62]. This enzyme deficiency arises from a somatic mutation within a pluripotent haemopoietic stem cell and subsequent clonal expansion and proliferation of populations of Tn+ red cells, platelets, granulocytes, and lymphocytes [63–65]. Tn-active red cells are not totally deficient in T transferase as some normal tetrasaccharides are present on the glycophorin molecules [66].

Tn-active red cells have depressed M and N antigens and T cryptantigen [56,67,68], and they have reduced sialic acid content [55,69]. Tn is destroyed by papain treatment of red cells [69,70].

The immunodominant monosaccharide of Tn is N-acetylgalactosamine, so it is not surprising that Tn-activated red cells are agglutinated by lectins that also agglutinate group A cells, such as *Dolichos biflorus* and *Helix pomatia* [59,69,70]. *Salvia sclarea* lectin is more specific for Tn (Table 31.2) [9]. Tn cells are more strongly agglutinated by human sera containing anti-A than those lacking it [69]. Many murine monoclonal Tn antibodies have been produced [26,27,58, 71–78], some of which cross-react with sialyl-Tn [78]. It should be remembered that all of these anti-Tn reagents, like the anti-Tn present in the serum of most adults, react only with the Tn+ population of cells, giving the characteristic mixed-field pattern of agglutination with red cells of individuals with Tn polyagglutination.

Tn polyagglutination is often associated with haemolytic anaemia, leucopenia, and thrombocytopenia [16,30] and, on occasion, is detected in healthy blood donors [16,69,79]. Although usually persistent, Tn polyagglutination has been known to recede [60]. There are three reports of transient Tn polyagglutination in newborn babies, possibly because of a late development of full T transferase activity [80–82]. Flow cytometry with monoclonal anti-Tn revealed less than 1×10^{-6} Tn red cells in the peripheral blood of healthy donors [76].

Reports of patients with Tn polyagglutination and concurrent acute myeloid leukaemia [60,83,84], or who subsequently developed leukaemia, led Ness *et al.* [83] to propose that Tn polyagglutination may represent a preleukaemic state and that careful clinical observation of individuals with Tn polyagglutination would be circumspect. Polyagglutination vanished during chemotherapy [60,83]. Tn-active cells were detected in five of 725 abnormal bone marrow aspirates: two in patients with new acute leukaemia and two in patients whose disease terminated in acute leukaemia [85]. Tn cells were detected in bone marrow 8–12 months before polyagglutination was apparent in peripheral blood. In some patients with acute leukaemia, the number of Tn-active red cells and granulocytes in the peripheral blood and in erythroid and granulocyte precursors in the marrow increased as the disease progressed [72,85]. Tn polyagglutination has also been associated with myelodysplasia [40,79].

31.2.3 T, Tn, and Tk in malignancy

T and Tn are cryptantigens on epithelial tissues, in the carbohydrate chains of glycoprotein and glycolipids. Springer and others have shown that T and Tn are exposed on about 90% of primary and metastatic carcinomas, probably as a result of incomplete biosynthesis [86]. Sialyl-Tn is also often expressed in carcinomas, although it also occurs in healthy tissue. Increased density of Tn over T is an indicator of high metastatic potential of the tumour. A correlation between malignancy and depression in titre of circulating anti-T has led to the development of diagnostic tests. Immunotherapy with a vaccine derived from T- and Tn-activated red cells has been successful in preventing recurrence of breast cancer and has a potential for wider application. This whole topic is thoroughly reviewed by Desai [87].

Monoclonal anti-Tk reacted with 48% of human colorectal carcinomas [42]. Vaccination of rats with

Tk-active red cells provided protection against growth of Tk+, but not Tk–, tumours.

31.3 Inherited polyagglutination

31.3.1 Sd(a++) (Cad)

Sd^a is a red cell antigen of incidence about 91% and of variable strength. Red cells of the very rare individuals with an extra strong form of Sd^a antigen (referred to as Sd(a++) or Cad) are polyagglutinable. The immunodominant structure of Sd^a is N-acetyl-D-galactosamine in β-linkage with galactose. Sd(a++) cells are agglutinated by *Dolichos biflorus* and *Helix pomatia* lectins, but can be distinguished from Tn cells by *Salvia sclarea* and *Leonurus cardiaca* (Table 31.2). Sd^a and Sd(a++) are described in detail in Chapter 29.

31.3.2 Congenital dyserythropoietic anaemia type II (HEMPAS)

Red cells of patients with the rare autosomal recessive syndrome, congenital dyserythropoietic anaemia type II (CDA II or hereditary erythroblastic multinuclearity with a positive acidified serum lysis test, HEMPAS) are agglutinated at 20°C, or lysed at 37°C, by complement fixing IgM antibodies in about one-third of normal sera [88,89]. CDA II cells have elevated i and depressed H antigens [88–91]. Over 250 cases of CDA II are reported, many involving patients of southern Italian ancestry [92].

The biochemical defects in CDA II may be abnormalities in N-acetylglucosaminyltransferase II or α-mannosidase II, giving rise to branching anomalies in the complex N-glycans of glycoproteins, particularly bands 3 and 4.5 (glucose transporter), which contain repeating N-acetyllactosamine units [93,94]. This reveals a cryptantigen responsible for the polyagglutination and abnormal complement activation, and also results in excess production of i-active linear N-acetyllactosaminylceramides. A defect in transcription factors regulating the genes encoding these enzymes might be responsible. A putative disease gene, CDAN2, has been localized to chromosome 20q11.2 by linkage to microsatellite markers in Italian families [95]. An Irish CDA II patient, however, was doubly heterozygous for splice site mutations in MII, a gene encoding an N-glycan processing enzyme and a British patient had very low levels of MII transcript [96]. CDA II is reviewed in [92,96].

31.3.3 NOR polyagglutination

NOR is a form of polyagglutination, found in two families, that appears to be inherited in a dominant manner [97,98]. Red cells of a total of nine individuals from two generations of each of the families were agglutinated by IgM antibody in 71–75% of ABO compatible adult sera, but were not agglutinated by cord sera. The reaction of NOR cells with human sera was enhanced by papain and sialidase, but reduced by α-galactosidase treatment of the cells. NOR polyagglutination was completely inhibited by hydatid cyst fluid and avian P1 substance, but NOR red cells had normal expression of P1 and P antigens. Thin-layer chromatographs of glycolipids from NOR cells revealed one major and several minor additional bands, compared with control cells, when stained with lectins specific for galactose (*Ricinus communis* I) and Galα1→3Gal (*Griffonia simpicifolia* IB4) [98]. NOR red cells appear to contain neutral glycolipids with an abnormal oligosaccharide structure, which probably terminates with α-galactosyl residues, shared with the P1 structure [98].

31.3.4 Hyde Park polyagglutination

Polyagglutination associated with a rare haemoglobin variant in a large South African family of mixed ethnicity remains a puzzle. Thirty-five members of the family were studied: 12 had the variant haemoglobin M-Hyde Park and polyagglutinable red cells; 23 had neither [99]. Polyagglutination had not been observed previously in association with haemoglobin M-Hyde Park. The name 'Hyde Park' was suggested for the polyagglutination.

Group O, N+ Hyde Park cells show the following serological characteristics [99,100]:

1 agglutination with a minority of normal human sera (7 of 40);

2 enhanced agglutination with *Vicia graminea* and *Ulex europaeus* lectins and with human anti-I and -i, but normal strength agglutination with rabbit and monoclonal anti-N;

3 agglutination by monoclonal anti-Tn, but not by Tn-specific *Salvia sclarea* lectin;

4 agglutination by *Glycine soja*, *Sophora japonica*,

and *Arachis hypogaea* (weakly), lectins that detect de-sialylated *O*-glycans; and

5 agglutination by the *N*-acetylglucosamine-specific lectins *Vicia hyrcanica* and GSII (weakly) (Table 31.2).

These serological characteristics, together with results of biochemical analyses, suggest that the polyagglutination is caused by two unrelated anomalies, one associated with heterogeneity of sialylation of the *O*-glycans of glycophorin molecules and the other associated with exposed *N*-acetylglucosamine residues on the *N*-glycans of bands 3 and 4.5 (glucose transporter) [100]. The nature of the relationship between these aberrations of glycosylation and the abnormal haemoglobin is obscure.

31.4 Polyagglutination of undetermined status

31.4.1 VA polyagglutination

VA polyagglutination is very rare. The red cells are not agglutinated by *Arachis hypogaea* or *Dolichos biflorus* lectins, but give a mixed-field agglutination with *Helix pomatia* lectin [101,102]; they also give a characteristic stippled appearance in immunofluorescence with *H. pomatia* lectin [102]. An associated depression of H antigen has led to the suggestion that microbial α-fucosidase could be responsible for VA exposure [101,103]. In the original case described by Graninger *et al.* [101,102], VA polyagglutination was persistent and associated with haemolytic anaemia. In the only other reported example, VA-active red cells were also Tk active [103].

31.4.2 Tr polyagglutination

Tr polyagglutination has been found in one individual [104]. Tr red cells gave a unique pattern of reactions with a panel of lectins (Table 31.2) and reacted with monoclonal anti-T+Tn and -Tk. Results of tests with lectins, reduced periodic acid–Schiff staining of glycophorins A, B, and C, and increased electrophoretic mobility of band 3 suggested a reduction in sialylation of both *N*- and *O*-glycans, exposing $\beta 1 \rightarrow 4$Gal and $\beta 1 \rightarrow 3$Gal residues. Reid *et al.* [104] suggested that Tr might result from a defective glycosyltransferase, probably an $\alpha 1,6$-sialyltransferase.

References

1 Bird GWG. Complexity of erythrocyte polyagglutinabiliy. In: JF Mohn, RW Plunkett, RK Cunningham, RM Lambert, eds. *Human Blood Groups, 5th Int Convoc Immunol, Buffalo NY.* Basel: Karger, 1977:335–43.

2 Bird GWG. Anti-T in peanuts. *Vox Sang* 1964;9:748–9.

3 Liew YW, Bird GWG. Separable anti-T and anti-Tk lectins from the seeds of *Vicia hyrcanica. Vox Sang* 1988;54:226–7.

4 Bird GWG, Wingham J. *Vicia cretica*: a powerful lectin for T- and Th- but not Tk- or other polyagglutinable erythrocytes. *J Clin Pathol* 1981;34:69–70.

5 Bird GWG, Wingham J. Lectins for polyagglutinable red cells: *Cytisus scoparius, Spartium junceum* and *Vicia villosa. Clin Lab Haematol* 1980;2:21–3.

6 Judd WJ, Beck ML, Hicklin BL, Shankar Iyer PN, Goldstein IJ. BSII lectin: a second hemagglutinin isolated from *Bandeiraea simplicifolia* seeds with affinity for type III polyagglutinable red cells. *Vox Sang* 1977; 33:246–51.

7 Bird GWG, Wingham J. 'New' lectins for the identification of erythrocyte cryptantigens and the classification of erythrocyte polyagglutinability: *Medicago disciformis* and *Medicago turbinata. J Clin Pathol* 1983; 36:195–6.

8 Bird GWG. Lectins in immunohematology. *Transfus Med Rev* 1989;3:55–62.

9 Bird GWG, Wingham J. Haemagglutinins from *Salvia. Vox Sang* 1974;26:163–6.

10 Bird GWG, Wingham J. Anti-Cad lectin from the seeds of *Leonurus cardiaca. Clin Lab Haematol* 1979;1:57–9.

11 Levene C, Levene NA, Buskila D, Manny N. Red cell polyagglutination. *Transfus Med Rev* 1988;2:176–85.

12 Bird GWG. Clinical aspects of red blood cell polyagglutinability of microbial origin. In: C Salmon, ed. *Blood Groups and Other Red Cell Surface Markers in Health and Disease.* New York: Masson, 1982:55–64.

13 Bird GWG. Erythrocyte polyagglutination. In: TJ Greenwalt, EA Steane, eds. *CRC Handbook Series in Clinical Laboratory Science. Section D. Blood Banking*, Vol. 1. Cleveland: CRC Press, 1977:443–54.

14 Judd WJ. Microbial-associated forms of polyagglutination (T, Tk and acquired-B). In: ML Beck, WJ Judd, eds. *Polyagglutination: a Technical Workshop.* Arlington: American Association of Blood Banks, 1980:23–53.

15 Judd WJ. Review: polyagglutination. *Immunohematology* 1992;8:58–69.

16 Beck ML. Blood group antigens acquired *de novo*. In: G Garratty, ed. *Blood Group Antigens and Disease.* Arlington: American Association of Blood Banks, 1983:45–65.

17 Vaith P, Uhlenbruck G. The Thomsen agglutination phenomenon: a discovery revisited 50 years later. *Z Immun-Forsch* 1978;154:1–14.

18 Horn KD. The classification, recognition and signifi-

cance of polyagglutination in transfusion medicine. *Blood Rev* 1999;13:36–44.

19 Beck ML. Red blood cell polyagglutination: clinical aspects. *Semin Hematol* 2000;37:186–96.

20 Friedenreich V. *The Thomsen Hemagglutination Phenomenon*. Copenhagen: Levin and Munksgaard, 1930.

21 Seger R, Joller P, Bird GWG *et al*. Necrotising enterocolitis and neuraminidase-producing bacteria. *Helv Paediatr Acta* 1980;35:121–8.

22 Seger RA, Kenny A, Bird GWG *et al*. Pediatric surgical patients with severe anaerobic infection: report of 16 T-antigen positive cases and possible hazards of blood transfusion. *J Pediatr Surg* 1981;16:905–10.

23 Rawlinson VI, Stratton F. Incidence of T activation in a hospital population. *Vox Sang* 1984;46:306–17.

24 Rahman AFR, Longenecker BM. A monoclonal antibody specific for the Thomsen–Freidenreich cryptic T antigen. *J Immunol* 1982;129:2021–4.

25 Seitz R, Fischer K, Poschmann A. Differentiation of red cell membrane abnormalities causing T-polyagglutination by use of monoclonal antibodies. *Rev Franc Transfus Immuno-Hémat* 1983;26:420.

26 Metcalfe S, Springer GF, Svvennsen RJ, Tegtmeyer H. Monoclonal antibodies specific for human Thomsen–Freidenreich (T) and Tn blood group precursor antigens. *Prot Biol Fluids* 1985;32:765–8.

27 Longenecker BM, Willans DJ, Maclean GD *et al*. Monoclonal antibodies and synthetic tumor-associated glycoconjugates in the study of the expression of Thomsen–Freidenreich-like and Tn-like antigens on human cancers. *J Natl Cancer Inst* 1987;78:489–92.

28 Clausen H, Stroud M, Parker J, Springer G, Hakomori S. Monoclonal antibodies directed to the blood group A associated structure, galactosyl-A: specificity and relation to the Thomsen–Freidenreich antigen. *Mol Immunol* 1988;25:199–204.

29 Písacka M, Stambergová M. Activation of Thomsen–Freidenreich antigen on red cells: a possible source of errors in antigen typing with some monoclonal antibodies. *Vox Sang* 1994;66:300.

30 Mollison PL, Engelfriet CP, Contreras M. *Blood Transfusion in Clinical Medicine*, 10th edn. Oxford: Blackwell Science, 1997.

31 Klein PJ, Bulla M, Newman RA *et al*. Thomsen–Freidenreich antigen in hæmolytic uræmic syndrome. *Lancet* 1977;ii:1024–5.

32 Seger R, Joller P, Baerlocher K *et al*. Hemolytic uremic syndrome associated with neuraminidase-producing microorganisms: treatment by exchange transfusion. *Helv Paediatr Acta* 1980;35:359–67.

33 Engelfriet CP, Reesink HW, Strauss RG *et al*. Blood transfusion in premature or young infants with polyagglutination and activation of the T antigen. *Vox Sang* 1999;76:128–32.

34 Hysell JK, Hysell JW, Nichols ME, Leonardi RG, Marsh WL. *In vivo* and *in vitro* activation of T-antigen recep-

tors on leukocytes and platelets. *Vox Sang* 1976;31(Suppl.1):9–15.

35 Bird GWG, Wingham J, Beck ML *et al*. Th, a 'new' form of erythrocyte polyagglutination. *Lancet* 1978;i:1215–16.

36 Sondag-Thull D, Levene NA, Levene C *et al*. Characterization of a neuraminidase from *Corynebacterium aquaticum* responsible for Th polyagglutination. *Vox Sang* 1989;57:193–8.

37 Wahl CM, Herman JH, Shirey RS, Kickler TS, Ness PM. Th activation of maternal and cord blood. *Transfusion* 1989;29:635–7.

38 Levene NA, Levene C, Gekker K *et al*. Th polyagglutination with fatal outcome in a patient with massive intravascular hemolysis and perforated tumour of colon. *Am J Hematol* 1990;35:127–8.

39 Herman JH, Shirey RS, Smith B, Kickler TS, Ness PM. Th activation in congenital hypoplastic anemia. *Transfusion* 1987;27:253–6.

40 Janvier D, Guignier F, Reviron M, Benbunan M. Concomitant exposure of Tn and Th cryptantigens on the red cells of a patient with myelodysplasia. *Vox Sang* 1991;61:142–3.

41 Bird GWG, Wingham J. Tk: a new form of red cell polyagglutination. *Br J Haematol* 1972;23:759–63.

42 Meichenin M, Rocher J, Galanina O *et al*. Tk, a new colon tumor-associated antigen resulting from altered O-glycosylation. *Cancer Res* 2000;60:5499–507.

43 Inglis G, Bird GWG, Mitchell AAB, Milne GR, Wingham J. Effect of *Bacteroides fragilis* on the human erythrocyte membrane: pathogenesis of Tk polyagglutination. *J Clin Pathol* 1975;28:964–8.

44 Doinel C, Andreu G, Cartron JP, Salmon C, Fukuda MN. Tk polyagglutination produced *in vitro* by an endo-beta-galactosidase. *Vox Sang* 1980;38:94–8.

45 Judd WJ. The role of exo-β-galactosidases in Tk-activation [Abstract]. *Transfusion* 1980;20:622.

46 Doinel C, Rufin JM, Andreu G. The Tk antigenic determinant studies of Tk-activated red blood cells with endoglycosidases. *Rev Franc Transfus Immuno-Hémat* 1981;24:109–16.

47 Inglis G, Bird GWG, Mitchell AAB, Wingham J. Tk polyagglutination associated with reduced A and H activity. *Vox Sang* 1978;35:370–4.

48 Andreu G, Doinel C, Cartron JP, Mativet S. Induction of Tk polyagglutination by *Bacteroides fragilis* culture supernatants: associated modifications of ABH and Ii antigens. *Rev Franc Transfus Immuno-Hémat* 1979;22:551–61.

49 Iyer PNS, Wilkinson KD, Goldstein IJ. An *N*-acetyl-D-glucosamine binding lectin from *Bandeiraea simplicifolia* seeds. *Arch Biochem Biophys* 1976;177:330–3.

50 Liew YW, Bird GWG, King MJ. The human erythrocyte cryptantigen Tk: exposure by an endo-beta-galactosidase from *Flavobacterium keratolycus*. *Rev Franc Transfus Immuno-Hémat* 1982;25:639–41.

51 Bird GWG, Wingham J, Seger R, Kenny AB. Tx, a 'new' red cell cryptantigen exposed by pneumococcal enzymes. *Rev Franc Transfus Immuno-Hémat* 1982;**25**:215–16.

52 Pisacka M, Karasova R, Prosicka M, Cermak J. Two cases of erythrocyte cryptantigen reactive with Arachis hypogaea in association with myelodysplastic syndrome [Abstract]. *VI Reg Eur Congr Int Soc Blood Transfus*, 1999:81.

53 Moreau R, Dausset J, Bernard J, Moullec J. Anémie hémolytique acquise avec polyagglutinabilitédes hématies par un nouveau facteur présent dans le sérum humain normal (anti-Tn). *Bull Mémoires Soc Med Hôp Paris*, 1957;**20 and 21**:569–87.

54 Dausset J, Moullec J, Bernard J. Acquired hemolytic anemia with polyagglutinability of red blood cells due to a new factor present in normal human serum (anti-Tn). *Blood* 1959;**14**:1079–93.

55 Dahr W, Uhlenbruck G, Gunson HH, van der Hart M. Molecular basis of Tn-polyagglutinability. *Vox Sang* 1975;**29**:36–50.

56 Sturgeon P, Luner SJ, Mcquiston DT. Permanent mixed-field polyagglutinability (PMFP). II. Hematological, biophysical and biochemical observations. *Vox Sang* 1973;**25**:498–512.

57 Dahr W, Uhlenbruck G, Bird GWG. Cryptic A-like receptor sites in human erythrocyte glycoproteins: proposed nature of Tn-antigen. *Vox Sang* 1974;**27**:29–42.

58 Kjeldsen T, Hakomori S, Springer GF *et al.* Coexpression of sialosyl-Tn (NeuAcα2→6GalNAcα1→O-Ser/Thr) and Tn (GalNAcα1→O-Ser/Thr) blood group antigens on Tn erythrocytes. *Vox Sang* 1989;**57**:81–7.

59 Bird GWG, Shinton NK, Wingham J. Persistent mixed-field polyagglutination. *Br J Haematol* 1971;**21**: 443–53.

60 Bird GWG, Wingham J, Pippard MJ, Hoult JG, Melikian V. Erythrocyte membrane modification in malignant diseases of myeloid and lymphoreticular tissues. *Br J Haematol* 1976;**33**:289–94.

61 Cartron J-P, Andreu G, Cartron J *et al.* Demonstration of T-transferase deficiency in Tn-polyagglutinable blood samples. *Eur J Biochem* 1978;**92**:111–19.

62 Berger EG, Kozdrowski I. Permanent mixed-field polyagglutinable erythrocytes lack galactosyltransferase activity. *FEBS Lett* 1978;**93**:105–8.

63 Cartron JP, Nurden AT. Galactosyltransferase and membrane glycoprotein abnormality in human platelets from Tn syndrome donors. *Nature* 1979;**282**:621–3.

64 Vainchenker W, Testa U, Deschamps JF *et al.* Clonal expression of the Tn antigen in erythroid and granulocyte colonies and its application to determination of the clonality of the human megakaryocyte colony assay. *J Clin Invest* 1982;**69**:1081–91.

65 Brouet J-C, Vainchenker W, Blanchard D, Testa U, Cartron J-P. The origin of human B and T cells from multipotent stem cells. *Eur J Immunol* 1983;**13**:350–2.

66 Blumenfeld OO, Lalezari P, Khorshidi M, Puglia K, Fukuda M. O-linked oligosaccharides of glycophorins A and B in erythrocytes of two individuals with the Tn polyagglutinability syndrome. *Blood* 1992;**80**: 2388–95.

67 Sturgeon P, Mcquiston DT, Taswell HF, Allan CJ. Permanent mixed-field polyagglutinability (PMFP). I. Serological observations. *Vox Sang* 1973;**25**:481–97.

68 Bird GWG, Wingham J. The M, N and N_{Vg} receptors of Tn-erythrocytes. *Vox Sang* 1974;**26**:171–5.

69 Mylleylä G, Furuhjelm U, Nordling S *et al.* Persistent mixed field polyagglutinability: electrokinetic and serological aspects. *Vox Sang* 1971;**20**:7–23.

70 Gunson HH, Stratton F, Mullard GW. An example of polyagglutinability due to the Tn antigen. *Br J Haematol* 1970;**18**:309–16.

71 Hirohashi S, Clausen H, Yamada T, Shimosato Y, Hakomori S. Blood group A cross-reacting epitope defined by monoclonal antibodies NCC-LU-35 and -81 expressed in cancer of blood group O or B individuals: its identification as Tn antigen. *Proc Natl Acad Sci USA* 1985;**82**:7039–43.

72 Roxby DJ, Morley AA, Burpee M. Detection of the Tn antigen in leukaemia using monoclonal anti-Tn antibody and immunohistochemistry. *Br J Haematol* 1987;**67**:153–6.

73 Springer GF, Chandrasekaran EV, Desai PR, Tegtmeyer H. Blood group Tn-active macromolecules from human carcinomas and erythrocytes: characterization of and specific reactivity with mono- and poly-clonal anti-Tn antibodies induced by various immunogens. *Carbohydr Res* 1988;**178**:271–92.

74 Takahashi HK, Metoki R, Hakomori S. Immunoglobulin G3 monoclonal antibody directed to Tn antigen (tumor-associated α-N-acetylgalastosaminyl epitope) that does not cross-react with blood group A antigen. *Cancer Res* 1988;**48**:4361–7.

75 Numata Y, Nakada H, Fukui S *et al.* A monoclonal antibody directed to Tn antigen. *Biochem Biophys Res Commun* 1990;**170**:981–5.

76 Bigbee WL, Langlois RG, Stanker LH, Vanderlaan M, Jensen RH. Flow cytometric analysis of erythrocyte populations in Tn syndrome blood using monoclonal antibodies to glycophorin A and the Tn antigen. *Cytometry* 1990;**11**:261–71.

77 King MJ, Parsons SF, Wu AM, Jones N. Immunochemical studies on the differential binding properties of two monoclonal antibodies reacting with Tn red cells. *Transfusion* 1991;**31**:142–9.

78 O'Boyle KP, Markowitz AL, Khorshidi M *et al.* Specificity analysis of murine monoclonal antibodies reactive with Tn, sialylated Tn, T, and monosialylated (2→6) T antigens. *Hybridoma* 1996;**15**:401–8.

79 Bird GWG, Wingham J, Richardson SGN. Myelofibrosis, autoimmune haemolytic anaemia and Tn-polyagglutinability. *Haematologia* 1985;**18**:99–103.

531

80 Wilson MJ, Cott ME, Sotus PC. Probable Tn-activation *in utero* [Abstract]. *Transfusion* 1980;**20**:622.

81 Schultz M, Fortes P, Brewer L, Miller A, Beck M. '*In utero*' exposure of Tn and Th cryptantigens [Abstract]. *Transfusion* 1983;**23**:422.

82 Rose RR, Skradski KJ, Polesky HF *et al.* Transient neonatal Tn-activation: another example [Abstract]. *Transfusion* 1983;**23**:422.

83 Ness PM, Garratty G, Morel PA, Perkins HA. Tn polyagglutination preceding acute leukemia. *Blood* 1979;**54**:30–4.

84 Baldwin ML, Barrasso C, Ridolfi RL. Tn-polyagglutinability associated with acute myelomonocytic leukemia. *Am J Clin Pathol* 1979;**72**:1024–7.

85 Roxby DJ, Pfeiffer MB, Morley AA, Kirkland MA. Expression of Tn antigen in myelodysplasia, lymphoma, and leukemia. *Transfusion* 1992;**32**:834–8.

86 Springer GF. T and Tn, general carcinoma autoantigens. *Science* 1984;**224**:1198–206.

87 Desai PR. Immunoreactive T and Tn antigens in malignancy: role in carcinoma diagnosis, prognosis, and immmunotherapy. *Transfus Med Rev* 2000;**14**:312–25.

88 Crookston JH, Crookston MC, Burnie KL *et al.* Hereditary erythroblastic multinuclearity associated with a positive acidified-serum test: a type of congenital dyserythropoietic anaemia. *Br J Haematol* 1969;**17**:11–26.

89 Crookston JH, Crookston MC, Rosse WF. Red-cell abnormalities in HEMPAS (hereditary erythroblastic multinuclearity with a positive acidified-serum test). *Br J Haematol* 1972;**23**(Suppl.): 83–91.

90 Bird GWG, Wingham J. The action of seed and other reagents on HEMPAS erythrocytes. *Acta Haematol* 1976;**55**:174–80.

91 Rochant H, Gerbal A. Polyagglutinabilité due à l'antigène Hempas. *Rev Franc Transfus Immuno-Hémat* 1976;**14**:239–45.

92 Wickramasinghe SN. Congenital dyserythropoietic anemias. *Curr Opin Hematol* 2000;**7**:71–8.

93 Fukuda MN. Hempas disease: genetic defect of glycosylation. *Glycobiology* 1990;**1**:9–15.

94 Fukuda MN, Masri KA, Dell A, Luzzatto L, Moremen KW. Incomplete synthesis of N-glycans in congenital dyserythropoietic anemia type II caused by a defect in the gene encoding α-mannosidase II. *Proc Natl Acad Sci USA* 1990;**87**:7443–7.

95 Gasparini P, Miraglia del Giudice E, Delaunay J *et al.* Localization of the congenital dyserythropoietic anemia II locus to chromosome 20q11.2 by genomewide search. *Am J Hum Genet* 1997;**61**:1112–16.

96 Fukuda MN. HEMPAS. *Biochim Biophys Acta* 1999; **1455**:231–9.

97 Harris PA, Roman GK, Moulds JJ, Bird GWG, Shah NG. An inherited RBC characteristic, NOR, resulting in erythrocyte polyagglutination. *Vox Sang* 1982;**42**: 134–40.

98 Kusnierz-Alejska G, Duk M, Storry JR *et al.* NOR polyagglutination and Stᵃ glycophorin in one family: relation of NOR polyagglutination to terminal α-galactose residues and abnormal glycolipids. *Transfusion* 1999;**39**:32–8.

99 Bird AR, Kent P, Moores PP, Elliott T. Haemoglobin M-Hyde Park associated with polyagglutinable red blood cells in a South African family. *Br J Haematol* 1988;**68**:459–64.

100 King MJ, Liew YW, Moores PP, Bird GWG. Enhanced reaction with *Vicia graminea* lectin and exposed terminal N-acetyl-D-glucosaminyl residues on a sample of human red cells with Hb M-Hyde Park. *Transfusion* 1988;**28**:549–55.

101 Graninger W, Rameis H, Fischer K *et al.* 'VA', a new type of erythrocyte polyagglutination characterized by depressed H receptors and associated with hemolytic anemia. I. Serological and hematological observations. *Vox Sang* 1977;**32**:195–200.

102 Graninger W, Poschmann A, Fischer K *et al.* 'VA', a new type of erythrocyte polyagglutination characterized by depressed H receptors and associated with hemolytic anemia. II. Observations by immunofluorescence, electron microscopy, cell electrophoresis and biochemistry. *Vox Sang* 1977;**32**:201–7.

103 Beck ML, Myers MA, Moulds J *et al.* Coexistent Tk and VA polyagglutinability. *Transfusion* 1978;**18**:680–4.

104 Reid ME, Halverson GR, Lee AH *et al.* Tr: a new type of polyagglutination [Abstract]. *Transfusion* 1998;**38**: 100S.

32 Blood group gene mapping

32.1 Introduction

Blood groups have had an important role as human gene markers. In 1951, when the Lutheran locus was shown to be genetically linked to the locus controlling ABH secretion, blood groups were involved in the first recognized human autosomal linkage and, consequently, the first demonstration of recombination as a result of crossing-over in humans [1–3]. Through this linkage, and that between *ABO* and the gene for nail–patella syndrome, came the first evidence that the rate of crossing-over in humans can be substantially higher in females than in males [4,5]. When in 1968 the Duffy blood group locus was shown to be linked to an inherited visible deformity of chromosome 1, it became the first human gene locus assigned to an autosome [6]. All blood group system loci have now been assigned to their chromosome, as have the genes encoding a few other blood group antigens (Table 32.1). In this chapter the chromosomal assignment of blood group loci are described chromosome by chromosome; Table 32.1 lists the blood group systems in their numerical order. Figure 32.1 is a diagrammatic representation of the human male karyotype showing regional localization of blood group gene loci.

32.2 Linkage analysis and chromosome mapping

32.2.1 Linkage

When genes are on separate chromosomes, or far enough apart on the same chromosome, they segregate independently; that is, alleles at the different loci assort independently in the formation of germ cells. However, if two loci are close together on the same chromosome they are linked; they do not assort independently and the characters they control will be inherited together more often than would be predicted by chance. For example, the loci for Lutheran and ABH secretion are linked. A doubly heterozygous *Lu^a/Lu^b Se/se* person with *Lu^a* and *Se in cis* (on the same chromosome) will pass either *Lu^a* together with *Se* or *Lu^b* together with *se* to most of their children; only an occasional child would receive *Lu^a* with *se* or *Lu^b* with *Se*. This recombination results from crossing-over at meiosis between the two loci.

The greater the distance between two loci on the same chromosome, the greater the probability of crossing-over occurring between them. This premise is the basis for measuring distances between linked genes. When two loci are far enough apart that the probability of crossing-over occurring between them reaches 0.5 (50% recombination), linkage is no longer detectable and the loci are not considered linked. The term used to describe unlinked loci on the same chromosome is syntenic. If, for example, in a series of families, recombination between two linked genes occurs in 8% of meioses, then the recombination fraction ($\hat{\theta}$) is 0.08 and the map distance between the genes is 8 centimorgans (cM).

Statistical methods for the estimation of linkage are available. The traditional method for blood groups involves the use of lod scores in which log probabilities of linkage at various recombination values ($\hat{\theta}$) are obtained for each family with a doubly heterozygous propositus [7]. For a series of families the log probabilities or lod scores for each value of ($\hat{\theta}$) can be summed. A total score of +3 or more at any value of ($\hat{\theta}$) is considered statistically significant evidence in favour of linkage and a score of –2 is considered significant evidence against linkage. When two loci are linked the recombination fraction with the highest lod score represents the genetic distance between the loci. Computer programs, such as LIPED for two-point analysis and LINKAGE and VITESSE for multipoint analysis, are

533

Table 32.1 Chromosomal assignment of blood group loci.

Blood group	Gene symbol	Cytogenetic location
ABO	ABO	9q34.1–q34.2
MNS	GYPA, GYPB, GYPE	4q28–q31
P	P1	22q11.2–qter
Rh	RHCE, RHD	1p36.2–p34
Lutheran	LU	19q12–q13
Kell	KEL	7q33
Lewis	FUT3	19p13.3
Duffy	FY	1q22–q23
Kidd	SLC14A1	18q11–q12
Diego	SLC4A1	17q12–q21
Yt	ACHE	7q22
Xg	XG, MIC2	Xp22.32, Yp11.3
Scianna	SC	1p36.2–p22.1
Dombrock	DO	12p13.3–p13.2
Colton	AQP1	7p14
Landsteiner–Wiener	ICAM4	19p13.2–cen
Chido/Rodgers	C4A, C4B	6p21.3
Hh	FUT1	19q13.3
Kx	XK	Xp21.1
Gerbich	GYPC	2q14–q21
Cromer	DAF	1q32
Knops	CR1	1q32
Indian	CD44	11p13
Ok	BSG	19p13.3
RAPH	MER2	11p15.5
John Milton Hagen	SEMA7A	15q22.3–q23
I-branching enzyme	GCNT2	6p24
Pᵏ (Gb3 synthase)		22q11.2–qter
P (globoside synthase)		3q25
Radin	RD	1p36.2–p34
Rh-associated glycoprotein	RHAG	6p21–qter
CD59	CD59	11p13
HLA (Bg)	HLA-A, -B, -C	6p21.3
Secretor	FUT2	19q13.3
LU suppressor	XS	Xp21.2–q21.1

Gene nomenclature and cytogenetic location obtained from the HUGO Gene Nomenclature Committee (http://www.gene.ucl.ac.uk/nomenclature/) and the Genome Database (http://www.gdb.org/).

available for calculating linkage from family data [8–12].

Linkage map distances do not represent true physical distances between loci. Crossing-over rates differ between males and females and different distances must be calculated according to the sex of the doubly heterozygous propositus. Crossing-over rates also vary in different regions of the chromosome.

Most of the blood group loci have been indirectly as-signed to an autosome through linkage to genes or other markers of known chromosomal location.

32.2.2 Chromosome banding patterns

Traditionally genes are mapped to chromosomes according to the metaphase banding patterns obtained by Giemsa (G-banding) and quinacrine (Q-banding) staining (Fig. 32.1) [13]. In recent years mapping has related more to positions relative to numerous genetic markers on the chromosome, yet terminology based on the banding patterns continues to be used. Soon all distances of genes from the centromere will be defined in terms of megabases. In the interim, banding pattern locations are used here.

32.2.3 Other methods used in chromosome mapping

32.2.3.1 Deletion mapping

Deletion of part of a chromosome can result in loss of an allele at a particular locus and, consequently, apparent homozygosity at that locus. If the chromosomal location of the deletion can be determined and apparent homozygosity occurs where, according to the parental blood groups, heterozygosity would be expected, then evidence for assignment of the affected locus is provided. Monosomy of part of an autosome may occur as a result of deletion or translocation; heterozygosity excludes any locus from a region of the genome known to be monosomic.

32.2.3.2 Exclusion mapping

Information from deletion mapping for a blood group locus, plus the chromosomal regions excluded by negative linkage information with a number of mapped loci, can be very informative for excluding the locus from much of the genome. Cook *et al.* [14] applied exclusion mapping to the MNS system and, as a result, accurately predicted an assignment of the *MNS* locus to a region of the long arm of chromosome 4 (Section 32.3.4.1).

32.2.3.3 Somatic cell hybridization

Under appropriate conditions, cultured human cells, usually fibroblasts, can be induced to fuse with cultured rodent cells. The resulting human–rodent hybrid cells are unstable and will randomly shed human chromosomes. By cloning hybrid cells, a variety of cell lines lacking different human chromosomes can be obtained. In some cases, hybrid cell lines may be produced that contain only a single human chromosome or only part of a human chromosome. If a collection of these cell lines is analysed for a human marker, such as a cell surface antigen, correlation of the presence or absence of the marker with that of a specific human chromosome can result in chromosomal assignment of the gene encoding that marker. When a gene has been cloned its presence in a somatic cell hybrid may be detected by the use of labelled DNA probes. Red cells cannot be cultured, so these techniques have only been applicable to blood group antigens present on cell types other than red cells. For example, somatic cell hybridization was used to map the genes controlling expression of Ok[a] and MER2 to chromosomes 19 and 11, respectively [15,16].

32.2.3.4 *In situ* hybridization

When a gene has been cloned and sequenced, DNA probes can be produced that will hybridize with the DNA of that gene in a preparation of intact chromosomes. If the probe is made visible by the use of radioactive or fluorescent labels, then its localization on a chromosome can be determined. By this technique the gene encoding glycophorin C, which carries the Gerbich blood group antigens, was assigned to the long arm of chromosome 2 [17].

32.3 Chromosomal assignment of blood group loci

32.3.1 Chromosome 1

32.3.1.1 Duffy (*FY*)

In 1963, *FY* was shown to be closely linked to a gene for zonular pulverant cataract (*GJA8*, gap junction protein alpha-8) [18]. When Donahue *et al.* [6] showed that *FY* is linked to a visible deformity on the long arm of chromosome 1, *FY* and *GJA8* were assigned to that chromosome. Regional assignment of *FY* to 1q22–q23 was achieved through studies of families with rearrangements of chromosome 1 [19,20], deletion mapping (two individuals with deletions of part of 1q were Fy(a+b+)) [21,22], detailed lod score analysis [23], and *in situ* hybridization with *FY* cDNA [24].

32.3.1.2 Rh (*RHCE* and *RHD*)

The second autosomal linkage reported in humans was that between the Rh blood group polymorphism (*RH*) and a gene for elliptocytosis [25–28]. This Rh-

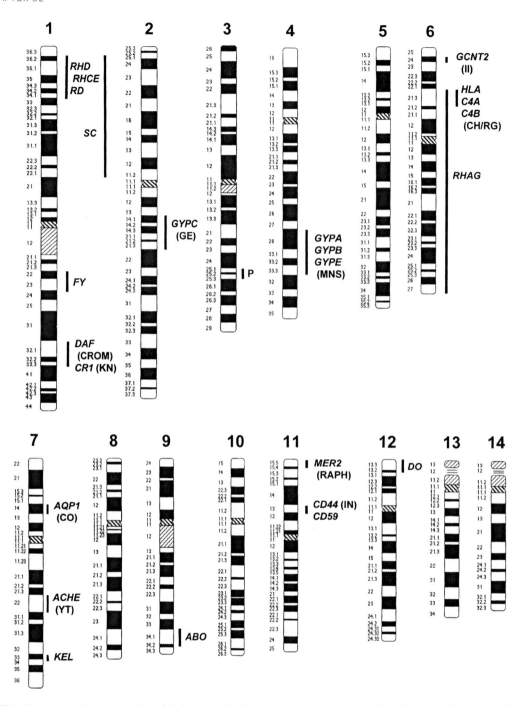

Fig. 32.1 Diagrammatic representation of the human male chromosomes showing regional localizations of blood group loci.

linked form of elliptocytosis is caused by mutations in *EPB41*, the gene encoding the cytoskeletal protein band 4.1 [29,30]. Linkage with other markers followed: 6-phosphogluconate dehydrogenase (*PGD*)

[31–33]; phosphoglucomutase 1 (*PGM1*) [33–35]; uridine monophosphate kinase (*UMPK*) [36]; and α-L-fucosidase (*FUCA1*) [37]. When the gene for peptidase C (*PEPC*) was assigned to chromosome 1 by

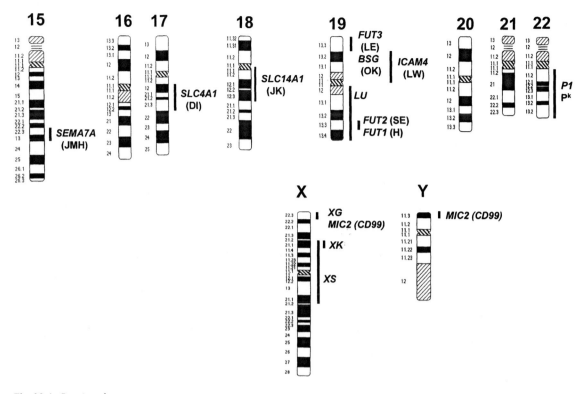

Fig. 32.1 *Continued*

somatic cell hybridization [38], it was already known to be syntenic with *PGM1*, *UMPK*, and *FUCA1*, so the linkage group containing the Rh genes was assigned to chromosome 1. The blood group locus *SC* and the gene controlling expression of the blood group antigen Rd are part of the same linkage group (see below); *FY* is not within direct measurable distance of *RH* [33,39,40]. There was a hint of linkage between *RH* and the dominant inhibitor gene *In(Lu)* [41].

In situ hybridization and somatic cell hybrid analysis with cDNA clones representing *RHCE* showed that this gene is located in the region 1p36.1 [42–44]. The two Rh genes are arranged in opposite orientation and are separated by *SMP1*, a gene for a small membrane protein of unknown function: *pter–5'RHCE3'–5'SMP13'–3'RHD5'–cen* [44,45].

32.3.1.3 Scianna (*SC*) and Radin (*RD*)

In 1976, analysis of families with the rare antigen Sc2 of the Scianna system (Chapter 13) demonstrated linkage between *SC* and *RH* with a male recombination fraction of about 0.10 [46,47]. Combined lod scores suggested linkage between *SC* and *PGM1* and *UMPK* [46,47] (see Section 32.3.1.2). The detection of linkage between *RH* and the gene governing the low frequency antigen Rd (700015) (*RD*), with a recombination fraction similar to that for *RH* and *SC*, led to speculation that Rd may be controlled by the *SC* locus [48]. Analysis of nine Swedish families with Rd+ propositi confirmed linkage of *RD* to *RH* and *PGM1* [49,50].

32.3.1.4 Cromer (*DAF*) and Knops (*CR1*)

Antigens of the Cromer blood group system are located on CD55, the complement regulatory glycoprotein decay accelerating factor (DAF) (Chapter 19); antigens of the Knops system have been located on CD35, complement receptor 1 (CR1) (Chapter 20). *DAF* and *CR1* belong to a cluster of genes, the regulator of complement activation (RCA) linkage group, localized to

537

1q [51–57]. Both *DAF* and *CR1* have also been assigned to 1q32 by somatic cell hybridization and by *in situ* hybridization [54,58].

32.3.2 Chromosome 2

32.3.2.1 Gerbich (*GYPC*)

Antigens of the Gerbich system are located on two glycoprotein isoforms, glycophorins C and D (GPC and GPD), encoded by a single gene, *GYPC* (Chapter 18). *GYPC* was localized to 2q14–q21 by *in situ* hybridization with a cDNA clone representing the 3′ untranslated region and almost the entire coding sequence of *GYPC* [17].

32.3.3 Chromosome 3

32.3.3.1 P (globoside) synthase

An expressed sequence tag (EST) localized to chromosome 3q25, initially considered to encode a β1,3-galactosyltransferase (β3Gal-T3) [59], was subsequently shown to encode the β1,3-*N*-acetylgalactosaminyltransferase (β3GalNAc-T1) that catalyses the synthesis of P antigen (globoside) from P^k (Gb3 or CD77) [60] (Chapter 4).

32.3.4 Chromosome 4

32.3.4.1 MNS (*GYPA*, *GYPB*, and *GYPE*)

The original suggestions that the genes controlling MNS were located either on chromosome 2 or 4 came as a result of studies on a mentally retarded boy with chromosome rearrangements involving 2q and 4q. He was M+N–S+s– (apparently *MS/MS*), while his father was M–N+S–s+ (apparently *Ns/Ns*) [61–63]. Assignment to chromosome 4 was demonstrated in 1979 on the basis of accumulated evidence. This included exclusion mapping, which showed that the MNS genes were about 45 times more likely to be on 4q28–q31 than on their next most likely site [14,64], and loose linkage with the gene for vitamin D-binding protein (*GC*), known to be on chromosome 4 [65]. Further linkage analyses on the MNS groups of families with chromosome 4 rearrangements supported assignment of *MNS* to 4q28–q31 [66].

MN and Ss antigens are located on glycophorins A and B, which are encoded by two very closely linked genes, *GYPA* and *GYPB* (Chapter 3). *GYPA* and *GYPE*, a third homologous gene of the cluster, were localized to 4q28–q31 by *in situ* hybridization [67,68], confirming the localization obtained by genetic linkage analysis.

32.3.5 Chromosome 6

32.3.5.1 Chido/Rodgers (*C4A* and *C4B*)

The genes controlling Ch and Rg expression were known to be linked to *HLA* before the Ch/Rg antigens were found to be determinants on the fourth component of complement (C4) (Chapter 17) [69,70]. With only rare exceptions, *C4A* and *C4B* produce Rg and Ch antigens, respectively. They are situated, together with genes for the complement factors C2 and properdin factor B (*BF*), in the Class III region of the major histocompatibility complex between *HLA-DR* and *HLA-B* on the short arm of chromosome 6 [71–74]. Strong linkage disequilibrium exists between the highly polymorphic *C4A*, *C4B*, *C2*, and *BF* genes, haplotypes being inherited as units known as complotypes [75]. *C4B* and *C4A* have at their 3′ ends the steroid 21-hydroxylase gene (*CYP21A2*) and pseudogene (*CYP21A1P*), respectively [76].

32.3.5.2 *HLA*

HLA antigens are not generally considered red cell antigens (Chapter 30) and will not be discussed in detail here. The major histocompatibility complex, which includes the *HLA* loci, is located on 6p21.3 [74].

32.3.5.3 Rh-associated glycoprotein (*RHAG*)

RHAG, the gene encoding a glycoprotein that co-immunoprecipitates with the Rh proteins and shares significant sequence homology with those polypeptides (Chapter 5), has been localized to 6p21–qter by somatic cell hybrid analysis [77] and to 6p21.1–p11 by *in situ* hybridization [78].

32.3.5.4 Ii (*II*)

GCNT2, a gene encoding a β-1,6-*N*-acetylglucosaminyltransferase, may be the branching enzyme responsible for converting i-active linear oligosaccharide chains to I-active branched chains (Chapter 25). *GCNT2* was initially assigned to chromosome 9q21 through *in situ* hybridization [79], but mapping of 39 ESTs to 6p24–p23, one of which was identical to *GCNT2*, has provided contradictory evidence regarding the location of this gene [80].

32.3.6 Chromosome 7

32.3.6.1 Colton (*CO*)

The absence of Colton antigens from red cells of some patients with monosomy 7 of the haemopoietic tissue (Section 15.5) provided the first indication that the Colton locus may be on chromosome 7. Zelinski *et al.* [81] demonstrated close linkage between CO and the 7p marker *ASSP11* (argininosuccinate synthetase pseudogene 11). The Colton polymorphism was subsequently shown to be encoded by *AQP1*, the gene for the water transport protein aquaporin-1, which had been located on 7p14 by *in situ* hybridization [82] (Chapter 15).

32.3.6.2 Kell (*KEL*)

In 1991, Zelinski *et al.* [83] demonstrated tight linkage between *KEL* and *PIP*, the gene for prolactin-inducible protein (detected by a *Taq*I polymorphism). *PIP* had previously been localized to 7q32–q36. Close linkage of *KEL* to three DNA markers, which are tightly linked to the cystic fibrosis gene (*CFTR*) [84], and *in situ* hybridization with cDNA encoding the Kell protein [85,86], confirmed the assignment of *KEL* to 7q33–q35.

Linkage between *KEL* and the locus for the Yt blood group system is discussed in Section 32.3.6.3.

32.3.6.3 Yt (*ACHE*)

An analysis of 31 families informative for segregation of *YT* and *KEL* revealed loose linkage between these loci with maximum likelihood of a recombination fraction of 0.26 [87]. Two years later, *KEL* was provisionally assigned to 7q through linkage to *PIP* [83] and close linkage between *YT* and two chromosome 7 markers, *COL1A2* and *D7S13*, was reported [88].

In 1992, the Yt blood group polymorphism was shown to represent a point mutation in the acetyl-

cholinesterase gene (*ACHE*) (Chapter 11). The same year, by *in situ* hybridization and by polymerase chain reacion (PCR)-based somatic cell hybridization techniques, *ACHE* was assigned to chromosome 7q22 [89,90].

32.3.7 Chromosome 9

32.3.7.1 ABO (*ABO*)

In 1955, Renwick and Lawler [91] showed that *ABO* is closely linked to a gene for nail–patella syndrome (*LMX1B*), a dominantly inherited disorder characterized by dystrophic nails and deformed patellae and elbow joints. A suggestion of linkage between *ABO* and the gene for adenylate kinase 1 (*AK1*) [92] was quickly confirmed [93–96]. *LMX1B* and *AK1* are closely linked [95].

In 1976, *AK1*, and hence the *ABO–LMX1B–AK1* linkage group, was assigned to chromosome 9 by the use of somatic cell hybrids in four separate laboratories [97–100]. Analyses of families with abnormalities of chromosome 9 showed that both *ABO* and *AK1* are localized to 9q34 [101,102] and the *ABO* localization has been confirmed by *in situ* hybridization [103].

32.3.8 Chromosome 11

32.3.8.1 Indian (*CD44*)

In[a] and In[b] antigens of the Indian system are located on the proteoglycan CD44 (Chapter 21). Testing of the original CD44 antibody with a panel of somatic cell hybrids showed that the determinant recognized was encoded by a gene on chromosome 11 [104]. This was subsequently confirmed with other similar antibodies [105,106] and CD44 was localized to 11p13 [107,108].

32.3.8.2 MER2 (*MER2*)

MER2 antigen of the RAPH system, polymorphic on red cells, is present on a variety of other cell types (Chapter 23). *MER2* was assigned to chromosome 11p15 by somatic cell hybridization [16].

32.3.7.3 CD59 (*CD59*)

The complement regulatory glycoprotein CD59 is present on red cells, but carries no blood group alloantigen (Chapter 19). CD59 has been assigned to 11p13 by somatic cell hybridization analyses and by pulsed field gel electrophoresis [109–111].

32.3.9 Chromosome 12

32.3.9.1 Dombrock (DO)

As a result of testing five informative families for 448 classical markers and 115 informative families for 80 markers, the gene encoding Do^a (DO), as determined by testing red cells with anti-Do^a, was excluded from all chromosomes except 12p [112]. Linkage between DO and three DNA microsatellite markers was analysed in 17 large families and confirmed the assignment of DO to 12p. Further analyses of families segregating for DO and for four anonymous DNA markers and for the von Willebrand factor gene (VWF) refined regional localization to 12p13.2–p12.3 [113]. DO was cloned as a result of analysing ESTs derived from chromosome 12p [114].

32.3.10 Chromosome 15

32.3.10.1 JMH (SEMA7A)

JMH antigen is the semaphorin CDw108 (Chapter 24), encoded by the gene SEMA7A. SEMA7A has been localized to 15q22.3–q23 by radiation hybrid mapping [115] and by fluorescence in situ hybridization [116].

32.3.11 Chromosome 17

32.3.11.1 Diego (SLC4A1)

Antigens of the Diego system are determined by missense mutations within SLC4A1 (solute carrier family 4, anion exchanger 1), the gene for band 3 glycoprotein (Chapter 10). SLC4A1 is located on chromosome 17q12–q21 [117]. Tight linkage, with no recombination, has been demonstrated between DI, as determined by the Di^a and Wd^a (DI5) antigens, and SLC4A1, as detected by a PstI restriction fragment-length polymorphism (RFLP) [118,119].

32.3.12 Chromosome 18

32.3.12.1 Kidd (SLC14A1)

In 1987 significant linkage data were obtained between JK and two chromosome 18 markers, D18S6 and D18S1 [120,121]. From previous reports of heterozygosity at the JK locus in individuals with deletions involving chromosome 18, the shortest region of overlap for JK is 18q11–q12 [122,123]. Early suggestions of linkage between JK and the locus for type 1 insulin-dependent diabetes mellitus [124] has not been supported [125–127]. However, there is evidence for a type 1 diabetes susceptibility locus, IDDM6, on 18q21, estimated to be 13 cM from JK [128,129].

The Kidd glycoprotein is a urea transporter (Chapter 9) encoded by SLC14A1 (solute carrier family 14, member 1). SLC14A1 and a gene encoding another urea transporter, SLC14A2, were both localized to 18q12–q21 by in situ hybridization [130,131].

32.3.13 Chromosome 19

Considering chromosome 19 is one of the smallest human chromosomes, it seems to carry an excess of blood group, or blood group-related, loci. The genes governing red cell expression of the Lutheran (LU), Lewis (FUT3), Landsteiner–Wiener (ICAM4), H (FUT1), and Ok^a (BSG) antigens, and those controlling secretion of H antigen (FUT2) in body fluids, are all on chromosome 19. FUT1 and FUT2, which encode α1,2-L-fucosyltransferases, are also known as H and SE, respectively; FUT3, which encodes an α1,3/4-L-fucosyltransferase is the Lewis gene LE.

32.3.13.1 Lutheran (LU), Secretor (FUT2), Lewis (FUT3), Hh (FUT1), and Landsteiner–Wiener (ICAM4)

In 1951, Mohr et al. [1–3] reported linkage between the Lutheran blood group locus (LU) and the locus (FUT2) governing secretion of ABH substances as detected by Le^a or Le^b expression on red cells (Chapter 2). This linkage was confirmed in numerous family studies and the recombination fraction estimated as 0.1 [132–135]. LU and FUT2 (SE) are closely linked to the gene for myotonic dystrophy (DMPK), a dominantly inherited neuromuscular disorder [3,136,137]. FUT3 (LE) was not found to be directly linked to LU or *FUT2*, but the *LU–FUT2–DMPK* linkage group was extended to include *FUT3* when *FUT3* and *DMPK* were shown to be loosely linked [138].

Linkage between the Lewis gene (*FUT3*) and the gene for the third component of complement (*C3*) was discovered in 1974 [139]. *C3* was assigned to chromosome 19 by analysis of somatic cell hybrids with a monoclonal antibody specific for human C3 and with a human C3 DNA probe [140], so *FUT3* was indirectly assigned to chromosome 19 together with *LU* and *FUT2* (*SE*) through their linkage to *DMPK*. *FUT2* was later shown to be linked to *C3* [141]. Southern blot analysis of somatic cell hybrids confirmed that *FUT3* is on chromosome 19 [142]. Analysis of families for Au^b (LU19) and an RFLP for the chromosome 19 marker *APOC2* revealed close linkage, providing further confirmation that *LU* is on chromosome 19 [143].

In the early 1980s Oriol, Le Pendu and their colleagues provided substantial evidence that the gene controlling the presence of A, B, and H substances in body secretions is a structural gene producing an α1,2-L-fucosyltransferase in secretory tissue (Chapter 2). A series of families with the rare deficiency of H antigen on their red cells caused by an absence of red cell α1,2-L-fucosyltransferase encoded by *FUT1* (*H*), demonstrated very close linkage between *FUT1* and *FUT2* [144,145]. Hence, *FUT1* joined the chromosome 19 linkage group. Localization of *FUT1* and *FUT2* on 19q13.3 has been confirmed by fluorescence *in situ* hybridization [146]. A 100-kb cosmid contig containing *FUT1*, *FUT2*, and a homologous pseudogene *Sec1* has been assembled and the order of the genes is *cen–Sec1–*12 kb*–FUT2–*35 kb*–FUT1–qter* [146,147].

The Lewis gene, *FUT3*, belongs to a cluster of α1,3/4-fucosyltransferase genes on 19p13.3: *pter–FUT6–*14 kb*–FUT3–*23 kb*–FUT5–cen* [147,148].

When *ICAM4*, the gene for the LW blood group, was shown to be closely linked to *C3* and *LU*, it became the latest blood group gene to join the chromosome 19 linkage group [149,150]. Location of *ICAM4* on 19p13.3 was confirmed by *in situ* hybridization [151].

From accumulated data the following gene order can be deduced: *pter–FUT3–C3–ICAM4–cen–LU–FUT2–FUT1–qter* [150,152,153].

32.3.13.2 Ok^a (*BSG*)

Identification of a monoclonal antibody with Ok^a specificity enabled Williams *et al.* [15] to show that this high incidence red cell antigen is present on all human cell types tested, but not on mouse cells. They exploited this species specificity by somatic cell hybridization techniques to demonstrate that Ok^a is produced by a gene on chromosome 19. Human chromosome 19 material is essential for Ok^a expression and a cell line with a translocation containing 19pter–p13.2 showed that this region was sufficient for antigen expression. Ok^a is located on the immunoglobulin superfamily molecule CD147, also known as basigin (*BSG*) (Chapter 22). In 1993, before the relationship of CD147 to Ok^a was known, *BSG* was mapped to 19p13.3 by fluorescence *in situ* hybridization [154].

32.3.14 Chromosome 22

32.3.14.1 P1 and P^k

P1, the gene controlling the P$_1$/P$_2$ polymorphism, was assigned to chromosome 22 when Eiberg *et al.* [155] showed that *P1* is linked to *TCN2*, the gene for transcobalamin II, and *TCN2* was assigned to chromosome 22 by the use of somatic cell hybrids and monosomic meningioma cells [156]. Linkage analyses with several loci localized *P1* to 22q11.2–qter [157–159].

Chromosome 22 was the first human chromosome to be sequenced [160]. As the *P1* gene product is predicted to be an α1,4-galactosyltransferase (Chapter 4), Steffensen *et al.* [161] searched chromosome 22q11.2–qter for sequence homologous to that of a bacterial α1,4-galactosyltransferase gene. An α1,4-galactosyltransferase gene was isolated, but while the encoded enzyme synthesizes P^k (Gb3) from lactosylceramide, it is unable to synthesize P1 antigen. This gene appears to be *P^k* and not *P1* (Chapter 4).

32.3.15 X and Y chromosomes

32.3.15.1 Xg (*XG*) and CD99 (*MIC2*)

Like most X-linked genes, *XG* was assigned to the X chromosome because of its characteristic mode of inheritance (Chapter 12). The first firm evidence that

XG is located near the tip of the short arm of X was provided by an Xg(a–) woman who had failed to inherit her father's *Xg^a* gene [162]: she had an X–Y translocation, 46,X,t(X;Y)(p22.3;q11), in which the distal segment of the short arm of one of her X chromosomes was missing and replaced by part of the long arm of a Y chromosome. X inactivation was random and so the *XG* locus must have been lost with the missing Xpter–p22.3 region. The woman's son, who had inherited the abnormal chromosome and was nullisomic for Xpter–p22.3, was also Xg(a–). He suffered from a generalized ichthyosis as a result of zero steroid sulphatase activity, locating the steroid sulphatase (*STS*) gene, known to be closely linked to *XG*, on Xpter–p22.3.

The relationship between *XG* and *MIC2*, the structural gene for CD99, is described in Chapter 12. Figure 12.1 shows that *MIC2* is within the X and Y pseudoautosomal regions in which the X and Y chromosomes pair at meiosis and crossing-over occurs. *MIC2* is close to the pseudoautosomal boundary (*PAB1*) and only recombines with X- and Y-linked genes in about 2% of male meioses [163]. *XG* spans the pseudoautosomal boundary.

32.3.15.2 Kx (*XK*)

XK governs expression of Kx antigen on red cells, absence of which is associated with impaired expression of Kell system antigens (McLeod phenotype) and a variety of muscular and neurological defects that collectively constitute McLeod syndrome (Chapter 7). *XK* was assigned to the X chromosome through the characteristic mode of inheritance of Kx and the McLeod phenotype. A male patient with McLeod syndrome, chronic granulomatous disease (CGD), Duchenne muscular dystrophy (DMD), and one type of retinitis pigmentosa (RP) was shown, both by DNA analysis and cytogenetics, to have an interstitial deletion of part of the short arm of the X chromosome at Xp21.1 [164]. Other patients, with smaller deletions at the same region, had McLeod syndrome and CGD, but not DMD; some also had RP [165]. This suggests that the *XK* locus is located at Xp21.1, very close to the genes for X-linked CGD (*CYBB*), DMD (*DMD*), and RP (*RPGR*). Bertelson *et al.* [166] sited *XK* between the loci for CGD and DMD. Physical mapping by pulsed field gel electrophoresis has limited *XK* to a 150–380 kb region of Xp21 [167].

Family studies suggested that *XK* and *CYBB* are linked to *XG* [168,169], but the physical distances between these genes on the X chromosome make this unlikely.

32.3.15.3 X-linked Lutheran suppressor (*XS*)

XS2, a very rare recessive allele at the X-linked *XS* locus, acts as a suppressor of expression of Lutheran system antigens (Chapter 6). Use of polymorphic DNA markers and of anti-Xg^a for analysis of the only known family with the X-linked type of Lu-null suggested close linkage of *XS* to *DXS14*, a DNA marker located near the centromere at Xp11 [170]. *XS* is likely to be situated near the centromere and, at least, between Xp21.2 and Xq21.1; it is unlikely to be close to *XG*.

References

1 Mohr J. A search for linkage between the Lutheran blood group and other hereditary characters. *Acta Path Microbiol Scand* 1951;28:207–10.

2 Mohr J. Estimation of linkage between the Lutheran and the Lewis blood groups. *Acta Path Microbiol Scand* 1951;29:339–44.

3 Mohr J. *A Study of Linkage in Man.* Copenhagen: Munksgaard, 1954.

4 Cook PJL. The Lutheran–Secretor recombination fraction in man: a possible sex difference. *Ann Hum Genet* 1965;28:393–401.

5 Renwick JH, Schulze J. Male and female recombination fractions for the nail–patella: ABO linkage in man. *Ann Hum Genet* 1965;28:379–92.

6 Donahue RP, Bias WB, Renwick JH, McKusick VA. Probable assignment of the Duffy blood group locus to chromosome 1 in man. *Proc Natl Acad Sci USA* 1968;61:949–55.

7 Maynard-Smith S, Penrose LS, Smith CAB. *Mathematical Tables for Research Workers in Human Genetics.* London: Churchill, 1961.

8 Ott J. Estimation of the recombination fraction in human pedigrees: efficient computation of the likelihood for human linkage studies. *Am J Hum Genet* 1974;26:588–97.

9 Falk CT, Walker ME, Martin MD, Allen FH. Autosomal linkage in humans (methodology and results of computer analysis). *Series Haematol* 1975;8:153–237.

10 Lathrop GM, Lalouel JM, Julier C, Ott J. Strategies for multilocus linkage analysis in humans. *Proc Natl Acad Sci USA* 1984;81:3443–6.

11 Attwood J, Bryant S. A computer program to make linkage analysis with LIPED and LINKAGE easier to perform

and less prone to input errors. *Ann Hum Genet* 1988;**52**:259.

12 O'Connell JR, Weeks DE. The VITESSE algorithm for rapid exact multilocus linkage analysis via genotype set-recoding and fuzzy inheritance. *Nature Genet* 1995;**11**:402–8.

13 Standing Committee on Human Cytogenetic Nomenclature. An international system for human cytogenetic nomenclature. *Cytogenet Cell Genet* 1978;**21**:309–404.

14 Cook PJL, Noades JE, Lomas CG, Buckton KE, Robson EB. Exclusion mapping illustrated by the MNSs blood group. *Ann Hum Genet* 1980;**44**:61–73.

15 Williams BP, Daniels GL, Pym B *et al.* Biochemical and genetic analysis of the Okᵃ blood group antigen. *Immunogenetics* 1988;**27**:322–9.

16 Daniels GL, Tippett P, Palmer DK *et al.* MER2: a red cell polymorphism defined by monoclonal antibodies. *Vox Sang* 1987;**52**:107–10.

17 Mattei MG, Colin Y, Le Van Kim C, Mattei JF, Cartron JP. Localization of the gene for human erythrocyte glycophorin C to chromosome 2, q14–q21. *Hum Genet* 1986;**74**:420–2.

18 Renwick JH, Lawler SD. Probable linkage between a congenital cataract locus and the Duffy blood group locus. *Ann Hum Genet* 1963;**27**:67–84.

19 Cook PJL, Robson EB, Buckton KE, Jacobs PA, Polani PE. Segregation of genetic markers in families with chromosome polymorphisms and structural rearrangements involving chromosome 1. *Ann Hum Genet* 1974;**37**:261–74.

20 Cook PJL, Page BM, Johnston AW, Stanford WK, Gavin J. Four further families informative for 1q and the Duffy blood group. Human Gene Mapping 4. *Cytogenet Cell Genet* 1978;**22**:378–80.

21 Estévez de Pablo C, García Sagredo JM, Ferro MT, Ferrando P, San Román C. Interstitial deletion in the long arms of chromosome 1: 46,XY,del(1)(pter→q22::q25→qter). *J Med Genet* 1980;**17**:483–6.

22 Schinzel A, Schmid W. Interstitial deletion of the long arm of chromosome 1, del(1)(q21→q25) in a profoundly retarded 8-year-old girl with multiple anomalies. *Clin Genet* 1980;**18**:305–13.

23 Collins A, Keats BJ, Dracopoli N, Shields DC, Morton NE. Integration of gene maps: chromosome 1. *Proc Natl Acad Sci USA* 1992;**89**:4598–602.

24 Mathew S, Chaudhuri A, Murty VVVS, Pogo AO. Confirmation of Duffy blood group antigen locus (FY) at 1q22→q23 by fluorescence *in situ* hybridization. *Cytogenet Cell Genet* 1994;**67**:68.

25 Chalmers JNM, Lawler SD. Data on linkage in man: elliptocytosis and blood groups. I. Families 1 and 2. *Ann Eugen* 1953;**17**:267–71.

26 Goodall HB, Hendry DWW, Lawler SD, Stephen SA. Data on linkage in man: elliptocytosis and blood groups. II. Family 3. *Ann Eugen* 1953;**17**:272–8.

27 Goodall HB, Hendry DWW, Lawler SD, Stephen SA. Data on linkage in man: elliptocytosis and blood groups. III. Family 4. *Ann Eugen* 1954;**18**:325–7.

28 Lawler SD, Sandler M. Data on linkage in man: elliptocytosis and blood groups. IV. Families 5, 6 and 7. *Ann Eugen* 1954;**18**:328–34.

29 Conboy J, Mohandas N, Tchernia G, Kan YW. Molecular basis of hereditary elliptocytosis due to protein 4.1 deficiency. *N Engl J Med* 1986;**315**:680–5.

30 McGuire M, Smith BL, Agre P. Distinct variants of erythrocyte protein 4.1 inherited in linkage with elliptocytosis and Rh type in three white families. *Blood* 1988;**72**:287–93.

31 Weitkamp LR, Guttormsen SA, Shreffler DC, Sing CF, Napier JA. Genetic linkage relations of the loci for 6-phosphogluconate dehydrogenase and adenosine deaminase in man. *Am J Hum Genet* 1970;**22**:216–20.

32 Weitkamp LR, Guttormsen SA, Greendyke RM. Genetic linkage between a locus for 6-PGD and the Rh locus: evaluation of possible heterogeneity in the recombination fraction between sexes and among families. *Am J Hum Genet* 1971;**23**:462–70.

33 Robson EB, Cook PJL, Corney G *et al.* Linkage data on Rh, PGM₁, PGD, Peptidase C and Fy from family studies. *Ann Hum Genet* 1973;**36**:393–9.

34 Renwick JH. The Rhesus syntenic group in man. *Nature* 1971;**234**:475.

35 Cook PJL, Noades J, Hopkinson DA, Robson EB, Cleghorn TE. Demonstration of a sex difference in recombination fraction in the loose linkage, Rh and PGM₁. *Ann Hum Genet* 1972;**35**:239–42.

36 Giblett ER, Anderson JE, Lewis M, Kaita H. A new polymorphic enzyme, uridine monophosphate kinase: gene frequencies and a linkage analysis. Human Gene Mapping 2. *Cytogenet Cell Genet* 1975;**14**:329–31.

37 Corney G, Fisher RA, Cook PJL, Noades J, Robson EB. Linkage between α-fucosidase and the rhesus blood group. *Ann Hum Genet* 1977;**40**:403–5.

38 Ruddle F, Ricciuti F, McMorris FA *et al.* Somatic cell genetic assignment of peptidase C and the Rh linkage group to chromosome A-1 in man. *Science* 1972;**176**:1429–31.

39 Sanger R, Tippett P, Gavin J, Race RR. Failure to demonstrate linkage between the loci for the Rh and Duffy blood groups. *Ann Hum Genet* 1973;**36**:353–4.

40 Lewis M, Kaita H, Giblett ER, Anderson JE. Data on chromosome 1 loci Fy, PGM₁, Sc, UMPK, Rh, PGD, and ENO1: two-point lods, R:NR counts, multipoint information, and map. Human Gene Mapping 4. *Cytogenet Cell Genet* 1978;**22**:392–5.

41 Shaw MA, Leak MR, Daniels GL, Tippett P. The rare Lutheran blood group phenotype Lu(a−b−): a genetic study. *Ann Hum Genet* 1984;**48**:229–37.

42 Chérif-Zahar B, Mattéi MG, Le Van Kim C *et al.* Localization of the human Rh blood group gene structure to

543

chromosome region 1p34.3–1p36.1 by *in situ* hybridization. *Hum Genet* 1991;**86**:398–400.

43 MacGeoch C, Mitchell CJ, Carritt B *et al*. Assignment of the chromosomal locus of the human 30-kDal Rh (Rhesus) blood group-antigen-related protein (Rh30A) to chromosome region 1p36.13→p34. *Cytogenet Cell Genet* 1992;**59**:261–3.

44 Suto Y, Ishikawa Y, Hyodo H, Uchikawa M, Juji T. Gene organization and rearrangements at the human Rhesus blood group locus revealed by fibre-FISH analysis. *Hum Genet* 2000;**106**:164–71.

45 Wagner FF, Flegel WA. *RHD* gene deletion occurred in the *Rhesus box*. *Blood* 2000;**95**:3662–8.

46 Lewis M, Kaita H, Chown B. Genetic linkage between the human blood group loci Rh and Sc (Scianna). *Am J Hum Genet* 1976;**28**:619–20.

47 Noades JE, Corney G, Cook PJL *et al*. The Scianna blood group lies distal to uridine monophosphate kinase on chromosome 1p. *Ann Hum Genet* 1979;**43**:121–32.

48 Lewis M, Kaita H. Genetic linkage between the Radin and Rh blood group loci. *Vox Sang* 1979;**37**: 286–9.

49 Lewis M, Kaita H, Philipps S *et al*. The position of the Radin blood group locus in relation to other chromosome 1 loci. *Ann Hum Genet* 1980;**44**:179–84.

50 Hildén J-O, Shaw M-A, Whitehouse DB, Monteiro M, Tippett P. Linkage information from nine more Radin families. Human Gene Mapping 8 [Abstract]. *Cytogenet Cell Genet* 1985;**40**:650–1.

51 Holers VM, Cole JL, Lublin DM, Seya T, Atkinson JP. Human C3b- and C4b-regulatory proteins: a new multigene family. *Immunol Today* 1985;**6**:188–92.

52 Reid KBM, Bentley DR, Campbell RD *et al*. Complement system proteins which interact with C3b or C4b: a superfamily of structurally related proteins. *Immunol Today* 1986;**7**:230–4.

53 Medof ME, Lublin DM, Holers VM *et al*. Cloning and characterization of cDNAs encoding the complete sequence of decay-accelerating factor of human complement. *Proc Natl Acad Sci USA* 1987;**84**:2007–11.

54 Lublin DM, Lemons RS, Le Beau MM *et al*. The gene encoding decay-accelerating factor (DAF) is located in the complement-regulatory locus on the long arm of chromosome 1. *J Exp Med* 1987;**165**:1731–6.

55 Rey-Campos J, Rubinstein P, de Cordoba SR. Decay-accelerating factor: genetic polymorphism and linkage to the RCA (regulator of complement activation) gene cluster in humans. *J Exp Med* 1987;**166**:246–52.

56 Carroll MC, Alicot EM, Katzman PJ *et al*. Organization of the genes encoding complement receptors type 1 and 2, decay-accelerating factor, and C4-binding protein in the RCA locus on human chromosome 1. *J Exp Med* 1988;**167**:1271–80.

57 Rey-Campos J, Rubinstein P, de Cordoba SR. A physical map of the human regulator of complement activation

58 Weis JH, Morton CC, Bruns GAP *et al*. A complement receptor locus: genes encoding C3b/C4b receptor and C3d/Epstein–Barr virus receptor map to 1q32. *J Immunol* 1987;**138**:312–15.

59 Amado M, Almeida R, Carneiro F *et al*. A family of human β3-galactosyltransferases. Characterization of four members of a UDP-galactose:β-N-acetyl-glucosamine/β-N-acetyl-galactosamine β-1,3-galacto-syltransferase family. *J Biol Chem* 1998;**273**:12770–8.

60 Okajima T, Nakamura Y, Uchikawa M *et al*. Expression cloning of human globoside synthase cDNAs. Identification of β3Gal-T3 as UDP-N-acetylgalactosamine: globotriosylceramide β1,3-N-acetylgalactosaminyl-transferase. *J Biol Chem* 2000;**275**:40498–503.

61 German JL, Walker ME, Stiefel FH, Allen FH. Autoradiographic studies of human chromosomes. II. Data concerning the position of the *MN* locus. *Vox Sang* 1969;**16**:130–45.

62 German J, Chaganti RSK. Mapping human autosomes: assignment of the MN locus to a specific segment in the long arm of chromosome No. 2. *Science* 1973;**182**: 1261–72.

63 German J, Metaxas MN, Metaxas-Bühler M, Louie E, Chaganti RSK. Further evaluation of a child with the M^k phenotype and a translocation affecting the long arms of chromosomes 2 and 4. Human Gene Mapping 5 [Abstract]. *Cytogenet Cell Genet* 1979;**25**:160.

64 Cook PJL, Noades JE, Buckton KE, Lindenbaum RH. Exclusion mapping of *MNS* and *GPT*. Human Gene Mapping 5 [Abstract]. *Cytogenet Cell Genet* 1979; **25**:143.

65 Bootsma D, McAlpine PJ. Report of the committee on the genetic constitution of chromosomes 2, 3, 4, and 5. Human Gene Mapping 5. *Cytogenet Cell Genet* 1979;**25**:21–31.

66 Cook PJL, Lindenbaum RH, Salonen R *et al*. The MNSs blood groups of families with chromosome 4 rearrangements. *Ann Hum Genet* 1981;**45**:39–47.

67 Rahuel C, London J, d'Auriol L *et al*. Characterization of cDNA clones for human glycophorin A. *Eur J Biochem* 1988;**172**:147–53.

68 Kudo S, Chagnovich D, Rearden A, Mattei M-G, Fukuda M. Molecular analysis of a hybrid gene encoding human glycophorin variant Miltenberger V-like molecule. *J Biol Chem* 1990;**265**:13825–9.

69 Middleton J, Crookston MC, Falk JA *et al*. Linkage of Chido and HL-A. *Tissue Antigens* 1974;**4**:366–73.

70 Giles CM, Gedde-Dahl T, Robson EB *et al*. Rg^a (Rodgers) and the HLA region: linkage and associations. *Tissue Antigens* 1976;**8**:143–9.

71 Carroll MC, Alper CA. Polymorphism and molecular genetics of human C4. *Br Med Bull* 1987;**43**:50–65.

72 Teisberg P, Åkesson I, Olaisen B, Gedde-Dahl T, Thorsby E. Genetic polymorphism of C4 in man and

gene cluster linking the complement genes *CR1*, *CR2*, *DAF*, and *C4BP*. *J Exp Med* 1988;**167**:664–9.

localisation of a structural C4 locus to the HLA gene complex of chromosome 6. *Nature* 1976;**264**:253–4.

73 Carroll MC, Campbell RD, Bentley DR, Porter RR. A molecular map of the human major histocompatibility complex class III region linking complement genes C4, C2 and factor B. *Nature* 1984;**307**:237–41.

74 Ziegler A, Field LL, Sakaguchi AY. Report of the committee on the genetic constitution of chromosome 6. Human Gene Mapping 11. *Cytogenet Cell Genet* 1991;**58**:295–336.

75 Alper CA, Raum D, Karp S, Awdeh ZL, Yunis EJ. Serum complement 'supergenes' of the major histocompatibility complex in man (complotypes). *Vox Sang* 1983; **45**:62–7.

76 Carroll MC, Campbell RD, Porter RR. Mapping of steroid 21-hydroxylase genes adjacent to complement component C4 genes in *HLA*, the major histocompatibility complex in man. *Proc Natl Acad Sci USA* 1985;**82**:521–5.

77 Ridgwell K, Spurr NK, Laguda B *et al*. Isolation of cDNA clones for a 50 kDa glycoprotein of the human erythrocyte membrane associated with Rh (Rhesus) blood-group antigen expression. *Biochem J* 1992; **287**:223–8.

78 Cherif-Zahar B, Raynal V, Gane P *et al*. Candidate gene acting as a suppressor of the *RH* locus in most cases of Rh-deficiency. *Nature Genet* 1996;**12**:168–73.

79 Bierhuizen MFA, Mattei M-G, Fukuda M. Expression of the developmental I antigen by a cloned human cDNA encoding a member of a β-1,6-N-acetylglucosaminyltransferase gene family. *Gene Dev* 1993; **7**:468–78.

80 Olavesen MG, Bentley E, Mason RVF, Stephens RJ, Ragoussis J. Fine mapping of 39 ESTs on human chromosome 6p23–p25. *Genomics* 1997;**46**:303–6.

81 Zelinski T, Kaita H, Gilson T *et al*. Linkage between the Colton blood group locus and *ASSP11* on chromosome 7. *Genomics* 1990;**6**:623–5.

82 Moon C, Preston GM, Griffin CA, Jabs EW, Agre P. The human Aquaporin-CHIP gene: structure, organization, and chromosomal localization. *J Biol Chem* 1993; **268**:15772–8.

83 Zelinski T, Coghlan G, Myal Y *et al*. Genetic linkage between the Kell blood group system and prolactin-inducible protein loci: provisional assignment of *KEL* to chromosome 7. *Ann Hum Genet* 1991;**55**:137–40.

84 Purohit KR, Weber JL, Ward LJ, Keats BJB. The Kell blood group locus is close to the cystic fibrosis locus on chromosome 7. *Hum Genet* 1992;**89**:457–8.

85 Lee S, Zambas ED, Marsh WL, Redman CM. The human Kell blood group gene maps to chromosome 7q33 and its expression is restricted to erythroid cells. *Blood* 1993;**81**:2804–9.

86 Murphy MT, Morrison N, Miles JS *et al*. Regional chromosomal assignment of the Kell blood group locus (*KEL*) to chromosome 7q33–q35 by fluorescence in situ

hybridization: evidence for the polypeptide nature of antigenic variation. *Hum Genet* 1993;**91**:585–8.

87 Coghlan G, Kaita H, Belcher E, Philipps S, Lewis M. Evidence for genetic linkage between the *KEL* and *YT* blood group loci. *Vox Sang* 1989;**57**:88–9.

88 Zelinski T, White L, Coghlan G, Philipps S. Assignment of the YT blood group locus to chromosome 7q. *Genomics* 1991;**11**:165–7.

89 Getman DK, Eubanks JH, Camp S, Evans GA, Taylor P. The human gene encoding acetylcholinesterase is located on the long arm of chromosome 7. *Am J Hum Genet* 1992;**51**:170–7.

90 Ehrlich G, Viegas-Pequignot E, Ginzberg D *et al*. Mapping the human acetylcholinesterase gene to chromosome 7q22 by fluorescent *in situ* hybridization coupled with selective PCR amplification from a somatic hybrid cell panel and chromosome-sorted DNA libraries. *Genomics* 1992;**13**:1192–7.

91 Renwick JH, Lawler SD. Genetical linkage between the *ABO* and nail–patella loci. *Ann Hum Genet* 1955; **19**:312–31.

92 Rapley S, Robson EB, Harris H, Maynard Smith S. Data on the incidence, segregation and linkage relations of the adenylate kinase (AK) polymorphism. *Ann Hum Genet* 1967;**31**:237–42.

93 Weitkamp LR, Sing CF, Shreffler DC, Guttormsen SA. The genetic linkage relations of adenylate kinase: further data on the *ABO–AK* linkage group. *Am J Hum Genet* 1969;**21**:600–5.

94 Wille B, Ritter H. Zur formalen Genetik der Adenylatkinasen (EC:2.7.4.3) Hinweis auf Kopplung der loci für AK und ABO. *Humangenetik* 1969;**7**:263–4.

95 Schleutermann DA, Bias WB, Murdoch JL, McKusick VA. Linkage of the loci for the nail–patella syndrome and adenylate kinase. *Am J Hum Genet* 1969; **21**:606–30.

96 Robson EB, Cook PJL, Buckton KE. Family studies with the chromosome 9 markers *ABO*, *AK₁*, *ACONₛ* and 9qh. *Ann Hum Genet* 1977;**41**:53–60.

97 Westerveld A, Jongsma APM, Meera Khan P, van Someren H, Bootsma D. Assignment of the *AK₁:Np:ABO* linkage group to human chromosome 9. *Proc Natl Acad Sci USA* 1976;**73**:895–9.

98 Povey S, Slaughter CA, Wilson DE *et al*. Evidence for the assignment of the loci *AK₁*, *AK₃* and *ACONₛ* to chromosome 9 in man. *Ann Hum Genet* 1976;**39**:413–22.

99 Grzeschik K-H. Assignment of human genes: β-glucuronidase to chromosome 7, adenylate kinase-1 to 9, a second enzyme with enolase activity to 12, and mitochondrial IDH to 15. Human Gene Mapping 3. *Cytogenet Cell Genet* 1976;**16**:142–8.

100 Van Cong N, Weil D, Finaz C *et al*. Assignment of the *ABO–Np–AK₁* linkage group to chromosome 9 in man-hamster hybrids. Human Gene Mapping 3. *Cytogenet Cell Genet* 1976;**16**:241–3.

101 Ferguson-Smith MA, Aitken DA, Turleau C, de

Grouchy J. Localisation of the human *ABO:Np-1:AK-1* linkage group by regional assignment of *AK-1* to 9q34. *Hum Genet* 1976;34:35–43.

102 Cook PJL, Robson EB, Buckton KE *et al.* Segregation of *ABO*, *AK₁* and *ACON₅* in families with abnormalities of chromosome 9. *Ann Hum Genet* 1978;41:365–77.

103 Bennett EP, Steffensen R, Clausen H, Weghuis DO, van Kessel AG. Genomic cloning of the human histo-blood group ABO locus. *Biochem Biophys Res Commun* 1995;206:318–25.

104 Goodfellow PN, Banting G, Wiles MV *et al.* The gene, MIC4, which controls expression of the antigen defined by monoclonal antibody F10.44.2, is on human chromosome 11. *Eur J Immunol* 1982;12:659–63.

105 Francke U, Foellmer BE, Haynes BF. Chromosome mapping of human cell surface molecules: monoclonal anti-human lymphocyte antibodies 4F2, A3D8, and A1G3 define antigens controlled by different regions of chromosome 11. *Somat Cell Genet* 1983;9:333–44.

106 Forsberg UH, Jalkanen S, Schröder J. Assignment of the human lymphocyte homing receptor gene to the short arm of chromosome 11. *Immunogenetics* 1989;29:405–7.

107 Couillin P, Azoulay M, Henry I *et al.* Characterization of a panel of somatic cell hybrids for subregional mapping along 11p and within band 11p13. *Hum Genet* 1989;82:171–8.

108 Couillin P, Azoulay M, Metezeau P, Grisard M-C, Junien C. The gene for catalase is assigned between the antigen loci MIC4 and MIC11. *Genomics* 1989;4:7–11.

109 Forsberg UH, Bazil V, Stefanová I, Schröder J. Gene for human CD59 (likely Ly-6 homologue) is located on the short arm of chromosome 11. *Immunogenetics* 1989;30:188–93.

110 Heckl-Östreicher B, Ragg S, Drerchsler M, Scherthan H, Royer-Pokora B. Localization of the human CD59 gene by fluorescence *in situ* hybridization and pulsed-field gel electrophoresis. *Cytogenet Cell Genet* 1993;63:144–6.

111 Bickmore WA, Longbottom D, Oghene K, Fletcher JM, van Heyningen V. Colocalization of the human CD59 gene to 11p13 with the MIC11 cell surface antigen. *Genomics* 1993;17:129–35.

112 Eiberg H, Mohr J. Dombrock blood group (*DO*): assignment to chromosome 12p. *Hum Genet* 1996;98:518–21.

113 Mauthe J, Coghlan G, Zelinski T. Confirmation of the assignment of the Dombrock blood group locus (*DO*) to chromosome 12p: narrowing the boundaries to 12p12.3–p13.2. *Vox Sang* 2000;79:53–6.

114 Gubin AN, Njoroge JM, Wojda U *et al.* Identification of the Dombrock blood group glycoprotein as a polymorphic member of the ADP-ribosyltransferase gene family. *Blood* 2000;96:2621–7.

115 Yamada A, Kubo K, Takeshita T *et al.* Molecular cloning of a glycosylphosphatidylinositol-anchored molecule CDw108. *J Immunol* 1999;162:4094–100.

116 Lange C, Liehr T, Goen M *et al.* New eukaryotic semaphorins with close homology to semaphorins of DNA viruses. *Genomics* 1998;51:340–50.

117 Solomon E, Ledbetter DH. Report of the committee on the genetic constitution of chromosome 17. Human Gene Mapping 11. *Cytogenet Cell Genet* 1991;58:686–738.

118 Zelinski T, Coghlan G, White L, Philipps S. The Diego blood group locus is located on chromosome 17q. *Genomics* 1993;17:665–6.

119 Zelinski T, Coghlan G, White L, Philipps S. Assignment of the Waldner blood group locus (WD) to 17q12–q21. *Genomics* 1995;25:320–2.

120 Geitvik GA, Hoyheim B, Gedde-Dahl T *et al.* The Kidd (JK) blood group locus assigned to chromosome 18 by close linkage to a DNA-RFLP. *Hum Genet* 1987;77:205–9.

121 Leppert M, Ferrell R, Kamboh MI *et al.* Linkage of the polymorphic protein markers F13B, C1S, C1R, and blood group antigen Kidd in CEPH reference families. Human Gene Mapping 9 [Abstract]. *Cytogenet Cell Genet* 1987;46:647.

122 Magenis RE, Overton K, Wyandt H *et al.* Exclusion gene mapping utilizing patients with chromosome imbalance: the HL-A system as a prototype. *Humangenetik* 1975;27:91–109.

123 Mulley JC, Bryant GD, Sutherland GR. Additions to the exclusion map of man. *Ann Génét* 1980;23:196–200.

124 Hodge SE, Neiswanger K, Spence PI *et al.* Close genetic linkage between diabetes melitus and the Kidd blood group. *Lancet* 1981;ii:893–5.

125 Dunsworth TS, Rich SS, Swanson J, Barbosa J. No evidence for linkage between diabetes and the Kidd marker. *Diabetes* 1982;31:991–3.

126 Hodge SE, Anderson CE, Neiswanger K, Sparkes RS, Rimoin DL. The search for heterogeneity in insulin-dependent diabetes mellitus (IDDM): linkage studies, two-locus models, and genetic heterogeneity. *Am J Hum Genet* 1983;35:1139–55.

127 Olivès B, Merriman M, Bailly P *et al.* The molecular basis of the Kidd blood group polymorphism and its lack of association with type 1 diabetes susceptibility. *Hum Mol Genet* 1997;6:1017–20.

128 Davies JL, Kawaguchi Y, Bennett ST *et al.* A genome-wide search for human type 1 diabetes susceptibility genes. *Nature* 1994;371:130–6.

129 Merriman Twells R, Merriman M *et al.* Evidence by allelic association-dependent methods for a type 1 diabetes polygene (*IDDM6*) on chromosome 18q21. *Hum Mol Genet* 1997;7:1003–10.

130 Olivès B, Mattei M-G, Huet M *et al.* Kidd blood group and urea transport function of human erythrocytes are carried by the same protein. *J Biol Chem* 1995;270:15607–10.

131 Olivès B, Martial S, Mattie M-G et al. Molecular characterization of a new kidney urea transporter in the human kidney. FEBS Lett 1996;386:156–60.

132 Sanger R, Race RR. The Lutheran-secretor linkage in man: support for Mohr's findings. Heredity 1958;12:513–20.

133 Lawler SD, Renwick JH. Blood groups and genetic linkage. Br Med Bull 1959;15:145–9.

134 Metaxas MN, Metaxas-Bühler M, Dunsford I, Holländer L. A further example of anti-Lu^b together with data in support of the Lutheran-secretor linkage in man. Vox Sang 1959;4:298–307.

135 Greenwalt TJ. Confirmation of linkage between the Lutheran and Secretor genes. Am J Hum Genet 1961;13:69–88.

136 Renwick JH, Bundey SE, Ferguson-Smith MA, Izatt MM. Confirmation of linkage of the loci for myotonic dystrophy and ABH secretion. J Med Genet 1971; 8:407–16.

137 Harper PS, Rivas ML, Bias WB et al. Genetic linkage confirmed between the locus for myotonic dystrophy and the ABH-secretion and Lutheran blood group loci. Am J Hum Genet 1972;24:310–16.

138 Simola K, de la Chapelle A, Pirkola A et al. Data on DM-Le linkage. Human Gene Mapping 6 [Abstract]. Cytogenet Cell Genet 1982;32:317.

139 Weitkamp LR, Johnston E, Guttormsen SA. Probable genetic linkage between the loci for the Lewis blood group and complement C3. Human Gene Mapping 1. Cytogenet Cell Genet 1974;13:183–4.

140 Whitehead AS, Solomon E, Chambers S et al. Assignment of the structural gene for the third component of human complement to chromosome 19. Proc Natl Acad Sci USA 1982;79:5021–5.

141 Eiberg H, Mohr J, Staub Nielsen S, Simonsen N. Genetics and linkage relationships of the C3 polymorphism: discovery of C3-Se linkage and assignment of LES-C3-DM-Se-PEPD-Lu synteny to chromosome 19. Clin Genet 1983;24:159–70.

142 Kukowska-Latallo JF, Larsen RD, Nair RP, Lowe JB. A cloned human cDNA determines expression of a mouse stage-specific embryonic antigen and the Lewis blood group α(1,3/1,4)fucosyltransferase. Gene Dev 1990; 4:1288–303.

143 Zelinksi T, Kaita H, Johnson K, Moulds M. Genetic evidence that the gene controlling Au^b is located on chromosome 19. Vox Sang 1990;58:126–8.

144 Oriol R, Danilovs J, Hawkins BR. A new genetic model proposing that the Se gene is a structural gene closely linked to the H gene. Am J Hum Genet 1981; 33:421–31.

145 Oriol R, Le Pendu J, Bernez L et al. International cooperative study confirming close linkage between H and Se. Human Gene Mapping 7 [Abstract]. Cytogenet Cell Genet 1984;37:564.

146 Rouquier S, Lowe JB, Kelly RJ et al. Molecular cloning

147 Reguigne-Arnould I, Couillin P, Mollicone R et al. Relative positions of two clusters of human α-L-fucosyltransferase in 19q (FUT1–FUT2) and 19p (FUT6–FUT–FUT5) within the microsatellite genetic map of chromosome 19. Cytogenet Cell Genet 1995;71:158–62.

148 McCurley RS, Recinos A, III Olsen AS et al. Physical maps of human α(1,3)fucosyltransferase genes FUT3–FUT6 on chromosomes 19p13.3 and 11q21. Genomics 1995;26:142–6.

149 Sistonen P. Linkage of the LW blood group locus with the complement C3 and Lutheran blood group loci. Ann Hum Genet 1984;48:239–42.

150 Lewis M, Kaita H, Philipps S et al. The LW:C3 recombination fraction in female meioses. Ann Hum Genet 1987;51:201–3.

151 Hermand P, Le Pennec PY, Rouger P, Cartron J-P, Bailly P. Characterization of the gene encoding the human LW blood group protein in LW+ and LW– phenotypes. Blood 1996;87:2962–7.

152 Zelinksi T, Coghlan G, Greenberg CR, McAlpine PJ, Lewis M. Evidence that SE is distal to LU on chromosome 19q. Transfusion 1989;29:304–5.

153 Ball SP, Tongue N, Gibaud A et al. The human chromosome 19 linkage group FUT1 (H), FUT2 (SE), LE, LU, PEPD, C3, APOC2, D19S7 and D19S9. Ann Hum Genet 1991;55:225–33.

154 Kaname T, Miyauchi T, Kuwano A et al. Mapping basigin (BSG), a member of the immunoglobulin superfamily, to 19p13.3. Cytogenet Cell Genet 1993;64:195–7.

155 Eiberg H, Møller N, Mohr J, Nielsen LS. Linkage of transcobalamin II (TC2) to the P blood group system and assignement to chromosome 22. Clin Genet 1986;29:354–9.

156 Arwert F, Porck HJ, Fräter-Schröder M et al. Assignment of human transcobalamin II (TC2) to chromosome 22 using somatic cell hybrids and monosomic meningioma cells. Hum Genet 1986;74:378–81.

157 McAlpine PJ, Kaita H, Lewis M. Is the DIA₁ locus linked to the P blood group locus? Human Gene Mapping 4. Cytogenet Cell Genet 1978;22:629–32.

158 Julier C, Lathrop GM, Reghis A et al. A linkage and physical map of chromosome 22, and some applications to gene mapping. Am J Hum Genet 1988;42:297–308.

159 Kaplan J-C, Emanuel BS. Report of the committee on the genetic constitution of chromosome 22. Human Gene Mapping 10. Cytogenet Cell Genet 1989; 51:372–83.

160 Dunham I, Shimizu N, Roe BA et al. The DNA sequence of human chromosome 22. Nature 1999;402:489–95.

161 Steffensen R, Carlier K, Wiels J et al. Cloning and

547

expression of the histo-blood group P^k UDP-galactose: Galβ1–4Glcβ1–Cer α1,4-galactosyltransferase. *J Biol Chem* 2000;**275**:16723–9.

162 Ferguson-Smith MA, Sanger R, Tippett P, Aitken DA, Boyd E. A familial t(X;Y) translocation which assigns the Xg blood group locus to the region Xp22.3→pter. Human Gene Mapping 6 [Abstract]. *Cytogenet Cell Genet* 1982;**32**:273–4.

163 Goodfellow PJ, Darling SM, Thomas NS, Goodfellow PN. A pseudoautosomal gene in man. *Science* 1986;**234**:740–3.

164 Francke U, Ochs HD, de Martinville B *et al.* Minor Xp21 chromosome deletion in a male associated with expression of Duchenne muscular dystrophy, chronic granulomatous disease, retinitis pigmentosa, and McLeod syndrome. *Am J Hum Genet* 1985;**37**:250–67.

165 Heyworth PG, Curnutte JT, Rae J *et al.* Hematological-ly important mutations: X-linked chronic granulomatous disease (second update). *Blood Cells Mol Dis* 2001;**27**:16–26.

166 Bertelson CJ, Pogo AO, Chaudhuri A *et al.* Localization of the McLeod locus (XK) within XP21 by deletion analysis. *Am J Hum Genet* 1988;**42**:703–11.

167 Ho MF, Monaco AP, Blonden LAJ *et al.* Fine mapping of the McLeod locus (XK) to a 150–380-kb region in Xp21. *Am J Hum Genet* 1992;**50**:317–30.

168 Marsh WL. Linkage relationship of the *Xg* and *Xk* loci. *Cytogenet Cell Genet* 1978;**22**:531–3.

169 Wolff G, Müller CR, Jobke A. Linkage of genes for chronic granulomatous disease and Xg. *Hum Genet* 1980;**54**:269–71.

170 Mulley JC, Norman PC, Tippett P, Beal RW. A regional localisation for an X-linked suppressor gene (*XS*) for the Lutheran blood group. *Hum Genet* 1988;**78**:127–9.

Index

Page references in *italics* refer to figures; those in **bold** refer to tables

Printed in the United Kingdom
by Lightning Source UK Ltd.
134381UK00001B/65-68/P